Essentials of
Nurse Anesthesia

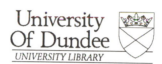

Essentials of Nurse Anesthesia

Laura Wild McIntosh, CRNA

Staff Certified Registered Nurse Anesthetist
Department of Anesthesiology
UMDNJ – Robert Wood Johnson Medical School
New Brunswick, New Jersey
Staff Certified Registered Nurse Anesthetist
Department of Anesthesiology
North Shore University Hospital Health Systems
Manhasset, New York

McGRAW-HILL
Health Professions Division

New York   St. Louis   San Francisco   Auckland   Bogotá
Caracas   Lisbon   London   Madrid   Mexico City   Milan   Montreal
New Delhi   San Juan   Singapore   Sydney   Tokyo   Toronto

McGraw-Hill

A Division of *The McGraw·Hill Companies*

Essentials of Nurse Anesthesia

Copyright © 1997 by The McGraw-Hill Companies, Inc. All rights reserved. Printed in the United States of America. Except as permitted under
the United States Copyright Act of 1976, no part of this publication may be
reproduced or distributed in any form or by any means, or stored in a data
base or retrieval system, without the prior written permission of the publisher.

1 2 3 4 5 6 7 8 9 0 MALMAL 9 8 7 6

ISBN 0-07-076537-5

The book was set in Times Roman by Digitype.
The editors were Martin J. Wonsiewicz and Peter J. Boyle;
the production supervisor was Clare Stanley;
the cover designer was Matthew Dvorozniak.
Malloy Lithographic, Inc. was printer and binder.

This book is printed on acid-free paper.

Library of Congress Cataloging-in-Publication Data

Essentials of nurse anesthesia / [edited by] Laura Wild McIntosh.
    p.   cm.
  Includes bibliographical references and index.
  ISBN 0-07-076537-5
  1. Anesthesiology.   2. Nurse anesthetists.   I. McIntosh, Laura
Wild.
  [DNLM: 1. Anesthesia—nurses' instruction.   WO 200 E785 1997]
RD82.E77   1997
617.9'6—dc20
DNLM/DLC
for Library of Congress   96-23810

Contents

Contributors*

Laura Baker, CRNA, MSN [23]
Staff Anesthetist
Columbia Presbyterian Medical Center
New York, New York

Charles R. Barton, CRNA, MEd [27,30]
Director
Graduate Anesthesia Program
The University of Akron
College of Nursing
Akron, Ohio

Minnette Beeson, CRNA, MSN [10,27]
Associate Director
Graduate Anesthesia Program
The University of Akron
College of Nursing
Akron, Ohio
Staff Nurse Anesthetist
Professional Anesthesia Services
Summa Health System
Akron, Ohio

Candace Brown, CRNA, MSN [13]
Staff Anesthetist
Baptist Hospital
Miami, Florida

John S. Burnett, MD [9]
Assistant Professor
Department of Anesthesiology
State University of New York
Syracuse, New York

Mark A. Caldwell, CRNA, MSN [4]
Clinical Instructor and Guest Lecturer
Nurse Anesthesia Track
University of Akron School of Nursing
Akron, Ohio

Thomas A. Davis, CRNA, MAE [1]
Assistant Professor
University of Kansas Medical Center
Nurse Anesthesiology Education
Lawrence, Kansas

Linda A. Downs, CRNA [25]
Staff Certified Registered Nurse Anesthetist
North Shore University Hospital Health Systems
Manhasset, New York

Dorothy Duffy-Gross, CRNA, MSN [6]
Staff Anesthetist
New York University – Tisch Hospital
New York, New York

Wayne Ellis, CRNA, ARNP, PhD [14,22]
Director, Nurse Anesthesia Program
University of Iowa
Iowa City, Iowa

Joan G. Fox, CRNA, MSN [26]
Staff Anesthetist / Clinical Instructor
Kaiser Permanente
Los Angeles Medical Center – Sunset
Los Angeles, California

Paula J. Goodman, CRNA, MSN [12]
Major, USAF NC
Chief Nurse Anesthetist
Beale AFB, California

Ekaterini Grivas-Mousouris, MS, RPh [3]
Staff Pharmacist
Memorial Sloan-Kettering Cancer Center
New York, New York

Carolyn G. Holland, CRNA [7]
Instructor, University of Cincinnati
College of Nursing and Health
Cincinnati, Ohio

Sherry Ikalowych, CRNA, MS [11]
Educational Coordinator
Columbia University
School of Nurse Anesthesia
New York, New York
Staff Anesthetist and Clinical Instructor
University of Medicine and Dentistry
Newark, New Jersey

John C. Kastor, CRNA [21]
Staff Anesthetist
Mercy Hospital
Janesville, Wisconsin

Terri E. Kole, CRNA [8]
President, Alternatives in Anesthesia
Director, Department of Anesthesia
Riverside Regional Medical Center
Newport News, Virginia

*The numbers in brackets following the contributor name refer to chapter(s) authored or coauthored by the contributor.

Leo A. LeBel, CRNA, MEd, JD [2]
Director, Nurse Anesthesia Program
Southern Connecticut State University
Director, Bridgeport Hospital Nurse Anesthesia Program
Bridgeport, Connecticut

William Gray McCall, CRNA, MHDL [11]
Assistant Professor
Associate Graduate Faculty Member
Murray State University
Murray, Kentucky
Program Coordinator
Trover Clinic Foundation
Murray State University Program of Anesthesia
Madisonville, Kentucky

Laura Wild McIntosh, CRNA, MSN [24,29]
Staff Certified Registered Nurse Anesthetist
Department of Anesthesiology
UMDNJ–Robert Wood Johnson Medical School
New Brunswick, New Jersey
Staff Certified Registered Nurse Anesthetist
Department of Anesthesiology
North Shore University Hospital Health Systems
Manhasset, New York

John Nagelhout, CRNA, PhD [5]
Assistant Professor of Anesthesia and Pharmaceutical
    Sciences
Wayne State University
College of Pharmacy
Detroit, Michigan

Colleen T. Ober, CRNA, MSN [24,32]
Staff Anesthetist
Memorial Sloan-Kettering Cancer Center
New York, New York

Vijayalakshmi U. Patil, MD [9]
Associate Professor
Department of Anesthesiology
State University of New York
Syracuse, New York

Cynthia K. Rau-Sobotka, CRNA, MSN [17]
Major, USAF NC
Chief Nurse Anesthetist
Vandenberg AFB Hospital
Vandenberg AFB, California

Laura Ricciardi, CRNA, MSN [28]
Staff Certified Registered Nurse Anesthetist
North Shore University Hospital Health Systems
Manhasset, New York

Nancy Smilen, CRNA, MS [31]
Staff Certified Registered Nurse Anesthetist
Department of Anesthesiology
Danbury Hospital
Danbury, Connecticut

Mary R. Steward, CRNA [15]
Staff Anesthetist
Medical Center of Delaware
Newark, Delaware

Celeste G. Villanueva, CRNA, MSN [18,19]
Assistant Professor
Associate Director, Nurse Anesthesia Program
Samuel Merritt College
Oakland, California

Rita Weiss, MD [20]
Adjunct Assistant Professor of Clincial Medicine
New York University
New York, New York
Assistant Attending
North Shore University Hospital
Manhasset, New York
Assistant Attending, Hematology / Oncology
St. Francis Hospital
Rosalyn, New York

Preface

When I was offered the opportunity to edit a review textbook for the certification examination for registered nurse anesthetists, I was delighted, both personally and professionally, to help satisfy the demand for a textbook in the profession of nurse anesthesia. In the time that has passed, I have had the pleasure of working with anesthetists in various settings and with a variety of interests and wide range of experience. What brings us together is a commitment to learn and foster learning in anesthesia.

The purpose of *Essentials of Nurse Anesthesia* is to provide the student with a practical and concise means of study for board preparation by offering fundamental information required in the daily practice of anesthesia. This text assumes prior study in the field of anesthesia and is meant to serve mainly as a review for the board certification candidate, but also as a source of reference for the practicing nurse anesthetist.

The contents are based on the CRNA Examination Content Outline, as determined by the Council on Certification of Nurse Anesthetists, and encompass every aspect of the field, from basic sciences to discussion of specific procedures. Although the range of information that may be covered on the exam is vast, each chapter provides a concise way to organize that information. Following each of the 32 chapters is a set of 20 practice questions that one might expect to find on the certification exam.

As the delivery of anesthetic care becomes more sophisticated, we always must remember the importance of the basic principles—while keeping current in the use of the latest anesthetic agents, techniques, and technology. The student nurse anesthetist must be willing to learn thoroughly all aspects of the profession in order to practice confidently and provide patients with the best care.

I believe CRNAs can and must make a contribution to the field of anesthesia.

Perhaps, too, we need to remember that growth in our work must be preceded by ideas, and that any conditions which suppress thought, must retard growth. Surely we will not be satisfied in perpetuating methods and traditions. Surely we shall wish to be more and more occupied with creating them.

M. Adelaide Nutting, 1925

I would like to thank Lisa Hughes Lynch, Iris Tsung, John Vickers, Mike DiPeri, Nalin Sudan, Joan Resnik, James Palma, Steven Johnson, and Claude Baconcini for their educational help. I would also like to thank everyone at McGraw-Hill, especially Peter Boyle and Edith Blume for their continuous assistance throughout this project. Finally, I thank my husband Daniel McIntosh for his love, support, and advice.

ONE

Professional Issues

1

Safety, Quality, and Legal Standards

Thomas A. Davis

Welcome to the profession of nurse anesthesia. As a nurse anesthetist, you are joining an elite group of specialty nurses with a tradition of over a century of quality, cost-effective anesthesia care for the world population. If we are competent providers of quality care, it is only because we have built our profession on the solid foundation established by those who came before us dedicating their lives to the pursuit of excellence. Therefore, to become full members of the professional community, we must have an appreciation for the rich history of anesthesia and the role played by nurse anesthetists. Knowledge of the historical basis for nurse anesthesia will enable the provider to defend the administration of anesthesia as a legitimate subspecialty of the practice of nursing.

☐ HISTORY OF ANESTHESIA

Pain has been a part of the human experience since the beginning of mankind. Efforts to control pain date back to the earliest recorded time. Some would argue that anesthesia is truly the "oldest profession" (". . . and God caused a great sleep to fall upon the man").[1] Use of the mandrake root for pain control dates back to 2000 BC and was described in *The Iliad* by Homer in 850 BC. Throughout the centuries, from prehistoric time to the mid 1800s, many techniques were used with varying degrees of success to control pain. Some of these techniques include the use of hypnosis, alcohol, herbs and extracts, local pressure, or ice. The Chinese are well known for the use of acupuncture and acupressure for pain relief. Although these techniques did not always produce complete pain relief, they were the best techniques available at the time.

The history of modern anesthesia begins with the discovery of the anesthetic properties of nitrous oxide and ether.

Nitrous oxide was discovered by Priestly in 1773 and ether may date back as far as the eighth century. It is certain that ether was produced by Cordus and Paracelsus in the 16th century. Sir Humphrey Davy is associated with extensive use of nitrous oxide and published a book about the use of the agent in 1800.[2] Although Davy hints that nitrous oxide might relieve pain, none of the early pioneers were truly aware of the anesthetic properties of nitrous oxide or ether.

EARLY PIONEERS OF ANESTHESIA

The decade of the 1840s should be remembered as the advent of modern anesthesia. It was during this time that the anesthetic properties of nitrous oxide and ether were fully appreciated, thus opening the door to painless surgery. On December 10, 1844, Horace Wells, a dentist, was in attendance at a public lecture regarding nitrous oxide. Members of the public were invited to come to the stage and inhale nitrous oxide to experience its euphoric effects. Dr. Wells noticed that a young man from the audience injured his leg while under the influence of nitrous oxide but did not feel the pain. Dr. Wells immediately saw the potential for pain relief in dentistry and the next day had one of his own teeth pulled while under the influence of nitrous oxide. The extraction was painless and the door was open for modern anesthesia. When a later demonstration failed at Harvard Medical School, Dr. Wells and nitrous oxide anesthesia were rejected by the audience.[3]

The first reported surgical use of ether was in 1842 by Dr. Crawford Long. Unfortunately, Dr. Long was a country doctor and did not publicly share his discovery with others in the medical community. Later, in 1846, Dr. William Morton demonstrated the anesthetic properties of ether by administering the agent for the removal of a neck tumor. In the years that followed the debate was heated, both in and out of court, as to who should be credited with the discovery of anesthesia. All three, Wells, Long, and Morton, claimed the honor. The famous Supreme Court Justice Oliver Wendell Holmes was brought into the debate and suggested that the term "anesthesia" be used to describe the state produced by the agents.[2]

The discovery of anesthesia was not universally accepted throughout the world. Many in the religious community believed that pain was sent from God and that this intrusion on God's will was blasphemy. Nowhere was the debate greater than in the obstetric community. It was not until Queen Victoria received chloroform anesthesia from Dr. Snow (recognized as the first true anesthesiologist) for the birth of Prince Leopold that relief of obstetric pain was accepted by the public.

Nurses as Anesthetists   In the first few years after the discovery of painless surgery, the administration of anesthesia was relegated to the junior person in the surgical theater. Usually this person was untrained and uninterested in anesthetic administration. The primary reason for being in attendance was to watch and learn from the surgeon. It rapidly became apparent that anesthesia posed a risk to the patient in and of itself. The safe administration of anesthesia became dependent on the presence of a reliable, competent anesthetist. This person was required to have anesthesia as his or her only interest and be willing to work for little monetary reward. Nurses were the perfect answer and have been safely administering anesthesia for well over a century.[3]

From the 1860s to the 1920s, nurses reliably and safely administered the vast majority of anesthetics delivered in the United States. Alice Magaw was the personal anesthetist for Dr. Charles Mayo who frequently referred to her as "the mother of anesthesia." Her work in the field of anesthesia drew more worldwide attention than any member of the Mayo Clinic group except the Mayo brothers themselves.[3] Nurses of the religious orders quickly became experts in the administration of anesthesia and were responsible for taking the art of anesthesia west as the railroads opened new territories.

By the 1920s, a number of anesthesia training programs existed throughout the United States. Nurse anesthetists were not organized as a group, and anesthesia education was not standardized. Agatha Hodgins envisioned the formation of a subspecialty group of nurse anesthetists. The purpose of this organization was to share knowledge and to standardize education. Due largely to her work, the National Association of Nurse Anesthetists was established in 1932. Education was a priority for the pioneers of the professional association with standards and guidelines for educational programs quickly adopted. Helen Lamb and Gertrude Fife were instrumental in establishing the first guidelines for educational standards. From the dedicated work of these insightful nurse anesthetists has evolved the professional organization that we know today as the American Association of Nurse Anesthetists (AANA).

☐ PROFESSIONALISM

ARE WE REALLY PROFESSIONALS?

The concept of professionalism historically was confined to a select group of occupations that placed the good of the public above personal needs and desires. The traditional professions include medicine, law, and the clergy. Early professionals were individuals who "professed" themselves to be accountable to a higher standard with a moral obligation to the public. However, in recent decades the concept of professionalism has been more loosely applied. To many, the term "professional" relates to that which we do to earn an income. Along that line, we now have professional athletes, salesmen, and gardeners to name but a few. If nurse anesthetists are to be more than day laborers in the field of anesthesia, they must be aware of the requirements of "professionalism."

In addition to the concept of duty to the public, other characteristics are common to professionals. Professionals master specific skills and knowledge arising from formal educational programs. Standards for education and entry to practice are defined by the professional organization. Professionals practice their art according to a strict code of ethics with the professional organization responsible for enforcing standards of practice. In addition, the professional makes decisions based on the best interest of the client, who is frequently in a dependent position. Duty to the patient supersedes any self-interest of the professional. This concept clearly separates the health care worker from those in the business community who operate from a "buyer beware" philosophy. Although the professional acts in accordance with standards and codes of the professional organization, the individual must be able to make decisions and act independently.[4] Are Certified Registered Nurse Anesthetists (CRNAs) professional? We are professional only to the extent that we follow the requirements described above. With the change to managed health care, the anesthetist must work for the payer whose monetary interest may be in conflict with the patient's health needs. In the managed care environment, the traditional duty to the patient becomes clouded, as does our professional status. When and if we become hourly day workers who require supervision and direction from a physician to practice in accordance with the mandates of the payer, our professional status will be in question.

THE AMERICAN ASSOCIATION OF NURSE ANESTHETISTS

The professional organization for nurse anesthetists is the American Association of Nurse Anesthetists (AANA). Although membership in the professional organization is optional, the AANA is highly respected because more than 90% of the nurse anesthetists in the United States are members. The AANA supports the practicing nurse anesthetist in many ways. The organization offers guidance to the anesthetist on a variety of practice issues ranging from consultation with other national organizations to the publication of a practice manual. In addition, the AANA represents the CRNA to the federal and state governments and actively lobbies on behalf of common interests of the members. Members are kept abreast of new developments in practice through publications and educational meetings sponsored by the AANA. The AANA conducts public awareness programs to promote the profession of nurse anesthesia. It also assists the member in areas such as group health insurance or professional liability insurance.[5] Finally, the AANA recruits new members into the organization and maintains education and membership records.

The AANA conducts its business through a president and board of directors elected by the membership. The board of directors consists of the president, president-elect, vice president, treasurer, and seven regional directors. This group is supported by full-time staff in the headquarters located in Park Ridge, Illinois. The headquarters and staff are the responsibility of the executive secretary who is a full-time employee of the AANA.[5]

Because federal antitrust law requires that individuals have the option to become certified to practice anesthesia without becoming members of the professional organization, autonomous councils exist. The councils for accreditation of educational programs, certification, recertification and public interest are autonomous bodies serving all CRNAs and not just those who are members of the AANA.

☐ QUALITY CARE

ASSESSING QUALITY

As a professional, the CRNA is expected to provide "quality" anesthesia that meets a "standard of care." The Joint Commission on Accreditation of Healthcare Organizations (JCAHO) requires that anesthesia departments establish a formal method to document the delivery of quality care. A problem that exists in meeting these expectations is that the terms "quality" and "standard of care" are poorly defined. By understanding the principles of quality assurance (QA), continuous quality improvement (CQI), and risk management (RM), the nurse anesthetist will be able to document the delivery of quality care and, at the same time, meet the requirements of JCAHO.

After World War II, two management philosophies emerged in the industrial sector of the world economy. The first philosophy was primarily adopted in the United States and held that the best way to run a business was that which would produce the largest profit. Management decisions were based entirely on enhancing corporate income. The second philosophy was promoted by W. Edwards Demming and was largely adopted by the Japanese industrial complex. According to Demming, the most cost-effective way to run a business was that which would produce the highest quality. Producing high quality meant that

less money would have to be spent fixing problems. In addition, quality products would lead to the development of a base of loyal satisfied customers who would ensure continued success. One has only to look at the automobile industry to validate the Demming concept of emphasis on quality. We are now learning that the same principles apply to the health care industry. Quality care is the most cost-effective care.

Although quality assessment for health care dates back to 1917, formal reviews of quality leading to hospital accreditation did not occur until 1951. Since 1951, JCAHO has been the nongovernmental organization responsible for hospital accreditation. Over the past four decades, the effort to ensure health care quality has shifted from QA to CQI. Therefore, it is imperative that the CRNA becomes familiar with the concepts of both QA and CQI.

QUALITY ASSURANCE

Quality assurance attempts to maintain quality care by stressing the performance of the individual health care provider. The QA approach is externally driven through institutional mandates and administered within each department. QA assumes that problems arise from mistakes made by the individual; therefore, the focus is on the individual provider. Benchmark indicators are identified and documentation is made when thresholds for indicators are exceeded. Occurrences with patient care are documented on the provider's personal record, and trends are monitored. This approach tends to have a negative effect on performance and tends to make the provider reluctant to report problems. Action is directed toward the provider under the assumption that correcting the individual will correct the problem.

Within the anesthesia department, it is common to have a formal QA review process with established indicators and thresholds. These programs frequently follow the JCAHO 10-step model. The 10 steps of the process are:[6]

1. Assign responsibility
2. Delineate scope of services
3. Identify important aspects of care
4. Identify indicators
5. Establish thresholds for evaluation
6. Collect data
7. Analyze data
8. Take action to improve services
9. Assess the impact of the action taken
10. Communicate results to the relevant components of the organization

The results obtained from the 10-step process are forwarded to staff, management, and administrative personnel. Following review of the information, budgetary priorities are established in accordance with the institutional strategic plan and steps are taken to correct any deficiencies identified by the QA process. The entire process is documented and reviewed by JCAHO at the time of hospital accreditation.

CONTINUOUS QUALITY IMPROVEMENT

Continuous quality improvement, as espoused by Demming, is more comprehensive than QA and looks beyond departmental indicators to review the entire process of health care. An assumption is made that even though care is good, there is always room for improvement. The CQI approach requires the institution to commit time, money, personnel, and training to the ongoing goal of quality care. Rather than individual departments seeking to improve their particular aspects of care, the entire process, from admission to discharge, is reviewed by a multidisciplinary group. A constant effort is made to enhance efficiency and effectiveness in support of institutional goals. CQI is patient and process oriented and makes the assumption that the staff is comprised of good people who sincerely want to do a good job. Under this philosophy, problems are viewed as arising from the institutional process rather than from the deficiencies of the individual. Bad process is thought to produce poor performance. The person accomplishing a task is in the best position to recommend change; therefore, grassroots suggestions for improvement are valued. With CQI, each individual is motivated to identify problems and work as a team to correct them. Action is directed at process improvement. CQI is committed to finding the right thing to do, doing it well, and continually improving patient care.[7]

RISK MANAGEMENT

A third aspect of department administration, *risk management*, is a process to identify and evaluate the potential for loss arising from a law suit. RM includes selecting the appropriate approach to reduce the risk, financing losses, and monitoring to determine program effectiveness. This summary is but a brief overview of the RM process. The individual anesthesia provider is encouraged to read *Risk Management Guide for the Certified Registered Nurse Anesthetist* published by the AANA.[8]

Risk management looks at the entire process of anesthesia delivery and asks two basic questions: Did the patient receive an anesthetic that met standard of care? Was the anesthetic care properly documented? When addressing the first question, one must consider the entire anesthetic process from preoperative evaluation through postoperative assessment. The preoperative interview affords the CRNA an opportunity to develop a relationship with the patient. In addition, the CRNA should review the current and previous medical charts and perform a basic examination of the patient. The CRNA should then conduct an interview with the patient to obtain information that might affect the choice of anesthetic delivery. The patient should have the opportunity to have questions answered and informed consent should be obtained. The entire visit must be documented on the medical record.

Vigilant monitoring of the patient with appropriate documentation is an essential part of risk management. Intraoperative monitoring must be in accordance with established standards or the case will not be able to be defended in a court of law. Both the AANA and the American Society of Anesthesiologists (ASA) have endorsed the standards for monitoring originally developed by the Department of Anesthesia at Harvard Medical School. These standards were approved by the ASA House of Delegates in 1986 and amended in 1990 for implementation in 1991.[9] Medical malpractice lawyers are familiar with monitoring standards and will attempt to convince a jury that deviation from the standards represents deficient anesthesia care. Briefly, the minimal standards for monitoring include:

1. Blood pressure and heart rate monitoring
2. Electrocardiogram monitor usage
3. Continuous monitoring of ventilation and circulation
4. Breathing system disconnection monitoring
5. Oxygen analyzer usage
6. Ability to monitor the temperature

The CRNA should be aware that carbon dioxide monitoring is rapidly becoming a standard of care. The prudent anesthetist will consider it to be a standard and incorporate carbon dioxide monitoring where appropriate. As with the preoperative visit, documentation of the care delivered is essential if the case is to be defended.

The postoperative visit gives the CRNA an opportunity to assess the patient and identify problems that might be related to the administration of anesthesia. The patient should be asked whether or not problems have occurred and be reassured that minor problems, such as sore throat, are transient in nature. Problems that have been identified should be appropriately treated and the entire visit should be documented. In the case of outpatients who are discharged shortly after surgery, a call to the home is an appropriate method of documenting the patient's postoperative status.

Equipment Failure Although machine failure is a rare event, anesthesia equipment must be checked for proper function before each case. The AANA endorses the use of the Food and Drug Administration (FDA) checklist as published in appendix B of the *Risk Management Guide for the Certified Registered Nurse Anesthetist*.[8] Because of the complexity of maintaining anesthesia equipment, each department is encouraged to adopt a strict "no fix" policy that prohibits maintenance by other than certified technicians. When individual providers are allowed to fix problems on the machine, defense attorneys will have the burden of proof that the repair did not contribute to the injury.

In the rare event that a patient is injured due to a machine malfunction, the CRNA should ensure that the machine or equipment in question is taken out of service immediately and kept out of service until the following have been achieved:

1. The cause of the malfunction is clearly identified.
2. The malfunction is reported to the manufacturer and regulatory agencies when required.
3. The hospital's risk manager or legal counsel has been advised of the equipment-related injury.

The continued use of defective equipment after an injury has occurred will be viewed by the jury as wanton neglect and may lead to the awarding of punitive damages. Detailed documentation of any equipment failure as well as steps taken to correct the problem are essential if the case is to be defended.

Documentation of Care Proper documentation of care is the foundation of any RM program. Regardless of the quality of care, the case may not be defensible if the care has not been properly documented. The following are essentials of quality medical records:

1. Timeliness
2. Meaningfulness
3. Authentication
4. Legibility

When these elements are not present, even good care can look bad and a case that actually met standard of care may not be able to be defended. In any case that goes to trial, the medical record will be regarded as the most valid documentation of patient care. All aspects of care from preoperative evaluation through intraoperative management and postoperative assessment must be documented.[8]

Correcting Charting Errors Despite our best intention, errors in charting can and do occur. What steps should be taken to correct errors in documentation? First and foremost, the record should never look as if it has been altered to hide or change information. When an error occurs, draw a straight line through the incorrect entry and write "error" above the entry. Write your initials so that it is clear who made the change. Some attorneys would also recommend writing the date when the change was made. If a long entry has been made in error, (preop note on the wrong chart) draw a line through the entire block of text and write "error" and then indicate the reason for the error ("wrong chart"). Sign your full name and date the note. When correcting anesthesia records where space is limited, draw a single line through the incorrect entry and write "error" and your initials. Next, make an asterisk and write the correction elsewhere on the form where it can be easily read.[8]

The following are common errors in documentation that make a case difficult to defend if litigation ensues.[8]

1. Illegibility
2. Abbreviations. Use only abbreviations authorized by the institution.
3. Unidentified entries
4. Advance charting. Never chart prior to the event.
5. Alterations. Lawyers assume the intent is to defraud.
6. Inconsistent timing of events. Make sure your times correlate with times recorded by surgical nurses and recovery nurses. Inconsistent times imply confusion and open the question of the accuracy of the remainder of the record.
7. Criticism of others. Never question a colleague in writing on the record.
8. Blank spaces. Mark all spaces on preprinted forms.

When problems arise, review your record to make sure that it accurately reflects the care that was given. Notify your risk manager of the possibility of litigation and make sure that your record can be defended in a court of law.[8]

☐ LEGAL ASPECTS OF ANESTHESIA CARE

LEGAL ISSUES IN NURSE ANESTHESIA PRACTICE

The student of nurse anesthesia dedicates considerable time and effort to master the technical skills and academic knowledge required for safe practice. Understanding the legal climate in which we practice is equally important but receives much less attention during the education process. To practice as a true professional, the individual anesthetist must understand the legal concepts that apply to the practice of nurse anesthesia. With this knowledge, the nurse anesthetist will be able to document that care has been delivered in a manner that can be defended in a court of law. In addition, the nurse anesthetist must have an understanding of the law if he or she is to defend the practice of anesthesia as a function of nursing. The following text is a brief overview of legal concepts that should be understood by the new graduate preparing for the Certification examination. The interested reader wishing a more comprehensive review of legal concepts is encouraged to read Chapter 13 "Understanding Malpractice Litigation" in *Professional Aspects of Nurse Anesthesia Practice*.[10] "Professional and Legal Issues of Nurse Anesthesia Practice" published by the AANA in the *Professional Practice Manual for the Certified Registered Nurse Anesthetist*,[11] and *The Nurse Anesthetist and the Law*.[12]

The Legal Basis for Nurse Anesthesia Registered nurses have administered the vast majority of anesthetics in the United States for over a century. It is only in the past two decades that the number of anesthetics administered by physician anesthesiologists has come close to the number administered by CRNAs. Even so, the legality of nurse anesthesia has been and continues to be challenged. Those entering the profession of nurse anesthesia should remain on guard, but be reassured that numerous court cases have affirmed the practice of nurse anesthesia as a function of nursing.

First and foremost, the courts in the United States have repeatedly recognized the delivery of anesthesia as a valid function of nursing. This legal standing is recognized in all 50 states and affirms the practice of nurse anesthesia in a wide variety of practice settings. The first case to affirm the practice of nurse anesthesia was *Frank v South* in 1917. A second case, *Chalmers-Frances v Nelson* in 1936 strengthened the finding of the earlier case and subsequent to these cases, the courts have repeatedly affirmed the practice of anesthesia as a function of nursing. The following is a brief summary of court findings regarding the legality of nurse anesthesia[11]:

1. CRNAs are independently licensed nurses who are authorized to practice within the scope of the Nurse Practice Act of the individual state.

2. Anesthesia is a recognized specialty of the practice of nursing and medicine. The fact that anesthesia is a specialty of medicine does not mean that it can not also be a specialty of nursing.

3. Nurses are expected to use judgment when following standing orders. Therefore, the fact that a nurse anesthetist uses judgment does not mean that the individual is practicing medicine.

4. When a physician (surgeon) prescribes an anesthetic, they are providing the required statutory supervisory function. There is no legal requirement that an anesthesiologist must supervise the nurse anesthetist.

5. The Board of Nursing of each state can determine what it believes to be within the realm of nursing. Nursing and medical practice acts clearly demonstrate that nursing and medicine overlap in the area of anesthesia.

Responsibility for the Acts of the Nurse Anesthetist When the practice of nurse anesthesia was upheld by the courts, those who would eliminate the profession attempted to convince surgeons that they would be held responsible for the negligent acts of the nurse anesthetist. The case of *Baird v Sickler* in 1981 had an extensive review of previous case law and found that there has never been a case upheld by an appellate court in which a surgeon was found liable for the negligent acts of the CRNA based solely on the requirement for supervision. This and numerous other cases have affirmed that liability is associated with control and that surgeons are not liable unless they control the conduct of the anesthetic. In cases where the surgeon provides only the required supervisory function but does not direct the actions of the CRNA, the liability for negligent acts related to the anesthetic remains solely with the CRNA. Similarly, when surgeons have directed physician anesthesiologists in the conduct of the anesthetic, they have shared responsibility for the outcome. Therefore, working with a CRNA does not add risk for the surgeon unless the surgeon actively directs the conduct of the anesthetic. Likewise, working with an anesthesiologist does not necessarily relieve the surgeon of responsibility. Clearly, legal responsibility goes to the person in control regardless of the type of license held.[11]

The question of whether or not the nurse anesthetist can legally administer regional anesthesia has also been debated in the legal system. Regional anesthesia is an accepted part of the practice of nurse anesthesia. Other medical specialties cannot restrict this practice solely to gain market control or prevent competition. When policies preventing CRNAs in California from administering regional anesthesia were put into place, the state Attorney General overturned the restric-

tion affirming regional anesthesia as a practice of nurse anesthesia. Currently, nurse practice acts in all 50 states allow CRNAs to perform regional anesthesia.

MEDICAL NEGLIGENCE

In addition to defending the right to practice, nurse anesthetists must have a working knowledge of the law if they are to reduce the risk of being named in a suit. Most commonly, when a nurse anesthetist (the defendant) is named in a law suit, the patient (plaintiff) alleges that the anesthetist was negligent. The term "malpractice" is often used; however, the legal concept that applies is negligence.

Elements of Negligence For negligence to be found, specific elements must be proven by the plaintiff:[10]

1. It must be established that the anesthetist had a *duty* to administer an anesthetic to the plaintiff taking reasonable care to prevent harm to the patient. There is no debate as to whether or not the anesthetist should prevent harm; however, the obligation to provide an anesthetic is often debated. If no relationship is established between the patient and the anesthetist, negligence does not apply.

2. There must be a *breach* of the appropriate standard of care in administering the anesthetic. This breach may involve a technical error or an error in judgment.

3. The breach must actually cause physical injury. This concept is termed *causation*. The plaintiff must prove that the injury was a direct result of the breach of the standard of care. Poor outcome does not in and of itself indicate negligence.

4. *Damage,* either economic or noneconomic, must have occurred to the patient.

Standards of care become important when determining whether or not negligence has occurred. "Standard of care" may be defined as a level of care generally practiced by members of the profession in the same or similar circumstances, a deviation from which represents a risk to the patient.[10] Standards arise from the professional organization, the community of providers, textbooks, journals, expert witnesses, statutes, and prior case law. When a case goes to court, expert testimony is essential for establishing the standard of care. Any competent anesthesia provider, nurse, or physician may be used as an expert witness in cases alleging negligence with regard to the administration of anesthesia.

Damages In a legal case, the plaintiff attempts to collect money to cover damages that have been incurred. *Economic damages* are assessed to cover the actual monetary loss the patient has incurred. This may include medical costs, lost wages, and projected expenses for ongoing medical care. *Noneconomic damages* cover intangible losses such as pain and suffering or loss of affection. Some states are attempting to place a limit on the amount of money that may be recovered for noneconomic damages. Within established policy limits, the anesthetist's malpractice insurance will cover these types of losses. Occasionally, the court will determine that the conduct was willful or wanton. In these cases, the court will punish the provider by assessing *punitive damages*. These damages are not covered by malpractice insurance and the anesthetist must pay from personal money. The individual may not declare bankruptcy to avoid paying punitive damages.[10]

PROTECT YOURSELF FROM A LAWSUIT

Hopefully, the anesthetist will be able to practice an entire career without being named in a lawsuit; however, that is not always the reality. In the unfortunate event that you are named in a lawsuit, the following steps are recommended[10]:

1. Note the date and time that you were notified of the suit and inform your insurance carrier immediately. Keep all documents from the court in a personal records file.
2. Do not speak to anybody about the case. Anybody you talk to may be drawn into the case as a witness.
3. Select an attorney to represent you. Usually your insurance carrier will appoint the attorney. If more than one person is represented by the attorney, make sure that your interests are guarded.
4. Cooperate with your attorney. Failure to cooperate with an attorney appointed by your insurance carrier may relieve the carrier of responsibility.
5. *Do not* conduct any investigations unless directed to do so by your attorney. Investigations directed by the anesthesia department may be used by the plaintiff.
6. Do not argue or accuse others named in the suit. When defendants fight, the plaintiff always wins.
7. Actively participate in the defense of the case. Prepare for depositions and court appearances.

In addition to the suggestions listed above, Simpson[10] recommends the following in an effort to avoid being named in a lawsuit:

1. Establish rapport with patients and their families before the surgical procedure and carry that relationship throughout the entire perioperative period.
2. When a problem arises, notify the family immediately and describe therapies and treatments planned to correct the problem.
3. Remain involved. Patients do not always sue based on outcome. Often it is the perception of lack of sensitivity that motivates the patient to file a suit.

RES IPSE LOQUITUR

When a patient is injured while under general anesthesia, he or she is unable to testify as to the negligent acts that caused the injury. In this case, the concept of *res ipse loquitur* applies. Literally translated, *res ipse loquitur* means "the thing speaks for itself." This concept makes the assumption that in-

jury would not have occurred in the absence of negligence. Therefore, the burden of proof shifts to the defendant who essentially becomes "guilty until proven innocent." For *res ipse loquitur* to apply, specific elements must be present[12]:

1. The injury must be of a type that does not normally occur in the absence of negligence.
2. The injury must be caused by an instrument within the exclusive control of the defendant.
3. The injury must not be a result of voluntary action or contributory action on the part of the plaintiff.

If any of the above elements are not present, the concept of *res ipse loquitur* does not apply and the burden of proof shifts back to the plaintiff in the negligence case.

CONSENT

A second legal concept that places the anesthetist at risk for a lawsuit is assault and battery. *Assault* is the threat to injure another with the apparent means to carry out the threat. *Battery* is the willful touching of another without the person's permission.[12] When anesthesia and surgery are performed without the consent of the patient, the concept that applies is assault and battery. Conversely, the best defense against assault and battery is informed consent.

The nurse anesthetist is responsible for ensuring that the patient has given consent before any touching or administration of anesthesia. Any adult who is competent may give consent for surgery and anesthesia. The doctrine of *informed consent* requires that the patient receive sufficient information to make a decision. The patient must be apprised of the risks, complications, and alternatives regarding the proposed anesthetic prior to giving consent.[12] Because it is impossible to apprise the patient of all possible risks, those that occur most frequently and those that have the most catastrophic effect must be revealed to the patient. Finally, consent must be in a written format that is signed by the patient and witnessed by a third person. Any person who may legally give consent has the right to withdraw that consent at any time.

Consent laws that apply to minors vary from state to state and anesthetists are advised to become familiar with their particular state law. Minors who are self-supporting and living as adults may give their own consent in most states under the concept of the *emancipated minor*.

Consent *implied in law* is assumed to exist in emergency situations. It is assumed that the unconscious patient would give consent to lifesaving treatment if he or she were able.

☐ REGULATION OF GASES AND EQUIPMENT

REGULATORY AGENCIES

Anesthesia providers, insurance carriers, and patients all have a vested interest in the reliability and safety of anesthesia. Education and vigilance are essential in the quest for zero complications. It is assumed that drugs and equipment used in the daily practice of anesthesia are safe and effective. That assumption is not always true. Equipment safety has evolved over decades of experience and continues to improve as new equipment is developed. Standards for safety have evolved both from within the anesthesia community and from regulatory agencies. The anesthetist must have an understanding of the agencies that regulate the drugs and equipment specific to the administration of anesthesia.

Compressed Gases   The compressed gases used in the delivery of anesthesia are regulated by federal agencies. The purity of the gases contained in the compressed gas cylinder must meet the specifications described in the *Pharmacopoeia of the United States* or the *National Formulary*.[13] The storage and transportation of compressed gases is regulated by the U.S. Department of Transportation (DOT). The DOT has numerous regulations regarding the manufacture of compressed gas cylinders as well as the manufacture and shipment of compressed gases. A cylinder used to contain a compressed gas must be stamped with a DOT code indicating that the cylinder was manufactured according to specifications. The service pressure of the cylinder must be stamped into the metal as well as the inspection date. Compressed gas cylinders must be inspected every 10 years and tested for structural integrity. At the time of testing, the cylinder must be able to withstand a pressure 1.66 times the working pressure to be certified as safe for use.

Fire Safety   The National Fire Prevention Association (NFPA) has been actively assisting in anesthesia safety for over 40 years. The specific interest of the NFPA is the prevention of fire within the hospital and the operating room. Many of the older anesthetic agents were flammable or explosive and posed a danger to the patient as well as to health care workers. In modern times, the NFPA remains concerned with fire safety in the operating room even though flammable agents are no longer in use. The NFPA has published a standard calling for the use of only nonflammable agents in the practice of anesthesia. *NFPA 99: Standard for Health Care Facilities* presents standards for pipeline gas sources and electric supply to the operating room.[14] Although these regulations are technically "voluntary," many states and local communities write NFPA standards into local codes, making them enforceable by law. A similar group, the Compressed Gas Association (CGA), also offers voluntary standards for the manufacture and delivery of compressed gases.

Equipment Safety   The development of new equipment and new applications for existing equipment has lead to breakthroughs in the practice of anesthesia and medicine. Unfortunately, new equipment does not always produce the desired results and, in some instances, may pose a safety threat to the patient. In the 1960s and 1970s it became apparent that thousands of injuries and hundreds of deaths were directly related to medical equipment. In 1976, the Medical

Device Amendments were put into law to supplement the authority of the Federal Food, Drug, and Cosmetic Act of 1938. These amendments authorized the FDA to regulate medical devices. Equipment was classified into categories according to their risk to the public. Class I equipment includes established technology known to be safe and effective. These devices are the controls to which new devices are compared. They must be registered but are under little control. Class II devices pose a greater risk to the public and are subject to compliance with established performance standards. Class III devices are those that pose a threat to life if malfunction should occur. These devices are subject to extensive regulation and must be tested and meet pre-market approval before they can be sold to the public.[14] A pacemaker would be an example of a class III device.

Prompted by patient deaths secondary to defective Foregger anesthesia machines in 1984, Congress reviewed the oversight of the FDA in the regulation of health care equipment. The Center for Devices and Radiological Health (CDRH), a subunit of the FDA, reviewed their policies and developed the medical device reporting system (MDR). This system requires that any death or serious injury related to a health care device be reported to the agency within 5 days of the event. MDR regulations allow the initial notification to be accomplished by phone with a complete written report to follow within 15 days. An attempt is then made to determine whether the injury resulted from a product defect or from user error.[14]

The Safe Medical Devices Act of 1990 was an attempt to further improve the safety of medical equipment. Under this act, notification of death or injury is required. Individual providers are encouraged to report potential problems or actual malfunction of equipment. In addition, manufacturers are required to report device malfunction information relayed to them by equipment users. This act permits the FDA to immediately halt the manufacture and recall any devices that prove to be harmful in the workplace. Finally, this act gives the FDA enforcement power in the form of civil penalties for noncompliance with the regulation.

In addition to federal regulation, many states are monitoring and controlling medical devices used within the state. Most states do not have extensive knowledge in assessing the safety of medical equipment; therefore, the most common approach is to accept standards produced by federal agencies or voluntary agencies and incorporate them into state law. Once this has been accomplished, violation of voluntary standards becomes a violation of state law. Individual anesthesia providers are encouraged to become familiar with state laws that regulate medical devices within the state in which they practice.

VOLUNTARY STANDARDS

Professional organizations and manufacturers have an interest in the safety of anesthesia. Both the AANA and the ASA have published standards for safe practice. In addition, other organizations interested in safety have proposed standards for manufacture and use of medical devices. The anesthetist should be aware that although these standards are categorized as "voluntary," in a court of law the plantiff's attorney will attempt to convince the jury that these are established standards of care. Standards have been developed over time in an attempt to protect the public. Voluntary standards tend to develop from experience and are more easily established than those arising through bureaucratic channels. The prudent anesthetist will follow established standards as closely as possible unless a specific circumstance mandates deviation from the standard.

The American National Standards Institute (ANSI) is a private organization founded over 70 years ago that is actively participating in the improvement of the safety of anesthetic equipment. It has published minimum safety and performance standards for all components of the anesthesia machine. The anesthesia provider would be remiss if he or she were to purchase and use anesthesia equipment that was not in accordance with ANSI standards.

The American Society for Testing and Materials (ASTM) has similar interests to ANSI. In 1983, the ASA switched from working with the ASTM to working with ANSI due to legal considerations. At the present time, ASTM publishes voluntary standards that apply to anesthesia machines. Both ANSI and ASTM agree on most standards. When reading the product information that accompanies the anesthesia machine, the anesthetist will see that machines sold in the United States comply with both ANSI and ASTM standards.

The Institute of Electrical and Electronics Engineers (IEEE) recognizes that new medical devices require more and more power for their operation. This organization writes standards used by electrical engineers when developing medical equipment. In addition, the IEEE is interested in developing systems of automated record keeping for anesthesia.

Established in 1951 as a private, nonprofit organization, JCAHO seeks to improve the quality of health care delivery in the United States. JCAHO establishes standards for quality health care in collaboration with health care professionals. Standards are published in the JCAHO *Accreditation Manual for Hospitals*. Although the standards are technically voluntary, many health care payers, including Medicare and Medicaid, require JCAHO accreditation as a prerequisite for reimbursement. The JCAHO manual provides standards for the operation of the entire hospital, including the operating room and the anesthesia department. A requirement of JCAHO that affects the anesthetist is the mandate for ongoing assessment of quality. A program is required that monitors outcomes, analyzes problems, and offers solutions. Indicators must be identified and monitored in an ongoing manner. Occurrences must be evaluated and steps taken to ensure that problems are not repeated. JCAHO also requires hospitals to have a safety management program that includes accident reporting, training, and education. An equipment management program is required to identify and control hazardous medical equipment. Assurance of electrical safety is a component of equipment management. Anesthetists interested in developing a broader knowledge of JCAHO requirements are encouraged to review the accreditation manual and to become involved on the local level with preparation for a JCAHO visit.

To summarize, the practice of anesthesia must follow established standards. Numerous professional and governmental organizations offer standards that are meant to improve patient safety. Although many of the standards are voluntary arising from private organizations, the anesthetist should attempt to follow all standards as closely as possible. In a court of law, the plaintiff's attorney will attempt to convince the jury that deviation from standards, whether mandatory or voluntary, constitutes a violation of standard of care.

☐ SAFETY IN THE OPERATING ROOM

ELECTRICAL SAFETY

Patient safety is a primary concern of every provider of anesthesia regardless of whether the individual is a nurse or a physician. The operating room presents an environment that is potentially hazardous to both the patient and the personnel who work there. Electricity poses two major threats: electrocution or burn. An understanding of basic electrical safety is essential for a safe operating room environment.

Characteristics of Current   The basic principles of electricity are described by Ohm's law: $E = I \times R$. In this equation, E is the electromotive force, which is measured in volts. I is the current, which is measured in amperes, and R is the resistance, which is measured in ohms. A useful analogy is the concept of blood pressure being equal to cardiac output times systemic vascular resistance. With electricity, blood pressure is represented by voltage, cardiac output is current, and systemic vascular resistance is the resistance.[15] Actual electrical power is measured in watts with a watt equal to the product of voltage times current. The amount of work done is measured in watt-seconds (joules).

Electrical current represents the flow of electrons. Any substance that permits the flow of electrons is classified as a *conductor*. If the flow of electrons is always in the same direction, it is classified as *direct current*. When the electrons alternate direction at regular intervals it is *alternating current*. The concept of resistance applies to direct current. When alternating current is present the concept of impedance applies. *Impedance* is defined as the sum of forces that oppose electron movement when alternating current is in use. Some equipment requires that a charge be stored and released at a later time (defibrillator). The term *capacitance* refers to the ability to store an electrical charge.[15] For current to flow, an electrical circuit must be present. A completed circuit allows the flow of current from the source, through the device requiring electricity and back to the ground.

Electrical Shock   Any time a person comes in contact with electricity, shock may occur. For shock to occur, an electrical circuit through the individual must be present. When electricity enters through the skin, passes through the body, and exits through the skin, macroshock has occurred. Current always follows the path of least resistance; therefore, muscle and blood vessels are most affected by shock through the body. Current may also enter the body through catheters or wires and directly enter the organs of the body. This type of shock is termed microshock. Obviously, much less current is required for microshock because the skin (which offers resistance to current flow) is bypassed. Seizures, cardiac arrest, or respiratory arrest are the three most common responses to shock.[16] A current of 1 milliamp (mA) produces the threshold for perception. A mild tingle will occur at this current. The "let go" current causes sustained muscle contraction and the individual is *unable* to let go of the source of electricity. A current of 10 to 20 mA produces the "let go" condition. A current of 100 to 300 mA will produce ventricular fibrillation but the respiratory center remains intact. A shock with current greater than 6000 mA is an immediate threat to life with damage to the heart and respiratory centers.[15]

Grounding and Line Isolation   Electrical safety in the operating room is based on prevention of allowing an electrical circuit to be completed through the patient. Operating rooms are designed with two safety features that greatly reduce the risk of shock. First, all electrical outlets and equipment plugs are grounded. This means that one of the wires to the equipment is intentionally in direct contact with the ground. The electric potential of the ground is zero. Because current follows the path of least resistance, any extraneous current will be diverted directly to the ground and will not pass through the relatively higher resistance of the patient or other personnel.

A second source of electrical safety in the operating room is the addition of a transformer to the system. A transformer is used to isolate the electrical system in the operating room. When an isolated electrical system is in use, there is a voltage potential between the live and neutral lines, but there is no voltage difference between the two working lines and the ground. When working properly, a circuit cannot be completed through the ground, thus reducing the risk of shock. If a short circuit occurs between the two working lines, potential develops between the lines and the ground, creating a potential for shock. When this occurs the condition is termed "first fault." Electrical systems that supply the operating room will alarm when a first fault condition is present. If the problem is not corrected and someone touches the faulty equipment, a circuit may be completed causing a "second fault" to exist and shock may occur. The *line isolation monitor* detects current leakage caused by the first fault and provides an audible warning for operating room personnel.[15] When this occurs, the source of the first fault must be immediately determined. Equipment should be unplugged in the reverse order (the last thing plugged in is the first thing unplugged) until the faulty equipment is found. The faulty equipment should immediately be taken out of service and not used until it has been repaired by qualified technicians.

Electrocautery   Electrocautery is commonly used to provide hemostasis in the surgical patient. When functioning properly, this device safely burns the area of bleeding without causing harm to the patient. Current passes from the tip of the cautery device through the tissue and back to the machine through a grounding pad and wire. Current density is focused at the tip of the cautery device causing a burn only at that precise spot. The grounding pad covers a large area and diffuses the current density so that a burn will not occur. An improperly placed grounding pad with a small area of contact may allow enough current density to develop to create a burn. The heart rhythm is not affected by electrocautery because the grounding pad is placed in an area where the heart is not directly between the surgical area and the grounding pad. In addition, very high or very low frequencies of current do not cause rhythm problems in the heart. The cautery device uses a frequency of 300 to 3000 kHz. This frequency is too high to produce cardiac or diaphragmatic electrocution.[16]

The patient with a pacemaker presents a special challenge regarding electrical safety and use of a cautery device. When cautery must be used in the patient with a pacemaker, the grounding pad should be at a site distant from the heart and in a location where the current will not pass through the heart en route from the cautery device to the grounding pad. The bipolar cautery device has current flow from point to point at the cautery site and current does not pass through the body. The bipolar cautery is preferred in the patient with a pacemaker.

LASER SAFETY

The use of lasers in the operating room has afforded the patient a new option for the treatment of disease. However, this wonderful new treatment modality is not without risk for both the patient and the health care worker. When lasers are in use, the patient is at risk for fire (especially in the airway) and the health care workers are at risk for eye damage. An understanding of laser technology and basic safety procedures is essential for the safe practice of anesthesia in the laser environment.

What Is a Laser?   The acronym *laser* stands for *Light Amplification of the Stimulated Emission of Radiation*. A laser is produced when an electric current is directed through a lasing medium and then focused on a target. When the electricity passes through the lasing medium, electrons are excited and change orbital patterns thus emitting energy in the form of light.[17] Laser light has three distinct characteristics. The light has *coherence*, which means that all light waves are in phase with each other. The light has *collimation* meaning that all light waves move in a parallel direction. Finally, laser light as *monochromaticity* meaning that all light waves have the same wave length.

Types of Lasers   Lasers are named for the lasing medium in use. For example, the carbon dioxide (CO_2) laser has CO_2 as the lasing medium. The type of lasing medium used determines the wavelength of light produced by the laser. Different wavelengths of laser energy have different effects on the tissues. Therefore, the surgeon can select the type of laser that has the characteristics most desired for the specific procedure being done. Lasers with a long wavelength are readily absorbed by water and thus affect most body tissues and pigments. Short wavelengths are strongly absorbed by hemoglobin and other pigments but pass readily through clear substances. Below is a summary of lasers commonly used in the operating room:[17]

1. The carbon dioxide (CO_2) laser has a wavelength of 10,600 and is absorbed by all tissues that contain water. This laser produces a very shallow depth of thermal penetration and the beam can be precisely focused. It is the most commonly used laser for ear-nose-throat procedures. It also has an application for neurosurgery, gynecologic, and plastic surgery when precision is important.

2. The neodynium-doped yttrium-aluminum-garnet (Nd:YAG) laser has a wavelength of 1064 and is absorbed by pigmented tissue. It is transmitted through clear substances and penetrates tissue to a depth of 2 to 6 mm. It is most commonly used for coagulation and debulking of tumors. This laser can be transmitted through fiberoptic cables to various sites within the body, including the trachea and bronchi.

3. The potassium titanyl phosphate (KTP) laser produces a wavelength of 532 and is visible with a color of emerald green. It is produced by passing a Nd:YAG laser through a KTP medium to shorten the wavelength. It is strongly absorbed by pigments and passes through clear substances. This laser has an effect between that of the CO_2 and the Nd:YAG with both precise focusing and good coagulation. The penetration depth is 0.5 to 2 mm and is suited for operations of the airway and neurosurgery.

4. The argon laser has a short wavelength of 488 to 515 and is absorbed by pigments and passes through clear substances. It has a shallow tissue penetration and is suited for eye procedures involving the retina. It may also be used for photocoagulation in plastic surgery and dermatology.

5. Helium-neon lasers produce a visible red light which is incorporated into the other lasers and functions as a aiming beam. This beam identifies the tissue which will be affected by the more powerful laser.

Eye Protection   Use of the laser in the operating room produces an environmental risk for the other health care workers who are in the room. The laser beam will cause damage to any tissue that it contacts regardless of whether it is intentionally directed toward the patient or inadvertently directed toward the health care worker. Eye damage presents the greatest risk to the health care worker in the laser environment. The specific risk depends on the type of laser in use. Therefore, the type of eye protection required depends

on the type of laser in use. Lasers with a long wavelength (CO_2) are absorbed by all surfaces and therefore affect the cornea and lens of the eye. Clear glasses will protect the eye from the CO_2 laser and colored lenses are not required. Lasers with a shorter wavelength (KTP and Nd:YAG) easily pass through clear substances and are absorbed by pigmented areas. These lasers will pass through the lens of the eye and damage the retina. Colored lenses are required to protect the eye from these types of lasers. Health care workers should wear eye protection when around lasers. In addition, the eyes of the patient should be protected from the laser beam. The patient's eyes should be closed and taped. Lubricant should be avoided due to the risk of fire should the laser beam contact the lubricant. A damp surgical sponge over the eyes will afford additional protection.[17] In addition to the risk of eye damage, the anesthetist should be aware that the use of the laser will vaporize tissue as well as any virus that may be present in the lesion. Special high filtration face masks should be worn by personnel in the operating room to prevent the inhalation of unwanted contaminants.

Airway Fires   The greatest risk to the patient receiving laser surgery is a fire within the airway. Three ingredients must be present for fire to occur. There must be a fuel, an oxidizing agent, and a source of ignition. In the case of laser surgery, the endotracheal tube is the fuel, the inspired oxygen is the oxidizing agent, and the laser is the source of ignition. If any one of these three is absent, fire will not occur. When an endotracheal tube is deemed necessary, a protected tube will reduce the likelihood of fire. Numerous commercially available laser tubes are on the market. Studies have shown various levels of success in actually preventing damage to protected tubes when exposed to the laser beam. The only tube that will absolutely not be damaged by the laser beam is a metal tube. Metal wrapping tape is available for use to protect conventional polyvinyl chloride (PVC) endotracheal tubes; however, some argue that the adhesive on the tape is flammable. Many authors recommend that the surgeon place a wet pledget over the base of the endotracheal tube when using the laser in proximity to the airway. The conventional PVC endotracheal tube is less dangerous when exposed to the laser than is the older red rubber endotracheal tube. The ink markings on the endotracheal tube and the colored barium strip along the channel to the endotracheal tube cuff increase the risk of ignition if hit by the laser beam. The best protection is not hitting the endotracheal tube with the laser beam. Filling the endotracheal tube cuff with saline may offer additional safety when lasers are in use.

Reducing the inspired oxygen concentration provides additional safety when lasers are used in the airway. Nitrous oxide should not be used during laser procedures. This gas supports combustion and diffusion hypoxia may develop if the patient suddenly must breathe room air. An inert gas such as helium is recommended to reduce the inspired concentration of oxygen. Helium has the characteristic of diffusivity, which means that it will carry more heat away from the surgical area than can be carried by the other gases commonly used in general anesthesia.[18] A helium concentration greater than 60% with an oxygen concentration less than 40% greatly reduces the risk of airway fire.[17]

If an airway fire should develop, the patient is in an immediately life-threatening position. Prompt action on the part of the anesthetist and the surgeon are required to save the life of the patient. The following are recommendations for management of an airway fire[17]:

1. Disconnect the tube at the Y piece and remove the tube immediately.

2. Turn off the oxygen.

3. Irrigate the site with water if it is still smoldering.

4. Ventilate the patient by mask or reintubate if possible. Attempt to maintain oxygenation and stabilized vital signs.

5. Perform laryngoscopy and bronchoscopy to evaluate the extent of damage.

6. Secure the airway by either intubation or tracheotomy as indicated.

7. Admit to the intensive care unit and monitor (including blood gas analysis) for at least 24 hours.

8. Use ventilators, steroids, and antibiotics as indicated.

REFERENCES

1. The Holy Bible, Genesis 2:21.
2. Calverly R. Anesthesia as a specialty: past, present and future. In: Barash P, Cullen B, Stoelting R, eds. *Clinical Anesthesia*. 2nd ed. Philadelphia: JB Lippincott; 1992:3–33.
3. Bankert M. *Watchful Care, a History of America's Nurse Anesthetists*. New York: Continuum; 1989.
4. Pellegrino E. What is a profession? *J Allied Health*. 1983;168.
5. Garde J, Foster S. The American Association of Nurse Anesthetists: the role of the professional organization. In: Foster S, Jordan L, eds. *Professional Aspects of Nurse Anesthesia Practice*. Philadelphia: FA Davis; 1994:35–48.
6. Lord J, Kraus G. Quality assessment and improvement for the 1990's. In: Foster S, Jordan L, eds. *Professional Aspects of Nurse Anesthesia Practice*. Philadelphia: FA Davis, 1994: 291–305.
7. Kraus G. The AANA quality assurance and risk management program and member services. In: Foster S, Jordan L, eds. *Professional Aspects of Nurse Anesthesia Practice*. Philadelphia: FA Davis; 1994:307–319.
8. American Association of Nurse Anesthetists. Risk management guide for nurse anesthetists. In: *Professional Practice Manual for the Certified Registered Nurse Anesthetist*. Park Ridge, IL: AANA; 1989.
9. Gravenstein J. Introduction to monitoring: clinical monitoring. In: Kirby R, Gravenstein N, eds. *Clinical Anesthesia Practice*. Philadelphia: WB Saunders; 1994:333–340.
10. Simpson J. Understanding malpractice litigation. In: Foster S, Jordan L, eds. *Professional Aspects of Nurse Anesthesia Practice*. Philadelphia: FA Davis; 1994:225–250.
11. American Association of Nurse Anesthetists. Professional and legal issues of nurse anesthesia practice. In: *Professional Practice Manual for the Certified Registered Nurse Anesthetist*. Park Ridge, IL: AANA; 1989.
12. Mannino J. *The Nurse Anesthetist and the Law*. New York: Grune & Stratton; 1982.
13. Dorsch J, Dorsch S. *Understanding Anesthesia Equipment*. 3rd ed. Baltimore: Williams & Wilkins; 1994.
14. Lees D. Standards and regulatory considerations. In: Ehrenwerth J, Eisenkraft J, eds. *Anesthesia Equipment*. St Louis: CV Mosby; 1993:521–533.
15. Ehrenwerth J. Lasers and electrical safety in the operating room. Part II: electrical safety. In: Ehrenwerth J, Eisenkraft J, eds. *Anesthesia Equipment*. St. Louis: CV Mosby; 1993:445–469.
16. Sommer R. Operating room safety: fire and electrical hazards. In: *Progress in Anesthesiology*. San Antonio, TX: Dannemiller Memorial Education Foundation; 1987:2.
17. Pashayan A. Lasers and electrical safety in the operating room. Part I: lasers. In: Ehrenwerth J, Eisenkraft J, eds. *Anesthesia Equipment*. St. Louis: CV Mosby; 1993:436–445.
18. Nilson J. Anesthetic considerations for laser surgery. In: Duke J, Rosenberg S, eds. *Anesthesia Secrets*. Philadelphia: Hanley & Belfus; 1996:479–482.

☐ QUESTIONS

1. Which of the following best describes quality assurance?
   a. The entire process of health care delivery is reviewed.
   b. Multidisciplinary groups work together on common problems.
   c. Each department establishes indicators and reports occurrences.
   d. It is focused on avoiding litigation.

2. Continuous quality improvement is based on the philosophy that problems arise from:
   a. Substandard provider education
   b. Poor institutional processes
   c. Defective equipment
   d. Unmotivated personnel

3. What is the goal of risk management?
   a. Identifying poor providers

b. Increasing the department budget
c. Reducing occupational hazards for the health care worker
d. Reducing the risk of lawsuits

4. Which of the following is *not* one of the basic elements of negligence?
   a. Duty owed to the patient
   b. Breach of duty
   c. Presence of a witness
   d. Occurrence of actual damage

5. The concept of *res ipse loquitur* makes the assumption that:
   a. The lawsuit is not valid
   b. The patient contributed to his/her injury
   c. Injury would not normally occur in the absence of negligence
   d. Consent for surgery was not valid

6. What is the legal concept that applies when anesthesia or surgery is performed without informed consent?
   a. Assault and battery
   b. Negligence
   c. Malpractice
   d. Emancipated minor

7. The patient must be advised of all of the following for informed consent to be present *except:*
   a. Required fees
   b. Risks
   c. Complications
   d. Alternatives

8. All of the following organizations regulate compressed gases *except:*
   a. Department of Transportation
   b. National Fire Protection Association
   c. American Society for Testing and Materials
   d. Compressed Gas Association

9. Cylinders used to store compressed gas must be inspected and certified every _____ years.
   a. 2
   b. 5
   c. 10
   d. 12

10. ANSI and ASTM offer voluntary standards for anesthesia equipment. The anesthetist should be aware that these standards:
    a. Should be followed because they will be presented as standard of care in a court of law
    b. Should be viewed as suggestions
    c. Have not improved safety
    d. Are only important on older machines

11. Electric current entering the body through a central catheter and exiting through the skin is called:
    a. Macroshock
    b. Microshock
    c. Impedance
    d. Thermal injury

12. The "let go" current is the current at which the person
    a. First becomes aware of a slight shock
    b. Is *able* to let go of the source of the shock
    c. Is *unable* to let go of the source of the shock
    d. Receives enough current to cause ventricular fibrillation

13. When a line isolation monitor alarms in the operating room, the correct first response would be to:
    a. Call plant management
    b. Initiate fire suppression procedures
    c. Continue with the case but be aware of the shock hazard
    d. Unplug equipment in the reverse order (last item plugged in is the first thing unplugged)

14. The routine use of electrocautery does not cause dysrhythmias because
    a. The electrocardiogram is not sensitive enough to detect the problem
    b. Grounding eliminates the risk
    c. The current frequency is too high to cause dysrhythmias
    d. The grounding pad prevents dysrhythmias

15. Clear glasses would be sufficient to protect the eyes from which type of laser?
    a. KTP
    b. Nd:YAG
    c. CO_2
    d. None of the above

16. Which of the following is true with regard to prevention of airway fire when laser surgery is performed on the larynx or trachea?
    a. A red rubber endotracheal tube is less likely to ignite.
    b. Using helium will increase the risk for fire.
    c. Protected laser tubes will always prevent fire.
    d. The fraction of inspired oxygen should be below 40%.

17. Which of the following lasers is most commonly used with ear-nose-throat surgery?
    a. Argon
    b. CO_2
    c. KTP
    d. Nd:YAG

18. In the event of an airway fire during a laser procedure, your *first* action should be to:
    a. Turn off the O_2 and immediately pull out the endotracheal tube
    b. Pour water into the airway
    c. Administer steroids
    d. Start a second IV and call for help

19. Which of the following gases is most recommended to reduce the fraction of inspired oxygen during laser surgery?
    a. Nitrous oxide
    b. Helium
    c. Nitrogen
    d. Hydrogen

20. Your patient has a pacemaker and will need cautery to control bleeding during the surgical procedure. Which of the following is *least* likely to cause dysrhythmias?
    a. Bipolar cautery
    b. Conventional cautery with the grounding pad near the heart
    c. Conventional cautery with the grounding pad distal from the heart
    d. All forms of cautery are contraindicated.

☐ ANSWERS

1. c	5. c	9. c	13. d	17. b
2. b	6. a	10. a	14. c	18. a
3. d	7. a	11. b	15. c	19. b
4. c	8. c	12. c	16. d	20. a

TWO

Basic Sciences

CHAPTER 2

Review of Chemistry, Biochemistry, and Physics

Leo A. Le Bel

☐ PHYSICS AND INORGANIC CHEMISTRY

The "basic sciences" encompass anatomy, physiology, pharmacology, pathophysiology, embryology, genetics, etc. However, the present review is limited to chemistry, physics, and biochemistry. Basic science knowledge makes up one of the largest components of the CRNA certifying examination. It is also the component most often responsible for a candidate failing that exam.

This review focuses on the most frequent and problematic areas students encounter in studying for the certifying exam. The reader is referred to standard texts for additional review. Topics rarely appearing on the exam or which are outdated are identified. Exam candidates should review them only briefly.

GENERAL

Basic Terms   Many basic concepts are common to both chemistry and physics, so it is sometimes hard to distinguish the two disciplines. The following are basic terms that the student should know, understand, and be able to identify or define.

Matter: Any material item possessing mass and occupying space. There are three *forms of matter*: gases, liquids, and solids:

  Gases have neither volume nor shape; they expand indefinitely (e.g., steam).

  Liquids have volume and assume the shape of their containers (e.g., water).

  Solids have volume and shape; they cannot be compressed (e.g., an ice cube).

Note: In each example, the substance is the same (water, H_2O), but the form differs (i.e., the physical properties change but not the chemical properties). The physical differences depend on the substance's molecular activity and the addition or loss of (heat) energy.

Element: Any basic substance made up of atoms of identical atomic (proton) structure, that cannot further be decomposed, and that loses its chemical properties by electromagnetic union with one or more other elements or through a nuclear reaction that changes its atomic (proton) configuration. The order of elements by atomic weight and electrical configuration is set out in the *Periodic Table of the Elements*. Key elements of the Table the examinee should know are listed below.

- Each element exists as discrete atoms of specific configuration.
- All matter is composed of one or more elements.
- Of 88 naturally occurring elements, 15 are commonly found in the human body. Non–naturally occurring elements are produced through nuclear reactions.
- The table of elements is based on the carbon-12 isotope.
- The name, abbreviation (symbol), atomic number* and atomic weight* of elements likely to be encountered on the certifying exam follow.

Name	Symbol	Atomic Number	Atomic Weight[a]
Bromine[b]	Br	35	79.9
Calcium	Ca	20	40.0
Carbon	C	6	12.0
Chlorine[b]	Cl	17	35.4
Fluorine[b]	F	9	18.9
Helium	He	2	4.0
Hydrogen	H	1	1.0
Iodine[b]	I	53	126.9
Iron	Fe	26	55.8
Nitrogen	N	7	14.0
Oxygen	O	8	16.0
Potassium	K	19	39.0
Sodium	Na	11	22.9
Sulfur	S	16	32.0

[a]Atomic weights are rounded to the most commonly used number. If actual atomic weights are provided on the exam, use them for any calculations.
[b]These four elements are among the five members of the *halogen (formerly called the salt-forming) group;* they have anesthesia uses. The fifth, astatine (As, atomic number 85; atomic weight 210), has no anesthesia use. Questions on halogens have been on the exam.

Compound: A substance made up of two or more chemically combined elements.

Mass: Any quantity of matter (usually expressed in weight units; e.g., pounds, kilograms)

Gravity: Force of attraction between two bodies. Varies inversely with the square of the distance between them. (Along with electrical, chemical, and mechanical = one of the natural forces.)

Weight: A measure of the forces of attraction between two bodies.

Note: The mass of an object differs in each frame of reference (the weight of a person on earth is greater than on the moon where gravity is less).

Force: A way of talking about energy (see "Energy"). The formula is

$$\text{Force } (f) = \text{mass } (m) \times \text{acceleration } (a)$$

Energy: The ability to do work or produce a change in matter. There are two forms of energy: (1) *kinetic energy,* or energy in motion, and (2) *latent energy,* or stored energy. Changing the form of matter involves the addition or removal of energy.

Note: Concepts of energy and mass are essential to understanding physics and chemistry. This is exemplified in Einstein's equation:

$$E \text{ (energy)} = m \text{ (mass)} \times c^2 \text{ (the speed of light squared)}$$

Work: Performed when a force is exerted over a distance (e.g., when 1 g is moved 1 cm or 1 lb is moved 1 ft). Work performed depends on the nature of the force (gravity, heat, electricity), and the manner in which it is applied. (For example, if one object hits a second, it changes the second object's direction—vector—or speed.)

The basic measures of force are as follows:

Dyne (dyn) = The force required to move a 1-g mass 1 cm in 1s

Erg = The amount of work done by a force of 1 dyne acting through 1 cm ($= 1 \text{ g/cm}^2/\text{s}^{-2}$, or 10^{-7} joules).

Newton (N) = The force required to move a 1-kg mass 1 m in 1 s.

Note: Movement per unit of time = *acceleration.*

Physical change: A substance undergoes a change in form but retains its essential properties.

Chemical change: A substance is changed into a new substance with new properties.

Law of conservation of energy: Energy can neither be created nor destroyed.

Note: Per Einstein's formula, mass and energy are interchangeable concepts, so all matter (theoretically) can be converted to pure energy, and any change in matter involves addition or loss of energy. As objects cool, their atoms move more slowly and their mass shrinks by about 1/273 for every degree Kelvin (see below) until, at absolute zero, or −273.16°C, all mass is converted to pure energy.

The foregoing definitions are covered in basic texts.

Scientific Measurement   Exam candidates should know the following basic and derived SI (Système Internationale) measurements:

BASIC SI UNITS

Measurement	Basic SI Unit	Symbol
Length	Meter	m
Mass	Kilogram	kg
Time	Second	s
Temperature	Kelvin	K

DERIVED SI UNITS

Measurement	SI Unit	Symbol
Frequency	Hertz	Hz
Force	Newton	N
Work/energy	Joule	J
Electrical resistance	Ohm	Ω
Pressure	Pascal	Pa

For both basic and derived units, prefixes derived from the metric system are used to indicate fractions or multiples of each unit: e.g., kilometer = 1000 meters, millimeter = 1/1000 meter.

Commonly, these measurements are expressed as powers of 10. Examinees should know at least the following common prefixes:

10^1 = deca (da) 10^{-1} = deci (d)
10^2 = hecto (h) 10^{-2} = centi (c)
10^3 = kilo (k) 10^{-3} = milli (m)
10^6 = mega (M) 10^{-6} = micro (μ)
10^9 = giga (G) 10^{-9} = nano (n)

Density: The relationship of a substance's weight to its volume.

$$\text{Density} = \text{weight} / \text{volume}$$

For example, if density = 150 grams/100 cubic centimeters, then density = 1.5. For most substances, density = grams per cubic centimeter; for gases, it is grams per liter.

Study hint: Exam questions on this topic either ask the examinee to calculate the density where weight and volume are provided (or to find any one factor when the other two are provided) or they ask the examinee to compare the densities of two or more substances and ask which is more/less dense.

Specific gravity: This expresses the ratio between the densities of two substances. The substance is usually compared to the density of water or, for gases, the density of air. The formula is as follows:

$$\text{Specific gravity} = \frac{\text{density of substance}}{\text{density of water (or air)}}$$

The number obtained is just a reflection of the ratio between the two. It is not expressed in discrete units. Specific gravity tells us whether a gas is heavier than air and thus can be used for gas inductions by flowing it over a patient's face.

ATOMIC AND MOLECULAR STRUCTURE AND ACTIVITY; THE THEORY OF OCTET

All elements are made up of discrete atoms of specific configuration. All atoms of an element are identical and each retains all of the element's properties, but if atoms of different elements are joined, either by electromagnetic means or nuclear reactions, a new substance with new properties is formed. Atoms of different elements differ in weight, size, chemical properties, and configuration. The *main elements of every atom,* which differ on the basis of mass and electric charge, are:

Protons: These have a positive charge.
Neutrons: These have no charge (i.e., they are electrically neutral).

Together, protons and neutrons make up the nucleus of each atom. They also have equal masses.

Electrons: These have a negative charge and a mass of approximately 1/1800th that of the nucleus; they circle the nucleus in various orbits of differing distances from the nucleus. These electron "orbits" are also called *energy levels* because the rate and vector of electron travel varies in distance and energy. The actual number of electrons in the atom's outer orbit varies and gives the atom its electrical properties, i.e., how readily it will donate, accept, or share electrons with other elements to form new substances. (See "The Theory of Octet," below.)

Note: Atoms (and molecules) have a great deal of freedom of movement, especially gases. Gases of single atoms can travel horizontally, vertically, and to and fro. Polyatomic atoms have even more freedom, being able to move in several directions at once and also being able to shrink or expand their overall size.

Atomic weight: This is equal to the masses of the protons and neutrons in the nucleus. Since protons and neutrons are equal in mass, they each represent one *atomic mass unit* (amu). *However: the electrical charge of the nucleus is determined by the number of protons. The electrical charge of the protons is balanced by the negative charges of the electrons, so that each atom is electrically neutral.*

Atomic number: This number refers to the number of protons or electrical charges of an atom. The number goes up as one proceeds up the periodic table from the simplest, most abundant of the elements, hydrogen. So where hydrogen has one proton, the next two elements, helium and lithium, have, respectively, two and three. The pattern continues as one proceeds to the heavier elements listed further down the periodic table. As elements go up in the number of protons, they are matched by a corresponding rise in neutrons and electrons.

The Theory of Octet   The theory of octet states that all elements tend to have an outer electron ring made up of exactly 8 electrons. Elements with exactly 8 outer electrons are highly stable. These include the so-called rare or noble gases. They are inert (i.e., they do not react readily with other elements).

Obviously, not all elements have 8 outer electrons; they may have any number from 1 to 8. Those having 4 outer electrons tend to share them readily with other elements. These are called *amphoteric substances.* Carbon is the best example. Its unique properties lie at the foundation of organic chemistry. (See the organic chemistry section below.)

Electrovalent Bonding   Metals and nonmetals react well together: metals with 1, 2, or 3 outer electrons (found on the left side of the periodic table) give them up to the outer orbits of elements with 5, 6, or 7 outer electrons (nonmetals, found on the right side of the periodic table, just before the inert, or noble, gases). Conversely, nonmetals, with 5, 6, or 7 outer electrons, tend to readily accept electrons from metal elements with 1, 2, or 3 outer electrons. In both cases, the elements are trying to achieve stability by providing 8 electrons for each element's outer orbit. *In every case, the bonding takes place in the most energy-efficient manner.* Such joinings produce an *electrovalent compound.* (This is also called *ionic bonding*.) Substances in the midportion of the periodic table (called *transition elements*), can behave as either metals or nonmetals.

Metals: Generally soft and shiny, metals are good conductors of electricity and heat and have low melting points.

Nonmetals: These vary widely in their properties; they can be liquids, gases, or solids. They are poor conductors of heat and electricity.

When electrons circle the nucleus (at varying distances and with varying energies), they tend to assume a recurring pattern (at least up to calcium, element 20). That pattern is:

- Two electrons in the first orbit
- Eight electrons in the second orbit
- Eight electrons in the third orbit

Beyond this point, elements tend to have outer electron rings wherein the electrons move about more freely, even changing orbits (energy levels).

This 2-8-8 configuration is repeated in nearly all elements. Exceptions are hydrogen, with only 1 electron, and helium, with a maximum of 2 outer electrons.

Electrovalent bonding of two or more elements depends on their atomic structures, especially the number of electrons in each element's outer orbits. Each element (atom), by itself, remains electrically neutral. But in bonding with other atoms, electrical neutrality is lost and the resulting particle is called an *ion.* If more protons remain than electrons, the ion will be positively charged—called a *cation;* if electrons are gained so that their numbers exceed those of the protons, the ion will carry a negative charge. This is an *anion.*

It is important to know that (1) the outer-orbit electrons determine how readily an atom interacts with other atoms and that (2) each element always "tries" to achieve an outer orbit configuration of eight electrons. If an element does not have 8 electrons of its own (as the inert elements do), it must get them by gaining, losing, or sharing its outer orbit electrons with those of other atoms. These two principles are essential to understanding both chemistry and physics because they explain how elements are combined to form new substances.

Naming Compounds   In order to *name compounds* that have been electrochemically bonded, the *general rule* is that the name of the metal is used first, followed by the name of the nonmetal—modified by the suffix *ide* to indicate that it is part of a compound—e.g., sodium chlor *ide.* (Most two-atom, or diatomic, compounds are named this way.)

Where one element cannot gain/lose the same number of electrons as the element with which it is combined, then two (or more) atoms of the element are needed to achieve an electrically balanced compound (i.e., one that is electrically neutral, with positive and negative charges being equal). An example of this type of compound is calcium chloride, ($CaCl_2$). Here, the formula indicates that two chlorine atoms have been joined to one atom of calcium. This is required for electrical balance because of calcium's *oxidation state.*

Oxidation numbers can reflect positive, negative, or neutral electrical balances. Positive oxidation numbers (= electrons given up) are indicated by a (+) sign; negative numbers (= electrons gained) are indicated by a (−) sign; neutral substances have neither signs nor numbers. *The numbers that accompany the (+) or (−) signs indicate the number of electrons that must be shifted to achieve electrical balance—e.g., +2 or −3. (The electrical algebraic sum of any compound must always total zero.)*

Note: The term *valence* means the same as oxidation number or oxidation state and is sometimes used in place of those terms.

Some elements can exist in several different oxidation states, therefore we must have some way to name them that distinguishes that state. The suffix *ous* is used for the lower oxidation state, while the suffix *ic* denotes the higher oxidation state. For example, one can have ferric oxide, where iron has a +3 oxidation state (Fe^{+3}) or ferrous oxide, where iron has a +2 oxidation state (Fe^{+2}). A few elements—e.g., tin (Sn) can have more than two oxidation states. The other is designated by a Roman numeral IV—e.g., tin (IV) chloride.

Radicals   Any group of atoms that have bonded together to act like an individual atom in chemical reactions are called radicals. Many are common to bodily reactions. Usually written within parentheses, they include:

Bicarbonate (HCO_3)	Hydroxyl (OH)
Phosphate (PO_4)	Ammonium (NH_4)
Sulfate (SO_4)	Carbonate (CO_3)
	Nitrate (NO_3)

Note: Radicals, too, can have different oxidation states, designated by the suffixes *ate* for the higher states and *ite* for the lower ones. The term *covalence* is sometimes used to denote the number of electron pairs that are shared in a compound.

It is always electrons that are lost or gained when compounds are formed, never protons or neutrons. An atom's nucleus can have an unequal number of protons and neutrons if it is a variant form of an element, call an isotope. Such an atom will have a different weight and retain the element's chemical properties, but its physical properties will differ. Any collection of elemental atoms will normally comprise both the basic atom and its isotopes.

Molecular Weight   Chemically combining atoms of different elements produces a *compound.* The smallest single component of a compound is a *molecule.* For example, the element sodium (atomic weight, 22.989) can be combined with chlorine (atomic weight, 35.453) to produce one molecule of common table salt, sodium chloride (atomic weight 58.442). The weight of a molecule of sodium chloride is the sum of its constituents. *To obtain the molecular weight of any compound, one simply adds the atomic weights of all the atoms that make up the molecule.*

Moreover, every compound is always made up of the same combination of atoms, in the same proportions and configuration. This is known as the *law of definite composition*. One gram's worth of a molecule is called the *gram molecular weight* (GMW), also called a *mole*. A GMW of any substance always contains 6.02×10^{23} molecules. This number is called *Avogadro's number*. Under standard conditions (0° C and 760 mm of mercury pressure), one GMW of a substance always occupies a volume of 22.4 L. This is known as the gram molecular volume (GMV).

Under standard conditions, equal volumes of two different molecules must always contain the same number of molecules and occupy the same amount of space.

These concepts, in turn, lead to other concepts important to anesthesia practice, especially the behavior of gases (i.e., pressure; volume) and how molecular forces can alter or be altered by heat and temperature (the laws of thermodynamics).

Volume The space occupied by an aggregate or collection of atoms or molecules is called the volume. Solids are measured by the cubic centimeter (cm^3 or cc), or the larger cubic meter (m^3); while liquids and gases are measured by the milliliter (mL), or liter (L). Collections of atoms or molecules (especially if contained in a closed container) exert pressures which, if great enough, can be measured. For example: the pressure exerted by the air molecules in our atmosphere can be measured. It averages (at sea level) about 760 mm of mercury pressure. Similarly, oxygen in an H size gas cylinder of the type used in anesthesia practice generates a pressure of 2200 psi when full. The pressure is registered on the cylinder's pressure gauge.

Pressure The force exerted by a collection of atoms or molecules is called pressure. This pressure is generated by two sources: (1) gravitational influences on the atoms or molecules and (2) the energy forces operating within the atoms or molecules themselves. Density plays a role also. Denser substances exert a greater pressure than less dense ones. For example, a column of mercury, being dense, exerts more pressure than a like column of (less dense) water.

Apart from density, the pressure generated by a collection of atoms or molecules relates to the *kinetic theory of matter*, which states that *all matter is made up of atoms or molecules in constant motion*. That is, all atoms/molecules are in constant motion and, as they move about and strike the sides of a container, they exert a certain force. The sum of forces exerted by a collection of molecules or atoms within a closed container can be read as the cylinder pressure. **The kinetic theory of matter is a critical concept. The reader must understand how atoms and molecules behave as they do, especially in response to changes in temperature caused by the addition or release (loss) of heat.** An understanding of this concept is critical to understanding how anesthetic gases (and vapors) behave.

The movement of molecules and the atoms of which they are made up is constant but not uniform. Their speeds (velocities), direction (vectors), and momentum (energy) vary continually. As intra-atomic or intra-molecular distances vary in *momentum*, heat will be lost or gained, and this will be accompanied by a rise or fall in temperature.

Momentum is also subject to the forces of the atoms or molecules interacting with their environment. That is, momentum is changed as the atoms/molecules strike each other—or the sides of the container that holds them. If atoms/molecules were to strike each other and be perfectly *elastic,* they would rebound with the same momentum as when they collided. But molecules are not perfectly elastic, since they exist in real space, where friction and other forces affect them. So when they do collide, there is a concomitant loss of energy (momentum) and a corresponding loss of heat. Conversely, if a cylinder of gas is heated, the increased temperature (heat) causes the molecules to travel with greater momentum. As a collection of atoms/molecules is heated or cooled and their activity is increased or decreased, there is a corresponding change in pressure. Depending on circumstances, the pressure exerted by a collection of atoms or molecules can be measured in kilopascals, pascals, pounds per square inch, millimeters of mercury, centimeters of water, or any other convenient method of measure.

In addition to the foregoing, other intermolecular interactions (forces) with which the reader should be familiar include the following:

Adhesion The interaction between unlike molecules; for example, water against the side of a glass. One particular application of adhesion is that of *capillary action,* where water or other fluid can be drawn up a clothlike dissimilar material. This phenomenon can be seen when blood spreads up a surgical drape or towel. It also is the principle that allows for use of a "wick" to pick up liquid anesthetic in draw-over vaporizers.

Cohesion The interaction between like molecules: for example, water molecules against other water molecules, as occurs when water flowing in the middle of a tube travels faster than the water against the container's sides. Cohesion influences the boiling points of liquids, their vapor pressure, viscosity, and surface tension, and the heat of vaporization (of anesthetics).

Surface Tension At a liquid-gas (air) interface, liquid molecules are pulled together by forces created by unequal intermolecular stresses. Cleaning agents work in part by altering water's surface tension.

Van der Waals Forces Also known as London dispersion forces, these occur where molecules interact strongly with each other electrically (at least over short distances). This causes polar molecules (i.e., those with a relatively positive and a relatively negative pole; called a *dipole molecule*) to line up with like molecules in forming a latticework of molecules. Water, H_2O, is the best example. Its latticework structure is best exemplified when the water turns to ice. (See "Hydrogen Bonding," below.)

Van der Waals forces, which increase the size of the molecules, are important because they affect boiling point, viscosity, the amount of energy needed to vaporize a liquid, etc.

TEMPERATURE SCALES AND TYPES OF HEAT

Heat is but one kind of energy, and its intensity is, by convention, measured by one of three temperature scales: Kelvin (K) or absolute zero scale; the centigrade (Celsius) scale; and the Fahrenheit scale.

Note: The examinee must know how to convert from one scale to another, especially if confronted by mathematical problems involving the gas laws.

The Kelvin scale begins at absolute zero ($-273.16°C$) and moves only in an upward direction. The centigrade scale was set based on the freezing and boiling points of water, allowing for $100°$ between the two to accommodate the decimal-based measurements of the metric system. Therefore, the scale was set at base $0°$ (water's freezing point) and, at the high end, a base of $100°$ (water's boiling point). In the Fahrenheit scale, water freezes at $32°$ and boils at $212°$, a difference of $180°$. The ratio (based on the freezing and boiling points of water) of the Fahrenheit scale to the centigrade scale is thus: $180°$ to $100°$, or a ratio of 1.8 to 1. This makes converting from one system to the other relatively easy, but one must remember to proceed from the Fahrenheit to centigrade scale and then to the Kelvin scale or, if necessary, to calculate them in the reverse order, using the following formulas.

To convert from Fahrenheit to centigrade temperatures:

$$°F = (°C \times 1.8) + 32$$

To convert from centigrade to Fahrenheit temperatures:

$$°C = (°F - 32) \div 1.8$$

To convert from centigrade to Kelvin scales:

$$°K = °C + 273.16$$

To convert from Kelvin to centigrade:

$$°C = K - 273.16$$

While the foregoing are measures of the intensity of heat, other terms are needed to discuss the amount of work done by heat or, conversely, the amount of heat lost by expending (heat) energy.

Small calorie, (or gram calorie): The amount of heat needed to raise the temperature of 1 g of water by $1°$ centigrade.

Kilocalorie: The equivalent of 1000 small calories.

Btu (British thermal unit): The amount of heat needed to raise the temperature of 1 lb of water $1°$ Fahrenheit.

Joule: A unit used to compare work done in various energy systems (e.g., electrical, mechanical).

Thermal heat capacity: The amount of heat needed to raise (at atmospheric pressure) the temperature of a given mass of substance by one degree unit (usually calories per gram per degree centigrade).

Specific heat: Ratio of the amount of heat required to raise the temperature of a given mass of substance $1°$ compared with that needed to raise the same mass of water $1°C$.

- Gases have two specific heats; one where volume is retained and one where pressure is retained.
- Generally, solids and liquids have high specific heats, but gases have low specific heats; so inhaled cold gases require external heat to raise their temperatures to that of the body, gaining heat from either the respiratory tract or from external heating devices. Similarly, vaporization will cease due to cooling unless additional external heat is applied to an anesthesia vaporizer. This too is partly due to the fact that gases/vapor have low specific heats. Water has a high specific heat.
- The rapidity with which heat is conducted between molecules varies. There are three possible mechanisms.

1. Transfer of heat directly from one molecule to another. This is called *conduction*.
2. Transfer of heat in electromagnetic waves, called *radiation* or radiant heat (e.g., microwave oven).
3. Transfer of heat by air currents. This is called *convection* heating.

Molal heat capacity: This is the amount of heat needed to raise, by $1°C$, the temperature of 1 mol of gas. It increases as the weight and number of atoms making up the gas increase, a process that makes the gas less susceptible to combustion. Inert gases, especially those with large thermal capacities, can cool an ignition source and keep it from igniting an otherwise combustible gas mixture. For this reason, gases with high molal heat capacities are often called *quenching agents.* Carbon dioxide is a notable example.

Converting the physical states of substances requires the loss or addition of heat. For example, converting 1 g of ice to water and then to steam requires not only 100 g calories but also the loss or gain of additional heat to effect the actual conversions from ice to water and from water to steam. (The latent heats for water amount to about 540 additional calories for each conversion.) These additional heats are referred to as *latent heats.*

Latent heat of melting: Serves to convert a solid object to a liquid.

Latent heat of vaporization: Serves to convert a liquid to a gas.

Latent heat of condensation: Serves to convert a gas to a liquid.

Latent heat of crystallization: Serves to convert a liquid to a solid.

- The first two types of latent heat involve adding heat, since molecules are being accelerated. The last two involve heat loss, causing steam to condense to water and then harden to ice.
- Questions dealing with latent heats (and other terms pertaining to heat and temperature) have appeared on past certifying examinations.

Actually, the contraction or expansion of molecules that accompanies a change in the physical state of matter depend on both temperature and pressure. Gases, because they have very high molecular velocities, cannot usually be liquified without first undergoing substantial cooling. As cooling proceeds, a point is reached where, if enough pressure is applied to the gas, it will be forced into the liquid state. However, there is a point (for all gases) above which they cannot be liquified regardless of the amount of pressure applied. This point is known as the *critical temperature*. Critical temperature and its associated concepts, which follow, have appeared as questions on the certifying examination.

Critical temperature: That temperature above which a gas cannot be liquified regardless of the amount of pressure applied.

Critical pressure: That pressure required to liquify a gas at its critical temperature.

Critical volume: The space occupied by one GMW of a gas at its critical temperature and pressure.

Critical density: The density of one GMW of a gas at its critical temperature and pressure.

Note: Cooling and pressurizing gases allows for their bulk storage (e.g., hospital oxygen supply).

WRITING CHEMICAL FORMULAS

Chemical formulas use symbols instead of words. They are a shorthand method of demonstrating the changes that take place in a chemical reaction. *Equations must take into account radicals, oxidation states, and electrical balances.*

There are four types of chemical reactions:

1. *Synthesis,* where reactants are combined
2. *Decomposition,* where a compound is broken down
3. *Single displacement,* where one of the reactants is replaced by another
4. *Double displacement,* where parts of both reactants are replaced by other substances

Another chemical reaction type is called an:

Oxidation/reduction reaction: Here atoms that are losing electrons are said to be oxidized while atoms gaining electrons are said to be reduced. These are often encountered in biochemical reactions occurring within the human body. For example, the body gains energy by oxidizing fats, carbohydrates, and proteins.

Writing chemical equations normally involves four steps: (1) Write down the reactants. (2) Write in and check the algebraic sum of the oxidation numbers to see if they total zero (e.g., $+1$ and $-1 = 0$, but a $+2$ and a $-1 \neq 0$). (3) If the algebraic sum is not zero, one must crisscross the oxidation numbers, a process analogous to obtaining an arithmetic least common denominator. The superscripts can then be erased. (4) Last, the equation must be balanced so that equal quantities of each element are present on both sides of the equation. An example of the four steps follows. The reactants are sodium and sulfate, (a radical). Remember, it is important to treat the radical as a single entity.

1. $Na \quad + \quad (SO_4) \quad \Rightarrow \quad ???$
2. $Na^{+1} \quad + \quad (SO_4)^{-2} \quad \Rightarrow \quad ???$ [algebraic sum $\neq 0$]
3. $Na^{+1}[1] \quad + \quad (SO_4)^{-2}[2] \quad \Rightarrow \quad Na_2(SO_4)$
4. $2Na \quad + \quad (SO_4) \quad \Rightarrow \quad Na_2(SO_4)$ [sodium sulfate]

In step (1) of the foregoing, a molecule (or atom) of sodium and a molecule of sulfate are to be joined to form sodium sulfate. In step (2), the oxidation numbers are placed as superscripts. Notice that because these are $+1$ and -2, the algebraic sum is not equal to zero. Reducing these to the (least common denominator) ratio of $[1]:[2]$, we must crisscross the two numbers in step (3) to balance the reaction. In step (4), we indicate that now *two* molecules of sodium must be combined with a single molecule of sulfate (to electrically balance the reactants). Joining these two sodium molecules and the sulfate molecule gives us an end product of sodium sulfate.

SOLUTIONS

Solutions are homogenous mixtures of two or more uniformly distributed substances that may or may not be in equal proportion. Solutions help some chemical reactions proceed more quickly. The term *solute* denotes the dissolved substance, while the substance into which the solute is placed is called the *solvent.*

Solutions can be solids in liquids, gases in liquids, gases in gases, or liquids in other liquids. The amount of solute dissolvable in a given amount of solvent depends on temperature. *Unsaturated solutions* permit the addition of more solute. *Saturated solutions* do not allow the addition or more solute without some of the solute precipitating out. Heating the solvent allows for addition of more solute, producing what is called a *supersaturated solution,* but the mixture then become unstable, so that mechanical disruption or a drop in temperature also causes the solute to precipitate.

Water   Water is but one type of "solution," though a very common one. Because it is abundant and because so many substances can be dissolved in or combined with it, water is called the *universal solvent.* In most circumstances, its *density is taken to be 1 g/mL,* though this may be altered by temperature and pressure. For example, as its temperature approaches 4°C, water expands, and this reduces its density somewhat. The expansion that water undergoes under such circumstances is not unlike that which human cellular water undergoes with frostbite.

Like other liquids, water is *subject to the forces of adhesion, cohesion, capillary action, and van der Waals forces.* Adhesive forces contribute to water's *"wetting" properties.* As with most liquids, water's adhesive forces often overcome its cohesive forces. That is why, in a water manometer, water's meniscus should be read at the bottom of the depression of water caused by the adhesive forces acting between the water and the sides of the glass tube of the manometer. This is in contrast to the meniscus of a mercury manometer; such a manometer should be read at the top because mercury's cohesive forces are strong enough to overcome its adhesive forces.

Water exerts a *vapor pressure of 47 torr.* As with any air-exposed liquid, some of its molecules leave the liquid state (because, as discussed earlier, molecules are in constant motion) and enter the air above it. If fully exposed to air, the liquid eventually evaporates. But *in a closed container containing a liquid, a point of equilibrium will eventually be reached where the number of molecules leaving and entering the liquid at the liquid/gas interface is equal.* This is the basic principle underlying the concept of *vaporization.* (Vaporization of liquid anesthetics is discussed below. It is a process that slowly, but continuously, occurs at any liquid/air interface.) When the number of molecules leaving and entering the liquid is equal, the liquid is said to be at its *boiling point.*

Hydrogen Bonding As mentioned earlier, water molecules are dipolar and thus can form latticework structures. This property is due to water's unique structure, which allows it to undergo *hydrogen bonding.* The two hydrogen molecules in water are not on a straight plane. Rather, *the hydrogens form an angle of 104.5° with respect to the oxygen molecule, giving the resulting water molecule a relatively dipolar configuration, that is, more positive at one end and more negative at the other;* as per:

$$O^-$$
$$H^+ \quad H^+$$
$$\angle = 104.5°$$

The molecule assumes this configuration because it joins the hydrogens and oxygen with great efficiency, (i.e., least expenditure of energy). The individual water molecules tend to line up one to the other in such as way as to allow some interaction between the positive and negative ends. For example:

Water's polarity makes it an excellent solvent for other polar compounds but not for nonpolar ones. Dissolving solutes such as salts into water creates anions, cations, and even undissociated substances such as radicals. It also changes water's physical properties, called *colligative properties* (e.g., water's freezing and boiling points). Water molecules can also be directly incorporated into the structure of crystalline compounds. Such combinations are called *hydrates.* An example is the (eight-water-molecule) octahydrate in barium hydroxide crystals used for carbon dioxide absorption in anesthesia machines. Where hydrates are dried by heating, an *anhydrate* remains. If a hydrate spontaneously yields its moisture on exposure to air, it is called *efflorescent.* Substances that absorb moisture from the surrounding air are called *hygroscopic compounds.* If hygroscopic compounds dissolve in the water they absorb, they are termed *deliquescent.* Calcium sulfate used to make plaster of Paris casts is such a compound.

Gases in Solution When gases are placed in solution, the amount of gas dissolved depends on the temperature, the solubility of the gas, and the nature of the solvent. When anesthetic gases are dissolved in blood, the gas is influenced by two physical laws: Boyle's law and Henry's law. Both of these are discussed below under "Gases and Gas Laws."

The amount of gas in a liquid solution can be measured in a number of ways. The two methods most frequently encountered in anesthesia are:

1. *The Ostwald solubility coefficient,* in which results are reported based on standard conditions of temperature and pressure.
2. *The Bunsen solubility coefficient,* in which the measurement results are reported under actual conditions (e.g., body temperature).

The solubility of gases in various body tissues is often of importance to anesthesia practitioners. These are expressed in terms of *partition coefficients;* e.g., blood/gas or blood/fat partition coefficients.

True solutions: These occur when the solute becomes fully dissolved in the solvent.

Suspensions: These are solutions wherein the solute cannot be dissolved in the solvent. They produce a milky appearing solution.

Colloidal solutions (colloids): Solutions that lie between true solutions and suspensions. In colloidal solutions the solute particles are too small to be suspended but too large to dissolve into a true solution. The solutes in colloidal solutions tend to move around in a zig-zag fashion termed *Brownian movement.* Colloidal solutions also disperse any light shining through the solution. This is called the *Tyndall effect.*

OSMOSIS

The process whereby water can move through semipermeable membranes (i.e., a membrane that selectively allows the passage of water to either side of the membrane). The process is vitally important to many bodily functions, such as urine formation. A semipermeable membrane consists of aqueous solutions on either side that each have their own concentrations of dissolved ions and molecules. The membrane allows the selective passage of water. *It is important to remember that the passage of water is always from the area of low solute concentration to the area of high solute concentration.* If the solute concentration on the two sides is equal, water flow ceases. If the solute concentrations change in strength, the flow of water can reverse. The pressure that moves the water across the membrane is called the *osmotic pressure.* This activity can be measured in *osmoles* (one GMW of a substance dissolved in 1 L = 1 osmol). However, osmoles are too large a quantity to express the concentrations found within the human body, so a smaller unit, the *milliosmole* (mosm, or 1/1000 osmol), is used. Osmolarity in humans generally averages 300 mosm. (See also the discussion on molarity, below.)

If two fluids exert the same osmotic pressure, they are said to be *isotonic*—that is, the solutions exert equal pressures, but in opposite directions. Solutions compatible with blood are isotonic. Solutions that exert a higher osmotic pressure are termed *hypertonic.* Because they have a higher solute (salt) load, they draw water from the surrounding red blood cells, causing them to shrink; a process called *crenation* or *plasmolysis.* Conversely, solutions having an osmotic pressure less than that of blood cause surrounding red cells to take in more water, enlarging and eventually rupturing (*hemolyzing*) them. These solutions are termed *hypotonic.*

Solution strength can be measured in various ways:

1. As the number of grams of solute per 100 mL of solution. This is called a *percent solution.* For example, a 0.9% solution of normal saline has 0.9 g of salt in each 100 mL of fluid.
2. Where a mole of a substance is placed in 1 L of solution, the result is said to be a one-molar solution; abbreviated 1 *M.* This concept is known as *molarity.* The concept holds also for both multiple molar solutions (e.g., 3*M*), and fractions of a mole (e.g., 0.3 *M*).

However, picking up from the earlier discussion on osmosis, it should be recognized that *osmolarity and molarity are equal only when the dissolved substance is an un-ionized one* (i.e., one that does not separate into two or more ions when placed in solution). *If the dissolved substance ionizes to two particles, then the same 1 L of solution will exert 2 osmols of pressure. The same will be true if the substance ionizes to three particles. The liter will then exert 3 osmols of pressure even though it is still a 1-M solution; i.e., 1 mol of the substance in 1 L of solution.*

Because the number of particles (not their weight/size) determines osmotic pressure, doubling/tripling particles requires a comparable increase in counterpressure if water is to be prevented from crossing the membrane. (See also "normality," below.)

Note: A molar solution and a *molal solution* are the same except that the latter is based on measurements made at 4° C, where, because of temperature-induced changes in the density of water (discussed above), 1 L of water is equal to 1000 g.

NORMALITY

Normality is a concept that *describes how an ionized substance interacts chemically with other substances.* It involves the concept of *equivalency.*

Equivalent weight: The substance's weight in grams needed to react with either 1 g of hydrogen or 8 g of oxygen. This is known as the *gram equivalent weight* (GEW). It is calculated by dividing the GMW by the substance's oxidation number. If the amount of dissolved substance in 1 L is doubled, it produces a 2-*N* (twice normal) solution. Similarly, if three times the amount of substance is dissolved, a 3-*N* solution is formed.

As with molarity, this measure is too large to express the concentrations found in the body, so a smaller measure, the milliequivalent (mEq; 1/1000 of an equivalent) is used.

For univalent cations and nonionizing substances such as sugars, the milliequivalent (mEq) and milliosmole (mOsm) are the same. But, for multivalent cations, the situation is different. For bivalent substances: 1 mEq of cation will equal 0.5 mOsm, while 2 mEq of cation will equal 1 mOsm. A similar relationship will hold for a trivalent substance: 1 mEq = 0.33 mOsm, while 3 mEq = 1 mOsm.

GASES AND GAS LAWS

Gases have a number of distinguishing characteristics. They expand easily and are readily compressed. Also, they have high velocities, weak intermolecular forces, and a high degree of random motion. These characteristics mean that gases can travel large distances quickly. Their ability to readily move about is called:

Diffusion: The process whereby gases move from an area of high concentration to areas of lower concentration.

Eventually, confined gases equilibrate throughout the confining area, whether it be a gas cylinder or a room. A mixture of gases will diffuse as readily and uniformly as a single gas, but *lighter gases diffuse more rapidly than heavy ones.* This is in keeping with:

Graham's law of diffusion: States that the rate of diffusion of a gas will vary with the square root of its molecular weight. Example: gas A has a molecular weight of 4 (square root = 2), while gas B has a molecular weight of 16 (square root = 4). Therefore, gas A will diffuse twice as quickly as gas B.

As gases move from high- to low-concentration areas, the large initial pressure difference speeds diffusion. But as the process continues, the pressure gradient diminishes and diffusion slows. This is in keeping with:

Fick's law: States that diffusion is proportional to the differences in partial pressure (e.g., at the start of inhalation anesthesia delivered concentration is high compared to the blood concentration. As the anesthesia proceeds, the pressure difference falls and the rate of diffusion into blood slows.)

The rate of diffusion of a gas also depends on its temperature, hotter gases diffusing more rapidly than cool ones. Also, each gas in a mixture (like the atmosphere we breathe) exerts its own independent pressure, called the *partial pressure.* The sum of all of those gases, at sea level, accounts for our atmospheric pressure (one atmospheric pressure = 760 mm of mercury, or 760 torr). This concept is defined in:

Dalton's law of partial pressures: The total pressure of a mixture of gases is the sum of all its individual (partial) gas pressures. The total pressure will always equal the atmospheric pressure, normally 760 torr at sea level, but varying somewhat with altitude.

Boyle's law: Expresses the compressibility of gases. At a constant temperature, gas volume varies *inversely* with pressure.

For the various gas laws, especially Boyle's, it is important to recognize the difference between ideal and real gases. *Ideal gases* can only exist in a rarified (vacuum) atmosphere and their molecules are not subject to intermolecular forces (e.g., friction, etc). Under those conditions, multiplying the gas volume by its pressure always equals a constant. But with *real gases,* these forces must be taken into account. *Van der Waals modification of Boyle's law* takes these factors into consideration. At low pressures and high temperatures, real gases behave more like ideal gases.

Charles's law: If pressure is held constant, the volume of expansion is proportional to the absolute temperature [i.e., temperature on the absolute zero (Kelvin) scale].

Gay-Lussac's law: when volume is held constant, gas pressure varies directly (proportionately) with absolute temperature. Charles's law and Gay-Lussac's law are similar in that they both serve to explain the effects of absolute temperature on gas volume and pressure.

The relationships expressed by Boyle's, Charles's, and Gay-Lussac's laws form the *general gas law: PV = nRT,* where *P* = pressure, *V* = volume, *n* = number of gas molecules, *R* = a constant that is the same for all ideal gases, and *T* = absolute temperature. It is useful for explaining the behavior of ideal gases.

Study hint: the general gas law for ideal gases has been modified for determining the effects of *P*, *V*, and *T* changes on real gases used in clinical practice. On the exam, five of six elements are given and the examinee must solve for the remaining element. Use the formula:

$P1 \quad V1 \quad A2 = P2 \quad V2 \quad A1$ (or "PVA 112 = PVA 221")

where $P1$ = initial pressure
$V1$ = initial volume
$A2$ = new temperature (in Kelvin degrees)
$P2$ = new pressure
$V2$ = new volume
$A1$ = initial temperature (in Kelvin degrees)

Three things are important to solve these problems correctly: (1) both volumes and both pressures have to be in the same measurements; (2) all non-Kelvin degrees must be converted to that scale (or sometimes the answer must be converted to that scale; the A in the formula is to remind one that temperatures must be in the Kelvin scale); and (3) the formula must be set up correctly. For example, finding P2 requires changing the formula to:

$$P2 = \frac{P1 \quad V1 \quad A2}{V2 \quad A1}$$

Henry's law: The solubility of a gas varies inversely with temperature.

Solubility (discussed above) varies with the nature of the solute and solvent and the temperature. For gases dissolved in blood, the amount of gas dissolved per unit of blood is directly proportional to the pressure of the gas in the alveoli. Another way to think of this is that the gas pressure over the gas/liquid interface (alveoli) is equal to the amount of gas pressure/tension in solution in the blood. In a mixture of gases, each gas will come to its own equilibration pressure. (The blood is regarded as the solvent and it is assumed that the gas does not physically combine with the blood.)

The number of gas molecules in solution changes directly with pressure, but, at a constant temperature, the volume of the dissolved gas will be independent of gas pressure—as per Boyle's law. Therefore, the gas "bubbles" must expand or contract as needed if the gas pressures in the blood are to be equal to the gas pressures in the alveoli. As body temperature rises, the gas expands and leaves the blood, i.e., comes out of solution. Conversely, as body temperature cools, more gas goes into solution. Therefore if a patient is allowed to become hypothermic during an anesthetic where the administered gas concentration remains constant, the amount of gas actually in solution increases and the depth of anesthesia can be inadvertently deepened. Patients with elevated temperatures are more difficult to anesthetize because it is more difficult for the gas to go into solution.

VAPOR PRESSURES AND VAPORIZATION

Vaporization: The conversion of a volatile liquid to a gas or vapor.

In anesthesia machine vaporizers, vaporization is typically made up of only two components: the vapor and the carrier gas (usually oxygen), and atmospheric pressure will equal 760 torr (at sea level).

Since everything coming out of the vaporizer must equal (total) 100% and 760 torr, every torr change in pressure will equal a 7.6% change in vapor concentration.

One therefore needs only to know the partial pressure of the agent at the temperature being used in order to determine what the percentages of vapor and carrier gas are.

For example, consider an agent, X, with a vapor pressure of 390 torr. This is half of the atmospheric pressure, therefore the vapor will constitute 50% of what comes out of the vaporizer and the carrier gas will constitute the other 50%, and each will contribute 390 torr of the total pressure.

Try working the three following problems:

1. Agent Y has a vapor pressure of 190 torr. What percent will this be of the total? What percentage will the carrier gas contribute?
2. Agent Z has a vapor pressure of 570 torr. What percent will this be of the total? What percentage will the carrier gas contribute?
3. The carrier gas exerts 60% of the atmospheric pressure. What percent of the total does this represent? What percent is represented by the vapor? What amount of pressure does the vapor produce?

Once one knows the amount of actual vapor being produced in milliliters for each 100 mL of carrier gas (which can be determined on a percentage basis from the foregoing approaches), one merely has to set the diluent flow at 100 × that amount to make setting the delivered concentration easy. For example, if 100 mL of carrier gas produces 30 mL of vapor, a 3000-mL (3-L) diluent flow makes changing calculations easy. If carrier flow is doubled to 200 mL, the delivered concentration will be 2%. If carrier flow is halved to 50 mL, delivered concentration falls to 0.5%. (One can also do the same thing by changing the diluent flow when the same 100 mL of carrier gas flow is still producing the same 30 mL of vapor. Now, reducing the diluent flow to 1500 mL (1.5 L) will double the delivered concentration. Doubling the diluent flow to 6000 mL (6 L) will halve the delivered concentration.

So delivered anesthesia concentrations can be calculated by the proportional methods just described.

However, the same principle is reflected in the traditional *formula for calculating delivered concentrations of anesthetic:*

$$\text{Concentration} = \frac{\text{VP}/(\text{AP} - \text{VP}) \times 100 \times 100}{\text{total flow}}$$

where VP = vapor pressure of the agent at the temperature being used
AP = atmospheric pressure (may vary with altitude) but is usually considered 760 torr sea-level pressure)
First 100 = a presumed carrier gas flow of 100 mL/min

Second 100 = a mathematical method for moving the decimal point in the fraction created by the ratio of vapor pressure to atmospheric pressure (i.e., the first part of the equation)

Total flow: Comprises vapor, carrier gas, and diluent flow; but for a shortcut method for making the calculations easy, only diluent flow is taken into consideration, though this is not as accurate. (For example: halothane's 243-torr vapor pressure at 20° C and with a 5-L diluent flow actually produces a concentration of 0.97%. But by using the shortcut method of calculating—i.e., dividing only by diluent flow, not total flow—one gets a concentration of 1%.) *Notice that the shortcut method is also safer in that the actual concentration is less than the calculated (shortcut) concentration.* This means that even if you use the shortcut method, you are not apt to overdose the patient.

If the temperature of use is changed (cooler or warmer), there will be a corresponding change in vapor pressure and delivered concentration. If a volatile liquid is cooled enough, vaporization will cease and the delivered anesthetic concentration will fall off drastically.

Also remember that gases with high vapor pressures (above 390 torr) produce high concentrations with little carrier-gas flow, while gases with low vapor pressures require very high carrier-gas flows in order to produce even minimal anesthetic concentrations. The best example of this was methoxyflurane (Penthrane; no longer used clinically). The maximum concentration possible with this agent was about 3.2%. For such agents to be useful, they must be very potent.

The principles of vaporization work with both main (non-agent-specific) vaporizers such as the Copper Kettle, Vernitrol, or side-arm Vernitrol anesthesia vaporizers *and* with agent-specific, temperature- and pressure-compensated out-of-circuit vaporizers such as the Tec variety.

Other points regarding vaporization:

- Too rapid a carrier gas flow can outpace vaporization.
- Cooling slows vaporization.
- Heating speeds vaporization.
- Contamination of wicks by water or other substances may hamper vaporization.
- "Back pressure" problems in the anesthesia circuit can cause sudden changes in delivered concentration—even draw liquid anesthetic into the circuit. Baffles and other protections built into the construction of such vaporizers minimize but do not completely eliminate these hazards.
- Vaporization even goes on in body cavities, etc.

THERAPEUTIC GASES

The following gases have therapeutic uses apart from their uses in anesthesia. The therapeutic uses generally rely upon some unique physical or chemical property of the gas. Important points are asterisked. Questions pertaining to the physical and chemical properties of these gases have appeared on the certifying examination.

Oxygen

Most widely used gas.
Colorless, odorless, tasteless.
One-fifth of atmosphere.
*Primarily used by body as oxidant for metabolic reactions.
Disease states interfere with delivery to tissues (e.g., sickle cell disease).
Other factors interfering with oxygen delivery include medications such as nitroprusside (cyanide in drug structure displaces oxygen from hemoglobin).
Three isotopes: O-16, O_2, and O_3.
Boiling point: $-183°C$; solidifies at $-217°C$.
*Is paramagnetic (useful in positron emission tomography).
*May form free radicals (superoxide anions) thought to be implicated with oxygen toxicity.
*Oxidizes metals and rancids acids; supports combustion; and forms peroxides.
Molecular weight: 32.
Density 1.4 at STP.
Specific gravity 1.105 compared to air.
Critical temperature: 118.4.
Has low specific heat and is readily soluble in water.
*In simple solution, 0.3 mL dissolves in each 100 mL of blood and 1.3 mL combines with each gram of hemoglobin.
High concentrations can result in retrolental fibroplasia (blindness of newborns).
Stored in green or green-and-white containers at 2000 to 2200 psi.

Nitrogen

An inert element.
Does not readily combine with other substances.
Prepared by fractional distillation of air.
Is odorless, colorless, tasteless.
Atomic weight is 14, but is diatomic, with a molecular weight of 28.
Density: 1.205 at STP.
*Specific gravity: 0.967, therefore lighter than air.
Can combine with hydrogen or oxygen.
*Five oxide configurations possible; one, nitric oxide (NO) is used to formulate nitric acid; another is nitrous oxide.
*Large amounts are in simple solution in the blood.
*Displacement = denitrogenation—used on induction of anesthesia.
Liquid nitrogen can produce "cold" burns.
Used as compressed gas to power tools in surgery.
Combined with oxygen, serves as breathing gas for deep-sea diving and flying.

Combined with oxygen, is stored in yellow containers. Nonmedical version stored in black-and-green cylinders.

Nitrous Oxide

Molecular weight: 44.02.
*Specific gravity 1.527; about 1.5 times heavier than air.
Colorless, has slight taste/odor, but is nonirritating.
Boiling point is $-89°C$ (the critical temperature).
Manufactured by decomposing ammonium nitrate.
Stored as liquid in blue containers.
*Cylinder pressures = 750 to 800, depending on local atmospheric conditions.
Moisture in outlet can cause condensation.
*Is insoluble in blood (blood solubility = 0.47).
*Expansion of the gas can create pressure problems in closed cavities—compare to sulfur hexafluorinium (SF6).
*MAC: 110 to 115%; therefore not a complete anesthetic.
Anesthesia requirements are generally 50 to 70%.
Is nonflammable, but because it contains oxygen, will support combustion.

Carbon Dioxide

An organic compound.
*Is the end product of respiration and is a respiratory stimulant in low concentrations.
*Carbon combines with oxygen to form either carbon monoxide or carbon dioxide.
*Forms 0.03% of atmosphere.
*Combines with water to form carbonic acid.
*Similar to nitrous oxide in molecular weight (44) and specific gravity (1.54).
Stored as compressed gas in liquid form in gray cylinders.
Is absorbed and neutralized by alkalies to form carbonates or bicarbonates.
*Has a high molal heat capacity, therefore is an excellent quenching agent.
Concentrations can be measured by infrared methods.
At 5% concentration, used as a respiratory stimulant.
Used for calibrating blood gas machines.

Helium

One of the rare gases, is inert.
*Used as a diluent for other gases.
Is the second lightest element known.
Atomic number 2, molecular weight 4.
*Diffuses three times faster than oxygen, therefore very useful in patients with respiratory disease.
Is colorless, tasteless, and odorless.
Liquifies at $-269°C$ (almost at absolute zero).
*Is quite insoluble at 0.87 mL/100 mL of blood at room temperature.
*Possesses a high degree of heat conductivity, therefore is also a quenching agent.

HUMIDITY

Humidity is mainly useful for personnel comfort in the O.R. and humidification of inhaled, cold, dry, anesthetic gases (usually by a humidifier). Water's vapor pressure: 47 torr.

Types of Humidity

Absolute: Maximum water saturation a volume of air can hold at a given temperature.
Relative: Actual saturation expressed as a percent of maximum possible saturation.
Dew point: Temperature at which, if a given volume of air is cooled, excess moisture precipitates.

The measurement of humidity is called *hygrometry. Barometers* are useful in measuring humidity because they measure changes in atmospheric pressure. Barometer types: *liquid* (water or mercury), usually in a closed "U" configuration; *anaeroid* (e.g., Bourdon gauges), used with blood pressure cuffs or on gas cylinders; and *electric.*

FLOW OF FLUIDS THROUGH TUBES AND ORIFICES

Fluids can be either liquids or gases. Their flow through tubes and orifices has numerous applications in anesthesia practice. For example, intravenous fluids flowing through tubing to the patient, gases flowing through the anesthesia delivery circuit, gases passing through the flowmeter tubes of anesthesia machines.

Tube: A pathway whose length is greater than its diameter.

Orifice: An opening that has diameter but not length.

Flow through tubes or orifices occurs when a pressure differential develops between the two sides of the tube or orifice. There are three types of flow:

Steady: Uniform (i.e., all molecules traveling in the same direction and at the same velocity).
Laminar: All molecules travel a parallel path within the tube.
Turbulent: Molecules travel in nonparallel paths, which gives rise to "eddy" currents.

Note: High flows increase velocity and create turbulence.

Velocity: Velocity varies with the cross-sectional area of the tube.

Volume flow rate (F): This *varies with* the *cross-sectional area* of the tube, tube *length,* and the *pressure differential* and *viscosity* of the fluid.

F is determined by *Poiseuille's law,* which states (for laminar flow in a cylindrical tube) that volume of discharge is directly proportional to the pressure gradient, inversely proportional to viscosity, inversely proportional to tube length, and directly proportional to the fourth power of the radius. (Some textbook sources state this incorrectly as the fourth power of the diameter.) Therefore, a doubling of the tube radius results in a 16-fold change in flow rate. Such changes are important in anesthesia circuits, intravenous tubing, etc.

By the same mechanism, doubling length halves the output. and halving the length doubles the output (i.e., output per unit of time).

However, for fluids *in confined pathways, Pascal's law* applies (i.e., any applied pressure is transmitted undiminished to all parts of the liquid).

Friction: Friction is opposition to flow; it accounts for a drop in pressure as fluid travels through a tube.

Friction *arises from two sources:* (1) adhesive forces arising from the difference between the molecules of the liquid and the molecules of the container wall, and (2) internal friction from the interaction of the molecules themselves. This latter friction is called *viscosity.* Viscosity of gases is measured by the *Reynold's number,* which is the ratio of the gas's viscosity to its density, but viscosity and density are not otherwise directly related. For example, carbon dioxide is heavier (more dense) than oxygen, yet it flows through a tube more readily.

- Mixing gases or liquids alters viscosity.
- Viscosity also is altered by changes in temperature; heated liquids lose viscosity while cooled liquids become increasingly viscous.

For any given liquid at any given temperature, a point exists beyond which flow cannot be laminar because the frictional forces keep the flow from being laminar. This point is known as the *critical flow rate.* It is analogous to the electrical resistance described by Ohm's law.

Bernoulli's law: When liquids flow through a tube, a pressure is exerted against the sides of the tube. The faster the flow rate, the less side pressure is generated. If the pathway is varied in cross-sectional area, then, at the point of greatest constriction, forward velocity is fastest and side pressure is least. This principle is exploited in the venturi tube, used for nebulizers and for creating vacuum systems.

If the venturi tube's angles are less than 15°, distal pressures return to what they were proximally. But at the point of greatest constriction, a tube can be inserted to allow influx of air or other liquids, as is done with atomizers and nebulizers (i.e., injectors, where the rate of aspirated fluid remains constant despite changes in the primary fluid flow—the so-called *Venturi effect*).

Summary *Flow through tubes is primarily dependent upon viscosity and hardly affected by density.*

Flow through orifices is primarily dependent upon density, with viscosity playing a minor role.

However, the picture becomes more complex in that orifices may be of two types, fixed and variable: In the former, the size of the opening remains *fixed* so that, as more gas arrives from the source, pressure builds on the proximal side. *Flow rate for any gas of given density will depend upon and be proportional to the square root of the proximal/distal pressure differential.*

So, the *flow will be proportional to the square root of the pressure difference on either side.*

Proximal Pressure	Flow Rate	Distal Pressure	Pressure Differential
1	1	1	1:1
4	$\sqrt{4} = 2$	1	4:1
16	$\sqrt{16} = 4$	1	16:1

When two different gases having dissimilar densities flow through the same fixed orifice, they will develop different pressure gradients, less pressure being generated by the lighter gas. The *pressure differential of two gases compared in this fashion will vary inversely with the square root of their densities.*

For example, hydrogen is 1/16 as dense as oxygen, or there is a ratio of 1:16. Taking the square root of the density differences tells us that oxygen, the heavier gas, will develop a fourfold pressure difference compared to hydrogen. Therefore, the proximal/distal pressure differences for these two gases will always be in a ratio of 1:4.

Flow rate will double with each fourfold increase in pressure differential of the two gases, but the actual flow rate for oxygen will always be double that of hydrogen due to the proximal/distal pressure differences of the two gases resulting from their different densities, as below:

	Proximal/distal Pressures	Flow Rate
Hydrogen	4/1	2
Oxygen	16/4	4

Flow rate per unit of time for less dense gases can, therefore, be accomplished through smaller orifices.

Last, if the proximal/distal pressure difference is kept constant, flow rate is directly proportional to the orifice diameter squared.

Bobbin Rotameters/Thorpe Tubes Bobbin-type Thorpe flowmeter tubes used on most anesthesia machines today have a double taper. As gas enters from the bottom (i.e., low flow rates), the ratio of bobbin length to the glass flowmeter is more tubelike. Gas flow is slight, and viscosity (gas density) is the major factor in determining flow rate (per Poiseuille's law).

At higher flows, the relationship of the bobbin to the glass Thorpe flowmeter tube is more orificelike (due to the ratio of the bobbin to the larger taper). Flows are higher and the proximal/distal pressure differences have a greater influence on flow rate. To accommodate a wide range of gas flows, the flowmeter tube is double-tapered. So, as the bobbin continues up the tube, there is, again, a change to a tube and then, once again, to an orifice.

However, Thorpe tubes are specifically designed so that, at higher flows, where the ratio of bobbin to glass tube is orificelike, the size of the orifice is changed *but the proximal/distal pressure differences are kept the same.* This provides a mechanical advantage in that all Thorpe tubes used on the anesthesia machine can be of roughly the same height. But owing to the differences in gas densities, one can never exchange a Thorpe tube and use it with another gas. Neither can one use a given glass tube with a different flow-rate scale—even with the same gas—because each glass tube is hand-blown and matched to its own scale. Due to slight differences inside the Thorpe tube that occur as a result of the hand-blowing process, flow rates on an unmatched scale will not be accurate because the scale no longer corresponds to the tube's shape. Each flowmeter and matched scale can be traced for accuracy back to the National Bureau of Standards.

CARBON DIOXIDE ABSORPTION

The absorption of carbon dioxide allows rebreathing of exhaled gases in anesthesia circuits by chemically removing exhaled carbon dioxide. Because carbon dioxide is a gaseous, nonmetal oxide, it combines readily with water to form carbonic acid. The acid then reacts with metal oxides, of which there are three types in soda lime (and one type in baralyme). The metal oxides then react with available water to form hydroxides that chemically neutralize the carbonic acid, converting the hydroxides to carbonates or bicarbonates.

Soda Lime

Lava-shaped; provides a large surface area for reactions.

Composed of three hydroxides: sodium (4%), potassium (1%), and calcium (76 to 81%) as well as water (14 to 19%) and a small amount of silica.

Size: 4 to 8 mesh (i.e., passes through a screen having 4 to 8 openings per square inch).

Hardness number 75 (after compressed mixing with metal ball bearings).

Peaking refers to the exhaustion of soda lime—as indicated by the color change of a dye (usually ethyl violet).

If, after peaking, the soda lime is allowed to stand outside the anesthesia circuit for many hours, the calcium and potassium carbonates are reconverted to hydroxides, allowing the soda lime to again be used in the anesthesia circuit for a limited period (until its complete exhaustion occurs). This process is known as *regeneration.* The dye color also reverses. (*Note:* barium hydroxide does not regenerate.) Regeneration is no longer clinically useful since most departments change the soda lime canister rather than regenerating it, but the examinee should know of the process for the exam.

Baralyme

Another agent used for carbon dioxide absorption.
Composed of 80% calcium hydroxide, 1% potassium hydroxide, and 19% barium hydroxide.
Pink in color.
Chemical formula: $Ba(OH)_2 \cdot 8H_2O$. Since this is an octahydrate, additional water is not required.
The indicator dye is Clayton yellow (the color changes to yellow).

Other Factors   Packing of granules is usually somewhat loose; this can lead to *funneling,* the funnel-shaped movement of gases through the canister; it can also lead to *channeling,* where gases passing through the canister take the path of least resistance, usually along its sides, where granules are less tightly packed. That is why changes in indicator dye occur first along the canister sides.

Other indicator dyes are ethyl orange, mimosa Z, and phenolphthalein. All work by reacting to the acidity/alkalinity (pH) of the soda or baralyme.

Steps in Carbon Dioxide Absorption

A. Carbonic acid is formed by exhaled carbon dioxide combining with available water:

$$CO_2 + H_2O \Rightarrow H_2CO_3$$

B-1. The carbonic acid forms ions of hydrogen and bicarbonate by dissociation:

$$H_2CO_3 \Rightarrow H^+ + HCO_3^-$$

B-2. The metal oxides (sodium, potassium, and calcium hydroxide) dissociate to their respective ions:

$$NAOH \Rightarrow Na^+ + OH^-$$
$$KOH \Rightarrow K^+ + OH^-$$
$$Ca(OH)_2 \Rightarrow Ca^{++} + 2OH^-$$

For baralyme, the dissociation occurs as:

$$Ba(OH)_2 \cdot 8H_2O \Rightarrow Ba^{++} + 2OH^- + 8H_2O$$

C. The hydroxides then react with carbonic acid to form carbonates:

$$2NaOH + H_2CO_3 \Rightarrow Na_2CO_3 + 2H_2O + heat*$$
$$2KOH + H_2CO_3 \Rightarrow K_2CO_3 + 2H_2O + heat*$$
$$Ca(OH)_2 + H_2CO_3 \Rightarrow CaCO_3 + 2H_2O + heat*$$

For baralyme, several reactions occur:
1. The baralyme reacts directly with carbon dioxide:

$$Ba(OH)_2 \cdot 8H_2O + CO_2 \Rightarrow BaCO_3 + 9H_2O + heat*$$

2. The water from (1) reacts with carbon dioxide to form carbonic acid:

$$9H_2O + 9CO_2 \Rightarrow 9H_2CO_3 + heat*$$

3 and 4. Carbonic acid reacts with the available potassium and calcium hydroxides:

$$2KOH + H_2CO_3 \Rightarrow K_2CO_3 + 2H_2O + heat*$$
$$9H_2CO_3 + 9Ca(OH)_2 \Rightarrow 9CaCO_3 + 18H_2O + heat*$$

*Water produced by these reactions liberates 13,700 calories of heat per mole of carbon dioxide absorbed.

D. Regenerative reactions (this only applies to potassium and sodium carbonates/hydroxides, which react with unused calcium hydroxide). Baralyme and calcium carbonates cannot be reconverted. Available calcium hydroxide is depleted by regenerative reactions, and the reactions add to the formation of calcium carbonate.

$$K_2CO_3 + Ca(OH)_2 \Rightarrow CaCO_3 + 2KOH$$
$$NA_2CO_3 + Ca(OH)_2 \Rightarrow CaCO_3 + 2NaOH$$

☐ ORGANIC CHEMISTRY

Organic chemistry was born in 1828, when Friedrich Wöhler, a German chemist, prepared urea (an organic substance) from ammonium cyanate, opening up a whole new branch of chemistry that depends on the unique structure and properties of carbon atoms.

Carbon has 6 protons and 6 neutrons in its nucleus. *Its 6 electrons are distributed per the theory of octet (see above) as 2-4. It is the 4 electrons in the atom's outer orbit that provides carbon's characteristics, since carbon shares those 4 outer electrons with other atoms, in pairs, through covalent bonds.* Carbon bonds readily with other elements, including other carbon atoms, and in particular with hydrogen which, by sharing its electrons with carbon, assumes the stable configuration of a helium atom. Compounds made up mainly of one or more carbon atoms with their respective hydrogen attachments are called *hydrocarbons.*

Hydrocarbons   The simplest form of an organic hydrocarbon is the gas methane, which has a single carbon atom attached to four hydrogen atoms:

$$
\begin{array}{c}
H \\
| \\
H-C-H \\
| \\
H
\end{array}
$$

Note that stripping one hydrogen from methane leaves one attachment point open for the carbon and its remaining three hydrogens. This (CH_3) is referred to as a *methyl group,* a common chemical group found in many organic substances including pharmacologic drugs. (The methyl group acts as a radical.)

The next most common hydrocarbon is ethane. It contains two carbon atoms that share an electron while the remaining electrons pair with hydrogen electrons:

$$
\begin{array}{c}
HH \\
|| \\
H-C-C-H \\
|| \\
HH
\end{array}
$$

Increasingly more complex hydrocarbons can be formed by linking successive carbon atoms in a chain. Such complex hydrocarbons are often envisioned (and drawn) as straight chain hydrocarbons. However, in reality, the chains may twist and turn in their spatial configuration.

In order after methane (1 carbon) and ethane (2 carbons), compounds are 3, 4, 5, 6 (etc.) carbon atoms compounds, *named progressively by using Latin/Greek stems with the -ane ending that indicates straight-chain hydrocarbons joined together by single bonds.* For example:

Hydrocarbon	Number of Atoms
Propane	3
Butane	4
Pentane	5
Hexane	6
Heptane	7
Octane	8
Nonane	9
Decane	10

These are the most commonly encountered straight-chain, single-bond compounds, also called the *alkane series.* The number of carbon atoms in the chain is almost limitless; though as the chain lengthens, the compound is more easily broken into smaller components.

As with the previously mentioned methyl group, other radicals can be made from the foregoing compounds by stripping away one hydrogen atom. Such radicals are named for the basic grouping, but the *-ane* ending of the parent compound is changed to *-yl,* so that one can have a propyl radical, a butyl radical, etc.

Alkanes with less than 5 carbon atoms are gases, those with 5 to 16 carbon atoms are liquids, and those with more than 16 carbons are solids. Alkanes are not very active chem-ically, but they do burn readily and react with halogens, especially bromine and chlorine—a fact that was important to the development of halogenated anesthetics.

Alkenes and Alkynes Where alkanes are straight-chain aliphatic (acyclic hydrocarbon) compounds with all chemical bonds occupied, it is possible to treat these hydrocarbons chemically not only to strip off hydrogen atoms but also to produce a situation where two carbon atoms are joined by either a double or a triple bond. Those with a double bond are called *alkenes;* those with triple bonds are *alkynes.* Because of their unsaturated states, these compounds tend to be highly reactive. They are named in the same manner as alkanes, but the endings are, respectively, *-ene* and *-yne.* The first compounds of each series are:

$$
\begin{array}{c}
HH \\
|| \\
C=C \\
|| \\
HH
\end{array}
\qquad \text{and} \qquad
\begin{array}{c}
HH \\
|| \\
C\equiv C
\end{array}
$$

C_2H_4; ethylene—a gas once used as an anesthetic.

C_2H_3; ethyne; also known as acetylene, a gas used in welding.

- All four bonds for each carbon atom are accounted for in each instance.
- Alkenes and alkynes are not the same as *-dienes* and *-trienes.* The latter are organic compounds that contain two or three double bonds within their structure, but they are not members of the alkene series, which contains only one double bond.

Isomers Compounds with identical molecular formulas but several alternate structures are called *isomers.* Carbon-based compounds facilitate isomer formation because *carbon has the unique ability to rotate its bonds around its central axis.*

Isomers are of *two* types:

1. *Structural isomers:* The two forms usually differ in chemical and physical properties:

   The straight-chain form is called the *normal isomer.*

   Where a methyl group, for example, is branched off the straight chain, the compound is called an *isoisomer.*

2. *Stereoisomers:* These have identical formulas but differ in their spatial arrangement.

   This class is further subdivided into optical and geometric isomers:

   Optical isomers occur when groups attached to the carbon atom differ from one another in such a way as to polarize (bend) light; those that bend light to the right are called *dextroisomers* and those that bend it to the left are called *levoisomers.* The two forms are "mirror images" of one another. Where there is a mixture of both dextro- and levoisomers, such that no bending of light occurs, the mixture is called *racemic.*

Geometric isomers occur when compounds contain two carbon atoms with a double bond; the double bond prevents axial rotation. *Two geometric forms can occur:* the *cis* isomer, where the groups are on the same side of the double bond, and the *trans* isomer, where the groups are located on opposite sides of the bond.

Note: Because the presence of the double bond prevents rotation, the spatial configuration of *cis* and *trans* isomers is always different.

$$C=C \begin{smallmatrix} C_2H_5 \\ \\ C_2H_5 \end{smallmatrix} \qquad \begin{smallmatrix} C_2H_5 \\ \\ C_2H_5 \end{smallmatrix} C=C \begin{smallmatrix} C_2H_5 \\ \\ \end{smallmatrix}$$

Cis isomer   *Trans* isomer

A variation of structural isomerism occurs when some of the atoms in the compound are able to shift around from one position to another. Such an ability is called *tautomerism,* and the isomers themselves are called *tautomers,* or *keto-enol isomers* because ketones are often able to shift a hydrogen bond from the carbon (keto) form to the carbonyl (enol) portion of the structure.

Example (where R represents any given radical):

$$\begin{matrix} & H & & \\ & | & & \\ R - C - H & & R - C - H \\ & | & & \| \\ R - C = O & & R - C - OH \end{matrix}$$

Keto isomer   Enol isomer

Some anesthesia drugs, notably the barbiturates, have tautomers in their structure.

Proteins can also temporarily rearrange their structure. Portions of the molecule change their spatial arrangements with respect to other parts of the molecule. Such alterations can be induced by either physical or chemical factors and are called *conformational changes.*

CLASSES OF ORGANIC COMPOUNDS

Organic compounds can be grouped by structure, which can be expressed by a general formula. In the formulas, R=any radical group; O=oxygen; H=hydrogen. The major organic groups are reviewed briefly below.

Halogen Compounds In these compounds, X can be any halogen atom (i.e., fluorine, chlorine, bromine, iodine, or astatine). Most of the inhalation anesthetic agents presently in clinical use fall into this class, derived from either aliphatic (straight-chain hydrocarbon) or ether compounds. Formula: R-X.

Alcohols These are derived from hydrocarbons; an OH group replaces a hydrogen atom (e.g., removing a hydrogen atom on methane leaves a methyl group, so when the hydrogen is replaced by the OH, the result is methyl alcohol). Alcohols easily enter into chemical reactions, burn easily, and have a unique taste. They are classed as *primary, secondary, or tertiary alcohols,* depending upon the position of the radicals attached to the carbon attached to the OH group. Alcohols are readily oxidized, typically to an aldehyde (see below), and can behave as weak acids. Formula: R-OH.

Aldehydes These are formed from oxidation of *primary* alcohols, which strips two hydrogens from the carbon atom to join with one oxygen (of O_2), forming water; the other oxygen attaches to the carbon with a double bond. Aldehydes are predisposed to polymerize, especially with other aldehyde compounds. Formula:

$$\begin{matrix} O \\ \| \\ -C-H \end{matrix}$$

Ketones These are formed from oxidation of *secondary* alcohols. Their general formula group is called a carbonyl group (see earlier discussion of keto and enol isomers). (For example, oxidizing isopropyl alcohol produces acetone. Also, diabetic ketoacidosis produces organic ketones.) Formula:

$$\begin{matrix} O \\ \| \\ -C- \end{matrix}$$

Organic Acids These are hydrocarbons in which a COOH (a combination of the carbonyl and hydroxyl groups) replaces one or more hydrogens. The hydrogen in the COOH ionizes to give the compound acidic properties. Organic acids play a role in forming body fats. Acetic acid (also known as ethanoic acid because it is derived from the oxidation of ethane) is important in bodily reactions—usually being further oxidized to acetaldehyde. Formula: COOH.

Esters These are made by interacting an alcohol with an acid. They are very volatile and often have very pungent odors (e.g., isoamyl nitrite, used to treat angina pectoris). Esters of para-aminobenzoic acid form a whole class of local anesthetic compounds. Formula: R-COO-R.

Ethers These are organic oxides composed of two radical groups joined by an atom of oxygen—which is the functional group. While the classic ether anesthetics (e.g., diethyl and divinyl ether) have long been abandoned because of their explosiveness, they have been replaced in part by nonexplosive halogenated ethers. One halogenated ether anesthetic, *methoxyflurane,* which once found wide use in obstetrics, was also later abandoned because of its association with high-output renal failure caused by renal interstitial accumulation of free fluoride ions. The anesthetics in current use are covered next.

Enflurane

This anesthetic (2-chloro-1,1,2-trifluorethyl difluoromethyl ether) is a nonflammable, sweet-smelling, chemically stable, preservative-free inhalation anesthetic. Like methoxyflurane, it too has been implicated as a cause of high-output renal failure on the basis of the same mechanism, but at a much lower incidence rate. Enflurane's use has fallen in recent years, due to the availability of newer and better agents, but it retains some clinical utility. Its chemical formula is:

$$
\begin{array}{ccccccc}
 & F & & F & & F & \\
 & | & & | & & | & \\
H- & C & - & C & -O- & C & -H \\
 & | & & | & & | & \\
 & Cl & & F & & F &
\end{array}
$$

Isoflurane

This (1-chloro-2,2,2-trifluoroethyl difluoromethyl ether) is clinically similar to enflurane, but with slightly shorter induction and recovery periods. Its formula is:

$$
\begin{array}{ccccccc}
 & F & & Cl & & F & \\
 & | & & | & & | & \\
F- & C & - & C & -O- & C & -H \\
 & | & & | & & | & \\
 & F & & H & & F &
\end{array}
$$

Note: Both enflurane and isoflurane are trifluororoethyl difluoromethyl ethers. The differences between the two drugs are the result of different halogen substitutions at various positions.

Study hint: If asked to distinguish these two agents when the structural formulas are given, remember that the *F* for Forane (the trade name for isoflurane) matches the three fluorines on the end carbon of the larger (ethyl) radical of the structure.

Desflurane

This anesthetic ((+/−) 1,2,2,2-tetrafluoroethyl difluoromethyl ether) is a volatile liquid that is minimally biotransformed in the liver. Only about 0.02% is recoverable in the urine. The minimum alveolar concentration of desflurane decreases with advancing age or administration of other neurologically depressing drugs, such as benzodiazepines and opioids. Its chemical structure is:

$$
\begin{array}{ccccccc}
 & F & & H & & F & \\
 & | & & | & & | & \\
F- & C & - & C & -O- & C & -H \\
 & | & & | & & | & \\
 & F & & F & & F &
\end{array}
$$

Sevoflurane

This ((fluoromethyl 2,2,2-trifluoro-1-[trifluoromethyl]) ethyl ether) is a fluorinated isopropyl methyl ether with a pleasant smell and a low blood/gas solubility. Questions about its safety have arisen with respect to its stability in the presence of soda lime (there may be toxic by-products) and as to the release of fluoride during biotransformation. These questions currently (March 1996) remain unresolved. Sevoflurane's chemical structure is:

$$
\begin{array}{l}
F \quad\quad \text{(sometimes written as CF3)} \\
| \\
F-C-F \\
| \\
H \\
| \\
H-C-O-C-H \\
| \\
F \\
| \\
F-C-F \\
| \\
F \quad\quad \text{(sometimes written as CF3)}
\end{array}
$$

Note: All currently used inhalation anesthetics are halogenated ethers with the single exception of halothane, which is covered here for convenient comparisons with the other agents. *Halothane is not a halogenated ether; it is a halogenated straight-chain hydrocarbon. (It is the only agent that does not follow the R-O-R formula for ethers.)*

Halothane

This (2-bromo-2-chloro-1,1,1-trifluoroethane) is a comparatively sweet-smelling agent widely used for pediatric gas inductions. Its structure is:

$$
\begin{array}{ccccc}
 & F & & Br & \\
 & | & & | & \\
F- & C & - & C & -H \\
 & | & & | & \\
 & F & & Cl &
\end{array}
$$

Amines   These are derivatives of ammonia (NH_3). Like alcohols, they can also be divided into primary, secondary, and tertiary types, depending on how many of the hydrogens are replaced by a radical. When attached to molecules, they make the molecule more water-soluble. Amines react with acids to form ammonium (NH_4) salts, with a benzene ring to form aromatic amines, and with water to form bases. Formula: ($R-NH_2$)

Quaternary Bases

Formed from $NH_4(OH)$ [ammonium hydroxide], they make up part of the structure of numerous anesthesia-related drugs, including muscle relaxants, cholinergics, and ganglionic blockers.

Amides   Amides are related to carboxylic acids; urea is the best example. They form another whole class of local anesthetics. Formula (sometimes written -$CONH_2$):

$$
\begin{array}{c}
O \\
\| \\
-C-NH_2
\end{array}
$$

Note: amines and amides are often confused. Remember, amines retain their hydrogens intact, whereas, in amides, hydrogens attached to the nitrogen are replaced by radicals.

Amino Acids   These contain an amino group (-NH_2) and an acid (-$COOH$); amino acids build proteins and hydrolysis splits proteins to amino acids. Amino groups also react with hydroxyls to produce acid amines in a reaction that forms water and peptides. Chains of peptides form polypeptides— a process that allows for formation of thousands of protein combinations. Of 20 fundamental amino acids, 10 are considered essential for life.

Because they contain both an amino and an acid group, amino acids are amphoteric and capable of self-neutralization. The process involves formation of a dipolar ion (zwitterion). This provides for both electrical neutrality and allows the amino acid to combine with other acids and bases.

Other Nitrogen-Containing Compounds   (1) Reacting nitrous acid with alcohols creates nitroso groups, ($-NO_2$), (also called nitrites), whereas (2) using nitric acid produces a nitro group, ($-NO_3$), (also called nitrates). (3) Heterocyclic ring structures containing nitrogen form the basis for pyridines, purines, pyrroles, and a number of alkaloids used in anesthesia practice (e.g., morphine, atropine, quinine, reserpine, codeine, and cocaine).

Thio (Sulfur Containing) Compounds (-S): are formed by replacing the oxygen in organic molecules with a sulfur atom (the functional group). Sulfur compounds are distinguished by a number of prefixes: thio-, sulfhydryl-, mercapto-, and purines.

Sodium Thiopental (Pentothal)
This drug is produced from malonic acid and thiourea; one of a class of short-acting barbiturates, all derived from the keto form of barbiturate acid.

Sodium thiopental

Note: The molecular structure of sodium thiopental is typical of the structure for ultra-short-acting thiobarbitures. The position (1) and (3) hydrogens are called *imide hydrogens;* they make the compound acidic. The position (2) oxygen characterizes oxybarbiturates. Substituting sulfur for this oxygen produces a thiobarbiturate; that is, it makes the compound shorter-acting. The two aliphatic (straight-chain hydrocarbon) compounds off the position (5) carbon (one of which is a short chain and the other of which is a long chain) confer hypnotic potency. The sodium (Na), which replaces the hydrogen at carbon position (2), makes the compound more water-soluble.

Aromatic Compounds   The ring configurations of which these are formed contain six (6) carbon atoms joined by three double bonds of oscillating electrons dispersed over the entire ring structure. The most basic configuration of this type is the benzene ring (C_6H_6), where each carbon has one attached hydrogen. For simplification, it is often drawn as a circle within a hexagon. Replacing hydrogens with radicals forms new compounds. If only one substitution is made, there is no need to distinguish the position, since each of the six carbons is identical. However, when two or more hydrogens are replaced, it becomes necessary to denote at which position a given radical lies. For this reason, three isomers are possible, their names and positions being:

> *Ortho:* The two radicals are at adjacent carbons.
> *Meta:* The radicals are separated by an intervening carbon.
> *Para:* The radicals are separated by two carbons.

Aromatic compounds are volatile, flammable, toxic, and insoluble in water. Several benzene rings can be joined to form *polynuclear aromatic compounds.* The same radicals found in straight-chain hydrocarbons can also be found in cyclic (aromatic) hydrocarbons. For example, replacing a single hydrogen with a hydroxyl group produces phenol, while replacing the hydrogen with the carboxylic acid radical produces benzoic acid.

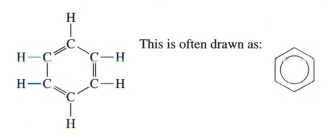

This is often drawn as:

GENERALIZATIONS REGARDING HYDROCARBON STRUCTURES

1. As molecular weight increases, volatility, flammability, and water solubility decrease.
2. The larger a compound, (i.e., the greater its molecular weight), the more likely it is to split into smaller, lighter compounds.
3. Lipid solubility increases with molecular weight as does a compound's oil/water distribution coefficient.
4. Potency of a compound increases with the degree of unsaturation as more potent substances generally react easily.
5. Hydroxyl replacement of hydrogen atoms typically reduces potency.

☐ BIOCHEMISTRY

Biochemistry is concerned with the chemical reactions needed for life. The *major substrates* for such reactions are water, carbohydrates, fats, and proteins as well as nucleic acids, enzymes, vitamins, and hormones. These reactions require energy, derived from biologic resources. Energy reactions are covered in the next section.

WATER

Constitutes 60 to 80% of weight of humans.
Serves as coolant, solvent, lubricant, and reactant for biochemical reactions.
Is mostly bound to cell constituents; some "free" water carries ions in solution.
Serves as transport system for bodily nutrients and wastes.
Dipolar configuration facilitates hydrogen bonding (see above).
Has limited ability to dissociate to H^+ and OH^-.
Plays role in acid-base balance.
Necessary for hydrolysis reactions.

CARBOHYDRATES (CHO)

Produced by plants through interaction of photosynthesis and light on carbon dioxide and water.
Are often long chains of carbon atoms to which hydrogen (H) and/or hydroxyl (OH) groups are attached—may also have aldehyde or ketone group, since sugars are derived from polyhydric alcohols.
Carbohydrates or sugars exist in four types: (1) mono-, (2) di-, (3) oligo-, and (4) polysaccharides.
Monosaccharides, the simplest sugars, cannot be further hydrolyzed; they can also be classed as trioses, pentoses, or hexoses, depending upon the number of carbon atoms present. Each monosaccharide may be further classed as an aldose or ketose, depending on which functional group is present (e.g., glucose is an aldose; fructose is a ketose).
Disaccharides, when hydrolyzed, produce two monosaccharides.
Oligo sugars yield two to six simple sugars when hydrolyzed.
Polysaccharides yield more than six simple sugars, which are often dextrins and starches.
Though saccharides are often drawn as straight-chain compounds, such a structure cannot account for all their properties, and x-ray diffraction studies show them to be bent-ring (chairlike) structures.
Oxidation of carbohydrates produces carbon dioxide, water, and energy. (This is covered in more detail below.)
Because of their structures, carbohydrates can also form isomerlike structures known as *anomers,* where groups on the first carbon become rotated, and *epimers,* where the hydrogen and hydroxyl groups on carbon atoms 2, 3, or 4 change positions.

Important Sugars

Monos
D-Glyceraldehyde, a triose sugar resulting from oxidation of glucose.

Oligos
Ribose and deoxyribose—both important to structure of RNA and DNA (both pentoses).

Polys
Also called hexoses.

1. *Glucose:* Always present in human blood; readily oxidized for energy.
2. *Galactose:* A glucose isomer produced from the hydrolysis of milk sugars.
3. *Fructose:* Obtained from the same sources and often interchangeable with glucose.
4. *Glycogen:* An amylopectinlike polysaccharide produced in the liver and stored both there and in muscle.
5. *Others:* Include *mucopolysaccharides* (e.g., heparin, dextran) and *glycoproteins,* which combine proteins and mucopolysaccharides. These contribute to tissue structure and are important biochemical constituents.

***Disaccharides: Sucrose, lactose, and maltose* are isomers of one another.**
Most mono- and disaccharides can be reduced by oxidizing agents (e.g., Benedict's or Fehling's solution). The oxidation of sugars for bioenergy is discussed below.

FAT (LIPIDS)

Fats: Are related to fatty acids, and have two distinguishing properties:

1. They are easily soluble in nonpolar solvents.
2. They are relatively insoluble in water.

Fats, oils, and waxes are included in this class.
Form emulsions when dissolved in water.
Are glistening and greasy to the touch.
Are the major constituents of adipose tissue.
Float on water, having a specific gravity of less than 1.
Are composed mostly of carbon, oxygen, and hydrogen (like carbohydrates) but also of nitrogen and phosphorus.
Hydrolysis produces even-numbered carbon, straight-chained fatty acids.
Are colorless, odorless, and tasteless.
Perform a multitude of functions in the body.
Are emulsified by bile in the intestines and carried to body cells in that fashion.
Saturated fats: Have no double bonds; name ends in *-anoic.*
Unsaturated fats: Have one or more double bonds; name ends in *-enoic.*
Are classified on the basis of their solubility and hydrolysis products.

Saturated lipids are classed as:

1. *Simple lipids:* Esters formed by reacting fatty acids with alcohols.
2. *Compound lipids:* Lipids containing another group in

addition to the ester. This group contains two special groups:

    a. *Phospholipids:* These—fatty acid, alcohol, and phosphoric acid residue—include a number of compounds important to the body; best example—surfactant needed to maintain alveolar surface tension.

    b. *Cerebrosides:* These—fatty acid, carbohydrate, and nitrogen, but not phosphoric acid—are found in large amounts in the brain and nervous system.

3. *Derived lipids:* These—fatty acids formed by hydrolyzing compound lipids—include ketones, aldehydes, sterols, and glycerols.

Unsaturated lipids are classed (on their degree of unsaturatedness) as:

1. *Monounsaturated acids* (e.g., oleic acid).
2. *Polyunsaturated acids* (e.g., linoleic, linolenic, and arachidonic acid). They have two or more double bonds. (*Note:* prostaglandins are derived from arachidonic acid.)

Alcohols in more complex lipids can include glycerol and cholesterol; triacylglycerols derived from glycerol form what are known as neutral fats or *triglycerides.* These can be oxidized for energy by most body cells except those of the brain.

Lipids may be split by "saponification," where a glyceride is split with a base to produce glycerol and the salt of a fatty acid.

Breakdown of fats leads to the formation of aldehydes and ketones, which are then acted upon by bacteria to produce butyric acid.

Danielli and Davson (1935) suggested that cell membranes were composed of a lipid bilayer sandwiched between proteins. In 1972, Singer and Nicolson suggested that the entire structure comprised a fluid "mosaic" capable of temporary restructuring to allow for entry of drugs and other substances into the cell. Current thinking supports the idea that both general and regional anesthetics work in this way. However, the actual mechanism by which anesthetics work remains uncertain.

PROTEINS AND NUCLEIC ACIDS

Are important to building and repairing tissue protoplasm.

Protein buffers maintain cellular, lymph, and body fluid pH.

Help maintain water balance in cells, lymph, etc.

Provide amino acids for synthesis of new nitrogen-containing compounds.

Can furnish energy when carbohydrates and fats are depleted.

Supply ingredients for building hormones, enzymes, and hemoglobin.

Are large molecules built by polymerization of amino acid combinations.

Generally contain hydrogen, oxygen, nitrogen, sulfur, and carbon.

Simplest amino acid; glycine.

Essential amino acids (10)—arginine, histidine, isoleucine, leucine, lysine, methionine, phenylalanine, threonine, tryptophan, and valine.

Nonessential amino acids (11)—alanine, aspargine, aspartic acid, cysteine, cystine, glutamic acid, glutamine, glycine, proline, serine, and tyrosine.

Can be classed as: *

    Simple: Hydrolysis produces only alpha-amino acids.

    Conjugated: Hydrolyze to other amino acid types.

Because of their asymmetrical carbon, amino acids can polarize light and thus form isomers, but all natural ones have the same levo (L) configuration.

Conjugated proteins consist of both a protein and a nonprotein (nucleic acids) portion, the latter being polymers of *nucleotides* (low-molecular-weight molecules that enter into a number of biochemical reactions). Nucleotides are comprised of *nucleosides* (a pentose sugar and a purine or pyrimidine ring) and *phosphate.*

*Proteins can also be classed by structure and by function (as structural proteins, hormones, enzymes, blood proteins, and contractile proteins).

Amino acids contain a basic amino group and an acidic carboxyl group, giving them an amphoteric nature.

In combining amino acids, a molecule of water is lost and the two are joined by the *peptide linkage* ($-CO-NH-$) (also known as the amide linkage) to form a dipeptide (replication of this process can be used to form polypeptides).

If the combining amino acids contain sulfur, the two may be joined in a *disulfide bond.*

Similarly, where ionic bonding occurs between an acid group and either a base or amino acid to form a salt, it is said to form a *salt bridge (bond).*

Also, hydrogen bonds may form between hydrogen and other parts of the protein structure.

Proteins tend to be high-molecular-weight compounds, often exceeding a weight of 1 million.

Their electrical charges, and the balance of positive and negative charges away from their baseline (isoelectric point), enable proteins to be identified by the process of electrophoresis.

Proteins can be destroyed by a number of mechanisms: hydrolysis by enzymes (proteases); heat and other sterilizing processes that denature the protein (*denaturation* physically disrupts the protein's structure).

Body cannot store proteins and has limited ability to build them, so nutrients must be constantly provided.

Upset of protein metabolism leads to elevated blood urea levels (uremia).

ENZYMES

Function as catalysts for various chemical reactions, a process that decreases the energy requirement for the reaction.

Each enzyme consists of two portions: an *apoenzyme* (protein portion) and a *coenzyme* (nonprotein portion).

Types of enzymes (6):

   oxidoreductases: Facilitate oxidation/reduction.

   transferases: Move chemical groups between substrates and water.

   Lysases: Help form double bonds.

   Isomerases: Help form isomers.

   Ligases: Break molecular couplings.

Important coenzymes: Adenosine mono-, di-, and triphosphate (AMP, ADP, ATP); cyclic adenosine monophosphate (cAMP); nicotinamide adenine dinucleotide with and without phosphate (NAD^+ and $NADP^+$); flavin adenine dinucleotide (FAD and coenzyme A (Co-A)).

Are important to electron transport and phosphate bond energy mechanisms.

Are named by the substrate and the type of reaction catalyzed, [e.g., cytochrome *c*; O_2 oxidoreductase (cytochrome *c* oxidase)]—*the suffix* -ase *identifies* enzymes.

Enzyme reactions are affected by temperature, pH, and the presence or absence of inhibitors (either competitive or noncompetitive).

VITAMINS

Exam questions on vitamins are rare. The most likely information follows:

Vitamin A: Needed for rhodopsin formation and eye function.

Vitamin D: Has role in mRNA and protein synthesis, important for calcium and phosphorus metabolism, needed for cholecalciferol and 1,25 dihydroxycholecalciferol—the metabolically active ingredients; excess intake of vitamin D can lead to formation of renal stones.

Vitamin E: lack causes hemolysis in premature infants; in adults, can lead to macrocytic anemia and altered erythrocyte survival; most important role—as antioxidant to scavenge oxide by-products such as peroxides.

Vitamin K: Most important role: to catalyze prothrombin synthesis in the liver; absence of vitamin K leads to hypoprothrombinemia and prolonged clotting times. It is also used to treat bleeding caused by excessive dicumarol administration.

Vitamin C (ascorbic acid): Found in large amounts in adrenal cortex; rapidly depleted with ACTH and thought to play a role in body's stress response.

Vitamin B_1 (thiamine): Coenzyme in glucose oxidation.

Vitamin B_2 (riboflavin): Coenzyme w/FMN and FAD in intracellular hydrogen transport.

Niacin: Helps form NAD^+ and $NADP^+$.

Vitamin B_6 (pyridoxine): Lack causes hypochromic macrocytic anemia, especially in infants and pregnant women.

Pantothenic acid: Part of coenzyme A; used in fatty acid oxidation.

Vitamin B_{12} (cyanocobalamin): Resembles a porphyrin (four reduced and substituted pyrrole rings around a cobalt atom); absorption from gut requires presence of hydrochloric acid (HCl) and intrinsic factor (IF), both of which are needed to prevent pernicious anemia, therefore vitamin B_{12} is often called the extrinsic factor.

Other B vitamins: Include lipoic acid, biotin, folic acid, inositol, and para-aminobenzoic acid). Have minimal biologic functions.

HORMONES

Act as the body's chemical messengers, supplementing neural pathways.

Produced by either *exocrine glands* (which secrete into ducts) or *endocrine glands* (which secrete directly into blood).

Chemically may be amino acids, polypeptides, proteins, or steroids.

Are secreted in minute amounts but have profound impact on growth, development, and survival.

Resemble enzymes and vitamins.

Their production is often autoregulated (by feedback mechanisms).

They catalyze reactions without engaging in them.

They often require conversion before they can exert their effects.

Cyclic adenosine monophosphate (cAMP) is an important mediator.

Impact can be influenced by mediators such as phosphodiesterase inhibitors and prostaglandins.

Hormones influence membrane transport, protein synthesis, enzyme and coenzyme activity, and numerous other biochemical reactions.

☐ BIOENERGETICS

Biochemical reactions result in energy changes, a process called *bioenergetics.* Nutrient substrates for biochemical reactions come from food. Nutrients are first absorbed through the gastrointestinal tract, where complex foods are reduced to substrates such as amino and fatty acids, sugars, etc. These are next reduced to chemical building blocks (e.g., acetyl groups, phosphoric acid, etc.).

Energy is derived from several pathways that use the same basic nutrients. *Glucose is the foremost energy substrate,* but fats and proteins can also contribute. As the glucose is oxidized for energy, its *end products* are carbon dioxide and water, while ATP (adenosine triphosphate) is continually replenished by metabolic processes. The *amount of energy produced depends on* the type of energy substrate, amount of free energy involved in the reaction, and electron transport.

FREE ENERGY

High-energy-bond compounds yield their excess energy when converted to low-energy compounds; the excess energy can be given off as body heat or transferred to "fire" other chemical reactions elsewhere in the body. *Types of reaction:*

exergonic, or reactions that give off excess ("free") energy, and *endergonic,* or reactions that take up excess energy. The two types of reactions are often coupled. *Amount of free energy produced depends on laws of thermodynamics:*

1. *law of conservation of energy:* Total energy in a chemical system (reaction) remains unchanged.
2. *extent of entropy:* Randomness of molecular activity *must increase* if spontaneous reactions are to occur.

Where reactions occur under constant temperature and pressure conditions, the relationship between free energy and randomness can be expressed by the *Gibbs equation:* ($\Delta G = \Delta H - T\Delta S$) (where G = amount of free energy change; H = the thermodynamic potential at constant pressure; and S = the change in randomness). If $G = 0$, the reaction is at equilibrium; if G is negative, a spontaneous reaction can occur and free energy will be liberated (an exothermic reaction); and if G is positive, more energy is needed for the reaction to proceed and thus it will be an endothermic reaction. Phosphate compounds are especially well suited for energy transfer, and the body has two such groups, a high-energy one and a low-energy one. ATP is halfway between the two in energy. Total free energy developed by a series of biochemical reactions = the algebraic sum of the free energy changes of each of the steps.

ATP

A nucleotide (composed of adenine, a ribose sugar, and three (3) phosphate units (bonds); it breaks down to ADP and a phosphate bond (P ~ P), which, in turn, can be broken down to AMP and a phosphate bond. When activated, ATP is part of a complex with magnesium.

Other biochemical reactions rely on substances similar to ATP: GTP (guanosine triphosphate): UTP (uridine triphosphate); and CTP (cytidine triphosphate). Each is degraded to its diphosphate form, and enzymes carry the phosphate bond from one nucleotide to another.

SIMPLIFIED STRUCTURES FOR ATP, ADP, AND AMP

FOUR PROCESSES CONTRIBUTING HIGH-ENERGY PHOSPHATE BONDS TO THE ATP/ADP CYCLE

1. Oxidative phosphorylation (occurs in mitochondria and is facilitated by enzyme: ATP synthetase).
2. Embden Meyerhof pathway (see below) (glucose is broken down to lactic acid; forms two high-energy phosphate groups per mole of glucose).
3. Citric acid cycle (see below).
4. Creatinine/arginine phosphate pathway (occurs in skeletal muscle).

OXIDATION-REDUCTION

Oxidation = loss of electrons; reduction = gain of electrons. One reaction is always matched by the other. Amount of free energy depends on ability of reactants to accept/donate electrons.

Biologically, *oxygen = prime electron acceptor* through an indirect process where flavins (pyridine nucleotides) carry the electrons—helping ADP and orthophosphate (P_i) combine to ATP (i.e., oxidative phosphorylation). The reduced forms transfer electrons to oxygen by means of an electron transport chain in the inner part of the mitochondrial membrane. The major electron carriers are NADH, NADPH, and $FADH_2$.

GLYCOLYSIS (THREE METABOLIC PATHWAYS OF GLUCOSE)

The Embden-Meyerhof (E-M) pathway (whereby glucose and other carbohydrates are metabolized to pyruvate or lactate) *is a non-oxygen-dependent series of reactions that can provide energy under anaerobic conditions but which usually feeds into the aerobic Krebs cycle, which serves as the final common pathway for oxidizing nutrients.* This is also known as the lactic acid cycle or Cori cycle.

Intermediate steps in the pathway have either six carbon substances (derived from glucose and fructose) or three carbon substances (derived from glyceraldehyde, glycerate, pyruvate, or dihydroxyacetone). These undergo a number of phosphorylative steps that result in phosphoryl groups with (ester or anhydride) linkages. The linkages can be split to allow for formation of water, transfer of the phorphoryl groups from ATP, interconnection of ketoses and aldoses, or splitting of aldol linkages. All of these steps allow substances to be recombined, broken down, or interconverted.

There are 10 steps in the glycolytic pathway; all take place in cell cytosol, and each step is facilitated by an enzyme. (Enzymes in the following are italicized)

1. Glucose combines with ATP; it is acted upon by *hexokinase* to form glucose 6-phosphate (G6P), ADP, and H^+.
2. *Phosphoglucose-isomerase* converts the G6P to fructose 6 phosphate (F6P).

3. F6P + ATP are acted upon by *phosphofructokinase* to form fructose-1,6 diphosphate, ADP, and H^+.

4. *Aldolase* acts on the fructose-1,6 diphosphate to produce dihydroxyacetone phosphate and glyceraldehyde 3-phosphate.

5. *Triose phosphate isomerase* acts on dihydroxyacetone phosphate to produce glyceraldehyde 3-phosphate.

6. Glyceraldehyde 3-phosphate + P_i + NAD^+ are acted upon by *glyceraldehyde 3-phosphate dehydrogenase* to produce 1,3 diphosphoglycerate + NADH + H^+.

7. 1,3 Diphosphoglycerate + ADP are acted upon by *phosphoglycerate kinase* to produce 3 phosphoglycerate and ATP.

8. *Phosphoglyceromutase* converts 3-phosphoglycerate to 2-phosphoglycerate.

9. *Enolase* converts the 2-phosphoglycerate to phosphoenol-pyruvate and water.

10. Phosphoenolpyruvate + ADP + H^+ are acted upon by *pyruvate kinase* to produce pyruvate and ATP.

The foregoing steps both produce and consume energy. Two ATP molecules are lost but four are produced by the pathway for a net gain of 2 ATP molecules.

The pyruvate produced can be converted either to lactate or to acetyl Co-A. If oxygen is limited, the pyruvate is reduced by NADH to form lactate (by the enzyme lactate dehydrogenase). This allows regeneration of NAD^+, which allows the pathway to proceed past the point where glyceraldehyde 3-phosphate is formed. If this were not possible, no ATP would be produced. Therefore pyruvate could produce energy only for a limited period—hopefully until oxygen became available. This mechanism provides a means for cellular survival under temporary anaerobic conditions. If or when oxygen becomes available, the lactate reconverts to pyruvate and any acidosis present resolves.

When the pyruvate combines with NAD^+ and Co-A, several substances are formed: carbon dioxide, NADH, H^+, and acetyl Co-A. The latter is then free to enter the citric acid cycle.

THE HEXOSE-MONOPHOSPHATE (H-M) SHUNT

This shunt generates ribose and NADPH. It is a series of aerobic, enzyme-dependent reactions. Three molecules of G6P join with six molecules of NADP to form three molecules of carbon dioxide, two molecules of F6P, six of NADPH, and a glyceraldehyde-3-phosphate molecule that is shared with the E-M pathway. The shunt is a direct oxidative pathway that operates mostly in the liver and only minimally in skeletal muscle. The shunt begins with oxidative reactions, but the sugars produced are enzymatically converted nonoxidatively. The required enzymes are in the cell cytosol. The shunt has two parts (A and B below):

(A)

1. Under the influence of the enzyme *G6P dehydrogenase*, G6P + $NADP^+$ is converted to 6 phosphogluconolacetone, NADPH, and H^+.

2. Under the influence of *lactonase*, 6 phosphogluconolacetone and water are converted to 6 phosphogluconate and H^+.

3. Under the influence of *6 phosphogluconate dehydrogenase*, 6 phosphogluconate + NADP is converted to ribulose 5 phosphate (R5P) and CO_2 and NADPH.

(B)

1. Under the influence of *phosphopentose isomerase*, R5P is converted to ribose-5-phosphate.

2. Under the influence of *phosphopentose epimerase*, R5P is converted to xylulose-5-phosphate.

3. Under the influence of *transketolase*, xylulose 5-phosphate and ribose-5-phosphate are converted to sedoheptulose-7-phosphate and glyceraldehyde-3-phosphate.

4. Under the influence of *transaldolase*, sedoheptulose-7-phosphate and glyceraldehyde-3-phosphate are converted to fructose-6-phosphate and erythrose-4-phosphate.

5. Under the influence of *transketolase*, xylulose-5-phosphate and erythrose-4-phosphate are converted to fructose-6-phosphate and glyceraldehyde-3-phosphate.

Because the two molecules of glyceraldehyde-3-phosphate can be recombined into a G6P molecule, the shunt pathway accounts for the complete oxidation of glucose. The shunt produces energy through its powers of reduction and not, as with the E-M pathway and Krebs cycle, through ATP production.

THE KREBS CYCLE (CITRIC ACID CYCLE, TRICARBOXYLIC CYCLE)

*Is the body's principal metabolic pathway.

*Combined with E-M pathway = aerobic glycolysis.

Enzymes for this pathway are located in the cristae of mitochondria.

The cycle begins with acetyl Co-A derived from pyruvate formed in the last stages of the glycolytic pathways.

In the cycle, hydrogen is lost in five reactions, mostly as NADH, which enters the electron transport chain. The hydrogen is passed between compounds to facilitate oxidation-reduction reactions and, eventually, ends up combining with oxygen to form water.

*Three ATP molecules are formed from each NADH molecule, but a total of 38 molecules of ATP are formed by the entire aerobic glycolysis process (4 from the E-M pathway; 6 from NADH release in the E-M pathway; 30 from the Krebs cycle's two pyruvic acids = 40, *less* 2 ATP molecules used in the E-M pathway = 38).

Study Hint: Past exams have had questions that focused on the amount and location of ATP formation.

*Important points often appearing on certifying exam.

THE CYCLE

Acetyl Co-A, water, and oxaloacetate, under the influence of *citrate synthetase,* produces citrate, Co-A, and H+.

Citrate, under the influence of *aconitase,* is converted to *cis*-aconitate and water.

Isocitrate and NAD^+, under the influence of *isocitrate dehydrogenase,* is converted to alpha-ketoglutarate, CO_2, and NADH (*Note:* formation of alpha-ketoglutarate here determines the overall functioning of the cycle.)

Alpha-ketoglutarate, NAD^+, and Co-A, under the influence of *alpha-ketoglutarate dehydrogenase complex,* is converted to succinyl Co-A, CO_2, and NADH.

Succinyl Co-A and Pi and GDP (guanosine diphosphate), under the influence of *succinyl Co-A synthetase,* produces succinate, GTP, and Co-A. (*Note:* in a set of dual reactions, the high-energy phosphate bond (Pi), associated with the succinyl Co-A, is released with the phosphorylation of the GDP but ends with the formation of GTP (guanosine triphosphate), which can be converted to ADP and then to ATP.)

Succinate and FAD, under the influence of *succinate dehydrogenase,* are converted to fumarate and $FADH_2$.

Fumarate and water, under the influence of *fumarase,* are converted to maltate.

Maltate and NAD^+, under the influence of *maltate dehydrogenase,* are converted to oxaloacetate, NADH, and H^+ (*Note:* Oxaloacetate is reformed from succinate to be reused in the first step of the cycle.)

GLYCOGENESIS

Glycogen, a polymerized form of glucose, is storable. Forming glycogen (glycogenesis) from excess glucose assures the continued function of the E-M, hexose-monophosphate, and Krebs cycle pathways during periods of starvation.

GLYCOGENOLYSIS

The breakdown of glycogen to glucose, *five steps:*

Glucose reacts with ATP under the influence of magnesium and the enzyme *glucokinase* to form ADP and G6P.

G6P is converted by *phosphomutase* to glucose-1-phosphate (G1P).

G1P reacts with UTP (uridine triphosphate; a uracil-containing nucleotide) under the influence of the enzyme *UDPG (uridinediphosphoglucose) pyrophosphorylase* to form UDP-glucose.

UDP-glucose is polymerized to glycogen under the influence of *UDPG-glycogen-transglucolase,* a reaction that releases UDP.

UDP reacts with ATP to form ADP and regenerates UTP (two ATP molecules are required for each glucose molecule stored).

Glycogenolysis is not merely the reverse process of glycogenesis. Rather, it is a highly accelerated process that involves a number of hormones (ACTH, glucagon, epinephrine), and a cascade where each step accelerates the following step 100-fold. This process, which occurs in the liver, provides large amounts of glucose immediately under conditions of stress or fear.

The glycogenolytic cascade:

1. Adenyl cyclase is activated by a hormone.
2. Adenyl cyclase converts AMP to its cyclic form, cAMP.
3. cAMP activates protein kinase.
4. Protein kinase activates phosphorylase kinase.
5. Phosphorylase kinase changes phosphorylase (b) to phosphorylase (a).
6. Phosphorylase (a) splits a G1P off the glycogen.
7. G1P is converted to G6P.
8. G6P is converted to glucose and either enters the blood or a glycolytic pathway.

SUGGESTED READINGS

Adriani J. *The Chemistry and Physics of Anesthesia.* 2nd ed. Springfield, Ill: Charles C. Thomas; 1962.*

Barker SJ, Tremper KK. Physics applied to anesthesia. In: Barash PG, Cullen BF, Stoelting RK, eds. *Clinical Anesthesia.* Philadelphia, Pa: Lippincott: 1992:141–82.

Cork RC. Physics in relation to anesthesia. In: Nunn JF, Utting JE, Brown BR Jr, eds. *General Anaesthesia.* London: Butterworths; 1989:310–319.

*Classic works.

Duffin J. *Physics for Anaesthetists.* Springfield, Ill: Charles C Thomas; 1976.*

LeBel LA. Principles of chemistry and physics in anesthesia. In: Waugaman WR, Foster SD, Rigor BM, eds. *Principles and Practice of Nurse Anesthesia.* 2nd ed. Norwalk, Conn: Appleton & Lange; 1992:57–84.

LeBel LA. Principles of organic chemistry and biochemistry in anesthesia. In: Waugaman WR, Foster SD, Rigor BM, eds. *Principles and Practice of Nurse Anesthesia.* 2nd ed. Norwalk, Conn: Appleton & Lange; 1992:85–104.

☐ QUESTIONS

1. Elements are distinguished from compounds in that:
    a. Although their atoms may be made up of subparts, they cannot be further divided without a loss of identity.
    b. They are composed of several different types of atoms.
    c. They only occur naturally.
    d. They can only exist as a single atom.

2. Atoms with two electrons in their outer shell are classified as:
    a. Transitional elements
    b. Inert elements
    c. Metals
    d. Nonmetals

3. Combining sodium and chlorine to produce sodium chloride is an example of a:
    a. Physical change
    b. Chemical change
    c. Biochemical change
    d. Isoelectrical change

4. Exerting a force over a distance, as in moving a 1-g weight a distance of 10 cm, defines the term:
    a. Energy
    b. Acceleration
    c. Momentum
    d. Work

5. One megavolt is equal to:
    a. A hundred volts
    b. A thousand volts
    c. A million volts
    d. Ten million volts

6. Gas X has a density of 3 g/L, gas Y's density is 1.5 g/L, and gas Z's density is 0.8 g/L. Therefore which of the following statements is true:
    a. Gas Y is twice as dense as gas X.
    b. Gas X is twice as heavy as room air.
    c. Gas Z will rise in room air.
    d. Gas Y constitutes half the molecules of gas X.

7. A temperature of 310°K is equivalent to:
    a. 100°F
    b. 98.6°F
    c. 90.3°F
    d. 39°C

8. Which following chemical compound exemplifies a "radical"?
    a. N_2O
    b. $Ca(OH)_2$
    c. Ca^{++}
    d. H_2O_2

9. Dissolving one molecular weight (1 mol) of a compound in one liter (1 L) of liquid produces a one-molar (1-M) solution, but dissolving one gram equivalent weight (GEW) of a compound in one liter (1 L) of liquid produces a one-normal (1-N) solution. The foregoing statement:
    a. Is completely true
    b. Is completely false
    c. Is partially true and partially false
    d. Cannot be determined to be true or false because not enough information is provided

10. Initially, compartment A contains 20 L of gas X and compartment B contains but 2 L of the same gas. When a partition between the two compartments is opened, the gas from compartment A rapidly diffuses to compartment B. Over time, the two compartments equilibrate, each containing the same amount of gas X. Now, the rate of diffusion between the compartments approaches zero. This change in the rates of diffusion is a function of:
    a. Charles's law
    b. Gay-Lussac's law
    c. Dalton's law
    d. Fick's law

11. A new anesthetic agent has a vapor pressure of 152 torr at 20°C. It is being used in a general-duty vaporizer (e.g., copper-kettle type) at that temperature and at sea-level pressure. What diluent flow should be used so that each 100 mL of oxygen carrier gas represents a 1% delivered anesthetic concentration?
    a. 10 L
    b. 6.5 L
    c. 4 L
    d. 2.5 L

12. Isoflurane's vapor pressure (238 torr at 20°C) means that:
    1. Isoflurane represents 31.3% of the output from the vaporizer
    2. The carrier gas, oxygen, represents the balance (68.7%), of the vaporizer's output
    3. Within the vaporizer, the carrier gas exerts 522 torr of pressure
    4. At higher temperatures, isoflurane will exert a greater proportion of the vaporizer output
       a. All but 4
       b. All of the above
       c. Only 2 and 4
       d. Only 1 and 2

13. A Thorpe tube–type of anesthesia machine flowmeter measures the flow rate of its gas at high flows by maintaining the same pressure difference on both sides of the orifice created by the ratio of the rotameter bobbin's cross-sectional area relative to the cross-sectional area of the glass tube that encloses it. Therefore flow rate in this flowmeter will be a function of:
   a. The density of the gas
   b. The viscosity of the gas
   c. The square of the orifice diameter
   d. The square root of the molecular weight of the gas

14. The soda lime used in anesthesia machine absorbers to neutralize exhaled carbon dioxide is made up of three metal oxides (sodium, calcium, and potassium hydroxide). As the three react with the carbonic acid (H_2CO_3) produced by the interaction of exhaled carbon dioxide and water, they are converted to their respective:
   a. Carbonates
   b. Halogens
   c. Nonmetal oxides
   d. Acids

15. This is the formula for a commonly used anesthetic.

$$F-\underset{\underset{F}{|}}{\overset{\overset{F}{|}}{C}}-\underset{\underset{Br}{|}}{\overset{\overset{Cl}{|}}{C}}-H$$

   Its structure identifies it as an:
   a. Ether
   b. Aldehyde
   c. Halogenated hydrocarbon
   d. Cyclic alkene

16. A compound has the following structural formula:

   The compound is:
   a. 1, 2, 10 Methyl decane
   b. 5, Di-butyl decane

   c. 2 Methyl decane
   d. Di-pento decane

17. The following identifies a _____ isomer (R1 = any radical).

$$\underset{}{\overset{R1}{\diagdown}}C=C\overset{}{\underset{R1}{\diagdown}}$$

   a. Cis
   b. Trans
   c. Iso
   d. Racemic

18. Amides, which include a whole class of local anesthetic compounds, are identified by which following functional group?

   a. $-\overset{\overset{O}{\parallel}}{C}-NH_2$

   b. $-\overset{\overset{O}{\parallel}}{C}-H$

   c. $-CO-NH-$

   d. $-\overset{\overset{O}{\parallel}}{\underset{\underset{O}{\parallel}}{S}}-$

19. In the first step of the Embden-Meyerhoff bioenergetic pathway, the enzyme hexokinase works on glucose and adenosine triphosphate (ATP) to produce adenosine diphosphate (ADP) hydrogen (H^+), and:
   a. A four-carbon sugar
   b. 2, 3, Di-phosphoglycerate
   c. Fructose-6-phosphate
   d. Glucose-6-phosphate

20. The net number of molecules of ATP (adenosine triphosphate) produced by the Krebs cycle is:
   a. 38
   b. 30
   c. 6
   d. 4

☐ ANSWERS

1. a	**5.** c	**9.** a	**13.** c	**17.** b
2. c	**6.** c	**10.** d	**14.** a	**18.** a
3. b	**7.** b	**11.** d	**15.** c	**19.** d
4. d	**8.** b	**12.** b	**16.** c	**20.** a

Principles of Pharmacology

Ekaterini Grivas-Mousouris

Pharmacology is a broad science that incorporates the knowledge of the origins, physical and chemical properties as well as the effects (pharmacologic and toxic) of drugs. The principles of pharmacokinetics and pharmacodynamics are valuable tools in the evaluation and comparison of drugs for their safe and effective use. *Pharmacokinetics* deals with the absorption, distribution, biotransformation, and excretion of drugs. *Pharmacodynamics* deals with the interaction of drugs and receptors and the conditions necessary to favor a pharmacologic response. In the perioperative setting, a nurse anesthetist must be concerned with the physical status of a patient as well as the effects of the many drugs administered simultaneously to induce and maintain anesthesia. An understanding of the basic principles of pharmacology is essential for the safe and effective use of all drugs.

☐ PHARMACOKINETICS

To exert a significant pharmacologic effect, a drug must be present in sufficient concentrations at its site of action. The dose of the drug administered—along with the rates and extent of absorption, distribution, tissue and receptor binding, biotransformation, and excretion—will determine the magnitude of drug effect.

A drug reaches the plasma either by absorption from enteral and parenteral sites of administration or by direct intravenous (IV) injection. Once in the systemic circulation, a drug can leave and penetrate various tissues, including its sites of action, metabolism, and excretion, or remain in the blood and become protein-bound. Metabolites formed by biotransformation of the drug may also enter the plasma and be distributed throughout the body (Fig. 3–1).

MOVEMENT OF DRUGS ACROSS MEMBRANES

The processes of absorption, distribution, biotransformation, and excretion involve the movement of drugs across biological membranes (e.g., plasma membrane, skin, intestinal epithelium, oral mucosa).

The cell membrane can be visualized as a flexible, mobile, mosaiclike structure. It is composed of globular proteins embedded either partially or completely in a lipid bilayer. Highly polar groups located on surface proteins render the structure impermeable to charged molecules.

Mechanisms of Membrane Transport Penetration is accomplished by (1) diffusion through membrane channels or pores (this is utilized by water and low-molecular-weight water-soluble substances such as urea); (2) dissolution and diffusion in the lipoprotein structure (molecules are moved across the membrane passively, across a concentration gradient); and (3) carrier-mediated transport and pinocytosis. These processes require energy. Compounds may be moved against an electrochemical or concentration gradient.

Factors Affecting Membrane Transport Movement of drugs across cell membranes is a function of the physicochemical properties of both the membrane and the drug molecules. The size of membrane channels and pores differs among the various biological membranes. Vascular capillary cells have large channels, allowing the passage of molecules such as albumin. Channels in red cell membranes, the intestinal epithelium, and cellular membranes of most tissues are up to ten times smaller, permitting only the passage of small molecules. The physicochemical properties of drugs that affect their membrane penetration are *lipid solubility, degree of ionization,* and *molecular size.*

47

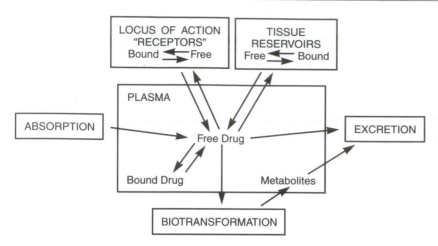

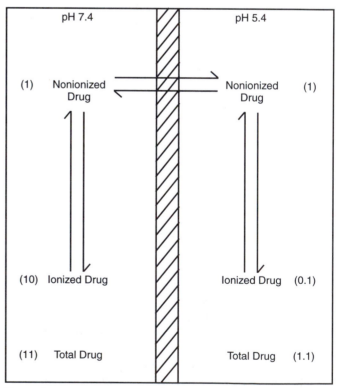

Figure 3–1 Schematic representation of the relationship between the absorption, distribution, binding, biotransformation, and excretion of a drug and its concentration at its locus of action. (Mayer SE, Melman KL, Gilman AG. *Goodman and Gilman's the Pharmacological Basis of Therapeutics.* 8th ed. New York: Macmillan; 1990. Reprinted with permission of McGraw-Hill.)

Lipid Solubility

Lipid solubility of drugs is expressed in terms of their lipid:water coefficient or partition coefficient. The greater the lipid:water coefficient, the more rapidly the drug can diffuse through the lipid components of cell membranes.

Degree of Ionization

Only a small number of drugs are completely ionized in solution (e.g., nondepolarizing neuromuscular blocking agents). Most drugs are weak acids and bases that are present in solutions as both ionized and nonionized molecules. The nonionized drug fraction is usually lipid-soluble and can cross biological membranes. The ionized fraction has a low lipid solubility and cannot penetrate membranes easily because it is repelled by similarly charged molecules on the surface of cell membrane proteins. Only the *nonionized* fraction of the drug can exert a pharmacologic effect, undergo reabsorption across renal tubules, and be susceptible to hepatic biotransformation (Table 3–1). Ionized fractions of drugs cannot be reabsorbed by renal tubules and are eliminated as unchanged drug.

The pKa (dissociation constant) and the pH of the surrounding fluid determine how much drug is in the nonionized form. The *pKa* is the pH at which half of a drug exists in the ionized form and half in the nonionized form. At an acidic pH, weak acids, such as barbiturates, exhibit a low pKa and remain in the nonionized form. At an alkaline pH, they dissociate readily to the ionized form. Weak bases, such as opioids and local anesthetics, tend to be ionized at an

acidic pH and nonionized at an alkaline pH. When the pKa of a drug and the pH are similar, small changes in the pH can cause a large change in the degree of ionization.

Since the nonionized form of a drug can penetrate a cell membrane, a concentration gradient can develop on two sides of a membrane separating fluids with different pHs (Fig. 3–2). The nonionized portion of drug will reach equilibrium, but the amount of ionized drug will be different on each side. This results in a very big difference in total drug concentration on each side of the membrane, which can be significant when one form of the drug exerts a greater pharmacologic effect than the other form.

Figure 3–2 A drug with a pKa of 6.4 is partially ionized as a weak acid in aqueous fluids separated by a membrane permeable only to the nonionized form of the drug. At steady state, the total quantity of drug is 10 times greater in one fluid than in the other, while the concentration of nonionized drug is the same. (Hug CC Jr. Pharmacokinetics of drugs administered intravenously. *Anesth Analg* 1978; 57: 704–723. Reprinted with permission of Williams & Wilkins.)

Table 3–1
CHARACTERISTICS OF NON-IONIZED AND IONIZED DRUG MOLECULES

	Non-ionized	Ionized
Pharmacologic effect	Active	Inactive
Solubility	Lipids	Water
Cross lipid barriers (renal tubules, GI tract, placenta, blood-brain barrier)	Yes	No
Renal excretion	No	Yes
Hepatic Metabolism	Yes	No

(Stoelting RK. *Pharmacology and Physiology in Anesthetic Practice.* 2nd ed. New York: Lippincott-Raven; 1991. Reprinted with permission.)

Differences in pH between two different body compartments can cause an accumulation of ionized drug in one compartment. This phenomenon is known as *ion trapping*. An example of this effect can be seen during the placental transfer of drugs from the mother to the fetus. In this case, the fetal pH is lower than the maternal pH. When a weak base, such as a local anesthetic, is administered to the mother and crosses the placenta, it is converted to a poorly lipid-soluble entity in the more acidic environment of the fetus. The ionized drug in the fetus cannot easily cross the placenta to return to the maternal circulation and thus becomes trapped in the fetus. Nonionized drug will continue to cross the placenta until it reaches equilibrium with the maternal circulation. At that time, the total drug concentration in the fetal plasma will exceed that in the mother's plasma. Accumulation of local anesthetics in the fetus has been associated with central nervous system (CNS) depression and bradycardia.

Molecular Size

A drug's molecular size will determine the mechanism necessary to transport it across a cell membrane. Ultimately, this can be manipulated to affect the rates of absorption, distribution, biotransformation, and excretion.

ABSORPTION

Bioavailability refers to the fraction of administered drug that reaches either its site of action or a biological fluid with access to the site of action. The factors affecting absorption (Table 3–2) determine bioavailability as well as the duration and intensity of drug action.

Factors Affecting Absorption   Regardless of the site of administration, drug absorption depends on *drug solubility*. Drugs in an aqueous solution are more rapidly absorbed than solids, suspensions, or oily solutions. For drugs in the solid form, the rate-limiting factor in their absorption is the rate of dissolution. The *concentration* of a drug also influences its rate of absorption. Highly concentrated solutions (oral or injectable) are absorbed more rapidly than those of a lower concentration. *Blood flow* to the site of absorption is an important factor. Increased blood flow, evoked by massage or local application of heat, enhances drug absorption. Decreased blood flow produced by vasoconstrictors or shock can delay absorption. Another important determinant of the rate of absorption is the *area of the absorbing surface*. Drugs are absorbed rapidly from large surface areas such as pulmonary alveolar epithelium and the intestinal mucosa. The absorbing surface is primarily determined by the *route of administration*.

Drugs absorbed from the gastrointestinal tract enter the portal venous blood and pass through the liver before entering the systemic circulation. Up to 90% of a drug can be extracted and rendered inactive. This phenomenon, known as the *first-pass effect*, can greatly decrease a drug's bioavailability. This accounts for the large differences between oral and intravenous doses seen with propranolol and lidocaine.

The oral route is the most convenient and economical route of administration. Disadvantages of this route include (1) irritation of the gastrointestinal mucosa by the drug, (2) destruction of the drug by digestive enzymes or acidic gastric fluid, and (3) changes in absorption caused by variations in gastric pH and gastrointestinal motility, and (4) the presence of food or other drugs. Drugs administered by the sublingual and buccal routes of administration are dissolved and absorbed in the mouth. As a result, first-pass effect and destruction by gastric enzymes is minimized. Rectal administration also bypasses the liver metabolism. Absorption from this route, while extensive, produces unpredictable plasma drug concentrations.

The subcutaneous and intramuscular routes produce rapid, predictable blood concentration, more so than after oral administration. The intravenous route places the drug directly into the systemic circulation, eliminating any obstacles to absorption. This is the fastest way to provide drug effect and is usually the route chosen during anesthesia. The inhalation route of administration is almost as fast as the intravenous route because the drug is exposed to the pulmonary circulation and the large absorptive surface of the alveoli.

Table 3–2
FACTORS AFFECTING DRUG ABSORPTION

Physicochemical properties of drugs
    Lipid solubility
    Degree of ionization
    Molecular size
Drug solubility
Rate of drug dissolution
Drug concentration
Blood flow to site of absorption
Area of absorbing surface
Route of administration
Local conditions at the gastrointestinal tract (for orally ingested
    drugs)
    Variations in gastric pH   ⎫
    Gastrointestinal motility   ⎬ Modify extent of
    Presence of food, drug, enzymes ⎪ absorption
    Gastrointestinal irritation   ⎭

DISTRIBUTION

Factors affecting distribution are lipid solubility, regional blood flow, tissue binding, and protein binding. Lipid-soluble drugs are rapidly distributed to highly perfused tissues (heart, brain, kidney, liver). When plasma concentrations of a drug decrease to a point below that in the highly perfused tissues, drug leaves the tissues and is redistributed to less perfused and poorly perfused areas such as skeletal muscles, bone, and fat.

When a drug binds to a tissue and does not yield a pharmacologic effect, that tissue has the potential to accumulate drug (i.e., to act as a reservoir). Binding to a nonresponsive tissue limits the magnitude of drug effect because the concentration of drug in the plasma—and, in turn, the sites of action—is decreased. Drugs stored in tissues that do not metabolize or excrete them retain their potential to exert a pharmacologic effect when they are redistributed to sites of action. If a reservoir for a drug fills rapidly, larger quantities of the drug are required to provide a therapeutic effect. Drugs can accumulate in a reservoir slowly, as in the case of fat tissue. When drug plasma concentrations decline due to metabolism, the reservoir releases drug into the systemic circulation slowly over a period of time, prolonging its duration of action. This accounts for the prolonged effects of anesthetics (e.g., impairment of cognitive function) seen for days after anesthesia.

Protein Binding   Plasma proteins, binding reversibly with drugs in blood, can function as drug reservoirs. The bound fraction of drug is *not* available to cross cell membranes, thus limiting distribution to tissues, access to hepatic metabolizing enzymes, and glomerular filtration.

Plasma albumin is the most important binding agent for weak acids and alpha$_1$-acid glycoprotein for weak bases. Binding of drugs to plasma proteins is nonselective. Many drugs with similar characteristics can bind to the same sites. Unlike some tissue reservoirs that may accumulate large amounts of drug, plasma proteins have a limited number of binding sites. When two drugs are administered together, they can compete for the same sites. This may not present a therapeutic problem unless the drugs are highly protein-bound (>95%), such as phenytoin and warfarin. If a drug, for example, is 98% protein-bound, a decrease in binding to 96% will double the plasma concentration. This is especially dangerous for drugs with a narrow therapeutic range.

Special Barriers   There are special considerations for the distribution of drugs to certain tissues. The *blood-brain barrier,* for one, consists of cerebral capillaries that limit the amount of drug entering the CNS from the plasma. Protein-bound drugs with a low lipid solubility, high degree of ionization and a large molecular size have limited access to the CNS. Conditions such as acute head injury, hypoxemia, and high fever can disrupt the blood-brain barrier and allow passage of normally restricted drugs.

Another special tissue barrier is the *placenta,* which restricts entry of certain drugs into the fetus. Two important factors determine the total amount of drug transferred from the mother to her fetus. One is the rate of penetration across the placenta. This is a function of the physicochemical properties of drugs and the integrity of the placenta. The other is the duration of exposure of the fetal circulation to drug in the mother's plasma. There is a greater risk of developing high drug plasma concentrations in the fetus from a continuous infusion or repeated administration of drugs to the mother than from single intravenous or bolus doses. Single doses cause a rapid rise and fall of plasma levels in the mother, limiting the exposure of drug to the fetal circulation.

VOLUME OF DISTRIBUTION

The volume of distribution (Vd) expresses the extent of distribution for a drug. It is calculated from the dose of drug administered intravenously divided by the resulting plasma concentration of drug. Protein-bound, ionized drugs with poor lipid solubility have limited access to tissues. They have high concentration in the plasma and a small calculated Vd. Examples of drugs with a small Vd, similar to extracellular fluid volume, are muscle relaxants. Lipid-soluble drugs with high tissue concentrations and low plasma concentrations have a large calculated Vd. Drugs such as thiopental and diazepam have large Vds that exceed total body water.

ELIMINATION

The elimination of drugs from the body usually involves two processes, biotransformation and excretion. Immediately after a drug is in the systemic circulation, it can be distributed to organs able to metabolize or excrete it. The liver is the main site of biotransformation and the kidneys are the main site responsible for excretion of noninhaled drugs.

Biotransformation   As described previously, only lipid-soluble drugs are readily absorbed and distributed to tissues. Drugs circulate to the kidneys, where they are filtered at the glomerulus and reabsorbed through the renal tubular cells. Small amounts of drug are excreted unchanged. Unless a drug becomes more water-soluble, allowing it to be eliminated in the urine, it will be reabsorbed and will reenter the systemic circulation over and over again.

The process of *biotransformation* converts lipid-soluble parent drugs to water-soluble metabolites. The water-soluble compounds have a smaller Vd and will not be reabsorbed readily. Metabolites may be active or completely inactive. Active metabolites may be more or less potent than the parent drug, exhibiting similar or different pharmacologic actions.

The four basic chemical reactions concerned in the biotransformation of drugs are (1) oxidation, (2) reduction, (3) hydrolysis, and (4) conjugation. Phase I reactions include oxidation, reduction, and hydrolysis. In phase II reactions, the parent drug or a metabolite reacts with an endogenous substrate, such as a carbohydrate or an amino acid, to form a water-soluble conjugate. While the liver is the major site of drug metabolism, biotransformation also occurs to a limited extent in the plasma, kidneys, lungs, and gastrointestinal tract.

Hepatic Microsomal Enzymes

Hepatic microsomal enzymes catalyze the reactions involved in the biotransformation of most drugs. They are primarily located in the hepatic smooth endoplasmic reticulum. These enzymes are also present in the kidneys and gastrointestinal epithelium. The term *microsomal enzyme* is derived from the fact that centrifugation of homogenized hepatocytes isolated fragments of the disrupted smooth endoplasmic reticulum in what was designated as the microsomal fraction. The microsomal fraction contains the cytochrome-P-450 mixed-function oxidase system. This is actually a large number of protein enzymes originally responsible for the metabolism of toxic substances.

Lipid solubility is an important requirement for a drug to be metabolized by the microsomal enzymes. A lipid-soluble drug can cross the cell membranes of enzyme-containing organs and bind with cytochrome-P-450. The rate of metabolism, as influenced by differences in microsomal enzyme activity, can vary sixfold or more among individuals.

Drugs or chemicals have the ability to increase enzyme activity. This unique property, known as *enzyme induction,* also occurs in the lungs, kidneys, and gastrointestinal tract. Phenobarbital induces microsomal enzymes by increasing the synthesis of cytochrome-P-450. This, in turn, leads to an accelerated metabolism of drugs administered with phenobarbital. Various environmental substances may also be responsible for enzyme induction in humans: pesticides, herbicides, industrial chemicals, alcohol, and tobacco smoke are but a few.

Nonmicrosomal Enzymes

Certain hydrolysis and conjugation reactions are catalyzed by *nonmicrosomal enzymes.* These enzymes are present primarily in the liver but can also be found in the plasma and gastrointestinal tract. An example of nonmicrosomal biotransformation is the hydrolysis of succinylcholine, atracurium, and esmolol by *plasma cholinesterase* and the *nonspecific esterases* found in the liver, plasma, and gastrointestinal tract. None of the nonmicrosomal enzymes are susceptible to enzyme induction. Their activity, however, is subject to genetic variation.

Factors Affecting Biotransformation

The rate of biotransformation of most drugs is determined by the concentration of drug at the sites of metabolism and by the intrinsic rate of the metabolism process. The concentration of drug at the site of metabolism is determined by its plasma concentration and blood flow to the liver through hepatic and portal vessels. The intrinsic rate of metabolism is influenced by enzyme activity and cofactor availability (e.g., genetics, enzyme induction).

First-Order Kinetics

Most drug biotransformation follows linear or *first-order kinetics,* with which a constant fraction of available drug is metabolized in a given time period. The fraction of total drug eliminated is not dependent on the plasma concentration of drug. However, the total amount of drug eliminated per unit time is dependent on the plasma concentration of drug. As the plasma concentration of a drug increases, so will the amount eliminated, but the fraction eliminated will remain the same.

Zero-Order Kinetics

Zero-order kinetics occur when the plasma concentration of drug exceeds the capacity of metabolizing enzymes. When the enzymes are saturated, only a constant amount of drug can be metabolized per unit time (e.g., 40 mg/h). The total amount of drug eliminated per unit time will remain the same, regardless of the drug's plasma concentration. The intrinsic activity of enzymes determines the constant amount of drug metabolized per unit time. The pharmacokinetics of ethanol, aspirin, and phenytoin exhibit zero-order metabolism.

Excretion   Drugs are excreted from the body either unchanged or as metabolites. Except for the lungs, excretory organs (i.e., kidneys, biliary system) eliminate water-soluble compounds more efficiently than lipid-soluble compounds. For this reason, the conversion, during biotransformation, of lipid-soluble drugs to water-soluble metabolites by the liver and other organs is very significant.

The kidney is the most important organ for the excretion of drugs and their metabolites. Fecal excretion is a key pathway for the removal of certain unabsorbed drugs or metabolites from the body. Drugs may also be excreted by other pathways, as by the intestine or lungs or via saliva, sweat, or breast milk. The overall contribution of these routes, however, is generally small.

The routes of excretion from breast milk and lungs, though minor, deserve mention. Excretion of drugs in breast milk is critical not for the amounts eliminated but for the potential of transmitting drugs and metabolites to a nursing infant. Pulmonary excretion is essential for the elimination of volatile anesthetics (Chap. 5).

Renal Excretion

The rate of excretion is determined by renal blood flow and by the rates of three renal processes: glomerular filtration, tubular secretion, and tubular reabsorption. Drugs that are not bound to plasma proteins pass through the glomerulus at a rate dependent on drug concentration and on the volume of glomerular filtrate. Tubular secretion involves active transport processes that are selective for certain drugs and drug metabolites, including protein-bound compounds. This process can be so efficient that both the free and protein-bound forms of the drug can be removed from the renal tubular plasma. Tubular reabsorption removes drug that has entered tubular fluid by glomerular filtration and tubular secretion. Reabsorption is most prominent for lipid-soluble drugs that are able to cross the cell membranes of renal tubular epithelial cells. The reabsorption of some drugs (e.g., thiopental) is so extensive that very little is excreted unchanged into the urine.

The rate of reabsorption from renal tubules is influenced by factors such as pH and rate of renal tubular urine flow. Passive reabsorption of weak acids and bases can be altered by urinary pH. Ionized drugs have a low lipid solubility and cannot cross renal tubular epithelial cells, thus enhancing their excretion. Urinary pH influences the fraction of drug that exists in the ionized form.

Creatinine clearance and serum creatinine are useful clinical indicators of the kidneys' ability to eliminate drugs. When either index increases significantly, the dose or frequency of a drug must be decreased to prevent accumulation of drug in the plasma and, ultimately, possible toxic effects of the drug.

Biliary and Fecal Excretion

Most of the metabolites of drugs formed in the liver are excreted in bile into the gastrointestinal tract. Often, these metabolites are reabsorbed from the gastrointestinal tract into the blood and ultimately excreted in the urine. Metabolites are actively transported into bile by carrier systems similar to those that transport them across the renal tubule. Substances excreted in the feces are mainly unabsorbed orally administered drugs or metabolites that were excreted in the bile and not reabsorbed from the gastrointestinal tract.

CLINICAL PHARMACOKINETICS

Pharmacokinetic principles describes the variation of plasma concentration of drug over time as a result of absorption, distribution, and elimination. Applied to therapy, pharmacokinetic principles help in the interpretation of measured serum concentration of drugs and in the selection and adjustment of drug dosage schedules. Commonly measured pharmacokinetic parameters of drugs are bioavailability, clearance, volume of distribution (Vd), and elimination half-time.

It should be noted that pharmacokinetic characteristics of drugs measured in healthy adults may be different in patients with chronic diseases (renal failure, cirrhosis of the liver, cardiac failure) and in various extremes of age, weight, hydration, nutrition, and skeletal muscle mass.

Two-Compartment Models   Pharmacokinetics has been simplified for many drugs by considering the body to comprise a limited number of compartments. The two-compartment model (Fig. 3–3) can be used to demonstrate the basic pharmacokinetic concepts that also apply to more complex models. In this model, the drug is introduced directly into the central compartment by an intravenous injection. The drug distributes to the peripheral compartment and returns to the central compartment, where elimination from the body occurs.

The central compartment consists of plasma and highly perfused tissues (lungs, heart, brain, kidneys, liver) into which uptake of drug is rapid. In adults, these highly perfused tissues receive almost 75% of the cardiac output but represent about 10% of the body mass. This central compartment is defined only in terms of its apparent volume (V1), which is estimated and does not necessarily correspond to actual anatomic volumes.

The plasma concentration of a drug is affected by its rate of distribution to the peripheral compartment and by its rate of elimination from the body. Distribution and elimination begin immediately after the drug enters the circulation. At first, both processes contribute to a gradual lowering of the plasma concentration of the drug. However, the effects of distribution on the decline of drug plasma levels are short-lived. This is because the exchange of drug between the central and peripheral compartments is an equilibrium process dependent on the concentration gradient of the drug. Initially, the movement of drug is from the central to the peripheral compartment at the maximum possible rate (k_{12}). With time, the gradient decreases as the concentration of drug builds up in the peripheral compartment and continues to decline in the central compartment. Eventually the net exchange of drug will be zero (equilibrium), and then the exchange will be reversed as the drug continues to be eliminated from the central compartment by biotransformation and excretion. Past the equilibrium point, the movement of drug from the peripheral compartment to the central compartment maintains rather than reduces plasma levels. If the rate of drug return from the peripheral compartment is slow (small k_{21}), it can limit the rate of elimination (k_e) of the drug from the body.

The peripheral compartment is also defined in terms of its apparent volume (V2). A large V2 suggests extensive uptake of drug by those tissues and organs composing the peripheral compartment. Any residual drug present in the peripheral compartment at the time of a repeat injection will diminish the effect of distributive processes on the reduction of drug levels in plasma and lead to more intense effects of the drug (i.e., drug accumulation).

Plasma Concentration Curves   For most drugs administered intravenously, a graphic representation of the change in plasma levels of a drug over time can be constructed by plotting the logarithm of the concentration on the ordinate against time on the abscissa (Fig. 3–4). Logarithms provide a convenient means for plotting the large range of plasma concentrations encountered in the plasma after an intravenous dose of a drug. They are also appropriate for depicting the processes of distribution and elimination, which can be described by first-order kinetics.

The typical graph is a biexponential curve and represents two distinct phases in the decline of the plasma concentration of a drug following a single intravenous dose. The initial portion of the curve is termed the distribution or *alpha phase*. As discussed, this phase begins immediately after intravenous injection of a drug and reflects that drug's distribution from the circulation (central compartment) to peripheral tissues (peripheral compartments). The terminal portion of the curve is termed the elimination or *beta phase*. This phase is linear and is distinguished by a more gradual decline in the drug

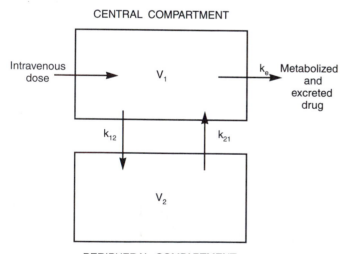

CENTRAL COMPARTMENT

PERIPHERAL COMPARTMENT

Figure 3–3   The two-compartment model of drug disposition. The intravenously administered drug equilibrates between the central and peripheral compartments but is eliminated only from the central compartment. K_e, rate constant for overall drug eliminate from body; K_{12}, rate constant for drug transfer from central to peripheral compartment; K_{21}, rate constant for drug transfer from peripheral to central compartment. (Hug CC Jr. Pharmacokinetics of drugs administered intravenously. Anesth Analg 1978; 57: 704–723. Reprinted with permission of Williams & Wilkins.)

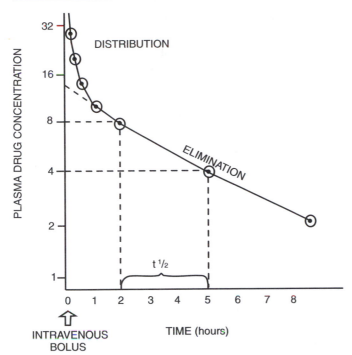

Figure 3–4 Plasma concentration curve. The plasma concentration curve depicts the decline in plasma concentration of a drug over time, following a single rapid intravenous injection into the central compartment. Using the figure above, drug X (250 mg) is administered intravenously and plasma samples are obtained to determine drug concentration. As drug distributes to the peripheral compartments (alpha phase), plasma drug concentration falls rapidly. When first-order elimination kinetics follow (beta phase), the plasma concentration declines gradually, as demonstrated by a straight line. When this line is extrapolated to time zero, 12 μg/mL represents the theoretical plasma concentration if distribution of the drug was instantaneous. This value is used to calculate Vd. The half-time of drug elimination can also be calculated. Once elimination began, 3 h was the time necessary for the plasma drug concentration to decline 50% (i.e., from 8 to 4 μg/mL). (Mayer SE, Melman KL, Gilman AG. *Goodman and Gilman's the Pharmacological Basis of Therapeutics.* 8th ed. New York: Macmillan; 1990. Reprinted with permission of McGraw-Hill.)

plasma concentration. This gradual decline exhibits the drug's elimination from the plasma (central compartment) by biotransformation and excretion.

Elimination Half-Time *Elimination half-time* is the time necessary for the plasma concentration of drug to decline 50% during the elimination phase (Fig. 3–4). *Elimination half-life,* in contrast to elimination half-time, defines the time necessary to eliminate 50% of the drug from the body following a rapid intravenous injection. Elimination half-time and elimination half-life can be equal unless the decrease in a drug's plasma concentration is not due to its elimination from the body. *Five elimination half-times are required for virtually complete (96.9%) elimination of the drug from the body.* For this reason, drug accumulation is predictable if dosing intervals are less than this period of time. Drug accumulation continues until the rate of elimination equals the rate of administration. As with drug elimination, the time necessary for a drug to achieve a steady-state

plasma concentration with intermittent dosing is about five elimination half-times.

Clearance Clearance (CL) is the volume of plasma (milliliters per minute) cleared of drug by renal excretion and/or metabolism in the liver or other organs. Clearance is a very important variable to consider when deciding on the rate of a continuous infusion. To maintain an unchanging plasma concentration of drug (steady state), the infusion rate must be equal to the rate of drug clearance by hepatic and renal mechanisms. If the rate of infusion exceeds CL, drug will start to accumulate in the plasma.

☐ PHARMACODYNAMICS

Once a drug has been delivered to the target organ, it can exert its pharmacologic effect. The most common mechanism by which this occurs is by the drug's interaction with a specific protein macromolecule in the lipid bilayer of cell membranes. This protein macromolecule is referred to as a *receptor.* Receptors exist for endogenous regulatory substances such as hormones and neurotransmitters. A drug-receptor interaction changes the conformation of a specific segment of the macromolecule and initiates or prevents a series of changes that characterize the pharmacologic effects of the drug.

Drugs that activate receptors are called *agonists. Antagonists* are drugs that bind to receptors without activating them while at the same time preventing agonists from binding and stimulating these same receptors. *Competitive antagonism* is present when increasing concentrations of an antagonist progressively inhibit responses to unchanging concentrations of agonist. High concentrations of agonist can overcome competitive antagonism. Noncompetitive antagonism is present when even high concentrations of agonist cannot completely overcome antagonism. A partial agonist is a drug that binds weakly to receptors and produces a minimal pharmacologic effect even though a maximal concentration is present.

RECEPTORS

Receptors are identified and subsequently classified (e.g., alpha, beta, histamine, mu) on the basis of how they respond to specific agonists and antagonists. Multiple subtypes of receptors (alpha$_1$ and alpha$_2$, beta$_1$ and beta$_2$, h$_1$ and h$_2$, mu$_1$ and mu$_2$) exist for many receptors. Most receptors are within the cell membrane with their binding sites facing outward. Substances with poor lipid solubility do not need to cross the cell membrane in order to exert their effect. Many endogenous substances (ligands), such as catecholamines and hormones, have poor lipid solubilities.

The concentration of receptors in the cell membrane is dynamic, either increasing *(upregulation)* or decreasing *(downregulation)* in response to drugs or endogenous substances. The response to a given concentration of drug may vary widely, depending on the status of receptors on the target cells. For example, prolonged treatment of asthma with a beta agonist may result in tolerance associated with a decrease in the concentration of receptors. On the other hand, chronic beta-antagonist therapy may result in increased numbers of receptors in cell membranes, such that an exaggerated response occurs if the blockade is abruptly stopped. The same concentration of endogenous catecholamines, now unopposed by an antagonist, is reacting with an increased number of receptors.

DOSE-RESPONSE RELATIONSHIPS

Dose-response curves portray the relationship between the dose of drug administered and the resulting pharmacologic effect (Fig. 3–5). Since a wide range of doses are studied, the logarithmic determination of dosage is frequently used. Four important parameters are considered in analyzing the dose-response curve: potency, slope, efficacy, and individual variation.

POTENCY

Potency is a statement of how much drug is required to produce a desired pharmacologic response. It is depicted along the dose axis of the dose-response curve. Factors that influence a drug's potency are absorption, distribution, metabolism, excretion, and affinity for the receptor. Lack of potency becomes a limiting factor only when so much drug is required to produce an effect that it is difficult to administer. Doses required to produce a specific response in 50% of patients are designated as the median effective dose, or ED_{50}.

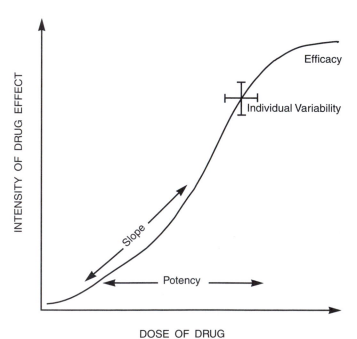

Figure 3–5 The log dose-response relationship. Dose-response curves illustrate four characteristic variables: potency, slope, efficacy, and individual variability. (Mayer SE, Melman KL, Gilman AG. *Goodman and Gilman's the Pharmacological Basis of Therapeutics.* 8th ed. New York: Macmillan; 1990. Reprinted with permission of McGraw-Hill.)

The lethal dose of a drug is expressed in similar terms. The LD_{50} is the dose of drug that is fatal to 50% of patients.

An inherently safe drug has an LD_{50} that is much greater than the ED_{50}. The therapeutic index is the ratio of the median lethal dose to the median effective dose, (LD_{50}/ED_{50}). Drugs have many therapeutic indices, depending on the therapeutic response being considered and the dose or drug necessary to evoke that response. For example, the therapeutic index for aspirin to exert an antiplatelet effect is very different from the therapeutic index to relieve the pain of severe rheumatoid arthritis.

SLOPE

The *slope* of the dose-response curve is related to the number of receptors that must be occupied to produce the pharmacologic effect. If a drug must occupy a large number of receptors before an effect is seen, the slope will be steep. This is demonstrated by the nondepolarizing neuromuscular blockers. A steep slope suggests that small increases in dose will produce large increases in pharmacologic effect. It is very likely that the difference between the therapeutic dose and the toxic dose will be small. Drugs with such narrow therapeutic indices require careful titration to achieve the desired effect and avoid toxic effects.

EFFICACY

The *efficacy* of a drug is the maximum pharmacologic effect that the drug can produce. It is depicted by the plateau in dose-response curves. Efficacy may be limited by the appearance of side effects below or within the dose range necessary to produce the desired effect. The efficacy and potency of a drug are not related.

Individual Variation Factors influencing pharmacokinetics (bioavailability, renal and hepatic function, age) and pharmacodynamics (genetic differences, receptor concentration), along with coexisting disease and drug interactions, account for the variability of patients' responses to drugs. Knowledge of the patient factors that alter responses allows the nurse anesthetist to adjust doses and choose agents that are least harmful to a specific patient.

TERMINOLOGY

Specific terms are used to describe drug responses in individuals and to define interactions among drugs administered together.

If a drug produces its usual effect at an unusually low dosage in a given patient, that individual is said to be *hyperreactive* or *hypersensitive*. The latter term is reserved for people who are allergic (sensitized) to a drug. If a drug produces its usual effect only at unusually large doses, the individual is said to be *hyporeactive*. Hyporeactivity acquired from chronic exposure to a drug is termed *tolerance*. Tolerance that develops rapidly after administration of only a few doses of drug is termed *tachyphylaxis*. The most important factor in the development of tolerance to drugs such as opioids and alcohol is neuronal adaptation, referred to as *cellular tolerance*. Other mechanisms of tolerance are enzyme induction and depletion of neurotransmitters caused by sustained stimulation. Reduced sensitivity is termed *immunity* when tolerance is the result of antibody formation. An unusual effect of a drug, regardless of dosage, that occurs in a small percentage of individuals is termed *idiosyncrasy*. Un-

usual effects of drugs should be described in terms of their underlying mechanism, usually as a result of drug allergy or genetic differences.

An *additive effect* means that a second drug acting with a first drug administered will produce an effect equal to an algebraic summation. *Synergistic effect* means that two drugs interact to produce an effect greater than an algebraic summation. *Antagonism* means that two drugs interact to produce an effect less than an algebraic summation.

SUGGESTED READINGS

Hardman JG, Goodman Gilman A, Limbird LE, eds. *The Pharmacological Basis of Therapeutics*. 9th ed. New York: McGraw-Hill; 1996.

Hug CC Jr. Pharmacokinetics of drugs administered intravenously. *Anesth Analg* 1978;57:704–723.

Longnecker DE, Murphy FL. *Introduction to Anesthesia*. 8th ed. Philadelphia: Saunders; 1992.

Stoelting RK. *Pharmacology & Physiology in Anesthetic Practice*. 2nd ed. New York: Lippincott; 1991.

Stoelting RK, Miller RD. *Basics of Anesthesia*. 3rd ed. New York: Churchill Livingstone; 1994.

☐ QUESTIONS

1. All statements regarding clearance are true *except* which of the following?
   a. Significant serum creatinine elevation may indicate the need to decrease the dose or frequency of a drug to prevent accumulation.
   b. A steady state occurs when the rate of clearance equals the rate of infusion of a drug.
   c. Clearance of a drug is not subject to individual variances.
   d. $CL = V_{dis}/T_{1/2B}$.

2. True statements regarding absorption of a drug include
   a. Rectal administration may yield unpredictable plasma drug concentrations.
   b. Massage or heat application may enhance drug absorption through increased blood flow.
   c. Administration via inhalation may be as fast as intravenous administration because of exposure to the pulmonary circulation and the large absorptive surface area of the alveoli.
   d. All are true.

3. Giving meperidine (Demerol) to a patient on isocarboxazid (Marplan) may result in all of the following *except*
   a. hypertensive crisis.
   b. increase in temperature.
   c. increased muscle weakness.
   d. convulsions.

4. Ionization of a drug
   a. may affect the drug's ability to cross membranes.
   b. may render a drug inactive.

   c. is a function of the pKa.
   d. All of the above.

5. Vessel-rich tissues include all *except*
   a. muscle.
   b. heart.
   c. liver.
   d. central nervous system.

6. When two drugs exhibit an additive effect
   a. one drug will prolong the action of the other.
   b. both drugs will have a more rapid onset.
   c. a second drug acting with the first drug will produce an effect equal to an algebraic summation.
   d. two drugs act together to produce an action greater than the algebraic summation.

7. The *most common* site of biotransformation is the
   a. plasma.
   b. kidneys.
   c. liver.
   d. gastrointestinal tract.

8. Highly protein-bound drugs include all *except*
   a. phenytoin.
   b. thiopental.
   c. warfarin.
   d. rocuronium.

9. A drug property that does *not* affect membrane penetration is
   a. degree of ionization.

    b. concentration gradient.
    c. molecular size.
    d. lipid solubility.

10. All statements are true *except* which of the following?
    a. Fentanyl tends to be nonionized at an alkaline pH.
    b. Fentanyl tends to be ionized at an acidic pH.
    c. At an alkaline pH, lidocaine will dissociate readily into an ionized form.
    d. Thiopental, with a low pKa, will remain nonionized in an acidic environment.

11. Volume of distribution
    a. equals the dose of a drug given divided by plasma concentration of the drug.
    b. is increased if the drug is highly protein-bound.
    c. is increased if the drug is highly ionized.
    d. cannot be calculated.

12. The first-pass effect
    a. is avoided by oral administration.
    b. explains the large differences between the oral and intravenous doses of propranolol.
    c. can greatly increase a drug's bioavailability.
    d. All of the above.

13. Examples of biotransformation via nonmicrosomal esterase hydrolysis include which of the following?
    a. atracurium, succinylcholine, propofol
    b. esmolol, atracurium, propofol
    c. succinylcholine, remifentanyl, esmolol
    d. enflurane, remifentanyl, mivacron

14. Drug Y is eliminated by first-order kinetics. If 40 mg of the drug is administered and 5 h later 20 mg has been metabolized, what is the total amount of drug that has been metabolized after 10 more hours?
    a. 30 mg
    b. 35 mg
    c. 40 mg
    d. 50 mg

15. Using the above question, how much of the drug will be left in the body 15 h after the drug was administered?
    a. 20 mg
    b. 10 mg
    c. 5 mg
    d. 2.5 mg

16. Zero-order kinetics
    a. occurs when plasma concentration of a drug exceeds the capacity of metabolizing enzymes.
    b. describes the most common drug biotransformation pathway.
    c. occurs when a constant fraction of a total drug is eliminated over time.
    d. a and c.

17. Which narcotic has the *lowest* Vd?
    a. Demerol (meperidine)
    b. Alfenta (alfentanil)
    c. Sufenta (sufentanil)
    d. fentanyl

18. A steep slope suggests that
    a. small increases in dosages will produce large increases in pharmacologic effect.
    b. the difference between the therapeutic dose and the lethal dose will be small.
    c. a drug must occupy a large number of receptors before an effect is seen.
    d. All of the above.

19. Zero-order kinetics describes all of the following *except* which one?
    a. the metabolism of thiopental
    b. the metabolism of ASA, alcohol, and phenytoin
    c. nonlinear elimination of drugs
    d. elimination in drug overdoses

20. The therapeutic index is the ratio of the median lethal dose to the median effective dose, (LD_{50}/ED_{50}). Is this statement true or false?
    a. True
    b. False

☐ ANSWERS

1. c	5. a	9. b	13. c	17. b
2. d	6. c	10. c	14. b	18. d
3. c	7. c	11. a	15. c	19. a
4. d	8. d	12. b	16. a	20. a

Pharmacology of Intravenous Agents

Mark A. Caldwell

☐ INTRAVENOUS ANESTHETIC AGENTS

BARBITURATES

Barbiturates are produced as highly alkaline solution (pH of 2.5% thiopental is 10.5). When injected, the 2.5% solution is not painful. The sedative-hypnotic properties of barbiturates result from substitutions at the 2 and 5 carbon atoms of barbituric acid. The more lipid-soluble thiopental comes from a substitution of a sulfur atom for the number 5 carbon; oxybarbiturates have an oxygen atom for the number 5 carbon. Methohexital has a short duration of action produced by placing a methyl group on the nitrogen of barbituric acid.

Mechanism of Action   One theory is that the inhibitory transmitter gamma-aminobutyric acid (GABA) has a decreased rate of dissociation from its receptors due to barbiturates causing a buildup of inhibitory transmitter. Anticonvulsant and anxiolytic effects are produced, but it is unknown whether the sedative-hypnotic effects occur in this manner.[1] GABA increases the passage of chloride ions through ion channels causing hyperpolarization of the postsynaptic neuron.

Depression of the reticular activating system appears to be another unique capability of barbiturates. Located in the brain stem, the reticular activating system controls consciousness. Barbiturates also suppress acetylcholine (Ach), an excitatory neurotransmitter.[2]

Anesthetic Concerns and Considerations   Barbiturates are used for the induction of anesthesia: thiopental 3 to 5 mg/kg and methohexital, 0.5 to 1.5 mg/kg. Unconsciousness is produced within 30 seconds as barbiturates rapidly enter the central nervous system (CNS). Barbiturates are considered short acting due to redistribution of the drug from the central compartment; however, the actual elimination half-life of thiopental is up to 12 hours.[1] The dose of thiopental for the elderly decreases with age, reflecting a slower passage from the central to peripheral compartment. Barbiturates can also be used as a supplement to an inhaled anesthetic during the course of anesthesia.[2]

Deposits of barbiturates after intravenous (IV) administration have been noted to cause venous thrombosis reflecting the difference in pH between barbiturates and blood. Because of the increasing diameter of veins, crystal formation and venous thrombosis are less hazardous. A more dilute solution helps to prevent this complication (thiopental 2.5% and methohexital 1%).[3] Accidental intra-arterial injection of barbiturates causes excruciating pain and vasoconstriction often leading to gangrene. Treatment involves use of phentolamine (an α blocker) 5 to 10 mg in 10 mL normal saline (NS) in local infiltration or in an injection of the artery. A dose of 10 mL 1% procaine can also inhibit smooth muscle spasm. Urokinase 75,000 IU may be used to lyse any emboli. A sympathectomy produced by a stellate ganglion block may also be necessary.[4]

Porphyria

Barbiturates are contraindicated in patients with porphyria. Porphyria is an inborn metabolic disorder manifested by the inability to metabolize porphyrin due to abnormal enzyme activity. It is believed that barbiturates stimulate enzymatic activity, which cannot be metabolized. This leads to severe pain and neurologic demyelination. All barbiturates should be avoided in susceptible patients.[5] Other anesthetic or related drugs that may precipitate the onset of porphyria include benzodiazepines, corticosteroids, etomidate, ketamine, and phenytoin. Safe anesthetics are believed to include anticholinesterases, anticholinergics, all muscle relaxants, droperidol, opioids, volatile anesthetics, and nitrous oxide. It should be noted that even with documented cases of porphyria, barbiturates and other suspected agents do not always cause attacks.

Cardiovascular

The blood pressure decreases and heart rate increases with a barbiturate induction dose. Barbiturates depress the medullary vasomotor center and decrease sympathetic stimulation from the CNS, causing vasodilation. This venous dilation decreases blood return to the heart. Patients who are hypovolemic or taking β-blocker therapy are prone to extreme decreases in blood pressure after barbiturates. Titration of induction dose and preoperative hydration reduce the chance of these problems in susceptible patients.[2]

Respiratory

The ventilatory response to hypercapnia is reduced due to barbiturate depression of medullary ventilatory centers. A brief period of apnea usually occurs after induction. A decreased rate of breathing and small tidal volume characterize spontaneous ventilation as the patient awakens. Laryngeal reflexes are maintained until large doses of barbiturates are given. Because airway reflexes are not reliably depressed, laryngospasm and bronchospasm can occur during induction.

Cerebral

Barbiturate-induced cerebral vasoconstriction creates a decrease in intracranial pressure (ICP), cerebral blood volume, and cerebral blood flow. Barbiturates can decrease cerebral metabolic oxygen requirements ($CMRO_2$) greater than the decrease they cause in cerebral blood flow. Consequently, areas of the brain with poor perfusion are thought to be protected when barbiturates are used.[4] Excitatory movement can be elicited by methohexital.[3]

Pharmacokinetics

Thirty seconds after IV administration maximal uptake of barbiturates occurs in the brain, causing induction of anesthesia. Redistribution of barbiturates from the brain to skeletal muscle and fat accounts for a quick regaining of consciousness. The typical time to awakening of the patient is 5 to 15 minutes.[3] Because over 80% of thiopental is protein bound, patients with low serum albumin will get a much greater brain concentration. The prolonged elimination of barbiturates depends almost entirely on metabolism. The elimination half-time for thiopental is 12 hours; for methohexital it is only 3.9 hours.[6]

PROPOFOL

Propofol (Diprivan) is a diisopropylphenol hypnotic agent used for the induction of anesthesia. It is available in a 1% solution and is administered in a dosage range of 1 to 2.5 mg/kg IV. Unconsciousness is produced within 40 seconds with a quicker awakening than with barbiturates.[3] Mainte-

nance of anesthesia can be obtained with a propofol infusion concurrent with 65% nitrous oxide.

Mechanism of Action   At a separate site on the GABA receptor from benzodiazepines or barbiturates, propofol may augment chloride ion channel function.[1]

Anesthesia Concerns and Considerations   The formulation for propofol is preservative free; therefore, good sterile technique must be observed. Pain is also noted to occur with propofol based on its formulation. Administration of lidocaine prior to propofol injection can attenuate this complication. There is less incidence of postoperative nausea and vomiting with propofol.

Cardiovascular

A decrease in systemic vascular resistance and cardiac output occurs after administration of propofol. The corresponding reduction in blood pressure is greater with propofol than with an induction dose of thiopental, but this is usually reversed with laryngoscopy and intubation. Hypotension with propofol can be magnified in patients with impaired left ventricular function, the elderly, and hypovolemic patients.[2]

Respiratory

Propofol is a respiratory depressant, and induction doses of propofol produce apnea.

Cerebral

Reduction in cerebral blood flow and ICP occurs with propofol. In the patient with elevated ICP, propofol reduces cerebral perfusion pressure.[2]

KETAMINE

Ketamine is a phencyclidine derivative that produces dissociative anesthesia with an induction dose of 1 to 2 mg/kg IV and 5 to 10 mg/kg intramuscularly (IM). Ketamine possesses a short duration of action (5 to 15 minutes) and a rapid onset; 30 seconds.[4]

The dissociative anesthesia produced by ketamine is actually a dissociation between the thalamus (which relays sensory input) and the limbic cortex (which involves awareness). In the clinical setting, the patient appears conscious (usually with rapid eye movement) even though the patient will not respond to outside stimulus.[2]

Anesthesia Concerns and Considerations   Ketamine may be used for an IM induction in mentally retarded patients and temperamental children. Its excellent analgesic properties and airway maintenance make it an ideal anesthetic for burned patients especially during dressing changes.

Cardiovascular

Ketamine causes sympathetic nervous system stimulation resulting in increases in heart rate, blood pressure, and myocardial contractility. Myocardial oxygen demand on the heart increases with ketamine; thus, patients with coronary artery disease are not good candidates for this drug.[1] Hypovolemic patients or those in cardiac failure may benefit from ketamine use.

Respiratory

Ketamine does not depress ventilation in subinduction doses. Because of sympathetic stimulation, the drug's bronchodilatory effects may benefit the patient in bronchospasm. Ketamine can be used for induction in an asthmatic patient because of its sympathetic stimulation to the airways. Increased airway secretions that occur with use of ketamine may be attenuated by the use of an antisialagogue.[4]

Cerebral

The $CMRO_2$ increases with ketamine. Ketamine also increases cerebral blood flow and ICP, which may compromise neurologic status.[2] For this reason, ketamine is an undesirable drug for the neurosurgical patient. Undesirable emergence delirium can be prevented by premedication with benzodiazepines. Do not use in a patient with a psychiatric history.

ETOMIDATE

Etomidate is a quick-acting induction drug with an onset less than 30 seconds. After a normal induction dose of 0.2 to 0.5 mg/kg, awakening occurs quickly without cumulative effects.[4]

Mechanism of Action Etomidate produces inhibitory effects in the brain by imitating GABA and depressing the reticular activating system.

Anesthesia Concerns and Considerations Etomidate causes adrenocortical suppression, preventing the production of cortisol for 4 to 8 hours.[7] Etomidate also produces pain on injection, which can be alleviated by prior injection of lidocaine. Subcortical disinhibition is the mechanism responsible for extrapyramidal activity seen with etomidate.

Cardiovascular

Etomidate possesses cardiac stability. Heart rate, cardiac output, and stroke volume are unaffected by etomidate.

Respiratory

Etomidate has less respiratory depression than barbiturates. Induction doses may not result in apnea unless opioids are also used.[2]

Cerebral

Cerebral blood flow, ICP, and $CMRO_2$ are reduced with etomidate. Myoclonic activity occurs as a side effect to etomidate in approximately one third of patients.[7]

OPIATES

Mechanism of Action Opiates are drugs that bind to specific opioid receptors in the CNS: mu_1, mu_2, kappa, sigma,

Table 4-1
OPIOID RECEPTOR AND EFFECT

Opioid Receptor	Effect
Mu_1	Supraspinal analgesia
Mu_2	Respiratory depression
	Physical dependency
	Most cardiovascular effects
Delta	Spinal analgesia
Kappa	Spinal analgesia
	Sedation
Sigma	Dysphoria
	Hallucinations

and delta. Mu_1 receptors are associated with supraspinal analgesia; kappa and delta receptors are significant at the spinal level (Table 4-1).[8] Endorphins are normally produced by the body and activate these receptors. Opioid potency is dependent on receptor affinity and specific receptor activation (i.e., kappa, mu_1, etc.).[2] Agonists bind to and activate opiate receptors; opiate antagonists competitively prevent opiates from binding to their receptors. Opiate agonists-antagonists have an affinity for select receptors while competitively blocking others.[8]

Substance P and Ach are excitatory neurotransmitters. Their release is inhibited by opiates.[2] These excitatory neurotransmitters play a role in signal transmission to the brain.

The *substantia gelatinosa* in the dorsal horn of the spinal cord and the *periaqueductal gray matter* in the midbrain are areas in which pain modulation occurs.

The uses and dosages of opioids are presented in Table 4-2.

Table 4-2
OPIOID DOSING

Drug	Use	Dosing
meperidine	Analgesia	0.5–2 mg/kg IV
morphine	Analgesia	2.5–15 mg IV
		0.05–0.2 mg/kg IV (children)—maximum dose 15 mg (children)
	Induction analgesia	1 mg/kg
fentanyl	Analgesia	0.7–2 μg/kg IV
	Induction	5–40 μg/kg IV
	Analgesia supplement	2–20 μg/kg IV
	Sole anesthetic	50–150 μg/kg IV(total dose)
alfentanil	Analgesia	5–10 μg/kg IV
	Induction	50–300 μg/kg IV
	Analgesia supplement	10–100 μg/kg IV
	Sole anesthetic	500–2000 μg/kg IV(total dose)
sufentanil	Analgesia	0.2–0.6 μg/kg IV
	Induction	2–10 μg/kg IV
	Analgesia supplement	0.6–4 μg/kg IV
	Sole anesthetic	10–30 μg/kg IV(total dose)

Anesthetic Concerns and Considerations

Cardiovascular

Opioids do not cause changes in myocardial contractility. Arterial blood pressure can fall with opiates (except meperidine) related to bradycardia and decreased venous sympathetic tone. Morphine and meperidine can cause a decrease in blood pressure secondary to histamine release. An increase in heart rate can occur with meperidine because it structurally resembles atropine.[2]

Respiratory

All opiates depress ventilation and produce a decreased response to the ventilatory stimulant effects of CO_2. The CO_2 response curve is shifted to the right. Respiratory rate is decreased with opiates, while there is a noncompensatory increase in tidal volume. Histamine release from morphine or meperidine can cause bronchospasm in some patients (i.e., asthmatics). Chest wall rigidity with fentanyl, alfentanil, and sufentanil may necessitate muscle relaxation for ventilation to occur.

Cerebral

Amnesia and unconsciousness cannot be reliably produced with opiates. Opiates cause decreases in ICP and cerebral blood flow. Normeperidine is an active metabolite of meperidine and can trigger convulsive activity.[9] A severe and potentially fatal reaction can occur if meperidine is given to a patient taking monoamine oxidase inhibitors.[4]

Opiates trigger the chemoreceptor trigger zone, producing emesis. A possible reason is the role opioids possess as partial dopamine agonists in the chemoreceptor trigger zone.[9] This can be aggravated by the decrease in gastrointestinal motility caused by opioids.

AGONIST-ANTAGONIST OPIATES

Pentazocine, butorphanol, nalbuphine, and buprenorphine are agonists-antagonists. These drugs possess strong kappa and weak mu receptor activation. Postoperative use of agonists-antagonists offers limited analgesia without respiratory depression.[8]

Antagonists   Naloxone is a competitive antagonist. Naloxone possesses a high affinity for mu receptors. Respiratory depression caused by opiates can be reversed with naloxone. If naloxone is titrated in incremental doses of 20 to 40 µg to the amount that alleviates respiratory depression, then some of the analgesic effects of opiates may be preserved.[8]

Side effects of naloxone include vomiting and a sympathetic response to sudden pain sensation. Elevated heart rate, elevated blood pressure, and pulmonary edema can accompany this sympathetic response.[4]

Nalmafene hydrochloride (Revex) is a newer opioid antagonist. This drug is available in two strengths: 100 µg/mL and 1 mg/mL. The 100 µg/mL concentration is available for treatment of postoperative opioid-induced respiratory depression. The initial dose is 0.25 µg/kg followed by 0.25-µg/kg

incremental doses at 2 to 5-minute intervals. Dosing is stopped once the desired effect is reached. A cumulative dose exceeding 1.0 µg/kg does not provide additional effects. Careful titration can reverse respiratory depression without diminishing the opioid's analgesic effects. The 1-mg/mL concentration is available to treat suspected opioid overdose. The recommended initial dose is 0.5 mg/70 kg with an additional dose of 1.0 mg/kg in 2 to 5 minutes if needed. Doses above 1.5 mg/70 kg are unlikely to have any additional effect. The half-life for Revex ranges from 30 to 60 minutes to many hours when doses of 1 mg/70 kg or greater are given. Even though Revex is the longest-acting opioid antagonist, a slight risk of renarcotization does exist. If this occurs, further incremental titration of Revex is required.

Nausea, vomiting, tachycardia, and hypertension were the most frequently noted side effects with Revex. As with all opioid antagonists, caution should be used when giving Revex to patients at high cardiovascular risk.[10]

BENZODIAZEPINES

Midazolam, diazepam, and lorazepam are the benzodiazepines used during surgery. Benzodiazepines produce the following positive pharmacologic attributes: amnesia, minimal circulatory or respiratory depression, and increased threshold for seizure activity.

Mechanism of Action   Benzodiazepines act on receptors in the CNS enhancing the inhibitory effects of GABA. GABA enhances chloride channel opening in the CNS, leading to quick hyperpolarization of the neuronal membrane.[2] Subsequently the cell membranes become resistant to other neuronal stimuli causing anxiolytic, hypnotic, anticonvulsant, and muscle relaxant effects.[11]

Anesthesia Concerns and Considerations   Benzodiazepines are highly lipid soluble, causing quick entrance into the CNS. Biotransformation occurs in the liver, converting benzodiazepines to water-soluble products.[2] Because of slow hepatic metabolism, diazepam has a longer elimination half-time than midazolam. Diazepam also has active metabolites that may prolong the drug's action.

Midazolam is water soluble at a low pH, but at body pH, the imidazole ring closes, allowing it to become highly lipid soluble. This accounts for the drug's quick onset. The short duration of action is caused by redistribution of this lipid-soluble drug to inactive tissue depots.[11] Sedative doses of midazolam IV (0.5 to 5 mg) and diazepam (2 to 10 mg) should be titrated slowly to desired effect.[4] Diazepam (0.2 to 0.3 mg/kg) or midazolam (0.1 to 0.2 mg/kg) can be used for anesthesia induction (Table 4-3). Awakening can be delayed with use of benzodiazepines for induction in comparison to barbiturates, a potential disadvantage to their use in induction. Benzodiazepines are extensively protein bound, which also increases the elimination half-time of these drugs.[11] Midazolam causes more amnesia than diazepam. Diazepam causes pain on injection related to its poor water solubility.

Table 4–3
BENZODIAZEPINE DOSING

	Induction Dose	Sedation Dose
midazolam	50–350 µg/kg	0.5–5 mg (IV) titrate slowly
diazepam	0.3–0.5 mg/kg (IV)	0.1–0.2 mg/kg (IV, IM, PO)
lorazepam	—	0.02–0.08 mg/kg (IV, IM)*

*Not for use with children.

Cardiovascular

There are minimal decreases in blood pressure, cardiac output, and systemic vascular resistance with benzodiazepines. A transient increase in heart rate does occur due to baroreceptor response. The increase in heart rate and decrease in blood pressure with an IV induction dose is greater with midazolam than diazepam.[11]

Respiratory

Depression of ventilation can occur with both midazolam and diazepam. Careful titration and vigilant monitoring are necessary with sedation because transient apnea may occur with benzodiazepines. Apnea risk increases when these drugs are given with other respiratory depressants. The ventilatory response to CO_2 is decreased with these drugs.[2]

Cerebral

Benzodiazepines are effective anticonvulsants due to the increased inhibitory performance of GABA in the limbic system.[11] Diazepam 0.05 to 0.2 mg/kg IV can abolish seizure activity.[4] ICP, cerebral blood flow, and $CMRO_2$ are reduced with benzodiazepines.

DROPERIDOL

Mechanism of Action Droperidol is a butyrophenone that acts on postsynaptic receptor sites to block the effects of dopamine. The medullary chemoreceptor trigger zone and the caudate nucleus are affected in the CNS.

Anesthesia Concerns and Considerations Because of droperidol's effect at the chemoreceptor trigger zone, it is used as an antiemetic in a dose of 1.25 mg.[12] Droperidol is also used in neuroleptanalgesia. Innovar is an available solution of droperidol and fentanyl in a 50:1 mix. Droperidol increases fentanyl's duration of action. Neuroleptanalgesia causes immobility (cataleptic state) and a state of intense analgesia.[13] Neuroleptanesthesia is the combination of Innovar with nitrous oxide, producing general anesthesia with a dissociative state. However, it is not widely used because of numerous reports of anxiety and fear associated with this technique.[2]

Cardiovascular

The mild α-blocking effects of droperidol can result in a decrease in blood pressure through vasodilation. The antidysrhythmic effect of droperidol may be related to this mild α blockade.[2]

Respiratory

Droperidol does not depress ventilation. In the patient with hypoxic ventilatory drive, the dopamine-blocking effect of droperidol at the carotid body may stimulate ventilation.[13]

Cerebral

Droperidol can produce extrapyramidal symptoms; therefore, patients with Parkinson's disease should not receive it.[4] Diphenhydramine can be used to treat the extrapyramidal effects. Droperidol is a cerebral vasoconstrictor reducing cerebral blood flow, but it does not affect the $CMRO_2$.[13]

☐ MUSCLE RELAXANTS

NEUROMUSCULAR JUNCTION PHYSIOLOGY

The neuromuscular junction contains a prejunctional motor nerve terminal, a postjunctional receptor on the muscle, and a narrow space between them called the synaptic cleft. Once the nerve impulse travels down to the nerve terminal, calcium moves into the terminal nerve membrane, and vesicles of acetylcholine move to the nerve terminal membrane.[14] At the membrane, Ach is liberated from the vesicles, crosses the synaptic cleft, and binds to the muscle end plate (Fig. 4–1).[15]

The Ach receptors contain five subunits: alpha (2), beta, gamma, and delta. The alpha subunits are identical.[15] The five receptor subunits are arranged in a cylindrical fashion (Fig. 4–2). One Ach binds the two alpha units, the cylinder is open and ions (Na and Ca into the cell and K out of the cell) move freely, generating an action potential to the muscle end plate.[14]

Neuromuscular blocking agents act by competitively binding to one or both alpha subunits, keeping the channel in the cylinder closed. Thus, an action potential will not occur.

Acetylcholine is broken down by acetylcholinesterase (Ach-ase) to acetyl and choline. Ach-ase is located in the muscle membrane near the motor end plate. Once Ach is broken down, the membrane is repolarized, preventing sustained depolarization.[14]

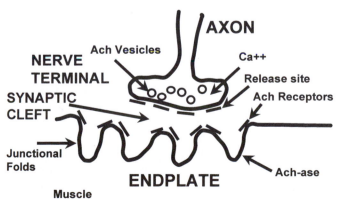

Figure 4–1 Neuromuscular junction.

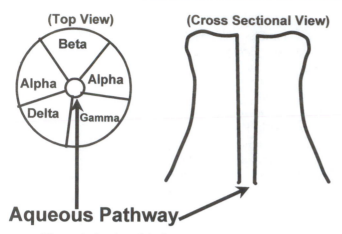

Figure 4-2   Acetylcholine motor endplate receptor.

DEPOLARIZING MUSCLE RELAXANTS

Mechanism of Action   Succinylcholine is a depolarizing muscle relaxant that structurally resembles Ach and binds to the Ach receptors. The usual doses are 0.7 to 1 mg/kg IV and 1 to 2 mg/kg in children. The onset time for succinylcholine is 0.5 to 1 minutes.[4] Succinylcholine generates an action potential, and it is broken down by *plasma cholinesterase*. Because succinylcholine is not broken down by Ach-ase, succinylcholine remains on the receptor longer, preventing the membrane receptor from repolarizing.[16] By preventing repolarization, the receptor's channel remains closed. Because no impulse can be generated by the receptor, the muscles remain relaxed. This is called a phase I block.[14]

A phase II block can occur when receptor exposure to succinylcholine is prolonged. The depolarizing block takes on nondepolarizing qualities: train-of-four (TOF) and tetanic fade. A prolonged paralysis occurs up to 30 to 60 minutes. This phase II block *can* be antagonized with neostigmine or edrophonium.[16] At a given point of time, varying degrees of phase I blockade and phase II blockade can coexist on the synaptic level because the majority of receptors shift from one blockade type to the other.

Plasma cholinesterase, which breaks down succinylcholine, originates in the liver. The rate that succinylcholine is broken down is related to the amount of plasma cholinesterase produced by the liver. A patient with a damaged liver may not generate as much plasma cholinesterase as a healthy adult; thus, the effect of succinylcholine would last longer.[14,15]

Anesthetic Concerns and Considerations   Some patients have an atypical plasma cholinesterase and lack the ability to hydrolyze succinylcholine. Patients are usually unaware of this rare problem until they experience prolonged paralysis after succinylcholine administration.[15]

Dibucaine is a local anesthetic that helps to identify people with this disorder. Eighty percent of normal plasma cholinesterase is inhibited by dibucaine, whereas the atypical enzyme in inhibited only 20%. The result of a dibucaine test is the dibucaine number that reflects the *quality* of the plasma cholinesterase rather than the quantity. A normal dibucaine number is 80, which confirms 80% inhibition of normal plasma cholinesterase. As the dibucaine number decreases, the longer succinylcholine will be effective in producing paralysis[15] (Table 4-4).

Potassium is elevated 0.5 to 1.0 mEq/L in the healthy patient due to normal muscle release following succinylcholine administration. Hyperkalemia leading to cardiac arrest can occur in patients with burns, spinal cord injury, and skeletal muscle injury. Extrajunctional receptors are thought to develop in these patients.[16]

Fasciculation occurs after giving succinylcholine. These unsynchronized contractions of muscle fibers are caused by depolarization. Patient complaints of myalgia may be related to this.

Succinylcholine also can cause increased intragastric and intraocular pressure. The injured eye may be further compromised by the use of succinylcholine.

Pretreatment with a nondepolarizing muscle relaxant may be protective against myalgias.[16] However, this is controversial.

Succinylcholine is a triggering agent for malignant hyperthermia.

Cardiovascular
Succinylcholine can imitate actions of Ach on postganglionic muscarinic receptors resulting in sinus bradycardia. Adults receiving more than one dose of succinylcholine are susceptible, as are children.[16] Atropine can be given prophylactically to children to prevent this problem.

Cerebral
Succinylcholine can transiently increase ICP. Pretreatment with a nondepolarizing muscle relaxant can prevent this phenomenon.

NONDEPOLARIZING MUSCLE RELAXANTS

Mechanism of Action   Nondepolarizing muscle relaxants (NDMRs, Table 4-5) compete with Ach for either one or both alpha subunits on the motor end plate receptor. Depolarization, which creates an open ion channel, will not occur if Ach is not allowed to bind with both alpha subunits.[15]

The NDMRs have difficulty crossing lipid-soluble membranes; therefore they do not affect the CNS.

Table 4-4
DEVIATIONS IN PLASMA CHOLINESTERASE ENZYME

Dibucaine Number	Succinylcholine Block Duration	Occurence
80	Normal	96%
40-60	Lengthened	1/480
20	Greatly lengthened	1/3200

Table 4–5
NONDEPOLARIZING MUSCLE RELAXANTS

Types	Onset (min)	Duration (min)
D-tubocurarine	<2	25–90
metocurine	<3	35–60
gallamine	1–2	25–90
rocuronium	0.75–1.5	15–150 (dose dependent)
vecuronium	<3	25–30
pipecuronium	<3	45–120
pancuronium	1–3	40–65
mivacurium	<2	6–16
atracurium	<3	20–35
doxacurium	<4	30–160

Anesthetic Concerns and Considerations

Cardiovascular

Several NDMRs are capable of releasing *histamine* to varying degrees: tubocurarine > metocurine > atracrium and mivacurium. Histamine released from mast cells can cause bronchospasm, hypotension, and cutaneous flushing.[2]

Pancuronium and gallamine have vagolytic side effects that block vagal muscarinic receptors to the sinoatrial node.[14] Heart rate and blood pressure increase as a result of this vagolysis.

Excretion and Metabolism

Several NDMRs are dependent or semidependent on renal excretion. Pancuronium, tubocurarine, vecuronium, pipecuronium, and doxacurium are all partially dependent on renal excretion; metocurine and gallamine are entirely dependent on renal excretion.[14] Patients with renal disease will have difficulty excreting these drugs and may have prolonged blocks. The drug of choice with renal disease is atracurium or mivacurium because their elimination does not depend on the kidney.[5] Atracurium is removed from the neuromuscular junction by *Hofmann elimination,* while mivacurium is rapidly broken down by *plasma cholinesterase.*

Hepatic metabolism plays a role in the breakdown of the NDMRs. Vecuronium and pancuronium depend on liver metabolism and patients with significant liver disease will have prolonged blockade.

Altered Response

Volatile agents *potentiate* NDMRs. Volatile agents alter postsynaptic membranes, depress the CNS, and decrease tone of skeletal muscle.[15]

Aminoglycoside antibiotics, lidocaine, and magnesium potentiate muscle relaxants by either decreasing Ach release or stabilizing postjunctional membranes.

The effects of an NDMR are impeded by a patient taking *phenytoin.* The dose of NDMR may need to be altered.[16]

Priming Principle

Onset of blockade by an NDMR can be accelerated by blocking the spare receptors that have no clinical effect on the pa-

tient. Adminstration of 10% of the Ed_{95} dose of an NDMR 4 minutes prior to giving two to three times the Ed_{95} dose can accomplish a quicker onset for the nondepolarizing drug.[15] However, it is prudent to warn patients of the impending generalized weakness that may result in eyelid heaviness.

Muscle Relaxant Evaluation

Peripheral nerve stimulators (PNS) are used to evaluate muscle relaxants through generating electrical stimuli. These stimuli (single twitch, TOF, tetanus, and posttetanic stimulation) are observed or evaluated visually, by recording or by touch (Fig. 4–3).

Gradual Ach depletion in the synaptic cleft can be evaluated by TOF or tetanus stimulation. Fade occurs as Ach is gradually depleted during prolonged stimulation. Posttetanic potentiation involves a greater twitch response after tetanus stimulation.[14]

The TOF involves a 2-Hz stimulus delivered four times in less than 10 seconds. Beyond four, further blockade is no longer discretely discernible. The four responses to these stimuli are then interpreted. As neuromuscular blockade progresses, the response to TOF stimulation begins to decrease in amplitude and in the total number of responses.[6] In a nondepolarizing block where only three responses are generated, up to 75% neuromuscular block is achieved. An 80%, 90%, or 100% block correlates with the absence of two, three, and all four responses.[17] Mechanical ventilation is ideal for patients with one to two responses. When only one or two responses exists to TOF stimulation, adequate surgical relaxation is achieved.[6]

Reversal of a nondepolarizing blockade should not occur until there is at least one response to TOF stimulation.[17] To regain performance of the neuromuscular junction, its function depends on the amount of spontaneous recovery prior to reversal, the effect of the anticholinesterase in reversing the block, and spontaneous recovery that occurs at the time reversal is given (possibly from clearance). Reversing the anti-

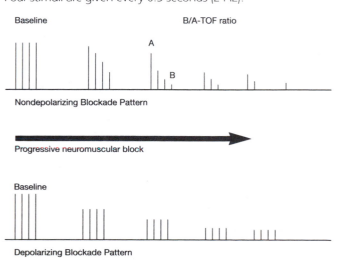

Figure 4–3   TOF response to PNS. Reproduced by permission from Smith and Barton.[6]

Table 4–6
TOF AND TETANIC RESPONSES TO PERIPHERAL NERVE STIMULATION

	Phase 1 TOF	Phase 2 TOF	Phase 1 Tetanus	Phase 2 Tetanus	Phase 1 PTF	Phase 2 PTF
Depolarizing Block					no	yes
	TOF	Tetanus	PTF			
Nondepolarizing Block			yes			

PTF, posttetanic fade; TOF, train-of-four

cholinesterase early does not help the spontaneous recovery factors needed for neuromuscular junction performance, and later reversal titration may be more difficult.[18]

A phase I depolarization block does not demonstrate posttetanic stimulation or fade, and this block may be *augmented* by anticholinesterase therapy.[19]

A phase II block, which occurs with nondepolarizers, can be seen with a depolarization block if enough depolarizing muscle relaxant is given. A phase II involves fade, posttetanic facilitation, and likely reversal with an anticholinesterase agent[19] (Table 4–6).

☐ CHOLINESTERASE INHIBITORS

MECHANISM OF ACTION

The NDMRs compete with Ach for the motor end plate receptor in the neuromuscular junction. Ach-ase is the enzyme responsible for breakdown of Ach. Blockade reversal relies on loss of NDMR from the neuromuscular junction from excretion, metabolism, diffusion, or specific reversal agent used.

Cholinesterase inhibitors are used to reverse NDMR because they bind Ach-ase indirectly allowing Ach to build up in the neuromuscular junction; consequently, neuromuscular transmission is regained.[20] A carbamyl-ester complex is formed at the esteratic site of the Ach-ase enzyme with neostigmine and pyridiostigmine. Edrophonium uses electrostatic attachment to the anionic site and hydrogen bonding at the esteratic site of Ach-ase[21]. Because edrophonium does not form a covalent bond with the acetycholinesterase enzyme, this bond is reversible, making edophonium a more unstable and, therefore, a shorter acting agent.[21]

ANESTHETIC CONCERNS
AND CONSIDERATIONS

Neuromuscular junctions are *nicotinic* receptors. Nicotinic receptors use Ach as their neurotransmitter between pregan-

glionic and postganglionic neurons in the parasympathetic and sympathetic nervous systems. These receptors are also found on skeletal muscle at the neuromuscular junction. *Muscarinic receptors* use Ach and are located between postganlionic neurons of the parasympathetic nervous system and receptors of effector organs. Muscarinic receptors are also located at postganglionic cholinergic neurons of the sympathetic system.[22] Cholinesterase inhibitors not only block Ach-ase at nicotinic receptors, but they also block it at muscarinic receptors. Muscarinic transmission is also reactivated when a cholinesterase inhibitor is given. Because muscarinic receptors affect bronchial smooth muscle, the heart, and salivary glands, undesired side effects of bradycardia and bronchoconstriction can occur.[23] To prevent these effects, an anticholinergic drug (atropine or glycopyrrolate) is given prior to or along with a cholinesterase inhibitor.

The choice of which anticholinergic to use with a cholinesterase inhibitor should be governed by comparable onset and duration of action of the drugs (Table 4–7).

Cholinesterase inhibitors are cleared via hepatic metabolism and renal excretion. Because NDMRs are cleared in the same manner, a patient with renal or liver problems will have an increased duration of action for both the NDMR and the cholinesterase inhibitor; therefore, the chance of paralysis recurring with the NDMR is greatly decreased.

Edrophonium is not recommended for reversal of an intense block because of the large dose required, variable response, and likelihood of an inadequate response.[18]

☐ LOCAL ANESTHETICS

NERVE ACTION POTENTIAL PROPAGATION

Nerves retain a negative resting membrane potential by maintaining extracellular sodium levels and a slight extracellular movement of potassium. Once a nerve impulse reaches the membrane, threshold potential is reached, causing influx

Table 4–7
CHOLINESTERASE INHIBITOR DOSING

	Dose	Duration (min)	Bonding	Max. Dose	Recommended Anticholinergic
neostigmine	0.05 mg/kg	40–60	Carbamyl ester complex at the esteratic site	5 mg	glycopyrrolate
pyridiostigmine	0.25 mg/kg	90	Carbamyl ester complex at the esteratic site	30 mg	glycopyrrolate
edrophonium	0.5–1 mg/kg	5–20	Electrostatic attachment to anionic site and hydrogen bonding at esteratic site (reversible)	40 mg	atropine

of sodium ions into the cell through sodium channels. This influx of sodium generates the beginning of an action potential along the nerve. As sodium fluxes inward, potassium moves out of the membrane. The sodium and potassium ion shift through the membrane propagates the action potential.

To restore the nerve's negative resting membrane potential, sodium channels are inactivated. The sodium–potassium pump returns intracellular and extracellular levels of sodium and potassium to normal. Thus, the negative resting membrane potential is reattained.

Mechanism of Action The local anesthetic molecule consists of a hydrophilic group usually containing a tertiary amine and a lipophilic group that consists of the benzene ring (Fig. 4–4). The intermediate hydrocarbon chain of this molecule possesses either an ester or amide linkage; hence, the division of local anesthetics into either amides or esters. Esters and amides differ on the site of metabolism and propensity to cause an allergic reaction. Amides are metabolized by the liver, whereas esters are broken down by pseudocholinesterase. One by-product of ester hydrolysis is *para-aminobenzoic acid*, which has allergic reaction potential.[23]

Sodium channels are blocked in the inactivated state by local anesthetics. By entering the aqueous pathway of the actual channel, the hydrophilic portion of the local anesthetic molecule binds to receptors rendering the sodium channel inactivated. The lipophilic portion of the molecule also participates in sodium channel blockade, gaining access to the channel through the lipid environment of the nerve membrane.[24]

Diffusion is necessary for a local anesthetic to enter a nerve. Diffusion is closely related to pK_a.[24] *Onset* of a local anesthetic is also dependent on the pK_a of a local anesthetic.[25] The *$pK_a 50$* is the pH at which the ionized and nonionized portions of the drug are in equal amounts. The nonionized portion is lipid soluble, whereas the ionized portion is water soluble. The higher the nonionized portion, the quicker the local anesthetic can penetrate a nerve membrane. Drugs with a pK_a close to body pH have a higher nonionized portion. This ability to penetrate nerve membrane leads to a quicker onset (Table 4–8).

The *potency* of a local anesthetic or its inherent ability to produce an effect is related to the drug's lipid solubility. Potency is measured by minimum concentration. Minimum concentration of a local anesthetic is the minimum amount of that local anesthetic that produces conduction blockade of a nerve impulse.[23]

Potency can be affected by how frequently a nerve is stimulated. Frequency-dependent blockade is the concept that the more frequently a nerve is used, the more times the sodium channel's aqueous pathway is opened. Thus, local anesthetics gain quicker access to the nerve whose sodium channels are open more often. Potency is also affected by the pH of the area where the local anesthetic is introduced, the nerve fiber size, the nerve fiber myelination, and the nerve fiber type.[23]

Duration of action is associated with protein binding. The greater the protein binding, the longer the duration[25] (see Table 4–8). As the unbound supply of local diffuses from the injection site, the proteins at the injection site release their depots. A drug's inherent vasodilatory quality also affects duration. Even though lidocaine structurally resembles mepivicaine, mepivicaine lasts longer than lidocaine because of lidocaine's vasodilatory effects.[26]

Anesthetic Concerns and Considerations

Epinephrine
Epinephrine has several clinical uses when used with local anesthetics including decreasing the potential for toxicity, increasing the duration of the block, and producing an antinocioceptive effect. By causing vasoconstriction in the area where the block is located, epinephrine prolongs local anesthetic block and decreases the potential for toxicity.[26] Anti-

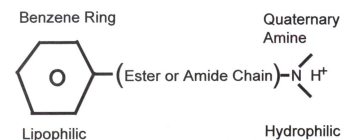

Figure 4–4 Local anesthetic structure. The charged quaternary amine exists in an acidic medium while the tertiary amine exists in an uncharged free-base form.[24]

Table 4-8
LOCAL ANESTHETICS

Name	Type	pK^a	Max. Dose (mg/kg)	Max. Dose with Epinephrine (mg/kg)	Duration/Protein Binding
bupivacaine (Marcaine)	Amide	8.1	3		Long/great
lidocaine (Xylocaine)	Amide	7.9	4.5	7	Moderate/intermediate
mepivacaine (Carbocaine)	Amide	7.6	4.5	7	Moderate/intermediate
prilocaine (Citanest)	Amide	7.8	8		Moderate/intermediate
etidocaine (Duranest)	Amide	7.7	4		Long/great
cocaine	Ester	8.7	3		Moderate/intermediate
procaine (Novacaine)	Ester	8.9	12		Short/minimal
chloroprocaine (Nesacaine)	Ester	9.1	12		Short/minimal
tetracaine (Pontocaine)	Ester	8.6	3		Long/great

nocioceptive receptors may be affected by epinephrine, possibly increasing the intensity of neural blockade.[24]

Epinephrine is also used in obstetric anesthesia as a component of a test dose. If an epidural catheter were accidentally placed in a blood vessel, 15 μg epinephrine would cause an increased heart rate within 25 seconds lasting 30 seconds.[24]

It is thought that the optimal concentration of epinephrine is 5 μg/mL when used with a local anesthetic. In higher concentrations toxicity may occur.

Epinephrine should not be used as a part of a local anesthetic when the patient has angina, dysrhythmias, hypertension, fetal distress, or uteroplacental insufficiency.[24]

Sodium Bicarbonate

To achieve better interneural penetration with a local anesthetic, sodium bicarbonate has been added to increase the nonionized portion of the drug. Onset is hastened with epidural anesthesia using bicarbonate with lidocaine.[24]

Toxicity

Toxicity can occur with local anesthetics caused by either accidental intravascular injection or administration of an excessive dose. CNS toxic effects depend on concentration. High concentrations may result in coma and death; low concentrations may result in circumoral numbness or lightheadedness.[24]

Local anesthetics can decrease myocardial contractility and rate of conduction of electrical impulses in cardiac tissue. Cardiovascular toxicity can occur with local anesthetics, especially Marcaine and etidiocaine. Although most local anesthetics dissociate during diastole, Marcaine and etidiocaine dissociate slowly allowing a buildup to occur. The decrease in heart muscle conduction leads to Marcaine being *70 times* more potent in blocking cardiac conduction than lidocaine.[24]

Treatment for systemic toxicity involves maintaining the airway, facilitating oxygen administration, and using pentathol or diazepam to suppress seizure activity.

Systemic absorption of local anesthetic is a factor in considering potential for toxicity. The rate of absorption depends on a body area's blood flow: intercostal > caudal > epidural > brachial plexus > sciatic/femoral.[27]

Prilocaine

Administration of excessive doses of prilocaine can lead to *methemoglobinemia*. A prilocaine derivative causes this problem when used in regional anesthesia in excess of 500 mg.[24] Methylene blue (1 to 2 mg/kg) is used to treat this problem because it reduces methemoglobin to hemoglobin.

Other Clinical Issues

Cocaine prevents reabsorption of norepinephrine from adrenergic nerve endings; thus, hypertension, tachycardia, and ventricular dysrhythmias can occur from the increased sympathetic outflow.[23]

Lidocaine is useful in the treatment of ventricular dyshythmias because it decreases automaticity especially in ischemic tissue. Reentrant dyshythmias may also be suppressed through lidocaine's ability to augment conduction in areas of the heart with a previous unidirectional block.[28]

Local anesthetics can be used as adjuncts to anesthesia. Prevention of sympathetic stimulation and increased ICP from intubation and relaxation of bronchial smooth muscle highlight some of the other clinical uses for local anesthetics.[23]

☐ ADJUVANTS TO ANESTHETIC PRACTICE

DIURETICS

Diuretics produce an increase in urine output in patients with functioning kidneys. Mannitol and furosemide are the two primary diuretics commonly used in anesthetic practice. Although these drugs both produce an increased urine output, their mechanisms of action are very different.

Mechanism of Action Mannitol is an osmotic diuretic. It is a sugar molecule that the gastrointestinal tract will not absorb, so it must be given IV. Mannitol is completely filtered through the glomeruli in the kidney without being reabsorbed. Therefore, it increases tubular osmolarity, dilutes the sodium concentration, and causes excretion of water, sodium, chloride, and bicarbonate.[29] The dose for mannitol is 0.25 to 1 g/kg with a peak effect in 1 hour and a duration of action of up to 8 hours.[4]

Furosemide inhibits the reabsorption of sodium and chloride in the ascending limb of the loop of Henle. The dose for furosemide is 0.1 to 1 mg/kg with 90% of the drug being protein bound.[29] The elimination half-time is 1 hour.

Ethacrynic acid is another example of a loop diuretic. The IV dose is 0.5 to 1 mg/kg.

Anesthetic Concerns and Considerations Mannitol is used for prophylaxis against acute renal failure, treatment of increased ICP, differential diagnosis of acute oliguria, and reduction of intraocular pressure.[29]

Because of the increase in intravascular volume produced by mannitol, it is *not* recommended for the heart failure patient with oliguria. In addition, rebound cerebral edema can occur if the blood–brain barrier is not intact.

Clinical uses for furosemide include mobilization of edema fluid, treatment for fluid overload, treatment of increased ICP, and differential diagnosis of acute oliguria.[29]

Furosemide can produce *ototoxicity* if given rapidly and in large doses. It can also induce hypokalemia and hypochloremia. Furosemide can potentiate the action of NDMRs.[29]

HISTAMINE BLOCKERS

Histamine is an amine that produces significant effects on the body. It is located within mast cells found in the skin, gastrointestinal tract, and lungs. Receptors for histamine are labeled H_1, and H_2.

Mechanism of Action H_1-receptor stimulation can produce bronchoconstriction, rhinitis, pruritus, and increased capillary permeability with ensuant edema formation. H_1 blockers are used to block these effects.[30]

The H_2-receptor antagonists are mainly used to prevent gastric acid secretion. H_2 blockers prevent histamine from combining with the H_2 receptor producing gastric acid. They are effective in patients with duodenal ulcers, peptic ulcers, and Zollinger-Ellison syndrome.[31]

Anesthetic Concerns and Considerations *Diphenhydramine* is the principal H_1 blocker. It is used to treat allergic reactions, rhinitis, and pruritus. The sedative side effect of many H_1 blockers is used to treat insomnia. The dose for diphenhydramine is 0.2 to 0.5 mg/kg IV with a peak effect in 1 to 3 hours.

Cimetidine and *ranitidine* are the principal H_2 antagonists used in anesthesia. They can be used as preoperative medications to decrease the chance of aspiration pneumonitis. The dose of cimetidine is 300 mg orally, IV, or IM and for raniti-

dine 150 mg orally and 50 mg IM or IV. The peak effect of cimetidine is 45 to 90 minutes and for ranitidine 2 to 3 hours.[4]

Cimetidine reduces hepatic blood flow and inhibits the P-450 oxidase system by binding to microsomal enzymes. Metabolism of drugs (lidocaine, diazepam, etc.) is slowed. Ranitidine does not alter metabolism of other drugs because it weakly binds to P-450 enzymes.[30]

Intravenous cimetidine produces hypotension after rapid infusion related to its vasodilatory effects. Nephritis, hepatotoxicity, and thrombocytopenia can occur with long-term use. Cimetidine can produce gynecomastia through an antiandrogen effect.[30] Cimetidine can cross the blood–brain barrier and side effects such as hallucinations, seizures, and agitation have been observed in the elderly.

METOCLOPRAMIDE

Metoclopramide is a dopamine antagonist that causes upper gastrointestinal tract motility while increasing lower esophageal sphincter tone.

Mechanism of Action Metoclopramide selectively stimulates gastric cholinergic receptors to produce its effects. It does not change gastric acid secretion. Metoclopramide's antiemetic effect results from antagonism of dopamine receptors in the chemoreceptor trigger zone.[3,32]

Anesthetic Concerns and Considerations Metoclopramide can be used as an antiemetic to decrease gastric fluid volume and to treat gastroparesis in diabetes.

The dose for metoclopramide is 10 mg orally, IV, or IM. The IV dose should be given over 1 to 2 minutes. IV onset is 1 to 3 minutes; oral, 30 to 60 minutes; and IM, 10 to 15 minutes. Dose should be adjusted in the patient with renal impairment because metoclopramide depends on renal excretion.[4]

Extrapyramidal side effects have occurred with administration of metoclopramide due to dopamine blocking effects. Metoclopramide is contraindicated in the patient with pheochromocytoma, epilepsy, and gastrointestinal hemorrhage and obstruction.[4] It is also contraindicated in patients receiving other drugs that may cause extrapyramidal reactions (butyrophenones and phenothiazines).[32]

☐ NONSTEROIDAL ANTI-INFLAMMATORY DRUGS

Nonsteroidal anti-inflammatory drugs (NSAIDs) are a group of drugs that principally block cyclooxygenase activity. Through this inhibition, prostaglandin synthesis is reduced. Prostaglandins magnify chemical and mechanical irritation to sensory pathways. Prostaglandins play a greater role in pain stimulus in inflamed and traumatized tissue.[33]

Ketorolac is a cyclooxygenase inhibitor that exhibits analgesic, anti-inflammatory and antipyretic activity.

Ketoralac is useful in the treatment of postoperative pain. The one-time IV dose is 30 mg. If the patient is over 65 years of age, has renal impairment, or weighs less than 50 kg, the IV dose is 15 mg.[34] The duration of action is 3 to 7 hours. The analgesic potency of 30 mg ketorolac IM is equal to 9 mg morphine.[4] An advantage to this drug is that it does not depress cardiovascular or respiratory function.[35] Ketorolac is also used to treat acute and posttraumatic pain.[35]

Inhibition of platelet aggregation resulting in a prolonged bleeding time occurs with ketorolac. It can also cause renal insufficiency by decreasing renal prostaglandin synthesis.

Renal failure may result from ketorolac if it is given to a patient with impaired renal function.[34]

Ketorolac is contraindicated in obstetric anesthesia, patients with active gastrointestinal lesions, patients with advanced renal impairment or renal failure, nursing mothers, patients at high risk for bleeding, and patients with a hypersensitivity to NSAIDs. Ketorolac should not be used preoperatively as it inhibits platelet aggregation. Ketorolac is contraindicated in intrathecal or epidural anesthesia because of its alcohol content.[34]

Ketorolac is metabolized through glucuronic acid conjugation. The elderly should receive a decreased dose because clearance is reduced.

REFERENCES

1. Fragen RJ, Avram MJ. Nonopioid intravenous anesthetics. In Barash PG, Cullen, BF, Stoelting RK, eds. *Clinical Anesthesia.* 2nd ed. Philadelphia: JB Lippincott; 1992: 385-412.
2. Morgan GE, Mikhail MS: *Clinical Anesthesiology.* East Norwalk, Conn: Appleton & Lange; 1992: 116-134.
3. Stoelting RK: *Pharmacology and Physiology in Anesthetic Practice.* Philadelphia: JB Lippincott; 1991: 102-117.
4. Omoigui S. *The Anesthesia Drugs Handbook.* St. Louis: CV Mosby; 1995.
5. Stoelting RK, Dierdorf SF: *Anesthesia and Co-Existing Disease.* 3rd ed. New York: Churchill-Livingstone; 1993: 375-378.
6. Smith JS, Barton CR. *Use of the Peripheral Nerve Stimulator in the Management of Neuromuscular Blockade.* Monograph. West Orange, NJ: Organon.
7. Stoelting RK. *Pharmacology and Physiology in Anesthetic Practice.* Philadelphia: JB Lippincott; 1991: 134-147.
8. Murphy MR: Opioids, In: Barash PG, Cullen BF, Stoelting RK, eds. *Clinical Anesthesia.* 2nd ed. Philadelphia: JB Lippincott; 1992: 413-438.
9. Stoelting RK: *Pharmacology and Physiology in Anesthetic Practice.* Philadelphia: JB Lippincott; 1991: 70-101.
10. *Physician's Desk Reference.* 48th ed. Montvale, NJ: Medical Economics Data; 1996: 1811-1813
11. Stoelting RK: *Pharmacology and Physiology in Anesthetic Practice.* Philadelphia: JB Lippincott; 1991: 118-133.
12. Moyers JR: Preoperative medication, In: Barash PG, Cullen, BF, Stoelting RK, eds: *Clinical Anesthesia.* 2nd ed. Philadelphia: JB Lippincott; 1992: 615-636.
13. Stoelting RK: *Pharmacology and Physiology in Anesthetic Practice.* Philadelphia: JB Lippincott; 1991: 365-383.
14. Morgan GE Mikhail MS: *Clinical Anesthesiology,* East Norwalk, Conn: Appleton & Lange; 1992: 135-148.
15. Stoelting RK: *Pharmacology and Physiology in Anesthetic Practice.* Philadelphia: JB Lippincott; 1991: 172-225.
16. Bevan DR, Donati F. Muscle relaxants. In: Barash PG, Cullen, BF, Stoelting RK, eds. *Clinical Anesthesia.* 2nd ed. Philadelphia: JB Lippincott; 1992: 481-508.
17. Shorten G. Neuromuscular blockade. In: Davison JK, Eckhardt WF, Perese DA, eds. *Clinical Anesthesia Procedures of the Massachusetts General Hospital.* 4th ed. Boston: Little, Brown; 1993: 151-170.
18. Silverman DG, Mirakhur RD. Reversal of nondepolarizing block. In: Silverman DG, ed. *Neuromuscular Block in Perioperative and Intensive Care.* Philadelphia: JB Lippincott; 1994: 217-238.

19. Silverman DG, Donati F: Neuromuscular effects of depolarizing relaxants. In: Silverman DG, ed. *Neuromuscular Block in Perioperative and Intensive Care.* Philadelphia: JB Lippincott; 1994: 239-254.
20. Morgan GE Mikhail MS: *Clinical Anesthesiology,* East Norwalk, Conn: Appleton & Lange; 1992: 149-155.
21. Stoelting RK: *Pharmacology and Physiology in Anesthetic Practice.* Philadelphia: JB Lippincott; 1991: 226-241.
22. Guyton AC. *Textbook of Medical Physiology.* 8th ed. Philadelphia: WB Saunders; 1991: 671.
23. Morgan GE Mikhail MS: *Clinical Anesthesiology,* East Norwalk, Conn: Appleton & Lange; 1992: 174-180.
24. Carpenter RL, Mackey DC: Local anesthetics. In: Barash PG, Cullen, BF, Stoelting RK, eds. *Clinical Anesthesia.* 2nd ed. Philadelphia: JB Lippincott; 1992: 509-541.
25. Sweitzer BJ. Local anesthetics. In: Davison JK, Eckhardt WF, Perese DA, eds. *Clinical Anesthesia Procedures of the Massachusetts General Hospital.* 4th ed. Boston: Little, Brown; 1993: 197-205.
26. Stoelting RK: *Pharmacology and Physiology in Anesthetic Practice.* Philadelphia: JB Lippincott; 1991: 148-171.
27. Tucker GT, Moore DC, Bridenbaugh PO, et al. Systemic absorption of mepivacaine in commonly used regional block procedures. *Anesthesiology.* 1972; 37:277.
28. Larach DR: Cardiovascular drugs. In: Hensley FA, Martin DE, eds. *The Practice of Cardiac Anesthesia.* Boston: Little, Brown; 1990: 114-115.
29. Stoelting RK: *Pharmacology and Physiology in Anesthetic Practice.* Philadelphia: JB Lippincott; 1991: 445-454.
30. Stoelting RK: *Pharmacology and Physiology in Anesthetic Practice.* Philadelphia: JB Lippincott; 1991: 393-406.
31. Morgan GE Mikhail MS: *Clinical Anesthesiology,* East Norwalk, Conn: Appleton & Lange; 1992: 181-188.
32. Stoelting RK: *Pharmacology and Physiology in Anesthetic Practice.* Philadelphia: JB Lippincott; 1991: 455-465.
33. Lebenow TR, McCarthy RJ, Ivankovich AD: Management of acute postoperative pain. In: Barash PG, Cullen BF, Stoelting RK, eds. *Clinical Anesthesia.* 2nd ed. Philadelphia: JB Lippincott. 1992: 1547-1578.
34. *Toradol Package Insert.* Nutley, NJ: Hoffman-LaRoche, 1995.
35. Stoelting RK: *Pharmacology and Physiology in Anesthetic Practice.* Philadelphia: JB Lippincott; 1991: 252-263.

☐ QUESTIONS

1. The pH of thiopental is:
   a. 2
   b. 7
   c. 10.5
   d. 4

2. The mechanism of action of barbiturates is:
   a. The inhibitory transmitter GABA is decreased.
   b. The inhibitory transmitter GABA's rate of dissociation is decreased at its receptors.
   c. Acetylcholine levels are increased.
   d. Stimulation of the reticular activating system

3. Which induction agent has myoclonic activity associated with it?
   a. Etomidate
   b. Thiopental
   c. Propofol
   d. Midazolam

4. Which set of induction agents have pain associated on injection?
   a. Propofol, thiopental
   b. Thiopental, etomidate
   c. Ketamine, thiopental
   d. Propofol, etomidate

5. Which opioid receptor is concerned with supraspinal analgesia?
   a. Mu_2
   b. Kappa
   c. Sigma
   d. Mu_1

6. The two areas in the central nervous system where pain modulation occurs are the:
   a. Medulla and cerebral cortex
   b. Thalamus and periaqueductal gray matter
   c. Substantia gelatinosa and the periaqueductal gray matter
   d. Substantia gelatinosa and the cerebellum

7. Two opiates that cause histamine release are:
   a. Morphine, meperidine
   b. Fentanyl, sufentanil
   c. Sufentanil, morphine
   d. Alfentanil, fentanyl

8. Pentazocine is an example of an:
   a. Induction agent
   b. Opioid
   c. Opioid antagonist
   d. Opioid agonist-antagonist

9. The only benzodiazepine that is water soluble is:
   a. Diazepam
   b. Midazolam
   c. Lorazepam

10. The ratio of droperidol to fentanyl in Innovar is:
    a. 1:1
    b. 25:1
    c. 100:1
    d. 50:1

11. A patient with a dibucaine number of 80 would be expected to have
    a. Normal length of block from succinycholine
    b. Slightly prolonged length of block from succinylcholine
    c. Greatly prolonged length of block from succinylcholine

12. One of the side effects of multiple doses of succinylcholine in the adult is:
    a. Sinus tachycardia
    b. Atrial fibrillation
    c. Premature atrial complexes
    d. Sinus bradycardia

13. The muscle relaxant that possesses a vagolytic effect is:
    a. Vecuronium
    b. Atracrium
    c. Pancuronium
    d. Succinylcholine

14. True statements include:
    a. A phase I blockade may be antagonized by an anticholinesterase drug.
    b. A phase II blockade will be enhanced by the administration of an anticholinesterase drug.
    c. A phase I and phase II neuromuscular blockade may coexist in varying degrees at a given time.
    d. All of the above are true.

15. Which local anesthetic is an ester?
    a. Tetracaine
    b. Bupivicaine
    c. Xylocaine
    d. Carbocaine

16. The pK_a of Marcaine is
    a. 7.1
    b. 6.1
    c. 9.1
    d. 8.1

17. Why is epinephrine sometimes used with local anesthetics?
    a. Decrease potential for toxicity
    b. Increase duration of block
    c. Antinocioceptive effect
    d. All of the above

18. The correct dose for mannitol is
    a. 0.25–1 mg/kg
    b. 0.1–0.2 mg/kg
    c. 0.25–1 gm/kg
    d. 0.1–0.2 gm/kg

19. Metoclopromide:
    a. Increases gastric emptying time
    b. Decreases gastric emptying time
    c. Antagonizes dopamine receptors in the chemoreceptor trigger zone
    d. Both a and c
    e. Both b and c

20. Contraindications to ketorolac include all of the following *except:*
    a. Obstetric anesthesia
    b. NSAID hypersensitivity
    c. Impaired renal function
    d. Treatment of postoperative pain

☐ ANSWERS

1. c	5. d	9. b	13. c	17. d
2. b	6. c	10. d	14. c	18. c
3. a	7. a	11. a	15. a	19. e
4. d	8. d	12. d	16. d	20. d

Inhalation Anesthetics

John Nagelhout

☐ CHEMISTRY

There are currently six inhalation anesthetic agents available in the United States. Their chemical structures are given in Fig. 5–1.

Despite their heterogeneous chemical structures, these agents are able to produce predictable levels of anesthesia with similar clinical results. The behavior of an individual agent is a reflection of its chemical structure. Some important physical-chemical properties of the anesthetics are listed in Table 5–1.

☐ PHARMACOKINETICS

UPTAKE, DISTRIBUTION, AND ELIMINATION

Numerous factors can influence anesthetic uptake. The efficacy of a particular agent is a reflection of the integration of these factors into a clinically useful compound which can produce a safe, pleasant anesthetic experience. Some of these are discussed below.

Blood/Gas Partition Coefficient   This numerical coefficient reflects the solubility of an anesthetic in the blood. The speed of an anesthetic is determined by its solubility in the blood and tissues and is expressed in the blood/gas solubility coefficient. The lower the blood/gas coefficient the faster an anesthetic works. A common method for expressing this relationship graphically is to plot the fraction of drug in the alveoli (FI) as related to the fraction of the drug inspired (FA) over time in minutes (Fig. 5–2). Simply put, the FA represents the concentration of the anesthetic achieved in the lungs in relation to the amount being administered from the vaporizer. Since the lung concentration is easily measured and is directly related to the amount in the brain, it is more convenient to relate the speed of onset of anesthesia to the alveolar concentration. For example, if you dial in 2% anesthetic gas on the vaporizer, the faster 2% anesthetic is achieved in the lungs (thus brain), the faster the patient achieves anesthetic minimum alveolar concentration (MAC). Thus the rate of rise of the alveolar concentration (FA) in relation to the amount you are giving (FI) over time is a main determinant of how fast the patient will "go to sleep." The lower the blood/gas coefficient, the faster the rate of rise of the anesthetic (FA) in the lungs. Desflurane and nitrous oxide, with their low blood/gas coefficients, exhibit the fastest rate of rise, whereas halothane exhibits the slowest. The same principles apply during emergence. The least blood-soluble agents leave the body more quickly than the more soluble drugs. A common clinical expression that amplifies this principle is "fast in, fast out — slow in, slow out."

The *MAC* is defined as the minimum alveolar concentration required to produce anesthesia in 50% of the population upon surgical stimulation.

The Oil/Gas Partition Coefficient   This is an indicator of *potency*. The higher the oil/gas coefficient, the more potent the drug and thus the lower the MAC.

Ventilation   As expected, increases in ventilatory rate and/or volume will increase uptake during induction and during elimination upon emergence.

Body Temperature   The lower the body temperature, the faster the patient tends to reach an anesthetic state. This is probably due to a lower dose requirement as a patient's temperature decreases.

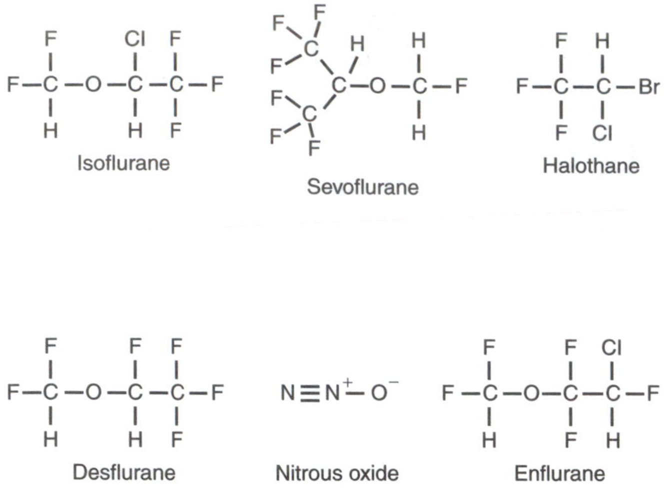

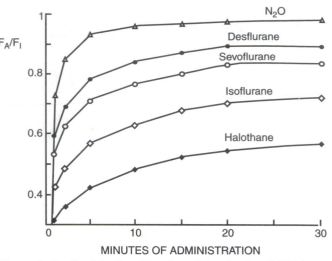

Figure 5–1 Chemical structures of the six inhalational agents currently available in the United States.

Figure 5–2 Graphic plot of fraction of drug in alveoli (FA) in relation to fraction of drug inspired (FI) over time.

Cardiac Output   Anesthetics initially diffuse into tissue with the highest perfusion. The body may be divided into various parts according to total mass and perfusion. The vessel-rich parts include the brain, heart, liver, kidney, and endocrine organs. Muscle groups are intermediate; adipose tissue receives less; and vessel-poor parts receive essentially none (Table 5–2).

Increases in cardiac output *slow* induction time by delaying the rise of the lung concentration as the drug becomes soluble in blood. This effect is most prominent with the agents that are more highly blood-soluble, such as halothane, and it diminishes as the case proceeds.

Second-gas Effect   When a second-gas—i.e., halothane, enflurane or isoflurane is given with the insoluble nitrous oxide, the alveolar concentration of the second gas will increase faster than if it were given in oxygen. This is due to the increase in alveolar ventilation produced by the rapid influx of nitrous oxide, as shown in Fig. 5–2. A high concentration of an insoluble agent is necessary to produce this action.

Concentration Effect   The higher the delivered concentration of anesthetic, the faster the concentration rises in the alveoli and brain.

Inflow Rates   The higher the total flow in liters (carrier and diluent gas) dialed on the machine, the faster the machine wash-in and alveolar uptake.

Ventilation Perfusion Deficit   Abnormalities in $\dot{V}/\dot{Q}$ slow the uptake of all anesthetics. The more soluble the anesthetic, the better you can compensate by increasing ventilation. With insoluble drugs (i.e., nitrous oxide) you have to increase concentration to compensate.

Diffusion Hypoxia   At the end of an anesthetic with high concentrations of the insoluble nitrous oxide, you may get a dilution of alveolar gases (O_2 and CO_2) as nitrous rapidly diffuses from the tissue through the lungs and out of the body. Compensate by giving 100% oxygen for approximately 5 minutes upon emergence.

Table 5–1
SELECT PHYSICAL CHARACTERISTICS AND PARTITION COEFFICIENTS OF INHALATION ANESTHETICS

Property	N_2O	Isoflurane	Enflurane	Halothane	Desflurane	Sevoflurane
Molecular weight	44	184.5	184.5	197.4	168	218
Boiling point, °C	-88.5	48.5	56.5	50.2	23.5	58.5
Specific gravity, 25°C	1.53[a]	1.5	1.52	1.86	1.45	1.5
Vapor pressure, 20°C, mmHg	38,770 (gas)	238	172	243	664	160
MAC in O_2, percent	105	1.28	1.58	0.75	4.6–6	1.71
Partition coefficients, 37°C						
Blood-gas	0.47	1.4	1.8	2.3	0.42	0.59
Oil-gas	1.4	99	98	224	18.7	50
Rubber-gas	1.2	62	74	120	20	30
Induction concentrations, percent	–	1.5–3	3.5–4.5	2–3	2.5 MAC (1–2 min)	1.8 MAC (1–1.6 min)
Maintenance concentrations, percent	–	1.0–2.5	1.5–3	.4–1.5	titrate to effect	titrate to effect

[a]Specific gravity for N_2O is for the gas relative to air, but for other anesthetics it is for the liquid relative to water.
MAC = minimum alveolar concentration.

Table 5–2
TISSUE GROUP CHARACTERISTICS

	Group			
	Vessel-Rich	Muscle	Fat	Vessel-Poor
Percentage of body mass	10	50	20	20
Perfusion as percentage of cardiac output	75	19	6	0

Table 5–4
FACTORS ASSOCIATED WITH HALOTHANE HEPATOTOXICITY

Repeat administration
Enzyme induction
Decreased liver blood flow
Upper abdominal surgery
Age (adult > children)
Female
Obesity
Eczema, allergy history
Immune susceptibility
Liver disease

METABOLISM

The metabolism of the anesthetics has been well documented and is fairly complex. Some important issues should be noted. The anesthetics are primarily metabolized by hepatic microsomal, mixed-function oxidase enzymes commonly referred to as $CYPA_{3A}$. The greater the metabolism, the higher the likelihood of toxicity. The extent of metabolism is listed in Table 5–3.

Halothane has long been associated with a rare but serious hepatotoxicity. Factors associated with this toxicity are listed in Table 5–4.

The metabolism of sevoflurane into fluoride ion may lead to renal toxicity, as discussed above. Nitrous oxide is metabolized in the gastrointestinal flora in trace amounts. No significant toxicity has been noted. Isoflurane and desflurane metabolism is minimal and metabolism related toxicity has not occurred.

Precautions and contraindications are summarized in Table 5–5.

☐ PHARMACODYNAMICS

ANESTHETIC MECHANISMS

The mechanism of action of the inhalation anesthetics remains unclear. Many chemicals including the inhalation anesthetics can produce loss of consciousness or anesthesia. The diversity of these compounds suggests that a single specific "anesthetic" receptor is unlikely. This does not rule out the possibility of a common mechanism for this heterogeneous group of drugs. In fact, a "unitary theory" has been proposed suggesting that these drugs act similarly.

One of the first properties of an anesthetic that could be correlated with a clinical effect was the lipid solubility of the individual drug. The Meyer-Overton rule of anesthetics states that anesthetic potency is directly related to lipid solubility. The more lipid-soluble a drug, the greater its anesthetic potency. It is likely that this is a pharmacokinetic phenomenon that allows for easier distribution into the central nervous system but does not address the actual mechanism of the anesthetics at the cellular level. The critical volume theory is an outgrowth of this concept in that once an anesthetic reaches a critical volume or concentration in the nerve cell, unconsciousness ensues. Many theories focusing on potential changes in membrane lipids have been postulated. The most widely discussed is the "lateral phase transition theory." It is proposed that the anesthetics induce changes in the conformation of the lipid layer of the cells, referred to as *disordering*, which changes the function of ion channels imbedded in these lipid layers and results in depression of activity. Recent evidence that changes in temperature or pressure produce a similar disordering effect without leading to anesthesia cast doubt in this theory as the sole explanation for the action of anesthetics. The exact mechanism of action of the anesthetics remains undefined. They produce complex changes in both the lipids and proteins of a cell, which disrupt neuronal transmission.

Table 5–3
PERCENT METABOLISM OF ANESTHETICS

Halothane	12–25%
Enflurane	2–5%
Sevoflurane	5%
Isoflurane	Trace
Desflurane	Trace
Nitrous oxide	Trace

Table 5–5
SPECIFIC ANESTHETIC PRECAUTIONS AND CONTRAINDICATIONS

Drug	Precaution/Contraindication
Enflurane	Seizure disorders
Isoflurane	Tachycardia respiratory initiation
Desflurane	Same as isoflurane
Sevoflurane	High fluoride levels, compound A, renal disease
Nitrous oxide	Pregnancy, expands closed spaces, bone marrow suppression

EFFECTS ON ORGAN SYSTEMS

All anesthetics, to varying degrees, depress the tissues in which they are distributed. Due to their high lipid solubility, the drugs are distributed, over time, throughout the body. It is helpful, in conceptualizing the general action of an anesthetic on an organ system, to place the effect of any individual agent in this context. Differences in the dynamics of the six agents are usually in degree of effect, although actions unique to a single agent do exist.

Central Nervous System   All anesthetics produce a dose-dependent depression of central nervous system (CNS) activity. The anesthetic state is produced by controlled, reversible, and measurable depression of CNS function. All anesthetics reduce cerebral oxygen consumption ($CMRo_2$), which is clinically beneficial in counteracting surgical stress. Anesthetics relax cerebral vessels, resulting in dilation, which increases cerebral blood volume. This becomes an issue in patients vulnerable to increases in intracranial pressure. Clinically, all anesthetics (nitrous oxide is controversial) raise intracranial pressure yet are still administered if carbon dioxide is lowered by hyperventilation. The low CO_2 will produce cerebral vasoconstriction and counteract the anesthetic effect. Enflurane is contraindicated in intracranial surgery due to the possibility of seizure-like activity. This effect is most likely with hyperventilation and deep levels of anesthesia ($> 2.5\%$). Both of these preconditions are common during cranial surgery. Given the number of choices available, avoiding enflurane in patients with a history of seizure is advised.

The effects of the inhalation anesthetics on the electroencephalogram (EEG) are dependent on depth and are at times similar to those changes produced by ischemia, epilepsy, cardiopulmonary bypass, hypotension, hypothermia, hyper- or hypocarbia, or other metabolic disturbances. Electroencephalographic monitoring may yield useful information as to the balance of cerebral oxygen supply and demand during procedures such as cartotid endarterectomy, where cerebral blood flow may be compromised, or during deliberate hypotension.

Although much variation is possible, depending on the doses and combinations of drugs used, a basic anesthesia-related EEG pattern has been noted. As the patient goes to sleep, the brain waves become larger in amplitude and slower in frequency. The alpha-EEG frequencies are seen in the frontal rather than the occipital leads. As noted below, at deep levels, total suppression of the EEG may occur.

Nitrous oxide, due to its low potency, produces little significant change in EEG patterns. Some amplitude decrease and alpha-wave dominance may occur. The more potent gases, when given in low doses, result in an active EEG with alpha and beta frequencies present. Isolated spike waves may occur as anesthetic depth increases. At 2 to 3 MAC, burst suppression is seen and virtually all intersuppression activity consists of large spike and wave discharges. Once a steady state of anesthesia is reached and maintained, the EEG pattern also stabilizes. As the anesthetic is deepened this fast activity changes, alpha and beta waves are abolished, and slower frequencies predominate. At very deep levels, the EEG amplitude decreases and eventually becomes flat or isoelectric. Enflurane may produce prominent epileptiform activity and, given the number of anesthetic choices available, should not be used when EEG monitoring is planned. Awakening usually results in the reappearance of higher-frequency beta patterns. Clinical monitoring of EEG is best when it is continuous, since you are looking for significant changes that may occur with surgical and anesthetic manipulations during the procedure and not an absolutely predictable and well-defined pattern from patient to patient.

Cardiovascular Effects   Anesthetics produce a dose-dependent depression of cardiac activity. Their effects on the components of cardiovascular function are outlined below.

Blood Pressure

The anesthetics decrease blood pressure in four major ways. They produce direct CNS, baroreceptor, and cardiac depression. Enflurane, isoflurane, sevoflurane, and desflurane also lower overall vascular resistance. Halothane and nitrous oxide do not. The effect of nitrous oxide is usually minimal.

Heart Rate

At or near equilibrium, the anesthetics tend to slow heart rate, although increases during the excitement stage are common. Isoflurane and desflurane can produce significant tachycardia in some patients as depth increases. Intravenous narcotics or beta blockers can control this effect in patients where transient tachycardia may be a problem. Again, the effect of nitrous oxide is minimal.

Other Cardiovascular Effects

Halothane sensitizes the myocardium to sympathomimetics. Injected epinephrine should be limited to no more than 0.1 mg in any 10-min period or 0.3 mg/h. If dysrhythmias occur, switching to another anesthetic and standard antidysrhythmic therapy may be necessary.

Right-to-Left Intracardiac Shunt

In the presence of a right-to-left intracardiac shunt, the rate of an inhalational anesthetic induction will theoretically be slowed because of a dilutional effect of shunted blood. This impact is greatest for N_2O because uptake of poorly soluble volatile anesthetics into pulmonary venous blood is minimal. Thus, the dilutional effect of the shunt on pulmonary venous anesthetic partial pressure is essentially unopposed. Yet the uptake of highly soluble volatile anesthetics is sufficient to partially offset the dilutional effect; therefore, a right-to-left intracardiac shunt will not have such a significant impact during induction with halothane.

Respiratory Effects   Anesthetics abolish respiratory drive as levels are deepened due to direct depression of the respiratory center. Tidal volume decreases faster than respiratory rate.

All anesthetics except nitrous oxide cause bronchodilation.

Halothane appears to be especially beneficial in asthmatics. Remember, however, that injecting bronchodilating sympathomimetics during halothane anesthesia may lead to dysrhythmias.

Isoflurane and desflurane are respiratory irritants; therefore deepening patients with intravenous agents prior to the administration of these drugs is advised.

The effects of the anesthetic gases on intrapulmonary shunting or the hypoxic pulmonary vasoconstriction (HPV) response are complex and may be influenced by lung disease, cardiac output, pH, pulmonary pressures, and other factors. Simply stated, the body consistently attempts to adjust and match circulatory and respiratory function in response to any number of environmental influences, so that efficient pulmonary oxygen and carbon dioxide exchange is possible. Hypoxia, for example, produces a redistribution of blood flow in the lungs from poorly ventilated to better ventilated areas in an attempt to maintain proper oxygenation. It is known that anesthetics, not surprisingly, depress pulmonary function and increase shunting. Changes in lung mechanics, pulmonary circulation, and pressures have been implicated. Clinically we compensate for these changes by administering a higher oxygen concentration of at least 30%. The effect of the anesthetics on HPV is not completely clear, but some general observations are possible. Nitrous oxide has little or no effect on this autoregulatory mechanism. The potent anesthetics agents depress the normal HPV response. With the possible exception of halothane, this effect appears to occur in a dose-related fashion. That is, the deeper the patient's anesthesia, the greater the depression. The clinical consequence is that certain patients, such as those with significant pulmonary disease and one-lung ventilation, require especially close monitoring for oxygen and carbon dioxide changes under anesthesia.

With anesthetic administration in the presence of an existing intrapulmonary shunt, blood emerging from unventilated alveoli will not contain anesthetic gases. This blood mixes with blood from adequately ventilated alveoli, producing a diluted arterial anesthetic partial pressure. As the uptake of volatile agent from the alveoli into pulmonary venous blood will be less than normal, transpulmonary shunt accelerates the rate of increase in F_A/F_I. With poorly soluble volatile anesthetics, such as N_2O, this shunt accelerates the increase in FA/FI only slightly. However, with highly soluble volatile agents such as halothane, the rate of increase in FA/FI is more significant.

Gastrointestinal and Renal Effects Anesthetics tend to depress and slow gastrointestinal function. Gastric emptying is delayed and hepatic blood flow altered. Function returns to normal soon after emergence and the clinical significance is minimal.

As the blood pressure decreases, renal blood flow is decreased by all agents except nitrous oxide. This leads to a decrease in glomerular filtration (GFR) and ultimately a decrease in urine output. Concentrating ability is unchanged. Clinical significance is minimal.

Sevoflurane may produce significantly elevated free fluoride ion levels, which have traditionally been associated with nephrotoxicity. Avoidance of sevoflurane in patients with renal disease is advised.

☐ ANESTHETIC-SPECIFIC EFFECTS

NITROUS OXIDE

The primary side effects with nitrous oxide administration are well known and easily avoided. Nitrous oxide expands closed gas spaces due to the difference in solubility with the nitrogen it replaces and the high concentrations required. Deleterious effects may occur in the following situations: pneumothorax, bowel obstruction, inner ear surgery, neurosurgical procedures with air injection, air embolism, gas injection in ocular surgery, and laparoscopy (rare). Expansion of endotracheal tube cuff volume and pulmonary artery catheter balloon have been reported. Controversy over the clinical significance of the depression of "bone marrow function" by nitrous oxide remains. Nitrous oxide depresses methionine synthetase, resulting in a decrease in vitamin B_{12} activity. It is associated with prolonged administration (6 to 12 h) in elderly or debilitated patients. Usual NPO restrictions produce similar effects. Standard use during routine surgery remains safe.

HALOTHANE

As noted earlier, halothane can sensitize the heart to catecholamines and related drugs. All types of dysrhythmias have been reported. Proper clinical patient selection can minimize their occurrence. Treatment is discontinuation of halothane and administration of appropriate antiarrhythmic drugs.

ENFLURANE

Seizure-like tonic-clonic movements occur under enflurane anesthesia when high MAC ($> 2.5\%$) and hypocarbia (hyperventilation) are instituted. The use of enflurane has declined with the introduction of newer anesthetics.

ISOFLURANE AND DESFLURANE

The clinical effects of these two drugs are similar. Respiratory irritation may occur with rapid initial administration. During induction, this may lead to tachycardia, which is especially common in younger, healthier patients. Narcotics, beta blockers, and close management of initial depth can control this effect in patients with heart disease, where tachycardia is a problem.

SEVOFLURANE

The breakdown of sevoflurane poses two major clinical problems. First, the drug breaks down in the carbon dioxide absorber of the anesthesia machine. Breakdown by-products have been termed compound A and compound B, among others. Compound A produces significant effects, including neurologic and pulmonary toxicity. Compound A production is greater in Baralyme than in soda lime. It also increases with duration of administration, heat, and low flows. The metabolism of sevoflurane (5%) produces significant increases in fluoride ion in the body. Due to past experience with methoxyflurane, renal toxicity is expected when free fluoride ion levels of 40 to 120 mmol/L are exceeded. Despite levels in this range, nephrotoxicity in healthy patients has NOT been reported. Deleterious changes in renal function in patients with renal disease have occurred. Levels would be expected to increase with duration of administration and increased metabolism by hepatic enzyme induction.

OBSTETRICS

All anesthetics except nitrous oxide are used during pregnancy. The anesthetics depress and thus relax the uterus. Administration of anesthesia during pregnancy is associated with an increased risk of postoperative miscarriage; however, no single agent has been implicated. This same risk has been linked to other anesthetic techniques. Low concentrations have minimal effects and are used with intravenous supplements to produce anesthesia in pregnant patients undergoing nonobstetric procedures. Uterine relaxation may also in-crease blood loss during intrauterine procedures. Nitrous oxide is teratogenic in animals and is contraindicated during pregnancy.

PEDIATRICS

The effect of the anesthetics in children are similar to those in adults. A few differences exist. The MAC of the anesthetics is higher in children and decreases with age. Despite their higher dose requirements, children achieve anesthetic concentrations faster due to higher respiratory efforts. Other differences exist in (1) blood/gas solubility of the anesthetics, (2) cardiac output distribution, and (3) body composition ratios. Children are also less vulnerable to the hepatoxic side effects of halothane, although the reason remains unclear.

SUMMARY

Anesthetic practitioners are among the few medical groups who administer drugs via the inhalation route. The pharmacokinetics of the anesthetic gases remain an important component of anesthesia practice. The six anesthetic gases have many similarities, but important differences exist. Proper selection of an anesthetic gas requires a thorough understanding of the pharmacokinetics and pharmacodynamics of these essential drugs.

BIBLIOGRAPHY

Nagelhout JJ. Uptake of distribution of the inhalation anesthetics. In: Nagelhout JJ, Zaglaniczny KL eds. *Nurse Anesthesia*. Philadelphia: Saunders; 1996, chap 17.

Kossick M. Inhalation anesthetics. In: Nagelhout JJ, Zaglaniczny KL eds. *Nurse Anesthesia*. Philadelphia: Saunders; 1996, chap 18.

Stevens WC, Kingston HG. Inhalation anesthesia. In: Barash PG, Cullen BF, Stoelting RK eds. *Clinical Anesthesia*. 2nd ed. Philadelphia: Lippincott; 1992.

Baden JM, Rice SA. Metabolism and toxicity. In: Miller RD, ed. *Anesthesia*. 4th ed. New York: Churchill-Livingstone; 1994, chap 8.

Stoelting RK. Inhaled anesthetics, In: *Pharmacology and Physiology in Anesthetic Practice*. 2nd ed. Philadelphia: Lippincott; 1991, chap 2.

QUESTIONS

1. Which anesthetic sensitizes the heart to the effect of catecholamines?
   a. enflurane
   b. halothane
   c. isoflurane
   d. sevoflurane

2. Which of the following parameters reflects the speed of an anesthetic?
   a. MAC
   b. vapor pressure
   c. blood/gas solubility coefficient
   d. oil/gas solubility coefficient

3. Which of the following drugs exhibits the fastest onset and emergence?
   a. sevoflurane
   b. isoflurane
   c. halothane
   d. desflurane

4. Which of the following drugs is contraindicated during pregnancy?

    a. nitrous oxide
    b. halothane
    c. sevoflurane
    d. enflurane

5. Which of the following enzymes is suppressed by prolonged nitrous oxide administration?
    a. cytochrome oxidase
    b. acetylcholinesterase
    c. methionine synthetase
    d. ALA synthetase

6. Which of the following agents undergoes the most metabolism?
    a. sevoflurane
    b. enflurane
    c. desflurane
    d. halothane

7. The increase in intracranial pressure produced by anesthetics is due to which of the following?
    a. decreased blood pressure
    b. release of CNS dopamine
    c. increase in cerebral volume
    d. increase in cerebral glucose utilization

8. Which of the following has the highest vapor pressure?
    a. halothane
    b. isoflurane
    c. sevoflurane
    d. desflurane

9. The MAC (dose) of an anesthetic is inversely related to which of the following?
    a. blood/gas solubility
    b. oil/gas solubility
    c. toxicity
    d. water/gas solubility

10. Which of these anesthetics is associated with seizure-like activity?
    a. enflurane
    b. halothane
    c. nitrous oxide
    d. sevoflurane

11. Increases in cardiac output during induction will _____ the onset of inhalation anesthetics?
    a. speed
    b. slow
    c. not affect
    d. affect only children in

12. The Meyer-Overton theory of anesthesia relates the anesthetic mechanism of action with
    a. lipid solubility.
    b. water solubility.
    c. neurotransmitter depression.
    d. membrane changes.

13. The toxic by-product of sevoflurane breakdown in carbon dioxide canisters is
    a. phosgene.
    b. carbon monoxide.
    c. compound A.
    d. compound B.

14. Sevoflurane is contraindicated in patients with
    a. hepatic disease.
    b. sickle cell disease.
    c. renal disease.
    d. COPD.

15. Which of the following is the most potent?
    a. desflurane
    b. isoflurane
    c. sevoflurane
    d. halothane

16. Which of the following is contraindicated in a patient with a pneumothorax?
    a. halothane
    b. nitrous oxide
    c. sevoflurane
    d. enflurane

17. Which of the following is associated with occasional significant tachycardia?
    a. desflurane
    b. halothane
    c. enflurane
    d. sevoflurane

18. Which of the following is not a mechanism for the decrease in blood pressure seen with anesthetics?
    a. CNS depression
    b. increase baroreceptor sensitivity
    c. cardiac depression
    d. vasodilation

19. Hepatotoxicity is an idiosyncratic reaction to
    a. sevoflurane.
    b. nitrous oxide.
    c. halothane.
    d. desflurane.

20. Which of the following is a respiratory irritant?
    a. isoflurane
    b. sevoflurane
    c. enflurane
    d. nitrous oxide

☐ ANSWERS

1.	b	**5.**	c	**9.**	b	**13.**	c	**17.**	a
2.	c	**6.**	d	**10.**	a	**14.**	c	**18.**	b
3.	d	**7.**	c	**11.**	b	**15.**	d	**19.**	c
4.	a	**8.**	d	**12.**	a	**16.**	b	**20.**	a

THREE

Anesthesia Equipment
and Monitoring

6

Intraoperative Patient Monitoring

Dorothy Duffy-Gross

☐ GOALS AND STANDARDS

The basic goal of intraoperative monitoring is patient safety. In 1974, the American Association of Nurse Anesthetists (AANA) developed Standards of Practice to facilitate patient safety.[1] The anesthetist has an obligation to the patient to practice such standards to provide safe consistent anesthesia care. The AANA Monitoring Standards apply to patients undergoing general, regional, or monitored anesthesia care for diagnostic or therapeutic procedures. Extensive monitoring may not be required in all cases, for example, epidural analgesia during labor and delivery or pain management therapy. Clinical judgment should be used by the anesthetist to differentiate such situations.

In fact, in the past, morbidity and mortality were as high as 1/10,000. It is important to keep in mind that not all mishaps are preventable. Nor are they caused by human error or equipment failure. Theoretically mishaps will be reduced with use of the Standards of Practice.

☐ ELECTROCARDIOGRAM MONITORING

An essential component of perioperative anesthesia care is electrocardiogram (ECG) monitoring. This standard monitor is required for the detection of dysrhythmias, conduction abnormalities, myocardial ischemia, pacemaker function, and electrolyte imbalances. Electrode pads with conductive gel connect the patient to the ECG machine. The conductive gel permits good electrical contact and lowers the skin's electrical resistance. Cleansing the site with alcohol before electrode placement can also help lower this resistance. The ECG pads should be applied to dry skin. This can especially be challenging when the operative field is in close proximity to lead placement. The electrical voltage signal measured from the ECG is small (approximately 1 mV), which causes electrical equipment with higher electrical voltage to induce electrical interference. Electrocautery is one example of such equipment. Different views of the electrical cardiac impulse, generated from myocardial cells, are recorded depending on the potential differences between two leads. Einthoven's triangle demonstrates the direction of potential electrical differences for the standard limb leads. The most commonly used intraoperative monitors are the three- or five-lead systems. Using the three-lead system (white, right arm; black, left arm; and red, left leg), lead I displays potential differences between the right arm to the left arm, lead II displays the potential differences between the right arm to the left leg, and lead III displays the potential differences between the left arm to the left leg (Fig. 6–1). Precordial leads can also be monitored with the three-lead system. Choice of lead monitoring should be individualized according to the patient's history. For example, in a patient with a history of *lateral wall ischemia*, V_5 lead monitoring would be preferred. If only a three-lead electrolyte system is available, a modified V_5 lead (Fig. 6–2) can be obtained by placing the right arm lead under the right clavicle, the left arm lead in the V_5 position, and the left leg lead as usual, while the monitor is in lead I setting. A five-lead system consists of a three-lead system with the addition of a right leg lead (green) and a precordial lead (brown). Simultaneous monitoring of leads II and V_5 is commonly used and can be accomplished with a five-lead system. One advantage of lead II monitoring is its increased sensitivity to inferior wall ischemia. Also, P waves are easily recognized in lead II and therefore can facilitate prompt diagnosis of *dysrhythmias*. On the other hand, lead V_5 views the anterior and lateral portions of the left ventricle. It is also

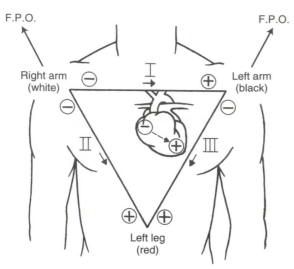

Figure 6-1 Einthoven's triangle. An electrical potential goes from a negative lead to a positive lead. Note lead I is a right arm lead to left arm lead, lead II is a right arm lead to left leg lead, lead III is a left arm lead to left leg lead.

commonly used for its detection of *myocardial ischemia.* The concurrent use of lead II and V_5 will increase the sensitivity for the detection of perioperative ischemia by 80% to 90%.[2] Tables 6-1 and 6-2 present further information on ECG leads.

A conscientious anesthetist should obtain a preinduction rhythm strip. This strip will act as a foundation for the detection of perioperative dysrhythmias and ischemic changes. Dysrhythmias can occur for various reasons. Tachycardia and bradycardia are the most common rhythm disturbances. Sympathetic stimulation during intubation, "light anesthesia," ketamine, Pavulon, gallamine, and hypovolemia are some causes of tachycardia. Bradycardia also has multiple causes—for example, vagal stimulation caused by carotid sinus stimulation, oculocardiac reflex, and traction on the mesenteric bed.

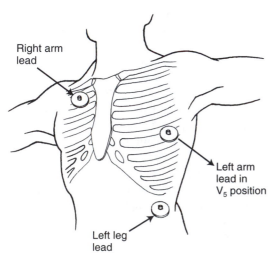

Figure 6-2 Modified V_5 lead monitoring. When only a three-lead system is available precordial leads can be monitored by manipulating leads, according to the lead monitoring desired.

Table 6-1
ELECTROCARDIOGRAM NOTES

Modified chest/ left arm lead (MCL_1):	Negative electrode on left arm and positive electrode in one chest lead position (e.g., V_6 or V_5)
Modified V_5:	Right arm lead (negative electrode) under right clavicle, left arm lead in V_5 position (positive electrode) and left leg lead in usual position, while monitoring lead 1
Rhythms:	Mobitz II—PR interval remains constant but there are occasional to frequently blocked QRS
	Mobitz I—progressive PR interval
	Complete heart block—P waves and QRS do not correlate; slow ventricular rate; PR interval not constant
QT interval:	Prolonged in congestive heart failure, myocardial infarction, ↓ Ca^{++}, myocarditis
	Shortened with digitalis, ↑ Ca^{++}, K^+ intoxication
Hyperkalemia ECG changes:	Peaked T waves, often with shortened QT interval, which progresses to widening of the QRS

Electrolyte abnormalities can also cause perioperative arrhythmias. Hyperkalemia is associated with "peaked" T waves. When levels of potassium continue to increase (>8.5 mEq/L), ventricular irritability occurs causing ventricular tachycardia and ventricular fibrillation. Patients with chronic renal failure, neuromuscular disease, burns, or those receiving potassium replacement are susceptible to hyperkalemia. Conversely, hypokalemia is commonly caused by respiratory alkalosis (hyperventilation), potassium-wasting diuretics, metabolic alkalosis (vomiting), and insulin administration. ECG changes manifest as an exaggerated U wave. Prolongation of the QT interval and inverted T waves are also seen with hypokalemia. These changes can have causes other than hypokalemia. Hypocalcemia is also associated with a prolonged QT interval. Hypercalcemia may cause a shortened QT interval although this abnormality is usually not evidenced until profound hypercalcemia occurs.

Medications such as digitalis, tricyclic antidepressants, and lithium have also caused ECG abnormalities.

Table 6-2
12-LEAD ECG IDENTIFICATION

Leads	Coronary Artery	Area Fed by Coronary Artery	Myocardial Area
II, III, aVF	Right	RA, RV, part of posterior LV	Inferior wall
I, aVL, V_{5-6}	Left	LA, LV, mainly anterior and lateral wall	Lateral wall
V_{1-4}	Left anterior descending	Anterior and lateral aspects of LV	Anteroseptal wall

LA, left atrium; LV, left ventricle; RA, right atrium; RV, right ventricle

☐ ARTERIAL BLOOD PRESSURE

Contraction of the left ventricle causes ejection of blood into the vasculature. Each contraction causes pulsatile blood flow and thus pulsatile arterial pressures. *Systole* correlates with the peak pressure within the vasculature, generated from myocardial contraction. Commonly the systolic pressure is used to evaluate normotension, hypertension, and hypotension. Systole also represents myocardial oxygen consumption because a high pressure is associated with high oxygen demands. An important calculation of myocardial oxygen demands is the rate-pressure product.

$$\text{Rate-Pressure Product} = \text{Systolic Blood Pressure} \times \text{Heart Rate}$$

A high heart rate and high systolic blood pressure create an increased workload on the heart and, therefore, an increase in myocardial oxygen consumption.

Mean arterial pressure (MAP) represents the driving pressure of blood flow causing organ perfusion. It can be estimated by the following calculations:

$$MAP = \frac{\text{Systolic BP} + 2\,(\text{Diastolic BP})}{3}$$

$$MAP = \text{Systolic BP} + \frac{\text{Pulse Pressure}}{3}$$

(Pulse pressure is systolic pressure minus diastolic pressure.)

Diastole represents left ventricular relaxation and, therefore, ventricular filling. Most of myocardial perfusion occurs during diastole, when the heart muscle is relaxed. When the heart muscle is contracting, as in systole, the muscle squeezes down and impedes blood flow through many of its own blood vessels (coronary arteries). Consequently, diastole is important for coronary perfusion.

NONINVASIVE PRESSURE MONITORING

Blood pressure monitoring is a standard requirement for anesthesia. Invasive verses noninvasive monitoring is dictated according to the type of surgery and the patient's medical history. Indications for invasive pressure monitoring are discussed later in this chapter. Whether invasive monitoring is used or not, a prudent anesthetist will utilize noninvasive monitoring (e.g., a Dinamap [device for indirect noninvasive automatic MAP]) as well. This additional monitor will help to verify a more accurate correlation in blood pressures. It will also act as a "backup monitor" in case the invasive arterial line is designated nonfunctional (e.g., the arterial line becomes clotted and is no longer working or unintentional intra-arterial line disconnection occurs).

Blood pressure should be determined every 3 to 5 minutes. More frequent monitoring should be avoided due to increased venous congestion within the limb caused by cuff inflation. This venous congestion can result in thrombus and nerve injuries. The extravasation of intravenous fluids has also been linked to overzealous use. The patient's medical history and type of surgery act as a guide for the need in frequency of measurements.

Techniques

Auscultation

Normally, blood flow is laminar. Blood pressures are commonly measured in the upper arm, but the thigh and calf can also be used. Initially, inflation of the pressurized blood pressure cuff should be 20 mm Hg above systolic or to approximately 170 mm Hg. Inflation of the cuff causes the blood vessels to collapse and cease arterial blood flow. While auscultating the median artery (assuming the upper arm is being measured), the cuff is slowly deflated and turbulent blood flow is ejected. This turbulence in flow is what is known as *Korotkoff's sounds*. As the cuff pressure is continually deflated, these Korotkoff's sounds can be heard until a muffling in the sound occurs. This muffling, which can also be a disappearance or a change in sound, is known as the diastolic pressure. The diastolic pressure is the sound heard once the artery is no longer occluded. The cuff should be deflated at a rate of 3 to 5 mm Hg/second. Rapid deflation will falsely lower the reading. Abnormal readings can also occur if the blood pressure cuff is not the proper size. If the cuff is too small, a falsely high reading will be auscultated and vice versa for too large a cuff. The width of the cuff should be 20% greater than the diameter of the limb. Pressure measurements can also be affected by alterations in the circulation. Auscultation of Korotkoff's sounds are difficult when the patient is hypotensive or in shock. These low flow states cause Korotkoff's sounds to be inaudible. Absence of pulsatile blood flow, as for example during cardiopulmonary bypass, also renders auscultation unattainable.

Palpation

A pressurized cuff is applied to a limb. Once an arterial pulse is palpated, the cuff is inflated causing cessation of the pulse. The cuff is then slowly deflated (at a rate of 3 to 5 mm Hg/second), until a palpable pulse is felt. This is considered the systolic pressure. A diastolic MAP cannot be palpated. This technique should only be used as a quick assessment because it is highly subjective and, consequently, inconsistent.

Oscillometry

Automated devices, such as a Dinamap operate on oscillometric methods. A pressurized cuff is applied to a limb. Initially, the cuff is inflated to 170 mm Hg. If the device senses that this pressure is below the patient's systolic pressure, the device will automatically reinflate the cuff to a higher value. The cuff then deflates at a rate of 3 mm Hg/second. A microprocessor analyzes the arterial pulsations that cause oscillations in the cuff. The systolic blood pressure is identified when a marked increase in the amplitude in oscillations occur. It is the point when blood begins to flow through the artery under the inflated cuff. MAP is identified as the average pressure at which maximal oscillations occur. The oscillations continue to decrease, and diastole is identified. A prudent anesthetist should use this technique with due precautions because systolic and diastolic readings do not always equal invasive measurements. Bradycardia, hypotension, and dysrhythmias should cause one to be more vigilant for possible inaccurate measurements. Motion artifact, electrocautery, and external pressure on the cuff (e.g., the resident leaning on the patient's arm), can cause erroneous readings.

Doppler Probe

This technique is especially useful for pediatric patients, obese patients, or patients with low flow states, such as shock. A pressurized cuff is applied to a limb and an arterial pulse is palpated distal to the cuff. Coupling gel is then applied to the arterial pulse and the Doppler is applied to that site. The cuff is then inflated until Doppler sounds have ceased. As the cuff is deflated, systole is recognized when the Doppler sounds resume. The ultrasonic Doppler device is sensitive to arterial wall motion and to arterial blood flow. It is important to recognize interference in readings caused by electrocautery and motion artifact.

INVASIVE PRESSURE MONITORING

Indications Invasive arterial blood pressure monitoring is indicated whenever continuous beat-to-beat analysis of blood pressure is required. Indications include coronary artery disease, chronic obstructive pulmonary disease, a history of critical illness, hypotensive anesthetic technique, pressure-supporting drug usage, cardiopulmonary bypass, major vascular surgery, intrathoracic procedures, major neurologic surgeries (e.g., aneurysm clipping or tumor resection), surgeries with anticipated large blood loss, or surgeries that require frequent blood sampling (e.g., activated clotting time monitoring). All of these are at the discretion of the anesthetist.

Contraindications Patients with poor perfusion, such as with peripheral vascular disease, are at risk for ischemic digits if good collateral blood flow does not exist. Blood dyscrasias, such as disseminated intravascular coagulation and idiopathic thrombocytopenic purpura, make insertion of an arterial line risky.

Potential Arterial Cannulation Sites and Risks
Radial Artery
The radial artery is the most common site used because it is easily palpable and is associated with adequate collateral blood flow in the majority of patients (Fig. 6–3). Adequacy of collateral blood flow can be assessed by an Allen test. It will help distinguish the dominant arterial vessel supplying the hand. In the awake patient, the patient is asked to tightly clench the fist, causing the skin to appear pallid. The anesthetist then occludes the patient's radial and ulnar arteries by compressing these arteries with the fingers. The patient is then asked to open the hand, and then compression of the ul-

nar artery is released. If adequate blood flow exists between the radial and ulnar arteries that feed the volar arch within the palm, the hand will flush and appear pink within 5 seconds. Inadequate collateral blood flow will delay the return of color or the hand will remain blanched. Allen's test can also be performed on the unconscious anesthetized patient. Apply a pulse oximeter to a finger on the hand being tested. Occlude both arteries with your fingers, but this time until you lose the pulse oximetry waveform on the patient's monitor. Wait approximately 5 seconds and release pressure on the ulnar artery. If the pulse oximeter waveform resumes within 5 seconds, good collateral blood flow is likely.

Ulnar Artery
Cannulation of the ulnar artery is similar to radial artery cannulation but may be technically more difficult because of its tortuous nature. It also lies deeper within the wrist. Caution should be used when placing a catheter within the ulnar artery because it may be the dominant artery. The ulnar artery is usually the primary supplier of blood flow to the hand. Allen's test can be performed to help distinguish the dominant artery, but this is not always a reliable test.

Dorsalis Pedis Artery
This is the second most common site used under anesthesia because of its low complication rate and easy accessibility. The systolic blood pressure will appear 20 to 30 mm Hg higher than in the radial artery because of its distance from the aorta. Diastolic pressures may appear 10 to 20 mm Hg lower than radial artery diastolic pressures. Allen's test can be performed to assess collateral blood flow within the foot.

Brachial Artery
Located within the antecubital fossa, the brachial artery is larger and more easily accessible than the radial artery. It is usually associated with reliable collateral blood flow. The awake patient is at risk of kinking the catheter because of its placement within the elbow.

Axillary Artery
The axillary artery is a large artery and is usually even palpable in low flow states such as extreme shock. However, because of its placement within the axillary plexus, neurologic consequences and nerve damage can occur. The cerebral circulation can be introduced with air or clots from the axillary artery because of its proximity to the aortic arch. The left axilla is preferred over the right because a right axillary catheter may lie within the innominate artery.

Technique The fluid-filled system should be aseptically set up and zeroed before arterial puncture is made. The system is comprised of a transducer that converts a pressure within the tubing to an electrical signal. This signal is amplified and exhibited on the monitor. The transducer is connected to rigid tubing that should be less than 4 feet long to prevent distortion in readings. A continuous flush device is also required to prevent clot formation of the catheter. The entire system should be flushed of air bubbles. The patient's wrist should be secured on a short padded armboard in the

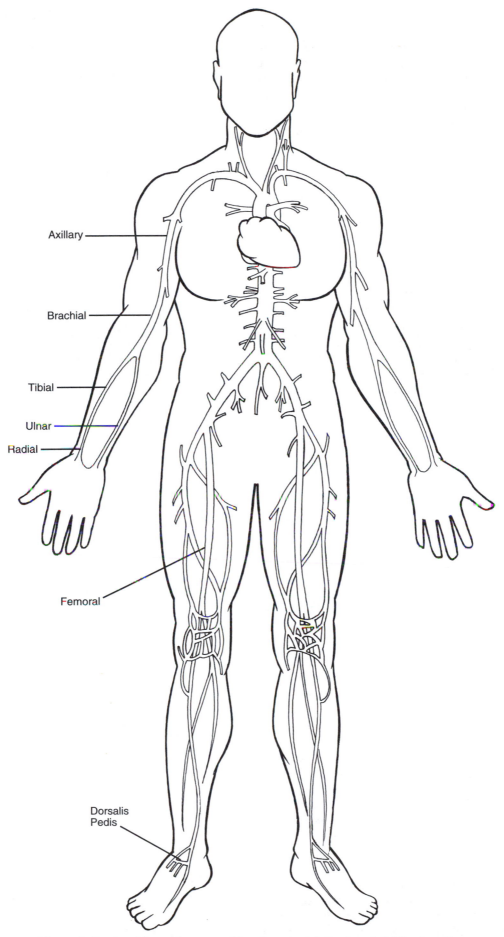

Figure 6–3 Arterial vascular system: Note the potential sites for arterial line insertion.

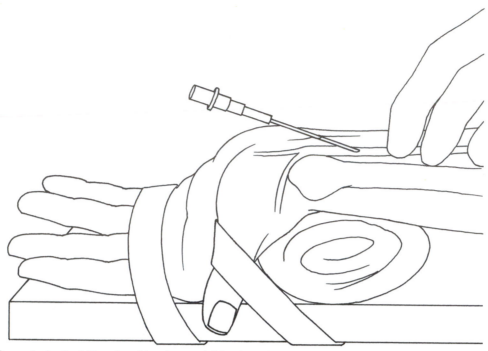

Figure 6-4 Dorisiflexed position for arterial line insertion. Notice the catheter is in at 45° to the artery.

dorsiflex position (Fig. 6-4). The patient's thumb is also taped back to help reduce the mobility of the artery. Dorsiflexion and extension of the wrist should not be extreme because it can distort or diminish the radial pulse. The radial pulse should be assessed after the wrist is secured and the thumb is taped back. The path of the radial artery is then palpated and the skin is sterilely prepped. In the awake patient, 1 mL 1% lidocaine is injected and a skin wheal is created, distal and along the path of the artery. A skin nick over the expected arterial puncture site is helpful to prevent deformation of the catheter tip, which is common with 22-gauge catheters. In infants, 22-gauge catheters are preferred; 20-gauge catheters are used for larger children. Adults generally receive 20-gauge catheters and if placement is extremely difficult, a 22-gauge catheter may be used. At a 30° angle and with the bevel up, the catheter is introduced through the nick in the skin made over the artery. The catheter is slowly advanced until a "flash" of arterial blood is seen at the back of the catheter. Once arterial blood is evidenced within the catheter, the catheter is lowered to a 5° to 10° angle. Blood should remain flowing into the back of the catheter once the angle has been lowered. The bevel of the needle should then be rotated 180° and advanced 1 cm to ensure its placement within the artery (Fig. 6-5). The catheter is slowly and freely advanced within the artery. The bevel is rotated 180° to prevent puncturing the posterior wall of the artery. If difficulty occurs advancing the catheter, the through-and-through technique can be performed. This technique consists of advancing the needle and catheter through the posterior wall of the artery (Fig. 6-6). Blood will cease to flow once the catheter is advanced through the posterior wall of the artery. The needle is then withdrawn from the catheter. The catheter is slowly withdrawn until free pulsating blood is spurted

from the back of the catheter. A 0.018-inch diameter guidewire is slowly passed through the catheter and the catheter can then be slowly readvanced over the guidewire, within the artery.

WAVEFORM INTERPRETATIONS

Valuable information can be obtained from the central (ulnar artery, central aorta, or femoral artery) arterial pressure waveforms (Fig. 6-7).

1. *Contractility* is represented by the sharp upstroke of the anacrotic limb (point A). If the upstroke is sharp and vertical in appearance, the ventricle is believed to have good contractility. If the upstroke is sloped or sluggish, poor contractility of the ventricle is noted.
2. *Systemic vascular resistance* (SVR) is reflected in the diacrotic limb (point B). The downstroke represents the fall in pressure at the aortic root as blood flows to the peripheral circulation. An elevated SVR will have a high diacrotic notch (point C) within the downward slope. Conversely, a low diacrotic notch will represent a low systemic resistance and thus, SVR.
3. *Aortic valve closure* is represented by the diacrotic notch. When ventricular pressure declines below the pressure in the aortic root, the aortic valve closes. The small upstroke is caused by blood flushing back against the aortic valve. This is when coronary perfusion occurs.
4. *Stroke volume* is represented as the area under the arterial pressure waveform (point D).

COMPLICATIONS

Mechanical errors, such as overdampening of the curve, can be caused by air bubbles within the tubing, a thrombus, or

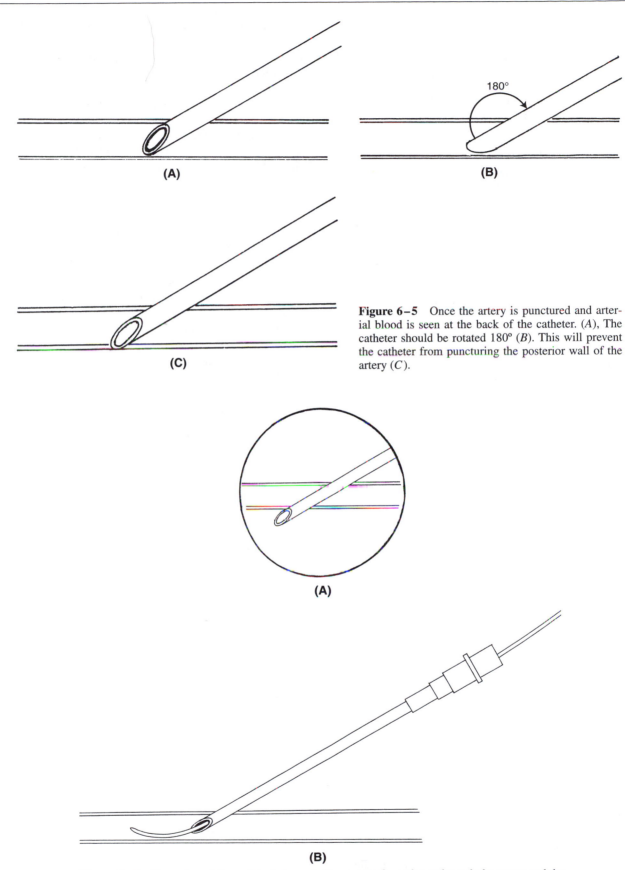

Figure 6–5 Once the artery is punctured and arterial blood is seen at the back of the catheter. (*A*), The catheter should be rotated 180° (*B*). This will prevent the catheter from puncturing the posterior wall of the artery (*C*).

Figure 6–6 Through-and-through technique. *A*. Represents the catheter through the artery and the stylet is removed. The catheter is slowly withdrawn until arterial blood pulsates from the back of the catheter. Once this occurs (*B*), the guidewire is advanced through the catheter, the catheter is advanced within the artery, and the guidewire is withdrawn. The catheter is then connected to pressurized tubing and transduced.

Normal arterial waveform

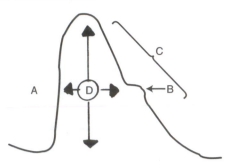

Figure 6–7 Point A represents ventricular contractility. Point B is at the diacrotic notch, which represents atrioventricular valve closure. Point C represents systemic vascular resistance and at point D, the area within the curve represents stroke volume.

the tip of the catheter infiltrating the arterial wall. It is important to periodically re-zero the line to prevent wandering. Also, double checking an abnormal pressure reading by cuffing a blood pressure (noninvasive method) will help avoid improper treatment with vasopressor medications for falsely lowered pressures. The transducer should be zeroed at the level of the right atrium, known as the *phlebostatic axis*. Ischemia, nerve damage, infection, thrombosis, fistula, or aneurysm formation are rare but possible complications.

☐ CENTRAL VENOUS MONITORING

INDICATIONS

Central venous pressure (CVP) monitoring represents right atrial pressures in patients without coexisting cardiovascular diseases. It is a poor indicator of left ventricular function. For example, a patient with left ventricular failure will have normal to elevated left arterial pressures, while right ventricular pressure will remain normal. As the left ventricle continues to fail, left atrial pressures will increase and cause the right ventricle to pump against an increasing afterload. Eventually, the right ventricle will also fail and cause an elevated CVP. Another instance in which right atrial pressures are not paralleled by CVP monitoring is in the patient with right ventricular infarction. The "stunned" and stiff right ventricle will have a decreased compliance. This decreased compliance causes increased pressures within the ventricle, which can be generated back up to the right atrium and therefore falsely increase CVP readings. Tricuspid disease also elevates CVP measurements (Table 6–3).

EQUIPMENT AND TECHNIQUE

Basic standard monitoring, such as ECG, a noninvasive blood pressure cuff, and pulse oximetry should be applied before placement of a CVP catheter. All equipment should be prepared before insertion of the CVP catheter and intravenous fluids that will be connected to the new CVP catheter should also be prepared. The electronic transducer should be

zeroed and pressurized tubing connected before insertion is started. In the awake patient, oxygen is applied and the procedure is briefly explained. (This procedure should be discussed with the patient preoperatively.) Several sites for cannulation are possible. The internal jugular vein, subclavian vein, external jugular vein, femoral vein, axillary vein, cephalic vein, and basilic vein are examples of central venous access sites. The most commonly used site is the internal jugular because it is easily accessible, has a high success rate and a low incidence of complications. The Seldinger technique is the most commonly used approach to insertion (Fig. 6–8). The patient's neck is slightly extended and turned to the left. Landmarks such as the mastoid process, the clavicle and the two heads of the sternocleidomastoid muscle are identified before sterile preparation is begun. Aseptic technique with betadine solution is required for central venous catheter placement. A triangle is formed by the sterile drapes and within the triangle the clavicle, the suprasternal notch, lower border of the mandible, and the lateral border of the sternocleidomastoid muscle are exposed. The patient is then placed in Trendelenburg's position to dilate the internal jugular vein and to reduce the risk of air entrainment and thus air embolus. A patient with a history of congestive heart failure or pulmonary hypertension may not tolerate Trendelenburg's position because of increased venous return to the heart. Common approaches to the internal jugular are the central, anterior, or posterior approaches. Identification of the external jugular vein should be made to avoid accidental puncture. In the awake patient, 1% lidocaine is infiltrated at the site of insertion, lateral to the carotid artery. With the left hand, the anesthetist should palpate the carotid artery. Once the carotid pulse is found, the 22- or 25-gauge finder needle is introduced lateral to the artery and at a 30° angle. Initially, the finder needle should be aimed at the ipsilateral nipple, but if venous blood is not aspirated, the anesthetist should carefully walk medially with the finder needle until venous blood is attained. This must be done carefully to avoid puncturing of the carotid artery. Once venous blood is aspirated, a larger 18-gauge needle is inserted at the exact angle and location of where the venous blood was aspirated. Easy aspiration of venous blood will occur once the internal jugular is located. The syringe is slowly removed from the needle without moving the needle placement. If there is doubt about the exact location of the catheter, it should be transduced to ensure its lo-

Table 6–3
INDICATIONS FOR CENTRAL VENOUS PRESSURE MONITORING

1. Guide for intravascular fluid monitoring
2. Access in patients with poor venous access
3. Administer vasopressor agents into the central circulation
4. Surgeries in which large blood loss or large volume shifts are expected
5. Remove air emboli
6. Access for transvenous pacing
7. Access for total parenteral nutrition or chemotherapeutic agents

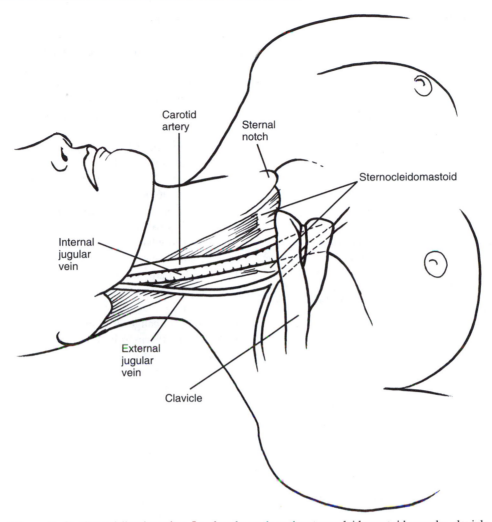

Figure 6–8 Central line insertion. Landmarks such as the sternocleidomastoid muscle, clavicle, mastoid process, etc, should be identified before sterile drapes are applied.

cation within the venous circulation before the guidewire is introduced. While the anesthetist listens to and watches the ECG monitor, a guidewire is advanced through the needle. Cardiac dysrhythmias can be witnessed if the guidewire enters the right ventricle. The 18-gauge needle is then removed over the guidewire. The skin is pierced with a number 11 blade to facilitate placement of the dilator. The dilator is gently and firmly advanced and then removed over the guidewire. With the distal tip of the guidewire in sight and secured, the multilumen catheter is passed over the guidewire. The guidewire is removed and blood is aspirated from all three ports. The infusion ports are then flushed with heparinized saline and the appropriate intravenous solutions are connected. The catheter can be sutured to the skin to secure placement. An occlusive dressing should be placed over the insertion site.

RISKS

A chest radiograph should be taken as soon as possible (usually after surgery in the recovery room) to rule out pneumothorax and verify the location of the radiopaque catheter.

Carotid artery puncture, cardiac puncture, air embolus, infection, hematomas, cervical nerve damage, vocal cord damage, tracheal laceration, endotracheal cuff rupture, and cardiac dysrhythmias are some of the possible complications that can occur with central venous catheter placement.

INTERPRETATION OF WAVEFORMS

Normal right atrial pressures are between 1 and 8 mm Hg. CVP readings are right atrial pressures. The normal CVP waveform (Fig. 6–9) consists of three ascending waves and two descending waves. The CVP waveform can be affected by various factors such as tricuspid valve function, heart rate, conduction disturbances, intrathoracic pressures and compliance of the right ventricle. The a wave represents *atrial contraction*. If no atrial contraction occurs, as with atrial fibrillation, the a wave does not appear in the waveform. During right atrial contraction, the tricuspid valve remains closed causing an increase in right atrial pressure. This increase in pressure is depicted by a sharp upstroke a wave. The atrium then relaxes, and right ventricular contraction occurs. Contraction of the right ventricle causes the tricuspid valve to

Central venous pressure waveform

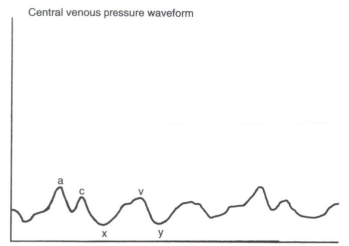

Figure 6-9   In the CVP waveform, a represents atrial contraction; c is tricuspid valve elevation during early ventricular contraction; x is downward displacement of the ventricle during systole; v is venous return against a closed tricuspid valve; and y is tricuspid valve opening during diastole.

bulge up toward the right atrium. This causes an increase in pressure within the right atrium and is known as the c wave on the CVP waveform. The *x wave* represents right ventricular ejection. This causes emptying of blood from the ventricles and therefore a rapid decrease in pressure. Immediately after, venous return to the right atrium causes an increase in right atrial pressure and a *v wave*. The tricuspid valve opens causing blood to flow into the ventricle and a decrease in pressure in the right atrium. This is known as the *y descending wave*.

Abnormal waveforms can be used to detect cardiac dysfunction. For example, a *giant v wave* can reflect tricuspid regurgitation. Atrioventricular dissociation, as with a mistimed pacemaker, can cause *cannon a waves*, which occur when the right atrium contracts against a closed tricuspid valve. Positive-pressure ventilation can falsely elevate pressures. For this reason, the ventilator should be off during CVP pressure reading. Also, end-expiration is the best time for reading CVP pressures. Conversely, negative pressures may be transmitted during inspiration in the spontaneously breathing patient.

☐ PULMONARY ARTERY PRESSURE MONITORING

INDICATIONS

The pulmonary artery catheter is used to assess right side intracardiac pressures, left side intracardiac pressures, cardiac output, and mixed venous blood saturations. It is indicated for patients whose perioperative care would benefit from these hemodynamic indices (Table 6-4).

EQUIPMENT

All equipment should be assembled and zeroed before insertion. The most commonly used catheters is a 7 F Swan-Ganz in adults and a 4 to 6 F Swan-Ganz in children. The polyvinylchloride 7 F Swan-Ganz catheter is typically 110 cm long. It consists of a proximal port for fluids, a distal port for fluids, a thermistor connector to connect to a thermodilution cardiac output machine, and a balloon valve port for inflation of air into the distal pulmonary capillary wedge pressure balloon. A ventricular infusion port (VIP) Swan-Ganz catheter has an additional port for infusion of fluids. Different variations of a pacing Swan-Ganz can also be used. The distal and proximal ports are connected to an electronic transducer to which a pressurized heparin-saline flush system is attached. The catheter is zeroed with the distal port at the level of the patient's mid axillary/mid right atrium. The cardiac output thermistor connector port is connected to a thermodilution cardiac output machine. The machine is capable of plotting a change in temperature as a function of time. It produces the thermodilution curve. The area under the curve is used by the computer to determine cardiac output. Typically, 10 mL (some computers require 2.5 or 5 mL) of iced or room temperature solution is injected into the right atrium. It is important to note that the injected solution is below normal blood temperature. The injected solution causes a change in the temperature of the blood, located at the distal portion of the thermistor output. The computer uses this information and plots a curve waveform over time. The area under the curve is used to calculate the cardiac output. A minimal temperature change will be evidenced with a high blood flow and cardiac output. Conversely, a large temperature change will be evidenced with a low blood flow and cardiac output.

The accuracy of cardiac output measurements depends on certain criteria. Electrocautery can cause a disruption in the electrical communication within the computer so the anesthetist should avoid obtaining measurements during electrocautery. The anesthetist should inject the exact and appropri-

Table 6-4
INDICATIONS FOR PULMONARY ARTERY PRESSURE MONITORING

1. Major surgery with large fluid shifts
2. Ventricular dysfunction and congestive heart failure
3. Severe coronary artery disease or recent myocardial infarction
4. Severe valvular disease
5. Conduction disturbances that might require a pacing Swan-Ganz catheter
6. Coronary artery bypass grafting, abdominal aortic aneurysm, liver or lung transplantation, valve replacements
7. Adult respiratory distress syndrome or severe chronic obstructive pulmonary disease
8. Septic or shock states
9. Acute burns over large body surface areas

ate volume that is set for the computer. A lower injected volume will cause a falsely higher cardiac output. Conversely, a higher injected volume will falsely lower the cardiac output. If the solution is injected slowly, a falsely low cardiac output will be determined. Rapid infusion of intravenous fluids through the distal, proximal, and VIP ports can also falsely obscure cardiac output readings because they can change the temperature of the injected solution. Intracardiac shunts and tricuspid regurgitation falsely alter cardiac output readings because only right ventricular output measurements are being made.

TECHNIQUE

The Seldinger technique, as described earlier, is commonly used to access the internal jugular vein for insertion of a pulmonary artery catheter. In place of a CVP catheter, an introducer sheath is threaded over the guidewire. The pulmonary artery catheter is threaded through the introducer's lumen. The right internal jugular is commonly used because it is easily accessible and has a low complication rate. The distal (pulmonary artery port) and proximal (CVP) ports are flushed with heparinized saline and are connected to an electronic transducer. The pulmonary artery catheter balloon is inflated with 1.5 cc of air to check patency and the symmetry of the cuffed balloon. The natural curve of the catheter is used to facilitate floatation of the catheter to the pulmonary artery. Through the introducer's lumen, the Swan-Ganz catheter is slowly advanced to the 20 cm marking (Fig. 6–10). The monitor will display right atrial pressures at the 20-cm marking. While the anesthetist watches for a change in the waveform on the monitor, the balloon is inflated and the catheter is slowly advanced until a right ventricular pressure waveform is seen. The right ventricular waveform is characterized by a sudden increase in the systolic pressure. This waveform should occur approximately at the 30 to 35 cm marking. Advancement of the catheter to approximately 40 to 45 cm will exhibit a pulmonary artery tracing. The pulmonary artery waveform is characterized as a sudden increase in the diastolic pressure. The catheter is advanced until another change in waveform is seen or to about 50 to 55 cm. This waveform should be a pulmonary capillary wedge pressure tracing. The balloon is then slowly deflated and a pulmonary artery waveform should appear. If it does not reappear, the catheter is slowly withdrawn until it does. The introducer is then sutured to the skin and an occlusive dressing applied. The normal pressures and distances for the right internal jugular are presented in Table 6–5.

RISKS

The most common complication of catheter insertion is cardiac dysrhythmias, especially when the tip of the catheter is located within the right ventricle. This causes ventricular irritability and dysrhythmias. Lidocaine (1 mg/kg) can be given

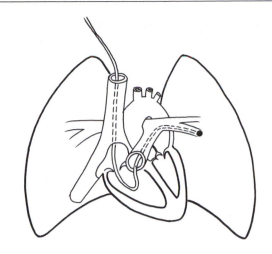

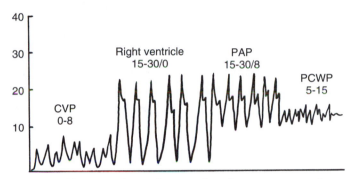

Figure 6–10   Normal waveforms as the pulmonary artery catheter is advanced to the pulmonary artery. CVP, central venous pressure; PAP, pulmonary artery pressure; PCWP, pulmonary capillary wedge pressure.

if the dysrhythmias do not resolve. A transient right bundle branch block may occur from insertion. Patients with a history of left bundle branch block or first-degree heart block are at increased risk for a complete heart block and risk-to-benefit ratio must be considered. Catheter kinking or knotting, right ventricular or pulmonary artery perforation, pneumothorax, air embolus, thoracic duct damage (occurs with

Table 6–5
NORMAL PRESSURES AND DISTANCES FOR RIGHT INTERNAL JUGULAR

		Pressure (mm Hg)	Distance (cm)
RA = RAP = RVEDP = CVP		1–8	15–20
RV = RVP	Systolic	15–25	30–35
	Diastolic	1–8	
PAP	Systolic	15–25	40–45
	Diastolic	8–15	
PW = PCWP = PaOP = LVEDP		6–12	50–55

CVP, central venous pressure; LVEDP, left ventricular end-diastolic pressure; PaOP, pulmonary artery occlusive pressure; PAP, pulmonary artery pressure; PCWP, pulmonary capillary wedge pressure; PW, pulmonary wedge; RA, right atrium; RAP, right atrial pressure; RV, right ventricle; RVEDP, right ventricular end-diastolic pressure; RVP, right ventricular pressure

left internal jugular approach), pulmonary infarction, bacterial, endocarditis, and pulmonary artery rupture are other rare but possible complications.

PHYSIOLOGY

A relationship between left ventricular end-diastolic muscle fiber length and left ventricular muscle function was established by Starling. He demonstrated that in a ventricle with normal compliance, left ventricular end-diastolic pressure will reflect left ventricular muscle length. Left ventricular end-diastolic pressures generate back up into the left atrium in the presence of a normal mitral valve. In the presence of a healthy pulmonary vasculature, left atrial pressures are generated back to the pulmonary artery. When the wedged balloon is inflated within the pulmonary artery, it reflects left atrial pressures, in the absence of pulmonary disease.

creatitis, carbon monoxide poisoning, portal caval shunt, cyanide poisoning, or a continuous wedged balloon. A decreased mixed venous O_2 may represent fever, hypoxia, low cardiac output, left ventricular failure, or anything that increases metabolic state.

☐ PULSE OXIMETRY

PHYSICS

The Lambert-Beer law exhibits how wavelengths of light are absorbed differently by oxyhemoglobin and deoxyhemoglobin. Pulse oximeters operate by using this law. Pulse oximeters consist of two light emitting diodes (LED) and a sensor. A pulsatile arterial bed, such as a finger, is placed between the sensor and the LEDs. The LED projects two different

right atrial pressure $\leftrightarrow$ pulmonary artery end-diastolic pressure $\leftrightarrow$ pulmonary capillary wedge pressure $\leftrightarrow$ pulmonary venous pressure $\leftrightarrow$ left atrial pressure $\leftrightarrow$ left ventricular end-diastolic pressure $\leftrightarrow$ left ventricular end-diastolic volume

INTERPRETATIONS

Important information can be obtained from a pulmonary artery catheter. The most commonly used hemodynamic parameters derived from the pulmonary artery catheter are listed in Table 6–6 and interpretations of pressure variations in Table 6–7.

Mixed venous oxygen saturation can also be obtained from the pulmonary artery catheter. Blood aspirated from the proximal port can be sent for blood gas analysis. Mixed venous saturation reflects oxygen consumption by the cell. Normal mixed venous oxygen saturation is between 68% and 70%. An elevated mixed venous O_2 can reflect sepsis, pan-

wavelengths, a red light at 660 nm and an infrared light at 940 nm, across the pulsatile arterial bed. A sensor on the other side of this bed computes the amount of red and infrared light absorbed. The ratio of the two is then analyzed by a microprocessor and the oxygen saturation is displayed on the monitor.

EQUIPMENT

The small sensors consist of two LED sources and a phototransistor detector. They can be applied to a finger, toe, ear, nose, or to the palm of a newborn. The anesthetist should test the pulse oximeter before it is used perioperatively.

Table 6–6
HEMODYNAMIC EQUATIONS DERIVED FROM PULMONARY ARTERY CATHETER

Parameter		Normal Value
Systemic vascular resistance (SVR)	$= \dfrac{MAP - CVP}{\text{Cardiac output}} \times 80$	900–1500
Cardiac index (CI)	$= \dfrac{\text{Cardiac output (L/min)}}{\text{Body surface area (m}^2\text{)}}$	2.8–4.2
Stroke volume (SV)	$= \dfrac{\text{Cardiac output (L/min)}}{\text{Heart rate}}$	60–90 mL/beat
Pulmonary vascular resistance (PVR)	$= \dfrac{\text{PAP (mean)} - \text{PCWP}}{\text{Cardiac output}} \times 80$	100–300 dynes/s/cm

CVP, central venous pressure; MAP, mean arterial pressure; PAP, pulmonary artery pressure; PCWP, pulmonary capillary wedge pressure

Table 6–7
INTERPRETATION OF PRESSURE VARIATIONS

Pressure Variation	Interpretation	Treatment
CVP ↑, CI ↑, PCWP ↑, PAP ↑	Hypervolemia Vasoconstriction	Diuretics ↓ fluids
CVP ↓, CI ↓, PCWP ↓, PAP ↓	Hypovolemia	Give volume
CVP ↑↓, CI ↓, PCWP ↑, PAP ↑	LV failure ↑ afterload	Inotropes α-adrenergic antagonists
CVP ↑, CI ↓, PCWP ↑, PAP ↑	Pulmonary edema	Diuretics
CVP ↑, CI ↓, PCWP ↓ or N, PAP ↓	RV failure ↑ preload	Vasodilators

CI, cardiac index; CVP, central venous pressure; LV, left ventricle; N, normal; PAP, pulmonary artery pressure; PCWP, pulmonary capillary wedge pressure; RV, right ventricle

Table 6–8
USING O_2 SATURATION TO PREDICT Pao_2

Pao_2:	10	20	30	40	50	60	70	80	90	100
Sao_2:	13	35	57	75	83	90	93	95	96	97

Table 6–9
MIXED VENOUS OXYGEN TENSION

Mixed venous oxygen tension depends on:
1. Cardiac output
2. Oxygen consumption
3. Hemoglobin concentration

INDICATIONS

Pulse oximetry is a standard monitor and is required for all intraoperative procedures. It is used to assess oxygen saturation. It can also assess tissue perfusion and measure heart rate (Table 6–8).

RISKS

Certain factors can alter the reliability of pulse oximeters. For example, a patient with carbon monoxide poisoning may have a falsely high/normal reading because the monitor is incapable of differentiating oxyhemoglobin from carboxyhemoglobin; both absorb light at 660 nm. Intravenous dyes, such as indigo carmine and methylene blue, can falsely lower readings. Artifact caused by electrocautery, shivering, the patient's movement, and ambient light can affect the reliability of pulse oximeters. Anemia, methemoglobinemia, and low perfusion states (hypotension, hypothermia, increased SVR from vasoconstrictive agents) can also cause an inaccurate reading. Oxygen saturation readings below 70% are also questionable. Conversely, *fetal hemoglobin* does not affect the reliability of pulse oximetry readings (Table 6–9).

☐ MASS SPECTROMETRY

PHYSICS

Airway gases from a sideport within the breathing circuit are drawn out into a vacuum chamber in the mass spectrometer. An electronic beam then ionizes these gases according to their molecular weight. This sample gas is then exposed to a magnetic field. The magnetic field has specific collecting plates for specific ionized gases. The ionized gas with the highest mass-to-charge ratio is least deflected and the ionized gas with the lowest mass-to-charge ratio is the most deflected. A predicted curve of deflection of each gas, therefore, results from their various mass-to-charge ratios.

ADVANTAGES

Mass spectrometry can monitor various gases, such as N_2, N_2O, O_2, and anesthetic agents. It can detect an air leak within the system or an air embolus because of its capability of monitoring N_2 within the system. It can also alert the anesthetist of an unintentional overdose due to a malfunctioning vaporizer. Misfilling of vaporizers can also be detected by

the mass spectrometer because each gas has its own specific mass to charge and is deflected to its own specific collecting plate.

DISADVANTAGES

Mass spectometry can only analyze gases it has collecting plates for. If a gas is included within the sample and the mass spectrometer does not have a collecting plate for it, the mass spectrometer will falsely overestimate the gases it is equipped to analyze. Also, because the mass spectrometer on average draws off 200 cc of sample gas, it can potentially decrease the amount of oxygen within a closed system circuit. When the patient has a small tidal volume or a valveless Mapleson system is in use, the potentially large entrainment of sampling gases can cause a hypoxic mixture within the circuit.

☐ CAPNOGRAPHY

PHYSICS

Measuring CO_2 levels in expired gas is an effective method of continuous monitoring of alveolar ventilation. The AANA standards recommend that the correct placement of an endotracheal tube must be verified by end-tidal CO_2 ($ETCO_2$) monitoring. It is the single best predictor of endotracheal placement of an endotracheal tube. The AANA recommends that other indicators of endotracheal placement, such as auscultation of breath sounds and chest wall excursion, also be used to verify accurate placement. A gradient between alveolar and arterial concentrations of CO_2 exists due to ventilation/perfusion mismatching. Typically, arterial concentrations of CO_2 are 4 to 6 mm Hg *higher* than alveolar concentrations. Therefore, the anesthetist should use the capnograph monitor as a method of following the trend in changes of arterial CO_2. It is important to keep in mind that $ETCO_2$ and arterial CO_2 gradients can change perioperatively due to changes in pulmonary blood flow, dead space, and ventilation/perfusion mismatching. It may be necessary to confirm arterial CO_2 ($Paco_2$) with arterial blood gas analysis (Fig. 6–11).

EQUIPMENT

The most popular method uses infrared spectroscopy, which consists of two wavelength beams of infrared light. The in-

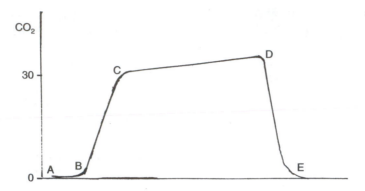

AB: Beginning of exhalation; dead space gas
BC: exhalation of gas from alveolar-capillary membrane; rapid sharp uprise
CD: end expiration, alveolar plateau
D: ETCO$_2$
DE: inspiration of gas, sharp downstroke to zero

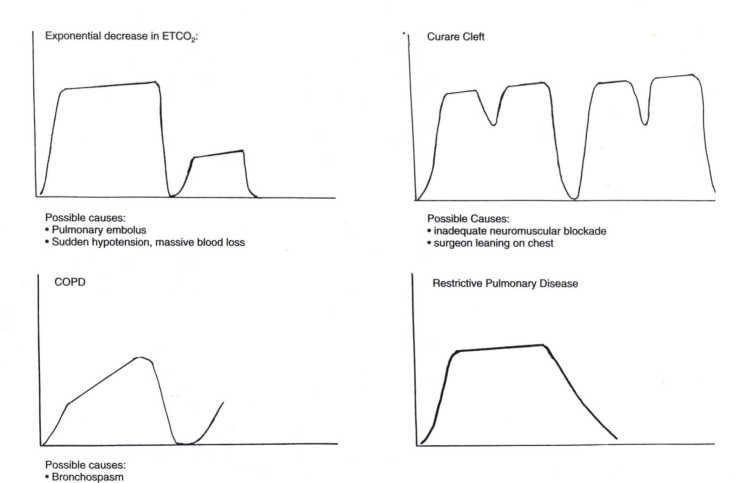

Exponential decrease in ETCO$_2$:

Possible causes:
• Pulmonary embolus
• Sudden hypotension, massive blood loss

Curare Cleft

Possible Causes:
• inadequate neuromuscular blockade
• surgeon leaning on chest

COPD

Possible causes:
• Bronchospasm

Restrictive Pulmonary Disease

Figure 6–11

frared light is passed through a sampled exhaled gas and a control calibrated CO$_2$ chamber. The quantity of light absorbed in both chambers is calculated and the ETCO$_2$ is displayed on the monitor. Samples of CO$_2$ can be obtained by a mainstream or a sidestream sampling method. Mainstream sampling consists of an in-line sampler in which CO$_2$ is mea-

sured by passing through an adapter placed in the breathing circuit. It is best placed at the end of the endotracheal tube and the connector of the circuit. This can lead to the inherent problems with this method such as adding extra weight and therefore potentiating a disconnection of the circuit. It also increases dead space within the circuit. This can be significant in a pediatric patient. Fresh gas flow should be increased to compensate for this additional dead space. Sidestream sampling, also known as an aspirating analyzer, continuously suctions gases from a small side port between the endotracheal tube and the connector to the circuit. Airway gases are transported via capillary tubing to a CO_2 sampling chamber for analysis. It adds no dead space to the circuit. However, it can cause a hypoxic gas mixture within a closed system circuit used commonly for pediatric patients. This can occur because it is capable of entraining fresh gas from the circuit. Again, increasing fresh gas flow will help to compensate for this problem. Another disadvantage of sidestream sampling is its potential for obstruction from water vapors and secretions.

INDICATIONS

Canography is used to confirm accurate placement of endotracheal intubations and adequate ventilation. It is also used to detect pathologic conditions such as pulmonary air embolus and malignant hyperthermia. Because a decrease in CO_2 (hyperventilation) causes a decrease in cerebral blood flow, $ETCO_2$ is frequently monitored during craniotomies or for the patient with increased intercranial pressure. It is important to look at the overall clinical picture when assessing increases and decreases in $ETCO_2$. For example, releasing a tourniquet can release metabolites and increase $ETCO_2$ readings. Laparoscopic procedures that use CO_2 to inflate the explored cavity can increase $ETCO_2$ (Table 6–10).

☐ NEUROMUSCULAR BLOCKADE MONITORING

NEUROMUSCULAR PHYSIOLOGY

An impulse at the prejunctional motor nerve ending causes an influx of calcium ions and an efflux of the neurotransmitter acetylcholine across the synaptic cleft to the postjunctional membrane (see Chap. 2). Peripheral nerve stimulators are used to stimulate the initiation of an impulse across the neuromuscular junction. Muscle relaxants are used to inhibit neuromuscular transmission and thus cause muscle relaxation. Therefore, utilizing this concept, muscle relaxants can be titrated to produce the desired effect of muscle relaxation.

INDICATION

Peripheral nerve stimulators should be used whenever depolarizing or nondepolarizing muscle relaxants are used to assess the depth of neuromuscular blockade. Timing of intubation after the administration of muscle relaxants is facilitated by peripheral nerve stimulators. Criteria for extubation require a peripheral nerve stimulator to assess adequate recovery and reversal of muscle relaxation. Early diagnosis of abnormal plasma cholinesterase levels are possible with a

Table 6–10
CHANGES IN END-TIDAL CARBON DIOXIDE

Cause of ↑ $ETCO_2$

1. Release of tourniquet from extremity
2. Right-to-left shunts
3. Exhausted soda lime
4. Faulty unidirectional valve
5. Kinking of inner tube with Bain's system
6. Inadequate fresh gas flow in Mapleson's system
7. Hypoventilation
8. Shivering
9. Laparoscopic surgeries
10. Sudden increase in pulmonary blood flow
11. Increased metabolic states such as malignant hyperthermia
12. Obstruction to expiration within the breathing circuit

Cause of ↓ $ETCO_2$

1. Hyperventilation
2. Pulmonary embolus
3. Disconnections in the breathing circuit
4. Cardiac arrest
5. Apnea
6. Esophageal intubations
7. Increased dead space

peripheral nerve stimulator use after a dose of succinylcholine.

EQUIPMENT AND TECHNIQUE

A pair of cutaneous electrodes or subcutaneous needles are placed over a motor nerve and attached to a battery-operated electrical current generator. Various frequencies of electrical current can be given according to the desired test required. The most common placement of the cutaneous electrodes is over the ulnar nerve, causing stimulation of the *adductor pollicis muscle*. Stimulation of the ulnar nerve will cause adduction of the thumb. Another commonly used site is placement over the facial nerve. Single twitch, train-of-four (TOF), tetanus, posttetanic, and double-burst stimulation are the five patterns used to assess neuromuscular blockade. Singe twitch consists of a supramaximal stimulus at .1 Hz which lasts only 0.1 to 0.2 seconds. It is generally used to assess neuromuscular blockade created by depolarizing muscle relaxants. Uniform depression of height in twitches is characteristic of single twitch. A *phase I blockade*, which is created by depolarizing agents, will exhibit a decreased response to a single twitch, a 75% blockade in TOF, a sustained tetanus, and no posttetanic facilitations. TOF stimulation involves four supramaximal stimuli at 2 Hz at 0.5-second intervals over 2 seconds. Progressive fade in twitches represents an increase in muscle relaxation. This is typical of a TOF blockade. It is used to monitor nondepolarizing muscle relaxants and it is based on the concept that acetylcholine is depleted with successive stimulation. TOF stimulation with no muscle relaxants given will cause four twitches equal in height. When the fourth (last) twitch has been eliminated, a 75% blockade is apparent. When the third twitch is eliminated, an 80% blockade is noted. When the second twitch is eliminated, a 90% blockade is exhibited. When the first twitch has disappeared, 100% blockade is noted. Clinically, surgical relaxation usually requires a 75% to 90% blockade. It is important to note that a phase II block can be created by depolarizing muscle relaxants. A *phase II block* resembles the fade in the TOF seen with nondepolarizing agents. Succinylcholine administered in doses greater than 2 to 4 mg/kg causes a phase II blockade. Doses of succinylcholine less than 2 mg/kg will not exhibit fade in TOF because a phase I blockade exists. Other characteristics of a phase II block are a decreased response to a single twitch, a unsustained tetanus, and posttetanic facilitation. A tetanic stimulus is delivered at 50 to 100 Hz for 5 seconds. It is a painful stimulus that causes the presynaptic release of acetylcholine. A nonsustained tetanus is seen with nondepolarizing agents and, thus, a phase II blockade is evidenced. Posttetanic stimulation is created when a single twitch is administered after a tetanic stimulus. An increase in twitch will be seen when a phase II block or a nondepolarizing agent is given. Depolarizing agents will not exhibit an increase in twitch. Posttetanic twitch indicates a residual neuromuscular blockade. Double-burst stimulation is produced by two 50-Hz stimuli. It also represents residual blockade.

RISKS

Reversal of neuromuscular blockade should be assessed with a peripheral nerve stimulator. Neglecting to use a peripheral nerve stimulator may result in significant residual neuromuscular blockade. It is important to use other clinical parameters, such as sustained head lift, a negative inspiratory effect greater than 20 cm H_2O, tidal volume and respiratory rate, and a strong hand grasp, when extubating a patient. Recovery of the adductor pollicus does not correspond with a full recovery of diaphragmatic muscles and a residual block may reside. Reversal of nondepolarizing muscle relaxants should not be attempted without a visible twitch as this may result in a prolonged neuromuscular blockade. Nerve stimulators can cause skin irritation, abrasions, and muscle pain at the site of electrode placement.

☐ RENAL FUNCTION

Depending on the type and length of surgery, and the patient's medical history, a Foley catheter may be indicated. Measuring urine output is a helpful guide for intravascular fluid volume and cardiac output. A decrease in urine output can be caused by sympathetic stimulation such as surgical incision and light anesthesia. Sympathetic stimulation causes the release of antidiuretic hormone (ADH). A low systolic blood pressure or a decreased cardiac output can also reduce urine output because autoregulation is not maintained by the

kidney under general anesthesia. Interventions should be taken if the urine output drops below 0.5 mL/kg per hour.

☐ TEMPERATURE MONITORING

Body heat can be lost through radiation, convection, conduction, and evaporation. *Radiation* refers to loss of heat that occurs with the release of infrared rays. The amount of heat lost is influenced by cutaneous vasodilation. In the adult, most of the body's (>50%) heat lost under anesthesia and surgery is through radiation. When warm air moves away cooler air takes its place. This loss in heat (warm air) is known as *convection*. During anesthesia, 12% of body heat is lost through convection. *Conduction* refers to the heat that is conducted from the patient to inanimate objects, such as the operating room table. *Evaporation* of water from the skin and the lungs (insensible losses) also results in heat loss. Burn patients lose most of their body heat through evaporation.

TECHNIQUE

Temperature can be monitored at various sites of the body. The most common site monitored under general anesthesia is the esophagus. Accurate placement of an esophageal probe requires the placement of the sensor at the lower third of the esophagus. Core temperature is reflected at this site. Rectal temperatures do not reflect core temperatures because of their slower response to change in temperature. Axillary and skin temperatures are also poor indicators of core temperature. During monitoring of axillary and skin temperatures, only trends should be followed and not the actual number. Tympanic membrane temperature monitoring reflects brain and cerebral blood temperatures.

METHODS

General anesthesia, muscle relaxation, cold operating rooms, infusion of cold intravenous fluids and blood, and open surgical wounds can all potentially cause hypothermia. Certain clinical situations may benefit from hypothermia, such as open heart surgery and neurosurgery. However, hypothermia is generally undesirable. The best way to prevent and minimize heat loss is to keep the room temperature above 21°C. Core temperature can be maintained above 36°C when room temperatures are as indicated. Heating blankets are ineffective and are the least effective method of preventing hypothermia.

An artificial nose or pall filter can be used to retain heat and moisture of the airway gases within the breathing circuit. Airway gases can also be heated and humidified to 35° to 37°C. Coverings such as plastic applied to the body will help maintain body heat. However, 60% of the body, including the head (most of the body's heat is lost through the scalp), needs to be covered to effectively maintain body heat. The best way to rewarm a patient is with an air warming system blanket, such as a bair hugger. Intravaneous fluids, blood, and irrigating solutions should also be warmed to preserve heat.

RISKS

Hypothermia slows the metabolic rate of the body. In certain situations a decreased cerebral blood flow and metabolic rate may be beneficial. However hypothermia can be detrimental. At temperatures between 28° and 30° C. ventricular irritability and fibrillation can occur. Hypothermia also decreases the metabolism of anesthetic agents by decreasing hepatic blood flow in addition to increasing agent solubility. This can prolong wake up and extubation of a patient.

☐ NEUROLOGIC MONITORING

PHYSICS

Electroencephalography (EEG) uses somatosensory stimulation to assess the integrity of the central nervous system. Somatosensory evoked potentials (SEPs) entail administering a small electrical current to a peripheral nerve, and simultaneously monitoring the brain wave responses. This allows the assessment of the neural pathways from the peripheral nerve to the spinal column up to the somatosensory cortex. It is important to point out that these evoked potential testing methods assess sensory pathways via the dorsal column and therefore are not reliable for assessing motor pathways via the ventral column. Motor pathways can be evaluated with motor evoked potentials (MEP) or with a wake-up test. Conversely, MEPs and the wake-up test are reliable modes of testing motor function only. However a potential complication of the wake-up test is recall. Brain stem auditory evoked potentials (BAEP) utilize a headset placed by the patient's ear. This projects an audible clicking that stimulates the eighth cranial nerve, which is then transmitted to the cerebral cortex. Visual evoked potentials (VEP) use a headset that administers flashing lights. This stimulates the optic nerve and is transmitted to the visual cortex within the occipital lobe.

INDICATION

Generally, EEG monitoring is used during surgical procedures that are associated with potential neurologic damage as a result of surgical manipulation. Carotid endartectomy, spinal cord surgery, aortic or thoracic aneurysm, and cerebral embolizations are examples of surgeries that use EEG testing.

WAVEFORMS

Delta waves (0 to 3 Hz) appear during deep anesthesia, ischemia, or pathologic states. Theta waves (4 to 7 Hz) appear during sleep or anesthesia. Alpha waves (8 to 13 Hz) appear during resting or awake states. Beta waves (above 13 Hz) are apparent during mental activity and awake states. Damage to the neuronal pathways is reflected as a decrease in amplitude and an increase in latency in EEG waves. Inhalation agents cause a dose-dependent increase in latency and a decrease in amplitude during SEP monitoring. BAEPs are the most resistant to anesthetic-induced changes.

REFERENCES

1. American Association on Nurse Anesthetists. Patient monitoring standards. *Journal of the American Association of Nurse Anesthetists.* 1992; 60:137.

2. London MJ, Hollenberg M, Wong MG, et al. Intraoperative myocardial ischemia: localization by continuous 12-lead electrocardiography. *Anesthesiology.* 1988;69:232-241.

SUGGESTED READINGS

Barash PG, Cullen BF, Stoelting RK. *Clinical Anesthesia.* Philadelphia: JB Lippincott; 1992.

Blitt CD. *Monitoring in Anesthesia and Critical Care Medicine.* New York: Churchill Livingstone; 1985.

Davison KJ, Eckhardt WF, Perese DA. *Clinical Anesthesia of the Massachusetts General Hospital.* Boston: Little, Brown; 1993.

Dorsch JA, Dorsch SE.: *Understanding Anesthesia Equipment: Construction, Care and Complications.* Baltimore: Williams & Wilkins; 1984.

Gravenstein JS, Paulus DA.: *Clinical Monitoring Practice.* Philadelphia: JB Lippincott; 1987.

Hensley FA, Martin DE: *The Practice of Cardiac Anesthesia.* Boston: Little, Brown; 1990.

Lake CL. *Clinical Monitoring for Anesthesia & Critical Care.* Philadelphia: WB Saunders; 1990.

Miller RD., et al.: *Anesthesia.* New York: Churchill Livingstone; 1990.

Morgan EG, Mikhail MS. *Clinical Anesthesiology.* East Norwalk, Conn: Appleton & Lange; 1992.

Ouellette RG. Comparison of four intraoperative warming devices. *Journal of the American Association of Nurse Anesthetists.* 1993; 61:394-395.

Sedlock S. Interpretation of hemodynamic pressures and recognition of complications. *Critical Care Nurse.* 1980; Nov/Dec: 39-54.

Stoelting RK, Miller RD. *Basics of Anesthesia.* New York: Churchill Livingstone; 1989.

☐ QUESTIONS

1. Mr. George Longobardi is 55 years old with a medical history of smoking; he is slightly overweight. He is scheduled to have an ethmoidectomy. Before induction, the patient states, "I feel like I'm having chest pain." You notice your patient's ECG monitor has ST elevations in V_5. You look at your patient's preoperative ECG again and it appears normal. You believe:
   a. Your patient is having a lateral wall myocardial infarction, which involves his left anterior descending artery.
   b. Your patient is having an anterior wall myocardial infarction, which involves his right coronary artery.
   c. Your patient is having a lateral wall myocardial infarction, which involves his left coronary artery.
   d. Your patient is having an anterior wall myocardial infarction, which involves his left anterior coronary artery.

2. Your patient's calcium level has rapidly climbed and now is at toxic levels. What ECG changes might you see?
   a. Prolonged QT interval
   b. Peaked T waves
   c. Shortened PR interval
   d. Shortened QT interval

3. What does the area within the arterial line waveform represent?
   a. Stroke volume
   b. Ventricular contractility
   c. Systemic vascular resistance
   d. Aortic valve closure

4. What does the downstroke on the arterial line waveform represent?
   a. Stroke volume
   b. Ventricular contractility
   c. Systemic vascular resistance
   d. Aortic valve closure

5. What does the c wave represent on the CVP waveform?
   a. Atrial contraction
   b. Tricuspid valve elevation, during early ventricular contraction
   c. Downward displacement of ventricle during systole
   d. Venous return

6. Mrs. Jean Gager is 70 years old with a history of a recent inferior wall myocardial infarction. She has no past medical history and takes no medications. She is scheduled for an emergency evacuation of a large cerebral hematoma. You decide that the safest way to monitor your patient is with an arterial line, a Swan-Ganz catheter and a 16-gauge angio catheter. Your patient's initial Swan readings are as follows: CVP,10; PCWP, 13; PAP, 45/25; CO, 6.5. You decide the best mode of treatment is:
   a. You believe your patient is hypovolemic and give a fluid challenge with 250 mL 5% albumin.
   b. You believe your patient is going into left ventricular failure and will administer α-antagonist agents.
   c. You believe your patient is in right ventricular failure and decide vasodilators may be necessary.
   d. You believe your patient is hypervolemic and decide to cut back on fluid administration.

7. Two days postop, you visit Mrs. Jean Gager for a follow-up visit. She states she "doesn't have pain, but just doesn't feel right." Her blood pressure is 165/88 and her heart rate is 65. CVP, 10; PCWP, 18; PAP, 48/25; CO 3.0. You believe:
   a. She is in pulmonary edema and needs diuretics.
   b. She is still behind in fluids and needs another fluid challenge.
   c. She is in left ventricular failure.
   d. These are normal readings for a patient with her history of a recent myocardial infarction and therefore no intervention is needed.

8. Mrs. Marianne R. Duffy is 45 years old and scheduled for a liver transplant. Her initial Swan-Ganz readings are: CVP, 2; CO, 3.0; PCWP, 4; PAP, 12/8. You believe:
   a. She is a hypervolemic and needs to remain hypervolemic to maintain perfusion to the kidneys.
   b. She is hypervolemic and needs diuresis.
   c. She is hypovolemic and needs volume replacement.
   d. She is hypovolemic and needs an inotropic agent.

9. The above patient's liver transplant was successful. She is currently in stable condition in the transplant ICU and this is post op day 1. She states "I have moderate incisional pain." Her current vital signs are: BP 150/86; HR, 98; CVP, 14; CO, 2.8; PCWP, 10; PAP, 13/7. You believe:
   a. She is hypovolemic and will benefit from a fluid challenge.
   b. She is hypervolemic and needs 10 mg Lasix.
   c. She is in left ventricular failure and needs inotrope agents.
   d. She has an elevated preload and needs 6 mg morphine for pain.

10. While visiting his mother in the hospital Mr. James J. Duffy passes out while the nurse was drawing blood from his mother. A code is called and you immediately

run to the code because you are in charge of the code beeper. Before you arrive, the nurse puts a pulse oximeter on James and his initial SaO_2 is 75%. You estimate his PaO_2 to be:

a. 60
b. 50
c. 40
d. 30

11. All of the factors below will alter the reliability of the pulse oximeter *except:*
a. Skin color
b. Venous pulsation
c. SaO_2 below 60%
d. Carbon monoxide poisoning

12. Ms. Eileen Cafasso is your patient. She is scheduled for a craniotomy in the sitting position. She has a medical history of COPD and is currently on 5 mg prednisone OD. The following statements are all true *except:*
a. The most sensitive indicator of venous air embolism is the transesophageal echocardiogram.
b. Mass spectrometry detects venous air embolism by detecting changes in $PECO_2$ and PEN_2.
c. Doppler ultrasound can detect as little as 0.5 mL air.
d. The mill-wheel murmur is the earliest indication of VAE.

13. After a single dose of vecuronium, your patient's peripheral nerve stimulator will exhibit:
a. Decreased response to single twitch, TOF ratio 0.7, sustained tetanus and no posttetanic stimulation
b. Increased response to single twitch, TOF ratio 0.7, sustained tetanus and no posttetanic stimulation
c. Decreased response to single twitch, TOF ratio 0.3, nonsustained tetanus, posttetanic stimulation
d. Decreased response to single twitch, TOF ratio 0.3, nonsustained tetanus, no posttetanic stimulation

14. After a single dose of succinylcholine, your patient's peripheral nerve stimulator will exhibit:
a. Decreased response to single twitch, TOF ratio 0.7, sustained tetanus and no posttetanic stimulation
b. Increased response to single twitch, TOF ratio 0.7, sustained tetanus and no posttetanic stimulation
c. Decreased response to single twitch, TOF ratio 0.7, non-sustained tetanus and no posttetanic stimulation
d. Decreased response to single twitch, TOF ratio 0.7, sustained tetanus and posttetanic stimulation.

15. Capnograph waveform: At what point is the $ETCO_2$ measured?
a. Point B
b. Point C
c. Point D
d. Point E

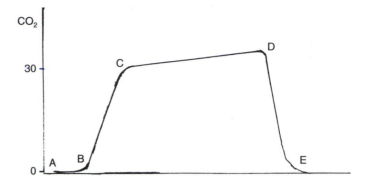

16. Capnograph waveform: From the $ETCO_2$ waveform, (below) your patient has:
a. COPD
b. Patient is fighting the ventilator
c. Right mainstem intubation
d. Restrictive disease

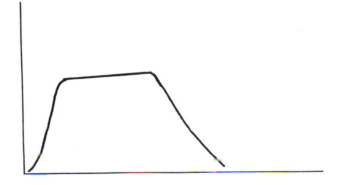

17. Capnograph waveform:
a. disconnection
b. bronchospasm
c. rebreathing
d. pulmonary embolism

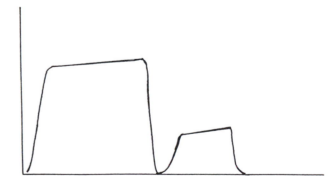

18. What is the best way to rewarm a patient?
a. Warming blanket
b. Bair hugger
c. Heat and humidify breathing circuit
d. Warm IV fluids and cover the patient's head with a plastic cap

19. How does a patient lose the majority of heat during surgery?
    a. Radiation
    b. Evaporation
    c. Conduction
    d. Convection

20. While inserting a Swan-Ganz catheter, you slowly advance the catheter to 40 cm and notice what waveform on the monitor?
    a. CVP
    b. Right ventricular
    c. PAP
    d. PCWP

☐ ANSWERS

1. c	5. b	9. d	13. c	17. d
2. d	6. d	10. c	14. a	18. b
3. a	7. a	11. a	15. c	19. a
4. c	8. c	12. d	16. d	20. c

Appendix to Chapter 6

AMERICAN ASSOCIATION OF NURSE ANESTHETISTS PATIENT MONITORING STANDARDS[1]

Basic to safe anesthesia care is the application of qualitative and quantitative monitoring which enables the anesthetist to administer anesthesia and evaluate its effect in a manner that optimizes desired responses while minimizing the risks of anesthesia. Fundamental to this endeavor is the use of multiple monitoring modalities which play vital roles in assisting anesthetists to provide conscientious care to patients receiving anesthesia.

These patient monitoring standards are intended to assist the CRNA practitioner in providing consistent, safe anesthesia care.

These standards apply to patients undergoing general, regional, or monitored anesthesia care for diagnostic or therapeutic procedures in designated anesthetizing locations. In extenuating circumstances, the CRNA must use clinical judgment in prioritizing and implementing these standards. All of these standards do not normally apply to epidural analgesia for labor or pain management therapy. The standards may be exceeded in any or all respects in any time at the discretion of the anesthetist, as required by individual patient needs.

While the standards are intended to encourage high quality patient care, they cannot insure specific patient outcomes. It is recognized that appropriately used monitoring modalities may fail to detect untoward clinical developments. Further, it is recognized by the AANA that under some circumstances certain monitoring standards may not be applicable. While this is a fact of practice, the omission of one or more monitoring standards should be documented and the reason stated on the patient's anesthesia record. Interruptions in monitoring may be unavoidable. Occasionally, the anesthetist must work at some distance from the patient because of an environmental hazard such as, but not limited to, radiation. Under such circumstances, provisions for monitoring the patient must be made and documented on the patient's anesthesia record.

Adequate facilities must exist to enable remote patient monitoring. The standards are subject to review and revision from time to time, as indicated by technology and practice.

☐ ANESTHESIA PROVIDERS

Continuous clinical observation and anesthetist vigilance are the bases of safe anesthesia care. The anesthetist, or nurse anesthesia student, shall be in constant attendance of the patient until the responsibility for care has been accepted by another qualified health care provider.

☐ PATIENT MONITORS

VENTILATION

Purpose: To assess adequate ventilation of the patient. (Standard in effect until October 1, 1992)

Standard: Ventilatory adequacy shall be assessed by continuous auscultation of breath sounds. Correct placement of an endotracheal tube must be verified by auscultation, chest excursion and end tidal CO_2 monitoring when available. Other quantitative ventilatory devices may be used in conjunction with auscultation, such as spirometry and ventilatory pressure monitors.

Breathing system disconnect monitor: When the patient is ventilated by an automatic mechanical ventilator, the integrity of the breathing system must be monitored by a device that is capable of detecting the disconnection of any component of the breathing system. Such a device shall be equipped with an audible alarm which is activated when its limited are exceeded.

(Standard to become effective October 1, 1992):

Standard: Intubation of the trachea shall be verified by auscultation, chest excursion and confirmation of carbon dioxide in the expired gas. Controlled or assisted ventilation during the anesthetic shall be monitored continuously with an end tidal carbon dioxide monitor. Additionally, spirometry and ventilatory pressure monitors may also be used.

Breathing system disconnected monitor: When the patient is ventilated by an automatic mechanical ventilator, the integrity of the breathing system shall be monitored by a device that is capable of detecting the disconnection of any component of the breathing system. Such a device shall be equipped with an audible alarm which is activated when its limits are exceeded.

OXYGENATION

Purpose: To assess adequate oxygenation of the patient.

Standard: Adequacy of the patient oxygenation shall be monitored continuously with pulse oximetry. In addition to pulse oximetry, oxygenation shall also be monitored by observations of skin color, the color of the blood in the surgical field and arterial blood gas analysis when indicated.

During general anesthesia, the oxygen concentration delivered by the anesthesia machine shall be monitored continuously with an oxygen analyzer with a low oxygen concentration limit alarm. An oxygen supply failure alarm system shall be operational to warn of low oxygen pressure to the anesthesia machine.

CIRCULATION

Purpose: To assess adequacy of the cardiovascular system.

Standard: Blood pressure and heart rate shall be determined and recorded at least every 5 minutes. The patient's electrocardiogram shall be monitored continuously during the course of the anesthetic.

Circulation also shall be assessed by at least one of the following measures: digital palpation of pulse, auscultation of heart sounds, continuous intra-arterial pressure monitoring, electronic pulse monitoring or pulse oximetry.

BODY TEMPERATURE

Purpose: To assess changes in body temperature.

Standard: Body temperature shall be intermittently or continuously monitored and recorded on all patients receiving general anesthesia; the means to monitor temperature shall be immediately available for use on all patients receiving local or regional anesthesia and used when indicated.

NEUROMUSCULAR FUNCTION

Purpose: To assess neuromuscular function.

Standard: The means to evaluate the patient's neuromuscular function by the use of a nerve stimulator shall be available immediately when neuromuscular blocking agents have been used.

☐ ANESTHESIA EQUIPMENT

A complete equipment safety check shall be performed daily and an abbreviated check of all equipment shall be performed before each anesthetic is administered.

All anesthesia machines and monitoring equipment shall conform to the appropriate national and state standards. An ongoing preventive maintenance program shall be established and enforced.

Anesthesia Equipment and Delivery Systems

Carolyn G. Holland

Since the introduction of ether anesthesia, patient safety remains the predominant factor in the evolution of anesthesia delivery systems. Dr. Jay Heidbrink described requirements for an ideal anesthesia machine in 1917 as one that would "accurately pass gases promptly, safely and economically."[1] Design of current anesthesia delivery systems continues refinement of these goals. The Standards for Nurse Anesthesia Practice section VIII state, "Appropriate safety precautions shall be taken to minimize the risks of fire, explosion, electrical shock and equipment malfunction."[2] Knowledge of the design and proper function of anesthesia equipment and delivery systems is necessary to recognize malfunction and minimize hazards. This chapter reviews the components of medical gas and vacuum systems and the anesthesia delivery system, explains the differences between the two major US manufacturers of anesthesia machines, and highlights safe use of anesthetic equipment.

☐ MEDICAL GAS AND VACUUM SYSTEMS FOR ANESTHESIA DELIVERY SYSTEMS

Anesthesia delivery systems receive the three major medical gases from a pipeline and cylinder supply.[3] Because medical gases flow directly to patients, they are drugs but are not sterile. The Emergency Care Research Institute (ECRI) compiled a listing of allowable contaminants after reviewing documents from the various organizations that have some role in gas purity determination. The values in this table are easy to obtain and are well below amounts considered to be hazardous to patients or staff[4] (Figure 7–1).

STORAGE OF COMPRESSED GAS SOURCE

After manufacture of medical gases, their storage as a gas or a liquid depends on the critical temperature of the gas. The definition of *critical temperature* is the temperature below which a gas is converted to a liquid form by pressure.[5] Each gas changes to a liquid at a known critical temperature by a known critical pressure. The critical temperature of oxygen is $-118°C$. Conversion of liquid oxygen from the gas requires a drop in temperature to slow the movement of molecules. Manufacturers accomplish this with temperature-controlled, insulated, and pressurized containers. Because the critical temperature of nitrous oxide is $36.5°C$, it exists as a liquid at room temperature.[5]

PIPELINE COMPRESSED GAS SOURCE

Oxygen and Nitrous Oxide Pipeline Supply Bulk supply systems incorporate large cryogenic containers or cylinder manifolds that store the compressed medical gases in a liquid form. A primary, secondary, and at least a 1-day reserve supply must be available.[4] An alarm panel informs hospital personnel of the integrity of the gas supply. The alarm panel warns of inadequate supply of oxygen, reserve supply status, and low or high pressure of each medical gas. End users constantly confirm adequate pipeline pressure via the anesthesia machine pipeline pressure gauges. Pressure is 50 to 55 psig for oxygen, nitrous oxide, and air.[6] The standard flow rate for oxygen and nitrous oxide is 100 L/min or greater, monitored by the maintenance department.[4]

Air Pipeline Supply Most medical air production occurs on site from ambient atmosphere using a mechanical compressor system. If the environment is excessively pol-

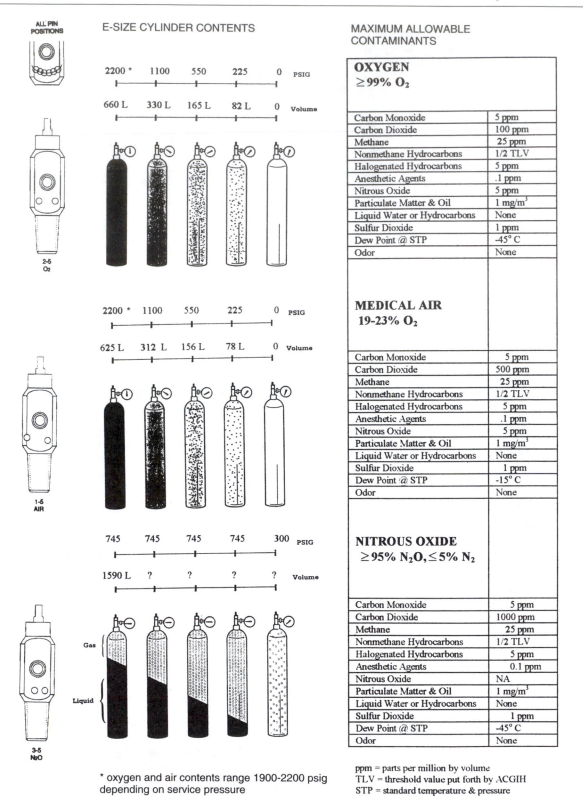

| ALL PIN POSITIONS | E-SIZE CYLINDER CONTENTS | MAXIMUM ALLOWABLE CONTAMINANTS |

OXYGEN
≥99% O₂

Carbon Monoxide	5 ppm
Carbon Dioxide	100 ppm
Methane	25 ppm
Nonmethane Hydrocarbons	1/2 TLV
Halogenated Hydrocarbons	5 ppm
Anesthetic Agents	.1 ppm
Nitrous Oxide	5 ppm
Particulate Matter & Oil	1 mg/m³
Liquid Water or Hydrocarbons	None
Sulfur Dioxide	1 ppm
Dew Point @ STP	-45° C
Odor	None

MEDICAL AIR
19-23% O₂

Carbon Monoxide	5 ppm
Carbon Dioxide	500 ppm
Methane	25 ppm
Nonmethane Hydrocarbons	1/2 TLV
Halogenated Hydrocarbons	5 ppm
Anesthetic Agents	.1 ppm
Nitrous Oxide	5 ppm
Particulate Matter & Oil	1 mg/m³
Liquid Water or Hydrocarbons	None
Sulfur Dioxide	1 ppm
Dew Point @ STP	-15° C
Odor	None

NITROUS OXIDE
≥95% N₂O, ≤5% N₂

Carbon Monoxide	5 ppm
Carbon Dioxide	1000 ppm
Methane	25 ppm
Nonmethane Hydrocarbons	1/2 TLV
Halogenated Hydrocarbons	5 ppm
Anesthetic Agents	0.1 ppm
Nitrous Oxide	NA
Particulate Matter & Oil	1 mg/m³
Liquid Water or Hydrocarbons	None
Sulfur Dioxide	1 ppm
Dew Point @ STP	-45° C
Odor	None

* oxygen and air contents range 1900-2200 psig depending on service pressure

ppm = parts per million by volume
TLV = threshold value put forth by ACGIH
STP = standard temperature & pressure

Figure 7–1   Pin-index safety system, cylinder contents, and ECRI-recommended maximum allowable contaminants of oxygen, air, and nitrous oxide. (Pin-index configuration reproduced by permission from Cicman and colleagues.[13] Cylinders reproduced by permission from Bowie and Huffman.[6] Cylinder contents data from Compressed Gas Association pamphlet P-2: *Characteristics and Safe Handling of Medical Gases*. CGA, Inc., 1235 Jefferson Davis Hwy., Arlington, VA. Contaminant information published in © 1994 ECRI. Reprinted with permission from *Health Devices*. 1994; Jan-Feb: 23(1–2).[4] All rights reserved.)

luted by Environmental Protection Agency (EPA) standards (carbon monoxide ≥ 9 ppm[4]), air is supplied from large cylinder manifolds or blended from supplies of oxygen and nitrogen through proportioning systems. Air production is more economical but more complex.[4] The final product is filtered for particulate matter and monitored for carbon monoxide and dew point (a measurement of the temperature at which water vapor in a gas is fully saturated and condenses to form liquid water) before entering the hospital pipeline system. Particulate matter leads to sludge formation in the piping system. Water vapor is minimized to prevent corrosion of the piping and colonization of bacteria and molds.[4]

Gas Outlet and Connector The pipeline supplies gas flows to the anesthesia machine via color-coded hoses with specific connectors to ensure correct coupling of gases. The wall outlet connection may be a quick connect type (Chemetron, Ohmeda, Oxequip, Puritan-Bennett, or Schrader) or a Diameter Index Safety System.[4] Each medical gas has a specific Diameter Index Safety connector at the anesthesia machine. By specifications of the Compressed Gas Association (CGA), oxygen is #1240, nitrous oxide is #1040, and air is #2040.[5] Inside the gas connector is a filter, a pipeline pressure gauge, and a check valve that prevents reverse flow of gases.[3] The filter protects particulate matter in the pipeline from entering the machine. The pressure gauge is upstream of the check valve.[7] The check valve floats freely in response to pressure. When using the pipeline supply, the pressure from the bulk supply (50 psig) pushes the check valve off its seat and gas flows into the machine. If pressure is greater inside the anesthesia machine than the pipeline supply pressure, the check valve closes. This is the reason cylinders should be closed when the pipeline is in use.[6] These check valves are designed so that the anesthesia machine will preferentially seek gas from the pipeline supply instead of the cylinder supply.[3] In the event of a pipeline contamination, the pipeline supply must be disconnected to allow the cylinder supply to serve the machine.

VACUUM SYSTEMS

The National Fire Protection Association (NFPA) 99 standard (refer to Chapter 1) dictates that vacuum pressure should be 12 mm Hg or greater and flow should be 85 L/min or more. Vacuum systems should maintain the indicated pressure and flow at the inlet farthest from the source under calculated system demand.[4] Alarm panels indicate the pressure of the vacuum system. A general rule of thumb that confirms adequate pressure and flow is the ability of the anesthetist's thumb to hold on to the suction tubing at waist height.[5] Vacuum connectors are also of the quick-connect type, are color coded white, and have a Diameter Index Safety #1220 by CGA standards.[5] A separate vacuum for the evacuation of anesthetic gases is preferable because it uses a liquid-sealed pump or a pump that is not damaged by the agents. The hospital vacuum system may not be equipped with this type of pump.[4]

HIGH PRESSURE COMPRESSED GAS SOURCE

Each anesthesia machine contains hangar yoke assemblies for the medical gases to serve as the emergency backup system.[3] Remember that the critical temperature of each gas determines how it is stored. At room temperature oxygen exists as a gas, nitrous oxide as a liquid with a gas phase above the liquid, and air is a blended gas. Because these gases are stored under high pressure, they are the *high pressure* component of the anesthesia machine.

Content Standards set forth by various agencies regulate the amount of gas safely stored in a cylinder (refer to Chapter 1). Figure 7–1 shows the contents of size "E" cylinders of oxygen, air, and nitrous oxide. At a constant temperature, the collisions between the molecules of a gas in a cylinder have a certain energy of motion and collide with the walls of the cylinder at a given frequency. *Boyle's law* states that at a constant temperature, the volume of a given mass of gas varies inversely with the absolute pressure.[8] It is from this relationship that the content of a cylinder is determined. If a known relationship exists between the volume of the cylinder in liters and the pressure that volume exerts, the volume is calculated from knowing the pressure ($P_1V_1 = P_2V_2$).[9] This is true with oxygen and air. The psig reading $\times .3$ provides an estimate of the amount of oxygen in liters.

Because air in a cylinder is a blended proportion of oxygen and nitrogen, *Dalton's law* applies. In a mixture of gases, each type of gas molecule contributes to the pressure exerted on the wall of the cylinder. Each molecule behaves independently of its neighbors. The pressure attributed to any one type of molecule is the same whether the other type of molecule is present or not. If two gases are combined, the total pressure exerted by the combination is additive (21 kPa O_2 + 79 kPa N_2 = 100 kPa absolute).[9] Because both oxygen and nitrogen exist as a gas at room temperature, it is easy to predict the contents of the air cylinder based on the pressure using Boyle's law ($P_1V_1 = P_2V_2$).

The volume of a cylinder of a gas stored as a liquid is not predictable until all of the liquid has vaporized and only gas remains. As the gas escapes from the cylinder, the liquid continues to vaporize into the space above the liquid. It exerts the same pressure on the wall of the cylinder until the liquid disappears. This vaporization requires heat and the liquid cools. This is an example of the *Joule-Thomson effect*. Together with Thomson, Joule found that the temperature of a gas falls when it expands without doing any work.[8] The only way to predict the contents of a cylinder of nitrous oxide is to weigh the cylinder. A full "E" cylinder of nitrous oxide weighs about 19 pounds. An empty cylinder weighs about 13 pounds[5]; therefore, the liquefied nitrous oxide in a full cylinder weighs about 6 pounds.[10]

The CGA specifies the service pressure of each medical gas cylinder. The *service pressure* is the maximum pressure to which the cylinder is filled at 70°F. A cylinder that contains a liquefied gas is filled not by a service pressure, as the same pressure is exerted by any amount of liquid. To prevent overfilling, the maximum amount of liquefied gas that can be in a cylinder is defined by its filling density. The *filling density* is defined as the percent ratio of the weight of the gas in the container to the weight of water that the container would hold at 60°F. The filling density for nitrous oxide is 68%.[5] This is not the same as the volume occupied by the liquid when the cylinder is full. The liquid in a full cylinder of nitrous oxide occupies 90% to 95% of the total cylinder volume. Because the molecules of the vapor phase of the nitrous oxide contribute to the total weight of the gas, it behaves differently than water in the cylinder and only contains 68% of the volume that water would fill.[5]

Because gases also obey Charles' law, it is necessary to strictly regulate the volume of medical gas cylinders. *Charles' law* states that at a constant pressure, the volume of a given mass of gas varies directly with the absolute temperature.[8] The service pressure of gases is specified at 70°F and the filling density of liquefied gas at 60°F. During transport, the ambient temperature may affect the volume of the gas contained in the cylinder.

Identification   Each cylinder is a specific color and has characteristic markings and labels to aid in identifying the content of the cylinder. In the United States, oxygen cylinders are kelly green, nitrous oxide cylinders are dark royal blue, air cylinders are bright yellow, carbon dioxide cylinders are gray, and helium cylinders are brown. The markings are permanently engraved on the cylinder and registered with the Bureau of Explosives. Typical markings include the serial number and test dates. A + indicates the cylinder can be 110% filled. A ★ indicates a 10-year retest interval.[11] The label identifies the contents, the manufacturer, and manufacturing information as well as the hazard class of the gas. A green diamond signifies a nonflammable gas; yellow, an oxidizer; and red, a flammable gas. A signal word (caution, warning, or danger) and a cautionary statement are included with the hazard classification.[5]

Cylinder Valve   The cylinders attach to the hangar yoke of the anesthesia machine with a valve via a pin-index safety system and the T handle. The pin-index system prevents misconnection of the medical gas cylinders. The system fails if pins are missing from the hangar yoke. Pin-index configurations are shown with each medical gas in Figure 7–1.[13] The cylinder valve contains a safety relief device located on the opposite side of the pin-index safety system. A safety relief device prevents rupture of the cylinder under extreme changes in temperature or pressure. This device is a: (1) fusible plug; (2) frangible disc; or (3) spring-loaded valve. A commonly used alloy in the fusible plug is *Wood's metal* that is composed of bismuth, lead, tin, and cadmium. It resembles a large diameter flat-head screw with a dull finish that melts at temperatures between 157° and 220°F.[5] A frangible disc consists of copper and bursts when pressure exceeds the service pressure by at least a factor of two.[10] A spring-loaded

safety relief valve opens in response to an increase in pressure and closes when the pressure is released.[5]

Hangar Yoke Connection   The hangar yoke assembly on the anesthesia machine is color-coded and labeled for each medical gas. There are two pin-index posts that correspond to the pin-index holes on the cylinder valve. A gasket resides between the gas outlet on the cylinder valve and the gas inlet on the anesthesia machine to prevent leakage. The T handle is securely screwed into the seat above the safety relief valve after the pins are correctly engaged. Inside the hangar yoke is a filter (100 μm maximum) for the entrapment of particulate matter. A check valve inside the hangar yoke prevents reverse flow of gases.[3] These check valves are free floating and respond to pressure. They prevent flow of gas from one cylinder to another when a second cylinder is turned on,[6] but they are not leak proof. The American Society for Testing and Materials (ASTM) allows a leak rate of 200 mL/min through these valves.[3] Each hangar yoke includes a pressure gauge to indicate the contents of the cylinder. The gauge has a pressure relief mechanism and a cover to prevent expulsion of the contents toward the anesthetist.[3] The most common pressure gauge used for high pressure compressed gas cylinders is the *Bourdon spring-type* pressure gauge.[11]

Safe Handling of Cylinders   Because medical gas cylinders exist at high pressures, care must be taken when handling to prevent personnel or patient injury. Cylinders are stored upright in holders in a cool, dry, clean, well-ventilated room with their protective caps on. They are held in a freestanding container when transported and protected from blunt trauma. Before placing on an anesthesia machine, they must be inspected for any visible signs of damage or decay and for appropriate cylinder markings and labels to confirm the contents.[5] They are "cracked" briefly before placement in the hangar yoke to clear dust, oil, or debris from the gas outlet. When the cylinder is opened while on the anesthesia machine, the valve is opened slowly.[5] This prevents *adiabatic compression ignition*. Experiments show that when a high pressure wave of oxygen rushes into a regulator it recompresses and raises the gas temperature. If dust, debris, or oil is in the gas outlet or in the piping on the way to the regulator, it self-ignites due to the rise in temperature and results in a fire in an oxygen-enriched environment.[4] Never transfill or cross-fill cylinders (filling small cylinders from large cylinders) because a risk of adiabatic compression ignition, overfilling, and possibly miss-filling exists.[5]

☐ COMPONENTS OF STANDARD ANESTHESIA DELIVERY SYSTEM

After compressed medical gases flow from either the cylinder or the pipeline, they supply the internal components of the anesthesia delivery system. The cylinder supply enters at a pressure dependent on the specific gas and cylinder volume. The pressure of a full oxygen or air cylinder is 1900 to

2200 psig and the pressure of a full nitrous oxide cylinder is 745 psig.[6] This is the high pressure portion of the machine. The pipeline supply enters at about 50 to 55 psig.[6] This is the intermediate pressure portion of the machine. The work of the anesthesia machine is to receive compressed gases at high or intermediate pressure, create a mixture of gases and anesthetic agents of a known concentration, and deliver a low pressure flow to the patient without causing injury. Preventing injury centers around preventing hypoxia, hypercarbia, inhalation overdose, barotrauma, or airway injury due to debris. Figure 7–2 shows the internal components of a standard anesthesia delivery system with oxygen, nitrous oxide, air, two vaporizers, an auxiliary oxygen flowmeter, and ventilator connector.

CYLINDER PRESSURE REGULATOR

The cylinder contents constitute the high pressure component of the anesthesia delivery system. After they connect to the hangar yoke via the pin-index safety system, their contents flow through a filter, past a check valve and to a Bourdon pressure gauge. Once inside the machine, this high pressure is reduced by the cylinder pressure regulator (the first stage regulator) (Figures 7–2 and 7–3). ASTM dictates that each gas supplied to the machine at high pressure have at least one pressure-reducing regulator. The pressure in the low pressure chamber of the regulator is set so that the machine preferentially seeks gas from the pipeline supply when the pipeline supply pressure is 50 psig or greater. Confirmation of the

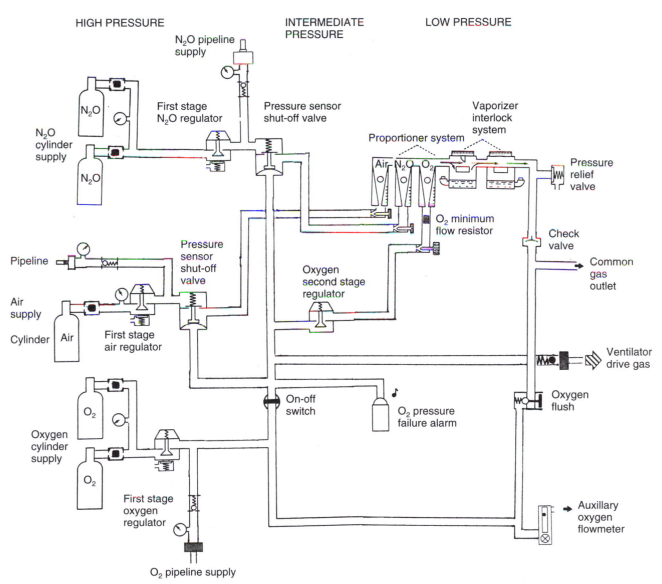

Figure 7–2 The internal components of an anesthesia delivery system with oxygen, air, and nitrous oxide, two vaporizers, and an auxiliary oxygen flowmeter. (Redrawn by permission from American Society of Anesthesiologists. *Check-Out: A Guide for Preoperative Inspection of an Anesthesia Machine,* 1987. ASA, 520 N. Northwest, Park Ridge, IL 60068-2573. Component parts reproduced with permission from Cicman and colleagues, courtesy of North America Drager.[13])

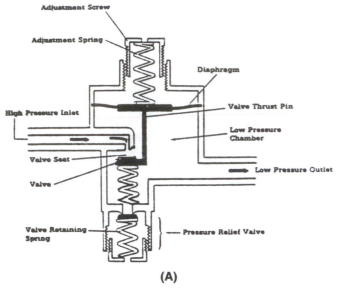

(A)

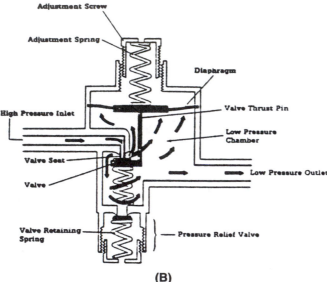

(B)

Figure 7–3 First stage regulator. It regulates the high pressure from the cylinders down to an intermediate pressure (50 psig). The springs and screws are set at the factory to control the amount of pressure in the low pressure chamber. There is a dynamic interplay between the valve thrust pin, the diaphragm, and the valve and valve seat to maintain a constant amount of pressure in the low pressure chamber. As the pressure reaches maximum, the valve seat closes (*B*). As the pressure declines, the valve moves off the valve seat to allow more high pressure gas in (*A*).[6] (Reproduced and redrawn by permission from Bowie and Huffman.[6])

function of the first stage regulator occurs when an oxygen flow of 2 L/min is restored to 2 ± 0.1 L/min within 2 seconds after each operation of the oxygen flush.[3] If the pipeline supply pressure decreases below 50 psig and the cylinders are open, the gas supply with the highest pressure services the machine. An acceptable forward flow through the regulator will be less than 10 mL/min when the outlet pressure is 50 psig.[3] Cylinder pressure regulators have safeguards to protect patients, personnel, and the anesthesia machine from barotrauma. A safety relief valve vents excessive pressure out of

regulator. This relief valve opens if the pressure exceeds four times the delivery pressure (4×50 to 55 psig) or if the cylinder pressure is 50% greater than normal. The diaphragm should rupture without causing hazard to the environment at 400 psig but should not rupture at 200 psig.[3]

AUXILIARY OXYGEN FLOWMETER

Contemporary anesthesia machines include an auxiliary oxygen flowmeter to administer oxygen during local, monitored anesthesia care (MAC), or regional anesthesia. The auxiliary oxygen flowmeter is operational when there is oxygen pressure supplied to the machine as it bypasses the on/off switch. The approximate fraction inspired oxygen (F_iO_2) is estimated by adding 3 percentage points to 21% for each liter delivered. For example, 1 L/min = 24% oxygen, 2 L/min = 27% and 3 L/min = 30% oxygen.[12] There are no ASTM standards for these flowmeters.

OXYGEN FLUSH VALVE

The oxygen flush valve is operational when the machine has a source of oxygen pressure. It is located in the *intermediate pressure* portion of the machine (Figures 7–2 and 7–4). ASTM standards originate from the ANSI Z-79 document. Oxygen flush valves are permanently marked and manually operated with self-closing construction. The actuating device has no more than one position when the valve is closed and is designed to prevent accidental activation. Operation occurs with a single rapid motion. When oxygen pressure is supplied at 50 psig, the output is *35 to 75 L/min*.[3] This flow rate was initially determined by what the machine could deliver and what the lung could tolerate (J.A. Dorsch, personal communication, 1991). The output flows to the common gas outlet without passing through a vaporizer during use. The pumping effect on the vaporizer should be minimized and pressure in the vaporizer should not increase more than 100 cm H_2O above its normal working pressure.[3] There is no allowable leak rate. Barotrauma has been reported from the oxygen flush and care should be taken in activating it when the reservoir bag is not included in the circle system.[5]

MASTER ON/OFF SWITCH

Components linked to the on/off switch include the O_2 sensor/shut off valve, the O_2 pressure failure alarm system, the second stage regulator (Ohmeda machines only), and the flow to the flowmeters.[13] Electronic alarms such as the oxygen analyzer, the airway pressure monitor, and the respiratory volume monitor connect to this switch.[3] The inclusion of the on/off switch prevents anesthetists from giving a hypoxic mixture without also turning on alarms to warn against hypoxia. Components that may be used without turning the machine on are the oxygen flush and the auxiliary oxygen flowmeter. ASTM standard requires the electronic alarms activated by the master switch to be either high, medium, or low priority. A high priority alarm requires immediate opera-

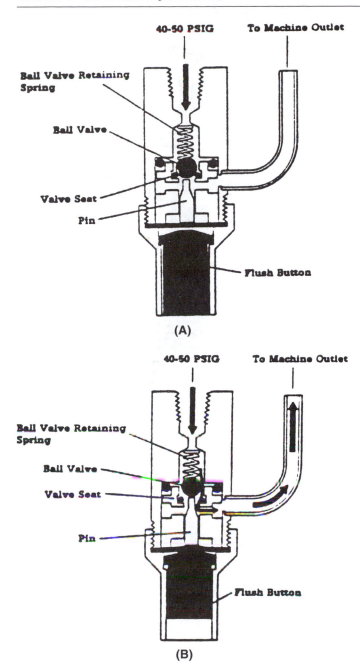

Figure 7–4 Oxygen flush valve. When the flush button is not activated, the 40 to 50 psig is kept behind the ball valve and valve seat (*A*). When the flush button is pushed, the pin pushes against the ball valve and this compresses the ball valve retaining spring. An opening is created around the O-rings to allow oxygen to flow to the machine outlet (*B*). When the anesthetist releases the button, the spring causes the oxygen to stop flowing.[6] (Reproduced by permission from Bowie and Huffman.[6])

tor response. A medium priority alarm requires prompt response. A low priority alarm requires operator awareness of a condition. Each different priority alarm has different visual and audible indicators. All audible indicators should be automatically reset when the alarm condition has resolved. Silencing a high or medium priority alarm is possible, but only for 120 seconds.[3]

VENTILATOR CONNECTOR

The oxygen in the intermediate pressure portion of the machine acts as the primary driving gas of the ventilator. Most modern ventilators require a pneumatic driving gas for bellows compression and electronics for the controls and alarms. These are enabled by the master switch as well as ventilator on/off switch. ASTM standards require that the ventilator connector have a check valve to prevent retrograde gas flow.[3]

SECOND STAGE REGULATOR

Ohmeda machines use second stage regulators for both oxygen and nitrous oxide. The oxygen second stage regulator reduces the intermediate pressure of 50 psig down to about 16 psig. The second stage nitrous oxide regulator reduces the intermediate pressure of 50 psig to about 26 psig. This occurs prior to the gases entering the flowmeters. Figure 7–2 contains a second stage regulator for oxygen only. Second stage regulators offer a more consistent supply of gas to the flowmeters and diminish bobbing of flowmeter floats as the pipeline pressure may vary.[6] ASTM defines second stage regulators as regulators in a series; therefore, the same standards apply as for first stage regulators. Because these regulators work at an intermediate to low pressure, there is no need for a safety relief valve. Second stage regulators, when they are present, divide the intermediate pressure portion of the machine from the low pressure portion of the machine. Drager machines do not use second stage regulators. The internal components of their machines exist at an intermediate pressure.

INTERNAL PIPING

The internal piping is usually metal and must withstand four times the intended service pressure without rupture (4×50 psig).[5] ASTM standards require that connections are either noninterchangeable or that the piping is labeled at each junction. Leakage should not exceed 10 mL/min at 50 psig (normal service pressure).[3]

PRESSURE SENSOR/SHUT-OFF VALVE

This component senses pressure (oxygen) and shuts off nitrous oxide or any other gases if there is inadequate (oxygen) pressure. It is the first component that makes the nitrous oxide or the air supply dependent on adequate oxygen supply (Figures 7–2 and 7–5). ASTM standards originate from the Z-79 document of the American National Standards Institute (ANSI). Whenever oxygen supply pressure is reduced from 'normal' and until flow ceases, the set oxygen concentration should not decrease at the common gas outlet. Each manufacturer of anesthesia machines must specify what 'normal' pressure is and must explain this device's performance in their operator manual.[3] This device is commonly called the 'fail-safe'. Remember that it senses pressure only. It does not

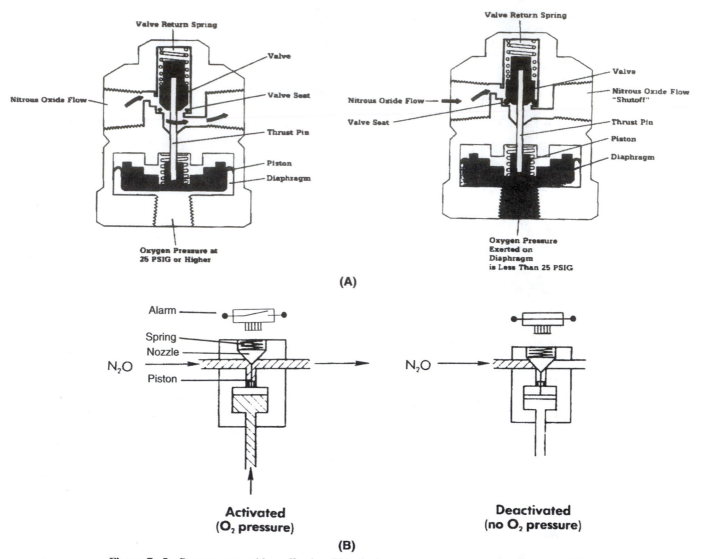

Figure 7–5 Pressure sensor/shut-off valve. This device connects oxygen to any other gas delivered to the anesthesia machine and will not allow other gases to flow unless there is sufficient oxygen pressure. In the Ohmeda device (*A*), the oxygen pressure pushes on a diaphragm, which pushes the pin up to allow N_2O to flow past the valve seat. If the oxygen pressure is less than 25 psig, the diaphragm falls. This causes the valve to rest on the valve seat and closes the channel where N_2O flows.[6] (Reproduced by permission from Bowie and Huffman.[6]) In the Drager device (*B*), the oxygen pressure pushes a piston up and causes the nozzle to compress the spring. If the oxygen supply pressure decreases, so does the piston. If there is no oxygen pressure, the nozzle closes the channel where N_2O flows. The electronic alarm system is also depicted. The alarm circuitry remains open when there is adequate oxygen pressure. If oxygen pressure is zero, the circuitry closes and activates an alarm.[13] (Illustration courtesy of North American Drager. Reproduced by permission from *Narkomed 2A Anesthesia System.* Technical Service Manual. Telford, PA: North American Drager; 1985 and Cicman and colleagues.[13])

sense oxygen. It does not sense flow. If another gas besides oxygen exerts 50 psig pressure in this device, its requirements are met and it allows nitrous oxide to flow to the flowmeters.

OXYGEN SUPPLY FAILURE ALARM

If oxygen supply pressure does decrease, there is an internal alarm to warn the anesthetist. This connects to the on/off switch and is pneumatically controlled with the oxygen sup-

ply. The Ohmeda device resembles a can of hairspray and is illustrated in Figure 7–6. The Drager alarm is electronic but is controlled by pneumatics. The electronic switch above the spring in Figure 7–5*B* illustrates the function of this alarm. When oxygen supply pressure is adequate, the electronic switch is open. If oxygen pressure is inadequate, the switch closes and an alarm message sounds and appears on the alarm panel.[13] ASTM standards require that whenever oxygen supply pressure decreases below a manufacturer's specified threshold, a medium priority alarm should enunciate

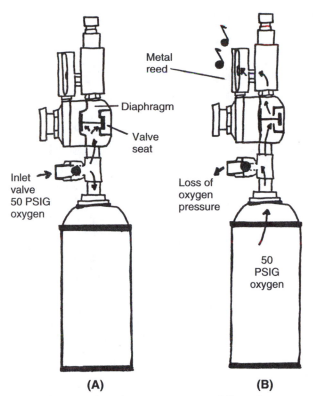

Figure 7–6   The Ohmeda oxygen pressure failure alarm system. When the machine is pressurized with 50 psig oxygen (*A*), the canister also fills via the inlet valve.[6] An equal pressure in the canister and the machine holds the ball bearing in equilibrium. The pressure also compresses the diaphragm that closes the channel at the valve seat. If oxygen pressure decreases in the machine (*B*), the higher pressure in the canister pushes the ball bearing to close the inlet valve. This decline in pressure relaxes the diaphragm and opens the channel at the valve seat. The high pressure oxygen rushes up through the valve seat and is released via a metal reed. This causes an audible alarm. (Redrawn by permission from Bowie and Huffman.[6])

within 5 seconds. That alarm can be silenced for 120 seconds, but it should automatically reset and resound if the condition is not remedied. It also resets after the restoration of oxygen supply pressure above the alarm threshold.[3]

FLOWMETERS

Flowmeters meter the flow of medical gases to the patient and are the beginning of the *low pressure* portion of the machine (Figure 7–7). They receive gas at either an intermediate pressure (Drager about 48 psig); or a low pressure (Ohmeda about 16 to 26 psig) depending on the presence of a second stage regulator.[10] Once compressed gas flows to the flowmeter, gas pressure changes to gas flow. The gas is still compressed in the flowmeter, but at a much lower value (2 to 5 psig for Ohmeda; 18 psig for Drager).[10] Flow is controlled by the flow control knob and measured in liters per minute. From this point on, flow is important and measurement of pressure will be in centimeters water.

Flowmeters used in anesthesia machines consist of a Pyrex glass tube called a Thorpe tube. It is pin indexed to a hand-calibrated scale and a socket in the flowmeter bank to ensure the proper tube and scale are matched to each medical gas. There is a specific float matched to the tube, scale, and gas based on the physical characteristics of the gas and the weight of the float.[5] The float may be an aluminum triangular device (Ohmeda) or a sapphire-coated ball type (Drager). The Ohmeda float is read at the top. The Drager float is read in the middle. There are 'stops' inside the Thorpe tube to stop the float from obstructing flow at either end, to prevent the float from damaging the tube, and to give the float a spot to rest to keep it in the correct orientation when there is no flow. There may be 'stops' on the flow control knob to stop anesthetists from turning the knob completely off.[6] This prevents damage to the Teflon needle valve and may provide a mechanism for minimum oxygen flow when the machine is turned on (Ohmeda).[6] Drager uses a resistor device to provide a minimum oxygen flow. The minimum oxygen flow is 150 to 250 mL/min.[13] Manufacturers incorporate this to prevent hypoxia. Any time the anesthesia machine is on, it will deliver at least basal metabolic oxygen for an adult.

The annular space exists between the float and the internal surface of the Thorpe tube. This is the area where gas flow occurs in the flowmeter. The anesthesia flowmeter is a variable orifice flowmeter because the annular space of the tube varies. The smallest annular space is at the bottom of the tube and the largest annular space is at the top. Because of the variable orifice, the annular space increases as the float rises higher in the tube, as it would in high flows. Because of this characteristic, these flowmeters are constant pressure flowmeters. The pressure drop (comparing P1 to P2) that occurs across the constriction (the float) is constant for all positions of the float.[5]

The characteristics that determine flow through the flowmeter differ for low and high flows. At low flows, gas flow is mainly laminar as the annular space has the characteristics of a tube (length greater than width). In laminar flow, gas flows from a region of higher pressure to lower pressure. The rate of flow depends on the pressure difference and the resistance to flow between the regions. The *Poiseuille-Hagan* formula explains the variables in flow of a long narrow tube (the tubular annular space). Flow is directly proportional to the pressure drop along the length of the tube and to the fourth power of the radius of the tube. Flow is inversely proportional to the length of the tube and to the viscosity of the gas.[14] The viscosity of the gas determines the resistance to flow. Because there are intermolecular forces operating within the gas, the velocity of flow of the layers of the gas are different. Gas flowing adjacent to the sides of the flowmeter has a decreased velocity due to frictional resistance of the tube. The gas flowing in the middle of the flow-tube has the greatest velocity because it encounters less resistance to flow. This gives the characteristic parabolic model of laminar flow. The resistance to flow varies for each medical gas because their viscosity values differ.[9]

As flow rate increases, the orderly parabolic laminar flow breaks down and the gas molecules start swirling in eddies and convert to turbulent flow. This change occurs at a point

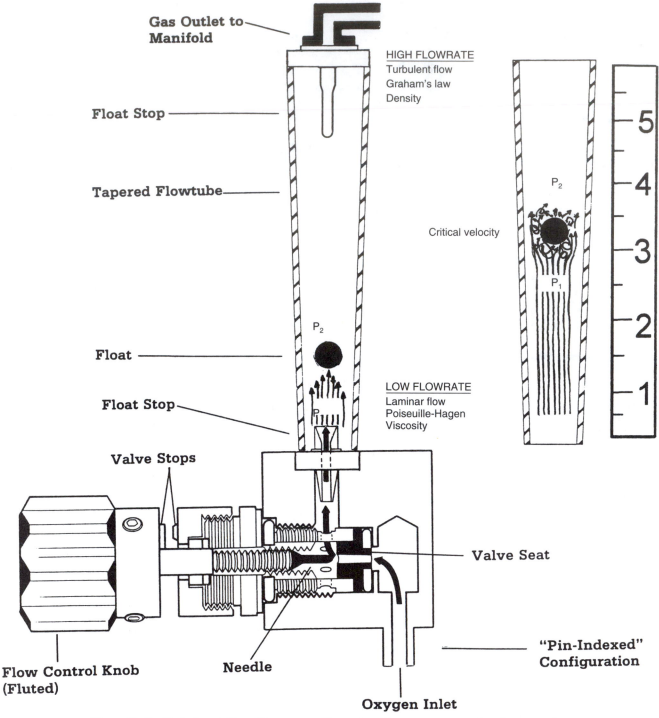

Figure 7–7 Typical variable orifice oxygen flowmeter. Flowmeters are made of a tapered Thorpe tube, are pin indexed, and have a hand-calibrated scale. Note the stops inside the tube and on the flow control knob. These are termed constant pressure flowmeters because the pressure drop (P1 compared to P2) across the constriction (the float) is constant for all positions of the float. This is due to the annular space increasing in size from the bottom to the top of the tube.[5,6] (Redrawn and reproduced by permission from Bowie and Huffman.[6] Schreiber P. *Safety Guidelines for Anesthesia Systems*. Telford, PA: North American Drager; 1985.)

called the *critical velocity*. The Reynolds number calculates the probability of turbulent flow. The variables in this calculation include the diameter of the tube, the velocity of the flow, the viscosity of the gas and the density of the gas.[9] When the float is high in the flowmeter, the annular space resembles an orifice (width greater than length) and the flow through it becomes turbulent. At higher flow rates, when flow is turbulent, the primary determinant of flow is the density of the gas. Graham's law explains that when flow is turbulent, the diffusion of a gas is indirectly proportional to the square root of the density of the gas. The density of a gas is a measure of the mass of a unit volume of the gas or the molecular weight of the gas.[14] The heavier a molecule is, the harder it is for it to flow. The density values for the medical gases differ; therefore, flowmeters are calibrated for each medical gas based on their viscosity and density.[9]

Accuracy varies from low to high flows. Up to a 70% deviation is possible at flows less than 1 L/min.[10] This is the reason for flowmeters in tandem. Flow control for up to 1 L/min is provided by a fine flowmeter. Then the flow overflows into the coarse flowmeter for higher flows. Accuracy decreases when dust or dirt accumulates on the float. This alters the annular space and causes increased resistance to flow, especially at low flows where the annular space is narrow. Static electricity has been reported in flowmeters with metal floats. Dirt or static electricity causes erratic movement or sticking of the float. Additional filters reside in the flowmeter housing to diminish dust accumulation from the nonsterile medical gases.[5]

Theoretically, changes in temperature affect both viscosity and to a lesser degree density of the gases. Both increase at low temperatures and decrease at high temperatures. Clinically, changes in room temperature do not significantly alter flowmeter accuracy.[5] Changes in atmospheric pressure affect the accuracy of flowmeters at high flows because at high flows, the density of the gas is the primary determinant of flow. Low flow rates are not affected by changes in atmospheric pressure because at low flows, flow is determined primarily by the viscosity of the gas. Flowmeters must be calibrated at the barometric pressure that they will operate in to be accurate.[15]

The ASTM standards require one, visible flow-control system for each medical gas adjacent to the gas flowmeter it controls. The flowmeter knobs are color coded and labeled with the name of the gas. The oxygen knob is fluted, larger and protrudes farther out than the round, knurled nitrous oxide and air knobs. The knobs design prevents disassembly when rotated. When the supply gas is 50 psig, flowmeters should be accurate to within ±10% of the setting or ±10 mL/min, whichever is greater. The leak rate should be no more than 5 mL/min.[3]

The oxygen flowmeter is closest to the patient (downstream), so there is a lower likelihood of a leak producing a hypoxic mixture.[16] Flowmeters are the most delicate component of the anesthesia machine and have a high incidence of leaks. The output of all the flowmeters communicate at the top of the flowmeter bank and a leak in one flowmeter will cause a leak in the whole machine.[16]

PROPORTIONING SYSTEM

Proportioning systems decrease the likelihood of delivery of a hypoxic mixture. Oxygen and nitrous oxide interface either mechanically or pneumatically with an electronic alarm so that the minimum oxygen concentration at the common gas outlet is not less than 25%. The ratio of nitrous oxide to oxygen should be approximately 3 : 1 (Figure 7–8). These devices are not completely protective against the possibility of a hypoxic mixture under the following conditions: (1) if a gas other than oxygen is present in the oxygen pipeline; (2) if

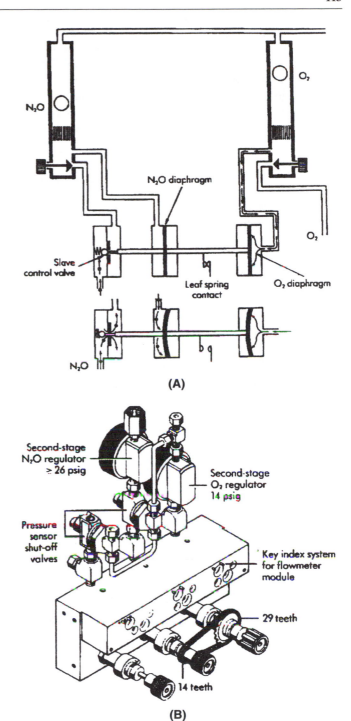

Figure 7–8 Schematics of proportioning systems. The Drager system (*A*) uses resistors in the oxygen and nitrous oxide flowmeters. These resistors cause a back pressure to be communicated to the oxygen and nitrous oxide chambers to compress the respective diaphragms. If oxygen pressure is adequate, the pin opens the nitrous oxide slave control valve and nitrous oxide is allowed to flow. If oxygen pressure is insufficient, the nitrous oxide slave control valve is closed and the leaf spring contact connects to cause an alarm.[13] The Ohmeda system (*B*) is a mechanical linkage of the flow control knobs of the oxygen and nitrous oxide. If the oxygen is decreased, the chain linkage decreases the nitrous oxide also. If the nitrous oxide is increased, the chain linkage also increases the oxygen.[10] (Reproduced by permission from Schrieber P. *Safety Guidelines for Anesthesia Systems*, Telford, PA: North American Drager; 1985. Ohmeda Link 25 Proportion Limiting System reproduced by permission from Ohmeda, A BOC Health Care Company, Madison, WI.)

the mechanical linkage or the resistors and diaphragms are defective, the ratio may not be maintained; (3) a leak downstream of these devices can exist; or (4) if a third gas such as helium, nitrogen, or carbon dioxide is administered, oxygen may be diluted. Presently, proportioning systems link only oxygen and nitrous oxide.[16] Failures of these devices have been reported.[17-20] The use of an oxygen analyzer cannot be overemphasized.

VAPORIZERS

A vaporizer accurately enriches the gas mixture with anesthetic agent that eventually reaches the brain and induces the anesthetic state. The partial pressure required to induce anesthesia varies with each agent as does the vapor pressure. For example, the $pMAC_1$ (the partial pressure in the brain at a concentration of 1 MAC) is 5.7 mm Hg for halothane, yet the vapor pressure of this agent at 20°C is 243 mm Hg[21] (Table 7-1). The *vapor pressure* is defined as the amount of pressure the vapor of a volatile liquid agent exerts on the walls of a closed container at 20°C and 760 mm Hg atmospheric pressure. When the vapor phase above the liquid contains all the molecules that it can hold at that temperature, it is saturated. If a closed container contains oxygen and isoflurane in equilibrium, the percent of isoflurane existing as a vapor is calculated by dividing the vapor pressure of isoflurane (239 mm Hg) by atmospheric pressure (760 mm Hg) or $239 \div 760 = 32\%$. The vapor pressure of each agent is *independent* of atmospheric pressure and depends only on the agents' physical characteristics and the ambient temperature.[22] As

the temperature rises, the vapor pressure rises. When the temperature rises, it is easier for the liquid molecules to escape to the vapor phase and exert pressure on the walls of the closed container. The vapor pressure of isoflurane at 20°C is 243 mm Hg, but at 30°C it is about 350 mm Hg.[23]

Anesthetic agents are volatile, meaning they change readily and rapidly into a vapor.[24] The process of converting a liquid into a vapor is called *vaporization*. It requires heat as the molecules of a liquid exhibit van der Waals' forces that cause attraction and cohesion.[8,9] The heat necessary for vaporization represents the energy necessary to overcome the van der Waals' forces. The *latent heat of vaporization* is defined as the number of calories required to change 1 gm of liquid into a vapor.[9] Without a source of heat, the liquid cools and vaporization ceases.[16]

Concepts Important in Design   Most of the concepts important in the design of vaporizers center on supplying heat for vaporization and compensating for temperature changes to maintain a constant vapor pressure. The *thermal heat capacity* of a substance is the amount of heat required to raise the temperature of 1 g of the substance by 1°C at atmospheric pressure. Another term often erroneously used interchangeably with thermal capacity is specific heat. The *specific heat* of a substance is the ratio of the quantity of heat required to raise the temperature of 1 g of the substance to the quantity required to raise the temperature of a unit mass of water 1°C.[22] The specific heat value for an inhalation agent is important because it indicates how much heat must be supplied to the liquid to maintain a constant temperature

Table 7-1
VAPORIZERS AND VAPORIZATION

	Halothane	Enflurane	Isoflurane	Sevoflurane	Desflurane
$pMAC_1$[†] (mm Hg) MAC × 760	.75 × 760 = 5.7 mm Hg	1.68 × 760 = 12.8 mm Hg	1.15 × 760 = 8.7 mm Hg	1.7 × 760 = 12.9[1] mm Hg	6.0 × 760 = 45.6[2] mm Hg 7.25 × 760 = 55.1[2] mm Hg
Vapor pressure @ 20° C ml vapor per ml liquid @ 20° C	243 mm Hg 226 mL	175 mm Hg 196 mL	238 mm Hg 195 mL	160 mm Hg 182 mL	664 mm Hg 207 mL
Splitting ratio* 1%	46:1 $\frac{98\%}{2\%}$	29:1 $\frac{96\%}{3\%}$	44:1 $\frac{98\%}{2\%}$	25:1 $\frac{96\%}{4\%}$	
2%	22:1 $\frac{95\%}{4\%}$	14:1 $\frac{93\%}{6\%}$	21:1 $\frac{95\%}{5\%}$	12:1 $\frac{92\%}{8\%}$	
3%	14:1 $\frac{93\%}{6\%}$	9:1 $\frac{90\%}{10\%}$	14:1 $\frac{93\%}{6\%}$	7:1 $\frac{88\%}{12\%}$	
Latent heat of vaporization cal/g	35 cal/g	41 cal/g	41 cal/g		

* $\frac{\%bypass - vaporizer}{\%vaporizing - chamber}$

[†]divided by 100 to eliminate volumes %.
[1]Katoh T, Ikeda K. The Minimum Alveolar Concentration (MAC) of Sevoflurane in Humans. *Anesthesiology* 1987;66:301.
[2]Rampil IJ, Lockhart SH, Zwass MS, et al. Clinical Characteristics of Desflurane in Surgical Patients: Minumum Alveolar Concentration. *Anesthesiology* 1991;74:429.

as heat is lost during vaporization.[16] Manufacturers select metals for vaporizer construction that have a moderately high specific heat to minimize the temperature changes during vaporization.[11,16] Materials with a high specific heat change temperature more gradually than those with a low specific heat.[5]

Some substances pass heat on from molecule to molecule more readily than others. This phenomena (conduction) is extremely important in vaporizers. The thermal conductivity is a measure of how quickly heat is conducted through a substance. It is measured as the quantity of heat in calories conducted through a square centimeter at a temperature difference of 1°C per second.[22] The higher the thermal conductivity, the better the substance conducts heat.[5] Vaporizers are constructed from metals chosen for their specific heat and thermal conductivity values, as well as their cost. Modern vaporizers are constructed of brass coated with copper and nickel with a chromium plating. Although other metals (silver and platinum) have more desirable specific heat and thermal conductivity, their cost is prohibitive.[11]

Because of the importance of temperature on the vapor pressure of an agent, the vaporizer's design incorporates a means for temperature compensation. Older Copper Kettle or Vernitrol vaporizers did not provide a mechanism for temperature compensation. Their design included a thermometer and anesthetists factored the vapor pressure as related to the ambient temperature in the equation for the vaporizer output.

A higher temperature means a higher vapor pressure in the vaporizing chamber. The anesthetist altered the vaporizer flow or the carrier gas flow to ensure correct output at the prevailing temperature. Compare the percent output concentration at different temperatures in the equations in Table 7–2. A higher temperature leads to more molecules in the vapor phase and therefore, a higher percent concentration output. This type of vaporizer is classified as a 'measured flow'[5] vaporizer because the method of regulating the output concentration is determined by the carrier gas flow and the measured flow through the vaporizer. A separate flowmeter flows to the vaporizer to bubble through the liquid agent, becomes saturated with the anesthetic, and then mixes with the carrier gas flow. The resulting output concentration depends on each of the variables in the equation.

Most contemporary vaporizers use an internal device for temperature compensation or supply heat to the vaporizer. A device for temperature compensation responds to changes in temperature and alters the flow of carrier gas to the vaporizing chamber. The vaporizing chamber is the reservoir where the liquid anesthetic resides. The area above the liquid is saturated with vapor molecules because the agent is a volatile liquid. As carrier gas enters the chamber, it flows over the liquid, becomes saturated with vapor, and carries the anesthetic out. This changes the equilibrium of molecules in the vaporizing chamber. More molecules of the liquid vaporize and saturate the area above the liquid. This process continues

Table 7–2
MEASURED FLOW VAPORIZER EQUATION

$$\% \text{ output concentration} = \frac{(PV)(FV)}{(Pb - PV)(Fd + FV)} \times 100^1$$

PV = vapor pressure of anesthetic (mm Hg)
Pb = barometric pressure (mm Hg)
FV = oxygen flow to the vaporizer (L/min)
Fd = diluent flow (total flow) (L/min)

Isoflurane vapor pressure @ 20° C = 238 mm Hg
Barometric pressure @ sea level = 760 mm Hg
Oxygen flow to vaporizer = 100 cc = .1 L/min
Total flow of carrier gas = 5 L/min

$$\% \text{ output concentration} = \frac{(238)(.1)}{(760 - 238)(5 + .1)} \times 100$$

$$\% \text{ output concentration} = \frac{23.80}{2662.20} \times 100$$

$$\% \text{ output concentration} = 1.0$$

The vapor pressure of isoflurane is approximately 350 mm Hg at 30° C. Substitute this vapor pressure in the equation to determine how the % output concentration will be affected by increases in temperature.

$$\% \text{ output concentration} = \frac{(350)(.1)}{(760 - 350)(5 + .1)} \times 100$$

$$\% \text{ output concentration} = \frac{35.0}{2091} \times 100$$

$$\% \text{ output concentration} = 2.0$$

SOURCE: Cooper JB, Newbower RS, Welch JP, Dedrick DF, Gevirtz CM: Preparation for anesthesia. In: Firestone LL, Lebowitz PW, Cook CE, eds. *Clinical procedures of the Massachusetts General Hospital.* Boston: Little, Brown and Company; 1988:97–127.

as long as energy is available for vaporization. This type of vaporizer is termed a 'variable bypass' – 'flow over'[5] vaporizer because the method for regulating the output concentration is determined by the amount of gas flow that bypasses the vaporizing chamber as compared to the amount of carrier gas that flows over the vaporizing chamber. It is also termed 'concentration calibrated'[5] as the output concentration is calibrated in volumes percent. This output concentration is stable over a range of ordinary room temperatures due to the temperature compensating device. If the temperature increases, the device decreases flow to the vaporizing chamber. This causes less vapor molecules to be carried out. If the temperature decreases, more carrier gas enters the vaporizing chamber, and carries more vapor out. The device is constructed of materials that change as the temperature changes (Figure 7–9). The most common types of temperature compensating mechanisms are: (1) the bimetallic strip[25] or (2) the bellows expansion element.[26] The temperature compensating mechanisms work by controlling the ratio of carrier gas flow that bypasses the vaporizer to the amount of carrier gas flow that enters the vaporizing chamber. This is termed the splitting ratio.[21] Temperature changes alter the splitting ratio to allow for accurate percent concentration output at variable temperatures.[10]

There are advantages to both types of vaporizers. Although a concentration-calibrated vaporizer may be simpler to use, it is agent specific because of the complexity of its design. The percent concentration output is different if it is incorrectly filled or if agents are mixed. The error is especially noticeable when an agent with a vastly different vapor pressure is introduced. For example, the error in percent concentration output is greatest when halothane or isoflurane is placed in an enflurane vaporizer or when enflurane is placed in a halothane or isoflurane vaporizer.[27,28] This is primarily due to the difference between the vapor pressure of enflurane as compared to halothane and isoflurane. This difference is estimated by dividing the vapor pressure of the liquid by the vapor pressure of the vaporizer and comparing to 1%. For example, if enflurane is put in an isoflurane vaporizer: $175 \div 239 = .7\%$. A lower concentration than expected results. If isoflurane is placed in an enflurane vaporizer: $239 \div 175 = 1.4\%$. A higher than expected concentration results. The new agent, sevoflurane, is closer to enflurane with regard to vapor pressure; therefore, the same error in percent concentration output would possibly occur between halothane or isoflurane and sevoflurane. In contrast, the older vaporizers are not agent specific. Because of their simple design, it is possible to use them to vaporize any anesthetic (except desflurane). Knowledge of each variable in the equation is all that is necessary to deliver a known percent concentration of the agent.

The amount of vapor picked up by the carrier gas flow depends on the vapor pressure of the agent and the efficiency of vaporization. When the vapor pressure is high, more molecules of anesthetic exist in the vapor phase and therefore, more are carried away. Efficiency of vaporization is increased by two factors: (1) increasing the surface area of the

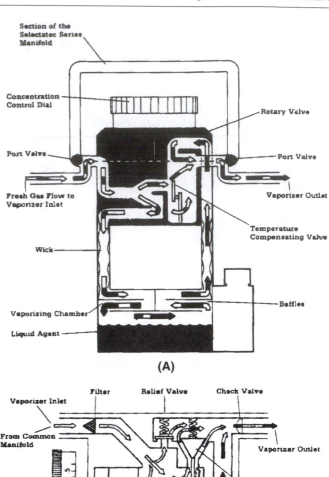

(A)

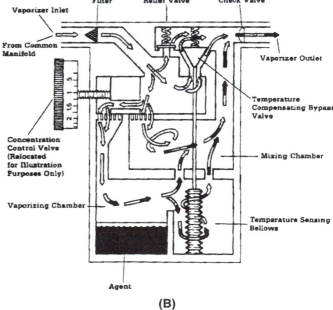

(B)

Figure 7–9 Temperature compensating devices. In *A*, the device is a bimetallic strip that bends in response to changes in temperature. In *B*, a bellows expansion unit expands or contracts due to changes in temperature. These changes alter the amount of gas bypassing the vaporizing chamber.[6] (Reproduced by permission from Bowie and Huffman.[6])

gas–liquid interface and (2) decreasing the velocity of the carrier gas flow.[5] The efficiency of the measured flow vaporizer increases when the liquid is deep and the gas bubbles are small. Both of these increase the surface area for vaporization. The efficiency of the concentration-calibrated vaporizer increases when wicks and baffles are in the vaporizer (see Figure 7–9A). The wicks typically hold 125 cc of agent. The carrier gas flows around the wicks and picks up more agent. The baffles take the carrier gas flow closer to the liquid where it can pick up the agent at the liquid–vapor surface. Baffles decrease the likelihood of liquid agent flowing out of the vaporizing chamber if the vaporizer is tipped. Liquid agent in the outflow tract leads to overdose as 1 cc of agent produces about 200 cc vapor. Efficiency of both types of vaporizers increases when the carrier gas flow velocity is decreased. Time is required to establish equilibrium between the liquid and the vapor. If the flow of gas is too fast, this equilibrium is not achieved and the percent concentration output is decreased.[5]

Because the carrier gas flow is compressed gas, the vaporizers are slightly pressurized. They are termed plenum for this reason.[5] They depend on a known smaller constant flow of compressed gas to overcome the resistance of the flow splitting valve and temperature compensating device. Typical pressure inside a plenum vaporizer is 22 cm H_2O at 5 L/min.[29]

Another type of vaporizer that is concentration calibrated and temperature compensated is called a drawover vaporizer. It is typically used in field anesthesia machines in war, natural disasters, or austere conditions. It is a low resistance vaporizer located in the breathing circuit. The patient's spontaneous breathing draws ambient air over the liquid anesthetic. It is also used with oxygen supplementation, a ventilator, and a scavenger.[30]

A vaporizer that defied standard classification systems was born with desflurane (Figure 7–10). The physical characteristics of desflurane demanded a vaporizer that could contain this highly volatile agent. With a boiling point close to room temperature (23.5°C) and a vapor pressure at 20°C close to one atmosphere (664 mm Hg), this agent wants to vaporize. To store desflurane in a closed container at room temperature requires pressure. The bottle of desflurane is pressurized up to 80 psig and has a spring-loaded opening device.[5] Heating the liquid maintains a constant vapor pressure and prevents condensation as the agent travels through the vaporizer. Pressurizing the agent keeps it in a liquid form. This pressure creates a condition in which desflurane becomes less volatile, less easily vaporized. Pressurization eliminates the possibility of desflurane boiling at clinically useful temperatures.[31]

Factors That Affect Vaporizer Output   Although temperature is the only factor that affects the vapor pressure of an agent, many factors affect the percent concentration output of a vaporizer. These include the carrier gas flow rate and composition, intermittent back pressure, and atmospheric pressure (Table 7–3).

The percent concentration output of variable bypass vaporizers is less than the dial setting at flow rates less than 250 mL/min. This is due to the high specific gravity (density) of the liquid agent. Low flows do not generate adequate pressure to reach the vaporizing chamber.[16] The gas–liquid surface area is decreased and less vapor is picked up. *The percent concentration output is less than the dial setting at flow rates greater than 15 L/min.* There is inadequate time for the flow rate to become saturated with vapor when the flows are

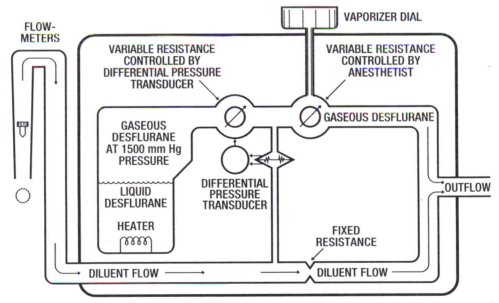

Figure 7–10   Schematic of the desflurane vaporizer. Diluent flow from the flowmeter enters and meets a fixed resistance. The resultant gas pressure is measured at the differential pressure transducer. The pressure difference controls the variable resistance and maintains a zero pressure differential between the desflurane and the diluent gas flow. The desflurane liquid is held in a heated and pressurized sump. The diluent gas flow does not enter the vaporizing chamber. The amount of desflurane vapor that exits the sump is controlled by the pressure regulating valve and the vaporizer dial. The anesthetist controls the vaporizer dial. The gaseous desflurane mixes with the diluent gas flow in the outflow tract. (Reproduced by permission from Eger EI. *Desflurane: A Compendium and Reference.* Liberty Corner, NJ: Anaquest, A BOC Health Care Company; 1993.)

Table 7–3
CHANGES IN ATMOSPHERIC PRESSURE AND CONCENTRATION CALIBRATED, VARIABLE BYPASS VAPORIZERS

For this exercise, halothane will be given at 20°C at 1% with a total flow of 4700 mL carrier gas. A comparison will be made between sea level (760 mm Hg), high altitude (500 mm Hg), and low altitude (2280 mm Hg).

1. Determine the splitting ratio for 1% halothane. This is 46:1. That means that there are 47 total parts entering the vaporizer. To deliver 1% halothane, 46 parts bypass the vaporizing chamber (4600 mL) and 1 part (100 mL) enters the vaporizing chamber and picks up the saturated halothane vapor. The vapor pressure of halothane at 20°C is 243 mm Hg.

Sea level 760 mm Hg	High altitude 500 mm Hg	Low altitude 2280 mm Hg

2. Calculate the volume percent of agent in the vaporizing chamber (Vapor pressure ÷ atmospheric pressure).

243 mm Hg ÷ 760 mm Hg = 32%	243 mm Hg ÷ 500 mm Hg = 49%	243 ÷ 2280 mm Hg = 11%

3. Calculate the volume percent of carrier gas in the vaporizing chamber (100 volume %–volume % agent).

100% − 32% = 68 volume %	100% − 49% = 51 volume %	100% − 11% = 89 volume %

4. Calculate the number of mL of agent in the carrier gas
   (100 mL ÷ volume % of carrier gas) × volume % of agent.

(100 mL ÷ 68 vol %) × 32 vol % = 47 mL	(100 mL ÷ 51 vol %) × 49 vol % = 96 mL	(100 mL ÷ 89 vol %) × 11 vol % = 12 mL

5. Calculate the total flow from the vaporizer in mL
   (mL in bypass chamber + mL in vaporizing chamber + mL agent leaving vaporizing chamber).

4600 + 100 + 47 = 4747 mL	4600 + 100 + 96 = 4796 mL	4600 + 100 + 12 = 4712 mL

6. Calculate the volume % halothane leaving the vaporizer (mL agent ÷ total flow leaving vaporizer).

47 mL ÷ 4747 mL = .009 = .99%	96 mL ÷ 4796 mL = .02 = 2%	12 mL ÷ 4712 mL = .0025 = .25%

7. Calculate the partial pressure of the agent in mm Hg leaving the vaporizer
   (% agent leaving vaporizer × atmospheric pressure).

.009 × 760 = 7.52 mm Hg	.02 × 500 = 10.0 mm Hg	.0025 × 2280 = 5.7 mm Hg

8. Calculate the actual anesthetic potency (partial pressure ÷ pMAC$_1$).

7.52 ÷ 5.7 = 1.3 MAC	10 ÷ 5.7 = 1.7 MAC	5.7 ÷ 5.7 = 1 MAC

Adapted from Eisenkraft JB.[23]

this high.[16] Most contemporary vaporizers are extremely stable at flows from 2 to 8 L/min while delivering up to 3% agent.[32,33]

The composition of the carrier gas flow influences the percent output concentration because the solubility of nitrous oxide is greater than oxygen or air. When nitrous oxide enters the vaporizing chamber, some dissolves in the liquid agent and the percent concentration output decreases until the liquid is saturated with nitrous oxide. If nitrous oxide is withdrawn, the nitrous oxide gas in the liquid comes out of solution and represents additional gas flow to the vaporizing chamber.[10] If the carrier gas flow is 100% nitrous oxide, the percent concentration output is approximately 10% less than the dial setting for about 15 minutes,[16] then it returns to normal.[10] Because nitrous oxide has lower viscosity than oxygen, there is less resistance to its flow through the vaporizer. When nitrous oxide is the carrier gas flow instead of oxygen, relatively more nitrous oxide flows through the bypass tract. This also results in a lower output concentration. However, at percent concentration outputs used clinically, this phenomenon is insignificant.[16]

Vapor pressure is independent of atmospheric pressure, but

changes in atmospheric pressure affect the percent concentration output of a vaporizer. Vaporizer output is measured clinically in volumes percent and this minimum alveolar concentration (MAC) value is expressed in volumes percent. Volumes percent expresses the relative ratio of gas molecules in a mixture of gases,[10] but this value is only indirectly related to patient uptake and the level of anesthesia.[5] *The amount of agent required in the brain to induce anesthesia is expressed in partial pressure (mm Hg).* This is difficult to measure clinically but important to understand especially when considering the effects of altitude on vaporizer output. The term $pMAC_1$ is used to express the partial pressure of an anesthetic agent at a concentration of 1 MAC. It is obtained by multiplying the MAC and the atmospheric pressure.[21] Anesthetic potency is directly related to partial pressure in the brain, and indirectly to the volumes percent dialed in at the vaporizer.

The following statements are true regarding variable bypass vaporizers and changes in altitude. High altitude (low atmospheric pressure) causes an increase in concentration measured in volumes percent but a less dramatic change in partial pressure measured as $pMAC_1$. Low altitude (high atmospheric pressure) causes a reduction in concentration measured in volumes percent but a less dramatic change in partial pressure measured as $pMAC_1$.[5,23] Changes in atmospheric pressure affect the density of gases and vapors but do not affect the viscosity.[15] Changes in density may affect the splitting ratio slightly.[21] When density increases at high atmospheric pressures, the gases flow less easily through the vaporizer. This causes a lower percent output from the vaporizer. When density decreases at low atmospheric pressures, the gases flow more easily through the vaporizer. This causes a higher percent output from the vaporizer. The effect on partial pressure is less dramatic.[5] Measured flow vaporizers respond to low atmospheric pressure by delivering an increased volumes percent and an increased partial pressure. When atmospheric pressure increases, they deliver a decreased volumes percent and a decreased partial pressure.[15]

The intermittent back pressure that occurs with positive-pressure ventilation and use of the oxygen flush can result in increased percent concentration output from a vaporizer. This is called the *pumping effect*. When this back pressure is transmitted to the vaporizer, it is believed that temporarily, a no-flow state exists in the vaporizer. During this interruption of flow, gas flows back to the bypass tract and the vaporizing chamber. Because the bypass has a smaller volume, more gas flows to the vaporizing chamber. While in the vaporizing chamber, more agent is picked up and therefore, the percent concentration output increases. Changes are more pronounced when there is a low level of agent in the vaporizer, low carrier gas flow (< 3 L/min), the dial setting is low, and the pressure fluctuations are high and frequent.[5]

Some vaporizers have a decreased percent concentration output with positive-pressure ventilation or oxygen flushing. The mechanism for this phenomenon is felt to be a pressurizing effect. Back pressure is transmitted to the vaporizer chamber where it compresses the carrier gas flow. This causes an increase in the number of molecules per milliliter

and pressurizes the vaporizer chamber. This increased pressure will not cause an increase in pick-up of vapor but perhaps a dilution of the carrier gas flow that is saturated with agent. Therefore, a decreased amount of vapor exits the vaporizer. This phenomenon is more common at high flow rates, low vaporizer settings, and large and frequent pressure fluctuations.[5] Perhaps the high flows do not allow adequate time for equilibrium to be achieved in the vaporizer. Between the two, the changes in vaporizer output are greater with the pumping effect and continue to be documented even in modern vaporizers at peak airway pressures above 60 cm H_2O.[34]

Manufacturers publish a specific maintenance schedule for each vaporizer in their operator manuals. These recommendations range from 1 to 5 years for a complete overhaul of the vaporizer with spot checks for accuracy of percent concentration output every 3 to 6 months.[35] It is common for halothane vaporizers to need more frequent cleaning due to the buildup of the preservative thymol. It is a waxy substance that clogs the wicks and reduces the surface area for vaporization. It may also gum up the control dial and possibly interfere with the temperature-compensating device.[29] Because thymol has a high boiling point it does not vaporize. It accumulates during successive fillings of the vaporizer.[11] These problems are eliminated by draining the vaporizer every 2 weeks.[29] Discoloration of halothane is likely caused by halothane free radicals produced by ultraviolet light and ambient ionizing radiation, not thymol. Enflurane and isoflurane have been found to be discolored without associated malfunction due to leaching of hydrocarbons from the plastic wick spacers.[11]

The ASTM standards for vaporizers include:

1. Location in the fresh gas circuit and concentration calibrated
2. Accept a total gas flow up to 15 L/min
3. Incorporate an isolation or interlock system
4. Fittings to demarcate correct flow through
5. Liquid level indicator
6. Agent-specific filling device
7. Anesthetic concentration less than 0.1% when OFF
8. Operator manual should state variation of ambient temperature, pressure, back pressure, input flow rates' effects on vaporizer performance, accuracy of calibration, and service intervals[3]

OUTLET CHECK VALVE

Because intermittent back pressure may increase or decrease the percent concentration output of vaporizers, anesthesia machines include a method to diminish this phenomenon. The device for compensation is included in the vaporizer or as a separate component of the anesthesia delivery system. Drager uses a coil system inside the vaporizer.[32] When intermittent back flow occurs, the gas does flow back into the vaporizer but encounters this coil and cannot reach the vaporizing chamber. Some Ohmeda vaporizers have a check valve at the outflow tract or incorporate an outlet check valve distal to

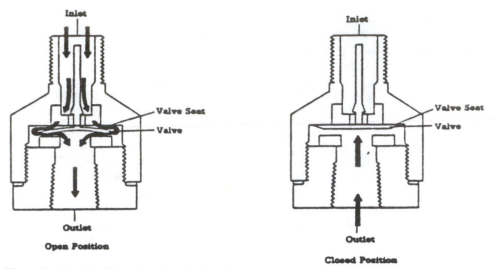

Figure 7–11 The Ohmeda outlet check valve to prevent intermittent back pressure to the vaporizer. Forward flow is allowed as the valve is pliable. Retrograde positive pressure closes the valve.[6] (Reproduced by permission from Bowie and Huffman.[6])

the vaporizers but prior to the common gas outlet (Figure 7–11).[6] This pliable valve responds to pressure in the piping of the anesthesia machine. Positive pressure closes it and forward flow of gases or negative pressure opens it. The presence of this check valve greatly influences the check-out procedure of the machine (Figure 7–12).[36]

PRESSURE RELIEF VALVE

Prior to the medical gases and anesthetic agents exiting the machine at the common gas outlet, there is a valve designed to open in the event of high pressure. Drager uses this inside the vaporizer and it opens at 18 psig.[21] Ohmeda has a separate component in the piping system designed to open between 2.3 and 2.9 psig or at 5 psig depending on the particular machine.[21]

☐ BREATHING CIRCUITS

The anesthesia delivery system's breathing circuit is the environment created by the anesthetist for the patient's respiratory exchange. The fresh gas flow from the anesthesia machine delivers known volumes percent of oxygen, nitrous oxide, air, and inhalation agents at a low pressure to the patient. Exhaled gases flow from the patient depending on the type of breathing circuit used. Although there is some disagreement as to how the breathing circuits are classified, this chapter compares open, semi-open, semi-closed, and closed systems.

OPEN SYSTEMS

This type of anesthesia is rarely used except in developing countries. Ether or halothane is dropped onto a gauze-covered mask and as the patient inhales, air acts as the carrier gas flow to vaporize the agent. Supplemental oxygen can be administered under the mask to diminish the likelihood of hypoxia because the agent dilutes the inspired oxygen content. If carbon dioxide is trapped under the mask, rebreathing becomes significant. A supplemental flow of oxygen helps minimize rebreathing. Insufflation is similar to open drop as it usually denotes blowing of anesthetic gases across a patient's face. High flows are required (> 10 L/min) and there is no rebreathing. Ventilation cannot be controlled and there is an unpredictable oxygen concentration.[37] The open drop and insufflation techniques have several disadvantages: (1) poor control of inspired gas concentration and depth of anesthesia; (2) inability to assist or control ventilation; (3) no conservation of exhaled heat or humidity; (4) pollution of the operating room with large volumes of waste gases.[37]

SEMI-OPEN SYSTEMS

The semi-open systems solve some of these problems by incorporating additional components into the breathing circuit. The location of the breathing tubes, fresh gas inlet, pressure relief valves, and breathing bag determine circuit performance with regard to rebreathing of carbon dioxide. High fresh gas flows based on the patient's weight prevent rebreathing of carbon dioxide. These systems can be used with a scavenger if the scavenging tubing is connected to the valve.[37] All Mapleson systems should incorporate an oxygen analyzer either with a manifold or at the common gas outlet.[38] When measuring end-tidal carbon dioxide ($ETCO_2$), the capnogram displays a plateau at a low value due to the high fresh gas flow. There may be an elevated baseline if any rebreathing of carbon dioxide is occurring.[39] To minimize the error, it is recommended to use a distal sampling site in the elbow connector, in the endotracheal tube adapter or as close to the patient as is possible.[40] Table 7–4 summarizes the semi-open systems.[37]

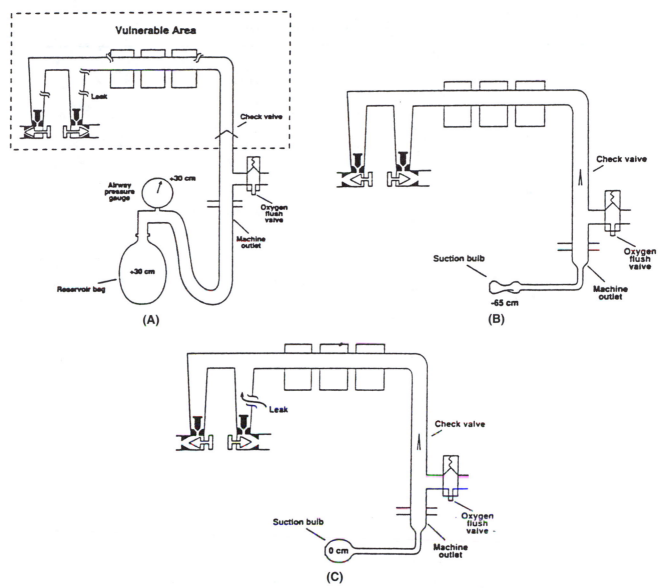

Figure 7–12 The vulnerable area where leaks may not be detected in an anesthesia machine with a check valve when only a positive pressure leak test is performed. Positive pressure in the reservoir bag (A) closes the check valve. Leaks in the vaporizer or flowmeters are not detected. In B, the negative pressure test is performed on a machine without leaks. The suction bulb stays compressed for approximately 15 to 30 seconds (depending on the machine). In C, the negative pressure test is performed on a machine with a leak in the flowmeter. The negative pressure opens the check valve, but the bulb does not stay compressed as flow from the leaking flowmeter fills it.[36] (Reproduced by permission from Andrews.[36])

None of the Mapleson systems are ideal for every situation. The relative order of merit in spontaneous ventilation is A, D, F, E and for controlled ventilation is D, F, E, B, C, A.[5] The circuits are simple, inexpensive, and easily assembled. Because there are minimal moving parts, they are easy to sterilize. Partial rebreathing results in some retention of heat and moisture, but the high fresh gas flows usually inhibit this slight advantage. Low resistance to breathing in spontaneously breathing patients led to their popularity in pediatrics. It was felt that the work of breathing was less with a Mapleson than with the circle system. This belief is being disputed and many have found that a pediatric circle system is equivalent to Mapleson systems.[5] The disadvantages include the costs of using extremely high fresh gas flows to ensure normocarbia and increased operating room pollution if scavenging is not used. It is sometimes difficult to change from spontaneous to controlled ventilation efficiently because some systems perform differently and may need different flowrates. Newer adaptations of semi-closed systems (Humphrey ADE and Multicircuit) allow choice of either spontaneous or controlled breathing with ease.[5] Semi-open systems allow a change in anesthetic concentration to occur quickly due to the high fresh gas flows used.

Table 7–4
SEMI-OPEN SYSTEMS

Mapleson Class	Other Names	Diagram[1]	REQUIRED FRESH GAS FLOWS	
			Spontaneous	Controlled
A	Magill		Equal to minute ventilation (≈ 80 mL/kg/min)	Very high and difficult to predict
B	Magill		2 × minute ventilation	2–2½ × minute ventilation
C	Magill		2 × minute ventilation	2–2½ × minute ventilation
D	Bain		2–3 × minute ventilation	1–2 × minute ventilation
E	Ayres T piece		2–3 × minute ventilation	3 × minute ventilation (I : E = 1 : 2)
F	Jackson-Reese		2–3 × minute ventilation	2 × minute ventilation

FGI , fresh gas inlet.
SOURCE: Reproduced by permission from Morgan and Mikhail.[37]

SEMI-CLOSED SYSTEM

The most commonly used breathing circuit is the semi-closed circle system (Figure 7–13). To remedy the disadvantages of Mapleson systems, the circle system uses components that make it more complex, but perhaps more efficient. This system diminishes the likelihood of rebreathing of carbon dioxide by adding unidirectional valves and a carbon dioxide absorber. This reduces the need for high fresh gas flows with the result being more heat and humidity at a lower cost. Operating room pollution is reduced by the incorporation of a waste gas scavenging system. The circle system can be used efficiently and easily in both spontaneous, assisted, and controlled ventilation. This is accomplished by the addition of an Adjustable Pressure Limiting (APL) valve and automatic ventilator. Monitoring the quality of the inspired mixture becomes possible with the mandatory oxygen analyzer, airway pressure gauge, and respiratory volume monitor.

Unidirectional Valves   Unidirectional valves are placed on the absorber housing so that gases flow in only one direction in the circle system. The inspiratory gas flows to the patient and the expiratory gas passes through the carbon dioxide absorbent. To prevent rebreathing of carbon dioxide, three conditions must be met: (1) a unidirectional valve must be located between the patient and the rebreathing bag on both the inspiratory and expiratory limbs; (2) the fresh gas flow cannot enter the circuit between the expiratory valve and the patient; (3) the APL valve cannot be located between the patient and the inspiratory valve. If these conditions are met, any arrangement of the other components will prevent

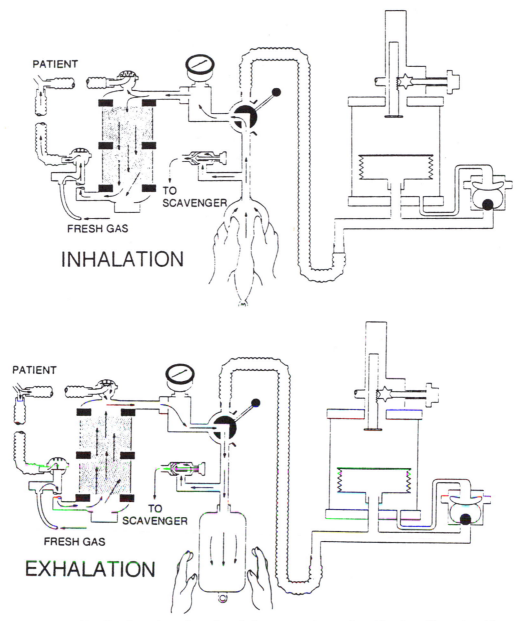

Figure 7–13   The flow of gas through a circle system using a rebreathing bag. (Reproduced by permission from Cicman and colleagues.[13])

rebreathing of carbon dioxide.[41] The integrity of these valves must be ensured to prevent rebreathing.[42] A faulty valve can lead to an elevated peak inspiratory pressure (PIP), an increase in $ETCO_2$, and an elevated baseline on the $ETCO_2$ waveform. Unidirectional valve disks increase resistance. They may be made of rubber, plastic or mica (similar to ceramic).[5]

The breathing circuit tubing is attached to ports that are connected to the unidirectional valves. This tubing is made of plastic or rubber and can be of various lengths. The length of the tubing does not affect the mechanical dead space or rebreathing in the circle system. Mechanical dead space is the space in the breathing circuit occupied by gases that are rebreathed without any change in composition. The dead space

begins at the Y piece at the partition and extends to any adapters or devices placed distal to the Y piece. Use of a Y piece with a septum decreases dead space. When inspiration or exhalation begin, the gases in the breathing tubes move in the opposite direction until stopped by closure of the unidirectional valves. This is called backlash. If the valves are competent, backlash is minimal and any increase in dead space is clinically insignificant.[5]

Carbon Dioxide Absorption   The inclusion of a carbon dioxide absorber allows the exhaled gases to be recycled after the carbon dioxide is removed. Carbon dioxide absorption is feasible when three requirements are met. The first is that it must not be toxic by itself or when combined with inhalation agents. Carbon dioxide granules cannot be used with trichloroethylene. In the presence of alkali and heat, trichloroethylene degrades into three toxic chemicals: (1) dichloroacetylene, a cranial neurotoxin that leads to cranial nerve lesions and encephalitis[43]; (2) phosgene, a potent pulmonary irritant that leads to adult respiratory distress syndrome[16]; and (3) carbon monoxide, which is formed when phosgene reacts with water.[43] Carbon dioxide granules cannot be used with chloroform. This combination also produces toxic chemicals that lead to phosgene and carbon monoxide.[5] These anesthetics are not commonly used.

Halothane, enflurane, isoflurane, desflurane and sevoflurane are degraded by absorbent to some extent.[5] When halothane reacts with soda lime, a metabolite BCDFE (2 bromo-2 chloro-1,1 difluoroethene) is formed. This is a specific nephrotoxin in rats. No nephrotoxicity has been reported in humans despite identifying the metabolite in the urine after exposure to halothane.[44] Enflurane reacts with soda lime to produce carbon monoxide, but only at (nonclinical) elevated temperatures.[43] Carbon monoxide buildup has been reported with the use of isoflurane, enflurane, and desflurane in both Sodasorb and Baralyme when the granules have been allowed to dry out. Dry granules occur more commonly with high fresh gas flows over long periods of time. Baralyme produces more carbon monoxide with desflurane, followed by enflurane and isoflurane.[45] Although the relationship of carbon monoxide poisoning to halogenated agents are still not entirely clear,[46] the Food and Drug Administration and the Centers for Disease Control and Prevention recommend that all soda lime that has been dormant in the anesthesia machine for more than 24 hours should be changed and dated. The anesthesia machine should also be flushed continuously with 100% oxygen for at least 1 minute before the first case of the day.[47] Daily behavior modification may be necessary to minimize the likelihood of carbon monoxide poisoning. Turning off the fresh gas at the end of each case and especially at the end of the day decreases drying of the granules. Changing the absorber canisters more frequently and especially prior to Monday morning diminishes the likelihood of this phenomenon.[48]

Sevoflurane reacts with the alkali in carbon dioxide granules to produce compound A (fluromethy-2,2-difluroro-1-trifluromethyl vinyl ether). This compound is nephrotoxic in rats, yet no cases in humans have been reported. Human blood levels of compound A increase for 1 to 2 hours after administration, plateau, then decline.[49] Most references recommend the use of higher fresh gas flows to flush the absorber of these toxic compounds (2 to 5 L/min),[48,49] yet not too high to prevent excessive drying of the granules.[45]

Water is contained both on the surface and inside the granules. The patient's exhaled carbon dioxide reacts with the water in and on the granules to form carbonic acid. This acid is then absorbed by the base (the hydroxide) of the granules to form a carbonate. Water and heat are the products of this chemical reaction.[5] Water helps to prevent absorption of the agent into the granules. When granules dry out, their pores open and more agent is absorbed.[11] Baralyme contains more water than Sodasorb as barium hydroxide is an octahydrate (contains 8 water molecules)[50] (A. Pinhaus, personal communication, 1995). USP standards recommend between 14% and 19% water content in carbon dioxide absorber granules.[11]

The second requirement for carbon dioxide absorption is that the carbon dioxide absorber have low resistance to airflow. The hydroxide granules used are precisely manufactured to minimize resistance to airflow while maximizing absorptive capabilities. The size of the granule can vary between 4 and 8 mesh. Mesh is a screen size and 4 mesh means that are $4\frac{1}{4}$ inch openings per linear inch. Eight mesh means there are $8\frac{1}{8}$ inch openings per linear inch.[5] The smaller mesh size allows more air space (less resistance) and the larger mesh size granules increase the surface area (more absorptive capability). Studies have shown that a blend of larger and smaller granules has the effect of minimizing resistance with little sacrifice in absorption efficiency. There is more resistance to airflow in the inner diameter of the canister than next to the walls of the canister. This is called the *wall effect* and is due to the air space distribution of the canister. There is less air space in the granule to granule space than the granule to smooth inner wall area.[5]

The third requirement involves efficiency of carbon dioxide absorption.[5] All the carbon dioxide that enters the canisters should be absorbed due to the chemical reaction between the carbon dioxide and the water on and in the granules. However, there is a point when the hydroxides no longer absorb the amount of carbonic acid they receive. Studies regarding carbon dioxide absorbers efficiency define the breakpoint and the exhaustion times. The *breakpoint* is defined as the time at which the first trace of unabsorbed carbon dioxide is detected in the inspiratory port of the absorber (approximately .1%). *Exhaustion* is the time at which the carbon dioxide level at the inspiratory port of the absorber reaches .5%.[51] The work of carbon dioxide absorption is accomplished by the composition and characteristics of the granules. The base that absorbs the acid is an alkali, a hydroxide. Both brands of carbon dioxide absorbent are composed of 80% calcium hydroxide in the inner core of the granule. Either sodium hydroxide (Sodasorb) or barium hydroxide (Baralyme) are on the surface of the granule.[5] It is difficult to separate potassium hydroxide from the sodium hydroxide and therefore, some potassium hydroxide is on the granule surface[50] (A. Pinhaus, personal communication, 1995). Typically, the surface reaction is fast, occurs first and acts as a catalyst for the reaction which occurs in the core of the granule. The internal reaction occurs more slowly.[5]

The efficiency of carbon dioxide absorption varies inversely with the hardness of the granules.[17] Silica is added to Sodasorb to prevent dust formation, yet it tends to clog the pores of the granule, so kieselguhr (diatomaceous earth) is added to make the granules harder.[5] The minimum desirable hardness is 80 on a scale of 100.[11] Measurements of efficiency of carbon dioxide absorbent vary according to the packing of the canister and the phenomena of channeling. *Channeling* occurs as the gases pass from the top of the absorber housing to the bottom. This flow is preferred to minimize the likelihood of dust reaching the patient's airway. The upper area receives the gas with the carbon dioxide first. Two areas along the sidewalls of the canister then receive gas flow due to the lower resistance near the smooth walls of the canister.[52] The last area to receive gas flow is the center lower canister. Channeling occurs in most canisters, but is more common with loosely packed granules.[11] The efficiency of carbon dioxide absorbent can be improved by using lower flow rates and minimizing high pressure fluctuations in the circle system.[11] The maximum amount of carbon dioxide that can be absorbed is approximately 26 L/100 g absorbent. However, due to the effects of channeling,[16] Sodasorb ranges from 14 to 23 L/100 g and Baralyme ranges from 9 to 18 L/100 g.[11]

Since the breakpoint and exhaustion of carbon dioxide granules may be hard to predict in the clinical area, manufacturers include a pH sensitive dye in the composition. This dye changes color from white to purple to signal that the chemical reaction is occurring and that gradually the granules are exhausting. Ethyl violet is the current dye used in both preparations.[5] Depending on this indicator dye to announce exhaustion is not completely reliable. It has been reported that ethyl violet is deactivated by fluorescent lights.[53] Anesthetists should rely on ETCO$_2$ monitoring as an indicator that carbon dioxide absorption is occurring, as well as the clinical signs of hypercarbia (hyperpnea and hypertension).[54] If rebreathing is suspected, the flow rate should be increased until the cause is determined.

Soda lime is reported to be more caustic to tissue than Baralyme. Dust from soda lime has been implicated in facial burns, bronchospasm, and irritation to mucous membranes.[11] The direction of gas flow through the absorber housing should diminish dust expulsion to the patient circuit. A dust cup or a drain is designed into the absorber housing to allow cleaning of dust particles and draining of water accumulation.[5]

Soda lime also exhibits the phenomenon of *regeneration* (also called reversion or peaking). After granules are exhausted, they should change color to purple. After a period of rest, (no carbon dioxide), the granules change from purple back to white. When a small amount of carbon dioxide reaches the previously exhausted granules, they very quickly revert to purple. This may be attributed to the solubility of sodium carbonate as compared to calcium carbonate and barium carbonate. It is reported that this reversion is less likely today as Sodasorb contains less silica and more potassium hydroxide. Baralyme has no regeneration capacity as barium hydroxide is insoluble.[16] Exhausted CO$_2$ canisters revert to normal color overnight.

Pressure Control and Monitoring   Pressure in the circle system is controlled by the anesthetist by various components in the absorber. The rebreathing bag acts as a reservoir

for the patient's exhaled gas and provides a means for assisted or controlled ventilation. A reservoir is necessary as the anesthesia machine cannot provide the peak inspiratory gas flow needed during normal respiration, which may range from 20 to 50 L/min.[43] It also acts as a buffer to protect the patient from excessive pressure in the breathing circuit.[5] Most bags are composed of rubber or neoprene. The ASTM standard for bags 1.5 L or smaller states that the pressure shall not be less than 30 cm H$_2$O or exceed 50 cm H$_2$O when the bag is expanded to four times its capacity. For bags that are larger than 1.5 L, the pressure should not be less than 35 cm H$_2$O or exceed 60 cm H$_2$O.[55] New bags develop higher pressures when they are initially overinflated than bags that have been overinflated several times or prestretched. It is considered good practice to overinflate the rebreathing bag prior to using it. Disposable plastic bags are inelastic and do not stretch after full inflation.[5] They may reach up to 100 cm H$_2$O pressure and rupture abruptly.[43]

The APL valve gives the anesthetist control of the amount of pressure in the circle system. It diverts excess gas to the scavenger system depending on its status. When fully open it scavenges excess gas when less than 1 cm H$_2$O pressure exists in the circuit. As the valve is closed, pressure builds in the circuit and less gas flows to the scavenger system. The resistance added to the circle system when the APL is fully open is variable and should be between 1 and 3 cm H$_2$O at 3 L/min.[5]

Absorbers incorporate a diaphragm-type pressure gauge to quantify the inspiratory and expiratory pressure in the breathing circuit. The pressure gauge only registers a pressure, it does not warn of any change. ASTM standards specify that airway pressure monitoring shall be used to detect and warn of conditions of high, sustained and subatmospheric pressure. The monitor should sound a high priority alarm in situations in which the pressure in the breathing circuit exceeds the limit set for continuing sustained positive pressure.[3]

Scavenger System

Guidelines for waste gas scavenging are published by the American Association of Nurse Anesthetists,[56] American Society of Anesthesiologists,[57] National Institute of Occupational Safety and Health,[58,59] and ANSI.[60] Until definitive studies resolve the effects of waste anesthetics in humans, it is prudent to ensure adequate room ventilation; a functioning scavenger; minimal allowable leak of the anesthesia machine; reasonable clinical habits; and periodic monitoring of the work environment.[61]

ENSURE ADEQUATE ROOM VENTILATION

The ventilation system is the single most important element to reduce personnel exposure to waste anesthetics. Unventilated operating rooms are four times more contaminated as those with ventilation systems that meet current standards.[61] Ventilation systems are either recirculating or nonrecirculating. A recirculating system partially recirculates filtered and conditioned stale with fresh air. This is more economical but does have the potential to contaminate 'clean' rooms with polluted air. Most operating rooms use a nonrecirculating ventilation system. Fresh air is continuously pumped into the room a number of times per hour and stale air is removed. The number of exchanges is 15 per hour for existing hospitals and 20 per hour for new facilities.[62]

USE OF SCAVENGER

The waste gas scavenger evacuates anesthetic gases from the anesthesia delivery system and vents them to the atmosphere (Figure 7–14). When a vacuum source is attached to the scavenger, the system is described as active.[5] Active systems are usually more effective in keeping waste gas levels low.[63] If a vacuum is not used, the system is described as passive and gas flows to the ventilation ducts where it will be evacuated to the atmosphere. Passive systems may not be as effective in lowering levels of waste gases.[5] When a passive system is used, it must be of the nonrecirculating type and supply at least 10 room air exchanges per hour. If a passive system vents directly through the wall to the outside (bypasses the ventilation system), it should be protected with a wire screen and should project downward.[61]

When the scavenger system interface valve has no open ports to the work environment, it is described as closed. Closed systems (see Figure 7–14A) contain positive and negative relief valves to ensure that excessive positive or negative pressure is not communicated to the patient circuit.[5] The positive pressure relief valve should open at 5 cm H_2O and vent to the room. The negative pressure relief valve should open at $-.25$ to -1.80 cm H_2O and draw in room air.[61] All ports of the interface valve should be covered for a closed system.

If the system has ports which are open to the work environment, it is described as open (see Figure 7–14B).[5] There are no positive or negative relief valves. The open ports provide a means of relief. Each type of scavenger system has a reservoir to hold the waste gases. All scavenger systems receive the waste gases from two sources: (1) the APL valve when using the rebreathing bag and (2) the pressure relief valve when using the ventilator. Waste gas scavenging is required for every type of breathing circuit[64] because the flow rates chosen by anesthetists typically exceed the patient's need.[65] When Mapleson systems are used, the scavenger should be connected to the exhalation port where most of the exhaled gases are vented.[61] The vacuum requirement of the scavenger changes if higher or lower flows are used. When a scavenger is used, the anesthetist must remember it may affect the pressure in the circle breathing system. *Any unexplained excessive positive or negative pressure may be due to malfunctioning positive or negative relief valves, inappropriately set vacuum or an obstructed route for waste anesthetic venting.*[61]

MINIMIZE ALLOWABLE LEAK OF ANESTHESIA MACHINE

No anesthesia machine is totally leak free.[66] Allowable leaks can be due to gas sampling technology (ETCO$_2$ or agent

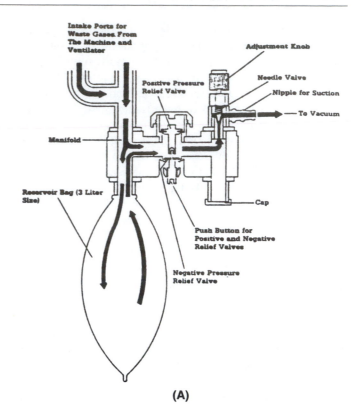

(A)

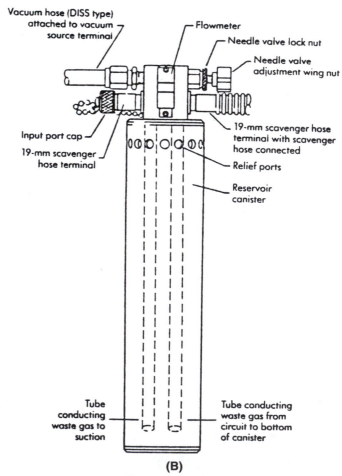

(B)

Figure 7–14 The Ohmeda active, closed scavenger system (A). The Drager active, open scavenger system (B). (Reproduced by permission from Bowie and Huffman[6] and North American Drager.)

analysis) or those specified by ASTM anesthesia machine standards. Gas sampling typically involves the aspiration of between 30 and 240 cc/min depending on the type of gas analyzer. This gas sample, once analyzed, should be scavenged unless it is returned to the circuit. The failure to include this sample in the scavenger can cause contamination of the operating room.[65] Leaks greater than 340 ml/min are considered excessive and are not allowed by ASTM standards.[3] Leaks less than 150 to 250 mL/min are difficult to document because the minimum oxygen flow masks these leaks. High pressure leaks in the cylinder system are common.

TECHNIQUE

Even if state of the art ventilation and scavenger systems are functioning, anesthetic technique can lead to operating room contamination.[67] Guidelines for reasonable clinical habits to decrease exposure should be incorporated into daily practice. NIOSH recommends "exposures as low as is technically feasible."[58]

MONITORING

It is recommended that operating rooms be monitored on a regular basis to meet the following objectives: (1) to determine that the ventilation system and current scavenger systems are functioning; (2) to determine if leak testing procedures are adequate and uncover unexpected leaks; (3) to document compliance with NIOSH recommendations and (4) to document safe working conditions as per Occupational Safety and Health Agency recommendations.[61] Monitoring should occur quarterly in locations where mixed anesthetic agents are used and whenever ventilation, anesthetic equipment or scavenging techniques are modified.[58] While most can detect the presence of inhalation agents in the room, nitrous oxide is odorless. The olfactory threshold for halothane is .005% to .01% (50 to 100 ppm).[68] Infrared analyzers or dosimeters are necessary to monitor the operating room.[61]

Ventilators The goal of mechanical ventilation is efficient oxygenation and carbon dioxide elimination without injury to the patient.[69] The most important feature of a ventilator is its ability to provide a consistent minute ventilation. It replaces the rebreathing bag and in actuality is an "educated hand" that allows the anesthetist to perform other responsibilities. Ventilators used in the United States are designed to function as volume preset devices as the anesthetist selects the minute volume. A safety valve or pressure limit (which may either be factory set or adjusted by the anesthetist) is incorporated so that the ventilator functions as a pressure limiting device. This pressure limit prevents patient injury by decreasing the likelihood of barotrauma. Therefore, most contemporary anesthesia ventilators are volume preset as well as pressure-limited devices.[69]

The term *double circuit* means there are two circuits in the ventilator (Figure 7–15). One circuit is the patient circuit (the oxygen/nitrous oxide/air and inhalation agent mixture) that is inside the bellows. The other circuit is the drive gas outside the bellows, but inside the bellows housing that pushes the bellows up or down and accomplishes ventilation.

Compressed gases provide the driving force behind this circuit. Therefore, ventilators are pneumatically driven. The pneumatic power can either be 100% oxygen (Ohmeda) or oxygen with room air entrained via a Venturi device (Drager).[16] The Venturi device draws in room air due to the fall in pressure at the narrowing of the tube based on Bernoulli's theorem.[9] The room air enters the ventilator and provides a larger volume of drive gas while using less compressed oxygen. Approximately 80% of the drive gas is room air when a Venturi is used[69] with the resultant FiO_2 being approximately 35%. Ohmeda ventilators use 100% oxygen but regulate the 50 psig down via two regulators prior to use as the drive gas.[10] Oxygen is chosen as the primary drive gas for several reasons. It is inexpensive, of high purity, free of particulate and water vapor and is readily available in operating rooms.[11]

The drive gas composition is important especially if a leak develops in the bellows. If the drive gas is 100% oxygen and it leaks into the patient circuit, the anesthetic mixture may be diluted. This may result in a decrease in the nitrous oxide concentration with the possibility of intraoperative recall as well as a higher FiO_2.[70,71] If the drive gas is supplemented with room air via a Venturi and a leak develops in the bellows, approximately 35% oxygen will be added to the patient breathing circuit. This may alter the FiO_2 and adds nitrogen to the circuit. If the gas analyzer has the ability to measure nitrogen, this occurrence could cause the anesthetist to suspect an air embolism.[69] Since both manufacturers drive, gas is compressed gas, a leak into the bellows can result in hyperventilation and possibly barotrauma.[72,73]

Anesthesia ventilators are time cycled. Initiation of inspiration is accomplished by a timing device. The timing device controls the flow of the driving gas. Inspiration occurs when the timing device causes the driving gas to fill the bellows housing. Inspiration stops when the driving gas stops flowing to the bellows housing. Exhalation begins when the driving gas is vented to the room and the patient's elastic recoil causes the bellows to refill. When the bellows are completely refilled, the excess anesthesia gas is vented to the scavenger.[16]

The bellows classification is determined by the direction of bellows movement during exhalation. Older, pneumatic ventilators use a weighted *descending bellows*. During exhalation, the bellows move down due to the patient's exhaled tidal volume as well as the weight. If the breathing circuit is disconnected, the bellows will continue to cycle up and down due to the action of the weight. For this reason, the disconnect may go unnoticed. Contemporary ventilators usually use *ascending bellows* (see Figure 7–15). During exhalation, the bellows move up due to the patient's exhaled tidal volume. There is no weight in the bellows. If the breathing circuit is disconnected, the bellows does not rise because there is no tidal volume being delivered. This type of bellows is considered safer as a disconnect is quickly noticed.[16] It has been shown that ascending bellows can continue to deliver a small tidal volume and aspirate up to 140 ml on expiration despite a disconnect.[74]

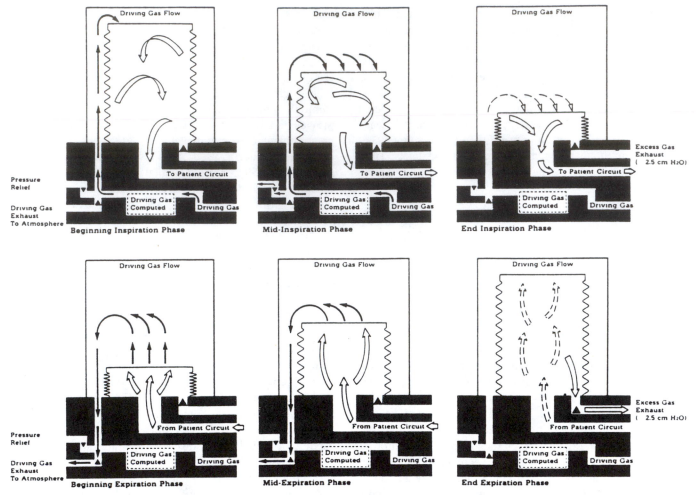

Figure 7–15 The functioning of an Ohmeda 7000 Series anesthesia ventilator during inspiration and exhalation. (Reproduced by permission from Ohmeda, A BOC Health Care Company, Madison, WI)

Pressure Limiting Valve

A pressure limiting valve is built into every ventilator for two purposes: (1) to vent the driving gas out to the room and; (2) to vent the patient's circuit out to the scavenger. Because the ventilator is a double circuit, both must be vented to prevent the possibility of barotrauma. The driving gas controls the inspiration; therefore, it must be vented during exhalation. The composition of the driving gas will be either 100% oxygen or 35% oxygen so it is not hazardous to vent it to the room. The driving gas will be vented at either a factory preset value (65 to 80 cm H_2O)[5] or at a value set by the anesthetist. Once this value is reached, the valve opens and inspiration ceases. The patient circuit must be vented because typically more flow is delivered than is needed. Because this circuit may contain nitrous oxide and halogenated agents, it should be vented to the scavenger to prevent room contamination. The patient circuit is vented when 2 to 3 cm H_2O is reached on an ascending bellows. Therefore, all ascending bellows will deliver 2 to 3 cm H_2O positive end-expiratory pressure. This is necessary to allow the bellows to fill.[75] At end-expiration, once 2 to 3 cm H_2O is sensed, the valve will vent the patient circuit to the scavenger. If the pressure relief valve malfunctions or the pilot tube becomes kinked or obstructed, excessive airway pressure is communicated to the patient circuit or hypoventilation results.[76–78] The actual functioning of the ventilator should be reviewed in Figure 7–15. Barotrauma may occur if the oxygen flush is used during the inspiratory cycle.[16]

Compression Factor

Some of the tidal volume set by the anesthetist is lost due to the compression factor of the machine and the breathing circuit. *The losses due to stretching and compression of the breathing circuit can be in excess of 6 mL/cm H_2O.* For example, a patient with a PIP of 20 cm H_2O can lose up to 120 mL due to the compression factor.[69] Plastic tubing tends to lose less than rubber tubing, but the actual amount lost can be unpredictable and depends on the particular ventilator, breathing circuit and PIP.[79] In all anesthesia ventilators, changes in compliance and resistance force some or all of the inspiratory volume to distend the breathing circuit hoses and compress the gas in the circuit. The anesthesia ventilator is designed to ventilate paralyzed patients with reasonable lung function. Patients with severe lung disease may not be efficiently ventilated. Some settings required in these patients are not available on anesthesia ventilators.[80]

Monitoring Ventilation

The delivery of gas to the patient is monitored to ensure that an adequate volume and oxygen content are being delivered and that carbon dioxide is eliminated. The quality of the inspiratory volume is documented by the oxygen analyzer and the expiratory volume is measured by a device on the absorber. This ensures that the gas delivered to the patient has been successfully returned to the circuit and that the entire ventilation system is operational. The vane anemometer is used by Ohmeda and a sealed volumeter by Drager.[81] A capnograph confirms carbon dioxide elimination.

Oxygen Analyzers The ASTM standard requires that anesthesia delivery systems include an oxygen analyzer that is enabled and functioning any time the machine is capable of delivering an anesthetic mixture.[3] Oxygen can be measured by various methods, but the most common method in anesthesia machines is either the polarographic electrode or the galvanic fuel cell. Since the mid-1980s, Drager and Ohmeda preferred the galvanic fuel cell for their oxygen analyzers.[11] Studies indicate that galvanic fuel cells provide reliable service with less frequent failures at a lower overall cost.[82] Both the polarographic electrode and the galvanic cell are electrochemical (sensors that convert energy from a chemical reaction into an electrical signal). Each obey Henry's law, which states that the volume of a gas that diffuses through a semipermeable membrane at a given temperature is directly proportional to the partial pressure of the gas in equilibrium.[9] Temperature must be kept constant to keep the voltage dependent on the number of molecules of oxygen only.[83]

Technical Limitations

Both types of oxygen analyzers depend on diffusion of oxygen molecules through a Teflon membrane. If water vapor is allowed to accumulate at the semipermeable membrane, the gas molecules are unable to accomplish this diffusion. The device should be kept upright to prevent this. Location of the oxygen analyzer in the inspiratory side of the circuit also keeps it drier. There is a protective grill over the membrane to prevent dirt or oil from decreasing the usable surface of the membrane.[5,11] Other gas molecules may also react with these electrochemical devices and affect their accuracy. Small amounts of halothane can be reduced by the polarographic sensor.[84] If the battery loses its charge in the polarographic, it will deliver less voltage to the cathode. As the battery fails, the voltage threshold is inadequate to reduce oxygen molecules, but is adequate to reduce nitrous oxide molecules.[85] A galvanic fuel cell's life will be reduced by exposure to carbon dioxide.[11] Temperature changes in the breathing circuit can affect the voltage output of the sensor cell,[86,87] as can extremes in airway pressure.[88] Increases in temperature and or pressure will favor diffusion across the membrane. Increases in airway pressure during mechanical ventilation can elevate the oxygen analyzer slightly.

Oxygen analyzers respond to the partial pressure of oxygen, but the output is measured in volumes percent. Therefore, their output will change if barometric pressure changes. At an altitude of 5000 feet, an analyzer calibrated to 21% at sea level will give a reading of 17.4%. At an altitude of 10,000 feet, it will read 14.2%. Under hyperbaric conditions, oxygen partial pressure will be much greater than at sea level.[15]

The life expectancy of an oxygen analyzer depends on the amount of oxygen molecules reduced by the device and the amount of active material at the anode. The amount of oxygen molecules that enter depends on the percent and the time of exposure. It is expressed as O_2% hours. Sensor lifetime usually ranges between 130,000 to 650,000 O_2% hours. A sensor exposed to 21% oxygen will last 12 to 15 months. The same sensor exposed to 100% oxygen will last 2 to 3 months.[11]

Failure

Polarographic analyzers fail more often than galvanic cells. Refilling the sensor with potassium chloride solution or changing the batteries may restore the analyzer. When the analyzer will not calibrate to 21% or will not hold calibration after the above measures have been taken, it usually means the silver anode is completely consumed and cannot give up any more electrons.[82] When galvanic cells fail, they cannot be repaired by adding solution or changing batteries. Most commonly the failure is due to exhaustion of the lead anode and the cell must be replaced. Four changes in performance were noted to precede exhaustion of the galvanic cell: (1) underreading high oxygen; (2) failure to remember calibration; (3) "blipping out" and (4) a color change of the electrolyte solution from clear to pink.[82]

Standards

The ANSI standards state that oxygen analyzers should be accurate to within ±3%. Interference from anesthetic agents must not exceed 4%. Once calibrated, they should be functional and enunciate a high priority alarm when the measured oxygen is below the user preset alarm. The alarm must activate within ±2% of the alarm setting.[89] The user should keep these tolerances in mind when setting the low alarm.

CLOSED SYSTEMS

Closed circuit anesthesia is a technique of extremely low flow anesthesia and a completely closed breathing circuit. The basic principle of closed circuit is maintenance of a constant anesthetic state by addition of gases and inhalation agent at the same rate that the body stores or eliminates them.[90] In the classic closed circuit approach, once a stable level of anesthesia is established with high flows, the APL valve is completely closed and the fresh gas flow rate is reduced to levels equal to the patient's metabolic need. Induction with a closed circuit is difficult for two reasons. The first involves the nitrogen in the body which dilutes the anesthetic gases in the system. This may result in hypoxia if nitrous oxide is administered along with the oxygen. It may also dilute the nitrous oxide and lead to recall. The second difficulty is the unpredictability of the dosage of anesthesia for each patient at induction. Due to the maximal uptake of anesthetic by the tissues and the time needed for equilibrium, inductions may be prolonged and stormy when using low flows. Once the anesthetic state is established and supposing the machine is totally leak free, there is little need for agent or nitrous oxide as they are rebreathed. The only gas that needs replenishing is oxygen as it is consumed during metabolism. The circuit should be opened every 1–3 hours and run at higher flows for 5–10 minutes.[91] This allows washout of the nitrogen that builds up during metabolism and eliminates any possible harmful substances that may build up in a completely closed system. Anesthetic concentrations do not change quickly unless the circuit is open and high flows are used. Due to the empirical calculations and fear of morbidity and mortality, the closed system lost its popularity; however, it is an excellent model for learning the uptake and distribution of inhalation agents.[92,93]

☐ CONCLUSION

The anesthesia delivery system has evolved into a complex piece of equipment. Critical incidents studies indicate 4% of incidents with substantive negative outcomes involved equipment failure. When human error was factored with anesthesia machine use, there was a 22% incidence of critical incidents. The most common factor contributing to the critical incidents was failure to check or inspect.[94] The importance of a preoperative check of the anesthesia equipment and delivery system cannot be overemphasized. The FDA checkout is a minimum requirement. It is through the checkout that problems with the anesthesia delivery system will be exposed before they are experienced by the patient. Anesthetists should know the current standards for anesthesia delivery systems.[3] Through knowing these standards for performance, one can set limits about equipment that should not be used or diagnose equipment that needs servicing. It is by having this knowledge and acting on it that nurse anesthetists can fulfill Standard VIII in our practice manual.

REFERENCES

1. Huffman L. Standards and safety components for anesthesia delivery systems. *AANA J.* 1987;55:559.
2. American Association of Nurse Anesthetists. *Guidelines and Standards for Nurse Anesthesia Practice.* Park Ridge, Ill; 1992.
3. American Society for Testing and Materials. *Standard Specification for Minimum Performance and Safety Requirements for Components and Systems of Anesthesia Gas Machines.* Philadelphia; 1989.
4. Anonymous. Medical gas and vacuum systems. *ECRI Health Devices* 1994;23:306. (ECRI address: 5200 Butler Pike, Plymouth Meeting, PA 19462-1298, USA).
5. Dorsch JA, Dorsch SE. *Understanding Anesthesia Equipment.* Baltimore: Williams & Wilkins; 1992.
6. Bowie E, Huffman LM. *The Anesthesia Machine: Essentials for Understanding.* Madison, WI: Ohmeda; 1985.
7. Lampotaug S. Pipeline pressure gauge location on modern anesthesia machines. *J Clin Monit.* 1994;10:277.
8. Microsoft USA. *Encarta Multimedia Encyclopedia.* 1994.
9. Parbrook GD, Davis PD, Parbrook EO. *Basic Physics and Measurement in Anesthesia.* East Norwalk, Conn: Appleton-Century-Crofts; 1986.
10. Eisenkraft JB. The anesthesia machine. In: Ehrenwerth J, Eisenkraft JB, eds. *Anesthesia Equipment.* St. Louis: Mosby-Yearbook; 1993:27–56.
11. Petty C. *The Anesthesia Machine.* New York: Churchill Livingstone; 1987.
12. Burton GW, Hodgkin JC. *Respiratory Care: A Guide to Clinical Practice.* Philadelphia: JB Lippincott, 1984.
13. Cicman J, Himmelwright C, Skibo V, Yoder J. *Operating Principles of Narkomed Anesthesia Systems.* Telford PA: North American Drager; 1993.
14. Rajala MM. Flowmeters: physics of gas flow. In: Faust RJ, ed. *Anesthesiology Review.* New York: Churchill Livingstone; 1991:191–193.
15. James MFM, White JF. Anesthetic considerations at moderate altitude. *Anesth Analg.* 1984;63:1097.
16. Andrews JJ. Anesthesia systems. In: Barash PG, Cullen BF, Stoelting RK, eds. *Clinical Anesthesia.* Philadelphia: JB Lippincott; 1989:505–541.
17. Lohmann G. Fault with an Ohmeda Excel 410 machine. *Anaesthesia.* 1991;46:695.
18. Gordon PC, James MFM, Lapham H, Carboni M. Failure of the proportioning system to prevent hypoxic mixture on a Modulus II Plus anesthesia machine. *Anesthesiology.* 1995;82:598.
19. Richards C. Failure of a nitrous oxide-oxygen proportioning device. *Anesthesiology.* 1989;71:997.
20. Khalil SN, Neuman J. Failure of an oxygen flow control valve. *Anesthesiology.* 1990;73:355.
21. Eisenkraft JB. Anesthesia vaporizers. In: Ehrenwerth J, Eisenkraft JB, eds. *Anesthesia Equipment.* St. Louis: Mosby-Yearbook; 1993:57–88.
22. Adriani J. *The Chemistry and Physics of Anesthesia.* Springfield, Ill: Charles C. Thomas; 1962.
23. Eisenkraft JB. Vaporizers and vaporization of volatile anesthetics. In: Eisenkraft JB, ed. *Progress in Anesthesiology,* vol 2. San Antonio: Dannemiller Memorial Educational Foundation; 1988.
24. *Webster's College Dictionary.* New York: Random House; 1991.
25. *Understanding the Tec 4 vaporizer.* Steeton, UK: Ohmeda; 1985.
26. *Operations and Maintenance Manual for Ohio Calibrated Vaporizers for Ethrane, Halothane and Forane.* Ohio Medical Products. Madison, WI.
27. Bruce DL, Linde HW. Vaporization of mixed anesthetic liquids. *Anesthesiology.* 1984;60:342.
28. Chilcoat RT. Hazards of mis-filled vaporizers: summary tables. *Anesthesiology.* 1985;63:726.
29. Davey A, Moyle JTB, Ward C. *Ward's Anesthetic Equipment.* London: WB Saunders; 1992.
30. Kingsley CP. Drawover anesthesia equipment for austere conditions. *Wellcome Trends in Anesthesiology.* 1992;10:3.

131

31. Weiskopf RB, Sampson D, Moore MA. The desflurane (Tec 6) vaporizer: design, design considerations and performance evaluation. *Br J Anaesth.* 1994;72:474.

32. *Anaesthetic Vaporizer.* Dragerwerk AG; 1991.

33. *Tec 5 Continuous Flow Vaporizer Operation and Maintenance Manual.* Ohmeda; Madison, WI: 1992.

34. Leob R, Santos B. Pumping effect in Ohmeda Tec 5 vaporizers. *J Clin Monit* 1995;11:348.

35. Huffman LM. Calibrated vaporizers: maintaining clinical performance. *AANA J.* 1990;58:119.

36. Andrews JJ. Understanding your anesthesia machine. *ASA Refresher Course* 161, 1995.

37. Morgan GE, Mikhail MS: *Clinical Anesthesiology.* East Norwalk, Conn: Appleton & Lange; 1992.

38. Kataria B, Maher J. A simple way to monitor inspired oxygen concentration in nonrebreathing circuits. *Anesth Analg.* 1987;66:1049.

39. Gravenstein JS, Paulus DA. *Clinical Monitoring Practice.* 2nd ed. Philadelphia: JB Lippincott; 1987.

40. Gravenstein N, Lampotang S, Beneken JEW. Factors influencing capnography in the Bain circuit. *J Clin Monit* 1985;1:6.

41. Eger EI II. Anesthetic systems: construction and function. In: Eger, EI II, ed. *Anesthetic Uptake and Action.* Baltimore: Williams & Wilkins; 1974.

42. Kim JM, Kovac AL, Mathewson HS. A method for detection of incompetent unidirectional dome valves: a prevalent malfunction. *Anesth Analg.* 1985;64:745.

43. Smith TC. Anesthesia breathing systems. In: Ehrenwerth J, Eisenkraft JB, eds. *Anesthesia Equipment.* St. Louis: Mosby-Yearbook; 1993:89–113.

44. Sharp JH, Trudell JR, Cohen EN. Volatile metabolites and decomposition products of Halothane in man. *Anesthesiology.* 1979;50:2.

45. Fang ZX, Eger EI II. Source of toxic carbon monoxide explained: CHF_2 anesthetic and dry absorbent. *APSF Newsletter* 1994;9(3):25.

46. Moon RE. Cause of CO poisoning relation to halogenated agents still not clear. *APSF Newsletter* 1994;9(2):13.

47. Lentz RE. Carbon monoxide poisoning during anesthesia poses puzzles. *APSF Newsletter* 1994;9(2):13.

48. Epstein RA. In my opinion: carbon monoxide, what should we do? *APSF Newsletter* 1994–95;9(4):37.

49. Kharasch ED. Inhalation anesthetic toxicity: current controversies. *ASA Refresher Course* 264, 1995.

50. *Catalog Handbook of Fine Chemicals.* Millwaukee, WI: Aldrich Chemical Company, Inc; 1994.

51. Baudendistel LJ: Performance comparison between prepacked canisters of Sodasorb and Baralyme. Unpublished report at St. Louis University Medical Center, March 27, 1987.

52. Conroy WA, Seevers MH. Studies in carbon dioxide absorption. *Anesthesiology* 1943;4:160.

53. Andrews JJ, Johnson RV, Bee DE, Arens JF. Photodeactivation of ethyl violet: a potential hazard of Sodasorb. *Anesthesiology* 1990;72:59.

54. Adriani J. Soda lime containing indicators. *Anesthesiology* 1944;5:45.

55. American Society for Testing and Materials. *Standard Specification for Anesthesia Reservoir Bags (F1204-88).* Philadelphia; 1988.

56. American Association of Nurse Anesthestists. *Management of Waste Anesthetic Gases.* Park Ridge, Ill; 1992.

57. American Society of Anesthesiologists. *Waste Anesthetic Gases in Operating Room Air: A Suggested Program to Reduce Personnel Exposure.* Park Ridge, Ill; 1980.

58. National Institute of Occupational Safety and Health. *Criteria for a Recommended Standard: Occupational Exposure to Waste Anesthetic Gases and Vapors. Publication no. 77-140,* Cincinnati, OH: US Department of Health, Education and Welfare; 1970.

59. National Institute of Occupational Safety and Health. *Guidelines for Health Care Workers.* Publication no. 88-119, Cincinnaati, OH: US Department of Health, Education and Welfare; 1988.

60. American National Standards Institute. *American National Standard for Anesthetic Equipment: Scavenging Systems for Excess Anesthetic Gases.* ANSI z79.11-1982. New York: ANSI; 1982.

61. Azar I, Eisenkraft JB. Waste anesthetic gas spillage and scavenging systems. In: Ehrenwerth J, Eisenkraft JB, eds. *Anesthesia Equipment.* St. Louis: Mosby-Yearbook; 1993:114–139.

62. American Institute of Architects Press. *Guidelines for Construction and Equipment of Hospitals and Medical Facilities.* 1-SBN-0-913962-96-11987 50-51. Washington DC: Author.

63. Gardner RJ. Inhalation anesthetics exposure and control, a statistical comparison of personal exposures in operating theatres with and without anaesthetic gas scavenging. *Ann Occup Hyg.* 1989;33:159.

64. Huffman LM. Common problems in waste gas management. *AANA J.* 1991;59:109.

65. Huffman LM. Understanding flow is important when monitoring respiratory gases. *AANA J.* 1989;57:311.

66. Anonymous. *Technology for Anesthesia.* Plymouth Meeting, Pa: Emergency Care Research Institute; 1991;12:5.

67. Whitcher CE, Siukola LVM. Occupational exposure, education and sampling methods. *Anesthesiology* 1979;(suppl 336):51.

68. Halsey MJ, Chand S, Dluzewski AR, et al. Olfactory thresholds: detection of operating room contamination. *Br J Anaesth.* 1977;49:510.

69. Grogono AW. Anesthesia ventilators: function, limitations and hazards. *ASA Refresher Course* 275, 1991.

70. Hillyer KW, Johnston RR. Unsuspected dilution of anesthetic gases detected by an oxygen analyzer. *Anesth Analg* 1978;57:491.

71. Feeley TW, Bancroft ML. Problems with mechanical ventilators. *Int Anesthesiol Clin.* 1982;20:83.

72. Waterman PM, Pautler S, Smith RB. Accidental ventilator-induced hyperventilation. *Anesthesiology.* 1978;48:141.

73. Rendall-Baker L, Meyer JA. Accidental disconnection and pulmonary barotrauma. *Anesthesiology.* 1983;58:286.

74. Gravenstein JS, Nederstigt JA. Monitoring for disconnection: ventilators with bellows rising on expiration can deliver tidal volumes after disconnection. *J Clin Monit.* 1990;6:207.

75. Schreiber P. *Anesthesia Systems.* Boston: Merchants Press; 1985.

76. Chaney MA. Delivery of excessive airway pressure to a patient by the anesthesia machine. *Anesth Analg.* 1993;76:1162.

77. Hensler T, Dhamee MS. Anesthesia machine malfunction simulating spontaneous respiratory effort. *J Clin Monit.* 1990;6:128.

78. Khalil SN, Gholston TK, Binderman J, Antosh S. Flapper valve malfunction. *Anesth Analg.* 1987;66:1334.

79. *Fluidically Controlled Anesthesia Ventilator Operation and Maintenance Manual.* Ohio Medical Products; Madison, WI: 1974.

80. Biddle C. Advances in ventilating the patient with severe lung disease. *AANA J.* 1993;61:170.

81. Raemer DB. Monitoring respiratory function. In: Ehrenwerth J, Eisenkraft JB, eds. *Anesthesia Equipment.* St. Louis: Mosby-Yearbook; 1993:779–802.

82. Meyer RM. Oxygen analyzers: failure rates and life spans of galvanic cells. *J Clin Monit.* 1990;6:196.

83. Duffin J. *Physics for Anaesthetists.* Springfield, Ill: Charles C. Thomas; 1976.

84. Severinghaus JW, Weiskopf RB, Nishimura M, et al. Oxygen electrode errors due to polarographic reduction of halothane. *J Appl Physiol.* 1971;31:640.

85. Piernan S, Roizen MF, Severinghaus JW. Oxygen analyzer dangerous-senses nitrous oxide as battery fails. *Anesthesiology.* 1979;50:146.

86. *Operation Maintenance. Model 5100 Oxygen Sensors.* Ohmeda; Madison, WI: 1985.
87. *Instruction Manual Oxymed PM.* Drager; Telford, PA: 1984.
88. Figallo EM, Smith RB, Pautler S, Reilly KR. Continuous oxygen analyzers in clinical anesthesia: A review. *Anesthesiol Rev.* 1978;5:25–31.
89. American National Standards Institute. *A National Standard: Requirements for Oxygen Analyzers for Monitoring Patient Breathing Mixtures.* Z-79.10. New York; 1979.
90. Philip JH. Closed circuit anesthesia. In: Ehrenwerth J, Eisenkraft JB, eds. *Anesthesia Equipment.* St. Louis: Mosby-Yearbook; 1993:617–635.
91. Kofke WA, Latta MB. Closed circuit anesthesia. In: Firestone LL, Lebowitz PW, Cook CE, eds. *Clinical Procedures of the Massachusetts General Hospital.* Boston: Little, Brown, 1982: 226–243.
92. Ernst EA, MacKrell TN, Pearson JD, et al. Patient safety: a comparison of open and closed anesthesia circuits. *Anesthesiology.* 1987;67:3A a474.
93. Petrella WK. Enhanced discovery of anesthesia related events: an analysis of 400 consecutive low flow and closed circuit cases. *The Circular* 1989;6:14.
94. Cooper JB, Newbower RS, Kitz RJ. An analysis of major errors and equipment failures in anesthesia management: considerations for prevention and detection. *Anesthesiology.* 1984; 60:34.

☐ QUESTIONS

1. The storage of medical gases is dependent on:
   - A. Critical temperature of the gas
   - B. Boyle's law
   - C. Dalton's law
   - D. Charles' law
     - a. A, B, C
     - b. B, C, D
     - c. C, D, A
     - d. None of the above
     - e. All of the above

2. Medical gases may contain the following contaminants:
   - A. Methane 25 ppm and sulfur dioxide 1 ppm
   - B. Nitrous oxide 5 ppm and anesthetic agent .1%
   - C. Particulate matter and oil 1 mg/m^3
   - D. Liquid water 1 mgH$_2$O/L and hydrocarbons 1 ppm
     - a. A, B, C
     - b. B, C, D
     - c. C, D, A
     - d. All of the above
     - e. None of the above

3. Medical air production is more economical than purchasing blended air in cylinders, but it must be tested for:
   - A. Carbon monoxide
   - B. Nitrogen
   - C. Carbon dioxide
   - D. Dew point
     - a. A, B, C
     - b. B, C, D
     - c. C, D, A
     - d. A and D
     - e. C and D

4. Which of the following statements are true?
   - A. An oxygen cylinder pin-index safety system is coded 2-3.
   - B. An oxygen cylinder pin-index safety system is coded 2-5.
   - C. An air cylinder pin-index safety system is coded 1-5.
   - D. A nitrous oxide pin-index safety system is coded 3-5.
     - a. A, B, C
     - b. B, C, D
     - c. C, D, A
     - d. A only
     - e. None of the above.

5. How long will an oxygen "E" cylinder with a service pressure of 2200 psig continue to supply oxygen for at a flow of 5 L/min?
   - a. 7 hours and 13 minutes
   - b. 4 hours and 50 minutes
   - c. 3 hours and 20 minutes
   - d. 2 hours and 12 minutes
   - e. 1 hour and 6 minutes

6. How long will a nitrous oxide cylinder registering 745 psig continue to deliver nitrous oxide at a flow of 2 L/min?
   - a. 6 hours and 30 minutes
   - b. 13 hours and 20 minutes
   - c. 2 hours and 20 minutes
   - d. Not predictable because nitrous oxide is stored as a liquid—must weigh the cylinder
   - e. Not predictable because liquid gas contents can never be known

7. A safety relief device on the cylinder valve may be:
   - A. Wood's metal that melts at a low and/or high range
   - B. Spring-loaded valve that opens at high pressure
   - C. Frangible disk that ruptures at high pressure
   - D. Rubber diaphragm that ruptures at high pressure or melts at high temperature
     - a. A, B, C
     - b. B, C, D
     - c. C, D, A
     - d. all of the above
     - e. none of the above

8. Devices incorporated on a contemporary anesthesia machine, which completely prevent hypoxia are:

A. Pin-index and diameter-index safety system
B. Pressure sensor shut-off valve
C. Second stage oxygen regulator
D. Oxygen/nitrous oxide proportioning system
   a. A, B, C
   b. B, C, D
   c. C, D, A
   d. All of the above
   e. None of the above

9. The oxygen sensor-shut off valve and oxygen failure alarm respond to:
   a. Flow of oxygen only
   b. Pressure of oxygen only
   c. Flow of supply gas only
   d. Pressure of supply gas only
   e. Percent of oxygen molecules

10. Which of the following statements are true?
   A. The first stage regulator reduces the pressure of the high pressure components of the anesthesia machine to an intermediate pressure.
   B. All anesthesia machines must have second stage regulators to reduce the intermediate pressure to low pressure to prevent barotrauma.
   C. The oxygen flush receives its supply of oxygen from the low pressure part of the anesthesia machine.
   D. The oxygen flush receives its supply of oxygen from the intermediate part of the anesthesia machine.
      a. A and B
      b. B and C
      c. C and D
      d. A and D
      e. None of the above

11. The on/off switch connects the following components of the anesthesia machine:
   A. Oxygen flush
   B. Oxygen sensor-shut off valve
   C. Oxygen flow to the flowmeters
   D. Oxygen failure alarm
      a. A, B, C
      b. B, C, D
      c. C, D, A
      d. All of the above
      e. None of the above

12. When the float is low in the flowmeter, flow is mainly laminar and is:
   A. Directly proportional to the pressure drop along the length of the tube
   B. Directly proportional to the 4th power of the radius of the tube
   C. Inversely proportional to the length of the tube
   D. Inversely proportional to the viscosity of the gas

   a. A, B. C
   b. B, C, D
   c. C, D, A
   d. All of the above
   e. None of the above

13. When the float is high in the flowmeter, flow is mainly turbulent. Which statements are true?
   A. The probability of turbulent flow is calculated by the Reynolds number. This includes the following variables: diameter of the tube, velocity of flow, viscosity and density of the gas.
   B. The annular space is similar to an orifice and diffusion of gas is dependent on the density of that gas.
   C. The annular space is similar to a tube and diffusion of the gas is dependent on the viscosity of the gas.
   D. The probability of turbulent flow can be predicted by calculating the kinematic viscosity, which is the viscosity ÷ density
      a. A, B, C
      b. B, C, D
      c. C, D, A
      d. A, B, D
      e. None of the above

14. Which of the following statements are true?
   A. The vapor pressure of each agent is independent of atmospheric pressure and depends only on the ambient temperature and the agents' physical characteristics.
   B. The specific heat is the amount of heat needed to overcome the van der Waals' forces in a volatile liquid.
   C. Vaporizers are constructed of metals chosen for their specific heat and thermal conductivity characteristics, as well as their cost.
   D. Temperature-compensation is accomplished by altering the splitting ratio in a variable bypass, concentration calibrated vaporizer.
      a. A, B, C
      b. B, C, D
      c. C, D, A
      d. All of the above
      e. None of the above

15. Check valves are incorporated in some anesthesia machines. Which statements are true?
   A. Check valves are incorporated to minimize the pumping effect to the vaporizer.
   B. Check valves are incorporated to minimize the pressurizing effect to the vaporizer.
   C. Check valves reduce the intermediate pressure of the machine to a low pressure.
   D. Check valves require a positive pressure leak test during check-out.
   E. Check valves require a negative pressure leak test during check-out.

　　　a. A, B, C
　　　b. B, C, D
　　　c. C, D, E
　　　d. D, E, A
　　　e. E, A, B

16. Which of the following statements are true regarding semi-open systems?
    A. Rebreathing of carbon dioxide is prevented with high fresh gas flows.
    B. A semi-open system cannot be used with a scavenger.
    C. Semi-open systems are convenient for use in either spontaneous or controlled ventilation.
    D. Semi-open systems are simple, inexpensive, easy to assemble and sterilize.
    E. They may offer lower resistance to breathing when patient is breathing spontaneously.
    　　　a. A, B, C
    　　　b. B, C, D
    　　　c. C, D, E
    　　　d. D, E, A
    　　　e. E, A, B

17. Which of the following statements are true regarding a semi-closed circle system?
    A. Rebreathing is minimized with the carbon dioxide absorber, but this adds the possibility of carbon monoxide accumulation and/or degradation of all the inhalation agents.
    B. Resistance to breathing may be increased due to the unidirectional valves, the granules in the absorber, and the APL valve.
    C. The rebreathing bag acts as a buffer to extremely high pressure in the system and will restrict pressure to 50 cm H_2O.
    D. Mechanical dead space is dependent on the length and diameter of the breathing circuit tubing.
    E. The compression factor is not significant as the design and strength of the tubing has improved.
    　　　a. A, B, C
    　　　b. B, C, D
    　　　c. C, D, E
    　　　d. D, E, A
    　　　e. E, A, B

18. Barotrauma can still be caused under which circumstances:
    A. Using the oxygen flush at end-expiration with the ventilator
    B. Using the oxygen flush at end-inspiration with the ventilator
    C. A leak in the bellows
    D. Obstruction of the scavenger vacuum
    E. Using the oxygen flush with the rebreathing bag
    　　　a. A, B, C
    　　　b. B, C, D
    　　　c. C, D, E
    　　　d. D, E, A
    　　　e. E, A, B

19. Which of the following statements are true regarding changes in atmospheric pressure?
    A. Changes in atmospheric pressure affect the accuracy of gas flow from flowmeter when the float is high in the flow tube, as the density of the gas is the main determinant of flow.
    B. Changes in atmospheric pressure affect the volume percent output of a concentration calibrated vaporizer, but a less dramatic change in the partial pressure measured as $pMAC_1$.
    C. Changes in atmospheric pressure affect the vapor pressure of a volatile agent in a concentration calibrated vaporizer.
    D. Changes in atmospheric pressure affect the high pressure pop-off of the safety relief valve of the anesthesia machine and the ventilator.
    E. Changes in atmospheric pressure affect the measured volume percent output of an oxygen analyzer, but this is of minor importance clinically.
    　　　a. A, B, C
    　　　b. B, C, D
    　　　c. C, D, E
    　　　d. D, E, A
    　　　e. E, A, B

20. A leak in the bellows of a ventilator that uses a Venturi for the drive gas causes which of the following:
    a. Altered FiO_2
    b. Increased peak inspiratory pressure
    c. Decreased percent agent and N_2O
    d. Increased nitrogen on gas analyzer
    e. All of the above

☐ ANSWERS

1. e	**5.** d	**9.** d	**13.** d	**17.** a
2. a	**6.** d	**10.** d	**14.** c	**18.** b
3. d	**7.** a	**11.** b	**15.** e	**19.** e
4. b	**8.** e	**12.** d	**16.** d	**20.** e

FOUR

Basic Principles of Anesthesia

CHAPTER 8

Patient Preparation and Preoperative Assessment

Terrie Kole

The roles of the patient interview, history, physical examination, and counseling are to obtain data necessary to planning effective risk: benefit-oriented anesthesia care and to provide opportunities for opening lines of communication between patients and anesthesia professionals, for the purpose of building the treatment partnership.

When a patient enters the hospital either for elective surgery or for emergency surgery, and anything other than local anesthesia is necessary, fear is a strong component of the preoperative mix. Several years ago, the American Association of Nurse Anesthetists (AANA) conducted a survey of its members and asked what was the greatest concern as expressed to them by the patients. The majority response was "afraid of not waking up." Not too far down the list was also the fear of "waking up too soon, while surgery is still in progress." These comments express fears of loss of personal control. Undergoing anesthesia means relinquishing control of one's self to someone else and trusting them to guard one's life as if it were her or his own.

☐ THE GOALS OF ANESTHESIA AND PREOPERATIVE ASSESSMENT

The four essential components of general anesthesia are unconsciousness, muscle relaxation, analgesia, and amnesia.[1,2] Without unconsciousness there may be learning, which may or may not have negative sequelae. Without muscle relaxation the surgical field may be inaccessible and the airway may not be patent. Total muscle relaxation without unconsciousness precipitates a terror "bound-and-gagged" scenario for patients, who cannot communicate their levels of pain or

fear. Without analgesia there is the perception of pain and the potential for disruption of the unconscious state. Without amnesia the perception, no matter how misconstrued, of intraoperative stimuli may be recalled and the potential for a learned response exists.

The purpose of the preoperative assessment and preparation is to gain enough information to develop a functioning anesthesia care plan that meets the goals and contains the four components of anesthesia. During this process, appropriate screening in a timely manner will yield patient selection information and will avoid delays and potential cancellations. Appropriate screening offers the potential to resolve some medical problems and anticipate or prevent others. The screening process can lead to tactics that will initiate corrective measures, minimize complications, and select and appoint optimal agents and techniques to ensure patient safety and optimal surgical results.

During the preoperative preparation, patient education is essential to compliance and to levels of understanding that ensure true informed consent. The anesthetist has a premium opportunity at this time to build patient rapport and trust, so that patient fears are allayed.

☐ THE PATIENT INTERVIEW

MEDICAL HISTORY

Patients may not always voluntarily provide a complete medical history. There are a variety of reasons for this omission, including but not limited to forgetfulness, intentional deletion, inappropriate prioritization, and denial. Depending on what the problem or diagnosis is, any patient may elect to withhold information. It is the role of the anesthetist to ferret out the appropriate information, sometimes by asking questions through several different approaches.

A recent study demonstrated that early preoperative assessment, such as that done at an outpatient clinic, reduces patient distress by reducing the number of preoperative tests performed and reducing late cancellations.[3]

Systems Review   It is essential to obtain pertinent information about past or current disease in the systems of the body, whether or not they are directly related to the condition for which the hospitalization occurs. They may have bearing on the selection and administration of anesthesia.

The anesthetist needs information on the following patient systems, described more fully in Table 8–1:

- Cardiovascular system
- Respiratory system
- Central and peripheral nervous system
- Gastrointestinal system
- Endocrine system
- Musculoskeletal system
- Urinary system
- Reproductive system
- Hematopoietic system/coagulopathy

Within the interview on each of these systems will be the opportunity to question the patient's history and any pertinent family history. Allergies to drugs, respiratory allergies, contact allergies, and previous idiosyncratic responses to drugs and anesthesia are of vital concern to the anesthesia professional and play a central role in decision-making for appropriate anesthesia care. As treatment for conditions within these systems, concomitant medications (even those taken within the previous month, if not being taken currently) may interact with anesthetics, a factor that should be considered for appropriate care planning and patient response to anesthetic agents. Any concomitant medication that affects the hemodynamic profile, the respiratory status, the metabolic process, musculoskeletal function, the central nervous system (CNS), and the inflammatory or healing process should be of primary interest to the anesthetist as these medications may change patient responses to anesthesia in some way.

Of concern also will be the patient's admitted (versus actual) use or abuse of chemical substances, tobacco, and alcohol. The circulatory, CNS, metabolic, and respiratory effects of these substances may complicate the patient's response to anesthesia. Everything from increased mucous production to circulatory collapse is possible when these substances are present in the tissues and anesthetics are introduced into the "mix." Obtaining accurate information on the use of these substances may be a problem because patients may feel either proprietary or guilty about disclosure. They may fear retribution. The interviewer must reassure patients that questions about the use of these substances are being asked for no other reason than to plan the correct anesthesia care. No

judgments will be made about the patients as a result of their responses. It should be explained to them that to withhold information on this topic could prove fatal at worst or could complicate both the operative process and the recovery at the least. In some instances, the automated form of preoperative health status questionnaire is a tool used to obtain information about the drug, alcohol, and tobacco consumption that may yield more honest answers to sensitive question.[4]

In some institutions, a preliminary "health quiz" is given to preoperative patients. Patients respond to questions posed on a computerized board or a printout. This does not eliminate the personal interview, but it is a trigger for additional questioning in areas of concern,[5] and may highlight areas of potential risk.[6,7] Participation in this form of interview implies the need for language skills and a cultural and educational background commensurate with the reading level of the questions. For patients with low literacy levels or whose ethnic or cultural language is not English, some institutions have developed videos to ask the same questions seen on the quizzes and to explain anesthesia procedures.[8,9] In one study, it was found that the video did not enhance patients' knowledge of the procedure, but their perceptions of the value of the preoperative visit improved with use of the video.[9]

Some patients will not be active participants in the preoperative interview. Patients who are seriously ill (i.e., in too much pain to concentrate or too toxic to understand the questions), sedated, too young to give answers, or cognitively disabled will not be of much help in obtaining information. Patients scheduled for emergency surgery may fall into this category. When this occurs, the anesthetist must rely on information from patients' families or significant others that could be potentially faulty or incomplete. For this reason, the physical examination findings and test results will comprise the principal portion of the "history" for these patients.

PHYSICAL EXAMINATION

When assessing the patient's preoperative status, the second stage is to conduct a physical examination. Vital statistics include heart rate, blood pressure, respiratory rate, height, and weight.

The anesthetist can review the preadmission physical conducted by the attending physician as a reference point. In addition, based on information gleaned from the patient history, the anesthetist may elect to revisit specific aspects of the physical examination, namely, those related to cardiovascular and respiratory status, airway patency evaluation, cognitive status and neurologic assessment, range of motion for torso and extremities, dentition, and wound site condition, if applicable. The presence of fever should also be noted. General nutritional status may be determined by direct observation of adipose tissue distribution, skin color and texture, gum and buccal mucosa color, and saliva fluid volume levels, and weight/height ratio. Further definition of nutritional status may require laboratory analysis (hematologic, electrolyte, and chemical profile).

Table 8–1
PATIENT HISTORY: SYSTEM REVIEW

Systems	Questions	Considerations

Cardiovascular	History of:
	  Myocardial infarct?
	  Congestive heart failure?
	  Stroke (TIA/CVA)?
	  Irregular beat?
	  Palpitations/fluttering?
	  Chest pain/arm radiation?
	  Hypertension?
	  Hypotension?
	  Blackouts?
	  Racing/too slow pulse?
	  Surgery on vessels/heart?
	  Pacemaker?
	  Congenital anomalies?
	  Calf pain when walking?
	  Extremity cold?
	  Extremity discoloration/blanching?
	  Pain or SOB on exertion?
	Medications?
	Previous diagnoses related to heart, vessels, or blood?
		Cardiac function
		Cardiac output
		Arterial patency/elasticity
		Venous return
		Thromboses/embolus potential

Respiratory	History of:
	  SOB?
	  Tightness in chest?
	  Pain/heaviness in chest?
	  Inhalant allergies?
	  Medication allergies producing respiratory
	    symptoms/other symptoms?
	  Tumor?
	  Pneumonia?
	  Emphysema?
	  Asthma?
	  Other lung disease?
	  Nasal congestion?
	  Sinus infections?
	  Deviated nasal septum?
	  Cervical lymphadenopathy?
	  Surgery?
	  Extremity discoloration?
	  Clubbing of fingers?
	  Hiatal hernia?
	  Diaphragmatic irregularities?
	Medications?
	Smoker/tobacco use?
		Tital volume
		Residual capacity
		Forced expiratory volume
		Clarity/airway patency
		Hypoxia potential

Neurologic	History of:
	  Epilepsy?
	  Tumor?
	  Blackouts?
	  Paralysis?
	  Head injury?
	  Numbness (any location)?
	  Back/leg or back/neck/arm radiculopathy?
	  Vertebral trauma?
	  Head/back/neck surgery?
	  Extremity discoloration/blanching?
	  Recurrent headaches?
	  Migraine headaches?
		Neuromuscular conductance factors
		Seizure potential
		Paresthesia
		Paralysis
		Cardiovascular innervation
		Respiratory innervation
		Response to pain
		Comparisons for postoperative evaluation
		  (range of motion/paralysis/paresthesia)
		Potential drug/drug interactions

(continued)

Table 8–1 (*continued*)
PATIENT HISTORY: SYSTEM REVIEW

Systems	Questions	Considerations
	Vision disturbances?	
	Glaucoma?	
	Cataracts?	
	Ophthalmic surgery?	
	Alzheimer's symptoms?	
	Alcohol consumption?	
	Chemical substance use/abuse?	
	Medications?	
Musculoskeletal	History of:	Frame support for respiration and positioning
	Fracture?	Comparisons for postoperative evaluation
	Loss of muscle tone?	(range of motion/paralysis/paresthesia)
	Amputation?	
	Tendonitis?	
	Bursitis?	
	Arthritis?	
	Gait irregularity?	
	Back pain?	
	Joint pain?	
	Loss of muscle strength?	
	Problems with grasp?	
	Multiple sclerosis?	
	Poliomyelitis?	
	Muscular dystrophy?	
	Amyotrophic lateral sclerosis?	
	Osteogenesis imperfecta?	
	Osteoporosis?	
	Postural deficiency (lordosis/kyphosis/scoliosis)?	
	Tendon injury/surgery?	
	Other surgery?	
	Dental status:	
	Caps, crowns, dentures, partial plates?	
	Overbite/underbite?	
	TMJ disease?	
	Nasoseptal defect or deviation?	
	Medications?	
Urinary	History of:	Detoxification and elimination capacity
	Kidney disease?	Comparisons for postoperative evaluation
	Kidney stones?	
	Prostate disease?	
	Bladder problems?	
	Hematuria?	
	Back pain?	
	Flank pain?	
	Bladder pain?	
	Urgency?	
	Frequency?	
	Dysuria?	
	Pyuria?	
	Medications?	
Gastrointestinal (GI)	History of:	GI tract patency
	Medication sensitivities producing GI symptoms?	Detoxification and elimination of anesthesia
	Ulcer?	Reflux/regurgitation/aspiration potential
	Diverticulitis?	Metabolic rate
	Reflux disease?	
	Hiatal hernia?	
	Inguinal hernia?	
	Bowel obstruction?	
	Hepatitis?	
	Pancreatitis?	
	Cholecystitis?	

Table 8–1 (continued)
PATIENT HISTORY: SYSTEM REVIEW

Systems	Questions	Considerations
	Gallstones?	
	Gallbladder disease?	
	Digestion problems?	
	Anorexia/bulimia?	
	General nutritional status?	
	Sudden weight gain or loss?	
	Current weight?	
	Abdominal pain/cramping?	
	Hemorrhoids?	
	Constipation?	
	Frequent diarrhea?	
	Dysphagia?	
	Food allergies or sensitivities?	
	Stomach stapling?	
	Surgery: (intra-abdominal/rectal)?	
	Medications?	
Endocrine	History of:	Systemic influences on hemodynamic profile
	Thyroid disease/surgery?	Hyper- or hypoglycemia
	Adrenal disease?	Decreased hepatic clearance/metabolism
	Pituitary tumors?	Potential for serum disease transfer
	Diabetes (mellitus or insipidus)?	Adhesion history delaying surgery
	Cirrhosis?	
	Hepatitis?	
	Digestive disorders?	
	Gallbladder disease?	
	Pancreatitis?	
	Medications?	
Reproductive	History of:	Pregnancy
	Prostate disease?	Coagulation disorders
	Testicular disease?	Thromboses/embolus potential
	Ovarian disease?	
	Uterine dysfunction?	
	Current pregnancy?	
	Para/gravida?	
	Menses onset/duration/cessation/menopause	
	Hormonal replacement therapy?	
	Birth control hormonal therapy?	
	Medications?	
Hematopoietic/ Coagulopathy	History of:	Serum disease transfer potential
	HIV status/high-risk behavior?	Hypoxia potential
	Anemias?	Coagulation disorders
	Leukemias/lymphomas?	Thromboses/embolus potential
	Hemophilia?	Chemical (controlled or chemotherapy) and
	Phlebitis?	anesthesia interaction
	Polycythemia vera?	Hemodynamic profile
	Leukocytosis?	
	Hyper/hypoglycemia?	
	Chemical/substance abuse?	
	Sickle cell disease?	
	Thromboses or embolus?	
	Septicemia?	
	Chemotherapy?	
	Medications?	
Other: Dermatologic	History of:	
	Allergies (adhesive tape, latex, detergents, etc)?	
	Infections/lesions?	
	Herpes?	
	Eczema?	

HIV, human immunodeficiency virus; SOB, shortness of breath; TIA/CVA, transient ischemic attack/cerebrovascular accident; TMJ, temporomandibular joint

LABORATORY TESTING

Newly developed automated preoperative health quiz reports that assess answers and record prompts for further exploration are also programmed to make recommendations regarding appropriate, relative preoperative testing. These programs reduce the use of extensive preoperative testing.

In one study, the general incidence of abnormal preoperative test results was low, even in a Veterans Administration medical center setting. The automation-assisted test selection that is based on patient response to the health questions will reduce the expense of preoperative testing with minimal compromise in the quality of patient care.[7] In this same study, the authors concluded that the cost of performing the protocol preoperative tests on 60 patients was over $15,000, whereas the combative cost of tests suggested by the automated interview were just over $7000. Results of only 16 of the 650 protocol tests were abnormal. The automated preoperative selection recommended conducting 13 of those 16 tests. Furthermore, none of the abnormal laboratory values derived from a test *not* recommended by the automated system required medical intervention.[7]

It stands to reason, however, that should the patient's preoperative status and proposed surgical procedure warrant, specific testing not normally included in standard protocols should be conducted (i.e., pulmonary function testing on the preoperative oat-cell carcinoma pneumonectomy candidate to determine baseline values for intraoperative ventilation and assessing remaining lung status). To this end, testing other than hemoglobin, hematocrit, complete blood count, limited chemical profile, urinalysis, and possibly chest x-ray for those patients whose respiratory status appears to be compromised (asthma, chronic obstructive pulmonary disease, emphysema, mediastinal lesion, etc.) must be evaluated on an individual, cost/benefit ratio. In some institutions, baseline electrocardiography is not included on all patients.[10] The University Hospital Consortium has made specific recommendations on indications for preoperative diagnostic evaluations.[11] Follow-up studies have shown these recommendations to be effective and cost saving without any effect on morbidity as evaluated by length of stay for elective surgery.[12]

If concomitant disease states warrant, specific testing may be ordered. For instance, patients with prescreen elevated fasting blood glucose levels who have not been diagnosed as diabetic may require an additional glucose analysis (glycosylated hemoglobin) to determine whether glucose levels were also elevated within the previous month, before the preadmission survey.

For asthmatic patients whose disease is in a state of flux, baseline peak expiratory flow readings should be compared to personal best or predicted values. Unless there is significant reduction (< 70% of predicted or personal best), pulmonary function studies may not be warranted. Chest x-rays for these patients may only be appropriate if significant reduction in respiratory function (< 70% of predicted) is accompanied by rales or rhonchi in the lungs. Asthmatic patients on theophylline may need a preoperative serum level assay as a baseline to ascertain optimal therapeutic effects going into surgery. Immediately preoperatively, pulse oximetry baseline values should be taken.

Patients with metabolic compromise in the form of liver, kidney, or thyroid disease may require additional testing to obtain more detailed profiles of electrolyte, chemical, coagulation, and oxygen-uptake status.

Cardiac risk assessment paradigms have been tested in many institutions. Extrapolations from these trials have been inconsistent because of irregularities in methodology and study design. The ability to predict with success subsets of patients for whom additional preoperative testing is needed and whose outcomes are then indicative of these additional precautions is desirable, so researchers continue to work on this problem.[13] Nonroutine diagnostic testing for preoperative cardiac risk factors may include, but are not necessarily limited to, exercise stress testing (electrocardiography and radionuclear), ambulatory electrocardiography, echocardiography (precordial, stress, and transesophageal), radionuclear ventriculography, dipyridamole-thallium scintigraphy, magnetic resonance imaging, and cardiac catheterization.[14]

☐ PREOPERATIVE PREPARATION

The American Society of Anesthesiologists (ASA) has developed a classification system to help the anesthesia professional determine the general status of a patient and the relative risk associated with administering anesthesia to that patient. Space in this chapter does not permit a full disclosure of the ASA classifications and their parameters. However, as an outline, the categories are: ASA I (lowest risk, generally health), ASA II (moderate risk, some complicating factors), or ASA III (high risk, several moderate-to-severe complicating factors/coexisting disease). ASA IV describes a severe systemic disturbance that may not be related to the reason for surgery. ASA Class V is reserved for the moribund patient with little chance of survival, even with surgery. Consult standard texts for definitive information on this subject.

A preoperative anesthesia checklist can be helpful (Table 8–2).

NPO STATUS

When determining what preoperative orders are required, the question of preoperative fasting becomes a consideration. The purpose for preoperative fasting was the belief that it allowed for complete gastric emptying before the administration of anesthesia. It has been the belief that this process limited the severity of the acid pneumonitis syndrome resulting from pulmonary aspiration. However, most studies agree that the time of ingestion of fluid intake bears little relation to the volume of gastric contents present at induction.[15–17] Also, the low incidence of acid pneumonitis (about 0.01%) makes the practice of preoperative fasting for prevention of this condition a matter of preference and of assessment of relative risk, rather than one of proven fact. Of consideration should be the timing of the ingestion of solid food on the day of surgery, assessment of the potential risk factor of allowing ingestion of clear

Table 8-2
CHECKLIST FOR ANESTHESIA PREOPERATIVE PREPARATION

Item/Procedure	DT Comp	Initials	Special Notes

Patient History/Documented
  System review:
  Allergies:
  Concomitant medications:			

Physical Examination
  Cardiovascular:
  Airway/Respiratory:
  Urinary:
  Hematopoietic:
  Dentition:
  Other:			

Preoperative Testing
  Hemoglobin/hematocrit:
  Complete blood count:
  Chemical profile:
  Coag times:
  Urinalysis:
  Radiography:
  Electrocardiography:
  Other:			

Informed consent/surgery:			
Patient counseling/discussion: NPO status/regimen:			
Patient counseling/discussion: Anesthesia plan/alternative/risks:			
Informed consent/anesthesia:			
Preoperative medication ordered:			
Other considerations:			

fluids until 2 hours preoperatively, restrictions on the amount of water ingested with oral preoperative medications, and the advisability of using an H_2-receptor antagonist for specific patients with known risks. For some patients, comfort preoperatively governs the use of preoperative fasting.

PREOPERATIVE MEDICATIONS

Analgesia, amnesia, anxiolysis and sedation, prevention of nausea in at-risk patients or for at-risk procedures, drying of airway secretions, reduction of anesthetic requirements, and prophylaxis against allergic reactions are the goals of preop-

erative medication.[18] Preoperative medication has its best results in patients who have been adequately prepared for the surgery, who feel empowered as a treatment partner, and who understand the purpose of, and events related to, the treatments used. When patients' fears are unabated, the stress response can counteract some of the effects of preoperative medication. So also may long-standing, preoperative behaviors (alcohol intake, substance or medication abuse, etc.) affects the results from preoperative medication. The anesthesia professional must take all of this into consideration when planning the preoperative sedation. The estimated duration of the proposed surgery and the potential for postoperative effects from cumulative action of the medications and anesthesia ancillary medications must also be considered. For instance, the addition of fentanyl intraoperatively to prevent cardiac stress response or irregularities precipitated by some inhaled anesthetics may have a cumulative effect with premedication that provides postoperative sedation for a longer period of time than premedications alone. In other cases, preoperative drugs may have predictable postoperative effects that the induction technique may or may not change.[19]

The preoperative regimen is determined by assessing patient condition and by considering the type of anesthesia planned, the estimated duration of the proposed surgery, and whether the patient is an outpatient or inpatient. Outpatients must be medicated in a way that permits timely discharge from the outpatient surgery unit and yet that serves the patient for efficacy and safety. Table 8–3 shows the basic categories of drugs and the standard selection of drugs in those categories from which are chosen the preoperative regimen for patients, both outpatient and inpatient.

Some patients should not be given depressants preoperatively, namely, those with little psychological reserve, those at the extremes of age, those who have head injury, or those who are hypovolemic.[18] Some surgical procedures require that the patient be sufficiently sedated to relieve anxiety but easily aroused, cooperative, and responsive to instructions. For these patients, the request to "not know anything that's happening" cannot be fulfilled. For these patients especially, psychological preparation is essential.

Many anesthesia professionals feel that the addition of an amnestic, such as midazolam, will help eliminate the potential for awareness and learning under anesthesia. However, research has determined the mean alveolar concentrations of inhaled anesthetics below which learning may occur, regardless of preoperative medications.[20]

In the prevention of postoperative nausea and vomiting, consideration is given to the patient's history of previous nausea and vomiting with anesthesia, the nature of the surgery planned (i.e., may occur more frequently with surgery of the abdomen), allergic or adverse event profiles of the drugs being used, and the type of anesthesia planned. The development of newer agents for perioperative antiemesis, such as ondansetron, and newer induction agents, such as propofol, has put more effective tools to prevent postoperative nausea and vomiting into the hands of anesthesia professionals.[21]

The use of barbiturates as preoperative medication is a tested practice of decades. However, as a class of drugs, the barbiturates carry with them a profile of side effects comprising the "hangover" syndrome within even an hour of administration. These agents lack specificity of action on the CNS and may have a lower therapeutic index than the benzodiazepines.[18]

Opioids are used in the preoperative regimen when analgesia before surgery is desirable. This includes the relief of existing pain, such as for those with orthopedic trauma or acute cholecystitis, or for the prevention of pain during the administration of regional anesthesia or the insertion of invasive monitoring. Caution should be exercised with elderly patients because they may have a reduced sensitivity to pain but

a heightened sensitivity to the effects of analgesics of this class[18] (see Table 8–3).

☐ COUNSELING PREOPERATIVE PATIENTS: INFORMED CONSENT

Research has shown that the principal fear of most surgical patients undergoing anesthesia (particularly general anesthesia) is the loss of self-control and the potential for "not waking up." The second strongest fear is that of "waking up too soon," while surgery is still in progress, and experiencing the shock and pain that event may entail.[22]

The first role of the preoperative interview is to obtain information, but other and equally important roles of the interview are to determine the patients' levels of understanding about the surgery and anesthesia planned. Additionally, the interviewer counsels patients about the plan and its risks while reassuring them of the standard of care they may expect, and the guardianship/patient advocate role of the anesthesia professionals involved.

Acknowledging the fears patients may have and empowering patients through information exchange, including the calm assurance that utmost care will be taken and that the anesthesia department staff are their best advocates during surgery, may help relieve the stress patients experience in these circumstances.[24] If levels of stress and fear go unabated, serious consequences may arise. Patients with precarious hemodynamic profiles have been seen to suffer catastrophic results in the operating room when fear and stress levels are too high, even before any anesthetic has been administered.

Any anesthesia may have risks for the patient. Some risks have more severe consequences than others. There is a great deal of controversy about how much to tell the patient to ensure true informed consent. Information about the risks of adverse reaction or interaction, awareness and learning under anesthesia, CNS and cardiac effects, and anaphylaxis may help the patient prepare and feel empowered or may further alarm the patient, raising stress levels and triggering negative response. There does not appear to be a concrete guideline to determining which patients will react which way, but in this day of frequent litigation, to err on the side of disclosure may be the safest route.[23,25] Some patients will ask many questions. Truthful answers without alarmist content will suffice for these patients. It is the patients who do not ask questions that the interviewer must prompt to participate more actively.

☐ SUMMARY

The anesthesia professional has a multifaceted role when interviewing and counseling the preoperative patient. The anesthetist, as patient advocate in the preoperative period, must be part detective, diagnostician, scientist, strategist, pharmacist, and counselor and must interact with the patient in the manner of both the physician and nurse. Physical, pharmacologic, sociocultural, and psychological aspects comprise the approach the anesthetist must take to the perioperative patient to combine appropriate care with preventive medicine.

Table 8–3
PROFILES OF SOME COMMONLY
USED PREOPERATIVE
MEDICATIONS, BY CLASS

Medication Class	Standard Medications*/Class	Comments
	Consult the prescribing information or the Physicians' Desk Reference on all medications before ordering or administering.	
Opioids	Opioid agonists: fentanyl, meperidine, morphine Opioid agonist-antagonists: butorphanol, pentazocine, nalbuphine	*Precautions:* Agonists— respiratory depression, bradycardia, asystole, arrhythmias, or orthostatic hypotension may result. Agonist-antagonists—reduce ventilatory side effects but may reduce analgesic effects of agonist postoperative pain therapy. Decrease doses for elderly.
Amnestics	Midazolam Diazepam Lorazepam Oxazepam	*Precautions:* Lengthy central nervous system depression may occur; may be pain at injection site with diazepam; nonanalgesic; agitation and restlessness may result instead of calm, especially in obstetric patients.
Anticholinergics	Atropine Glycopyrrolate	*Precautions:* Potential to increase risk of aspiration pneumonitis due to relaxation of gastroesophageal junction; does not reduce gastric acid content or gastric fluid pH
Tranquilizers/Sedative/ Hypnotics	Barbiturates: secobarbital, pentobarbital Butyrophenone: droperidol Hydroxyzine Diphenhydramine Phenothiazines: promethiazine, promazine, perphenazine Chloral hydrate	*Precautions:* Barbiturates unlikely to produce sedation in presence of pain; disorientation may occur; very low doses are antianalgesic. Droperidol may promote appearance of calm but dysphoria, restlessness, and death anxiety may occur. Hydroxyzine and diphenhydramine are additive with opioids but do not produce amnesia, have antihistaminic and anticholinergic actions. Chloral hydrate use limited due to use of benzodiazepines.
Antiemetics	Ondansetron Butyrophenone: droperidol Metoclopramide Domperidone	*Precautions:* May mask progressive ileus or gastric distention in abdominal surgery.
H_2-antagonists	Cimetidine Ranitidine	*Precautions:* Do not rely on these to affect gastric fluid volume or gastric emptying time.

*Doses are individualized within ranges and are not given in this table. Consult prescribing information for appropriate dosing information on all medications listed in this table.
Adapted from Moyers,[18] *Physicians' Desk Reference*,[26] and Koda-Kimble and Young.[27]

REFERENCES

1. Cooney GF. Drugs used in anesthesia: their effects on awareness and recall. *Anesthesia Today.* 1991;3(1):7–9.
2. Desiderio DP, Thorne AC. *Acta Anaesthesiol Scand.* 1990; 34(suppl 92):48–50.
3. Golden BA, McCarrol SM, Doyle ME, Donovan FM, Walsh CM. Preoperative assessment—the benefit of an anaesthetic assessment clinic. *Anesth Analg.* 1996;82(2S):S134. Abstract.
4. Smith I, White PF. Anesthesia for ambulatory surgery. *Current Reviews for Nurse Anesthetists.* March 1994;16(lesson 20): 171–178.
5. Lutner RE, Roizen MF, Stocking CB, et al. The automated interview versus the personal interview. *Anesthesiology.* 1991; 75:394–400.
6. Lutner RE, Roizen MF, Stocking CB, et al. The automated interview versus the personal interview. Do patient responses to preoperative health questions differ? *Anesthesiology.* 1991; 75(3):394–400.
7. Fu ES, Scharf JE. Assessment of computer-assisted preoperative test selection. *Anesthesiology.* 1995;83(3A):A434. Abstract.
8. Kaplan EB, Sheiner LB, Boeckmann AJ, et al. The usefulness of preoperative laboratory screening. *JAMA.* 1985;253(24): 3576–3581.
9. Zvara DA, Mathes DD, Brooker RF, McKinley AC. Video as a patient teaching tool: does it add to the preoperative anesthetic visit? *Anesthesiology.* 1995;83(3A):A1012. Abstract.
10. Paraskos JA. Who needs a preoperative electrocardiogram? *Arch Intern Med.* 1992;152:261–263.
11. University Hospital Consortium (UHC): *Technology Assessment: Routine Preoperative Diagnostic Evaluations.* Oak Brook, Ill: UHC; 1994.
12. Collins SL, Chendrasekhar A. Coordination of routine preoperative testing affects change in practice pattern. *Anesthesiology.* 1995;83(3A):A1038. Abstract.
13. Mangano DT. Preoperative risk assessment: many studies, few solutions—is a cardiac risk assessment paradigm possible? *Anesthesiology.* 1995;83:897–901. Editorial.
14. Mangano DT. Perioperative cardiac morbidity. *Anesthesiology.* 1990;72:153–184.
15. Crawford M, Lerman J, Christensen S, Farrow-Gillespie A. Effects of duration of fasting on gastric fluid pH and volume in healthy status. *Anesth Analg.* 1990;71:400–403.
16. Schreiner MS, Triebwasser A, Keon TP. Ingestion of liquids compared with preoperative fasting in pediatric outpatients. *Anesthesiology.* 1990;72:593–597.
17. Soreide E, Holst-Larsen K, Reite K, et al. Effects of giving water 20–450 mL with oral diazepam premedication 1–2h before operation. *Br J Anaesth.* 1993;71:503–506.
18. Moyers JR. Preoperative medication. In: Barash PG, Cullen BF, Stoelting RK, eds. *Clinical Anesthesia.* Philadelphia: JB Lippincott; 1989:485–503.
19. Malviya S, Green W, Huntington J, Stewart M, Voepel-Lewis T. Effects of anesthetic technique on side effects associated with fentanyl oralet premedication. *Anesth Analg.* 1996;82(2S): S290. Abstract.
20. Dwyer R, Bennett HL, Eger EI II. Learning and responsiveness at subanesthetic concentrations of isoflurane and nitrous oxide. *Anesthesiology.* 1991;75(suppl 3A):A334. Abstract.
21. Joshi S, Shevde K, Sanghvi M, Trivedi SM, Khan MA, Tyagaraj C. Comparison of ondansetron (O) and propofol (P) in the prevention of postoperative nausea and vomiting. *Anesth Analg.* 1996;82(2S):s210. Abstract.
22. AANA Survey—RE: Questions most asked by anesthesia patients (circa 1990). Internal survey; data on file at American Association of Nurse Anesthetists.
23. Ghoneim MF, Block RI. Learning and consciousness during general anesthesia. *Anesthesiology.* 1992:76:279–305.
24. Moerman N, van Dam FSAM, Muller MJ, Oosting A. The Amsterdam preoperative anxiety and information scale (APAIS). *Anesth Analg.* 1996;82:445–451.
25. Roizen MF, Klock A, Klaft J. How much do they really want to know? Preoperative patient interviews and the anesthesiologist. *Anesth Analg.* 1996;82:443–444.
26. *Physicians' Desk Reference,* 50th ed. Montvale, NJ; Medical Economics: 1996.
27. Koda-Kimble MA, Young LY, eds. *Applied Therapeutics: The Clinical Use of Drugs,* 5th ed. Vancouver, Wash: Applied Therapeutics; 1992.

ACKNOWLEDGEMENT

The author acknowledges the assistance of Judith B. Paquet, RN, for literature search and editorial review.

☐ QUESTIONS

1. What are the four components of general anesthesia?
   a. Analgesia, amnesia, drying of respiratory secretions, and hemodynamic stability
   b. Unconsciousness, muscle relaxation, analgesia, and amnesia
   c. Airway patency, unconsciousness, muscle relaxation, and amnesia
   d. Hemodynamic stability, unconsciousness, analgesia, and amnesia

2. Which one of the following is *not true?*
   a. Early preoperative assessment, done at an outpatient clinic, is too premature to be of use at the time of surgery.
   b. Patients may not always provide a complete medical history voluntarily.
   c. Patient education goes on simultaneously, as part of the patient interview.
   d. There are a minimum of nine body systems about which the patient interview should provide information.

3. Which one of the following is *true?*
   a. Except for cardiac, diabetic, and oncologic history, information about the patient's parents' or siblings' diseases is not necessary.
   b. Information about concomitant medications the patient is taking/has taken is only pertinent if they have taken them within the previous 24 hours.

c. Substance or chemical/pharmacologic abuse information is only important to include in the interview if the patient is an obstetric patient.

d. Some institutions use an automated health quiz to elicit patient interview information.

4. Which one *best* describes primary triggers for the anesthetist in preparing to do the physical examination?
   a. Patient and family historical risk factors, vital sign deviations, fever/pain, and systems at risk from anesthetics
   b. Patient risk factors only and general observation of the patient's overall condition
   c. Patient request for information about specific system status and hemodynamic profile
   d. Complaints of pain, fever, and vital signs deviations

5. Which one of the following best cites issues of *primary* concern to the anesthetist in the information gleaned from the physical examination?
   a. Intestinal patency, kidney function, pulse rate/volume, and pulse oximetry
   b. Vital signs, cardiovascular status, airway patency, and extremity range of motion
   c. Liver function, kidney function, respiratory status, and intestinal function
   d. Fever, vital signs, cognitive status, and general nutritional status

6. A 36-year-old female with no surgical or medical history is scheduled for an emergency craniotomy related to a subarachnoid hemorrhage. Upon arrival she is unconscious and hemodynamically stable. Which ASA physical status classification best describes this patient?
   a. ASA I E
   b. ASA II E
   c. ASA III E
   d. ASA IV E

7. Patients with asthma, whose disease is unstable, should have which one of the following done preoperatively, as a first option?
   a. Spirometry twice
   b. Chest computed tomography scan
   c. Histamine challenge pulmonary function study
   d. Peak expiratory flow rate baseline readings

8. In most hospitals, nonroutine preoperative cardiac risk factor testing includes which one of the following?
   a. ECG baseline, exercise stress testing, and magnetic resonance imaging
   b. Pulse oximetry, echocardiography, and chest computed tomography scan
   c. Exercise stress testing, echocardiography, and cardiac catheterization
   d. ECG baseline, echocardiography, and cardiac enzyme profile

9. 12-hour NPO status:
   a. Guarantees emptying of gastric fluids
   b. Is a cardinal component of all preoperative orders
   c. Is unnecessary, for all patients
   d. Must be individualized to the patient, and may be modified

10. Preoperative medications:
    a. Are necessary to provide total obfuscation of sensation for the patient
    b. Can include antiemetics and anxiolytics, as well as analgesics
    c. Rely on the patient's lack of anxiety in order to be effective
    d. Have no interaction with substance/chemical abuse agents if these agents were not taken within the previous 12 hours

11. Which patient should *not* be given depressants, preoperatively?
    a. The 52-year-old cholecystectomy patient
    b. The 24-year-old cranial trauma patient
    c. The 67-year-old knee joint replacement patient
    d. The 10-year-old appendicitis patient

12. Barbiturates have more specificity of action on the central nervous system than do benzodiazepines. *True* or *False?*
    a. True
    b. False

13. True informed consent includes a discussion, with patient comprehension, of all possible adverse events related to the proposed anesthesia and anesthesia/surgery interactions. *True* or *False?*
    a. True
    b. False

14. Which one best describes some of the impact of patient's neurologic status may have on the planned anesthesia?
    a. Seizure potential, peripheral vascular innervation, neuromuscular response to blockade
    b. Frame support for respiration, tidal volume capacity, hypoxia potential
    c. Airway patency, analgesia override, detoxification and elimination
    d. Metabolic rate, hemodynamic stability, seizure potential

15. What disease/condition is more likely to alter the hematopoietic system status negatively?
    a. Hypertension
    b. Septicemia
    c. Hiatal hernia
    d. Inflammatory bowel disease

16. The drugs in which class, of those listed in Table 8–3, are more likely to cause gastroesophageal reflux?
    a. Barbiturates
    b. Antiemetics
    c. Anticholinergics
    d. Amnestics

17. Butorphanol:
    a. Is an anticholinergic
    b. Is likely to cause pain on injection
    c. Is a potentially antagonistic to opioid analgesia
    d. Is an antacid modifier of gastric pH

18. Diazepam:
    a. Is an anticholinergic
    b. Is likely to cause pain on injection

c. Is likely to mask progressive ileus in abdominal surgery
d. Is an antiemetic

19. Very low doses of barbiturates:
    a. Are standard practice
    b. Promote gastric emptying
    c. Stimulate agitation
    d. Are antianalgesic

20. Which preoperative concomitant medication regimen may alter the hematopoietic profile negatively?
    a. Birth control/hormonal therapy
    b. One ASA tablet per day for patients after bypass surgery
    c. Theophylline therapy
    d. Antibiotic therapy

☐ ANSWERS

1.	b	**5.**	b	**9.**	d	**13.**	a	**17.**	c
2.	a	**6.**	d	**10.**	b	**14.**	a	**18.**	b
3.	d	**7.**	d	**11.**	b	**15.**	b	**19.**	d
4.	a	**8.**	c	**12.**	b	**16.**	c	**20.**	a

CHAPTER
9

Airway Management

John S. Burnett
Vijayalakshmi U. Patil

This chapter provides the essential information to safely practice airway management, with emphasis on direct laryngoscopy and endotracheal intubation. Topics discussed include airway anatomy, equipment, assessment, mask ventilation, direct laryngoscopy, endotracheal intubation, special situations and alternative techniques, extubation strategies, and complications.

☐ ANATOMY OF THE AIRWAY

A working knowledge and appreciation of the anatomy of the airway is a prerequisite for safe clinical practice.[1,2] The upper airway will be divided into four anatomic sections: nasopharynx, oropharynx, hypopharynx and larynx, and trachea (Figs. 9-1, 9-2, and 9-3).

NASOPHARYNX

The nasopharynx begins at the opening of the nares and continues posteriorly joining the oropharynx inferior to the soft palate. Mucosa lining the nasopharynx is highly vascular and prone to bleeding from relatively minor trauma. Drugs applied topically or injected submucously will produce rapid absorption and immediate blood levels simulating an intravenous injection. Topically applied local anesthetics may quickly produce signs and symptoms of local anesthetic toxicity. Trauma and bleeding from the mucosal surface can be minimized by using gentle technique, liberal lubrication, and a topical vasoconstrictor. Sensory innervation is diffuse and is supplied by the nasopalantine nerves and the anterior ethmoidal nerves, both branches of the trigeminal nerve. Topically applied local anesthetics provide effective sensory anesthesia for airway manipulation in conscious patients.

Pretreatment with a drying agent and a topical vasoconstrictor will decrease dilution of local anesthetics with secretions and enhance sensory anesthesia.

OROPHARYNX

The oropharynx begins at the opening of the oral cavity at the teeth and gums and courses posteriorly terminating at the base of the tongue or the vallecula, just superior to the epiglottis. The hard palate and soft palate separate the oropharynx from the nasopharynx. Injuries to the lips, teeth, and gums are common complications of laryngoscopy. The tongue, hard palate, soft palate, and anterior and posterior tonsilar pillars are used to evaluate the airway. Sensory innervation is supplied to the majority of the oropharynx by the glossopharyngeal nerve. The glossopharyngeal nerve can be blocked with local anesthesia injected medial to the base of the anterior tonsilar pillar. Topical local anesthetics also provide satisfactory sensory anesthesia to the oropharynx.

HYPOPHARYNX AND LARYNX

The hypopharynx begins at the base of the tongue and includes the epiglottis, glottic opening, larynx, and a small portion of the upper esophagus. The subglottic region refers to the larynx inferior to the glottic opening or vocal cords. The larynx consists of three single cartilages (epiglottic, cricoid, thyroid) and three paired cartilages (cuneiform, corniculate, arytenoid). The epiglottis is a cartilaginous structure that closes over the glottic opening during swallowing, preventing aspiration. Anterior to the epiglottis is the hyoid bone. The thyroid cartilage, cricothyroid membrane, and cricoid cartilage are inferior to the hyoid bone. The cricoid cartilage differs from tracheal rings in that it is a complete ring. Tracheal

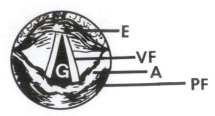

Figure 9–2 Anatomy at the level of the glottis. E, epiglottis; A, aryepiglottic fold; G, glottis; PF, pyriform fossa; VF, vocal folds.

rings are incomplete on their posterior surface. *External pressure applied to the cricoid cartilage will compress the esophagus against the body of the fifth or sixth cervical vertebra.* Cricoid pressure can prevent gastric distention and regurgitation during mask ventilation. The glottic opening is triangular in shape and, in young nonsmokers, the vocal cords appear pearly white during laryngoscopy. The larynx is a midline structure immediately inferior to the epiglottis and anterior to the esophagus. Sensory innervation to the anterior surface of the epiglottis is supplied by the glossopharyngeal nerve. Below the epiglottis the vagus nerve provides sensation to the airway structures. The internal branch of the superior laryngeal nerve, a branch of the vagus nerve, supplies sensory innervation to the posterior surface of the epiglottis and the larynx. The internal laryngeal nerve can be blocked easily as it passes between the cornu of the hyoid bone and thyroid cartilage. Local anesthetics can be applied topically by various methods. The external branch of the superior laryngeal nerve supplies motor innervation to the cricothyroid muscle; the recurrent laryngeal nerves innervate all other laryngeal muscles. The *posterior cricoarytenoid* muscles are responsible for ab-

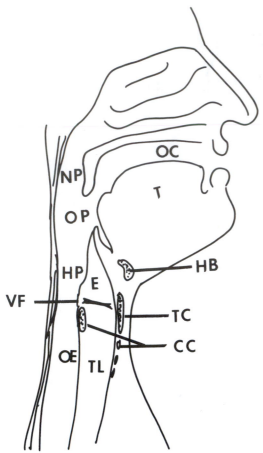

Figure 9–1 The sagittal section of the airway. OC, oral cavity; T, tongue; NP, nasopharynx; OP, oropharynx; HB, hyoid bone; E, epiglottis; HP, hypopharynx; TC, thyroid cartilage; VF, vocal folds; CC, cricoid cartilage; OE, esophagus; TL, tracheal lumen.

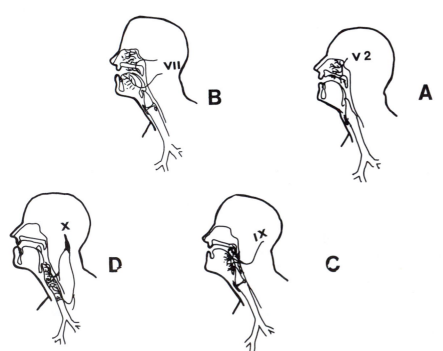

Figure 9–3 Sensory innervation of the airway. *A.* Maxillary branch of the trigeminal nerve — V2. *B.* Facial nerve — VII. *C.* Glossopharyngeal nerve IX. *D.* Vagus nerve X.

duction of the cords (remember *p*ull *c*ords *a*part). The lateral cricoarytenoid muscles primarily adduct the vocal cords.

TRACHEA

The trachea begins inferior to the cricoid cartilage and continues until it bifurcates at the carina into the left and right mainstem bronchi. The cricoid cartilage is at the level of the sixth cervical vertebra and the carina is at the fifth thoracic vertebra. An endotracheal tube positioned between these vertebrae as seen on a radiograph, can be assumed to be located correctly within the trachea. The angle of the bifurcation of the trachea is such that a deep endotracheal tube (ETT) will tend to enter the right mainstem bronchus. Stimulation of the carina with an ETT will induce coughing. Sensory innervation of the trachea is provided by the recurrent laryngeal nerve, a branch of the vagus nerve. The recurrent laryngeal nerve is not easily accessible to nerve block. Sensory anesthesia of the trachea is usually produced with topical local anesthetics.[3-7]

ADULT VERSES PEDIATRIC ANATOMY

Several significant anatomic differences are apparent between the adult and pediatric airway (Table 9–1; Fig. 9–4). *The larynx is shaped like a funnel in children because the smallest diameter is not at the vocal cords as in adults but at the cricoid cartilage.* ETT cuffs are not necessary in children because the cricoid cartilage acts like an anatomic cuff. Submucosal edema and postintubation croup can occur in adults but are more common in children.[8,9] Excessive pres-

Table 9–1
ADULT AND PEDIATRIC AIRWAYS

Infant	Adult
Large head relative to the body	
Large tongue	
Epiglottis—omega-shape close to the base of the tongue and more horizontal	Flat, flexible, more erect
Hyoid bone—close to the thyroid cartilage	Separate
Aryepiglottic folds—prominent	
Vocal folds—at C-3 to C-4	At C-4 to C-5
Vocal folds—inclined inferiorly	Horizontal
Cricoid—funnel shaped	Vertical
Narrow part of the airway is at cricoid ring	Narrow part is at vocal folds
Tracheal lumen circular in cross section	Tracheal lumen is horseshoe shape
Right and left main bronchi bifurcate at same angle	Right main bronchus bifurcates at a much smaller angle than the left
Lip to carina distance—13 cm	Lip to carina distance 24 cm—female 28 cm—male
Carina level—T-5	Carina level—T-4 to T-6

sure from a large uncuffed ETT or an overinflated ETT cuff is the cause. Because of the smaller diameter, any subglottic swelling has a large impact on airway resistance in the pediatric trachea. In severe cases of edema, tracheal intubation with a smaller than normal ETT may be required.

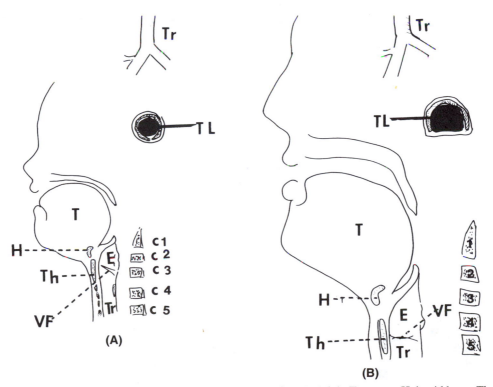

Figure 9–4   Airway anatomy in sagittal section. *A.* Infant. *B.* Adult. T, tongue; H, hyoid bone; Th, thyroid cartilage; VF, vocal folds; E, esophagus; TL, tracheal lumen; Tr trachea.

☐ EQUIPMENT USED

Equipment commonly used with mask ventilation, direct laryngoscope, and endotracheal intubation is discussed. Equipment used in special situations and for alternative techniques is discussed in a later section.

MASKS

Masks are available in a variety of sizes and materials. Transparent masks provide earlier warning of regurgitation and aspiration than opaque masks. Each institution usually has a variety of masks. Become familiar with several different masks at your institution.

Positive-pressure ventilation can only be achieved when a tight seal is maintained with a mask. Obtaining and maintaining a tight seal may be difficult in edentulous patients or those with thick beards. Maintaining a tight mask fit around the bridge of the nose is difficult for beginners. Dilution of anesthetic gases and a reduction in the inspired oxygen concentration also occurs with a leaky mask fit.

ARTIFICIAL AIRWAYS

Artificial airways are basically of two types, nasal or oral, (Fig. 9–5). Each type has a variety of subtypes. Artificial airways are commonly used to create a patient airway in unconscious patients. Unconscious or semiconscious patients are susceptible to upper airway obstruction from loss of muscle tone and collapse of the tongue and soft palate against the posterior oropharynx. Elevation of the tongue with an artificial airway may be necessary when simple maneuvers such as jaw thrust or neck hyperextension fail. Selection of the correct size is important because an incorrect size may worsen upper airway obstruction (Fig. 9–6). In sedated patients, nasal airways are tolerated better than oral airways. Stimulation of the hy-

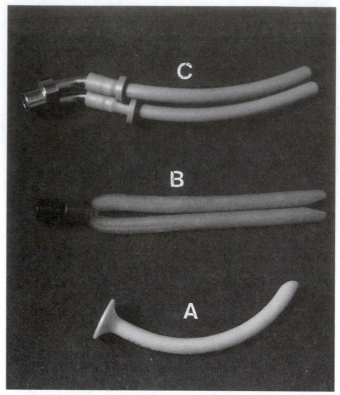

Figure 9–5   *A.* Nasal airway. *B* and *C.* Binasal airways.

popharynx may induce larynospasm or vomiting in lightly anesthetized patients.

LARYNGOSCOPES

Laryngoscopes are instruments designed to view the opening of the larynx directly. Laryngoscopes and blades are available in many shapes and sizes. Two commonly used blades are the straight (Miller) blade and curved (Macintosh) blade[9]

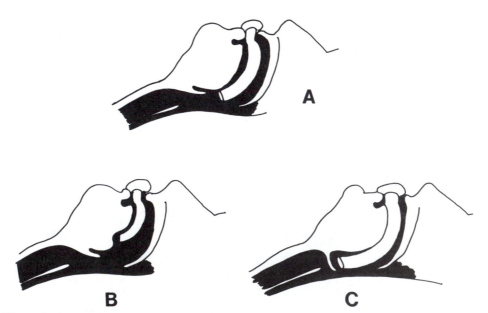

Figure 9–6   Oral airway. *A.* Appropriate size. *B.* Small size causes obstruction to the airway by displacing the tongue into the oral cavity. *C.* Large size obstructs the airway by pushing the epiglottis against the glottic opening or laryngospasm.

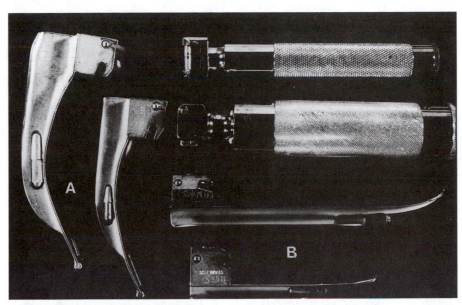

Figure 9–7   Laryngoscope blades. *A.* Macintosh. *B.* Miller.

(Fig. 9–7). Choice or blade depends on personal experience, training, and patient anatomy. Most clinicians, however, prefer to use straight blades in children and those with an anterior larynx. The blade of the laryngoscope is used to elevate the tongue and soft tissues in obtaining a direct view of the larynx. The tip of the straight blade is positioned immediately posterior to the epiglottis and lifts the epiglottis with laryngoscope. The tip of the curved blade is positioned in the vallecula superior to the epiglottis. Because the epiglottis is not stimulated during laryngoscopy, the curved blade is tolerated better in awake patients and bradycardia is less likely.

The use of an intubation stylet with the curved blade assists in successful endotracheal intubation, especially in patients with a slight anterior larynx.

ENDOTRACHEAL TUBES

Endotracheal tubes are made of sterile, nonirritating plastic. The manufacturer's markation of Z-79 indicates that the ETT is made of material tested and found to be nontoxic to tissues. They are available in a variety of sizes and shapes (Fig. 9–8). Selection of the correct size avoids

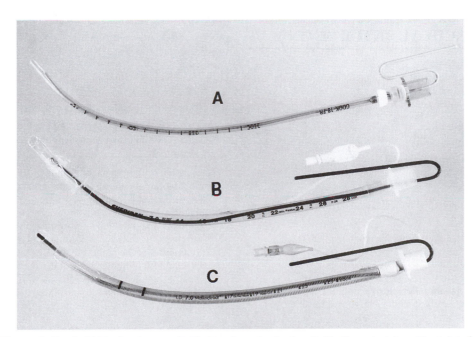

Figure 9–8   *A.* 18 F tube changer. *B.* No 7 endotracheal tube. *C.* No 7 anode tube with stylets for anticipated difficult intubation.

complications. Cuffed ETTs are generally not used in pediatric patients. Selection of the correct size for pediatric patients is at best difficult; several sizes should be immediately available.

INTUBATION STYLETS

Intubation stylets are malleable metal guides used to shape ETTs. If a stylet is used, ensure that it does not protrude from the end of the ETT or from the Murphy eye. Lubrication eases their removal after successful endotracheal intubation.

SUCTION EQUIPMENT

Suction equipment should always be immediately available. Stimulation of the gag reflex may induce vomiting lin a sedated or lightly anesthetized patient. Secretions or blood can interfere with vision during laryngoscopy and may occlude a patent airway. Both Yankauer and flexible catheters should be immediately available (Table 9–2).

☐ ASSESSMENT OF THE AIRWAY

Assessment of the airway begins with a thorough history and physical examination, particularly to evaluate possible difficulties with either mask ventilation or direct laryngoscopy.

Table 9–2
BASIC EQUIPMENT FOR ENDOTRACHEAL INTUBATION

1. Face mask—variable sizes
2. Oral airway—variable sizes
3. Nasal airway—variable sizes
4. Endotracheal tube—variable sizes
5. Stylet
6. Syringe
7. Tape
8. Laryngoscope blade—curved and straight
9. Large-bore IV catheter
10. Suction catheter—soft and rigid
11. Magill's forceps
12. Pillow or towel
13. Stethoscope
14. Water-soluble lubricant
15. Tongue depressor
16. Oxygen saturation probe
17. End-tidal CO_2 detector
18. Endotracheal tube position detector
19. Alternative techniques equipment—laryngeal mask airway, combitube, jet ventilator

Table 9–3
CONDITIONS ASSOCIATED WITH DIFFICULT DIRECT LARYNGOSCOPY

Difficult airway is anticipated in patients with:
1. Congenital anomalies
2. Short neck and thick neck, anterior larynx, prominent and overriding teeth, microstomia, macrognathia, macroglossia, receding chin, and narrow mandibular space
3. Tumors in and around the airway
4. Infection
5. Trauma
6. Pathology in temporomandibular joint and cervical spines

HISTORY

After a personal interview carefully review all available medical records especially old anesthetic records. Details of any history of airway difficulties should be noted and respected. To dismiss past difficulties as a result of either a lack of skill or experience should be discouraged. To repeat past mistakes that may result in serious morbidity or mortality is inexcusable.

Conditions associated with possible difficult direct laryngoscopy are also evaluated (Table 9–3).

PHYSICAL EXAMINATION

Physical examination of the airway provides additional information. Physical findings associated with difficulties with direct laryngoscopy are limited extension of the neck to less than 35°, mouth opening limited to 3 cm or less, and thyromental distance less than 6.5 cm with neck in full extension (Table 9–4; Figs. 9–9 and 9–10).

A thorough history and physical examination may not reliably predict difficulties with mask ventilation or direct laryngoscopy. Therefore, regardless of the initial assessment,

Table 9–4
FACTORS THAT LIMIT LARYNX VISUALIZATION

Visualization of the larynx is limited with one or more of the following factors present in adult patients:
1. Limited mouth opening—<3 cm
2. Inability to see the uvula and soft palate when the mouth is wide open and tongue is protruding in a sitting position
3. Extension of the neck is limited—<35°
4. Symphysis of the mandible to mandibular angle—<10 cm
5. Distance from inner border of the mandible at the symphysis menti to thyroid notch in patients with head in full extension—<6.5 cm
6. Rigid larynx—inability to move side to side or upward and backward

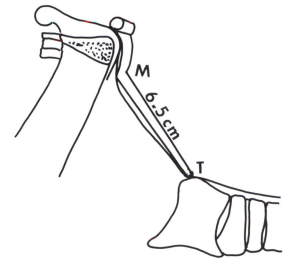

Figure 9-9   The degree of difficulty with endotracheal intubation is predicted if the distance between the lower border of the mandible (M) to the thyroid notch (T) is less than 6.5 cm with head in full extension.

when planning primary management technique, alternative techniques should be immediately available in case unexpected difficulties occur.[10-17]

☐ MASK VENTILATION, DIRECT LARYNGOSCOPY, AND ENDOTRACHEAL INTUBATION

Direct laryngoscopy and endotracheal intubation are usually performed after the induction of anesthesia. Rapid sequence intubation is a special technique using direct laryngoscopy

Table 9-5
INDICATIONS FOR AWAKE INTUBATION

1. Inability to maintain patent airway before insertion of endotracheal tube
2. Prone to aspiration of gastric contents or blood
3. Assess for nerve damage during intubation
4. Any factor indicating possible difficult intubation

for endotracheal intubation in patients at high risk for aspiration and is discussed in a later section. Intubation before the induction of general anesthesia by direct laryngoscope or by an alternate technique is done in patients in whom difficulties are anticipated. Appropriate use of intravenous sedation and local anesthesia facilitates intubation in awake patients (Table 9-5). Techniques other than direct laryngoscopy and endotracheal intubation for airway management are discussed in a later section.[18]

MONITORING

Monitoring of the patient during airway management increases patient safety and reduces complications. Precordial stethoscopes provide early warning of difficulties with ventilation including wheezing, airway obstruction, hypoventilation, or apnea. Pulse oximeters can detect early or unrecognized hypoxemia by providing noninvasive measurements of arterial oxygen saturation. End-tidal carbon dioxide monitoring is reliable in detecting esophageal intubation. An oxygen analyzer in the anesthesia circle system confirms that the inspired gas mixture contains adequate oxygen.

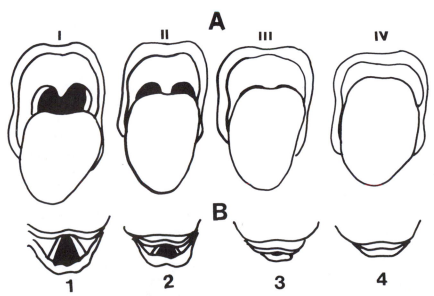

Figure 9-10   *A.* Samsoon and Young modification of the Mallanpati airway classification. *B.* Cormack and Lahane's grading of laryngoscopic view of the larynx.

PREOXYGENATION

Before the induction of anesthesia, patients may be preoxygenated with 100% oxygen. Preoxygenation replaces nitrogen in the functional residual capacity with 100% oxygen. This reserve of oxygen prolongs the time to the development of hypoxemia after induction. Preoxygenation is always done before a rapid sequence induction. Patients breathe 100% oxygen normally for 3 to 5 minutes or four vital capacity breaths.

MASK VENTILATION

Mask ventilation is an important skill to acquire and maintain. Hazards to avoid include the use of excessive pressure in maintaining a tight seal. This may cause pressure necrosis or nerve injury. Positive-pressure ventilation greater than 20 to 30 cm H_2O may lead to gastric distention. Gastric distention interferes with ventilation by impeding movement of the diaphragm and may cause regurgitation of gastric contents. Proper use of jaw thrust, neck extension, oral or nasal artificial airways, and cricoid pressure assists in maintaining normal gas exchange and decreases gastric distention.

After induction of anesthesia adequate mask ventilation should be demonstrated before proceeding with the administration of muscle relaxants and endotracheal intubation. Difficulties with mask ventilation may contraindicate the use of muscle relaxants to assist endotracheal intubation. Muscle relaxants will prolong the apnea caused by induction. If endotracheal intubation is then difficult, the clinical situation may deteriorate to the "can't ventilate or intubate" scenario. Patients who are difficult to mask ventilate after induction may be allowed to awaken after spontaneous ventilation returns. Airway management or anesthetic technique may then safely be altered[19,20] (Table 9–6).

ENDOTRACHEAL INTUBATION

The primary indication for endotracheal intubation is to maintain a continuous patent airway. Endotracheal intubation is commonly performed to facilitate positive-pressure ventilation and protect against aspiration (Table 9–7).

Endotracheal intubation with laryngoscopy may be done

Table 9–6
ALTERNATIVE TECHNIQUES FOR DIFFICULT VENTILATION

1. Oral, nasal, and binasal airways
2. Two-person mask ventilation
3. Esophageal tracheal combitube
4. Laryngeal mask airway
5. Transtracheal jet ventilation
6. Surgical airway access

Table 9–7
INDICATIONS FOR ENDOTRACHEAL INTUBATION

Medical indications

1. Ensure airway patency
2. Provide mechanical ventilatory support
3. Prevent aspiration
4. Treat respiratory failure
5. Perform cardiopulmonary resuscitation
6. Conduct pulmonary toilet

Anesthesia indications

1. Maintain airway patency in anesthetized patient
2. Ventilation with face mask is difficult
3. Facilitate positive-pressure ventilation
4. Extensive monitoring required
5. Patient prone to aspiration
6. Undergo prolonged surgical procedures

Surgical indications

1. Site of surgery—head, neck, and in the back
2. Muscle relaxation required
3. Intrathoracic or intra-abdominal surgery
4. Surgery performed in other than supine position

either orally or nasally. The choice usually depends on the site of surgery. With either case, it is generally performed with the patient in the sniffing position. The sniffing position (Fig. 9–11) facilitates direct vision of the glottic opening during laryngoscopy by aligning the oral, oropharyngeal, and tracheal axis. The beginner often neglects this detail making laryngoscopy more difficult and often more traumatic than necessary. With mask ventilation, neck extension is preferred. The sniffing position, however, allows flexion of the neck and extension of the atlanto-occipital joint. Use of lubrication, a topical vasoconstrictor, and gentle technique will decrease bleeding with a nasal intubation. Further complications of nasal intubation include eustachian tube obstruction, epistaxis, bacteremia, dislodgement of pharyngeal tonsils (adenoids), and maxillary sinusitis. Nasal intubation is usually not performed in children. Children often have hypertrophied adenoids prone to avulsion and bleeding. The use of curved forceps such as Magill forceps will facilitate introducing the ETT into the glottic opening. An intubating stylet assists oral endotracheal intubation especially when the entire larynx is not clearly seen during laryngoscopy.

Verifying Endotracheal Intubation Occasionally the esophagus is accidentally intubated. If recognized, immediate reintubation after a brief period of mask ventilation avoids serious morbidity or mortality. If unrecognized, death may result. Therefore, after any endotracheal intubation attempt, it is imperative to verify correct placement. Lack of a

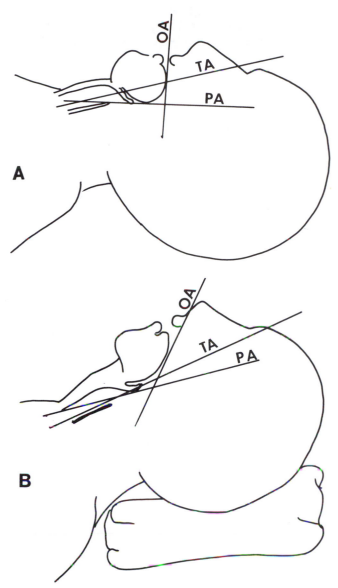

Figure 9–11 Position of the head for tracheal intubation. OA, oral axis; TA, tracheal axis; PA, pharyngeal axis in neutral position (*A*) and sniffing position (*B*) .

normal and sustained end-tidal carbon dioxide tracing indicates esophageal placement. Other techniques such as noting exhaled vapor or measuring exhaled volume are not as sensitive or specific as end-tidal gas monitoring for detecting esophageal intubation.[21–23] Direct laryngoscopy can confirm endotracheal intubation by visualizing the ETT in the glottic opening; fiberoptic examination through the ETT can confirm intratracheal placement if tracheal rings are seen. Changes in arterial oxygen saturation may be delayed with esophageal intubation especially after preoxygenation. Transmitted gastric sounds may be interpreted to be breath sounds with gastric ventilation. Listening for bilateral breath sounds establishes tracheal verses endo-

Table 9–8
ALTERNATIVE TECHNIQUES FOR DIFFICULT INTUBATION

1. Laryngoscopy with variable blades
2. Fiberoptic endoscopic intubation
3. Retrograde intubation
4. Light wand
5. Digital (tactile) intubation
6. Blind nasotracheal or oral intubation
7. Rigid bronchoscope
8. Surgical airway access

bronchial intubation, which cannot be detected with end-tidal gas monitoring.

☐ SPECIAL SITUATIONS AND ALTERNATE TECHNIQUES

Numerous alternatives, techniques, and equipment for direct laryngoscopy and failed endotracheal intubation are available (Table 9–8).

RAPID SEQUENCE INTUBATION

Rapid sequence intubation is used when the risk of aspiration is high. Anesthetic agents are chosen and administered to produce rapid loss of consciousness and onset of muscle paralysis. Direct laryngoscopy is used to view the vocal cords for endotracheal intubation. Preoxygenation and cricoid pressure are used to prevent hypoxia and regurgitation. Patients are not ventilated after induction to avoid stimulation of the gag reflex, gastric distention, and aspiration. A rapid sequence intubation is contraindicated when direct laryngoscopy is expected to be difficult.

BLIND NASAL INTUBATION

Blind nasal intubation is an alternative to laryngoscopy for endotracheal intubation when difficulties are expected or discovered. Listening to spontaneous ventilation through the ETT during intubation assists in guiding the ETT into the trachea. Although it is possible to blindly intubate an apneic patient, it is extremely difficult. Proper preparation of the patient with adequate local anesthesia or general anesthesia, with spontaneous ventilation, to avoid laryngospasm and swallowing, eases intubation.[20,24]

FLEXIBLE FIBEROPTIC LARYNGOSCOPY

A flexible fiberoptic laryngoscope is a versatile tool for endotracheal intubation (Fig. 9–12). It can be used in conscious and unconscious patients. Because of its flexibility it can

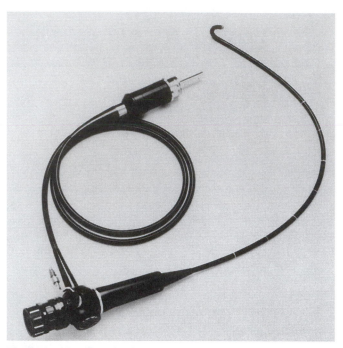

Figure 9–12   Flexible fiberoptic laryngoscope (Courtesy of Welch Allyn, Skaneatlas Falls, NY)

adapt to any anatomic abnormality, congenital or acquired. Most fiberoptic scopes contain a suction port through which secretions can be suctioned, local anesthetics administered, or oxygen insufflated.

A successful fiberoptic intubation depends on preparation, patience, and practice (Tables 9–9 and 9–10).

Fiberoptic intubation is technically easier in awake patients in the sitting position (Fig. 9–13). Loss of muscle tone and blood or secretions interferes with endoscopy. The sitting position aids in draining secretions and should be used with caution after general anesthesia. Local anesthesia and a dry-

Table 9–10
FIBEROPTIC LARYNGOSCOPY IN THE PATIENT WITH A DIFFICULT AIRWAY

1. Discuss the problems and formulate a plan with the surgeon.
2. Administer an antisialagogue preoperatively.
3. Use fiberoptic endoscopy initially when difficulty is anticipated.
4. Use equipment with which you are most familiar.
5. Have available conventional laryngoscopes with various blades, resuscitation equipment, cricothyrotomy needle, a tracheostomy set, rigid bronchoscopes, and light sources.
6. Ascertain that the endoscope and light sources are functional.
7. Induce anesthesia only after all equipment and personnel are prepared.
8. Allow sufficient time for anesthesia.
9. Arrange for an assistant to monitor patient.
10. Ask for help from another endoscopist when needed.

ing agent aid awake fiberoptic intubation. Various masks and artificial airways have been designed to aid endoscopy in anesthetized patients (Figs. 9–14 and 9–15). Flexible fiberoptic intubation requires experience and practice. Intubation of patients with normal anatomy under controlled conditions allows one to gain experience and confidence and maintain required skills.

Clinical indications for fiberoptic use are numerous (Table 9–11). The fiberoptic scope is useful in aiding and verifying correct placement of a double-lumen ETT. Visualizing the tip of a single-lumen ETT above the carina verifies midtracheal placement. Patency of airways can also be checked or cleared if found blocked.

Table 9–9
KEYS TO SUCCESSFUL FIBEROPTIC LARYNGOSCOPY FOR ENDOTRACHEAL INTUBATION

1. Check endoscope and light source.
2. Apply antifog agent to lens.
3. Focus lens prior to use.
4. Lubricate insertion tube (avoid lens).
5. Remove connector of endotracheal tube (ETT) and cut tube to correct length.
6. Insert endoscope into ETT.
7. Introduce endoscope into pharynx, maintain in midline, and advance 8–10 cm.
8. Look into endoscope and identify structures.
9. Flex tip of endoscope upward to visualize larynx.
10. Rotate distal end of insertion tube toward midline if necessary.
11. Enter vocal cords, return tip of endoscope to neutral position, and advance.
12. Position endoscope just above carina and thread ETT.

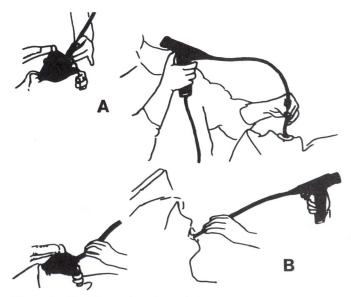

Figure 9–13   Fiberoptic endoscopic intubation is performed at the head of the patient (*A*), with the patient in the sitting position (*B*).

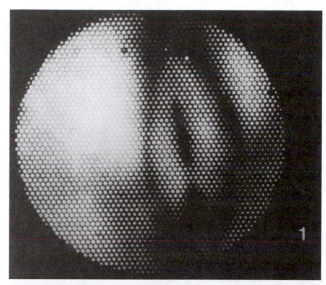

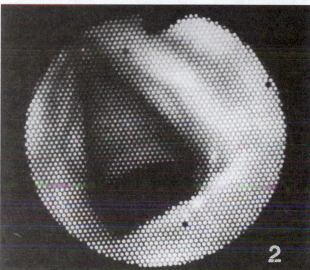

Figure 9–14 Endoscopic view of the glottis. Closed glottic opening (*1*), open glottic opening (*2*).

Table 9–11
CLINICAL APPLICATIONS OF FIBEROPTIC ENDOSCOPY

1. Evaluating airway pathology
    *   Congenital anomalies
    *   Trauma
    *   Tumor
    *   Inhalation injury
    *   Infection
    *   Nerve injury
    *   Difficult, traumatic, or prolonged intubation
2. Performing endotracheal intubation in difficult situations
    *   Receding mandible, anterior larynx
    *   Obesity
    *   Rheumatoid arthritis
    *   Cervical spine fracture
    *   Temporomandibular joint ankylosis
    *   Distortion due to surgery, radiation, burns
3. Assisting endotracheal intubation through laryngeal mask airway
4. Guiding endotracheal tube during retrograde intubation
5. Confirming tube placement
    *   Endotracheal
    *   Endobronchial
    *   Double-lumen
    *   Tracheostomy
6. Positioning endobronchial tube
7. Positioning selective segmental blockers
8. Changing endotracheal tubes
9. Performing tracheobronchial toilet
10. Placing nasogastric tubes

BULLARD LARYNGOSCOPE

An alternative to the flexible fiberoptic laryngoscope is the Bullard laryngoscope (Fig. 9–16), which combines a rigid, nonflexible fiberoptic scope with a specially designed laryngoscope. Intubation is accomplished by guiding an ETT with

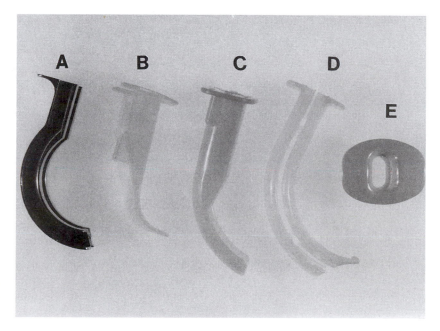

Figure 9–15 Endoscopic airways. *A*. Patil Syracuse airway. *B*. Ovassapian airway. *C*. Williams airway. *D*. Burman airway. *E*. Bite block.

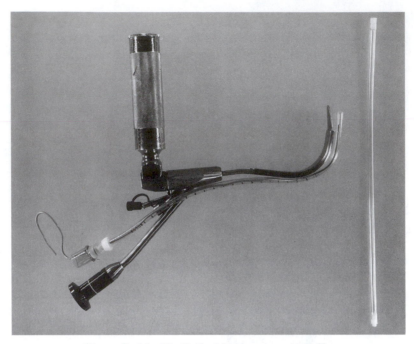

Figure 9–16   The Bullard laryngoscope (ACMI)

a specially designed intubating stylet or by passing a small catheter through the suction port into the trachea. An ETT can then be passed blindly over the catheter into the trachea. As with the flexible fiberoptic laryngoscope, blood and secretions can interfere with visualization. Because intubation can be done with ease with minimal mouth opening or neck flexion, it is a safe technique in managing cervical spine injuries.

LARYNGEAL MASK AIRWAY

The laryngeal mask airway (LMA) is an alternative to mask ventilation and endotracheal intubation for general anesthesia (Fig. 9–17; Table 9–12). Unlike a cuffed ETT, the LMA does not protect against aspiration. After induction of anesthesia, the LMA is inserted without the use of a laryngoscope

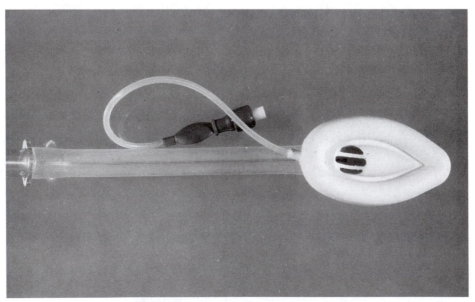

Figure 9–17   Laryngeal mask airway with inflated cuff.

Table 9-12
USES OF LARYNGEAL MASK AIRWAY

1. Administer anesthesia
2. Manage difficult airway to intubate trachea or recover from anesthesia
3. Intubate trachea through laryngeal mask airway as a conduit with endotracheal tube, gum elastic Bougie or fiberoptic endoscope
4. Perfom laryngoscopic examination
5. Perfom laryngoscopic procedures
6. Maintain airway to perform tracheostomy, retrograde intubation, or nasal intubation

Table 9-13
TECHNIQUE OF LARYNGEAL MASK AIRWAY (LMA) INSERTION

1. Choose appropriate size.
2. Inflate the cuff fully and deflate on a flat surface with glottic surface down.
3. Lubricate pharyngeal surface generously.
4. Hold the LMA like a pencil with index finger between the cuff and the tube.
5. Allow adequate depth of anesthesia.
6. Position the patient head in a sniffing position.
7. Insert the LMA against the hard palate.
8. Advance with steady pressure against the palate following the natural curve of the oropharynx.
9. Hold the LMA with the left hand and remove the right hand gently.
10. Advance the LMA until resistance is felt.
11. Inflate the cuff.
12. Attach the LMA to the anesthesia circuit and confirm position.

or muscle relaxants. Although positive-pressure ventilation is possible, with pop-off pressures usually between 15 and 20 cm H_2O, spontaneous ventilation is preferred. The LMA may be useful in the "can't ventilate or intubate" situation. It may provide a temporary means of oxygenation and ventilation or provide a guide for blind or fiberoptic intubation (Fig. 9-18). Insertion requires minimal training and is quick, usually requiring less than 10 seconds (Table 9-13). Stimulation is less than with endotracheal intubation and is equivalent to insertion of an artificial airway. Cricoid pressure is controversial because the tip of the airway is positioned immediately posterior to the cricoid cartilage. Cricoid pressure may dislodge the mask, obstructing the airway, or may partially compress the esophagus. Stimulation of the hypophar-

ynx in a lightly anesthetized patient may cause laryngospasm.[20,21,23,33-36]

ESOPHAGEAL COMBITUBE

The combitube is the combination of an ETT and an esophageal obturator airway.[37-42] It is used as an alternative airway management technique in the "can't ventilate

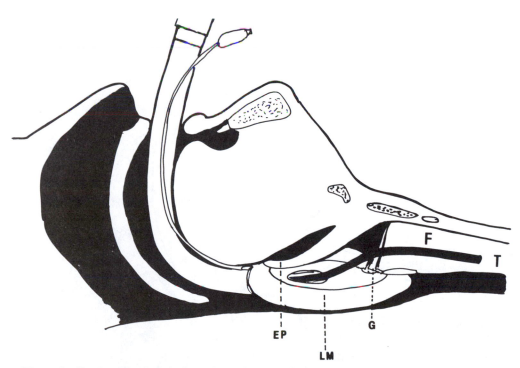

Figure 9-18 Laryngeal mask airway is used as a conduit to intubate trachea with fiberoptic endoscope. EP, epiglottis; LM, laryngeal mask; G, glottic opening; F, fiberoptic endoscope; T, tracheal lumen.

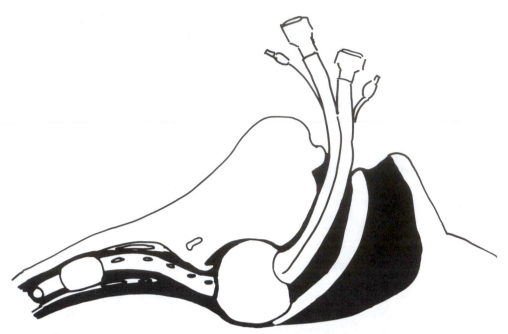

Figure 9–19   Combitube in the trachea lumen, functions like an endotracheal tube.

or intubate" situation. It is inserted blindly, without the aid of a laryngoscope. If inserted into the trachea, it is used as an ETT (Fig. 9–19). If inserted into the esophagus, it is used as an esophageal obturator airway (Fig. 9–20). As an esophageal obturator airway, ventilation and oxygenation have been reported to be as adequate as an ETT under a variety of clinical situations such as thoracic surgery, intra-abdominal surgery, or cardiac arrest and cardiopulmonary resuscitation. Removal from the esophagus may induce regurgitation or vomiting.

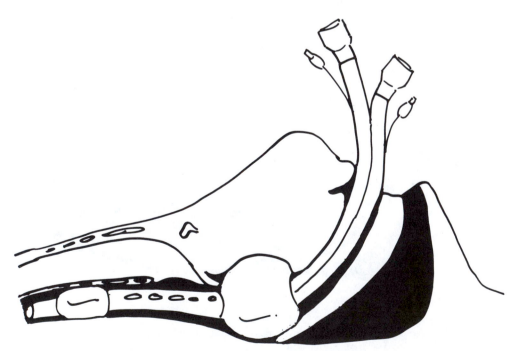

Figure 9–20   Combitube in the esophagus, functions like an esophageal obturator.

PERCUTANEOUS TRANSTRACHEAL JET VENTILATION

Percutaneous transtracheal jet ventilation is used when ventilation or oxygenation cannot be established by an alternative technique and is urgently needed. It is an alternative to a tracheostomy, requiring less time to perform and no surgical training. A temporary airway is created by passing a small catheter through the cricothyroid membrane. Usually a 14-gauge catheter or larger is inserted in a caudal direction at a 45° angle to the cricothyroid membrane. Aspiration of air confirms intratracheal placement. A high-pressure source is required for ventilation. Pressures of 50 psi are generally required and can be generated from any standard wall oxygen outlet, E cylinder of oxygen, or most modern anesthesia machines through flush valve (Fig. 9–21; Table 9–14). Complications can be life threatening. It is not uncommon for subcutaneous emphysema to form around a correctly placed catheter. To prevent dislodgment of the catheter it should be held firmly against the skin and secured snugly with sutures. If the catheter does become dislodged into the subcutaneous tissues, massive subcutaneous emphysema may obscure normal landmarks, making tracheostomy or even repeat percutaneous catheter placement virtually impossible.[43,44]

RETROGRADE INTUBATION

Retrograde intubation uses a catheter or wire passed cephalad through the cricothyroid membrane and retrieved

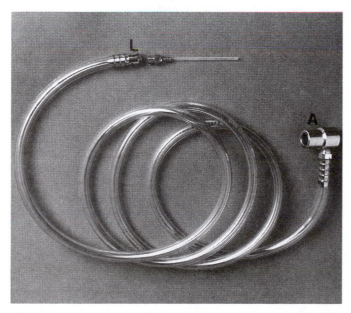

Figure 9–21 A rigid tubing with (L) Luer-lok connector and (A) 15-mm adapter to ventilate by connecting to the O_2 outlet.

Table 9–14

POTENTIAL COMPLICATIONS WITH TRANSTRACHEAL JET VENTILATION

1. Catheter kink
2. Catheter dislodgement
3. Pneumothorax
4. Pneumomediastinum
5. Subcutaneous emphysema
6. Bleeding
7. Barotrauma
8. Tracheoesophageal fistula
9. Subcutaneous fistula
10. Infection
11. Hematoma
12. Perforation of the esophagus
13. Damage to the surrounding arteries and nerves

through the mouth or nose. An ETT is then passed over the guide, blindly into the trachea. An alternative method is to retrieve the wire through and directly guide endotracheal intubation with a fiberoptic laryngoscope. Specialized kits have been developed that provide all the necessary equipment (Fig. 9–22). With the proper training and practice, this technique, although somewhat invasive, may offer a quick and effective alternative method of endotracheal intubation.[45-50] Bleeding disorders and pathology or infection in the airway contraindicate the retrograde technique (Table 9–15). Complications have been reported.

LIGHT WANDS

Light wands are basically malleable intubation stylets with an illuminating tip. Light wands are passed posterior to the epiglottis with the aid of a laryngoscope or blindly. Correct position is confirmed by transilluminating the thyrohyoid membrane. A preloaded ETT is then gently threaded into the trachea[51-53] (Figs. 9–23 and 9–24).

INTUBATION CATHETERS AND TUBE CHANGERS

Intubation catheters and tube changers are used in difficult intubations or to exchange ETTs. In exchanging ETTs, an intubation catheter is passed through the existing ETT. The intubation catheter is secured in place while the ETT is removed. A new ETT is then passed blindly over the catheter using it as a guide. A hollow two-part intubation catheter comes equipped with two rapid-fit connectors allowing the catheter to easily connect to the anesthesia circle system or a resuscitation bag via a 22-mm connection and to a jet ventilator via a Luer-lok

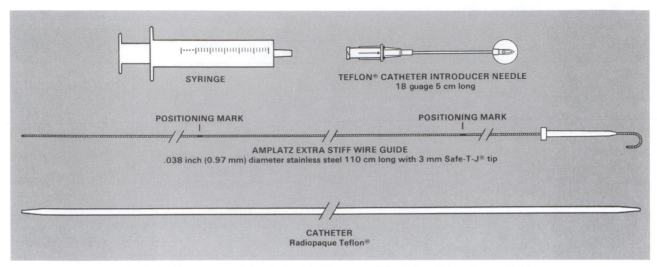

Figure 9–22   Retrograde intubation kit (Courtesy of Cook, Inc., Bloomington, Ind.)

Table 9–15
CONTRAINDICATIONS FOR RETROGRADE TRACHEAL INTUBATION

1.   Unable to retrieve the guidewire
2.   Distorted neck anatomy
3.   Pathology in the airway
4.   Bleeding disorders
5.   Infection in and around the airway
6.   Not for emergency airway access

connector. If difficulty is encountered on passing the new ETT into the trachea, oxygenation and ventilation can be quickly established using the intratracheal-located intubation catheter with these rapid-fit connectors.[54–56]

☐ EXTUBATION MANAGEMENT

Because the majority of patients require endotracheal intubation to facilitate positive-pressure ventilation and protect against aspiration, most patients can be extubated soon after the completion of surgery when the effects of anesthetic agents and muscle relaxants have been sufficiently reversed. Patients should demonstrate the ability to maintain oxygenation and ventilation independently. Adequate return of consciousness, protective airway reflexes, and muscle strength should also be well demonstrated. Prior to extubation, patients should be preoxygenated and the oropharynx adequately suctioned. In selected patients, particularly those at high risk for aspiration, a catheter should be passed into the

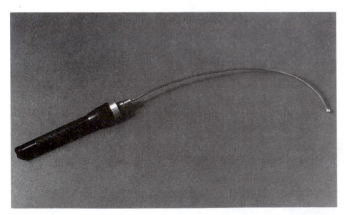

Figure 9–23   Lighted fiberoptic stylet (Courtesy of Anesthesia Associates, San Marcas, California)

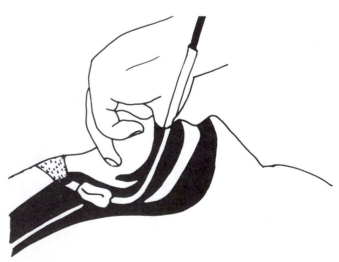

Figure 9–24   Position and the shape of the light wand required to elicit transillumination of the soft tissues of the neck for successful endotracheal intubation.

Table 9–16
COMPLICATIONS OF ENDOTRACHEAL INTUBATION

Immediate Complications

1. Trauma to lips, teeth, gums, and eyes
2. Trauma to oropharynx, larynx, trachea, and esophagus
3. Hypoxia, hypertension, tachycardia, bradycardia, and dysrhythmia
4. Increased intracranial pressure
5. Esophageal intubation
6. Laryngospasm
7. Bronchospasm
8. Pneumothorax
9. Subcutaneous emphysema
10. Aspiration
11. Airway obstruction, kink, foreign body
12. Dislocation of arytenoids and temporomandibular joint
13. Submucosal dissection (nasotracheal intubation)
14. Epistaxis
15. Sore throat

Delayed Complications

1. Ulceration
2. Granulomas
3. Webs
4. Stenosis
5. Infection
6. Pressure necrosis

stomach to remove excess contents and decompress the stomach. After extubation, patients should be monitored closely for signs and symptoms of airway obstruction, respiratory distress, hypoventilation, apnea, and respiratory failure. Supplemental oxygen should be administered until the patient demonstrates the ability to protect the airway adequately to prevent diffusion hypoxia. Suction equipment and equipment needed to quickly intubate the trachea should be immediately available. Trained personnel able to detect and respond to airway emergencies must remain with the patient until discharged from the postanesthesia care unit.

Extubation of the patient who had a difficult airway or acquired a potentially compromised airway may require a special approach. The best approach would be to keep the patient intubated until there is no doubt that the airway can be maintained without intubation or mechanical ventilation. However, this may be unpleasant and dangerous for some patients.

☐ COMPLICATIONS OF AIRWAY MANAGEMENT

Appropriate training and technique will minimize airway complications. Complications can result in minor morbidity or major mortality (Table 9–16). Trauma to the teeth and gums is the most common complication related to airway management. Sore throat, a common complaint after general anesthesia, may certainly be related to endotracheal intubation. It may also be related to the use of unhumidified gases or trauma with the laryngoscope, insertion of artificial airways, or suctioning the oropharyngeal cavity prior to extubation.

☐ SUMMARY

Mismanagement of the airway is a cause of major morbidity and mortality directly related to anesthesia. In an attempt to assist in guiding airway management decisions, the American Society of Anesthesiologists has recommended an algorithm to follow when managing the expected or unexpected difficult airway. Common errors when managing the unexpected difficult airway are; not correctly assessing the situation, not calling for appropriate help early, and persisting with a difficult laryngoscopy. It is best to use only practiced and familiar techniques, especially when difficulties arise. Therefore, become familiar with emergency airway management techniques and be prepared to use them appropriately.

Equipment used in emergency airway management should be stored in a mobile cart in an accessible location. All members of the anesthesia care team should be familiar with the location and use of this cart.

When a difficult airway is discovered, details should be documented in the medical record for future referral. The patient should be informed directly, preferably in writing. A letter detailing the difficulties allows the patient to directly share this information with future health care providers. Finally, patients should be encouraged to wear a Medical Alert bracelet.

REFERENCES

1. Finucane BT, Santora AH. *Principles of Airway Management.* Philadelphia: FA Davis; 1988.
2. Benumof JL. *Clinical Procedure in Anesthesia and Intensive Care.* Philadelphia: JB Lippincott; 1992.
3. Ellis H, Felman S. *Anatomy for the Anesthetists.* 6th ed. Oxford: Blackwell Scientific; 1993.
4. Roberts J. Functional anatomy of the larynx. *Int Anesthesiol Clin.* 1990; 28:101 (review).
5. Williams P, Warwick R, Dyson M, et al. *Gray's Anatomy.* 37th ed. New York: Churchill Livingstone; 1989; 1248–1286.
6. Pectu LP, Sasaki CT. Laryngeal anatomy and physiology. *Clin Chest Med.* 1991; 12:415.

7. Norton ML, ed. *Atlas of the Difficult Airway*. St. Louis; CV Mosby; 1991.

8. Pulleritis J, Holzman R. Anesthesia equipment for infants and children. *Int Anesthesiol Clin*. 1992;30:3.

9. Borland LM. The pediatric airway. *Int Anesthesiol Clin*. 1992; 30:4.

10. Bellhouse CP, Dore C. Criteria for estimating likelihood of difficulty of endotracheal intubation with the Macintosh laryngoscope. *Anaesth Intensive Care*. 1988; 16:329.

11. Wilson ME, Spiegelhalter D. Robertson JA, Lesser P. Predicting difficult intubation. *Br J Anaesth*. 1988; 61:211.

12. Frerk CM. Predicting difficult intubation. *Anaesthesia*. 1991; 46:1005.

13. Mallampati SR. Clinical sign to predict difficult tracheal intubation (hypothesis). *Can Anesth Soc J*. 1983; 30:216.

14. Mallampati SR, Gatt SP, Gugino LD, et al. A clinical sign to predict difficult tracheal intubation: a prospective study. *Can Anaesth Soc J*. 1985; 32:429.

15. Patil VU, Stehling LC, Zauder HL. *Fiberoptic Endoscopy in Anaesthesia*. Chicago: Year Book Medical Publishers; 1983.

16. Samsoon GLT, Young JRB. Difficult tracheal intubation. A retrospective study. *Anaesthesia*. 1987; 42:487.

17. Frerk CM. Predicting difficult intubation. *Anaesthesia*. 1991; 46:1005.

18. Reed AP. Preparation of the patient for awake flexible fiberoptic endoscopy. *Chest*. 1992; 101:244.

19. Benumof J. Management of the difficult adult airway. *Anesthesiology*. 1991; 75:1087.

20. Benumof JL: *Airway Management Principles and Practice*. St. Louis: Mosby-Yearbook; 1996.

21. Murray IP, Modell JH. Early detection of endotracheal tube accidents by monitoring carbon dioxide concentration in respiratory gas. *Anesthesiology*. 1983; 59:344.

22. Dunn SM, Mushlin PS, Lind LJ, et al: Tracheal intubation is not invariably confirmed by capnography. *Anesthesiology*. 1990; 73:1285.

23. Wafai Y, Salem MR, Baraka A, et al. Effectiveness of the self-inflating bulb for verification of proper placement of the esophageal tracheal Combitube. *Anesth Analg*. 1995; 80:122.

24. Carlson RC, Sadove MS. Guided non-visualized nasal endotracheal intubation using a transtracheal Fogarty catheter. *Illinois Medical Journal*. 1973; 143:364.

25. Patil V, Stehling L, Zander H, et al. *Fiberoptic Endoscopy in Anesthesia*, Chicago: Year Book Medical Publisher; 1983.

26. Roberts JT. Fiberoptics in anesthesia. *Anesth Clin North Am*. 1991; 9.

27. Watson CB. Fiberoptic endoscopy and anesthesia in a general hospital. *Anesth Clin North Am* 1991; 9:129.

28. Ovassapian A. Fiberoptic tracheal intubation. In: *Fiber Airway Endoscopy in Anesthesia and Critical Care*. New York: Raven Press; 1990:57–79.

29. Borland LM, Casselbrant M. The Bullard laryngoscope: a new indirect oral laryngoscope (pediatric version). *Anesth Analg*. 1990; 70;105.

30. Paterson SJ, Byrne PJ, Molesky MG, et al. neonatal resuscitation using the laryngeal mask airway. *Anesthesiology*. 1993; 79:A983.

31. Verghese C, Smith TGC, Young E. Prospective survey of the use of the laryngeal mask airway in 2359 patients. *Anesthesia*. 1993; 48:58.

32. Vertesi L. The paramedic ambulance: a Canadian experience. *Can Med Assoc J*. 1978; 119:25.

33. Zagnoev M, McCloskey J, Martin T. Fiberoptic intubation via the laryngeal mask airway. *Anesth Analg*. 1994; 78:813.

34. Brain AIJ. The laryngeal mask airway—a possible new solution to airway problems in the emergency situation. *Arch Emerg Med* 1984;1:229.

35. Brain AIJ. The laryngeal mask—a new concept in airway management. *Br J Anaesth*. 1983; 55:801.

36. Brimacombe J. Cricoid pressure and the laryngeal mask airway. *Anaesthesia*. 1991; 46:986.

37. Frass M, Frenzer R, Zdrahal F, et al. The esophageal tracheal combitube: preliminary results with a new airway for CPR. *Ann Emerg Med*. 1987; 16:768.

38. Frass M, Roder S, Frenzer R, et al: Esophageal tracheal combitube, endotracheal airway and mask: comparison of ventilatory pressure curves. *J Trauma*. 1989; 29:1476.

39. Frass M, Frenzer R, Mayer G, et al. Mechanical ventilation with the esophageal tracheal combitube (ETC) in the intensive care unit. *Arch Emerg Med*. 1987; 4:219.

40. Staudinger T, Brugger S, Watschinger B, et al. Emergency intubation with the combitube: comparison with the endotracheal airway. *Ann Emerg Med*. 22(10):15B-5 1993 Oct.

41. Banyai M, Falgers S, Roggla M, et al. Emergency intubation with the combitube in a grossly obese patient with bull neck. *Resuscitation*. 1993; 26:271.

42. Bigenzahn W, Pesau B, Frass M. Emergency ventilation using the combitube in cases of difficult intubation. *Eur Arch Otorhinolaryngol*. 1991; 248:129.

43. Cote CJ, Eavey RD, Todres ID, Jones DE. Cricothyroid membrane puncture: oxygenation and ventilation in a dog model using an intravenous catheter. *Crit Care Med* 1988; 16:615.

44. Benumof JL, Scheller MS. The importance of transtracheal jet ventilation in the management of the difficult airway. *Anesthesiology*. 1989; 71:769.

45. Guggenberger H, Lenz G. Training in retrograde intubation. *Anesthesiology*. 1988; 69:292 (letter).

46. Gupta B, McDonald JS, Brooks HJ, et al. Oral fiberoptic intubation over a retrograde guidewire. *Anesth Analg*. 1989; 68:517.

47. Barriot P, Bruno R. Retrograde technique for tracheal intubation in trauma patients. *Crit Care Med*. 1988; 16:712.

48. Bourke D, Levesque PR. Modification of retrograde guide for endotracheal intubation. *Anesth Analg*. 1974; 53:1013.

49. Butler FS, Cirillo AA. Retrograde tracheal intubation. *Anesth Analg*. 1960; 39:333.

50. Audenaert SM, Montgomery CL, Stone B, et al. Retrograde-assisted fiberoptic tracheal intubation in children with difficult airways. *Anesth Analg*. 1991; 73:660.

51. Hung OR, Stevens SC, Morris I, et al. Clinical trial of a new lightwand device for intubating surgical patients. *J Anesth* 1994; 8(suppl):A708.

52. Hung OR, Stevens SC, Pytka S, et al. Clinical trial of a new lightwand device for intubation in patients with difficult airways. *Anesthesiology*. 1993; 79:A498.

53. Macintosh R, Richards H. Illuminated introducer for endotracheal tubes. *Anaesthesia* 1957; 12:223.

54. Doyle DJ, Sandler AN. The difficult airway II. *Anesthesiol Clin North Am*. 1995; 13(3):697.

55. Sandler AN, Doyle DJ. The difficult airway I. *Anesthesiol Clin North Am*. 1995;13(2).

56. Benumof JL: Additional safety measures when changing endotracheal tubes. *Anesthesiology*. 1991; 75:921.

☐ QUESTIONS

1. The distance from the lips to the carina is:
   1. 13 cm in the infant
   2. 26 cm in the adult male
   3. 28 cm in the adult male
   4. 24 cm in the adult female
      a. 1,3
      b. 1,3,4
      c. 2,4
      d. All of the above are true

2. Cricoid pressure applied during rapid sequence induction:
   a. Compresses the cricoid cartilage against the inferior border of the hyoid bone
   b. Pinches the esophagus closed between the cricoid cartilage and third vertebra
   c. Compresses the trachea between the vertebral column and the cricoid cartilage
   d. Compresses the esophagus against the body of the sixth cervical vertebra in the adult patient

3. Potential complications of nasotracheal intubation include all *except:*
   a. Eustachian tube obstruction
   b. Epistaxis
   c. Palatine tonsil dislodgment
   d. Maxillary sinusitis

4. What nerve (nerves) are blocked by the use of cocaine pledgets in the nasal passage?
   a. The glossopharyngeal nerve
   b. The facial nerve
   c. The nasopalatine nerves and the anterior ethmoidal nerves, both branches of the trigeminal nerve
   d. The internal laryngeal nerve, a branch of the vagus nerve

5. The primary muscles of the larynx responsible for cord abduction are the lateral cricoarytenoids. True or false.
   a. True
   b. False

6. In which patients would a difficult airway be anticipated?
   1. A 23-year-old woman scheduled for I+D with Ludwig's angina
   2. A 22-year-old man scheduled for an elective hernia repair with a thyromental distance of 5.5 cm with full neck extension
   3. A 75-year-old woman on the emergency schedule for repair of a fractured hip with mouth opening limited to 3.5 cm
   4. A full-bearded 45-year-old man with a Mallanpati airway classification I
      a. 1,3
      b. 2,4
      c. 1,2,4
      d. All are correct

7. Which statements regarding the innervation of the airway are correct?
   1. The vagus nerve supplies sensory innervation only to the airway.
   2. The recurrent laryngeal branch of the vagus provides sensory innervation to the larynx below the vocal cords and to the trachea.
   3. Only the cricothyroid muscle receives motor innervation from the external branch of the superior laryngeal.
   4. The recurrent laryngeal nerve supplies motor function to all other laryngeal muscles.
      a. 1,3
      b. 2,4
      c. 2,3,4
      d. All are correct

8. In the adult the trachea bifurcates at what level?
   a. C-6
   b. T-1
   c. T-3
   d. T-5

9. A healthy 60-year-old man with an uneventful anesthetic history is induced with 75 mg lidocaine, 140 mg propofol IV, and 60 mg Zemuron IV. Ventilation is not possible despite multiple attempts with and without oral and nasal airways. Alternative techniques include all *except:*
   a. Two-person mask ventilation
   b. Laryngeal mask airway insertion
   c. Allow the patient to resume spontaneous respiration
   d. Surgical airway access

10. Clinical applications of fiberoptic intubation include:
    1. Assess actual or suspected nerve injury
    2. Confirmation of endobronchial tube placement
    3. Temporomandibular joint ankylosis
    4. Placement of nasogastric tubes
       a. 1,2,3
       b. 2,4
       c. All of the above
       d. None of the above

11. The cartilages of the larynx
   1. Are formed by four paired cartilages: the cuneiforms, epiglottics, corniculates, and the arytenoids, and by two single cartilages: the thyroid, and the cricoid
   2. Are formed by three paired cartilages: the cuneiforms, corniculates, and the arytenoids, and by three single cartilages: the thyroid, epiglottic, and the cricoid
   3. Are complete rings except for the cricoid and thyroid cartilages
   4. Are all incomplete except for the cricoid cartilage
      a. 1,3
      b. 2,4
      c. 1,2,3
      d. 4 only

12. What is the level of the larynx in the adult?
   a. C-3 to C-4
   b. C-4 to C-5
   c. C-5 to C-7
   d. C-7 to T-1

13. During morning M&M conference you learn that a patient you anesthetized 2 days ago developed a bilateral superior laryngeal nerve palsy. In this patient, examination would reveal:
   a. Mild hoarseness without airway concerns
   b. Taut midline vocal cords
   c. Stridor and complete loss of voice
   d. No appreciable signs

14. While on call you are paged to the emergency room to evaluate a 28-year-old fireman rescued from a burning building 4 hours ago. Recently, he has developed significant respiratory effort and you notice presence of singed nasal hairs and sooty sputum. Your best course of action is to:
   a. Have a tracheostomy performed stat
   b. Administer 100% O_2 via face mask with nebulizer treatment
   c. Intubate
   d. Administer high-dose steroids

15. In which of the following would you consider a standard induction?

   a. Pierre Robin syndrome
   b. Acromegaly
   c. Rheumatoid arthritis
   d. Epiglottis

16. The blood supply to the larynx includes:
   a. Inferior thyroid artery
   b. Superior thyroid artery
   c. All of the above
   d. None of the above

17. All of the following are true statements *except:*
   a. The left bronchus branches off at a 45° angle.
   b. The right bronchus branches off at a 25° angle.
   c. Accidental endobronchial intubations are more likely on the left side.
   d. The carina is the bifurcation of the trachea into left and right bronchi at the angle of Louis.

18. Difficulties of inserting the laryngeal mask airway (LMA) include:
   1. Curling up of LMA tip against the hard palate
   2. Insufficient seal on inflation
   3. Esophageal intubation
   4. Potential airway trauma
      a. 1,3
      b. 2,4
      c. 1,2,4
      d. All of the above

19. What does the Z-79 marking on the endotracheal tube indicate?
   a. Manufacturer's identification number
   b. Tube has been tested and found to be nontoxic to tissue
   c. Maximal pressure allowed
   d. None of the above

20. When endotracheal cuff pressures exceed capillary hydrostatic pressure in the trachea, mucosa ischemia may occur. At what pressure will this occur?
   a. 22 mm Hg
   b. 32 mm Hg
   c. 38 mm Hg
   d. 42 mm Hg

☐ ANSWERS

1. b	**5.** b	**9.** c	**13.** a	**17.** c
2. d	**6.** c	**10.** c	**14.** c	**18.** c
3. c	**7.** c	**11.** b	**15.** c	**19.** b
4. c	**8.** d	**12.** b	**16.** c	**20.** b

Positioning

Minnette Beeson

Positioning is an important part of the comprehensive intraoperative care of a patient. Under general anesthesia or regional blockade a patient is not able to make the normal compensatory position changes that an unanesthetized individual would make in response to sustained pressure or pain to skin, subcutaneous tissue, muscle, nerves, and bone. Nor are they able to respond to discomfort caused by extension of joints beyond their normal limitations. However, the need for adequate surgical exposure may require the stabilization of a particular static position or an extension of a normal position for longer than normally tolerable.

☐ CONSEQUENCES

Careful positioning and monitoring often seem to go unrewarded. However, compromises in alignment or inattentive intraoperative monitoring can leave the patient with injuries ranging from transient paresthesias and cutaneous injuries to lifelong disabilities. These compromises can lead to serious problems that contribute to pain and discomfort, loss of function, and delayed recovery for unsuspecting patients.

Safe and effective patient positioning requires continuity of care and a team approach. The focus of perioperative positioning should be on prevention of injuries. The anesthesia care provider must have an understanding of the operation to be performed and the specific problems that the surgeon and anesthesia team might face during the procedure. In addition, consideration should be given to how operative positioning might affect vascularity, nerve transmission, ventilation/perfusion ratios, venous return, monitoring of vital signs, and the ability to have emergency access to the patient's airway and invasive line insertion sites.

VASCULAR ISCHEMIA

Stretch, compression, or obstruction can lead to interruption in blood flow to skin, subcutaneous tissue, muscle, nerves, and bone.[1] The subsequent ischemia is the principal mechanism of injury to these tissues. Progressive ischemia can lead to necrosis of local and regional tissues. Compression over a smaller surface area increases the potential for tissue injury. The duration of pressure seems to be more important than the intensity.[2]

PERIPHERAL NERVE INJURY

Peripheral nerves can be damaged from ischemia or mechanical distortion of the nerve membrane, cytoplasm, or myelin sheath.[3] The severity of the injury varies according to the degree of distortion ranging from transient failure of impulse conduction and pain, to permanent neurologic injuries.

Brachial Plexus The brachial plexus is the second most injured nerve bundle. It passes under the clavicle, over the first rib, under the pectoralis minor muscle and branches into the short lateral, medial, and posterior cords. The main tributary of the posterior cord is the radial nerve, which branches under the humerus. The median nerve runs close along the biceps brachii, and the ulnar nerve runs a long superficial course down the axilla (Figure 10–1). This nerve plexus can be injured in many different ways in many positions.

Shoulder braces placed tightly against the base of the neck can injure the nerve root. Compression between the clavicle and first rib can occur if the shoulder is allowed to move dorsally or if the supine patient shifts cephalad while the upper extremity is secured. Damage can occur when the brachial

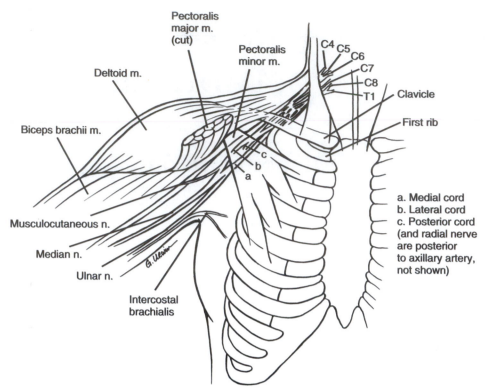

Figure 10–1 The brachial plexus. The brachial plexus and divisions in relation to muscle and bone.

plexus is stretched when the arm is abducted, extended, and externally rotated, and the head is deviated to the opposite side (Figure 10–2). Long thoracic nerve damage has been reported from position-related compression. The long thoracic nerve branches out from C-5, C-6, C-7 and sometimes C-8.[4] Injury to the nerve results in serratus anterior muscle dysfunction (Figure 10–3).

Ulnar Nerve   The distribution of the nerves that branch from the brachial plexus down the arm is shown in Figure 10–4. The ulnar nerve is the most commonly injured nerve in the anesthetized patient.[5] The ulnar nerve may be injured when it is compressed against the posterior aspect of the medial epicondyle of the humerus[6] at the elbow against the armboard (Figure 10–5) or the side of the bed (Figure 10–6). The ulnar nerve may also be injured when the elbow is flexed greater than 90° for a prolonged period of time. The extent and severity of nerve damage will vary with the location and the extent of the lesion.[7] However, rapid assessment can identify an acute injury if a pin prick cannot be felt in the little finger[8] (see Figure 10–4).

Radial Nerve   Other nerves injured in the upper extremity include the radial and median nerve (see Figure 10–4). The radial nerve can be injured if compressive force is ap-

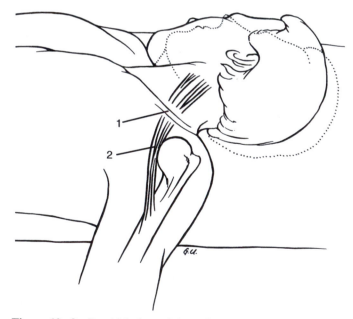

Figure 10–2 Brachial plexus injury. Compression of the brachial plexus can occur (1) between clavicle and first rib if the shoulder moves dorsally, if the patient shifts cephalad while the arms are secured, or when shoulder braces are placed incorrectly; or (2) against the head of the humerus when arms are extended greater than 90°, externally rotated, or if the patient's head is deviated to the opposite side.

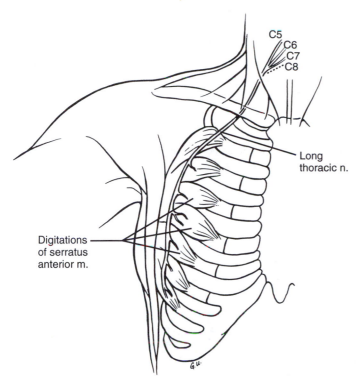

Figure 10–3 Long thoracic nerve injury. Serratus anterior muscle dysfunction has been reported and is thought to be caused by long thoracic nerve compression.

plied on the upper arm trapping the radial nerve against the spiral groove of the humerus by an object such as an anesthesia ether screen or excessive cycling of an automatic blood pressure cuff[9] (Figure 10–7). Symptoms include a wrist drop, weakness of abduction of the thumb, inability to extend the metacarpophalangeal joints, and loss of sensation in the web space between the thumb and index finger[10] (see Figure 10–4).

Median Nerve The median nerve runs along the medial cubital and basilic veins in the antecubital fossa (see Figure 10–4). It is most likely to be injured, not from malpositioning, but from iatrogenic infiltration of intravenous drugs or fluid. Injury to the nerve manifests as an inability to oppose the thumb and little finger and decreased sensation on the palmar surface of the thumb, index, and long fingers, as well as the radial side of the ring finger.[11]

Other Peripheral Nerves The most commonly injured nerves in the lower extremities are the common peroneal and saphenous nerve. These nerve injuries will be discussed in the lithotomy position section. (Figure 10–20, 10–21)

Compression damage to the pudendal, sciatic, anterior tibial, femoral, and obturator nerves has been reported. Other nerves have been injured by misaligned anesthesia airway equipment or injections. They include the phrenic nerve, stellate ganglion, lumbar spinal, optic and supraorbital, facial, abducens, and trigeminal nerves.

ALTERED VENTILATION/PERFUSION AND PULMONARY FUNCTION

In the lungs, inspired oxygen is transported to alveoli (ventilation) that permits its diffusion to red blood cells. These cells carry the necessary element to tissues, otherwise known as perfusion. In the ideal situation, all inspired oxygen should be available for diffusion and subsequent perfusion. However, the matching of ventilation to perfusion (V/Q) occurs in a precise manner.[12]

In zone 1, alveolar pressure exceeds either arterial or venous pressure and perfusion of the blood is minimal. In zone 2, arterial pressure exceeds alveolar pressure, and the alveolar pressure exceeds venous pressure. Perfusion occurs as a result of fluctuating balance between arterial and alveolar pressures. In zone 3, perfusion is determined by the difference between arterial pressure and venous pressure because

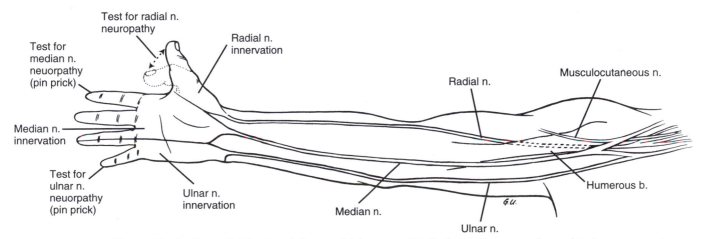

Figure 10–4 Nerve distribution of the arm. Major nerve distribution in the arm and associated neuropathies.

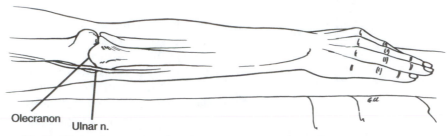

Olecranon   Ulnar n.

Figure 10–5   Ulnar nerve compression: *Incorrect* arm placement. The ulnar nerve may be injured when the arm is abducted and pronated on an extended armboard, causing the nerve to be compressed in the ulnar groove against the medial epicondyle.

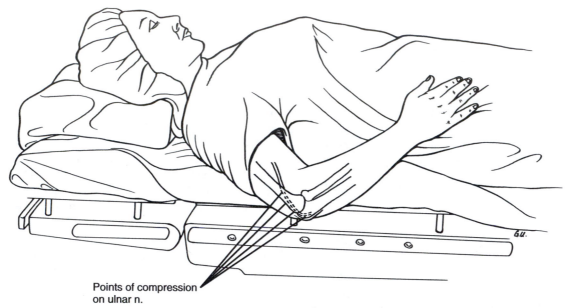

Points of compression
on ulnar n.

Figure 10–6   Ulnar nerve compression: *Incorrect* arm placement. The ulnar nerve can be compressed between the distal portion of the humerus and the side of the operating room table.

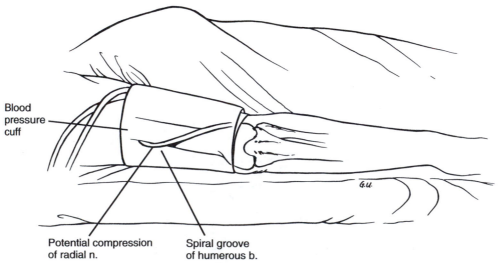

Blood
pressure
cuff

Potential compression   Spiral groove
of radial n.   of humerous b.

Figure 10–7   Radial nerve injury. The radial nerve can be injured if compressive force is applied to the lateral aspect of the upper arm, trapping the radial nerve in the spiral groove of the humerus.

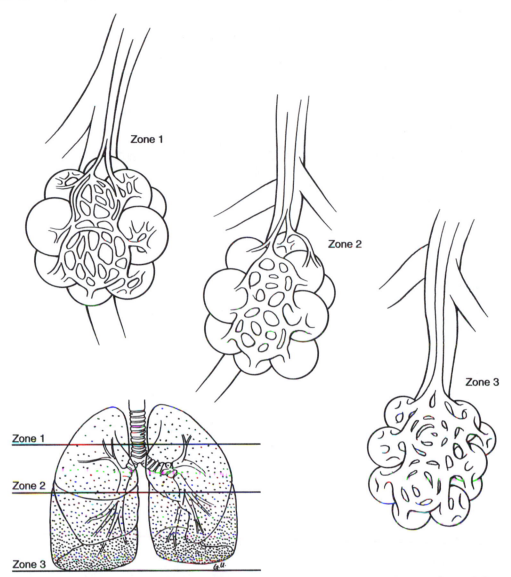

Figure 10–8 An illustration of ventilation-perfusion variability in the various portions of the lung.

of increased hydrostatic forces and subsequent venous congestion (Figure 10–8).

Alteration of V/Q and pulmonary function that may occur during the intraoperative period is varied and complex. Body position and control of respiration significantly affect V/Q matching. Pulmonary blood flow will normally increase in gravity-dependent areas of the lung (zone 3), whereas ventilation is greatest in nondependent areas (zone 1). However, the specific area of the lung receiving the increased ventilation or increased perfusion varies with the specific position. Figure 10–9 summarizes the effects of both in the erect, lateral, and supine positions.

In the lateral position the dependent lung is compressed, forcing ventilation to the nondependent lung. Perfusion increases to the dependent lung and decreases to the nondependent lung.

In the supine position, gravity increases perfusion to dorsal portions of lung and ventilation to ventral portions, creating V/Q differences from the normal erect position.[13]

Unlike an anesthetized patient, a spontaneously breathing individual is able to compensate partially by increasing diaphragmatic contraction strength, increasing ventilation to the gravity dependent areas of the lung, and providing an improved V/Q match.

Other pulmonary changes caused by positional changes include changes in lung volumes and diaphragmatic displacement specific for each position. Functional residual capacity (FRC), the amount of air remaining in the lungs after a normal expiration, acts as a reservoir providing additional oxygen in time of need. FRC is reduced by general anesthesia, muscle paralysis, most surgical positions, and further still in the postoperative period. During anesthesia, the reduced FRC can contribute to airway closure and to compression atelectasis. Then, postoperatively when intermittent spontaneous deep breathing (sighing mechanism) is reduced or prohibited, the alveolar volume is again reduced, contributing to airway closure and decrease surfactant distribution. Both can lead to hypoxemia and infection.[14]

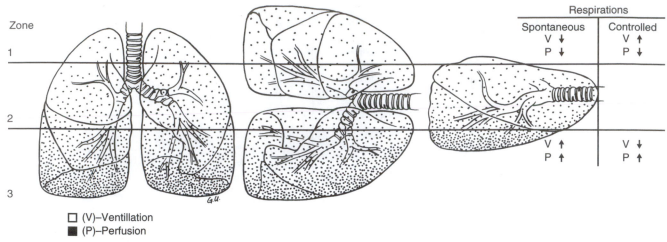

□ (V)–Ventillation
■ (P)–Perfusion

Figure 10–9 Altered ventilation/perfusion. Body position and controlled ventilation significantly effect ventilation/perfusion matching in various surgical positions when compared to the erect spontaneously breathing patient.

Postoperative pulmonary complications are the single leading cause of morbidity and mortality in the postoperative period. Abdominal procedures report 4.5% to 76% (average of 11%) pulmonary complication incidence. Most are thought to be caused by atelectasis, or collapse of the alveoli, started during the intraoperative period.[15]

COMPROMISED VENOUS RETURN

Position affects venous return. Blood will pool in distensible veins, especially when lower extremities are below the level of the heart, reducing the effective blood volume, cardiac output, and systemic perfusion.[16] Venous return can also be inhibited by inferior vena cava compression (i.e., gravid uterus, tumor, direct compression), and increased abdominal pressure (i.e., improper padding, positioning, or retraction).

VITAL SIGN MONITORING

Position can alter vital sign monitoring. Pressures have been shown to change by 2 mm Hg for each 2.5 cm that a given point varies in vertical height above or below the level of the heart.[17] Noninvasive or invasive blood pressure monitoring should be recorded at the level of the right atrium (phlebostatic axis).

LIMITED PATIENT ACCESS

Some positions and procedures limit ready access to patients for repositioning pulse oximetry probes, checking blood pressure cuffs, electrocardiographic leads, and so forth. More importantly, emergency access to the airway or to sites for insertion of invasive monitoring should be considered and a contingency plan developed should the need arise.

☐ PATIENT VULNERABILITY

Vulnerability also increases in patients with concurrently existing disease states as their tissues and systems have less resistance to the compromises surgical positioning imposes. These disease processes need to be identified and managed intraoperatively because they compromise regional blood flow leading to increased risk of ischemia.

LENGTH OF SURGERY

Risk of injury increases with prolonged surgical times that can lead to excessive or sustained pressure to skin, muscle, nerves, and bony prominences that are specifically outlined for each of the various positions. These specific dependent areas should be padded and protected for any surgical procedure.

ALTERATIONS IN CARDIAC FUNCTION

The effect of low or interpreted low blood perfusion pressure increases patient risk because of decreased preload and subsequent decreased cardiac output. The effect is more pronounced in patients with lowered reserves, as in those with arteriosclerosis, anemia, hypovolemia, fever, and infection, because the patient is less able to compensate further for decreases in cardiac output and increases in sympathetic nervous stimulation.

ALTERATIONS IN RESPIRATORY FUNCTION

Patients with altered respiratory function (obstructive or restrictive lung disorders) have baseline physiologic ventilation/perfusion mismatching. The degree to which V/Q is altered varies for specific disease processes, but the mismatching leads to degrees of relative hypoxia.[18] The patient with existing pulmonary compromise is less able to compensate to the challenges imposed by various positions redistributing normal ventilation and blood flow, and those caused by general anesthetics.

ALTERATIONS IN MUSCULOSKELETAL FUNCTION

Patients undergoing surgery and anesthesia could have many musculoskeletal conditions that would alter their compensatory mechanisms and increase their risk for vascular and neurologic ischemia.

Osteoarthritis and Rheumatoid Arthritis   Osteoarthritis (degenerative joint disease) is the most common musculoskeletal disease. It is characterized by a progressive loss of articular cartilage accompanied by changes in joint structure and subchondral bone. It becomes more prevalent with increasing age. Biomechanical, biochemical, inflammatory, and immunologic factors may all be involved in its development.[19]

Rheumatoid arthritis is a systemic inflammatory disease process speculated to be viral in origin.[20] Early in the disease process there is breakdown of the microvascular structures with subsynovial tissue edema. Later in the disease process, the synovium becomes edematous and projects into the joint cavity. As microvascular disease progresses, the resulting venous distention and capillary obstruction are of primary concern during positioning.[21]

Other Musculoskeletal Abnormalities   Many other musculoskeletal and neuromuscular disease processes alter the patient's ability to move muscles and joints normally. Among them are systemic inflammatory processes including systemic lupus erythematosus, polymyositis, and dermatomyositis. Systemic sclerosis (scleroderma) alters vascularity of skin, blood vessels, synovium, skeletal muscles, and internal organs.[22]

Duchenne-type muscular dystrophy is a degenerative disorder that first attacks skeletal muscle and proceeds to loss of ambulation, respiratory, and cardiac dysfunction and early death.

All present challenges for uncomplicated intraoperative positioning.

DIABETES MELLITUS

Diabetes mellitus is an endocrine disorder that eventually affects multiple organ systems. The vascular and neuropathic complications are of major concern for safe and effective positioning of the diabetic patient intraoperatively.

Microvascular changes that accompany the disease are caused by a thickening in the capillary basement membrane leading to retinopathies, nephropathies, and neuropathies.

Macrovascular complications of diabetes mellitus include cardiovascular disease, stroke, and peripheral vascular disease.[23] All preexisting peripheral neuropathies in the diabetic patient should be noted on the patient's chart appropriately.

CACHEXIA, EMACIATION, AND MALNOURISHMENT

Cachexia, emaciation, and malnourishment will lead to a combination of symptoms including weight loss, muscle wasting, and weakness. Protein and vitamin deficiencies are common. Existing alterations in skin integrity are likely. Patients with this existing disease process will most likely have difficulty responding to the stress of surgery and anesthesia, as well as maintaining vascularity to dependent areas during sustained positions.

OBESITY

In the obese patient, excess weight compressing the chest, abdomen, and diaphragm imposes a restrictive ventilation defect. Expiratory reserve volume, vital capacity, and FRC are reduced.[24] Morbid obesity has also been known to complicate positioning normally used for specific procedures because beds and equipment are not always adaptable to the patient's increased size.

☐ POSITIONING: GENERAL CONCERNS

The most common positions used in the operating room are supine (horizontal, reverse Trendelenburg, Trendelenburg), lithotomy, sitting, lateral decubitus, prone (horizontal, on a horizontal frame, jackknife, sitting-like, knee-chest), with some variations in arm position and knee flexion or extension. Each position has special concerns and considerations for patient safety.

SURGICAL TABLE

The design of the surgical table (Figure 10–10) allows a great range of positions, at varying heights for different size and shape patients. However, it has a few potential hazards as well.

Precautions   Missing or broken parts can compromise patient safety. The table parts must be checked to verify they are present and in working order. Ignoring proper inventory can pose a threat to the patient. Lateral table edges should be padded to prevent compression of the skin, nerves, blood vessels, tendons, and other vital structures. The patient should be protected from projections and insulated from metal surfaces. Arm boards should be properly padded. If the table is electric, it should be properly oriented to the patient and properly grounded.

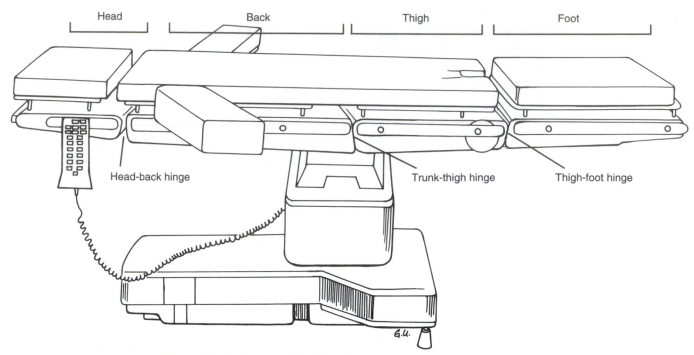

Figure 10–10   The surgical table. The surgical table's sections and hinges.

REPOSITIONING AND JOINT PROTECTION

Turning and positioning the anesthetized patient are potentially dangerous. The patient's autonomic compensatory mechanisms are obtunded by volatile anesthetics, narcotics, and muscle relaxants. In addition, the anesthetized patient has lost muscle tone and the sensation of pain that would ordinarily protect the joints. The preoperative assessment should include information concerning sore or stiff joints and range of motion limitations. All joints should be protected and kept within their limitations intraoperatively. Position changes should be anticipated and done gradually, allowing the body time to adjust. Fluids may need to be administered to prevent hypotension.

Patients should be "log rolled" into position. Head, neck, and hips should remain in anatomically correct alignment. Improper alignment during turning could result in severe spine injuries.

CHARTING

Notations concerning existing preoperative neuropathies, paresthesias, or range of motion limitations should be documented on the anesthetic record preoperatively. Positions used during anesthesia and specific comments about special protective measures provided, such as eye care and pressure point padding, should also be noted intraoperatively.[25]

☐ PRESSURE POINTS, COMMON NERVE INJURIES, AND PHYSIOLOGIC CHANGES

SUPINE

Horizontal   In the standard horizontal supine position (Figure 10–11), the patient lies on the back with both arms supinated and placed on padded arm boards at less than 90° abduction, or properly padded at the patient's side. The supine patient may be completely horizontal or in varying degrees of Trendelenburg (head up or head down).

In the supine position, pressure is exerted over the occiput, scapula, olecranon, ulnar nerve, sacrum, ischial tuberosities, and calcaneus areas. These bony prominences are the most likely areas to sustain obstructive or pressure-related injury to the skin and deeper tissues. They need to be well padded and monitored.

Nerve injuries in the supine position are relatively uncommon. The greatest cause for concern would be for the ulnar nerve caused by compression (see Figure 10–5) and the brachial plexus caused by stretching (see Figure 10–2). Other reported injuries include focal alopecia (hair loss) after long procedures from compression to the occiput, especially when hypothermia or hypoperfusion occurs concurrently. Use of an inflatable wedge or soft support in the lumbar sacral curve decreases the incidence of postoperative backache[26] thought to be caused from the stretch of relaxed spinal

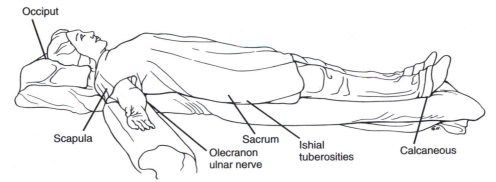

Figure 10–11   The horizontal supine position and pressure points.

muscles and ligaments during general anesthesia. The feet should not be allowed to hang over the end of the table because compression of the Achilles tendons could result in postoperative gait impairment.

In the horizontal supine position the influence of gravity to the cardiovascular system is minimal. As the abdominal contents shift more cephalad, they can displace the diaphragm, reducing lung volumes. Gravity-induced changes in pulmonary circulation increase blood flow to the dorsal portions of the lung (see Figure 10–9). Compliance is reduced, and passive ventilation tends to distribute gases preferentially to substernal units where pulmonary blood volume is reduced. To reduce V/Q imbalance during controlled ventilation, the tidal volume is increased to more than normal spontaneous ventilation.

Reverse Trendelenburg   In the head-up supine position, or reverse Trendelenburg (Figure 10–12), the head is elevated and the lower extremities are below the level of the heart. Blood can pool in dependent vessels. Mean arterial pressure in the brain could be significantly lower than the mean blood pressure as measured by oscilloscope at the right atrium or phlebostatic axis (i.e., 24 mm Hg for 12 inches). Direct arterial monitoring transducers should be zeroed at the highest point on the skull.[27]

Lawnchair   Variations of the supine position include the "lawnchair" modification (Figure 10–13). This position refers to a contoured supine posture.[28] The trunk–thigh hinge is slightly flexed (approximately 15°) and the foot is angulated a similar amount in the opposite direction.

Sitting Position   Venous air embolism (VAE) is considered to be a major complication of the sitting position (Figure 10–14) used in posterior cervical or occipital surgery. The incidence has been reported to be as high as 30% although not always responsible for major complications or increased morbidity and mortality.[29,30]

Areas of compression include the occiput, scapula, olecranon and ulnar nerve, sacrum and ischial tuberosities, and calcaneous.

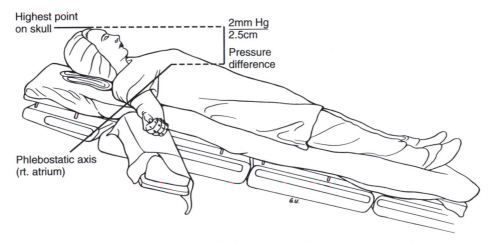

Figure 10–12   The supine reverse Trendelenburg position. Cerebral mean arterial pressure (used to estimate cerebral perfusion pressure) could be significantly lower than the mean blood pressure measured by oscilloscope or transducer at the level of the heart (phlebostatic axis) by 2 mm Hg for each 2.5 cm (1 inch). (Transducers should be zeroed at the highest point on the head.)

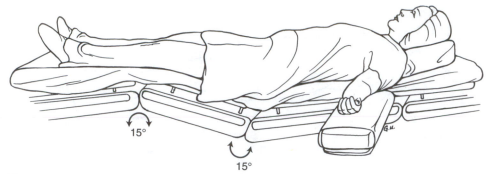

Figure 10–13 The supine contoured sitting "lawnchair" position. The trunk–thigh hinge is flexed 15° and the foot is angulated a similar amount in the opposite direction.

Other physiologic changes that occur include pooling of venous blood in the lower extremities, lessened by placing elastic support stockings (TED hose) on the patient preoperatively. Variances will exist between mean arterial blood pressure measured on the upper arm by oscilloscope and the actual mean arterial cerebral pressure.

Trendelenburg In the head-down or Trendelenburg position (Figure 10–15), cerebral circulation and venous pressure are increased. Extreme effects can lead to cerebral edema, facial congestion, retinal detachment, and changes in blood pressure by baroreceptors in carotid and aortic bodies; decrease pulmonary compliance, FRC, and vital capacity; and increase the incidence of atelectasis. Obese patients are often unable to tolerate this position because of already compromised FRCs. In these patients ventilation must be controlled or assisted.

Lithotomy In the lithotomy position (Figure 10–16), the patient lies on the back with legs and thighs flexed. The use of proper fitting equipment is essential to minimize risk

of injury. Lower extremity nerve damage is significant in this position. Risk of developing a significant lower extremity neuropathy (persistent foot drop or leg weakness requiring either prosthetic or ambulatory support) is even higher (45%) when the position is sustained for more than 4 hours or the patient is thin or a smoker.[31]

The lower extremity nerve distribution is diagrammed in Figures 10–17, 10–18, and 10–19.

The legs should be elevated together and flexed together. If stationary "knee-padded" stirrups are used, excessive pressure may be placed on the popliteal space[32] (see Figure 10–16). Common peroneal injuries can occur if the legs are compressed against the stirrups on the lateral aspects of the legs and are the most common injuries to the lower extremities. The common peroneal nerve is a branch of the sciatic and branches along the head of the fibula where it can be compressed against the lateral braces used in the lithotomy position (Figure 10–20). Injury manifests as a foot drop, inability to dorsally extend the toes, and inability to evert the foot.[33]

Saphenous nerve injuries can occur if the medial aspects

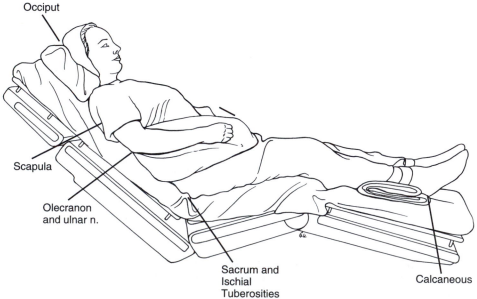

Occiput

Scapula

Olecranon and ulnar n.

Sacrum and Ischial Tuberosities

Calcaneous

Figure 10–14 The supine sitting position and pressure points. (Example shown for shoulder surgery).

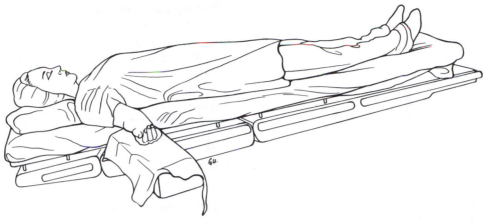

Figure 10–15   The supine Trendelenburg position. The supine Trendelenburg position increases cerebral circulation and venous pressure and decreases pulmonary compliance, functional residual capacity, and vital capacity.

of the calf rest on the stirrups (Figure 10–21), compressing this branch of the femoral nerve against the medial tibial condyle. Numbness in the lateral thigh (meralgia paresthetica) is caused by injury to the lateral femoral cutaneous nerve, which branches off the L2 and L3 vertebraes running a long course transversely through the pelvis posterior-laterally, exiting under the inguinal ligament anteriorly.

Bilateral tibial compartment syndromes have been reported during longer procedures arising from compression of nerves and muscles.[34–36] Bilateral compartment syndrome is a grave complication, which if unrecognized, may result in severe neurovascular damage and permanent disabilities.

Brachial plexus injuries can occur if shoulder braces are used incorrectly. Care should be exercised to keep the shoulders in neutral alignment throughout table adjustments. Fingers should be protected from table hinges to prevent injuries caused by the foot section being returned to the normal position (Figure 10–22).

In the anesthetized patient total lung volume can be decreased by 15% with 20° head-down tilt. Ventilation is best maintained with assisted or controlled mode. Circulatory effects can occur rapidly as the blood pressure decreases with sudden lowering of legs.

LATERAL DECUBITUS

Horizontal   Areas at risk for pressure related injuries include the dependent eye, cheek and ear acromion process, iliac crest, greater trochanter, lateral knee, femur, fibula, peroneal nerve, and malleolus (Figure 10–23).

The spine should be in an anatomically correct position without twisting. The trunk should be stabilized to prevent rolling forward or back. The dependent thigh should be flexed with a pillow between the legs to decrease pressure on bony prominences. An axillary role placed slightly caudad to

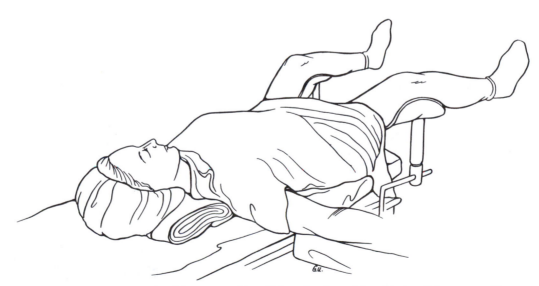

Figure 10–16   The supine lithotomy position. This patient is positioned in low lithotomy position with popliteal support.

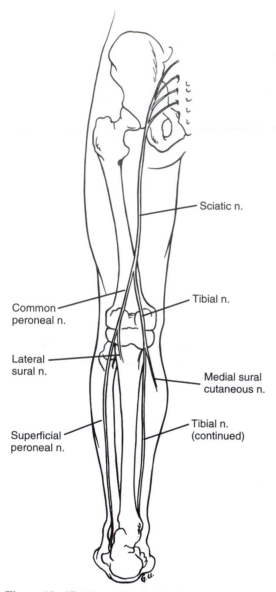

Figure 10–17   Nerve distribution in the posterior leg.

Kidney Rest   The "kidney rest" or "gallbladder rest" is one of the potentially most dangerous items on the operating room table. When placed in its upward position (Figure 10–24), it can impair ventilation, dangerously contort the thoracolumbar spine, decrease FRC, and compromise venous return due to compression and elongation of the vena cava and thereby decrease cardiac output. Extreme flexion should be avoided. The patient must be positioned with the iliac crest over the kidney rest.

PRONE

Horizontal   In the horizontal prone position (Figure 10–25), the patient is placed on the ventral side (ventral de-

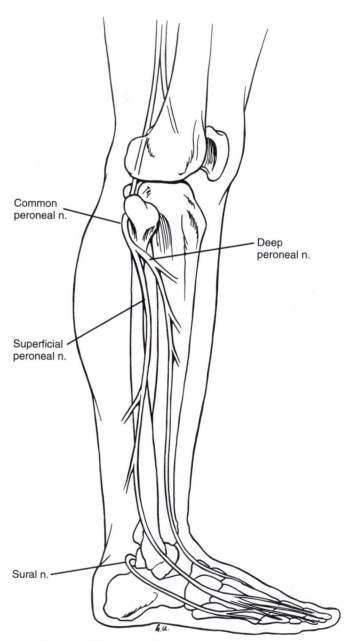

Figure 10–18   Nerve distribution in the lateral lower leg.

the dependent axilla prevents neurovascular compression. Forearms should be flexed at the elbows and supported. The head should be kept in anatomic alignment in a "neutral position" and placed on an appropriate-sized head rest or pillow.

Some of the more serious complications reported with the lateral decubitus position include the "crush syndrome" with injuries from sustained pressure to the contralateral side (in one case the gluteal compartment[37]) involving paresthesias, massive swelling of the thigh with myonecrosis, acute renal failure secondary to myoglobinuria, and arterial insufficiency resulting in a below-the-knee amputation.[38]

In the lateral decubitus position physiologic changes occur in the mechanically ventilated patient. This position decreases FRC and increases airway resistance. The pulmonary blood flow is greater in the dependent lung, and ventilation is increased in the nondependent lung.

crease risk of pressure injuries. If the procedure, position, and patient condition allow, limbs can be taken through a modified range of motion and the head and neck can be repositioned intraoperatively at convenient times to decrease risk of ischemic injury.

Elaborate measures may be needed to keep the head in a safe position and to prevent neck injury. A serious complication of prone positioning recently reported has been unilateral blindness.[39] The patient's head was placed on a padded Mayfield head rest. This may not be appropriate for all patients because exophthalmus or a flattened nasal bridge may allow transmission of pressure to the globe of the eye, causing blindness. An unexplained intraoperative occurrence of bradyarrthythmia or conduction disturbance may signal increased intraorbital pressure.

Ears can be folded back and pressure can be exerted by the weight of the head. Elastic cartilage is easily damaged and is

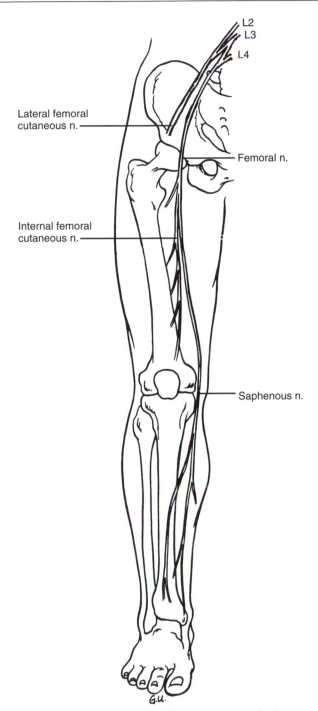

Figure 10–19   Nerve distribution in the anterior leg.

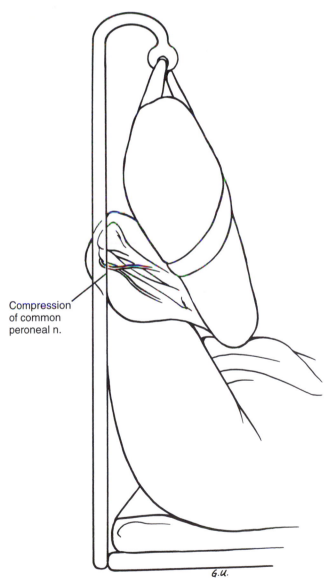

Figure 10–20   Common peroneal nerve injury. Compression of the common peroneal nerve against *lateral* braces.

cubitus) and is best supported with two padded rolls that extend from the clavicle to the iliac crest freeing the abdominal wall and anterior thoracic wall to improve ventilation and increase venous return.

Neurologic injuries from improper prone positioning can cause injuries to the eyes, ears, cheeks, acromion process, clavicle, iliac crests, patella, toes, and dorsum of the feet. All of these pressure points must be padded and well protected. Pressure points should be massaged, if at all possible, every 20 to 60 minutes to improve regional blood flow and de-

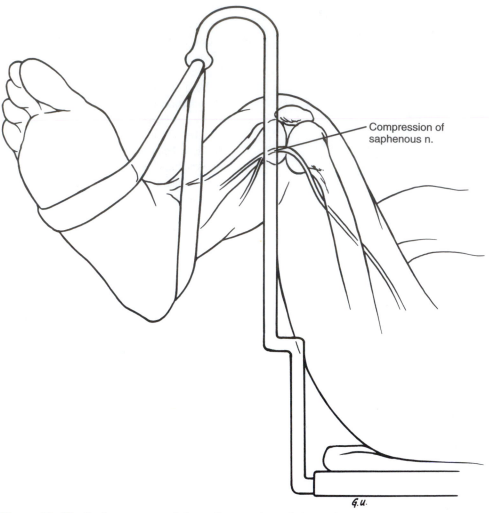

Figure 10–21 Saphenous nerve injury. Compression of the saphenous nerve against *medial* braces.

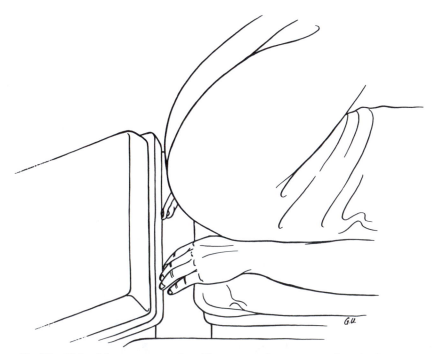

Figure 10–22 Risk of finger compression. Fingers may be compressed as the foot section is returned to normal position after a procedure performed in the lithotomy position.

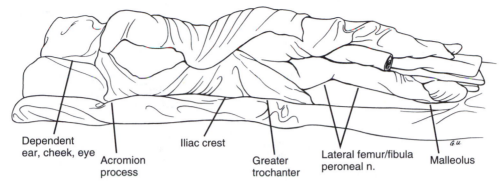

Figure 10–23   Lateral decubitus position and pressure points.

slow to heal because all cartilage receives little blood supply.[40] Brachial plexus neuropathies can occur if arms are extended above shoulders secondary to stretching. The female breasts can be injured if pushed, pulled, or twisted from their normal anatomic position. Care should be taken to limit the compressive forces exerted on any pendulous soft tissue. Male genitalia should be protected by ensuring that the patient is not lying on them and that they are not caught between patient and table; the electrosurgical ground pad should be well away from the area. The nerves and tendons of the dorsum of the foot can be injured if the foot rests on the metal edge of the table.

In the horizontal prone position diaphragmatic movement is restricted and the tidal volume may be limited by the weight of the body. Increased intra-abdominal pressure may compress the inferior vena cava, resulting in a decrease in venous return and reduced blood pressure.

Pressure in the carotid area must be avoided. Compression of a carotid artery can cause reduced intracerebral blood flow. Compression of carotid sinuses can cause reflexive hypotension and dysrhythmias. In certain neurosurgical procedures head tongs are used to stabilize the head and maintain the neck in a neutral position.

Prone Horizontal with Frame (Wilson)   The Wilson frame is a contoured apparatus that when placed over a flat operating table, allows a patient to be rolled over into a flexed prone position. Its principal advantage, when properly used, is that it permits venous return from lower extremities.

Disadvantages include potential for eye and facial compression, brachial plexus stretching as arms are placed overhead, ulnar nerve compression, and increased intra-abdominal pressure.

Prone Jackknife   The prone jackknife position (Figure 10–26) was developed to achieve specific exposure for anal and rectal surgery. The operating table is flexed with the pelvis at flexed point or body flexed over a large roll. The head is turned to one side and the arms are abducted up and away from the body.

Prone Sitting (Andrew's Frame)   The Andrew's frame maintains a prone sitting-like position (Figure 10–27). The kneeling position decreases operative time and intraoperative blood loss when compared to the prone position in the patient undergoing lumbar disk surgery.[41] However, there have been reports of complications associated with its use. Anterior tibial compartment syndrome resulting from sustained pressure to nerves and muscles is one of the more serious.[42]

Knee-Chest   The knee-chest position (Figure 10–28) has been used for anal and gynecologic procedures. When the patient's ischial spines and sacrum are supported by adjunct devices, lumbar surgery can be performed. Although it may appear uncomfortable, it provides specific surgical exposure with less cardiovascular and respiratory compromise compared to other prone positions. Adequate padding must be provided to all dependent body areas.

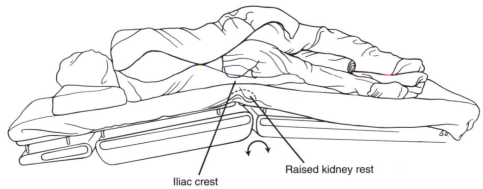

Figure 10–24   Flexed lateral decubitus position with kidney rest. *Correct position* of iliac crest in relation to flexion point in flexed lateral decubitus position with kidney rest raised.

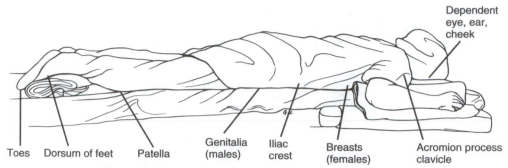

Figure 10–25   Horizontal prone position and pressure points.

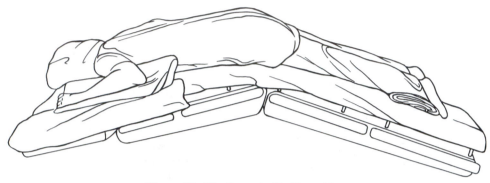

Figure 10–26   Prone jackknife position.

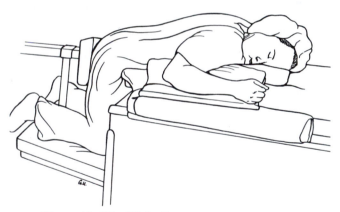

Figure 10–27   "Sitting" prone position on Andrew's frame.

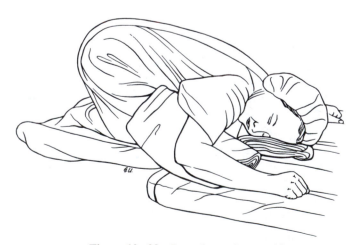

Figure 10–28   Prone knee-chest position.

□ SUMMARY

Intraoperative positioning is a big responsibility that necessitates a thorough understanding of related physiologic and pathophysiologic concepts. Patients depend totally on their caregivers to provide and protect their well-being during the intraoperative period. This can be a challenge. Consistently delivering this high standard of quality care requires knowledge, vigilance, and an uncompromising attitude toward patient safety.

REFERENCES

1. Waugaman WR, Foster SD, Rigor BM, *Principles and Practice of Nurse Anesthesia.* 3rd ed. East Norwalk, Conn: Appleton & Lange; 1992.

2. Gruendemann BJ. *Positioning Plus.* Chatsworth, Calif: Educational Department of Devon Industries; 1987: 21.

3. Alexander CM. Perioperative ulnar nerve injury. *Current Reviews for Nurse Anesthetists.* 1995; 18(13): 115–121.

4. Martin JT. Patient positioning. In: Bararsh PG, Cullen BF, Stoelting R, eds. *Clinical Anesthesia.* 2nd ed. Philadelphia: JB Lippincott; 1992; 717.

5. Kroll DA, Caplan RA, Pasner K, Ward RJ, Cheney FW. Nerve injury associated with anesthesia. *Anesthesiology.* 1990; 73: 202–207.

6. Stoelting RK, Miller RD. *Basics of Anesthesia.* 3rd ed. New York: Churchill Livingstone; 1994: 195–196.

7. Chusid JG. *Correlative Neuroanatomy and Functional Neruology.* Los Altos, Calif: Lange Medical Publications; 1985:149.

8. McAlpine FS, Seckel BR. Peripheral nervous system complications. In: Martin JT, ed. *Positioning in Anesthesia and Surgery.* 2nd ed. Philadelphia: WB Saunders; 1987:303.

9. Bickler PE, Schapera A, Bainton CR. Acute radial nerve injury from use of an automatic blood pressure monitor. *Anesthesiology.* 1990; 73:186.

10. Chusid JG. *Correlative Neuroanatomy and Functional Neurology.* Los Altos, Calif: Lange Medical Publications; 1985:145.

11. Stoelting RK, Miller RD. *Basics of Anesthesia.* 3rd ed. New York: Churchill Livingstone; 1994: 198.

12. West JB, Dollery CT, Naimark A. Distribution of blood flow in isolated lung: relations to vascular and alveolar pressures. *J Appl Physiol.* 1964; 19:713.

13. Martin, JT. Patient positioning. In: Bararsh PG, Cullen BF, Stoelting R. *Clinical Anesthesia.* 2nd ed. Philadelphia: JB Lippincott; 1992: 711.

14. Hedenstierna G. Mechanisms of postoperative pulmonary dysfunction. *Acta Chir Scand Suppl.* 1989; 550:152–158.

15. Drain C. Postanesthesia care of the surgical patient. In: Waugamann WR, Rigor BM, Katz LE, Bradshaw HW, Garde JF, eds. *Principles and Practice of Nurse Anesthesia.* 2nd ed. East Norwalk, Conn: Appleton & Lange, 1988: 643.

16. Martin JT. Patient positioning. In: Bararsh PG, Cullen BF, Stoelting R. *Clinical Anesthesia.* 2nd ed. Philadelphia: JB Lippincott; 1992; 709.

17. Enderby GEH. Postural ischemia and blood pressure. *Lancet* 1954; 1:185.

18. Stoelting RK, Dierdorf SF. *Anesthesia and Co-existing Disease.* 3rd. ed. New York: Churchill Livingstone, 1993.

19. Copstead LC. *Perspectives on Pathophysiology.* Philadelphia: WB Saunders; 1995.

20. Harris E. Pathogenesis of rheumatoid arthritis. In: Kelley W. Harris E, Ruddy S. Sledge D, eds. *Textbook of Rheumatology.* Philadelphia: WB Saunders; 1985:886–903.

21. Ishikawa H, Ziff M. Electron microscopic observations of immunoreactive cells in the rheumatoid synovial membrane. *Arthritis Rheum.* 1976; 19:1–14.

22. Medsger TA. Systemic sclerosis (scleroderma), eosinophilic fasciitis, and calcinoses. In: McCarty D, ed. *Arthritis and Allied Conditions.* 10th ed. Philadelphia: Lea & Febiger; 1985: 994–1036.

23. Siegel J. Diabetes mellitus. In: Copstead LC, ed. *Perspectives in Pathophysiology.* Philadelphia: WB Saunders; 1995.

24. Stoelting RK, Miller RD. *Basics of Anesthesia.* 3rd ed. New York: Churchill Livingstone; 1994: 325.

25. Martin, JT. Patient positioning. In: Bararsh PG, Cullen BF, Stoelting R. *Clinical Anesthesia.* 2nd ed. Philadelphia: JB Lippincott; 1992: 709.

26. O'Donovan N, Healy TE, Faragher EB, Wilkens RG, Hamilton AA. Postoperative backache: the use of an inflatable wedge. *Br J Anaesth* 1986; 53:280–283.

27. Bendo AA, Kass IS, Hartung J, Cottrell JE. Neurophysiology and neuroanesthesia. In: Bararsh PG, Cullen BF, Stoelting R, eds. *Clinical Anesthesia.* 2nd ed. Philadelphia: JB Lippincott; 1992.

28. Martin JT. *Positioning in Anesthesia and Surgery.* 2nd ed. Philadelphia: WB Saunders; 1987.

29. Young ML, Smith DS, Murtagh F, Vasquez A, Levitt J. Comparison of surgical and anesthetic complications in neurosurgical patients experiencing venous air embolism in the sitting position. *Neurosurgery.* 1986; 18(2):157–61.

30. Black S, Ockert DB, Oliver WC Jr, Cucchiara RF. Outcome following posterior fossa craniectomy in patients in the sitting or horizontal positions. *Anesthesiology.* 1988; 69(1): 49–56.

31. Warner MA, Martin JT, Schroeder DR, Offord DP, Chute CG. Lower extremity motor neuropathy associated with surgery performed on patients in a lithotomy position. *Anesthesiology.* 1994; 8:6–12.

32. Gruendemann BJ. *Positioning Plus.* Chatsworth, Calif: Educational Department of Devon Industries, 1987; 53.

33. Khalil M. Bilateral compartmental syndrome after prolonged surgery in the lithotomy position. *J Vasc Surg.* 1987; 5: 879–881.

34. Moses TA, Kreder KJ, Thrasher JB. Compartment syndrome: an unusual complication of the lithotomy position. *Urology.* 1994; 43:746–747.

35. Schwartz LB, Stahl RS, De Cherney AH. Unilateral compartment syndrome after prolonged gynecologic surgery in the dorsal lithotomy position. A case report. *J Reprod Med.* 1993:38(6):469–471.

36. Rommel FM, Kabler RL, Mowad JJ. The crush syndrome: a complication of urological surgery. *J Urol.* 1986; 135:809–811.

37. Smith JW, Pelluci PM, Sharroch N, Mineo R, Wilson PD. Complications after total hip replacement: the contralateral limb. *J Bone Joint Surg.* 1989; 71:528–535.

38. Wolfe SW, Lospinuso MF, Burke SW. Unilateral blindness as a complication of patient positioning for spinal surgery. A case report. *Spine* 1992; 17:600–605.

39. Banasik JL. Genetic control—inheritance. In: Copstead LC.

Perspectives in Pathophysiology. Philadelphia: WB Saunders; 1995.

40. Bostman O, Hyrkas J, Hirvensalo E, Kallio E. Blood loss, operating time, and positioning of the patient in lumbar disc surgery. *Spine* 1990; 15:360–363.

41. Geisler FH, Laich DT, Goldflies M, Shepard A. Anterior tibial compartment syndrome as a positioning complication of prone-sitting position for lumbar surgery. *Neurosurgery* 1993; 33: 1117.

☐ QUESTIONS

1. Numbness in the lateral thigh is caused by injury to the:
   a. Lateral femoral cutaneous nerve
   b. Saphenous nerve
   c. Peroneal nerve
   d. Pudendal nerve

2. Which one of the following parameters does not increase patient vulnerability to position-related injuries?
   a. Induced hypotension
   b. Use of a modern operating room table
   c. Length of surgery
   d. Hypothermia

3. Injury to the radial nerve from compression of the ether screen during a long case could cause which of the following symptoms?
   a. Ulnar deviation of fourth and fifth digits
   b. Unable to oppose thumb and little finger
   c. Wrist drop
   d. Third finger weakness

4. Which one of the areas listed would not be a primary concern for prone positioning?
   a. Risk of injury to female breasts and male genitalia
   b. Positioning of bolsters from clavicle to iliac crests to improve ventilation and venous return
   c. Unilateral blindness and/or damage to supraorbital area
   d. Popliteal nerve damage

5. The most commonly injured nerve during intraoperative procedures is the:
   a. Brachial plexus nerve
   b. Ulnar nerve
   c. Saphenous nerve
   d. Radial nerve

6. What nerve could be injured by antecubital intravenous infiltration or placement?
   a. Radial nerve
   b. Ulnar nerve
   c. Musculocutaneous nerve
   d. Median nerve

7. Which nerve is the most commonly injured nerve of the lower extremities?
   a. Common peroneal
   b. Femoral nerve
   c. Pudendal nerve
   d. Saphenous nerve

8. The primary reason for respiratory compromise with general anesthetics, position changes, or in compromised patients is caused by:
   a. Poor diffusion
   b. Poor ventilation
   c. Ventilation/Perfusion mismatching
   d. Poor circulation

9. The primary reasons why patients with a history of diabetes mellitus are at increased risk for intraoperative positioning injuries include all *except:*
   a. History of macrovascular changes such as increased cardiovascular disease, incidence of stroke, and peripheral vascular disease
   b. Capillary basement membrane thickening and microvascular changes
   c. Existing neuropathic complications of their disease
   d. Articular cartilage degeneration

10. Pressure exerted over the acromion process, iliac crest, greater trochanter, peroneal nerve, and malleolus is characteristic for which position?
    a. Supine-sitting
    b. Lateral decubitus
    c. Supine-horizontal
    d. Prone Wilson's frame

11. The incidence of venous air embolism associated with the sitting position has been reported to be as high as:
    a. 30%
    b. 10%
    c. 3%
    d. 50%

12. Common peroneal injuries can occur if the legs are compressed _____ against the leg stirrups used for the lithotomy position
    a. Inferiorly
    b. Medially
    c. Superiorly
    d. Laterally

13. Which of the following is not a complication of brachial plexus root injury?
    a. Long thoracic nerve injury and scapular winging
    b. Compression between clavicle and first rib
    c. Inability to oppose thumb and little finger
    d. Dorsal extension and lateral flexion of the head to the opposite side

14. Which position can be associated with injuries to the operative contralateral side?
    a. Lateral decubitus
    b. Sitting position
    c. Prone position
    d. Lithotomy position

15. Which single item on the operating table is considered to be the most dangerous?
    a. Leg stirrups
    b. Kidney rest
    c. Mayfield head rest
    d. Reorientation option

16. Neurologic injuries from improper _____ position include damage to the eyes, ears, cheeks, acromion process, clavicle, iliac crests, patella, and dorsum of the feet.
    a. Sitting
    b. Lateral decubitus
    c. Prone
    d. Reverse Trendelenburg

17. If during a laparoscopic cholecystectomy the patient is in a reverse Trendelenburg position, at a 20° angle elevating the head 14 inches above the level of the right atrium, and experiences a hypotensive episode the mean cerebral pressure will be:
    a. 14 mm Hg higher than oscilloscope reading
    b. 40 mm Hg lower than oscilloscope reading
    c. 28 mm Hg higher than oscilloscope reading
    d. 28 mm Hg lower than oscilloscope reading

18. What is the primary mechanism of injury related to perioperative positioning?
    a. compression
    b. ischemia
    c. obstruction
    d. stretching

19. What is the second most injured nerve bundle?
    a. Radial nerve
    b. Femoral nerve
    c. Sciatic nerve
    d. Brachial plexus root

20. Injury to the median nerve manifests as:
    a. Wrist drop
    b. Scapular winging
    c. Inability to oppose thumb and little finger
    d. Loss of sensation to pin prick of little finger.

☐ ANSWERS

1.	a	5.	b	9.	d	13.	c	17.	d
2.	b	6.	d	10.	b	14.	a	18.	b
3.	c	7.	a	11.	a	15.	b	19.	d
4.	d	8.	c	12.	d	16.	c	20.	c

11

Fluid Management and Blood Replacement

W. Gray McCall

One of the multiple perioperative tasks of the anesthesia provider is to maintain fluid balance for the patient. The overall purpose of this chapter is to review the physiologic basis of fluid management and blood replacement during the perioperative period.

The goals of fluid therapy are to avoid or correct a hypovolemic state, restore intravascular volume, and maintain the oxygen-carrying capacity of the intravascular volume. Successful achievement of these goals should foster hemodynamic stability and physiologic balance necessary for optimum tissue perfusion. If these goals are not met, the hypoxic cellular sequence leading to damage of end organs such as the kidneys could result.

☐ BODY FLUID COMPARTMENTS

Total body water, which is approximately 42 L (60% of body weight) in the 70-kg patient, is the primary component of the human body. Total body water is divided into two major compartments. The intracellular volume is the fluid contained within the cells, which is approximately 40% of body weight or 28 L. The extracellular volume, which constitutes 20% of body weight, is subdivided into intravascular volume at 3 L and interstitial volume at 11 L.[1]

FLUID DYNAMICS

The main forces affecting the physiologic movement of fluid at the capillary level include capillary hydrostatic pressure, interstitial fluid pressure, plasma colloid osmotic (oncotic) pressure, and interstitial fluid colloid pressure.

Capillary hydrostatic pressure has its greatest effect at the arterial side of the capillary. It is estimated that capillary pressure at the arterial end of the capillaries is 25 mm Hg while pressure at the venous end of capillaries is 10 mm Hg resulting in a mean capillary hydrostatic pressure of approximately 17 mm Hg.[1] Looking at this parameter alone, the increased hydrostatic pressure on the arterial side of the capillary in the systemic circulation is responsible for the majority of fluid movement out of the capillary. As the pressure increases, either by overinfusion of crystalloid solution, decreased renal function, cardiac failure, or numerous other factors, the rate of diffusion out of the capillary is increased. *Edema* occurs when the rate of diffusion results in more fluid leaking out of the capillary compared to the ability of the lymphatic system to transport the excess away.

Another factor causing fluid movement out of the capillary is the *interstitial fluid pressure*. By indirect measurements, it is estimated that average interstitial fluid pressure is 3.0 mm Hg.[1] This negative pressure is generated by the tendency of the capillaries to absorb fluid from the interstitial spaces, which results in compacting of the interstitial spaces. When tissues lose this negative interstitial fluid pressure, fluid accumulates in the spaces, manifesting as edema. Once significant edema formation has occurred, the increased distance between the cells and capillaries will decrease the effectiveness in meeting the metabolic needs of the cell.

The *plasma colloid osmotic pressure* tends to draw fluid from the interstitium back into the capillary. Colloid osmotic pressure is primarily generated by the presence of protein molecules within the plasma volume. A special effect, called the Donnan equilibrium, causes the colloid osmotic pressure to be about 50% greater than that caused by proteins alone.[1] With protein molecules possessing a negative charge (anions), a large number of positively charged cations, mainly sodium ions, are necessary to balance the charges generated by the protein molecules. In other words, the total osmotic pressure across the membrane is generated by both colloid molecules and electrolytes, although it is measured as *colloid osmotic pressure.* The pressure generated by the proteins is termed *oncotic pressure* and the force generated by the electrolytes is termed *osmotic pressure.* Normal plasma osmolality is generally 285 mOsm/kg (or approximately twice the Na$^+$), a value determined almost entirely by small molecules and positively charged ions. Due to the lower number of protein molecules compared to ions, the oncotically active molecules of protein contribute only about 1 mOsm/kg. The albumin molecules are larger, but there are few of them compared to the ions. Large reductions in colloid osmotic pressure must occur to effect water movement in or out of the capillaries, especially through the blood–brain barrier.

Interstitial fluid colloid osmotic pressure, generated by a small protein concentration in the interstitial fluid, causes movement out of the capillary. The average interstitial fluid colloid osmotic pressure is 8.0 mm Hg.[1] The majority of the capillary pores, which allow free movement of water and ions between intravascular and interstitial fluid, have a diameter smaller than the size of protein molecules. However, small amounts of plasma proteins do leak into the interstitial spaces. The concentration of the protein in the interstitial fluid is only a little more than one-fourth that in plasma or about 1.8 to 2.0 g/dL. If capillary permeability increases due to multiple etiologies, more albumin is allowed to enter the interstitium and the potential for edema will greatly increase.

The mean forces causing fluid movement both in and out of the capillary are listed in Table 11–1.[1] A slight imbalance of forces at the capillary membranes causes slightly more filtration of fluid into the interstitial spaces than reabsorption. This slight excess of filtration is called net filtration, and it is balanced by fluid return to the circulation through the lymphatics.

Table 11–1
FORCES CAUSING CAPILLARY FLUID MOVEMENT

	mm Hg
Mean forces tending to move fluid outward:	
Mean Capillary Pressure	17.3
Negative interstitial free fluid pressure	3.0
Interstitial fluid colloid osmotic pressure	8.0
TOTAL OUTWARD FORCE	28.3
Mean forces tending to move fluid inward:	
Plasma colloid osmotic pressure	28.0
TOTAL INWARD FORCE	28.0
Summation of mean forces:	
Outward	28.3
Inward	28.0
NET OUTWARD FORCE	0.3

SOURCE: Reproduced by permission from Guyton AC. The microcirculation and the lymphatic system: capillary fluid exchange, interstitial fluid and lymph flow. In: *Textbook of Medical Physiology.* 8th ed. Philadelphia: WB Saunders; 1991:179.

The primary means by which substances are transported between the intravascular space and the interstitial fluids is by *diffusion.* (For the purpose of this discussion, the capillary beds in the cerebral, hepatic, and renal circulation are excluded.) Water molecules diffuse through the capillary membranes via two routes. Partial water diffusion occurs through the pores of the endothelial cellular membranes into the endothelial cells and then out of the membrane on the other side of the cell. Little net water movement occurs by this route because of the small surface area of the endothelial cells and the establishment of a concentration gradient by electrolytes and proteins, which are unable to diffuse through the cellular membrane. This results in a strong osmotic gradient that immediately pulls the water molecules back through the membrane. The bulk of water diffusion occurs primarily through the slitlike pores between the endothelial cells. The width of these slitlike pores is approximately 20 times the size of a water molecule or 60 to 70 Å (6 to 7 nm). The molecular diameter of different substances will effect their permeability through the capillary pores. Plasma protein molecules are slightly larger than the pores, as well as other substances such as sodium and chloride ions which have intermediate diameters.

☐ FLUID TYPES

CRYSTALLOID SOLUTIONS

Maintenance solutions are designed to replace insensible fluid losses including obligatory water losses from the respiratory mucosa, sweat, stool, and urine. The adult loses approximately 1.5 mL/kg/h or 2.5 L/d from these sources. If correcting for only this fluid loss, the use of maintenance solutions would be appropriate. The most common examples of maintenance solutions are 5% dextrose in water and 5% dextrose in half normal saline. However, most clinicians agree the deficit incurred while NPO prior to surgery can be corrected with polyionic, nearly isotonic crystalloid solutions, commonly called replacement fluids. This is due to the composition of 5% dextrose in water not being isotonic and a large bolus of dextrose can cause a rebound hypoglycemia.

Replacement solutions are formulated to correct body fluid deficits caused by loss of nearly isotonic body fluids. Losses may be external, such as gastric drainage, fistula drainage, weeping from raw surfaces, and pleural or ascitic fluid. Loss may also be internal; for example, the acute sequestered edema that occurs as a result of tissue injury from trauma, infections, burns, or a host of other conditions. Because the losses are nearly isotonic, the replacement fluids should be polyionic and nearly isotonic. Multiple types of polyionic, nearly isotonic solutions are available today.

Replacement solutions should be given to replace external and internal losses that occur progressively during the surgical procedure. The amount will depend on the severity of surgical trauma and the duration of the procedure. For this purpose, surgical procedures should be classified according

Table 11–2
GUIDELINES FOR INTRAOPERATIVE CRYSTALLOID THERAPY

Insensible fluid losses	2 mL/kg/h
Surgical Trauma	
Minimal	3–4 mL/kg/h
Moderate	5–6 mL/kg/h
Severe	7–8 mL/kg/h

Replace 1 mL of blood loss with 3 mL of crystalloid solution
Monitor vital signs and maintain urine output (0.5–1 mL/kg/h)

SOURCE: Reproduced by permission from Stoelting RK, Miller RD. *Basics of Anesthesia.* 3rd ed. New York: Churchill Livingstone; 1994:238.

to the severity of surgical trauma as minimal, moderate, or extreme. Table 11–2 lists recommended guidelines for intraoperative crystalloid therapy for both maintenance replacement and surgical trauma, commonly referred to as third-space loss.

A recent study revealed that patients can require up to 10 to 15 mL/kg/h in addition to replacement for blood loss during major surgery (Table 11–3).[3]

COLLOIDS

The role of colloids in fluid management of surgical patients is to help maintain the colloid osmotic pressure and to avoid administering large amounts of crystalloid solutions. The most commonly used colloid solutions in fluid management are 5% albumin and 6% hydroxyethyl starch. Albumin, a naturally occurring plasma protein, provides approximately 80% of the intravascular colloid osmotic pressure in normal subjects.[4] A 5% albumin solution has a colloid osmotic pressure of approximately 20 mg Hg. The albumin molecule, due to its molecular weight of 69,000, is relatively impermeable to the capillary membrane under ordinary circumstances. The

Table 11–3
INTRAOPERATIVE FLUID REQUIREMENTS

1. Basic formula
   a. Deficit: baseline hourly fluid requirement

4 mL/kg/h	1–10 kg
2 mL/kg/h	11–20 kg
1 mL/kg/h	21 up

   b. Maintenance: crystalloid solution such as Ringer's lactate at a rate of 5–15 mL/kg/h
   c. Losses: Ringer's lactate can be used if hematocrit remains above 30% at 3 mL/mL of blood loss.
2. Overall formula (rough estimates) for fluid replacement

10 mL/kg	first hour
7 mL/kg	second hour
5 mL/kg	third hour
3 mL/kg	fourth hour

SOURCE: Reproduced by permission from Jordan LM. Fluid and electrolyte therapy. In: Waugaman WR, Foster SD, Rigor BM eds. *Principles and Practice of Nurse Anesthesia.* East Norwalk, Conn: Appleton & Lange; 1992:296–297.

intravascular half-life of infused albumin is approximately 24 hours and hemodynamic improvement after 5% albumin infusion persists for approximately 24 to 36 hours.[5] Six percent hydroxyethyl starch is a synthetic colloid consisting of a hydroxyethyl-substituted branched chain amylopectin with a number of average molecular weight of 69,000.[6] Particle sizes, however, range from molecular weights of 10,000 to 1 million. The colloid osmotic pressure of 6% hydroxyethyl starch solution is 32 mg Hg.[7] Hydroxyethyl starch is cleared from the body by several different routes. The low molecular weight particles either penetrate the vascular membrane and enter the interstitial space or can be excreted directly in the urine and are cleared quickly.[8] Because of this, it has been suggested hydroxyethyl starch should be avoided in patients with significant renal disease. Larger particles are enzymatically degraded in the liver followed by clearance in urine and stool. The largest particles are phagocytized by the reticuloendothelial system. Approximately 90% of the 6% hydroxyethyl starch dose is eliminated from the body with a half-life of 17 days with the remaining 10% having a half-life of approximately 48 days.[8] In clinical use, infused 6% hydroxyethyl starch continues to expand the plasma volume for 24 to 36 hours, with approximately 40% of the maximum plasma expansion still present at 24 hours.[8] During the acute resuscitative period, 1 L of 6% hydroxyethyl starch or 5% albumin significantly increases the plasma colloid osmotic pressure of patients with hypovolemic shock.[9] Hydroxyethyl starch produced a 36% increase compared to an 11% increase with albumin with 1 L of saline producing a 12% decrease in colloid osmotic pressure. In addition, patients who received the colloid solutions continued to have significant elevations of plasma colloid osmotic pressure for 2 days from the onset of resuscitation in those receiving polyionic, nearly isotonic crystalloid fluids. Patients who received normal saline continued to have lower colloid osmotic pressures compared to baseline values for up to 5 days.

COLLOID VERSUS CRYSTALLOID

The controversy between the use of crystalloid solutions and colloid solutions continues. Elements involved with this controversy include expense, replacement of third-space loss, plasma volume expansion, peripheral edema, pulmonary edema, coagulopathy, and effects on intracranial pressure.

The cost of 1 L of polyionic, nearly isotonic crystalloid solution is approximately 10% of that for 6% hydroxyethyl starch (500 mL) or 4% of that for 5% albumin (250 mL). Major surgical procedures cause tissue trauma, blood loss, and "third spacing" as plasma and blood cellular elements move from the intravascular space. This acute sequestered edema is formed at the expense of healthy interstitial fluid, intracellular fluid, and plasma fluid. Half or more than half of the intravascular albumin can be lost by third spacing.[10] This loss of albumin results in lowered plasma colloid osmotic pressure and hypovolemia. The fluid sequestered in the new edema space is isotonic and should be replaced with polyionic, nearly isotonic crystalloid solutions. In 48 to 72 hours the patient will enter the resolution phase of the healing process and will mobilize the fluid sequestered in the edema space and excrete the excess fluid in the urine. A patient with a significant history of heart disease, specifically congestive heart failure, will require close monitoring to avoid the potential for the development of congestive failure.

Colloids are more effective as plasma expanders than crystalloids. At the end of infusion of 1 L Ringer's lactate, the plasma volume will expand by less than 200 mL.[11] This increase in volume expansion is usually abated after 20 minutes. Infusion of 500 mL albumin results in expansion of the plasma volume by 500 mL or more. The infusion of 500 mL of 6% hydroxyethyl starch expands the plasma volume 500 mL or a 1:1 ratio. Colloids draw approximately 20 mL within the circulatory system per gram of colloid given.[2] The fluid status and disease process of the patient will alter the plasma expansion of both these colloid solutions. In a recent study, Kröll and colleagues investigated the changes in plasma volume following an infusion of 500 mL 6% hydroxyethyl starch versus 500 mL Ringer's lactate.[12] After a 30-minute infusion period of 6% hydroxyethyl starch, the plasma volume increased 702 mL. After 60 minutes, the increase was 815 mL. Ringer's lactate increased the plasma volume 380 mL and 100 mL, respectively. The increment in plasma volume will be gradually reduced as colloid redistributes throughout extracellular volume. In summary, crystalloid solutions are ineffective plasma expanders. As a result of extravascular redistribution, three to four times the volume has to be administered for every volume of whole blood lost, which may place the patient at risk for pulmonary edema. In addition, volume replacement with crystalloid solutions cannot correct the deficiency of oxygen-carrying capacity caused by loss of red cell mass and hemoglobin.

☐ COMPLICATIONS OF FLUID THERAPY

PERIPHERAL EDEMA

Peripheral edema is the presence of excess interstitial fluid in peripheral tissues. As long as interstitial fluid pressure remains negative, edema does not occur. Edema is usually not detectable in tissues until the interstitial fluid volume has risen to 20% to 30% above normal. Increased capillary hydrostatic pressure results in filtration of fluid in excess of reabsorption. Most often, this increase in capillary hydrostatic pressure is due to impaired venous return, as seen in cardiac failure. Another source of peripheral edema is a decrease in plasma concentrations of protein, which lowers the colloid osmotic pressure (the force pulling fluid back into the capillary), resulting in the predominance of capillary hydrostatic pressure. It is estimated that edema begins to appear when the plasma colloid osmotic pressure declines to between 11 and 20 mm Hg.[2,10] Peripheral edema is common during prolonged surgical procedures when a large amount of crystal-

loid is used to maintain urine output. Peripheral edema will be observed before the development of pulmonary edema in patients who do not suffer from chronic or an acute cardiovascular compromise. Peripheral lymph flow can only increase its ability to carry away excess fluid by a factor of three while the lymph flow within the lung has a greater ability to increase its ability to move excess fluid. Peripheral edema may result in problems with healing and infection although others feel it is of cosmetic importance only.[13] Peripheral edema is not associated with colloid administration due to reverse distribution. Eighty percent of the volume of colloid infused remains intravascular while 20% moves to the interstitial space if the integrity of the capillary remains intact.[13] An increase in vascular permeability allows a greater amount of albumin and synthetic colloids to enter the interstitial compartment. This is seen with sepsis, venom poisoning, in some drug overdoses, in anaphylactoid reactions, surgical trauma, and traumatic injuries.[10] It has been recommended that colloid solutions be used during operations involving bowel resection to decrease the risk of anastomotic dehiscence.[14] One consideration is to use both colloid and polyionic, nearly isotonic crystalloid solutions to lessen the formation of peripheral edema.

PLASMA COLLOID OSMOTIC PRESSURE AND PULMONARY EDEMA

The center of controversy about crystalloid versus colloid is pulmonary edema. What causes it? Dissolved proteins of the plasma and sodium ions are primarily responsible for the osmotic pressure that develops at the capillary membrane. Pulmonary artery wedge pressure is normally 6 to 12 mm Hg and is equivalent to pulmonary capillary hydrostatic pressure. Colloid osmotic pressure has a mean average of 28 mm Hg. If the difference between these two pressures approaches 6 mm Hg, the incidence of pulmonary edema increases dramatically.[13] Low colloid osmotic pressure has been implicated as a causative factor in pulmonary edema. Puri and coworkers concluded that infusion of large volumes of crystalloid in patients with low albumin contributed to the persistence of low oncotic pressure and pulmonary edema.[15]

As a result of extravascular redistribution, when using polyionic, nearly isotonic fluid, three to four times the volume has to be administered for every volume of whole blood lost, placing the patient at risk for pulmonary edema. Most investigators agree that neither crystalloid or colloid has specific advantages or disadvantages concerning pulmonary edema. In fact, the lungs remain unaffected by large amounts of fluid and a wide variation in colloid osmotic pressure due to the ability of the lymphatic drainage to increase by as much as 400%.[16] After reviewing the advantages and disadvantages of each, it has been suggested that either crystalloids or colloids may be safely given as resuscitative fluids if appropriate monitoring is performed.[16] Pulmonary edema can also occur when the pulmonary capillary wedge pressure exceeds 25 mm Hg due to overzealous fluid replacement with crystalloid or colloid solutions. Basically, the capillary hydrostatic pressure will exceed the colloid osmotic pressure, thus favoring flow out of the capillary.

Another cause of pulmonary edema is an increase in pulmonary capillary permeability. This can be seen with septic shock, vasoactive agents, and bacterial toxins. *The consequence of pulmonary edema is an increase of the alveolar-arterial gradient due to an increase in distance between the pulmonary capillary endothelium and the alveolar wall.* The rate of diffusion of oxygen between two points is inversely proportional to the distance between the cells (alveolar wall) and capillaries. The end result is a drop in the PaO_2, which ultimately results in a decrease in oxygen availability at the cellular level. Tanaka and colleagues, in their investigation using the dog model, concluded that hetastarch may have a protective effect on alveolar flooding after acute lung injury and low pressure pulmonary edema.[17]

COAGULOPATHY

Hydroxyethyl starch affects coagulation somewhat in a dose-related manner. Most effects of coagulation observed when blood or plasma were mixed with 6% hydroxyethyl starch in vitro were trivial and simply reflected as dilution.[18] In vivo, hydroxyethyl starch alters coagulation in a dose-related fashion by three main mechanisms. First, hydroxyethyl starch causes the conversion of fibrinogen to fibrin to be accelerated resulting in a less stable thrombus consequently more prone to lysis. Second, an acquired von Willebrand's syndrome may develop, with reduced levels of factor VIII activity. Third, hydroxyethyl starch macromolecules coat the platelets, thus decreasing the adhesiveness of platelets and resulting in prolonged bleeding times. Moderate doses of 6% hydroxyethyl starch (20 mL/kg) exert minor effects on coagulation.[19] Platelet count is unchanged or temporarily decreased but remains in excess of levels required for normal hemostasis.[19] Bleeding time remains normal. The coagulation cascade also remains normal or shows mild to moderate increases in prothrombin time (PT) and partial thromboplastin time (PTT) and decreased fibrinogen.[19] As the dose of hydroxyethyl starch increases, factor VIII coagulant activity decreases. The exact mechanism by which hydroxyethyl starch reduces factor VIII activity remains unknown.[19] It does not appear to be due to dilution because other clotting factors diluted to the same degree do not show the same decrease in activity.[20] Massive doses of 6% hydroxyethyl starch (> 30 mL/kg) are associated with decreased platelet count, decreased platelet adhesion, and decreased concentration of clotting proteins.[16] Gold and coworkers concluded hydroxyethyl starch at 1 g/kg or less is safe to use as a volume expander in patients undergoing abdominal aortic aneurysm repair.[19]

EFFECTS ON INTRACRANIAL PRESSURE

Colloid solutions were traditionally used in neurosurgery because of the concern that reductions in colloid osmotic pressure will cause brain edema.[21] The question of whether the patient for intracranial procedures should receive crystalloids or colloids has not been settled. The goal of fluid therapy for intracranial procedures is the maintenance of normal cerebral perfusion pressure and for the patient undergoing an intracranial procedure is to remain isovolemic, iso-osmotic, and iso-oncotic.[22]

The key determinant of water movement across the blood–brain barrier is plasma osmolality, rather than colloid osmotic (oncotic) pressure. This is due to the differences in the permeability of the cerebral capillaries versus peripheral capillaries. The pores of the endothelial layer of the capillary are much smaller in the cerebral capillaries, approximately 8 Å in diameter. In fact, the blood–brain barrier has been defined as a series of tight junctions between capillary endothelial cells that are impermeable to most ions (relatively impermeable to sodium ions) and to the larger molecules of colloid solutions.[23]

Another factor concerning the effects on intracranial pressure is the interstitial compliance in the brain. In the periphery, the interstitial pressure is low and compliance is very high. As a result, there are few impediments to the movement of fluid into that space and it is hence easy for edema to form. By contrast, the brain interstitium is made up of a tightly interwoven matrix of glial cells and neurons that are noncompliant. This acts to limit fluid influx.[24] Furthermore, any increase in intracranial volume will increase intracranial pressure, thus impeding movement of fluid even more. Both of these factors inhibit the formation of cerebral edema unless the forces driving fluid out of the vasculature are very large. One of the reasons for edema to form in the brain following a craniotomy is the increase in compliance due to decompression of the intracranial space. In summary, the colloid osmotic pressure is not the predominant factor in movement of water in the brain, but the total osmolality of the intravascular fluid.

Albumin binds about 90% of the protein-bound fraction of calcium. Total serum calcium consequently depends on albumin levels. In general, an increase or decrease in albumin of 1 g/dL is associated with a parallel change in total serum calcium of 0.8 mg/dL. The concentration of free calcium ions is of critical importance in regulating skeletal muscle contraction, coagulation, neurotransmitter release, endocrine secretion, and a variety of other cellular functions.[24] Carlson and colleagues investigated the effect of infusing albumin and the effect on ionized calcium.[25] The conclusion of this investigation revealed that albumin infusion in patients does not lower ionized calcium or adversely affect hemodynamics.

ALLERGIC REACTIONS

There are no reports of allergic reactions to crystalloid solutions. Allergic reactions to albumin are rare, less than 0.011%.[26] Transmission of hepatitis B virus by albumin is also rare and only occurs secondary to accidents in its preparation.[2] The incidence of anaphylactoid reactions to hydroxyethyl starch has previously been reported as 0.085% in a large (16,405 infusions) prospective clinical study.[26] This incidence of allergic reactions was not statistically different from albumin. Cullen and Singer, in England, reported on a severe anaphylactoid reaction to hydroxyethyl starch in 1990.[27] Kreimeier and associates recently reported a case of anaphylaxis due to hydroxyethyl starch reactive antibodies.[28]

FLUID RESUSCITATION

Hypovolemic (hemorrhagic) shock is a clinical state in which tissue perfusion is rendered relatively inadequate by loss of blood or plasma after injury to the vascular tree.[29] The primary objective in the management of hypovolemic shock is maintenance of tissue oxygenation with restoration to normal values.

Assessment of the adequacy of intravascular volume begins with palpation of a peripheral pulse. The pulse should be assessed for rate, rhythm, and character. Systolic blood pressure can be estimated via determination of the presence of palpable pulses. If a radial pulse is palpable, a minimal systolic blood pressure of 80 mm Hg is present; 70 mm Hg if a palpable femoral pulse is present; and 60 mm Hg if a carotid pulse is palpable. Simultaneously the general skin condition and mental status should be assessed. The seriously volume-depleted trauma patient will have cool, moist, pallid, or cyanotic skin, especially at the extremities. If the blood volume is at least 70% to 80% of normal, external jugular veins can be appreciated. A confusing clinical picture may arise in the setting of cardiac tamponade or tension pneumothorax, which of themselves may lead to venous distention.

Initial fluid resuscitation is usually followed by definitive treatment (including surgery). If the patient has lost more than 750 mL blood, clinical presentation will assist in the decision to replace with crystalloid or colloid or blood.[30] The site of hemorrhage should be considered carefully when cannulation is undertaken. If significant injury has occurred in the pelvis or lower abdomen, cannulation of the femoral vein should be avoided. If the patient has suffered significant penetrating chest trauma, a peripheral IV access in the arm or cannulation of the internal or external jugular may need to be reconsidered. All fluids should be infused through fluid warmers. A decrease in resuscitation time plus an increase in unexpected survival has followed rapid infusion of normothermic fluids.[31]

ROLE OF CRYSTALLOID AND COLLOID DURING RESUSCITATION

The quantity of the fluid chosen is based on the severity of hemorrhage, surgical trauma, and the duration of the procedure. The fluid loss incurred with a mild class I blood loss of less than 750 mL or 15% of the blood volume can usually be replaced with polyionic, nearly isotonic solutions.[30]

The role of colloids in fluid management of trauma patients, exclusive of replacing blood loss, is to help maintain the colloid osmotic pressure, circulating blood volume, and perfusion of the microcirculation. Funk and Baldinger found that volume replacement with artificial colloids yielded he-

modynamic stability and adequate tissue oxygen supply in the hamster model, whereas administration of crystalloids alone jeopardized tissue perfusion and oxygenation.[32] Lowell and colleagues found that patients who were resuscitated with albumin, blood, or hypertonic crystalloid solutions had less weight gain, less intrapulmonary shunting, and better tissue oxygenation than patients treated with less concentrated crystalloids.[33]

When significant blood loss occurs, the initial fluid replacement should be aimed at restoring blood volume and extra- and intracellular loss. Crystalloid or colloid can be used for urgent volume expansion. Which fluid to administer—colloid or crystalloid—is one of the long-standing debates of modern medicine. Proponents of the use of colloids contend that, because the deficit occurs initially in the vascular space, a colloid solution that remains in the vascular space should be given. Proponents of colloids also point out that large-volume infusion of crystalloid will result in a decrease of colloid osmotic pressure, potentially increasing the risk of systemic, cerebral, and pulmonary edema. Crystalloid proponents contend traumatic injuries, burns, infections, and many surgical conditions lead to a transfer of healthy or functional extracellular fluid into a "third space," creating deficits in many spaces, including the vascular space.

To estimate the effects of fluid infusion on plasma volume (PV) the following formula has been used:[34]

$$PV\ increment = volume\ infused \times PV \div distribution\ volume$$

Example: A traumatized, 70-kg patient has suffered an acute blood loss of 2 L, or 40% of blood volume. To replace loss blood volume, i.e., expand the PV by 2 L, using 5% D_5W, which distributes throughout total body water, would require an infusion of 28 L.

2 L = volume infused $\times$ 3 L $\div$ 42 L	3 L = PV
= 42 L $\times$ 2 L	42 L = Total Body
3 L = 28 L volume to be infused	Water

If lactated Ringer's solution, which distributes only throughout the extracellular volume, were chosen, a 2-L PV increment would require infusion of approximately 9.33 L.

2 L = volume infused $\times$ 3 L $\div$ 14	3 L = PV
= 14 L $\times$ 2 L	14 L = Extracellular
3 L = 9.33 L volume to be infused	Volume

Excerpted from Prough DS, Perioperative fluid management: crystalloid, colloid and hypertonic solutions. ASA Refresher Course Lectures, #261, October 1991. A copy of the full text can be obtained from ASA, 520 N. Northwest Highway, Park Ridge, IL 60068-2573.

FLUID RESUSCITATION AND INTRACRANIAL PRESSURE

Although laboratory investigations have difficulty demonstrating superiority of colloid over crystalloid after cerebral trauma, many clinicians feel cerebral edema is more severe after crystalloid resuscitation. Others suggest that the use of crystalloid or colloid does not matter. The goals of fluid resuscitation in a patient with cerebral trauma include preservation of an iso-osmotic and iso-oncotic state, fluid replacement to normovolemia, and maintenance of normal cerebral perfusion pressure.[21,35] Overzealous therapy with either colloids or crystalloids will ultimately give rise to the formation of edema. Glucose-containing solutions are contraindicated because an elevated blood glucose has been demonstrated to worsen cerebral ischemic injury.[36] Hypertonic crystalloid solutions may be beneficial in the future.[36] Czinn, Salem, and Crystal investigated the influence of isovolemic hemodilution on vasoconstriction responses in the brain and spinal cord during hypocapnia in dogs.[37] In the control group, the hematocrit was maintained at 42% and in the isovolemic hemodilution group, the hematocrit was lowered to 19% with 5% dextran 40. Hypocapnia (22 $\pm$ 1 mm Hg) was induced in both groups. Hemodilution either attenuated or completely abolished vasoconstrictor responses within the brain and spinal cord. These findings suggested that induced hypocapnia may be less effective as a clinical maneuver to reduce increased intracranial pressure during hemodilution.

HYPEROSMOTIC RESUSCITATION SOLUTIONS

Studies have demonstrated hyperosmotic saline solutions effectively restore hemodynamics, even when infused in volumes much smaller than the original shed blood volume.[38,39] Recent data suggest the primary mechanism by which hyperosmotic saline increases venous return is by plasma volume expansion, potentially via loss of the intracellular fluid compartment.[40,41] The term "small-volume resuscitation" has been used to describe an intravenous bolus infusion of 4 mL of hypertonic saline per kilogram of body weight.[42] Halvorsen suggested 7.5% NaCl/12% dextran 70 was the optimal hypertonic/hyperosmotic solution and could be safely administered as a 4 mL/kg bolus.[43] Investigations have revealed restoration of cardiac filling pressures and cardiac output plus an increase in systemic pressure following "small-volume resuscitation" although some feel it is short-lived.[41,42,44] Krausz reported that to date no significant improvement in mortality has been demonstrated by either hypertonic saline or when hypertonic saline is combined with dextran.[45] It has been observed that hypertonic saline treatment of controlled hemorrhagic shock resulted in an increase in both blood pressure and cardiac output, whereas hypertonic saline treatment of uncontrolled hemorrhagic shock led to increased bleeding from injured blood vessels, hemodynamic deterioration, and increased mortality.[45,46] The etiology of the increase in bleeding was felt to be due to vasodilatation and this has been reported if hypertonic fluid is administered within 15 minutes of injury.[47]

Hyperosmotic saline solutions have been used in the resuscitation of burn patients. Recent studies have questioned the actual advantage of these fluids compared to conventional crystalloid solutions.[48]

Resuscitation of the patient with the combination severe closed head injury and hypovolemic shock remains controversial.[49–57] In situations where there is mechanical injury to the brain, brain edema will occur irregardless of the fluid used. Potential complications following the use of hypertonic saline include hypernatremia, hyperchloremia, hyperosmolarity, hypokalemia, metabolic acidosis, intracellular dehydration, cerebral hemorrhage, inhibition of lipolysis, hyperosmolar coma, and central pontine myelinolysis.[55–57]

☐ BLOOD REPLACEMENT

COMPATIBILITY

When time is available, complete compatibility testing will avoid an antigen–antibody reaction in the recipient. Blood from both the donor and recipient blood is typed in the red cell surface ABO and Rh systems plus the sample is screened for antibodies to other cell antigens. Red cells have either A, B, AB, or no surface antigens. If the A or B surface antigen is missing on the red cells within the patient's sample, then antibodies will be produced against it. Type B blood will have anti-A antibodies. A patient who is type O, which means there is neither A nor B surface antigens present, will have anti-A and anti-B antibodies present. A person with type AB does not have antibodies to either type A or type B and can receive blood from any blood type. The universal red cell donor is type O because neither A nor B surface antigens are present. Another test evaluating blood compatibility is for the presence of a Rh surface antigen. Eighty-five percent of patients are Rh positive.[58]

MINIMAL ACCEPTABLE HEMOGLOBIN

How low should a patient's hemoglobin be allowed to drop before administering blood? Healthy Jehovah's Witnesses have tolerated hemoglobins in the 3 g/dL range.[59] The physiologic rationale for blood transfusion is the lowered oxygen-carrying capacity that accompanies a decreased hematocrit versus resistance to flow of the less viscous blood. The ideal hematocrit of the traumatized patient remains controversial. It has been recommended in patients without ischemic heart disease, the minimal acceptable hematocrit is 20% to 25%.[60,61] The heart has been considered the organ determining the limit at which anemia is tolerated. Initially, stroke volume compensates with hematocrits down to about 20%, then at lower hematocrits the heart rate begins to increase.[61] If there is concern for risk factors of cardiac disease or the myocardium is suspected of being impaired due to hypoperfusion or blunt trauma, a minimal hematocrit of 30% would be indicated.[60,61] Another component on "when to transfuse" is the total body oxygen consumption and oxygen delivery. A 70-kg man at rest has a total body oxygen consumption of 250 mL and an oxygen delivery of 1000 mL/m for an oxygen extraction of 25%. An oxygen extraction ratio of greater than

Table 11-4
CALCULATION FOR ALLOWABLE BLOOD LOSS

Patient is a 75-kg man with a hematocrit of 42% and an estimated blood volume of 70 mL/kg.

Estimated Blood Volume (EBV)	= wt (in kg) × blood volume (per kg) = 75 × 70 = 5250 mL blood volume
Estimated Red Cell Mass (ERCM)	= EBV × hematocrit = 5250 × 0.42 = 2205 mL
Estimated Red Cell Mass Desired (ERCMd)	= EBV × Desired hematocrit = 5250 × .25 = 1312 mL
Allowable Red Cell Loss (ARCL)	= ERCM − ERCMd = 2205 − 1312 = 893 mL
Allowable Blood Loss (ABL)	= 2 × ARCL = 2 × 893 = 1786 mL

Table 11-5
CHANGES THAT OCCUR DURING STORAGE OF WHOLE BLOOD IN CITRATE-PHOSPHATE DEXTROSE

	Days of Storage at 4°C			
	1	7	14	21
pH	7.1	7.0	7.0	6.9
PCO_2 (mmHg)	48	80	110	140
Potassium (mEq/L^{-1})	3.9	12	17	21
2, 3Diphosphoglycerate ($\mu M/m1^{-1}$)	4.8	1.2	1	1
Viable platelets (%)	10	0	0	0
Factors V and VIII (%)	70	50	40	20

SOURCE: Reproduced by permission from Fluid and Blood Therapy in Stoelting RK, Miller RD: *Basics of Anesthesia*, 3rd ed. New York: Churchill Livingstone, 1994;240.

50% to 60% is an indication for transfusion to increase oxygen-carrying capacity.[62] One commonly used formula to calculate allowable blood loss is contained within Table 11-4.

Whole blood is the ideal replacement in patients with major hemorrhage. Limitations of supply may dictate that concentrated red cells are used and diluted to normal values of packed cell volume by concurrent transfusion of either normal saline, Ringer's lactate, or hydroxyethyl starch. Dilution of packed red blood cells with crystalloid solutions will not speed the infusion time of the red cells themselves.[63] Dilution is indicated in patients needing both an increase in intravascular volume and red cells. The use of calcium-containing solutions is not contraindicated. Ringer's lactate solution causes little clot formation when less than a 1 : 1 ratio is used during rapid infusion. There is no evidence the clot formation occurring with Ringer's lactate causes any pathophysiologic sequelae during or after blood transfusion.[64,65]

Trauma centers should retain a small number of relatively fresh units of O negative blood for immediate transfusion in cases of severe, life-threatening hemorrhage. Once the patient receives more than 2 units of type O uncrossmatched whole blood, he or she should continue to receive type O through the resuscitative period.[66] If the patient is switched to crossmatched, type-specific blood hemolysis could occur due to the mixing of type-specific donor blood with the blood previously transfused with anti-A and anti-B antibodies. Blood transfused rapidly should be warmed before infusion to maximize flow rates and to minimize the risk of cardiac dysrhythmias and core hypothermia. The use of microaggregate blood filters is probably only beneficial in those patients with a history of febrile reactions.[66]

COMPONENT THERAPY

Even though relatively fresh whole blood is the ideal replacement for lost blood during a surgical procedure, blood component therapy has evolved into the accepted technique. The three most frequently used blood components acquired from a unit of whole blood consists of packed red blood cells, fresh-frozen plasma, and platelets. The most common component of blood therapy is packed red cells. Packed red cells have a hematocrit of between 70% and 80%. A unit of packed red blood cells contains approximately 190 to 390 mL, with 155 to 270 mL consisting of erythrocytes. *One unit of packed red blood cells is felt to raise the hemoglobin in a 70-kg man 1 g or the hematocrit by 3%.* Citrate-phosphate-dextrose-adenine (CPDA)-1 packed red blood cells have a shelf life of 35 days when stored at 4°C (Table 11-5).

AUTOLOGOUS REPLACEMENT

Autologous blood transfusion is, in principle, a safe and effective method for avoiding exposure to allogeneic blood in appropriate circumstances. Both blood ordering and blood procurement practices in autologous blood donation programs are important factors in blood conservation efforts to minimize allogeneic blood exposure.[67] Patients should be screened before preoperative donation for anemia, ischemic heart disease, cerebral vascular disease, recent seizures, cardiac dysrhythmia, chronic heart failure, valvular or congenital heart disease, symptomatic dyspnea, insulin-dependent diabetes, and or current therapy with two or more antihypertensive medications.[68] If proper precautions are taken, the patients at high risk with some preexisting medical conditions can safely donate autologous blood as well as blood for homologous transfusion. The most common cause for incomplete autologous blood collection is late referral or anemia.[69] Although autologous transfusion decreases the incidence of postoperative infections and other complications, the question of cost effectiveness of this therapy has not been fully answered.[70,71]

Perioperative autotransfusion of shed blood also decreases the incidence of homologous transfusion. The amount of autologous blood reinfused during perioperative autotransfusion ranges from 4.65 U during cardiac surgery to 1.05 U in orthopedic surgery.[72] An investigation by Clugston and colleagues found that in reduction mammoplasty procedures, autologous blood did not make a difference.[73] Postoperative hemoglobin values were actually lower in the autologous group, even in patients who received their blood during surgery or during the immediate postoperative period. In patients with severe thoracic or abdominal injuries "clean" blood may be aspirated from the cavity, anticoagulated, and returned to the patient through an IV cannula using a "cell-saver" system. Autologous blood or intraoperative salvage and reinfusion is valuable in patients with major vascular injuries of the thorax and abdomen and in those with a ruptured liver or spleen. This source of blood cannot be used in patients with abdominal trauma who have a ruptured bowel or in those with thoracic trauma who have esophageal or lung damage. In addition, this blood does not contain functioning platelets or coagulation factors due to the washing of the shed blood prior to reinfusion.[61,74] The reinfusion of salvaged blood has several advantages which include red cells with normal 2,3-diphosphoglycerate levels, pH, and potassium levels plus the blood is normothermic.[75]

COAGULOPATHY AND BLOOD TRANSFUSIONS

Coagulation problems can occur in patients with massive blood loss because of the dilutional effects of blood and blood substitutes. The main cause of nonsurgically remediable hemorrhage can be traced to massive blood transfusions of greater than 1.5 times the blood volume and the fact that coagulation factors deteriorate rapidly in stored blood (within 24 to 48 hours).[76,77] Moreover, tissue destruction releases various products that inhibit the normal coagulation process. The clotting process should be monitored by regular screening and deficiencies treated definitively rather than by infusion of fresh-frozen plasma and platelets on an arbitrary basis.

Fresh-frozen plasma is prepared from fresh blood and frozen within 6 hours. To maintain the labile plasma coagulation factors, fresh-frozen plasma is stored at $-18°C$ or lower. Fresh-frozen plasma is indicated when multiple coagulation deficiencies have occurred. Specifically, fresh-frozen plasma contains factor V, factor VIII, and fibrinogen. If it is impractical to measure laboratory results due to the rapidity of blood loss, the administration of 1 U fresh-frozen plasma per 10 U blood is felt to be acceptable.[78] If the patient is known to have a factor deficiency, for example from warfarin therapy, liver disease, disseminated intravascular coagulation, or following major trauma, the threshold for transfusion of fresh-frozen plasma should be lowered. Fresh-frozen plasma should be infused within 30 minutes following thawing. Volume expansion and nutritional support are not indications to transfuse fresh-frozen plasma.

Platelets are necessary for normal bleeding times and can be administered as a component of blood therapy. If the platelet count is above 100,000/mm³, hemostasis is usually adequate. A platelet count less than 50,000 to 75,000/mm³ may indicate platelet function is compromised and this low count is considered minimally acceptable for surgery.[76] If allowed to decrease to 10,000/mm³ the likelihood of spontaneous bleeding is increased. If platelet dysfunction is suspected, a bleeding time is indicated. It should be less than 10 minutes. The addition of 1 U of platelets will raise the platelet count by 5000 to 10,000 mm³.[76,79] If platelets are infused within 24 hours of being drawn, they are viable in the blood for as long as 8 days.[79] Random donor platelet concentrate can be stored for 72 hours at room temperature and 48 hours at 4°C.[80] A standard 170-μm blood filter set should be used when administering platelets.

COMPLICATIONS OF BLOOD TRANSFUSIONS

Multiple potential complications are related to blood transfusion therapy. They may be due to incompatibility, allergy or, rarely, bacterial contamination of the blood product. Among the more serious complications of such therapy are hepatitis and acquired immunodeficiency syndrome. As the number of transfused units increases, other complications (Table 11–6) that can arise include development of metabolic acidosis due to the lowered pH of the anticoagulant preservative in the bank blood, hypo- or hyperkalemia, hypothermia, low levels of plasma proteins, decreased ionized magnesium and ionized calcium.[81] Agarwal and colleagues reported the infec-

Table 11–6
COMPLICATIONS OF BLOOD THERAPY

Transfusion reactions
  Febrile
  Allergic
  Hemolytic
Metabolic abnormalities
  Acidosis
  Accumulation of potassium
  Decreased 2, 3-disphosphoglycerate
Citrate intoxication
  Alkalosis
  Hypocalcemia
Transmission of viral diseases
Microaggregates
Hypothermia
Coagulation disorders
  Dilutional thrombocytopenia
  Dilution of factors V and VIII
  Disseminated intravascular coagulation
Immunosuppression

SOURCE: Reproduced by permission from Fluid and Blood Therapy in Stoelting RK, Miller RD: *Basics of Anesthesia*, 3rd ed. New York: Churchill Livingstone, 1994;241.

tion rate was elevated significantly as the number of units of blood transfused increased.[82] The best prevention of any type reaction to blood transfusion is to administer blood products only when necessary and giving attention to eliminating clerical errors, which are responsible for many hemolytic reactions.[83] In addition to the use of autologous blood, intraoperative hemodilution, hypotensive anesthetic techniques, and postoperative blood salvage decrease the need for allogeneic blood.

☐ MONITORING VOLUME REPLACEMENT

No individual parameter best indicates the adequacy of intravascular fluid volume replacement. Urine output is the most commonly used monitor and minimal urine output is 0.5 mL/kg/h. If the urine output is over 100 mL/h, the patient is probably receiving too much fluid. The use of urinary output and vital signs to guide initial burn resuscitation may lead to suboptimal resuscitation. Invasive cardiorespiratory monitoring may be necessary to optimize resuscitation of seriously burned patients.[84] Additional methods to determine the adequacy of fluid therapy in addition to urine output are arterial blood gases (specifically looking at the base deficit or metabolic acidosis), tachycardia, and the occurrence of large fluctuations in blood pressure during positive-pressure ventilation.

Metabolic acidosis signifies hypoperfusion in the periphery leading to anaerobic metabolism and the production of lactic acid. The base deficit can be used as an indicator of the severity of the shock state and the efficacy of resuscitation when invasive monitoring is impractical or not available. Studies in the animal model have demonstrated that the base deficit was more reflective of the true volume deficit during compensated shock than other physiologic variables.[85] Resolution of acute metabolic acidosis implies that perfusion has been substantially improved. If the patient is adequately anesthetized, hemoglobin levels are within normal limits, and malignant hyperthermia is not suspected, hypovolemia is usually the cause of tachycardia. Large fluctuations in the blood pressure during positive-pressure ventilation are easily observed during hypovolemia if an arterial line is in place. Hypovolemia causes the width of the arterial waveform to narrow and the dicrotic notch will begin to descend down the anacrotic limb of the arterial wave form. Other monitors used to assess fluid therapy are pulmonary artery catheters and mixed venous oxygen monitoring.

Clinical parameters commonly used in monitoring volume replacement during resuscitation include character and frequency of pulse rate, arterial pressure, central venous pressure, and urine flow rates. Volume replacement should be continued until an adequate arterial pressure and urine flow is established. In using central venous pressure values, a sustained increase of more than 3 cm H_2O in response to a rapid infusion of 200 mL indicates that hypovolemia is being corrected. Failure to maintain the improved values indicates continuing loss and requires further transfusion and possibly early surgery. If the patient does not respond satisfactorily to rapid volume replacement, the rate of loss is exceeding the fastest possible rate of intravenous replacement. This is usually associated with major thoracic, abdominal, or pelvic injuries. In such instances the patient must be taken to the operating room for immediate thoracotomy or laparotomy and bleeding controlled with clamps or packs, or both, to allow time for rapid volume replacement.

☐ CONCLUSION

The intent of this chapter is not to empirically state which solution is better. However, by reviewing the physiologic basis of fluid management and looking at specific advantages or disadvantages of each solution, the anesthesia provider will be able to use the appropriate solution in the appropriate manner at the appropriate time. Today the question is not whether the anesthesia provider prefers either crystalloid or colloid or blood component therapy, but what is the appropriate combination to facilitate optimal hemostasis care for the anesthetized patient.

REFERENCES

1. Guyton AC. The microcirculation and the lymphatic system: capillary fluid exchange, interstitial fluid and lymph flow. In: Guyton AC, ed. *Textbook of Medical Physiology,* 8th ed. Philadelphia: WB Saunders;1991:172–179.
2. Stoelting RK, Miller RD. *Basics of Anesthesia,* 3rd ed. New York: Churchill Livingstone;1994;238.
3. Campbell IT. I.V. fluids during surgery. *Br J Anaesth.* 1990;65:726–729.
4. Tullis JL. Albumin. *JAMA.* 1977;237:(4)355–360
5. Rothschild MA, Bauman A, Yalow RS, et al. Tissue distribution of I^{131}-labeled human serum albumin following intravenous administration. *J Clin Invest.* 1955;34:1354–1357.
6. Metcalf W, Papadopoulous A, Tufaro R, et al. A clinical physiologic study of hydroxethyl starch. *Surg Gynecol Obstet.* 1970; 131:255–267.
7. Haupt MT, Rackow EC. Colloid osmotic pressure and fluid resuscitation with hetastarch, albumin, and saline solutions. *Crit Care Med.* 1982;10:159–162.
8. Rackow EC, Falk JL, Fein IA, et al. Fluid resuscitation in circulatory shock: a comparison of the cardiorespiratory effects of albumin, hetastarch, and saline solutions in patients with hypovolemic and septic shock. *Crit Care Med.* 1983;11:839–850.
9. Haupt MT, Rackow EC. Colloid osmotic pressure and fluid resuscitation with hetastarch, albumin, and saline solutions. *Crit Care Med.* 1982;10:159–162.
10. Haynes GR. Colloid osmotic pressure as a guide for the anes-

thesiologist in directing fluid therapy. *South Med J.* 1989;82:618–623.

11. Shoemaker WC. Comparison of the relative effectiveness of whole blood transfusions and various types of fluid therapy in resuscitation. *Crit Care Med.* 1976;4:71–78.

12. Kröll W, Gerner P, Colombo T, et al. Einfluss von 6% HES 200/0.6 auf plamavolumen und blutgerinnung. *Infusionstherapie.* 1992;19:171–180.

13. Davies MJ. Crystalloid or colloid: does it matter? *J Clin Anesth.* 1989;1:464–471.

14. Prien T. Effect of intraoperative fluid administration and colloid osmotic pressure on the formation of intestinal edema during gastrointestinal surgery. *J Clin Anesth.* 1990;2:317–323.

15. Puri VK, Weil MH, Michaels S, Carlson RW. Pulmonary edema associated with reduction in plasma oncotic pressure. *Surg Gynecol Obstet.* 1980;151:344–348.

16. Funk W, Baldinger V. Microcirculatory perfusion during volume therapy. *Anesthesiology.* 1995;82:975–982.

17. Tanaka H, Dahms TE, Bell E, et al. Effect of hydroxyethyl starch on alveolar flooding in acute lung injury in dogs. *Am Rev Respir Dis.* 1993;148:852–859.

18. Strauss RG. Review of the effects of hydroxyethyl starch on the blood coagulation system. *Transfusion.* 1981;21:299–302.

19. Gold MS, Russo J, Tissot M, et al. Comparison of hetastarch to albumin for perioperative bleeding in patients undergoing abdominal aortic aneurysm surgery. *Ann Surg.* 1990;211:482–485.

20. Sanfelippo MJ, Suberviola PD, Geimer NF. Development of a von Willebrand-like syndrome after prolonged use of hydroxyethyl starch. *Am J Clin Pathol.* 1987;88:653–655.

21. Domino KB. Fluid management for the neurosurgical patient. *ASA Refresher Course Lectures #246.* Park Ridge, Ill: American Society of Anesthesiologists;1989.

22. Craen RA, Gelb AW. The anaesthetic management of neurosurgical emergencies. *Can J Anaesth.* 1992;39(pt II):R29–R34.

23. Todd M. Fluid therapy for the patient with brain injury. *ASA Refresher Course Lectures #422.* Park Ridge, Ill: American Society of Anesthesiologists;1990.

24. Graf G, Rosenbaum S. Anesthesia and the endocrine system. In: Barash PG, Cullen BF, Stoelting RK, eds. *Clinical Anesthesia.* 2nd ed. Philadelphia: JB Lippincott;1992:1243.

25. Carlson RW, Rattan S, Haupt MT. Fluid resuscitation in conditions of increased permeability. *Anesth Rev.* 1990;17:14–24.

26. Ring J, Messmer K. Incidence and severity of anaphylactoid reactions to colloid volume substitutes. *Lancet.* 1977;328:466–469.

27. Cullen MJ, Singer M. Severe anaphylactoid reaction to hydroxyethyl starch. *Anaesthesia.* 1990;45:1041–1042.

28. Kreimeier U, Christ F, Kraft D, et al. Anaphylaxis due to hydroxyethyl-starch-reactive antibodies. *Lancet.* 1995;346:49–50.

29. Guyton AC. Circulatory shock and physiology of treatment. In: Guyton AC, ed. *Textbook of Medical Physiology.* 8th ed. Philadelphia: WB Saunders, 1991:263–271.

30. Baskett JF. Management of Hypovolemic Shock. *Br J Med.* 1990;300:1453–1457.

31. Buchman TG, Menker JB, Lipsett PA. Strategies for trauma resuscitation. *Surg Gynecol Obstet.* 1991;172:8–12.

32. Funk W, Baldinger V. Microcirculatory perfusion during volume therapy. *Anesthesiology.* 1995;82:975–982.

33. Lowell JA, Schifferdecker C, Driscoll DF, et al. Postoperative fluid overload: not a benign problem. *Crit Care Med.* 1992;18:728–733.

34. Prough DS. Perioperative fluid management: crystalloid, colloid and hypertonic solutions. *ASA Refresher Course Lectures #261.* Park Ridge, Ill: American Society of Anesthesiologists;1991.

35. Frost EAM. Anesthesia for neurosurgical emergencies: central nervous system trauma. *Anesth Rev.* 1991;18:21–26.

36. Drummon JC. Changing practices in neuroanesthesia. *Can J Anaesth.* 1990;37(pt II):39–51.

37. Czinn EA, Salem R, Crystal GJ. Hemodilution impairs hypocapnia-induced vasoconstrictor responses in the brain and spinal cord in dogs. *Anesth Analg.* 1995;80:492–498.

38. Velasco IT, Pontier V, Rocha E, et al: Hyperosmotic NaCl and severe hemorrhagic shock. *Am J Physiol.* 1980;239:H664–H673.

39. Pascual JM, Watson JC, Runyon AE, et al. Resuscitation of intraoperative hypovolemia: a comparison of normal saline and hyperosmotic/hyperoncotic solutions in swine. *Crit Care Med.* 1992;20:200–210.

40. Schertel ER. Influence of 7% NaCl on the mechanical properties of the systemic circulation in the hypovolemic dog. *Circ Shock* 1990;31:203–214.

41. Ratner LE, Smith GW: Intraoperative fluid management. *Surg Clin North Am.* 1993; 3:229–241.

42. Kreimeier U, Messmer K. Use of hypertonic NaCl solutions in primary volume therapy. *Zentralbl Chir.* 1992;117:532–539.

43. Halvorsen L, Gunther RA, Dubick MA, et al. Dose response characteristics of hypertonic saline dextran solutions. *J Trauma.* 1991;31:785–794.

44. Prough DS, Whitley JM, Taylor CL, et al. Small-volume resuscitation from hemorrhagic shock in dogs: effects on systemic hemodynamics and systemic blood flow. *Crit Care Med.* 1991;19:364–372.

45. Krausz MM. Controversies in shock research: hypertonic resuscitation—pros and cons. *Shock* 1995;3:69–72.

46. Gross D, Landau EH, Klin B, et al: Treatment of uncontrolled hemorrhagic shock with hypertonic saline solution. *Surg Gynecol Obstet.* 1990;170:106–112.

47. Krausz MM, Landau EH, Lin B, et al. Hypertonic saline treatment of uncontrolled hemorrhagic shock at different periods from bleeding. *Arch Surg* 1992;127:93–96.

48. Huang PP, Stucky FS, Dimick AR, et al. Hypertonic sodium resuscitation is associated with renal failure and death. *Ann Surg.* 1995;221:543–554.

49. Feldman JA, Fish S. Resuscitation fluid for a patient with head injury and hypovolemic shock. *J Emerg Med* 1991;9:465–468.

50. Schmoker JD, Zhuang J, Shackford SR. Hypertonic fluid resuscitation improves cerebral oxygen delivery and reduces intracranial pressure after hemorrhagic shock. *J Trauma.* 1991;31:1607–1613.

51. Battistella FD, Wisner DH. Combined hemorrhagic shock and head injury: effects of hypertonic saline 7.5% resuscitation. *J Trauma* 1991;31:182–188.

52. Whitley JM. Rebound intracranial hypertension following resuscitation with hypertonic saline from hemorrhagic shock accompanied by an intracranial mass lesion. *Anesthesiology* 1991;75:319–327.

53. Wisner DK, Schuster L, Quinn C. Hypertonic saline resuscitation of head injury: effects on cerebral water content. *J Trauma* 1990;30:75–78.

54. Vassar MJ, Perry CA, Gannaway WI, et al. 7.5% sodium chloride/dextran for resuscitation of trauma patients undergoing helicopter transport. *Arch Surg* 1991;126:1065–1072.

55. Carvajal HF, Parks DK. Optimal composition of burn resuscitation fluids. *Crit Care Med.* 1988;16:695–700.

56. Cross JS, Briber DP, Burchard KW, et al. Hypertonic saline fluid therapy following surgery: a prospective study. *J Trauma.* 1989;29:817–826.

57. Griffel MI, Kaufman BS. Pharmacology of colloids and crystalloids. *Crit Care Clin.* 1992;8:235–253.

58. Jordan LM. Fluid and electrolyte therapy. In: Waugaman WR, Foster SD, Rigor BM, eds. *Principles and Practice of Nurse Anesthesia.* East Norwalk, Conn: Appleton & Lange; 1992:301.

59. Wong DHW, Jenkins LC. Surgery in Jehovah's Witnesses. *Can J Anaesth.* 1989;36:578–585.

60. Bainton C. Anaesthesia for trauma and emergencies. In: Healy

TE, Cohen PJ, eds. *A Practice of Anaesthesia,* 6 ed. London: Arnold;1995:1015.

61. Murray JR, Tremper KK. Alternatives to homologous blood transfusions: strategies for the 1990s. *Semin Anesth* 1993;12: 268–275.

62. Symposium Report. Blood and blood substitutes: methods of reducing blood loss and non-blood substitutes. *Can J Anaesth.* 1991;38:595–612.

63. Boisvenu G, Warriner CB, Haley LD, et al. Effects of saline dilution and IV catheter size on the infusion of packed red blood cells. *Can J Anaesth.* 1990;37:S85.

64. Dickson DN, Gregory MA. Compatibility of blood with solutions containing calcium. *South Afr Med J* 1986;57: 785–787.

65. Edwards MP, Clark DJ, Mark JS, et al. Compound sodium lactate solution. Caution: risk of clotting. *Anaesthesia.* 1986;41: 1053–1054.

66. Crosby ET. Perioperative haemotherapy: II. risks and complications of blood transfusion. *Can J Anaesth.* 1992;39:822–837.

67. Goodnough LT, Vizmeg K, Verbrugge D. The impact of autologous blood ordering and blood procurement practices on allogeneic blood exposure in elective in orthopedic surgery patients. *Am J Clin Pathol.* 1994;101:354–357.

68. Hillyer CD, Hart KK, Lackey DA 3rd, et al. Comparable safety of blood collection in "high-risk" autologous donors versus not-high-risk autologous and directed donors in a hospital setting. *Am J Clin Pathol.* 1994;102:275–277.

69. Howard MR, Chapman CE, Dunstand JA, et al. Regional transfusion centre preoperative autologous blood donation programme: the first two years. *BMJ.* 1992;305:1470–1473.

70. Healy JC, Frankforter SA, Graves BK, et al. Preoperative autologous blood donation in total-hip arthroplasty. A cost-effectiveness analysis. *Arch Pathol Lab Med.* 1994;118: 465–470.

71. Toy MU. Autologous transfusion: current trends and research issues. National Heart, Lung, and Blood Institute Autologous Transfusion Symposiuum Working Group. *Transfusion* 1995; 35:525–531.

72. Giordano GF, Giordano DM, Wallace BA, et al. An analysis of 9,918 consecutive perioperative autotransfusions. *Surg Gynecol Obstet.* 1993;176:103–110.

73. Clugston PA, Fitzpatrick DG, Kester DA, et al. Autologous blood use in reduction mammoplasty: is it justified? *Plast Reconstr Surg.* 1995;95:824–828.

74. Glover JL, Broadie TA. Intraoperative autotransfusion. *World J Surg.* 1987;11:60–64.

75. McShane AJ, Power C, Jackson JF, et al. Autotransfusion: quality of blood prepared with a red cell processing device. *Br J Anaesth.* 1987;59:1035–1039.

76. Irving GA. Perioperative blood and blood component therapy. *Can J Anaesth.* 1992;39:1105–1115.

77. Petrovitch C. Perioperative coagulation: an approach to the bleeding patient. *Semin Anesth.* 1993;12:132–141.

78. Boysen PG. Anesthetic considerations for thoracic surgery. In: Kirby RR, Gravenstein N, eds. *Clinical Anesthesia Practice.* Philadelphia: WB Saunders;1994:1230.

79. Nuttal GA. Indications and risks of platelet transfusion. In: Faust RJ, ed. *Anesthesiology Review.* New York: Churchill Livingstone;1994:482.

80. Jordan LM, Dosch MP. Coagulation and blood component therapy. In: Waugaman WR, Foster SD, Rigor BM, eds. *Principles and Practice of Nurse Anesthesia.* East Norwalk, Conn: Appleton & Lange;1992:304.

81. Wilson RF, Binkley LE, Sabo FM, et al. Electrolyte and acid base changes with massive blood transfusions. *Am Surg.* 1992; 58:535–544.

82. Dabrow MB, Wilkins JC. Hematologic emergencies. Management of transfusion reactions and crises in sickle cell disease. *Postgrad Med.* 1993;93:183–190.

83. Agarwal N, Murphy JG, Cayten CG, Stahl WM. Blood transfusion increases the risk of infection after trauma. *Arch Surg.* 1993;128:171–176.

84. Dries DJ, Waxman K. Adequate resuscitation of burn patients may not be measured by urine output and vital signs. *Crit Care Med.* 1991;19:327–329.

85. Davis JW, Shackford SR, Holbrook TL. Base deficit as a sensitive indicator of compensated shock and tissue oxygen utilization. *Surg Gynecol Obstet.* 1991;173:473–476.

☐ QUESTIONS

1. Total body water is divided into the intracellular volume and the extracellular volume. The extracellular volume is divided into the interstitial volume which comprises 11 L and the intravascular volume which constitutes:
   a. 3 L
   b. 5 L
   c. 8 L
   d. 10 L

2. The water molecule can easily traverse the slitlike pores located between the capillary endothelial cells. However, a protein molecule of average size can traverse the slitlike pores:
   a. 1/100 that of a water molecule
   b. 1/1000 that of a water molecule
   c. 1/10,000 that of a water molecule
   d. 1/100,000 that of a water molecule

Mr. White, a 32-year-old man has been admitted through the emergency room following a gunshot wound to the upper abdomen. His past medical history is essentially negative. Chest x-ray is clear and no hemothorax is suspected. On arrival to the OR, his pulse rate is 100 and his blood pressure is 90/60. Mr. White is conscious and a preanesthetic evaluation is completed prior to induction. Due to the difficulty in locating a vein, Mr. White is sent to the operating room without an IV. Questions #3 through #8 apply to this scenario.

3. On arrival, the radial pulse of Mr. White is palpable. His minimal systolic pressure would be expected to be:
   a. 60 mm Hg
   b. 70 mm Hg
   c. 80 mm Hg
   d. 90 mm Hg

4. Which of the following sites for venous cannulation would be least desirable for this patient?
   a. Internal jugular
   b. Femoral vein
   c. Basilica vein located on back of hand
   d. Subclavian vein

5. A decision is made to use crystalloid solution for the initial fluid management of Mr. White. Of the following crystalloid solutions, which would be the most appropriate.
   a. 5% dextrose in water
   b. 5% dextrose in ½ normal saline
   c. Ringer's lactate
   d. 7.5% sodium chloride

6. The anesthetic technique consists of ketamine for induction, rocuronium for facilitation of intubation plus muscle relaxation, and fentanyl/midazolam for maintenance. Once induction is completed and the surgery begins, a volatile agent, of .75 MAC is added to the technique due to an increase in heart rate. Within a few minutes, the blood pressure begins a significant decrease. The abdominal cavity has not been entered at this time. The most appropriate choice would be to:
   a. Administer a vasopressor, such as norepinephrine
   b. Administer a 1000-mL bolus of 6% hetastarch
   c. Maintain current technique until the abdominal cavity is entered
   d. Turn the volatile agent off until the abdominal cavity is entered in an attempt to quantify blood loss

7. Following induction, a Foley catheter is inserted atraumatically into his bladder. Minimal urine requirements for this patient would be:
   a. 0.1 mL/kg/h
   b. 0.5 mL/kg/h
   c. 1.5 mL/kg/h
   d. 2.5 mL/kg/h

8. On entering the bladder, 500 mL blood is aspirated by the surgeon. On his initial exploration, the surgeon notes the bullet penetrated the large bowel at several locations. The patient's blood pressure and pulse are acceptable at this time. Your first reaction would be to:
   a. Calculate the blood volume of Mr. White and administer blood if greater than 5% of blood volume has been lost
   b. Capture the blood in a cell-saver system and return the blood back to Mr. White
   c. Administer a 1000-mL bolus of crystalloid
   d. Maintain current technique and continue close surveillance of patient's vital signs

9. If 1 L of polyionic, nearly isotonic crystalloid solution is administered to a patient, the plasma volume will expand approximately:
   a. 200 mL
   b. 400 mL
   c. 600 mL
   d. 800 mL

10. A main focus of the crystalloid/colloid controversy centers around pulmonary edema. Which of the following statements is correct concerning this issue?
    a. Pulmonary edema will not occur during sepsis due to the decrease in pulmonary capillary permeability.
    b. Either crystalloid or colloids may be safely given as resuscitative fluids if appropriate monitoring is performed.
    c. The administration of colloid solutions will decrease oncotic pressure and contribute to pulmonary edema.
    d. Pulmonary edema will occur if the gradient between plasma oncotic pressure and pulmonary capillary pressure approaches 16 mm Hg.

11. Hydroxyethyl starch has been found to affect coagulation somewhat in a dose-related manner. Which of the following statements is correct concerning hydroxyethyl starch?
    a. Hydroxyethyl starch slows the conversion of fibrinogen to fibrin.
    b. An acquired von Willebrand's syndrome may occur, representing reduced levels of factor VIII activity.
    c. The adhesiveness of platelets will increase, resulting in prolonged bleeding times.
    d. Hydroxyethyl starch facilitates hypercoagulability following abdominal surgery.

12. While administering an anesthetic for a traumatized patient, the surgeon states that bleeding occurs everywhere he touches the patient. A complete blood count reveals the platelet count having decreased to 15,000. Which of the following would be an appropriate therapy?
    a. Administer no blood product at this time due to the chance of transmitting an infection to the patient.
    b. Administer 5 U fresh-frozen plasma.
    c. Administer 6 U platelets and repeat the platelet count.
    d. Administer several units of packed red blood cells to increase the platelet count.

13. Which of the following is a clinical sign of hypovolemia?
    a. Increasing base deficit value on a blood gas report
    b. Increasing pulse pressure of systemic blood pressure
    c. Increase in width of arterial pressure waveform
    d. Loss of fluctuations of the height of systolic pressure peaks coinciding with the inspiration phase of the ventilator

14. In patients without heart disease, the minimal acceptable hematocrit before elective surgery is:
    a. 10%–12%
    b. 15%–18%
    c. 20%–25%
    d. 30%–35%

15. On arrival to the operating room, the patient is hemor-rhaging profusely. Uncrossmatched blood is sent up from the blood bank. This blood must be quickly administered. Of the blood types, which is the universal donor?
    a. Type A
    b. Type B
    c. Type O
    d. Type AB

16. Going back to question #15, which of the following is an appropriate statement.
    a. Due to the severity of the patient, forget about blood filters and run the blood through a straight intravenous set.
    b. Administer all blood through a 170 micropore blood filter.
    c. Avoid diluting blood with Ringer's lactate during rapid infusion due to the increased incidence of clot formation.
    d. Attempt to warm all fluids administered to this patient.

17. Packed red cells have a hematocrit of:
    a. 30%–40%
    b. 50%–60%

    c. 70%–80%
    d. 90%–100%

18. The most common cause for incomplete autologous blood collection is:
    a. Recent seizures
    b. Valvular heart disease
    c. Insulin-dependent diabetes
    d. Anemia

19. In using central venous pressure values, a sustained increase of more than _____ in response to a rapid infusion of 200 mL indicates that hypovolemia is being corrected.
    a. 1 cm H_2O
    b. 2 cm H_2O
    c. 3 cm H_2O
    d. 10 cm H_2O

20. Currently, the ideal manner in which to replace an acute fluid loss following trauma is:
    a. With crystalloid solutions alone
    b. With colloid solutions alone
    c. With whole blood replacement
    d. An appropriate combination to facilitate optimal hemostasis care for the patient

☐ ANSWERS

1. a	5. c	9. a	13. a	17. c
2. c	6. d	10. b	14. c	18. d
3. c	7. b	11. b	15. c	19. c
4. b	8. d	12. c	16. d	20. d

CHAPTER
12

Electrolytes and Acid–Base Balance

Paula J. Goodman

Illness, anesthesia, and surgery can place huge demands on the fluid, electrolyte status, and acid–base balance of the patient. These problems may be subtle or dramatic, but the ability to diagnose and manage them is critical to the safe practice of anesthesia. This chapter gives you an overview of the physiology of water and electrolytes and their imbalances along with a brief review of acid–base balance.

☐ TOTAL BODY WATER

Water is the most abundant compound in the body. It is a key player in regulating cellular volume, removing waste products, and transporting nutrients and electrolytes. In the average 70-kg adult, water makes up approximately 60% of the total body weight (600 mL/kg). Termed total body water (TBW), the amount varies with age, gender, and weight. Lean body mass contains more water than fat; therefore, the young male has a greater percentage of TBW than the female, elderly, or obese person. Infants have a higher body fluid content than adults. The weight of a premature infant is composed of 90% TBW, whereas the full-term infant TBW weighs in at 70% to 80%. During the first year of life, TBW gradually decreases to 65%.[1-3]

Total body water is distributed either within the cell membrane or outside the cell membrane. Intracellular fluid (ICF) is the water found within the cell membrane. It composes 40% of the TBW (400 mL/kg). Skeletal muscle contains the greatest amount of ICF.[2]

Extracellular fluid (ECF) is water found outside the cell membrane, totaling 20% of the TBW (200 mL/kg). The ECF volume is greater in young males and less in the elderly and female population. In the infant, one half of the TBW is contained within the ECF, making the infant more vulnerable to fluid volume deficit. ECF is subdivided into two volume compartments, intravascular volume or interstitial volume. The intravascular volume, or plasma, is the noncellular portion of the blood and has a higher concentration of protein than interstitial fluid. The interstitial volume is comprised of lymph and transcellular fluids (pleural, cerebrospinal, joint, intraocular, peritoneal).

Water and electrolyte balance is regulated by several homeostatic mechanisms. Some of these are antidiuretic hormone (ADH), aldosterone, parathyroid hormone (PTH), calcitonin, thirst, and normal renal function.[3]

WATER BALANCE

Body fluid is in a constant state of flux. Water balance is easily maintained in the healthy individual through daily food and fluid intake. Metabolic rate dictates the daily water requirement. As the metabolic rate increases, so does the need for water. Water losses through the skin and respiration, termed insensible losses, can account for as much as 30% of the daily water requirement. Sensible water losses occur via the urine, gastrointestinal tract, and perspiration. The average adult urine output is 1.5 to 2 L/d.

Hypovolemia
Hypovolemia ensues when there is a volume deficit in the ECF and circulating blood volume. Gastrointestinal losses, fever, blood loss, burns, peritonitis, fluid shifts, diuretics, and inhalation of dry gases are common contributing factors. Physical signs of volume depletion include tachycardia, orthostatic hypotension, flat jugular neck veins when supine, decreased central venous pressure (CVP) and urine output, and dry mucous membranes. Cardiovascular collapse and renal failure may occur if the volume depletion occurs rapidly or goes undetected by the health care provider and is not cor-

rected in a timely manner. Compensatory mechanisms seen in the healthy adult during a hypovolemic episode are abolished by anesthesia. Therefore, fluid management is a critical component of the anesthesia plan.

Hypervolemia

Volume excess, or hypervolemia, occurs when the fluid intake exceeds the fluid output. The increase in ECF volume may be precipitated by excessive isotonic intravenous fluids, congestive heart failure, renal failure, long-term use of corticosteroids, and Cushing's syndrome. Some common physical findings are distended neck veins, peripheral edema, dyspnea, pulmonary edema, hypertension, increased CVP, polyuria, and cyanosis. Laboratory values show a decreased serum and urine osmolality, decreased urine specific gravity, lowered serum albumin, and hemodilution. Treatment includes diuretics, fluid and sodium restriction, and oxygen and cardiovascular support.

☐ ELECTROLYTES

Water and electrolytes are the fundamental components of body fluid. An electrolyte can be defined as matter that develops an electrical charge when dissolved in water. The charged particles are called ions. Positively charged ions are called cations. Sodium, potassium, calcium, and magnesium are examples of cations. Anions, such as chloride and bicarbonate, are ions that have a negative charge.

The electrolyte compositions of the ECF and ICF differ substantially. It is customary to measure the electrolytes in the ECF, namely the plasma. Within the ECF the principal cation is sodium and the principal anion is chloride. Potassium is the major cation in the ICF, with proteins and organic phosphates the major anions. Serum electrolytes are measured in milliequivalents per liter (mEq/L), indicating the chemical reactivity of the ion.

Electrolyte abnormalities are associated with many disease processes. The clinical picture is often confusing because several electrolyte imbalances may occur together and have similar clinical presentations. Treatment for electrolyte imbalances initiated preoperatively may need to be continued intraoperatively as well as postoperatively. Because anesthesia often obliterates the signs and symptoms of impending imbalances, serum electrolyte levels must be closely monitored.

ELECTROLYTE IMBALANCES

Sodium   Sodium is the predominant cation in the ECF with a normal concentration of 135 to 145 mEq/L. The sodium ion plays a critical role in the regulation of extracellular osmolality and intravascular volume.[1] It also maintains the active transport mechanism in conjunction with potassium and aids in the transmission of neuromuscular impulses. Sodium regulation is directed by the kidney and the secretion of aldosterone and ADH.

Hyponatremia

Hyponatremia is defined as ECF sodium concentration less than 135 mEq/L. Sodium depletion may be caused by gastrointestinal losses and fluid shifts from burns and peritonitis. Addison's disease is an aldosterone deficiency precipitated by an adrenal cortex disorder. Hyponatremia develops because the lack of aldosterone prevents the reabsorption of the sodium ion from the kidney tubules.[2] The syndrome of inappropriate antidiuretic hormone (SIADH) is caused by a persistent release of ADH from the hypothalamus, pituitary, or an ectopic focus. This may occur in patients with pulmonary, intracranial, or endocrine disease. Laboratory findings indicative of SIADH are hyponatremia and low serum osmolality combined with a high urine osmolality.[3]

More often, hyponatremia results from excess water retention rather than a sodium ion deficiency. Causative factors are usually tied to renal failure, congestive heart failure, and overhydration with electrolyte-free solutions. One example of water overload is the intravascular absorption of large amounts of electrolyte-free irrigation fluid during transurethral resection of the prostate (TURP syndrome).

Clinical findings of hyponatremia are muscle weakness, cramping of lower extremity muscles, nausea, vomiting, agitation, confusion, and visual disturbances. Cardiac dysrhythmias, hypotension, widening of the QRS complex, ST segment elevation, pulmonary edema, coma, and seizures are associated with a serum sodium concentration less than 115 mEq/L.[2,4]

Therapeutic management is based on the rate of development of hyponatremia, correction of the causative factor, and sodium replacement. If the onset of the hyponatremia occurs over a period of days or weeks and the patient is asymptomatic, conservative medical management with water restriction, oral sodium intake, and intravenous normal saline may suffice. Rapid development of symptomatic hyponatremia is a life-threatening emergency and requires aggressive management. Treatment modalities may include intravenous hypertonic saline (3%), respiratory and cardiovascular support, and diuresis. Sodium serum concentrations are measured every 1 to 2 hours during rapid correction. Central pontine myelinolysis is a complication associated with rapid correction of hyponatremia.[4,5]

Hypernatremia

A serum sodium concentration greater than 145 mEq/L denotes a surplus of sodium ions in the ECF. Hypernatremia is seen when there is excessive water loss or inadequate replacement of water. Resuscitation events where sodium bicarbonate therapy is overused is a common cause of hypernatremia.[2] Clinical signs are thirst, flushed skin, mental status changes, hypotension, hypovolemia, shock, and myoclonus. Treatment includes restricting sodium intake, administering sodium-free intravenous solutions, and diuretics.

Potassium   Potassium is the major intracellular cation. It is often considered the most essential ion for normal cellular function. Potassium is crucial for the transmission of nerve impulses; promotes myocardial, skeletal, and smooth muscle contraction; and aids in the regulation of acid–base balance. Dietary intake, aldosterone secretion, insulin production, and renal excretion of 50 to 100 mEq/d regulate potassium balance. Imbalances are usually associated with renal dysfunction, diuretics, dietary intake, vomiting, diarrhea, and sweating. Normal serum concentration is 3.5 to 5.0 mEq/L.

Hypokalemia

Hypokalemia is probably the most frequently encountered electrolyte abnormality. It is commonly associated with the chronic use of diuretics without potassium supplements. Hypokalemia may occur in a variety of clinical settings, such as the loss of gastrointestinal fluids, prolonged use of digitalis, excessive steroid administration, alkalosis, and hypomagnesemia. Increased aldosterone secretion from a tumor or a diseased adrenal cortex (Cushing's syndrome) are more insidious causes. Clinical signs are paralytic ileus, hyporeflexia, anorexia, muscle cramps and weakness progressing to paralysis, lethargy, and confusion.

The cardiac effects of hypokalemia are the most dramatic findings. The appearance of a U wave on an electrocardiogram (ECG) may be normal in some patients, but it can be an early indicator of low potassium concentration. As the potassium depletion increases, the U wave becomes more prominent, the T wave flattens out or may invert, and the ST segment becomes depressed. The U wave may be accentuated in the digitalis toxic patient.[6] Untreated hypokalemia can produce life-threatening cardiac dysrhythmias. Premature ventricular contractions, ventricular tachycardia, and atrial dysrhythmias are not uncommon findings.

The therapeutic management of hypokalemia requires close monitoring by the provider. Oral potassium supplements along with an increase in dietary potassium may be all that is required to correct the hypokalemia. More acute cases may require intravenous potassium replacement therapy. Intravenous potassium is extremely irritating to the peripheral vein and is best given through a central line in a very dilute solution. The rate of replacement in adults is recommended to be no greater than 40 mEq in 100 mL fluid over 1 hour through the central line, even less through a peripheral line.[5] Magnesium sulfate supplements should also be considered in patients with severe hypokalemia who are nonresponsive to intravenous potassium supplements.

Hyperkalemia

Hyperkalemia results from the redistribution of potassium ions from the ICF to the ECF. A patient with a serum potassium concentration that exceeds 5.5 mEq/L is considered to be hyperkalemic.

The etiology of hyperkalemia can usually be attributed to numerous concurrent factors. Laboratory error due to hemolysis of the patient's blood sample must be ruled out. Once this is done, the health care provider should consider other possible causes of hyperkalemia. These include renal failure, acidosis, adrenal insufficiency, excessive dietary intake of potassium salts, hyponatremia, hypocalcemia, traumatic crush injuries, burns, and the rapid administration of a large

volume of stored blood. Hyperkalemia can also be attributed to the administration of certain drugs. Penicillin G potassium, excessive administration of intravenous potassium chloride, potassium-sparing diuretics as triamterene, and aldosterone antagonists as spironolactone are known agents.[7] An induction dose of succinylcholine increases serum potassium 0.5 mEq/L in patients with normal renal function.[8] Although this rise is transient, an even greater effect may be seen in the presence of neuromuscular disease and renal failure.

Signs and symptoms of hyperkalemia include muscle weakness progressing to paralysis and paresthesia. Cardiac dysrhythmias are common. ECG changes correlate well with serum potassium concentration. The earliest sign of hyperkalemia on the ECG is a change in the T wave. At a concentration of 6 to 7 mEq/L, the T wave is described as tall, narrow, peaked, or tenting. As the potassium level rises, changes occur first in the atrial portion of the complex, then in the ventricular portion. At 8 mEq/L, the P wave flattens, widens, and may disappear entirely. At 10 mEq/L, the QRS begins to widen. Ventricular fibrillation and death can occur at serum potassium levels of 10 to 12 mEq/L.[7]

Treatment is directed toward lowering the serum potassium concentration. In the chronic hyperkalemic patient, restricting potassium intake, administering ion exchange resins, and dialysis are useful measures in decreasing total body potassium content. When the rise of serum potassium is rapid and life threatening, emergency treatment is focused on driving the potassium ion intracellularly. The first line of defense is the intravenous administration of calcium gluconate or calcium chloride.[3] Within 1 to 2 minutes, myocardial contractility is revived for a brief time. Glucose-insulin infusion, β agonists, and sodium bicarbonate are effective at promoting the extracellular-intracellular shift of potassium over a longer time period.[9] Hemodialysis is the preferred method of treatment in extreme cases. Calcium salts are contraindicated in the patient receiving digitalis.

Chloride   Chloride is a principal anion in the ECF. The normal serum concentration of chloride is 98 to 108 mEq/L. The primary function of chloride is to preserve the acid–base balance. Chloride also works in conjunction with sodium to maintain the body osmolality and water balance.

Hypochloremia

A serum chloride concentration less than 98 mEq/L is termed hypochloremia. Prolonged gastric suctioning and diuretic therapy precipitate a chloride deficiency and metabolic alkalosis. Patients with small-bowel obstruction or pyloric stenosis frequently are hypochloremic.[5] Clinical findings are hypoventilation, hypotension, and muscle excitability. Treatment includes intravenous sodium chloride with potassium chloride and stopping the loss of chloride ions.

Hyperchloremia

A serum chloride concentration greater than 108 mEq/L is considered hyperchloremia. It is usually associated with metabolic acidosis, but can also be caused by overadministration of chloride-containing products. Treatment is aimed at restricting the intake of chloride ions.

Calcium Calcium is an important electrolyte that helps to regulate normal cellular function. It is essential for maintaining the integrity of the cell membrane, initiation and propagation of electrical impulses, myocardial contractility, and blood coagulation. Most of the calcium is found in the bony skeleton. The normal serum calcium level is 4.5 to 5.3 mEq/L (9 to 10.5 mg/dL). Two forms of calcium are found within the blood, free ionized calcium and nonionized protein-bound calcium. Only the ionized form of calcium is physiologically active.[1] PTH, calcitonin, and vitamin D play vital roles in the regulation of calcium. PTH increases reabsorption of calcium from the bone, vitamin D is necessary for the absorption of calcium from the gastrointestinal tract, and calcitonin suppresses bony calcium reabsorption. Calcitonin is more effective and precise at regulating calcium concentration than is the PTH.[1]

Hypocalcemia

A serum calcium concentration less than 4.5 mEq/L is referred to as hypocalcemia. The most common cause of hypocalcemia is a low serum albumin level.[9,10] Other related causes include chronic renal failure, hypoparathyroidism, hypomagnesemia, acute pancreatitis, malabsorption syndromes, liver failure, alkalosis, and transfusion of a large volume of citrated blood. Clinical findings are circumoral paresthesia, muscle weakness, tetany, seizures, hypotension, and pathologic fractures. A prolonged QT interval due to a lengthening in the ST segment is seen on the ECG. The presence of Chvostek's (lightly tapping the facial nerve causes facial muscle twitching) or Trousseau's (carpal spasm is elicited when the arm circulation is constricted) sign is indicative of hypocalcemia.[1] In anesthesia, the potential for postoperative laryngospasm secondary to hypocalcemia is a major concern. Hypocalcemia may occur if the parathyroid glands are damaged or inadvertently removed during a thyroidectomy or radical neck procedure.[2]

The treatment for hypocalcemia is the administration of calcium gluconate or calcium chloride. Calcium chloride is very irritating to the peripheral vein and should be given via a central line. Calcium gluconate may be given either peripherally or centrally. The routine use of calcium during cardiopulmonary resuscitation is no longer recommended because an excess of calcium may worsen the myocardial reperfusion injury. Calcium infusions during cardiac arrest should be considered in known cases of citrate toxicity, hyperkalemia, or calcium antagonist toxicity.[10]

Hypercalcemia

An excess of calcium ions in the ECF is termed hypercalcemia. The most common causes of hypercalcemia are neoplasms, hyperparathyroidism, and immobilization. Clinical findings include renal calculi, hypertension, anorexia, fatigue, and lethargy. A shortening of the QT interval is seen on the ECG.[6] Therapeutic management of hypercalcemia is focused on treating the underlying cause and lowering serum calcium levels by increasing urinary calcium excretion. This can be accomplished through intravenous and oral hydration and loop diuretics.

Magnesium Magnesium is a major intracellular cation that plays a significant role in activation of cellular enzymes systems, cell membrane excitability, and potassium regulation. It is a key factor in oxidative phosphorylation and the production of adenosine triphosphate (ATP).[9] Magnesium is described as a physiologic calcium antagonist because of its role in regulating calcium ion release at the nerve ending. A normal serum magnesium concentration is 1.5 to 2.5 mEq/L. The glomerular filtration rate of the kidney controls the excretion of magnesium.

Hypomagnesemia

A serum magnesium concentration less than 1.5 mEq/L is termed hypomagnesemia. It may be caused by chronic alcoholism, malabsorption syndromes, protracted vomiting or diarrhea, hyperaldosteronism, and theophylline toxicity. Hypomagnesemia leads to increased neuromuscular irritability. Clinical signs are agitation, confusion, exaggerated deep tendon reflexes, tremors, spasticity, tetany, and tachycardia. Supraventricular and ventricular dysrhythmias are seen in patients with a magnesium deficiency. ECG findings consist of a prolonged PR interval, widened QRS complex, and flattened T wave. Most symptomatic patients also have hypocalcemia, hypokalemia, and hypophosphatemia, which complicates the clinical picture.[10]

Severe hypomagnesemia in the patient with normal renal function is treated with intravenous magnesium sulfate or magnesium chloride. Intravenous calcium chloride or calcium gluconate should be readily available in case the hypomagnesemia is overcorrected.

Hypermagnesemia

A serum magnesium concentration that exceeds 2.5 mEq/L is called hypermagnesemia. Chronic renal failure and diabetic ketoacidosis are known to trigger hypermagnesemia. In obstetrics, hypermagnesemia is induced in the toxemic patient to prevent convulsions by parenteral administration of magnesium sulfate. Magnesium sulfate is a central nervous system depressant and skeletal muscle relaxant. It can cross the placenta and cause neonatal hypotonia, hyporeflexia, and respiratory depression. The therapeutic magnesium level in this case is 4 to 6 mEq/L.[9,10]

Clinical findings are associated with the suppressed neuromuscular function and sedative effects of an elevated serum magnesium level. These signs include sedation, lethargy, bradycardia, hypotension, and respiratory depression. Respiratory depression is caused by the magnesium-induced neuromuscular blockade. When the serum magnesium concentration exceeds 10 mEq/L, deep tendon reflexes are lost. Heart block and respiratory muscle paralysis occur when the magnesium concentration is greater than 12 mEq/L. Hypermagnesemia enhances the effect of depolarizing and nondepolarizing neuromuscular blockers and requires close patient monitoring.

Emergency management of severe hypermagnesemia is to provide respiratory and cardiovascular support. Intravenous calcium chloride or calcium gluconate may help to antagonize the effect of the magnesium. Hemodialysis may be required in the patient with renal failure.

Phosphate Phosphate is an intracellular anion that is similar to calcium. The bony skeleton contains 70% to 80% of the body's store of phosphate. It is a key factor in energy metabolism, maintenance of acid–base balance, and an essential element in protein structure. Serum phosphate is regulated primarily by the kidneys. Nearly all of the phosphate absorbed by the gut is excreted by the kidneys. PTH acts on the proximal renal tubules to modulate the absorption of phosphate. The normal phosphate serum concentration is 1 to 2 mEq/L (3 to 4.5 mg/dL) for adults with a higher value (4 to 7 mg/dL) for children. This difference may be attributed to renal maturity and the fast rate of bone growth.[11]

Hypophosphatemia

A serum phosphate concentration below 1.5 mg/dL is called hypophosphatemia. It may be caused by alcoholism, diabetic ketoacidosis, malabsorptive syndrome, salicylate overdose, sepsis, and the administration of drugs such as epinephrine and corticosteroids. Acute hypocalcemia and acute hypomagnesemia worsen hypophosphatemia by increasing the renal excretion of phosphate ions by promoting parathyroid hormone secretion.

Clinical findings are related to depleted intracellular ATP levels impairing the energy-driven cardiovascular and neuromuscular systems. Hypotension, impaired platelet function, muscle weakness, seizures, rhabdomyolysis, and cardiorespiratory failure are associated with severe hypophosphatemia.[1] Treatment with intravenous phosphate supplements is usually reserved for severe hypophosphatemia. Parenteral phosphate solutions are hypertonic and should be diluted prior to use or given via a central line. Calcium supplements will precipitate with phosphate additives if mixed together.

Hyperphosphatemia

A serum phosphate concentration greater than 4.5 mg/dL in adults is defined as hyperphosphatemia. Causative factors include increased intake (excessive administration of phosphate supplements, laxatives), redistribution of ions into the extracellular space (tissue necrosis, massive cell lysis), and reduced renal excretion (renal failure, hypoparathyroidism). Treatment is elimination of phosphate in the diet or parenteral fluids and promoting the excretion in the urine with diuretics. Aluminum-based antacids bind phosphate secreted into the gut.[3]

☐ ACID–BASE BALANCE

Acid–base balance is determined by the hydrogen ion concentration within the body which, in turn, determines the pH of the blood. Even the slightest change challenges normal cellular function. The pH is defined as the negative logarithm of the hydrogen ion concentration. An increase in the hydrogen ion concentration lowers the pH, making the solution more acidic. In contrast, a decrease in the hydrogen ion concentration raises the pH, rendering the solution more alkaline. Three factors can regulate the hydrogen ion concentration to maintain the body's pH within the narrow, physiologic range of 7.35 to 7.45. These factors are chemical buffers, respiratory mechanisms, and renal mechanisms.[12]

Three chemical buffers can neutralize any acid or base produced within the ECF almost instantaneously. Intracellular buffering may require several hours. The bicarbonate system is the largest chemical buffer in the body. It consists of sodium bicarbonate and carbonic acid in a ratio of 20:1. As long as this ratio remains stable, the pH of the blood will remain normal. The extracellular operation of the bicarbonate buffer is important. It excretes excess hydrogen ions via respiration and converts excess base into bicarbonate, which is excreted by the kidneys. The second chemical buffer is the phosphate system. It allows the kidney to excrete hydrogen ions in the renal tubules. The third buffer system is protein. The high protein concentration within the cell makes it the most potent intracellular buffer. Hemoglobin is part of the protein buffer system, but its buffering capability depends on the degree of oxygenation.[12,13]

The kidney dominates the process of pH maintenance.[12] It regulates the bicarbonate ion by making the pH of the urine more acid or basic. Also, the kidney can adequately compensate for any weaknesses in the respiratory or chemical buffer systems.

The respiratory, or ventilatory, response can respond to any change in hydrogen ion concentration within 1 to 5 minutes.[13] The rate of ventilation increases to eliminate excess carbonic acid, an end product of metabolism, from the body (for further discussion see Chap. 16).

An acid–base disturbance is categorized as acidosis or alkalosis. Acidosis occurs when the hydrogen ion concentration in the blood increases, driving the serum pH below 7.35. Alkalosis occurs when the hydrogen ion concentration in the blood drops, raising the serum pH above 7.45. The imbalance can be further categorized according to the causative agent, such as respiratory alkalosis or metabolic acidosis. Compensation describes the physiologic responses that help to restore the pH to a normal level (Table 12–1).

Respiratory acidosis is caused by any factor that reduces alveolar ventilation resulting in a decreased pH and an elevated $Paco_2$. Drugs, anesthesia, or intrinsic pulmonary disease can cause respiratory acidosis. Respiratory alkalosis is the result of alveolar hyperventilation, causing excessive elimination of carbon dioxide. This results in an increased pH and a decreased $Paco_2$. Etiology may be related to pregnancy, hysteria, overenthusiastic mechanical ventilation, fever, pain, and high altitude.[13]

Metabolic acidosis occurs when there is an accumulation of the acidic end products of metabolism decreasing the pH and bicarbonate level. Renal failure, ketoacidosis, and diarrhea are some causative factors. Metabolic alkalosis is generally related to a loss of hydrogen ions or an accumulation of

Table 12–1
INTERPRETATION OF ACID–BASE IMBALANCES

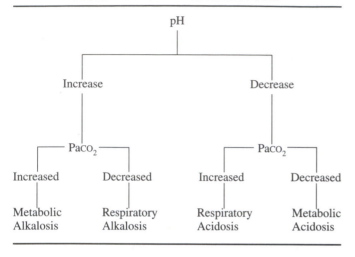

bicarbonate resulting in an increase in pH and bicarbonate. The most common causes are related to chloride depletion from vomiting, gastric suctioning, and diuretic therapy.

When analyzing acid–base imbalances, it is helpful to refer to the sodium bicarbonate (HCO_3^-) and the base excess levels. A normal plasma concentration of HCO_3^- is 24 ± 2 mEq/L. Derivations beyond this range are indicative of acidemia or alkalemia of primary metabolic disturbances. The base excess is a numerical value that predicts the amount of acid or base necessary to return blood pH to 7.40 and Pa_{CO_2} to 40 mmHg. A positive base excess indicates metabolic alkalosis, whereas a negative base excess signifies a metabolic acidosis.

The conclusions and opinions expressed are those of the author and do not reflect the official policy of the Department of the Defense, the Department of the Air Force, or other Departments of the US Government.

REFERENCES

1. Skeie B, Askanazi J, Khambatta H. Nutrition, fluid and electrolytes. In: Barash PG, Cullen BF, Stoelting RK, eds. *Clinical Anesthesia.* Philadelphia: JB Lippincott; 1989:738–751.
2. Jordan LM. Fluid and electrolytes. In: Waugaman WR, Rigor BM, Katz LE, et al, eds. *Principles and Practice of Nurse Anesthesia.* East Norwalk, Conn: Appleton & Lange; 1988:387–393.
3. Tonnesen AS. Crystalloids and colloids. In: Miller RD, ed. *Anesthesia.* 4th ed. New York: Churchill Livingstone; 1994:1602–1606.
4. Malhotra V. Anesthesia and the renal and genitourinary systems. In: Miller RD ed. *Anesthesia.* 4th ed. New York: Churchill Livingstone; 1994:1957–1958.
5. McGough EK, Kirby RR. Fluids and electrolytes. In Kirby RR, Gravenstein N, ed. *Clinical Anesthesia Practice.* Philadelphia: WB Saunders; 1994:722–727.
6. Dubin D. *Rapid Interpretation of EKGs.* 4th ed. Tampa, Fla: Cover Publishing; 1989.
7. Brensilver JM, Goldberger E. *A Primer of Water, Electrolyte and Acid-Base Syndromes.* 8th ed. Philadelphia: FA Davis; 1996:238–249.
8. Prough DS, Foreman AS. Anesthesia and the renal system. In Barash PG, Cullen BF, Stoelting RK, eds. *Clinical Anesthesia.* Philadelphia: JB Lippincott; 1989:1093.
9. Stoelting RK. *Pharmacology and Physiology in Anesthesia Practice.* Philadelphia: JB Lippincott; 1987:536–545.
10. James MFM. Calcium and magnesium in anaesthesia. In: Healy TE, Cohen PJ, eds. *A Practice of Anaesthesia.* London: Edward Arnold; 1995:316–321.
11. Siegel NJ, Carpenter T, Gaudio KM. The pathophysiology of body fluids. In: Oski FA, DeAngelis CD, Feigin D, et al, eds. *Principles and Practice of Pediatrics.* Philadelphia: JB Lippincott; 1990:75–76.
12. Brensilver JM, Goldberger E. *A Primer of Water, Electrolyte, and Acid-Base Syndromes.* 8th ed. Philadelphia: FA Davis; 1996:119–136.
13. Stoelting RK. *Pharmacology and Physiology in Anesthesia Practice.* Philadelphia: JB Lippincott; 1987:734–740.

☐ QUESTIONS

1. In the average 70-kg adult, water makes up approximately what percentage of total body weight?
   a. Less than 25%
   b. Less than 50%
   c. Less than 70%

2. The relationship between obesity and total body water is:
   a. Linear
   b. Sine
   c. Inverse

3. An anion is a:
   a. Positively charged ion
   b. Negatively charged ion
   c. Isoelectric ion

4. Hypovolemia may be attributed to:
   a. Cushing's syndrome

  b. Peritonitis

  c. Long-term use of corticosteroids

5. Regulation of water and electrolyte balance falls under the auspices of:
  a. Angiotensin and renin
  b. Aldosterone and oxytocin
  c. Antidiuretic hormone and thyroid-stimulating hormone

6. The predominate cation in the extracellular fluid is:
  a. Chloride
  b. Potassium
  c. Sodium

7. Resuscitation events where sodium bicarbonate therapy is overused is a common cause of:
  a. Hypernatremia
  b. Respiratory alkalosis
  c. Ventricular fibrillation

8. During a routine transurethral resection of the prostate, your patient with a stable T-10 spinal level suddenly complains of poor vision, becomes agitated and hypotensive. Your *best* response is to:
  a. Administer oxygen by mask, notify the surgeon to stop the procedure as soon as possible, treat the hypotension, and draw stat serum electrolytes.
  b. Administer oxygen by nasal cannula, change the intravenous fluid to normal saline, draw routine serum electrolytes, and slowly titrate midazolm intravenously.
  c. Administer oxygen by nasal cannula and administer 1 L of lactated Ringer's solution.

9. Rapid correction of acute hyponatremia is believed to predispose the patient to:
  a. Ventricular dysrhythmias
  b. Seizures
  c. Central pontine myelinolysis

10. The electrocardiogram on a preoperative patient reveals a U wave and a flat T wave. A laboratory result may show:
  a. Serum potassium is less than 3.2 mEq/L.
  b. Serum potassium is greater than 5.5 mEq/L.
  c. Serum calcium is less than 3 mEq/L.

11. What drug should be considered if the serum potassium concentration in a severely hypokalemic patient is not responding to intravenous potassium supplements?
  a. β agonists
  b. Magnesium sulfate
  c. Insulin drip

12. Life-threatening hyperkalemia is initially treated by the intravenous administration of:
  a. Calcium chloride
  b. Glucose-insulin drip
  c. β agonists

13. The earliest sign of hyperkalemia noted on an electro-cardiogram is:
  a. The presence of a U wave
  b. A tall, narrow T wave
  c. A widened QRS complex

14. Hypochloremic alkalosis is commonly seen in patients with:
  a. Paget's disease
  b. Renal failure
  c. Pyloric stenosis

15. Calcium is physiologically active only when it exists in the:
  a. Ionized form
  b. Nonionized form

16. Accidental removal of the parathyroid glands during a radical neck procedure may:
  a. Precipitate laryngospasm and hyperactive deep tendon reflexes postoperatively
  b. Produce a peaked T wave on the electrocardiogram
  c. Require periodic interscalene blocks to relieve the severe postoperative pain

17. The most common cause of hypocalcemia is:
  a. Chronic alcoholism
  b. Hyperparathyroidism
  c. Reduced serum albumin level

18. Magnesium is a major:
  a. Intracellular anion that plays a significant role in the acid–base balance
  b. Intracellular cation that is a key factor in oxidative phosphorylation
  c. Extracelluar cation that is integral to the structure of proteins

19. If hypomagnesemia is overcorrected in a patient with normal renal function, intravenous _____ should be considered.
  a. Calcium gluconate
  b. Potassium chloride
  c. Sodium bicarbonate

20. The clinical effects of hypophosphatemia is due to:
  a. Decreased secretion of aldosterone
  b. Increased production of vasopressin
  c. Low levels of intracellular adenosine triphosphate

☐ ANSWERS

1. c	**5.** a	**9.** c	**13.** b	**17.** c
2. c	**6.** c	**10.** a	**14.** c	**18.** b
3. b	**7.** a	**11.** b	**15.** a	**19.** a
4. b	**8.** a	**12.** a	**16.** a	**20.** c

CHAPTER
13

Regional Anesthesia

Candace Brown

Regional or conduction block anesthesia includes spinal, epidural, caudal, and various peripheral nerve blocks. Some advantages of regional anesthesia are:

1. The patient is allowed to remain awake, removing the need to manipulate the airway and to undergo the stress of general endotracheal anesthesia.
2. It provides excellent surgical conditions with profound skeletal muscle relaxation
3. It can often be continued to provide postoperative pain control.

☐ PATIENT PREPARATION

Preoperative evaluation is essentially the same as that for general anesthesia. These patients should also be evaluated for signs of infection in the area that is to be anesthetized. Adequate landmarks required to perform the regional technique need to be identified and documentation of normal coagulation studies should be obtained.

Preoperatively, apprehensive patients need to be assured that they can be sedated during the procedure and that intraoperatively they will not feel the pain of surgery. Preoperative medication should be administered to alleviate some of the anxiety and discomfort associated with the technique while still allowing the patient to cooperate and provide feedback. An intravenous line should be in place before any regional anesthesia is administered, and appropriate resuscitation equipment should be readily available. Fluid needs to be administered as indicated.

☐ ANATOMY AND PHYSIOLOGY

The safe and effective administration of regional anesthesia requires a thorough understanding of the anatomy and physiology of the spinal cord, vertebrae, and nerve pathways.

BONY STRUCTURES

Twenty-four individual vertebrae make up the bony spinal column, divided into 7 cervical, 12 thoracic, and 5 lumbar vertebrae. The sacrum and coccyx are distal segments formed by fused vertebrae early in life. Each individual vertebra contains a body (with two pedicles anteriorly and two laminae posteriorly) and an arch (located posteriorly and attached to the body via the pedicles). The transverse process joins the two lamina. The spinous process is the most dorsal portion of the lamina and is a major landmark in identifying where to place the needle for regional anesthesia blocks in the back. Between each vertebrae is the intervertebral disk (Fig. 13–1).

The vertebral column has a natural curve that forces the spinous processes to come off at different angles, depending on the level at which they are located. When administering a spinal or epidural block it is important to note that the spinous processes at the lumbar level are nearly horizontal; therefore, the needle can be introduced perpendicular to the spinal column. From T-3 to L-1, however, the spinous processes come off at a caudad angle so the needle needs to be directed more cephalad to enter the space between spinous processes (Fig. 13–2).

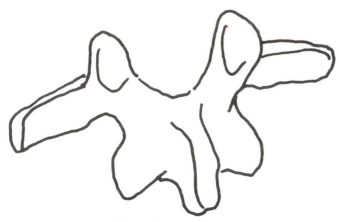

Figure 13–1   Lamina

LIGAMENTS

The anterior and posterior longitudinal ligaments support the vertebral bodies. The supraspinous, the interspinous, and the ligamentum flavum connect the dorsal spines and can be identified with experience, as the needle passes through them

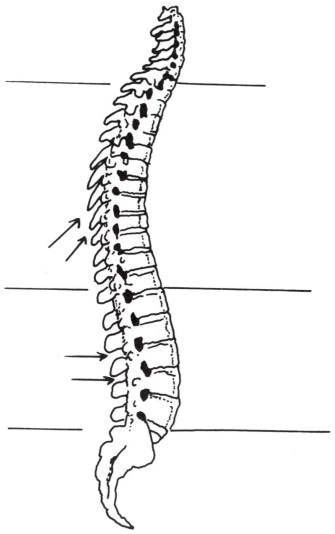

Figure 13–2   Spinal column

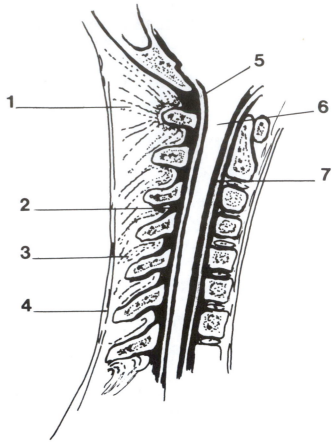

Figure 13–3   1. Ligament 2. Ligamentum flavum 3. Intraspinous ligament 4. Supraspinous ligament 5. Subarachnoid space 6. Cerebral spinal fluid 7. Epidural space

on the way to a spinal or epidural block. The supraspinous ligaments connect the most dorsal part of the spinous process. The intraspinous ligaments connect the spinous processes to each other. The ligamentum flavum connects the laminae. These three posterior ligaments are thickest in the lumbar region (Fig. 13–3). If a *paramedian* approach is used, the supraspinous and intraspinous ligaments will not be encountered because they are located medially between the vertebrae.

SOFT TISSUES AND NERVES

Inside the bony vertebral column sits the spinal canal and the spinal cord. The dura mater, the arachnoid mater, and the pia mater surround the spinal cord and its nerves. The outermost layer, the dura mater, forms a continuous covering, starting at the intracranial dura and extending as the dural sac to the second sacral vertebrae in the average adult. Adjacent to the dura mater is the arachnoid mater. It is between the dura mater and the arachnoid mater, known as the subarachnoid space, that spinal anesthetics are administered. The cerebrospinal fluid (CSF) is located here. The volume of CSF is 150 mL in the average adult. At body temperature the specific gravity is 1.003 to 1.008. The pH is physiologic. The pia mater directly surrounds the spinal cord, which originates at the foramen magnum and ends at the L1-2 interspace. *In the infant, the spinal cord ends at L-3 until it rises up to the L-1 level by the end of the first year.* The level of the spinal cord is especially important to note when administering thoracic level epidurals or spinals because of the potential for cord injury. Below L-1 to L-2, the nerves coming off the cord are referred to as cauda equina.

Spinal nerves exit off the spinal cord and travel through openings in the intervertebral spaces called intervertebral foramina. Each nerve ends at a specific dermatome or skeletal muscle (Fig. 13–4). Preganglionic sympathetic nerves come off the cord at T-1 through L-2. For example, *cardiac accelerators* originate at T-1 through T-5. Therefore, profound sympathetic nervous system blockade with high level

spinal and epidural anesthesia can occur with hypotension and possible bradycardia.

The epidural space exists between the ligamentum flavum and the dura. It is a potential space created by injecting fluid into it. It consists of connective fat tissue and venous plexi. The epidural space is narrowest at the lower cervical/upper thoracic level and the lower thoracic/upper lumbar region due to bulging spinal cord neural tissue in the areas. At the end of the spinal cord, L-2 level, the space widens.

The three types of nerve fibers that are affected by regional anesthetic blocks are sympathetic, motor, and sensory. Close to the surface of the nerve are the small diameter, unmyelinated sympathetic nerve fibers. These shallower sympathetic nerve fibers absorb the local anesthetic *first* and are bathed in

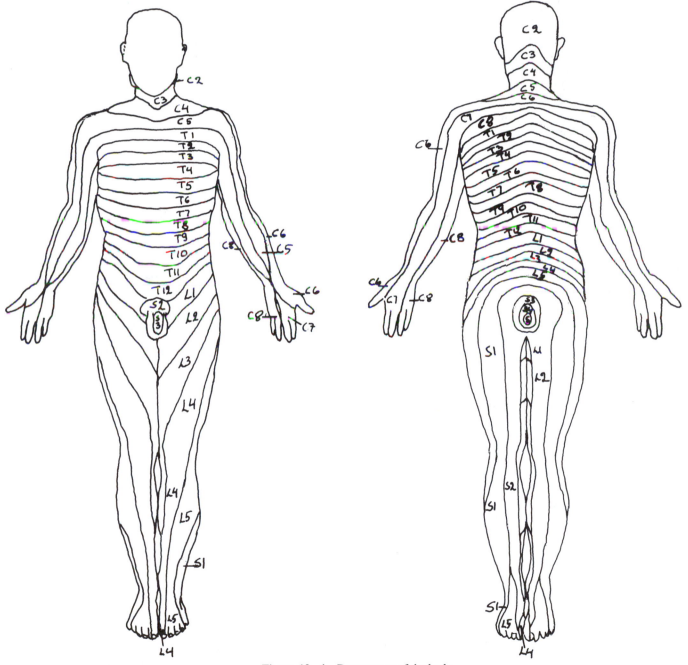

Figure 13–4 Dermatones of the body

it for a longer period of time. Therefore, sympathetic blockade is seen before sensory and motor blockade. Specifically, sympathetic block is usually two segments higher than sensory block, which is in turn two segments higher than motor block. This is important for assessing the level of blockade for surgery.

□ SPINAL BLOCK

TECHNIQUE

The two basic approaches to spinal anesthetic blockade are midline and paramedian. The patient can be placed in the lateral decubitus or sitting position. Sick or heavily sedated patients are easiest to handle in the lateral decubitus position. The operative side should be positioned downward if possible, to allow for gravitational flow of local anesthetic to the surgical site. The knees should be bent and the neck flexed downward, putting the patient in a "fetal" position with the back arched like the letter C, an angry cat, or a cooked shrimp. Spinal blocks may also be administered with the patient in the sitting position. The sitting position is especially useful in patients with narrow interspaces from calcified ligaments and stenotic spines. It is also helpful if a low level of spinal anesthesia is required for lower extremity or vaginal surgery.

Most spinal anesthetics are administered at the L-2 to L-3 or L-3 to L-4 level. A line drawn between the iliac crests crosses the spine at the L-4 vertebra. Thus, one or two interspaces above are most commonly used. Remember, the spinal cord ends at L-1 to L-2, so most anesthetics are administered into the area surrounding the cauda equina. Commercial kits are available containing all the necessary equipment, needles, and local solutions.

Administering spinal anesthesia is a sterile procedure and appropriate care should be taken. The anesthetist first dons sterile gloves; the area is then washed with a Betadine solution. Care is taken not to get Betadine on the sterile gloves, and after the wash sterile gauze is used to wipe off all Betadine from the skin. (Betadine is toxic to nerve tissue.) The local anesthetic for the block is prepared and placed within easy reach. A dilute solution of local anesthetic to produce a skin wheal and infiltration of superficial tissue is administered subcutaneously at the midline. A 3-inch 22- or 25-gauge needle and stylet is introduced through the skin wheal at a slightly cephalad angle (10° to 30°). If the needle is beveled, the bevel should be sideways to facilitate entrance into the longitudinal dural fibers. After passing through the subcutaneous tissues, the needle will meet the supraspinous ligament, the interspinous ligament, and the ligamentum flavum. These ligaments are identified as increased resistance against the needle. A loss of resistance is felt at the epidural space, and a "pop" is felt as the needle punctures the dura and enters into the subarachnoid space. The stylet is withdrawn and free flowing CSF confirms proper placement. The needle should never be advanced without the stylet securely

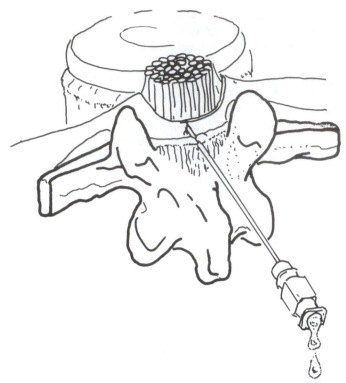

Figure 13–5 Spinal anesthesia

in place as this may cause inadvertent bone biopsy and subsequent clogging of the needle with bone tissue. Next the syringe of local anesthetic is attached to the spinal needle carefully so as not to dislodge it. A small amount of CSF withdrawn into the syringe at this point confirms that the needle has not been displaced. The local anesthetic should be injected slowly, and placement of the needle should be confirmed at least once by withdrawing a small amount of CSF into the syringe during the injection (Fig. 13–5).

The differences between 22- and 25-gauge needles for spinal anesthesia are clear. The 22-gauge needle carries a much higher risk of postspinal block headache. Younger people are much more susceptible to this phenomenon, so 22-gauge needles should be used only for older patients. The 22-gauge needles are stronger and less pliable than 25-gauge needles. Using 25-gauge needles can make it difficult to feel the resistance on the needle necessary for distinguishing the discrete tissue layers as the subarachnoid space is approached. Many clinicians use a short, large-bore 22- to 18-gauge needle as an introducer for the 25-gauge spinal needle. It is placed into the supraspinous ligament, and the 25-gauge spinal needle is placed through it to provide necessary stability. Finally, because of the small bore of the 25-gauge spinal needle, free-flowing CSF may not be as apparent and gentle aspiration with a syringe may be necessary to confirm placement. Still, most spinal anesthetics can be administered through a 25-gauge spinal needle and on younger patients it is usually the needle of choice.

Spinal anesthesia can also be administered using a paramedian approach bypassing the ligaments in the midline. The paramedian approach is especially useful for patients who cannot assume a good flexed position or have calcified liga-

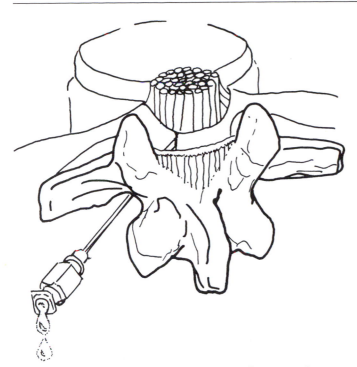

Figure 13–6   Spinal anesthesia paramedian approach

ments midline. The technique is the same as that for the midline approach but the needle is inserted lateral to the midline at the level of the spinous process below the interspace to be entered. The needle is then directed slightly cephalad and toward the midline bringing it into the ligamentum flavum, the epidural space, the dura, and the subarachnoid space where the local anesthetic can be administered (Fig. 13–6).

DURATION OF SPINAL BLOCKADE

The duration of spinal blockade is primarily determined by the specific local anesthetic used, the dosage chosen, and whether or not epinephrine is added to the solution.[1] The local anesthetics used for spinal anesthesia are procaine, lidocaine, tetracaine, and bupivacaine. Lidocaine and tetracaine are used most frequently. Local anesthetics vary in duration due to *lipophilic properties*. Tetracaine, which is highly lipophilic, has a duration of 60 to 90 minutes. Bupivacaine has a similar duration. Lidocaine, which is less lipophilic, has a duration of 45 to 60 minutes. Procaine, the least

lipophilic, lasts only 30 to 45 minutes. The use of epinephrine, 0.1 to 0.2 mL of a 1:1000 solution, adds to the duration of the local anesthetic by causing vasoconstriction in the area of administration. The constriction of nearby blood vessels limits systemic absorption of the local anesthetic by allowing it to bathe the nerve root for a longer period of time before it is absorbed into the systemic circulation. The use of epinephrine with a tetracaine spinal, for instance, increases the duration from 60 to 90 minutes to 120 to 180 minutes (see Table 13–1). Choosing the dosage of local anesthetic is important in determining duration as well as level of spinal blockade. Specifically, the larger doses are reserved for higher levels of blockade and longer surgeries. Another factor to consider when choosing dosage is the volume of the subarachnoid space or the height of the patient. A shorter person does not need as large a dose of local anesthetic as a tall person to achieve a similar level of spinal blockade.

LEVEL OF SPINAL BLOCKADE

The level of spinal blockade is primarily determined by the baricity of the solution and the position of the patient at the time of injection and for several minutes after.[1] Local anesthetics for spinal blocks are mixed with different types of solvents to create hyperbaric, hypobaric, and isobaric solutions. *Baricity* refers to the density of the local anesthetic solution relative to the density of the CSF.

Hyperbaric solutions are the most commonly used because of the widespread belief that they provide levels of spinal blockade that are predictable and easy to control. Hyperbaric solutions are prepared by mixing local anesthetic with 10% dextrose, which makes the solution heavier than the CSF. The solution will flow with gravity to the most dependent position in the subarachnoid space. In the supine position a hyperbaric spinal anesthetic solution administered above L-3 will spread cephalad to the T-6 area because of the spinal curvature. If the hyperbaric spinal solution is administered below L-3, it will spread caudad because of an opposite curve in the spine at this level (see Fig. 13–2). A slight head-up or head-down position will also aid in the spread of a hyperbaric solution to the desired level. In the sitting position, spread of a hyperbaric solution follows gravity in a caudad direction. The sitting position is effective for spinal blockade below L-2 to L-3, for instance, for anal, vaginal, or foot

Table 13–1
DURATION OF SPINAL BLOCKADE

Type of Local	Dosage for T-10 Level (mg)	Duration with Epinephrine (min)	Duration without Epinephrine (min)	Dosage for T-4 Level (mg)
Procaine 5%	100–150	60–75	30–45	150–200
Lidocaine 5%	30–50	60–90	45–60	75–100
Tetracaine 0.5%	6–10	120–180	60–90	12–16
Bupivacaine 0.5%	6–10	90	90	12–16

SOURCE: Adapted with permission from Stoelting RK, Miller RD. *Basics of Anesthesia*. 3rd ed. New York: Churchill Livingstone; 1994.

surgery. Hyperbaric solutions are also used for unilateral blocks such as hip surgery. In these instances spinal anesthetic is administered with the operative site down. The patient is then kept in this position for several minutes before being positioned for surgery.

Isobaric solutions are prepared by withdrawing CSF and mixing it with equal volumes of local anesthetic. This creates a solution that is equal in density to that of the CSF. The solution remains in the area that it was injected. Isobaric spinal blockade is useful because it can be administered in any position and the level will not be altered by moving the patient to the desired position required for surgery.

Hypobaric solutions are prepared by mixing sterile water with the local anesthetic. This creates a solution that is lighter than the CSF. Therefore, it will float to the least dependent area of the subarachnoid space. Patients having anal surgery in the jacknife position or unilateral hip surgery benefit from this technique. The spinal anesthetic is administered with the surgical site upward, and the patient does not have to be moved after the block is administered. The head needs to be maintained below the lumbar sacral area to avoid cephalic spread of the hypobaric solution. Less local anesthetic and greater volume (4 to 8 mL) are required for hypobaric solutions (Table 13–2).

COMMON COMPLICATIONS AND TREATMENT

Hypotension seen in spinal anesthesia is directly related to a decrease in sympathetic vascular tone occurring in the venous system to a greater extent than in the arteries. Venous return to the heart is decreased, causing a reduction in cardiac output and subsequent fall in blood pressure. The level of spinal blockade and the volume status of the patient will determine the severity of the hypotension. Treatment of hypotension consists of fluid replacement and positioning of the patient slightly head down. Sympathomimetics with both vasoconstrictor and positive inotropic effects such as ephedrine are also used. Care must be taken not to overhydrate because hemodilution can lower the hematocrit, compromising the myocardial oxygen supply.

Bradycardia can occur if there is a blockade of the cardiac accelerators that exit the cord at the T-1 to T-5 levels. Bradycardia is best treated with atropine.

Nausea is thought to be caused by hypotension severe enough to affect cerebral perfusion. Treatment with ephedrine usually corrects the problem. Another possible cause is unopposed vagal stimulation that occurs from the selective sympathetic blockade of the gastrointestinal tract. Atropine should be used to correct nausea of this origin. Backache caused directly from the administration of a spinal anesthetic is rare. It is usually caused by malpositioning of overrelaxed skeletal muscles and should be treated symptomatically.

Urinary retention after spinal anesthesia occurs because of the blockade of the nerves responsible for bladder control. It is usually a short-lived problem although administration of large amounts of fluids may distend the bladder, requiring catheterization before bladder function returns. Urinary retention is seen more commonly with spinal than with epidural anesthesia.

High spinal blockade is accompanied by severe hypoten-

Table 13–2
LEVEL OF SPINAL BLOCKADE

Level	Type of Surgery	Baricity of Solution	Position of Patient	Estimated Dosage
S-2 to S-5 (perineal)	Rectal surgery Hemorrhoidectomy	Hyperbaric	Sitting	Lidocaine 50 mg
S-2 to S-5 (perineal)	Rectal surgery Hemorrhoidectomy	Hypobaric	Jackknife (head down)	
L-2 to L-3 (knee)	Foot surgery	Hyperbaric	Sitting	Tetracaine 6 mg
L-1 (inguinal ligament)	Lower extremity	Hyperbaric	Sitting	Tetracaine 6 mg
T-10 (umbilicus)	Hip surgery	Hyperbaric	Operative side down	Lidocaine 50–75 mg
	Hip surgery	Hypobaric	Operative side up	
	TURP, prostate, vaginal delivery	Hyperbaric	Sitting or lateral decubitus for administration and supine immediately after	Tetracaine 6–10 mg
T-6 (xyphoid process)	Lower abdominal	Hyperbaric	Sitting or lateral decubitus for administration and supine immediately after or slight head down as tolerated	Lidocaine 75–100 mg
T-4 (nipple)	Upper abdominal	Hyperbaric	Sitting or lateral decubitus for administration and supine immediately after or slight head down as tolerated	Tetracaine 12–16 mg

TURP, transurethral resection of the prostate.
SOURCE: Adapted with permission from Stoelting RK, Miller RD. *Basics of Anesthesia.* 3rd ed. New York: Churchill Livingstone; 1994.

sion, nausea, difficulty breathing, or apnea and profound sensory and motor blockade. The patient may require respiratory and circulatory support and should be intubated and given fluid and vasopressors as needed.

Systemic toxicity from the local anesthetics is rare in spinal blocks because of the low dosages and small volumes that are used.

Postspinal headache can occur with spinal anesthesia although it is more common with accidental subarachnoid puncture during epidural anesthesia. When it occurs, the headache is severe and postural. Treatment is bed rest.

Hematoma causing nerve injury has been reported but is rare in patients with normal coagulation status.

CONTRAINDICATIONS

There are a few absolute contraindications to spinal anesthesia:

1. Any open sores or infected lesions at or very near the site of needle placement can increase the risk of infection intrathecally.
2. Increased intracranial pressure and any dural puncture carries the possibility of herniation of the brain.
3. Patients with blood clotting abnormalities or taking anticoagulants should not have spinal blocks because of the possibility of intrathecal hematoma formation with subsequent nerve damage.
4. Uncooperative, agitated patients or those who refuse spinal anesthesia should not undergo spinal blocks for obvious reasons.
5. Cardiovascular lesions such as aortic stenosis or idiopathic hypertrophic subaortic stenosis may contraindicate the use of spinal anesthesia depending on the severity of the disease. These patients often cannot tolerate the hypotension associated with a regional block.

☐ EPIDURAL BLOCK

TECHNIQUE

The midline approach is used most often for epidural anesthesia. It is generally easy to identify the midline ligaments and avoid the epidural veins that lie paramedially. Most commonly L2-3 or L3-4 interspaces are used. The patient is placed in the lateral decubitus or sitting position and is draped and prepped. Sterility is maintained. A skin wheal is made with a low-dose local anesthetic such as 1% or 2% lidocaine. Prepackaged sterile kits with all equipment necessary are available. An epidural needle is used to locate the epidural space. A 17- to 18-gauge Tuohy needle especially designed for this purpose is used. A Tuohy needle has a blunt tip designed to lessen the chance of dural puncture and a beveled opening on the side used to direct the epidural catheter cephalad or caudad. The needle and stylet are inserted through the skin wheal, through the supraspinous and interspinous ligaments, and into the ligamentum flavum. These structures are identified as increasing resistance against the needle. At this point the stylet is removed and a syringe is attached to the hub of the needle. (The needle should never be advanced without the stylet as this may lead to inadvertent bone biopsies if bone is encountered.) Resistance is checked by gentle pressure on the plunger or the syringe as the needle is advanced very slowly. As the needle passes through the ligamentum flavum and moves into the epidural space a distinct loss of resistance is felt. Air from the syringe is easily injected into the epidural space. Some anesthetists use the "hang drop" technique whereby entrance into the epidural space is confirmed by watching a drop of saline at the hub of the needle as it is sucked into the negative pressure of the epidural space. Once position of the needle is confirmed, a small amount of local anesthetic is injected through the needle to ensure the ease of injection found in the elastic epidural space. If a single-shot epidural is desired, 3 mL of local anesthetic is injected at this time as a test dose and then the total amount of local anesthetic required for the block is injected through the needle; the needle is withdrawn. If a catheter is being placed it should be threaded through the needle approximately 2 to 5 cm into the epidural space. The needle is withdrawn as the catheter is held in place with firm pressure. The catheter should never be pulled back through the needle because shearing of epidural catheters in the epidural space has been reported. Before injecting local anesthetic into the epidural space, a test dose is required. The test dose rules out placement of the catheter into an epidural vein or accidental puncture of the dura placing the catheter in the subarachnoid space (Fig. 13–7). If CSF is noted at any time, either through the epidural needle or through the catheter, the procedure needs to be repeated at a different interspace.

LOCAL ANESTHETICS USED

Many local anesthetics have been used successfully for epidural anesthesia. The most common drugs are chlorprocaine, lidocaine, and bupivacaine. Procaine and tetracaine are rarely used for epidural blocks because of their prolonged onset of action. Chlorprocaine has a relatively fast onset of action although its short duration limits its use for surgery. Lidocaine has an onset of action of 5 to 10 minutes and bupivacaine of 10 to 20 minutes. Generally, dosages required for epidural blocks are 1 to 1.5 mL of local anesthetic per segment to be blocked. Stronger concentrations of solutions and slightly greater volumes may be needed for solid motor blockade.

LEVEL AND DURATION

Unlike spinal blockade, the level of epidural blockade does not depend as much on position of the patient or the baricity of the solution given. Instead, level of epidural block depends on the dose, the volume, the concentration, whether or not epinephrine is used, and the actual level at which the

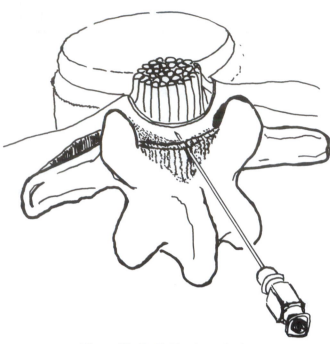

Figure 13–7 Epidural anesthesia

medication is injected.[1] If injected in the lumbar region, the medication tends to spread cephalad. Adequate volume (1 to 1.5 mL/segment) is required, and if high levels of block are necessary or specific levels desired, it may be more effective to administer the anesthetic at the thoracic or even the cervical level of the epidural space, remembering that the cord could be injured with dural puncture at these levels. Individual local anesthetics have varying duration. Nesacaine has a short duration, lidocaine is intermediate, and bupivacaine has the longest duration. As with spinal blocks, the use of epinephrine in the solution will extend the duration of the anesthetic. Duration of the anesthetic is not a major concern with epidural anesthesia because the epidural catheter allows continuous infusion or redosing as needed.

COMPLICATIONS AND TREATMENT

Hypotension associated with epidural blocks is similar in magnitude to that seen with spinal anesthesia but slower in onset so it may not be as profound in normovolemic patients. Ephedrine or Neosynephrine and fluids provide effective treatment as needed. *Nausea* presumably occurs because of hypotension and decreased cerebral blood flow. Resumption of normal blood pressure corrects the problem. *Urinary retention* occurs secondary to denervation of the bladder combined with filling from the extra fluids administered to maintain blood pressure. As with spinal blockade, catheterization may be necessary.

Postdural puncture headache (PDPH) occurs in many of the patients who receive an accidental dural puncture with a large-bone epidural needle. It is due to CSF leaking through the hole in the dura. As CSF pressure lowers, this results in

traction on meningeal nerves and vessels. It is always postural in nature and is exacerbated when the patient assumes the upright position. It often lasts a few days and can be treated with bed rest, analgesics, and fluids. Occasionally, however, it is persistent and incapacitating and requires an *epidural blood patch* to close the hole. An epidural needle is placed at the same level as the initial epidural and 10 to 15 mL of the patient's own blood is injected epidurally under sterile technique. The pain relief is usually instantaneous. Epidural blood patch is 90% to 95% successful in treating the PDPH.

High spinal and accidental intravascular injection of local anesthetic can occur with malplacement of epidural catheters and needles. Properly placed catheters can migrate even when taped securely. Each time local anesthetic is injected into an epidural catheter, negative aspiration of blood and CSF needs to be ensured. If an epidural vein is entered, the basic test dose of local anesthetic will produce *tinnitis* and *circumoral numbness* with a metallic taste. The large doses of local anesthetic required for epidural anesthesia will cause *seizures* and *cardiovascular collapse* if injected into an epidural vein. Treatment for accidental intravascular injection of local anesthetic is symptomatic. Typically the patient will experience neurologic symptoms such as tinnitis, slurred speech, confusion, and possible seizure activity. Benzodiazepines, which raise the seizure threshold, should be administered. Cardiovascular depression and total collapse can occur and resuscitative measures are taken as necessary. A local anesthetic with epinephrine added for a test dose helps rule out venous injection by causing an increase in heart rate and blood pressure within a few minutes after injection, which alerts the anesthetist to the problem.

If the catheter migrates through the dura and into the subarachnoid space, the test dose of 2 to 4 mL of local anesthetic would cause sensory and motor blockade within 3 to 5 minutes. The large doses of local anesthetic required for epidural anesthesia injected into the subarachnoid space would cause high spinal blockade with sympathetic disruption requiring vasopressors and cardiac and respiratory support. When administering a test dose, 3 to 4 mL of local anesthetic injected into the proper epidural space should not cause any sensory, motor, or cardiovascular symptoms at all. Unlike spinal anesthesia, the large volumes and high doses of local anesthetics used for epidural anesthesia cause some systemic absorption of local anesthestic. For instance, it is not uncommon to see increases in heart rate if a local anesthetic with epinephrine is used for a long period of time. Generally speaking, systemic absorption of local anesthetics through a properly placed epidural catheter is not enough to cause toxicity.

Contraindications for epidural anesthesia are the same as those listed for spinal anesthesia.

☐ CAUDAL BLOCK

Occasionally it is difficult to achieve adequate analgesia in the S-1 to S-2 region from a lumbar epidural. Connective tissue covering the nerve roots at this level may be the cause of the ineffective blockade. Some anesthetists prefer to administer a caudal block to achieve anesthesia for rectal and genital surgery and for the final stages of labor. The caudal space is an extension of the epidural space.

TECHNIQUE

The patient is placed in the prone or lateral decubitus position. The lower sacral vertebrae are fused, so a caudal anesthetic must be administered through the sacral hiatus. The sacral cornu are located about 5 cm above the coccyx, and the sacral hiatus is a midline opening between the cornu. A $1\frac{1}{2}$ - to 2-inch needle is inserted perpendicularly through the skin into the sacral hiatus until it meets the coccygeal ligament. At this point the needle is lowered to a 45° angle. Further advancement will bring the needle into the sacral canal. The canal can be identified by a distinct pop and loss of resistance. The needle is further advanced until it meets the sacrum. Then the needle is withdrawn slightly and redirected at an angle parallel to the skin. It is inserted 1 to 2 cm into the canal. The dural sac extends to S-2 in most adults but can extend lower, so careful aspiration for CSF and blood is necessary. Larger doses of local anesthetic may be required caudally.[1]

☐ PEDIATRIC REGIONAL

CONSIDERATIONS

Administering regional anesthesia to the pediatric patient requires a knowledge of the anatomical variances, drug dosages, indications, and contraindications for this method. In the child, *minimal hemodynamic* response will be seen with a regional induced sympathectomy. Hypotension is rarely encountered until the age of eight.

When choosing a regional anesthetic, patients will offer little or no assistance in determining whether or not the block is adequate, so *loss of motor ability* and *lack of reaction* to painful stimulus is conclusive. (Not infrequently, a regional anesthetic will be administered after general anesthesia is induced.) Because the spinal cord ends at a higher level in the pediatric patient, needle entry site may differ.

When choosing a regional technique for the pediatric patient, whether direct local infiltration, nerve block, or epidural or SAB, the utmost care must be given to proper doses of local anesthetics and epinephrine and to maximum levels.

Advantages to pediatric regional include use in high-risk premature infants where postoperative apnea is a concern. This assumes intraoperative sedation is avoided. As stated, infants are relatively free from hemodynamic side effects. Other advantages include a decreased sympathetic stress response to surgery and postoperative pain management. No longer is it an accepted belief that pediatric patients experience less pain than adults. Disadvantages include block failure, inability to hold child in quiet position for administra-

tion, and postoperative respiratory depression with epidural or intrathecal narcotics. The most serious potential complication is an intravascular injection.

Contraindications are the same as with adults, and also include parent refusal. Any preexisting condition such as spina bifida, meningocele, hydrocephalus, and other neurological disorders may preclude the use of spinal or epidural anesthesia.[2,3]

CAUDAL

The caudal epidural space requires relatively large volumes of anesthetic agent. Therefore, careful monitoring should be available and toxic dosages must be familiar to the anesthetist. This technique is appropriate for surgical procedures on the lower extremities in addition to those below the umbilicus, such as herniorrhaphies. (See the section in this chapter on caudal anesthesia.) Urinary retention is possible. The general dosage is 0.25% bupivacaine 1mL/kg or 1.0% xylocaine 1mL/kg.[2,3]

EPIDURAL

As with adults, the midline approach is most common. Positioning can be sitting or lateral decubitus. Because the spinal cord ends lower in children less than one year, the L4 to L5 or L5 to S1 interspace is preferred. The epidural space can be identified as the needle meets increased resistance at the ligamentum flavum (though considerably more subtle in children than adults), followed by a sudden loss of resistance as the epidural space is entered. Thoracic epidural, though unusual, may also be administered following the same technique as with adults. The depth from skin to epidural space is less than that of the adult and varies with age. Upper limit dosages are 3–5 mg/kg of bupivacaine and 7–10 mg/kg of lidocaine. A test dose with epinephrine is recommended to rule out intravascular injection.[2,3]

SPINAL

Intrathecal administration of anesthesia is particularly useful in the high-risk premature infant. Infants have CSF volume doubled from that of adults, 4mL/kg as compared to 2mL/kg. When administering a spinal, anesthetic dosages must be adjusted for the *shorter duration* of action seen in the pediatric patient. In the premature infant, spinal lidocaine lasts no longer than 45 minutes and bupivacaine lasts 60 to 75 minutes. Dosages are based on weight. See Table 13-3. Spinal anesthesia is administered in either the sitting or lateral decubitus position.[2,3] In infants, a 22-gauge, 1.5-inch spinal needle can be used, while in older children a 25-gauge needle is appropriate.

☐ PERIPHERAL NERVE BLOCKS

Peripheral nerve blocks provide an opportunity for profound sensory and motor blockade directed at a specific area of the

Table 13–3
SPINAL ANESTHESIA DOSAGES*

Weight	Bupivacaine (0.5%)	Tetracaine (1%)	Lidocaine (5%)
<5 kg	0.5mg/kg	0.5mg/kg	2.5mg/kg
5–15 kg	0.4mg/kg	0.4mg/kg	2mg/kg
>15 kg	0.3mg/kg	0.3mg/kg	1.5mg/kg

*Dosages based on hyperbaric solution.

body. Knowledge of anatomy, location of nerve plexi, and distribution of distal branches is necessary for successful blockade. Time is involved to administer successful peripheral nerve blocks, and cooperation of the patient is often necessary. As with all regional anesthetic techniques an intravenous line should be placed prior to blockade and adequate resuscitation equipment should be readily available.

TECHNIQUE

Several techniques are used to ensure proper placement of the needle for peripheral nerve blocks. Often it is necessary to elicit paresthesia. A cooperative patient is able to verbalize proper needle placement after experiencing the paresthesia that occurs as the needle passes through the peripheral distribution of a nerve. Injection involves placement of a needle into the sheath surrounding the nerve and not the nerve tissue itself. If a patient complains of immediate and excruciating pain with injection of only a small amount of local anesthetic, chances are the needle is in direct contact with the nerve and needs to be pulled back slightly. Bony landmarks can also serve to identify nerves that lay adjacent. Often it is only necessary to place the needle on a bony prominence to anesthetize the nerve. Loss of resistance as the needle meets the sheath of the nerve and passes through it can provide positive feedback to the experienced anesthetist of proper needle placement for nerve block. Nerves can also be located adjacent to arteries, so aortic pulsations, or needles actually passing through an artery, can confirm proper needle placement. Direct stimulation by low-voltage nerve stimulators provides objective confirmation of needle position near the nerve and are used successfully by many clinicians.

CERVICAL PLEXUS BLOCK

Anatomy The cervical plexus is formed via communicating nerves originating from C-1 to C-4 vertebrae. The deep cervical plexus passes under the vertebral artery and forms the paravertebral region of the second, third, and fourth cervical vertebrae. These nerves supply cutaneous dermatomes through the lesser occipital, greater auricular, and suprascapular nerves.[4] These nerves also supply motor function to the skeletal muscles of the neck and the phrenic nerve. For surgery on subcutaneous layers only, it is possible to do a superficial cervical plexus block. The superficial

branches of the cervical plexus merge about midway and posterior along the sternocleidomastoid muscle. Injection of local anesthetic to these superficial branches provides analgesia to the C-2, C-3, and C-4 dermatomes. A superficial cervical plexus block will anesthetize the skin of the neck, the base of the skull and mandible, and the shoulder and clavical areas.[4] Superficial cervical plexus blocks do not give muscle relaxation. Deep cervical plexus blocks are therefore used for procedures such as carotid endarterectomy. Here profound skeletal muscle relaxation of the neck is achieved while an awake patient, through ongoing communication, alerts the surgeon to problems with blood flow to the brain during carotid manipulation.

Technique Two techniques are commonly used to administer deep cervical plexus blocks. The classic three-needle technique is performed with the patient supine on the table with the face turned away from the anesthetist. The cornu of the transverse process of the second, third, and fourth cervical vertebrae are identified. They lie just posterior to a line drawn between the tip of the mastoid process and the point of insertion of the sternocleidomastoid muscle on the clavical. About 1 inch below the mastoid process, a skin wheal is made. A 2-inch needle is inserted over the cornu of C-2, which is about $\frac{1}{2}$ to $1\frac{1}{2}$ inches medial depending on the thickness of the neck tissue. A slight caudad direction prevents the needle from popping through the vertebra into the epidural or subarachnoid space. Local anesthetic, 3 to 5 mL, is injected. Care must be taken to ensure aspiration is negative for CSF or blood, remembering the vertebral artery is nearby. Next, needles are inserted similarly $\frac{1}{2}$ to 1 inch apart to locate cervical plexus nerves at the C-3 and C-4 levels (Fig. 13–8). The most superficial contact with the bone is the cornu. Needles can also come in contact with the more distal transverse processes next to the cornus. Local anesthetic injected here can cause an unsuccessful cervical plexus block.

The single-needle technique uses the same positioning and bony landmarks; however, only the C-3 or C-4 level transverse process is located and 8 to 10 mL of local anesthetic is injected here. Because the bulk of the cervical plexus is located here, a large amount of local anesthetic injected will cause a deep block. Again, careful aspiration for CSF and blood is necessary prior to injection.[4]

For superficial cervical plexus blocks the patient is placed in the supine position and the head is turned away. The sternocleidomastoid muscle is identified by asking the patient to raise his head against slight resistance. A skin wheal is raised midway and posterior to the muscle. Local anesthetic solution, 10 mL, is administered through a 2-inch needle as it is advanced 1 or 2 inches superior and inferior along the edge of the muscle.[4]

Drugs Used Choice of local anesthetic largely depends on the personal preference of the anesthetist, the type and duration of anesthesia required, and physical status of the patient. Lidocaine, Marcaine, mepivacaine, and various combinations have all been used successfully. As with all local

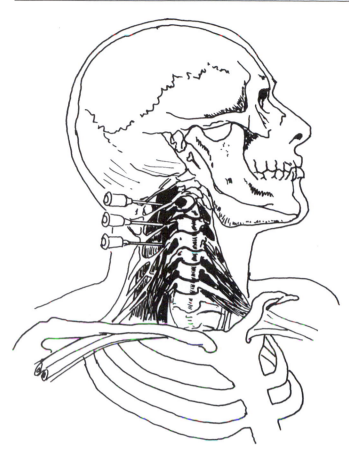

Figure 13–8   Cervical plexus block

anesthetics, the addition of epinephrine prolongs the duration of the cervical plexus block. Because of the relatively small volume of local anesthetic used in cervical plexus blocks, maximum safe dosages do not apply.

Complications   Complications from cervical plexus block occur when the needle is accidently placed into the vertebral artery or into the cervical epidural or cervical subarachnoid space. If local anesthetic is injected intra-arterially, systemic toxic convulsion occurs. As with any intravascular toxic reaction to local anesthesia, 100% oxygen is administered and, if necessary, control of the airway is maintained. Barbiturates or benzodiazepines are administered as needed. If epidural or subarachnoid injection occurs, the complications include high or total spinal anesthesia; cardiovascular and ventilatory support may be indicated. Deep cervical plexus blockade can produce *Horner's syndrome* (ptosis, enophthalmos, miosis, and anhidrosis) and hoarseness can occur if the recurrent laryngeal nerve is blocked.

Contraindications   If motor-blocking concentrations of local anesthetic are used, the phrenic nerve can be blocked. The diaphragm is only innervated in the center by the phrenic nerve and laterally by the intercostal nerves. Patients with well-developed intercostals usually are not bothered by

unilateral phrenic nerve paralysis. Patients who depend on phrenic nerve innervation of the diaphragm for respiration may be compromised by cervical plexus blocks. Therefore, cervical plexus blocks are contraindicated in patients with high level cord injury or severe respiratory compromise.

BRACHIAL PLEXUS BLOCK

Anatomy   The brachial plexus and its branches innervate the upper extremities. It originates from the anterior rami of C-5 to C-8 and T-1. The nerves are located paravertebrally at these levels. They join together between the anterior and middle scalene muscles, and then pass over to the first rib and under the midpoint of the clavicle on the way to the apex of the axilla.[1] The three most common ways to administer brachial plexus blocks are by the interscalene, supraclavicular, and axillary approaches.

Technique
Interscalene
The interscalene approach to the brachial plexus block can be used to provide anesthesia from the shoulder level to the hand. The object is to reach the nerve roots of the brachial plexus in the groove between the middle and anterior scalene muscles. The patient is placed supine, head turned away. The groove is then identified. It is located laterally from the cricoid cartilage at the C-6 level. The lateral edge of the sternocleidomastoid is identified at the C-6 level. The fingers are moved laterally until they roll onto the anterior scalene muscle. If the fingers move more laterally still, at the C-6 level, the groove between the anterior and middle scalene muscles will be appreciated as a slight depression. A skin wheal is made and a needle is inserted into the groove between the muscles. The needle is directed parallel to the muscles and at a right angle to the skin in a slight caudad direction. The anesthetist advances the needle $\frac{1}{2}$ to 1 inch deep, redirecting slightly until paresthesia is apparent to the patient. Remember, the transverse process is superficial at the C-6 level. Any paresthesia of the shoulder and upper arm confirms placement in the brachial plexus. After careful aspiration, negative for CSF and blood, 30 to 40 mL of local anesthetic is injected. Horner's syndrome can occur and often some degree of phrenic nerve paralysis is apparent. If surgery is planned on the upper levels of the arm and below, the patient can be placed at a 45° angle and pressure with the fingertips applied at the C-4 or C-5 transverse processes to avoid cephalad spread to the cervical plexus. If surgery is planned on the shoulder joint itself, cephalad spread can be encouraged with the patient remaining supine, allowing the cervical plexus to be blocked also.[4] (Fig. 13–9).

Supraclavicular
The supraclavicular approach is designed to reach the brachial plexus as it passes over the first rib and under the midpoint of the clavicle. The patient is positioned supine. The landmarks that need to be identified are the clavicle, the

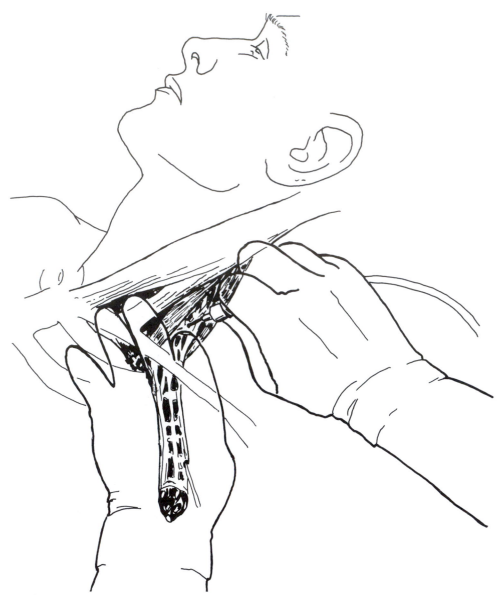

Figure 13–9   Interscalene approach to brachial plexus block

anterior and midscalene muscles, the subclavian artery, and the first rib. The midpoint of the clavicle is identified by an attempt to locate the subclavian artery. The subclavian artery lies in the middle of the clavicle, between the midscalene and anterior scalene muscles. A needle is inserted between the muscles and directed toward the subclavian artery. It is advanced slowly until paresthesia is elicited, or a depth of $1\frac{1}{2}$ inches is reached. If no paresthesia is identified and no rib or artery is encountered, then the landmarks should be reevaluated. After proper placement, 15 to 25 mL of local anesthetic solution is injected.[4] Pleural cavity entrance and pneumothorax are the most common complications with a 1% occurrence even in the most skilled hands. Phrenic nerve paralysis can occur. Absolute contraindications are rare but patients with severe chronic obstructive pulmonary disease may not be the best candidates for supraclavicular blocks because of increased risk of pneumothorax.

Axillary

The axillary approach to brachial plexus block attempts to reach the brachial plexus by perivascular infiltration of the axillary sheath. It provides good anesthesia to the forearm and hand. The axillary sheath surrounds the neurovascular complex of the axilla. The patient is placed supine with the arm extended to 90° or placed behind the head. The axillary artery is identified and compressed. A $1\frac{1}{2}$-inch needle is inserted as high up into the axilla as possible just over the compressed artery, and a skin wheal is made. The needle is then directed toward the artery. As it enters the nerve sheath a popping sensation is noted and pulsations can be felt through the needle. Some clinicians attempt to elicit paresthesia at this point. Paresthesia at the wrist or fingers indicates median and ulnar nerve contact. After careful aspiration, 30 to 40 mL of local anesthetic is injected slowly. An alternative technique uses the axillary artery as a landmark. It is palpated and the needle is allowed to pass through the artery, confirmed by aspiration of blood, and 15 to 20 mL of local anesthetic is administered just posterior to the artery when aspiration of blood becomes negative. The needle is then pulled back out through the artery, and the additional 15 to 20 mL of local anesthetic is administered just superficial to the artery. Careful aspiration of blood into the syringe and then aspirating negative for blood is necessary to avoid intravascular injection.[4]

The musculocutaneous nerve exits the axillary sheath just proximal to the injection of local anesthetic during axillary blocks. It innervates the radial side of the forearm and is often missed with axillary block anesthetics. Digital pressure applied over the site of injection for several minutes can help the spread of local to reach the nerve. The nerve can be blocked directly, also, as it emerges below the biceps and brachialis muscles proximal to the elbow crease. Injecting a small amount of local anesthetic subcutaneously proximally and medially in the axilla blocks the intercostal brachial nerve, which innervates the skin in the axilla and medial border of the arm allowing analgesia for application of a tourniquet.[1]

Drugs Used As with other peripheral nerve blocks, the choice of local anesthetics and dosages for brachial plexus blocks are determined by the personal preference of the anesthetist, the type and duration of anesthesia required, and the physical status of the patient.

When administering the large doses of local anesthetic needed for brachial plexus blocks, care must be taken not to exceed maximum allowable doses. Procaine can be used up to 7 mg/kg, and lidocaine 1% to 2% up to 4.5 mg/kg. Chlorprocaine can be administered in doses up to 20 mg/kg due to rapid hydrolysis by pseudocholinesterase.[5]

Complications and Contraindications Complications resulting from brachial plexus blocks involve accidental epidural or spinal injection, and intra-arterial injection of large amounts of local anesthetic. Resuscitative equipment should be available. It is important to remember that large amounts of local anesthetic are required for brachial plexus block and signs of systemic toxicity need to be recognized. Horner's syndrome, blockage of the recurrent laryngeal nerve, and phrenic nerve paralysis can occur, and therefore brachial plexus blocks may be contraindicated in patients who depend on phrenic nerve function to maintain respiration.

☐ INTERCOSTAL NERVE BLOCKS

ANATOMY

Twelve pairs of intercostal nerves innervate the intercostal and abdominal wall skeletal muscles and the skin of the abdominal wall. Intercostal nerve blocks are generally reserved for postoperative pain control after thoracic or abdominal surgery, intercostal pain as with rib fracture, and neuritic

conditions (e.g., herpes) in the area. Intercostal nerve blocks in conjunction with other blocks are necessary if surgical anesthesia is required. The intercostal nerves T-1 to T-12 follow a circumferential path around each rib, inferiorly. The nerves are a part of a bundle containing nerve, vein, and artery. The lateral cutaneous branches of the nerves that innervate anterior and laterally come off at the midaxillary line. Therefore, a posterior approach is effective in reaching these nerves.

TECHNIQUE

The patient is positioned prone. The nerves are best blocked 6 to 8 cm laterally from the midline. The arms are placed above the head allowing for access to the ribs at T-4 to T-6 levels if necessary. A skin wheal is made at the site. A 22-gauge short bevel 4-cm needle is inserted until it meets the periosteum. Then it is redirected caudally and walked off the inferior border of the rib until it enters the intercostal muscle. A loss of resistance confirms placement and the needle is advanced 3 to 5 mm. After negative aspiration for blood, 3 to 5 mL local is injected. The technique is repeated at other ribs to achieve the desired level of intercostal blockade (Fig. 13–10).

DRUGS AND DOSAGES

Many drugs have been used successfully in intercostal nerve blocks and the choice depends on the individual preference of the clinician. Local anesthetics of longer duration are used for postoperative pain relief.

COMPLICATIONS AND CONTRAINDICATIONS

Intercostal nerve blocks provide greater systemic absorption and higher circulating blood levels of local anesthetic than any other nerve block. Toxic levels of local anesthetic can occur and manifest in the form of convulsions. Pneumothorax is also a possibility because of the proximity of the pleural space to the intercostal nerves. Patients with severe respiratory compromise may not be able to tolerate the loss of the intercostal muscle groups, and intercostal nerve blocks may be contraindicated in these patients.

☐ LOWER EXTREMITY BLOCKS

ANATOMY

The lower extremities are innervated from the sciatic nerve originating in the sacral plexus and the group of nerves that originate from the lumbar plexus, the femoral, the obturator, and the lateral femoral cutaneous. These nerves are located far from each other as they enter the thigh, and many clinicians prefer to administer epidural or spinal anesthesia rather than to block many individual nerves. It is possible to block the whole lumbar plexus, and in that case a separate block is

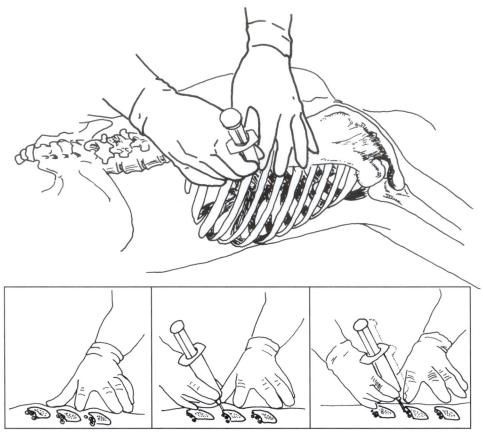

Figure 13–10   Intercostal nerve block

necessary if the sciatic nerve is also to be anesthetized. Drugs and dosages for lower extremity blocks depend on the personal preference of the anesthetist.

SPECIFIC BLOCKS

Sciatic Nerve Block   The sciatic nerve is the largest nerve in the body and it originates from L-4 to L-5 and S-1, S-2, and S-3. The sciatic nerve innervates the lateral aspect of the foot and the lateral three toes as it divides into the tibial and common peroneal nerves. If combined with a femoral nerve block, it can be used for surgery below the knee.[4] The sympathetic fibers are located along the sciatic nerve and therefore sciatic nerve block is also used for pain diagnosis and therapy.

The patient is placed in the lateral decubitus position, the side to be blocked upward. A line is drawn between the greater trochanter and the posterior iliac spine. Midway between the line and 5 cm caudad, a skin wheal is raised. A needle is inserted perpendicular to the skin until paresthesia occurs. Paresthesia to the thigh confirms close proximity to the sciatic nerve but paresthesia to the lower leg or foot (slightly deeper in) is mandatory. For adequate sciatic blockade 10 to 15 mL of local anesthetic is injected.

The nerve should not be probed excessively because this could lead to damage. Hematoma formation is also a possibility and should be treated symptomatically.

Femoral Nerve Block   The femoral nerve originates in the lumbar plexus by the posterior divisions of L-2, L-3, and L-4. It provides innervation to the muscle of the anterior thigh and the quadraceps and the skin of the anterior thigh. It continues down to form the saphenous nerve, which supplies the extremity below the knee. Combined with the sciatic nerve block it can be used for surgery below the knee.

Landmarks are the femoral artery and the inguinal ligament. The patient is placed supine. The femoral artery is located and palpated as it passes below the inguinal ligament. A needle is inserted and a skin wheal is raised just lateral to the femoral artery just below the inguinal ligament. A loss of resistance is felt and paresthesia is elicited. If no paresthesia occurs, 15 mL of local anesthetic is injected medially and laterally. If paresthesia occurs, 8 to 10 mL of local anesthetic is enough to provide a block.[4]

A possible complication is accidental vascular injection in the groin area. Cardiovascular support and airway protection are used as needed.

Lateral Femoral Cutaneous Block   The lateral femoral cutaneous nerve arises from the L-2 and L-3 levels. It supplies only sensory innervation from the proximal lateral thigh down to the knee. It is blocked primarily for pain control from paresthesia in the area.

The patient is placed supine. The identifying landmarks are the anterior superior iliac spine and the inguinal ligament. About 2 cm medial and just inferior to the inguinal ligament a needle is inserted and a skin wheal is raised. The needle is advanced 1 to $1\frac{1}{2}$ inches perpendicular to the skin and paresthesia is obtained. Five to 8 mL of local anesthetic is injected. The lateral femoral cutaneous block is usually used in conjunction with other lower extremity blocks. It can be used for muscle biopsies and tourniquet discomfort.

Obturator Nerve Block   The obturator nerve arises from the ventral branches of L-2, L-3, and L-4. It supplies the motor nerves of the adductor muscle of the thigh. There is a branch to the hip and a cutaneous branch that varies in its innervation of the lower, medial border of the thigh. It is used to diagnose hip joint pain and in conjunction with sciatic and femoral nerve blocks for surgery of the knee.

The patient is placed supine. A skin wheal is placed 1 inch lateral and inferior to the pubic tubercle. The area is infiltrated with several milliliters of local anesthetic because this can be a painful block to administer. A 3-inch needle is then inserted until the pubic bone is touched. It is withdrawn slightly and directed cephalad and lateral. Ten to 15 mL of local is administered. Successful block causes paresis of the abductor muscles.[1] Complications occur with systemic injection of local anesthetic into the vascular pubic area. Other complications include failed block and discomfort during insertion.

☐ ANKLE BLOCKS

ANATOMY

An ankle block refers to anesthetizing the nerves supplying the foot as they cross at the ankle. These nerves include the superficial and deep peroneal, the sural, the posterior tibial, and the saphenous. The tibial, sural, and peroneal nerves are all branches of the sciatic nerve. The saphenous is the terminal branch of the femoral nerve. The posterior tibial and the sural nerves are located posteriorly on the ankle, and the peroneal and saphenous nerves are located anteriorly.

SPECIFIC BLOCKS

Posterior Tibial Nerve Block   At the ankle, the tibial nerve arises between the Achilles tendon and the medial malleolus. It divides here into the medial and plantar nerves. It supplies the skin of the toes 1 through 4, and sensation to the medial side of the sole of the foot. The posterior tibial nerve is found by locating the posterior tibial artery, which lies just anterior to the nerve. The patient is either prone or lateral. The artery is located and the needle is inserted, posterior and lateral to the artery at the level of the medial malleolus. Local anesthetic, 5 mL, is injected here. Paresthesia may be elicited before bone is contacted. If no paresthesia occurs, the needle is withdrawn from the bone approximately $\frac{1}{2}$ inch, and 5 mL of local anesthetic is injected (Fig. 13–11).

Sural Nerve Block   The sural nerve is a branch of the posterior tibial nerve. It is located behind the lateral malleolus

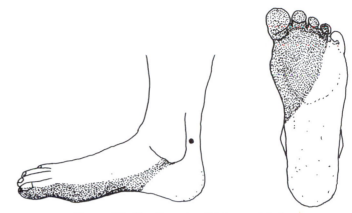

Figure 13–11   Posterior tibial nerve block

and between the lateral malleolus and the Achilles tendon. It provides skin sensation on the posterior lateral heel and lateral aspect of the foot to the base of the toe. To block the sural nerve, a needle is inserted just lateral to the Achilles tendon and directed to the posterior surface of the lateral malleolus. Paresthesia should occur. If not, bone is located and 5 mL of local anesthetic is injected on the way out[4] (Fig. 13–12).

Superficial Peroneal and Saphenous Nerve Blocks   The saphenous and superficial peroneal nerves are responsible for supply to the dorsum of the foot. The saphenous nerve can be accessed just anterior to the medial malleolus. The superficial peroneal nerves run along the lateral part of a line drawn joining the medial and lateral malleoli.

The patient is supine and local anesthetic is injected across the dorsum of the foot from the medial to the lateral malleolus (Fig. 13–13).

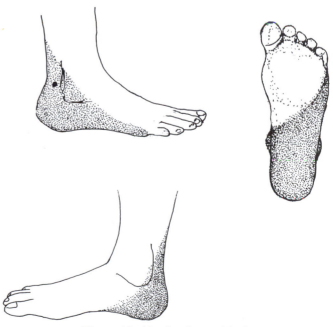

Figure 13–12   Sural nerve block

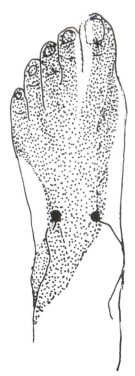

Figure 13–13 Superficial peroneal and saphaneous nerve block

Deep Peroneal Nerve   The deep peroneal nerve supplies the area of the skin between the first and second toes and the extensor muscles of the tarsal and metatarsal joints.

The deep peroneal nerve is accessed by locating the tibialis anterior tendon and the anterior tibial artery. At the level of the medial malleolus, the deep peroneal nerve lies lateral to the artery and medial to the tendon. A needle is inserted here, and 5 to 8 mL is injected. Paresthesia may or may not be elicited (Fig. 13–14).

Complications encountered with nerve blocks in the ankle are few and generally not significant. Occasionally it is difficult to get the desired levels of anesthesia, and alternative choices of anesthesia should be available. Epinephrine

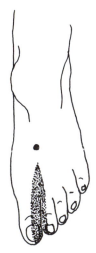

Figure 13–14 Deep peroneal nerve bloc

should *not* be added because of the possibility of severe vasoconstriction and ischemia to the small arteries of the foot.

☐ INTRAVENOUS REGIONAL ANESTHESIA

Intravenous regional anesthesia, or Bier block, as it is commonly referred to, is a relatively easy, very effective means of providing anesthesia to an arm or a leg for short surgical procedures.

TECHNIQUE

An intravenous line is placed in the limb that is to be anesthetized. The arm or leg is exsanguinated. A tourniquet is applied to the limb proximal to the site of surgery and is inflated to 50 mm Hg above the systolic pressure. The limb is then injected through the intravenous line with a weak concentration of local anesthetic, 25 to 55 mL for the arm and 100 to 200 mL for the leg. A double tourniquet can be used to cover the tourniquet pain. A second tourniquet more proximal than the first is applied and inflated first. When the patient begins to complain of tourniquet pain, the distal tourniquet closer to the operative site and over a now anesthetized part of the arm is inflated and the other one is deflated.

CHOICE OF DRUGS

Optimal choices of local anesthetics for intravenous regional block are drugs that carry a low risk for toxicity with systemic absorption. Common local anesthetics used are 0.5% lidocaine or prilocaine. Chlorprocaine is not used because of a hypothesized risk of thromboembolism, and bupivacaine is not recommended because of the irreversible effects of toxic systemic absorption.[5]

COMPLICATIONS

The biggest risk with intravenous regional anesthesia is systemic absorption of the intravenous administration of local anesthetics. This can occur when the tourniquet is deflated and local anesthetic enters the systemic circulation. A full 20 minutes of tourniquet time decreases this risk. Many anesthetists will deflate the tourniquet slowly or intermittently to avoid large boluses of local anesthetic. In reality the systemic absorption generally does not produce clinically significant complications. Still, cardiovascular complications can occur, usually in the form of bradycardia. Contraindications exist for very obese patients where a tourniquet cannot be applied effectively and diabetic patients with peripheral nerve damage where a tourniquet can further injure the nerves. It is wise to avoid oversedating the patient before injection so the patient can warn of systemic absorption of local anesthetic.

REFERENCES

1. Stoelting RK, Miller RD. *Basics of Anesthesia*. 3rd ed. New York: Churchill Livingston; 1994.
2. Dalens BJ. Regional anesthesia in children. In: Miller RD, ed. *Anesthesia*. Vol. 2, 4th ed. New York: Churchill Livingstone; 1994:1565–1594.
3. Martin TW. The pediatric patient. In: Kirby RR, ed. *Clinical Anesthesia Practice*. Philadelphia: WB Saunders; 1994: 1060–1061.
4. Katz J. *Atlas of Regional Anesthesia*. East Norwalk, Conn: Appleton & Lange; 1993.
5. Hardman JG, Goodman Gilman A, Limbird LE. *The Pharmacological Basis of Therapeutics*. 9th ed. New York: McGraw-Hill; 1996.

☐ QUESTIONS

1. The spinal cord ends at L-1 to L-2 in the _____?
   a. Average adult
   b. Child
   c. Premature infant

2. Of the three types of nerves to be blocked during spinal anesthesia, which is the last to return to normal function?
   a. Sympathetic
   b. Sensory
   c. Motor

3. Of the three types of nerves blocked by spinal anesthesia, _____ is blocked two levels higher than _____, which is two levels higher than _____.
   a. Sensory, motor, sympathetic
   b. Sympathetic, sensory, motor
   c. Motor, sympathetic, sensory

4. What two factors are most important in determining the level of spinal blockade?
   a. Dosage of local anesthetic chosen and patient's position
   b. Baricity of the solution and position of patient at time of injection
   c. Size of the patient and baricity of solution
   d. Position and size of the patient

5. When doing rectal or vaginal surgery in the lithotomy position what is the best choice of local anesthetic?
   a. Tetracaine hyperbaric in the sitting position
   b. Lidocaine hypobaric in the lateral position
   c. Lidocaine isobaric in the sitting position

6. Why does epinephrine added to a local anesthetic increase the duration of action of the drug?
   a. Causes local vasodilatation thereby increasing systemic absorption of the drug
   b. Changes the pH of the solution thereby decreasing systemic absorption of the drug
   c. Causes local vasoconstriction of blood vessels thereby decreasing systemic absorption
   d. Causes local vasodilatation thereby decreasing systemic absorption

7. Bradycardia after spinal blockade is most likely due to:
   a. Vagal stimulation secondary to vasodilatation
   b. Calcium channel blockade directly in the myocardium
   c. High level of spinal anesthesia affecting the cardiac accelerators T-1 to T-5
   d. Myocardial depression resulting from local toxicity

8. Urinary retention is seen more frequently after spinal anesthesia than epidural anesthesia. True or False?
   a. True
   b. False

9. Which local anesthetic has the shortest duration?
   a. Lidocaine
   b. Bupivacaine
   c. Tetracine
   d. Procaine

10. What is the shortest-acting local anesthetic?
    a. Chlorprocaine
    b. Lidocaine
    c. Bupivacaine
    d. Tetracaine

11. Which is *not* a treatment for postdural puncture headache?
    a. Fluids
    b. Steroid administration
    c. Flat bed rest
    d. Blood patch

12. What is the initial volume of local anesthetic required for epidural anesthesia?
    a. 3 to 4 mL per dermatome
    b. 4 to 5 mL per dermatome
    c. 1 to 1.5 mL per dermatome
    d. 2 to 3 mL per dermatome

13. Superficial cervical plexus block can be used for carotid endarterectomy surgery. True or False?
    a. True
    b. False

14. During deep cervical plexus block, hoarseness occurs if what nerve is blocked?
    a. Recurrent laryngeal nerve
    b. Superior laryngeal nerve
    c. Internal laryngeal nerve
    d. Inferior laryngeal nerve

15. Which is *not* a common way to administer a brachial plexus block?
    a. Intercostal
    b. Interscalene
    c. Supraclavicular
    d. Axillary

16. What is the maximum amount of lidocaine without epinephrine that can be administered during anesthetic blocks?
    a. 2 mg/kg
    b. 3.5 mg/kg
    c. 4.5 mg/kg
    d. 10 mg/kg

17. Which type of block allows for the greatest systemic absorption of local anesthesia?
    a. Cervical plexus block
    b. Epidural block
    c. Brachial plexus block
    d. Intercostal nerve block

18. When doing peripheral nerve blocks, what symptom would you expect to see with a direct intraneural injection?
    a. Total paralysis of the nerve injected
    b. Seizure
    c. Tinnitus and circumoral numbness
    d. Immediate and excruciating pain on injection of only a small amount of local anesthetic

19. What area of the foot is blocked with a successful posterior tibial nerve block?
    a. Skin of toes 1 to 4 and sensation to the medial side of the sole of the foot.
    b. Posterior lateral heel, lateral aspect of the base of toe
    c. Dorsum of the foot
    d. Skin between the first and second toe and the extensor muscle of the tarsal and metatarsal joints

20. Which scenario could safely use intravenous regional anesthesia?
    a. 5-minute procedure for removal of infected nail
    b. Severely obese patient undergoing procedure on forearm
    c. 25-minute procedure of finger
    d. Brittle diabetic for amputation of infected finger

☐ ANSWERS

1. a	**5.** a	**9.** d	**13.** b	**17.** d
2. a	**6.** c	**10.** a	**14.** a	**18.** d
3. b	**7.** c	**11.** b	**15.** a	**19.** a
4. b	**8.** a	**12.** c	**16.** c	**20.** c

FIVE

Anatomy, Physiology, and Pathophysiology: Applied Priniciples of Anesthesia

CHAPTER
14

The Central Nervous System

Wayne E. Ellis

□ ANATOMY

The central nervous system (CNS) is contained within the bony structures of the cranial vault and the spinal column. Within the cranial vault or cranium are the (1) brain and linings, (2) cerebrospinal fluid (CSF), and (3) vascular structures as well as the blood supplying the tissues of the brain and linings. The brain and linings continue caudad through the spinal canal, as the spinal cord and linings, to the termination of the spinal canal at the level of the fifth sacral vertebra.[1–7]

SUPRATENTORIAL STRUCTURES

The *cerebrum* is considered a supratentorial structure; it is located in the anterior and middle fossae and separated by the longitudinal fissure into right and left hemispheres. Each hemisphere is further divided into four lobes identified as the frontal, parietal, temporal, and occipital. Cerebral dominance is discussed in relation to "right" or "left" brain dominance in the control of body activities. Many functions of the opposite side of the body are represented in both hemispheres; however, some functions are existent in only one hemisphere. Language is relegated to only one hemisphere, with the left hemisphere dominance being the significant control in 99% of right-handed persons and 95% of left-handed persons. Language dominance may not be present until the end of the first or second year of life in the majority of individuals.[1–7]

The largest lobe of the brain is the *frontal lobe*. This lobe encompasses approximately one third of the surface of the hemisphere. It extends from the anterior border adjacent to the frontal bones to the rolandic (central) sulcus or fissure. The precentral gyrus is identified as the primary motor cortex of the brain. In the motor and sensory cortex, there is consistent anatomic distribution of the body areas from those areas supplied by sacral nerves closest in the depths of the longitudinal sulcus to those supplied by the cervical nerve roots along the midportion of the surface of the lobe. Areas supplying other portions of the body are identified in other areas of the motor and sensory cortex from this point to the inferior portion of the motor and sensory cortex. *Broca's center* is located in the inferior area of the motor strip in the dominant hemisphere. This area is responsible for the motor component of speech. When a lesion develops in this area of the brain, the individual will be able to know and recognize a word but will be unable to articulate the words correctly. The anterior portion of the frontal lobe is involved with memory, mood, personality, and emotion.[1–7]

The *parietal* lobe extends from the central sulcus to the parieto-occipital sulcus. The postcentral gyrus is the primary somatosensory cortex of the brain. The other parts of the parietal lobe provide integration of sensory input and permit one to discriminate sensory input based on elements of size, shape, and texture.

The *temporal* lobe is inferior to the lateral fissure of Sylvius and extends posteriorly to the occipital and parietal lobes. The dominant temporal lobe is responsible for language function. Posteriorly, on the inner surface of the temporal lobe, are the transverse gyri of Heschl. These make up the primary auditory cortex. At the junction of the temporal and parietal lobes is located Wernicke's speech area. *Wernicke's speech area* is involved in the perception of language. Lesions developing in this area may result in the inability to perceive language (receptive aphasia). The medial portion (uncus) of the temporal lobe contains the olfactory cortex.[1–7]

The occipital lobe begins at the parieto-occipital sulcus and extends posteriorly, resting on the tentorium cerebelli. It contains the visual cortex. This area of the brain is responsible for the integration of the visual system.

CORPUS CALLOSUM

Connection between the two hemispheres of the cortex are maintained by way of the *corpus callosum*. The fibers within this structure make possible the exchange of "information" between the two hemispheres. The anterior temporal lobes and the amygdala are connected through fibers that pass through the anterior commissure.[1-7]

STRUCTURES OF THE POSTERIOR FOSSA

The *posterior fossa* is formed anteriorly by the tentorium cerebelli and posteriorly by the occipital bones and the foramen magnum. The cerebellum, pons, and medulla are located in the posterior fossa. The cerebellum lies dorsal to the pons and medulla and is the largest structure in the posterior fossa. The cerebellum forms the roof of the fourth ventricle. Integration of motor coordination and equilibrium occur in the cerebellum. The pons and medulla constitute the *brainstem*. The brainstem contains the ascending and descending neural pathways to the cerebral cortex. The respiratory, cardiovascular, and important autonomic control centers are located in the brainstem. The nuclei for cranial nerves III through XII are located within the posterior fossa. All cranial nerves except I and II exit the brainstem in the posterior fossa. Injury to structures in the brainstem may result in difficulties in swallowing, controlling secretions, and protecting the airway. Due to the relatively small space of the posterior fossa and the containment of cardiovascular and respiratory centers in the area, lesions in this area produce symptoms sooner than those in the supratentorial areas.[1-7]

CRANIAL NERVES

The *cranial nerves* arise in the brain and innervate the motor and sensory functions of the head and neck. These nerves also supply parasympathetic innervation to most of the body. Cranial nerves I (olfactory) and II (optic) arise in the middle fossa, while the rest of the cranial nerves arise from the posterior fossa.

Cranial nerve I is the olfactory nerve. It is a tract composed of axons that extend from the uncus of the temporal lobe to the olfactory bulb, where they synapse with processes from olfactory neurons. The olfactory neurons are located in the olfactory mucosa and the axons project through the cribriform plate.

Cranial nerve II is the optic nerve. Ganglion cells from the retina converge bilaterally to form the optic nerve, which then enter the cranial vault through the optic foramina. There is a partial decussation of the nerve at the hypothalmus in the optic chiasm. The fibers from the nasal aspects of the retinas cross to the opposite side. Following the crossing of the fibers of the optic nerves, the nerves become tracts synapsing in the geniculate bodies. The nasal retina receives light stimulation from the temporal visual fields. If a lesion develops that results in either actual or physiologic cutting of the optic chiasm, bitemporal heteronymous hemianopsia results.

Cranial nerve III is the oculomotor nerve. It supplies motor innervation to the superior rectus, inferior rectus, medial rectus, and inferior oblique muscles. It supplies the levator palpebrae, the voluntary elevator of the eyelid. Parasympathetic innervation of the pupil and the lens arise in the Edinger-Westphal nucleus, where narcotic receptors are located. Stimulus of these receptors will result in *pupillary constriction*.

Cranial nerve IV is the trochlear nerve. It supplies innervation to the superior oblique extraocular muscle. This muscle is responsible for the eye's ability to look downward.

Cranial nerve V is the trigeminal nerve. It supplies sensory innervation to the face and motor innervation to the muscles of mastication. It has *three divisions:* the ophthalmic, maxillary, and mandibular branches. The ophthalmic branch is responsible for sensation in the forehead and cornea. The maxillary branch is responsible for sensation in the maxillary area of the face. The mandibular branch transmits sensation from the mandibular area of the face and provides motor innervation to the muscles of mastication.

Cranial nerve VI is the abducens nerve. It provides motor innervation to the lateral rectus extraocular muscle. This muscle is responsible for lateral movement of the eye. This nerve has the longest intracranial course of any of the cranial nerves. It arises in the posterior fossa, crosses the tentorium into the middle fossa, and exits the skull through the superior orbital fissure. Because of the long course of the nerve, it can be subject to stretching. It may become dysfunctional as a result of multiple pathophysiologic conditions including the *reduced intracranial pressure that accompanies postdural puncture headaches.* Dysfunction of the abducens nerve results in medial deviation of the eye and diplopia.

Cranial nerve VII is the facial nerve. It provides innervation to the muscles of facial expression. Additionally, it provides the parasympathetic innervation of the submandibular, sublingual, and lacrimal glands. Taste in two-thirds of the tongue is also transmitted by the facial nerve.

Cranial nerve VIII is the auditory nerve. It provides innervation to the semicircular canals and the cochlea of the ear. This nerve is responsible for hearing and balance.

Cranial nerve IX is the glossopharyngeal nerve. It provides sensory innervation to the pharynx, tongue, carotid body, and sinus as well as taste to the posterior one-third of the tongue.

Cranial nerve X is the vagus nerve. It supplies motor innervation to the soft palate, pharynx, and larynx as well as sensory innervation to the pharynx, larynx, and abdominal and thoracic viscera. The vagus nerve is responsible for taste in the posterior pharynx and provides parasympathetic innervation to thoracic and abdominal viscera. The branches of the vagus nerve provide innervation to anatomic structures significant to the anesthesia practitioner. The superior and recurrent laryngeal nerves are branches of the vagus nerve. The superior laryngeal nerve becomes the internal and external branches. The internal branch of the superior laryngeal nerve penetrates the thyrohyoid membrane and provides sensory innervation to the epiglottis, base of the tongue, arytenoepiglottic fold, and most of the larynx. The external branch of the superior laryngeal nerve provides innervation to the cricothyroid muscle and the inferior constrictors of the pharynx. There is a minor contribution to sensory innervation of laryngeal structures by the superior laryngeal nerve. The recurrent laryngeal nerve innervates all of the intrinsic muscles of the larynx except for the cricothyroid muscle. Branches of the recurrent laryngeal nerve supply the mucosa of the trachea and the esophagus.

Cranial nerve XI is the spinal accessory nerve. It supplies motor innervation to the sternocleidomastoid and trapezius muscles. The nerve arises from the upper five cervical cord segments, ascends the spinal canal, enters the cranium by way of the foramen magnum, and then exits the skull through the jugular foramen. Thereafter it follows its course to the sternocleidomastoid and trapezius muscles.

Cranial nerve XII is the hypoglossal nerve. It provides motor innervation to the tongue.[1-7]

BLOOD SUPPLY

The brain and linings receive their blood supply from paired carotid and vertebral arteries. The vertebral arteries fuse at the level of the pons and medulla and form a single basilar artery. The basilar artery forms the posterior boundary of the circle of Willis, while the internal carotid arteries become the anterior segments of the circle of Willis. Together, the three vessels provide anastomotic connections between the arteries to provide continuous blood supply to vital cranial structures. The circle of Willis surrounds the pituitary stalk. The internal carotid artery branches into the middle and anterior cerebral arteries on each side of the cerebrum. The basilar artery bifurcates into the two posterior cerebral arteries. Under most "physiologically normal" conditions, there is little mixing of blood through the circle of Willis. The middle cerebral artery supplies the ipsilateral cerebral hemisphere. The flow through the basilar arteries supplies the posterior fossa and the posterior cerebral arteries. Unlike other vascular beds within the body, the extracranial and large arteries of the brain make up 25% to 50% of the vascular resistance found.[1-7]

THE LININGS OF THE BRAIN AND SPINAL CORD

There are three linings within the CNS. They are the *dura, arachnoid,* and *pia mater.* The pia mater is made up of a minute plexus of blood vessels held together by a fine areolar tissue. The pia mater contributes to the formation of the choroid plexus. The arachnoid mater is the second layer. It is extremely thin and delicate and has the appearance of spiderwebs. The space between the arachnoid and pia maters is the subarachnoid space. The space between the arachnoid and dura maters is the subdural space. The dura is a thick dense and inelastic membrane that is the exterior lining of the brain

and lies against the skull and spinal canal. The dura forms the internal periosteum of the brain. This layer acts as a protective barrier to the CNS.[1-7]

BLOOD-BRAIN BARRIER

The internal environment of the brain is separated from the circulating blood by a tissue barrier identified as the *blood-brain barrier.* The vascular endothelium is formed with "tight junctions" between individual cells. Substances may leave the intravascular space; however, they must pass through the endothelium. The endothelial cells permit minimal transport by *pinocytosis.* There is also an enzymatic barrier in the cerebral vessels. High levels of monoamine oxidase (MAO) and catechol *O*-methyltransferase (COMT) are present. This results in degradation of the catecholamines that pass through the endothelium, leading to reduced extraction of circulating catecholamines to approximately 5% by the brain. The precursors of the catecholamines may pass freely across the blood-brain barrier. The postrema, pineal body, choroid plexus, and portions of the hypothalamus are deficient with regard to the blood-brain barrier. For development of the blood-brain barrier, astroglial cells and the blood vessels must be in contact. Acute hypertension, hypoxia, and trauma may cause a disruption of the blood-brain barrier, and tumor vessels are deficient in their blood-brain barrier. Additionally, tumor vessels do not autoregulate normally. The most highly developed blood-brain barrier is found in the small arterioles and capillaries.[1-7]

CEREBRAL BLOOD FLOW

The brain accounts for approximately 2% (approximately 1400 g) of the body's total weight and receives approximately 15% of the cardiac output. The oxygen consumption of the brain represents approximately 20% of the body's oxygen consumption. The cerebral blood flow is approximately 700 mL/min. The average cerebral blood flow averages 50 mL/100 g/min. This is divided between the gray matter (80 mL/100 g/min) and white matter (20 mL/100 g/min). One of the concerns of the anesthesia practitioner is to preserve cerebral blood flow in an effort to maintain normal cerebral function. With the patient's temperature, oxygenation, hematocrit, and carbon dioxide levels maintained within normal limits, changes can be detected in the electroencephalogram (EEG) as the blood flow is reduced. When the total cerebral blood flow is reduced 20 to 24 mL/100 g/min, slowing of the EEG occurs. If the cerebral blood flow is further reduced to 15 to 19 mL/100 g/min, flattening of the EEG occurs. When the cerebral blood flow is reduced to < 10 mL/100 g/min, irreversible damage to brain cells occurs.

In the spinal cord, the average blood flow is 50 mL/100 g/min. The white matter receives approximately 15 to 20 mL/100 g/min. Blood supply to the gray matter is approximately 60 to 100 mL/100 g/min.

Total cerebral blood volume equals approximately 50 mL, or 4 mL/100 g. This is regionally distributed to the gray matter (4 to 6 mL/100 g) and white matter (1.2 to 2.5 mL/100 g). Changes in cerebral blood flow will cause changes in intracranial pressure. Changes in volume normally parallel blood flow; however, as the cerebral perfusion pressure falls, autoregulation induces vasodilation to maintain flow at a constant level. This results in an increase in cerebral blood volume.[1-7]

☐ REGULATION OF BLOOD FLOW

Autoregulation is the physiologic process that maintains a constant cerebral blood flow through a wide range of cerebral perfusion pressures. *Cerebral perfusion pressure* (CPP) is calculated by subtracting the intracranial pressure from the mean arterial pressure* (CPP=MAP–ICP). This formula remains constant as long as the cranial vault is intact. However, once the dura is opened, CPP equals mean arterial pressure. Because of the physiologic differences that exist from one person to another, there is great variability in autoregulation among individuals.

Autoregulation will maintain cerebral blood flow at a relatively constant rate between CPPs of 50 and 150 torr (Fig. 14–1). Below 50 torr, the cerebral blood flow falls linearly in relation to perfusion pressure. Reductions in cerebral blood flow can occur because of either increases in intracranial pressure or decreases in mean arterial pressure. The end result of either event is a decrease in the cerebral blood flow. If CPP exceeds 150 torr, cerebral blood flow begins to increase linearly as the pressure increases. If the CPP is increased above approximately 200 torr, disruption of the blood-brain barrier will occur, and the result is cerebral edema. With marked increases in the CPP, arterioles will passively dilate. The changes in arteriolar dilation will not resolve for several hours following a reduction in CPP. The speed of autoregulation is dependent on the degree of change in the cerebral perfusion pressure and normally ranges from 10 to 120 s.

There are significant changes in regional blood flow with changes in CPP. As flow is reduced, flow to the cortex and medulla will be maintained. In the presence of a marked increased CPP, the flow is distributed to attenuate the increase to the brainstem. The sympathetic nervous system plays a significant role in CPP.

In the presence of intense *sympathetic stimulation,* the curve of autoregulation shifts, so that autoregulation occurs at higher perfusion pressures. This has been suggested as one of the mechanisms that provides cerebral protection to the patient with hypertension. In the presence of an alpha blockade or cervical sympathectomy, a shift to the left of the lower limit of the autoregulation curve occurs.

The mechanisms of autoregulation are not completely understood; however, several theories have been suggested to explain the results that the clinician sees in evaluating patients. Autoregulation is said to be *myogenic.* It is an intrinsic response to changing arterial wall tension by the smooth muscle of the arterial wall. As the smooth muscle is stretched by increased flow, the muscles contract and restrict flow. When there is less flow and thereby reduced wall tension, the arterial wall relaxes, permitting increased flow in the arteries. Blood flow is regulated by metabolic mechanisms. As metabolism increases, the products of metabolism produce vasodilation in the vessels. There is also a neurogenic component to cerebral blood flow. Both vasodilator and vasoconstrictor nerves supply the blood vessels. However, this effect may be minimal within the normal range of autoregulation.

Autoregulation can be abolished with relative ease. The *loss of autoregulation* can occur with hypoxia, severe hypercapnia, head trauma, and the use of potent inhalation agents in anesthesia. The effects of agent-related inhibition result with increasing doses of the inhaled agent. There is a shift in the curve, with both upper and lower limits shifting together and the shape of the curve becoming more positive.

In the hypertensive patient, the curve may be normal in shape; however, it is shifted to the right. Once the systemic blood pressure returns to normal, the autoregulatory curve will return to "prehypertensive" levels over a 6- to 8-week period of time.

Blood flow in the spinal cord is probably regulated over the same range as the cerebral blood flow. However, the proliferation of arterial blood supply to the cranial structures is not duplicated in the spinal cord. The spinal cord receives most of its blood supply from regional *radicular arteries.*

The cerebral blood flow varies with changes in carbon dioxide content in a relatively linear fashion between 20 and 80 torr (Fig. 14–2). There is an approximate change of 1.5 to 2 mL/100 g/min for each 1-torr change in the arterial carbon

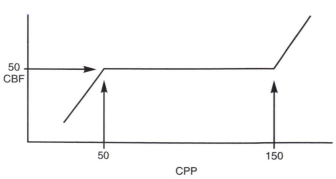

Figure 14–1 Regulation of blood flow.

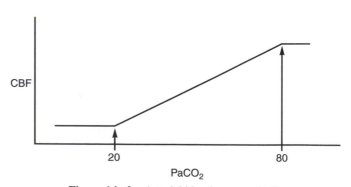

Figure 14–2 Arterial blood gases and pH.

dioxide level. Responses to these changes are dependent on preexisting flow, with areas receiving higher flows demonstrating a steeper response curve. These changes occur relatively quickly within less than 1 min.

Extravascular pH will mediate changes in cerebral vascular tone. *Carbon dioxide* readily crosses the blood-brain barrier and will then alter extracellular pH and then the pH of the CSF. Bicarbonate and fixed acids *do not* cross the blood-brain barrier, and they will not alter the pH in the brain. Alterations in the bicarbonate level can occur locally in the brain; however, this process takes up to 24 h. As the pH of the brain is corrected, the effects of carbon dioxide are negated. Other factors may be involved in the responses to carbon dioxide. Nitric oxide (NO) production by nonendothelial sources may be responsible for mediating some of these responses. Inhibitors of prostaglandin synthesis can blunt the responses to carbon dioxide. Once adaptation to a lower pH has occurred, the brain will respond to changes that bring the pH back to normal values as hypercarbia, with a resulting increase in ICP. Following extended periods of hyperventilation, the carbon dioxide should be normalized slowly.

The response to carbon dioxide appears to be *preserved* during potent inhalation anesthesia. Medications such as thiopental can blunt or lessen the responsiveness to increases in carbon dioxide. This action is dependent on the amount of flow reduction resulting from the anesthetic. Other factors such as aging, head injury, stroke, cardiac arrest, subarachnoid hemorrhage, and brain tumors will also blunt the response to carbon dioxide.

Measurable changes in cerebral blood flow (CBF) do not occur until the oxygen content falls below 50 torr. At this point, the CBF increases with vasodilation. With the increase in blood flow, there is a concomitant increase in cerebral blood volume. Oxygen content is apparently the driving factor in increasing flow. The physiologic mediator may be adenosine. This is produced from the breakdown of adenosine triphosphate (ATP) without resynthesis. With inhalation of 80% to 100% oxygen, there can be a 10% to 12% reduction in cerebral blood flow.

The CBF parallels local cerebral metabolism. This *flow-metabolism coupling* occurs, but the mechanism of its occurrence is not presently identified. Regional acidosis may be a factor; however, changes in flow have been demonstrated prior to measurable changes in pH. When neurons are depolarized, they release NO which produces vasodilation. The modulation in flow may occur because of changes in glucose consumption. Local neurogenic influences may have a role in local changes in CBF. Cerebral blood vessels are innervated with adrenergic, cholinergic, and multiple nonadrenergic, noncholinergic nerves.

Blood flow will remain relatively constant when the hematocrit is between 30% and 50%. When the hematocrit falls below 30% progressive vasodilation occurs. This is directly related to the reduction in oxygen delivery to the cerebral tissues. With a high hematocrit, the flow is reduced because of the increased viscosity of the blood.

With changes in body temperature, there are significant changes in CBF. *Oxygen consumption* changes 6% to 7% for each degree centigrade that the temperature changes. As an example, at a temperature of 28°C, cerebral blood flow and cerebral oxygen consumption are reduced by 50%. The electroencephalogram (EEG) will become isoelectric when the core temperature reaches 20°C. At 18°C, the oxygen consumption is approximately 10% of the normothermic baseline. Hyperthermia also inflicts problems and injury upon cerebral tissues. At temperatures above 42°C, there is marked reduction in the CBF. This is most likely related to the toxic effects of hyperthermia on the enzyme systems of the brain.[1–7]

☐ CEREBRAL METABOLISM

The brain is responsible for approximately 20% of the total body oxygen consumption at rest. This is approximately 1.3 to 1.6 μmol/100 g/min (3.0 to 3.5 mL/100 g/min). There are regional differences, with the cortex being the highest consumer of available oxygen resources. The most important process requiring oxygen is the reduction of oxygen by the electron transport chain. Fifty percent of the oxygen consumption is for the generation of electrical activity. *The practitioner must be aware of and constantly vigilant to maintain cerebral oxygen content and CBF because there are no oxygen reserves within the brain.* Consciousness is lost at an oxygen level of 30 torr. Once oxygen delivery to the brain ceases, consciousness is lost in 5 to 11 s.

The normal glucose consumption is 0.27 μmol/g/min (5 mg/100g/min). More than 90% is consumed aerobically; however, anaerobic metabolism occurs normally in the presence of adequate oxygenation. Lactic acid is produced during anaerobic metabolism, and lactate metabolism may be increased during times of oxygen stress. During periods of starvation, the brain can metabolize both acetoacetate and beta-hydroxybutyrate. These are the only substances that can support metabolism in the absence of glucose.[1–7]

☐ INTRACRANIAL PRESSURE

The total intracranial volume in an adult is approximately 1200 to 1500 mL. This is made up of the brain, blood volume, and CSF. The contents of the brain include 168 g of solid and 1092 g of water. The blood volume is approximately 50 mL. The CSF volume averages 75 mL. *Normal intracranial pressure is 10 torr or less.*

As intracranial pressure (ICP) increases, compensatory mechanisms arise to help maintain the pressures as near normal as possible. There is displacement of CSF into the spinal subarachnoid space, increased rate of CSF absorption, decreased CSF production, or decreased cerebral blood volume from venous compression. Only when compensatory mechanisms have been exhausted will the ICP begin to rise. The rapidity of decompensation is directly related to the rapidity of the volume increase. This would be similar to comparing a slow-growing tissue mass to the development of a hematoma.

If the practitioner has the ability to monitor the intracranial pressure, several waveforms may be seen that may be correlated to specific events relative to the status of decompensation within the cranium. *"A" waves* are plateau waves that are sustained, marked increases in the ICP lasting 5 to 10 min. These waves are considered life-threatening. They represent preterminal decompensation of ICP in patients with limited ability to compensate for increases in intracranial volume; they are initiated by increases in arterial pressure, pain, and coughing. *"B" waves* are smaller, sharper waves that occur at the rate of 0.5 to 2 per minute and may coincide with Cheyne-Stokes respirations. These "B" waves may be precursors to "A" waves. *"C" waves* are small, rhythmic oscillations with a frequency of 4 to 8 per minute; they are related to changes in arterial pressure.

The anesthesia practitioner must be constantly prepared to provide interventions to mediate the potentially negative results of severe intracranial hypertension. The patient with *intracranial hypertension* may present with *arterial hypertension* and *bradycardia*. These clinical signs are identified as Cushing's triad. When events designed to reduce the arterial pressure are initiated, cerebral ischemia may be further aggravated because of a concurrent reduction in cerebral perfusion pressure. Reductions in intracranial pressure can better promote cerebral perfusion while lowering systemic blood pressure.[1–7]

CEREBROSPINAL FLUID

Cerebrospinal fluid (CSF) is formed at a rate of 0.35 mL/min; the total CSF in the adult is 130 to 150 mL. The specific gravity of CSF ranges from 1.002 to 1.009. The pH of the CSF is regulated to maintain the steady-state pH at 7.32. Changes in arterial carbon dioxide content can effect changes in the CSF; however, over time, the movement of bicarbonate ions will return the pH to 7.32. Most CSF is formed at the capillary endothelium and some is derived from the water of oxidative metabolism. There is a reduction in secretion with decreased choroidal blood flow and choroidal capillary hydrostatic pressure, decreased body temperature, increased serum osmolality, and increased intraventricular hydrostatic pressure. *Medications* such as furosemide, vasopressin, spironolactone, and acetazolamide inhibit the formation of CSF. Ouabain and corticosteroids inhibit the Na^+, K^+-ATPase and thus inhibit the formation of CSF.

Cerebrospinal fluid flows into the fourth ventricle and out the medial foramen of Magendie and the lateral foramina of Luschka and into the cerebromedullary cistern (cisterna magna). From here, the flow continues into the subarachnoid space. Spinal subarachnoid circulation is slow compared to circulation in the cranial subarachnoid space. Obstructions to

flow will cause an increase in ICP and the development of the clinical condition known as *hydrocephalus.*

The majority of the CSF is reabsorbed by the *arachnoid villi.* Some 10% to 15% of the CSF is directly absorbed in the spinal subarachnoid space. The meningeal lymphatics reabsorb a small amount of CSF. Reabsorption is affected by venous pressure. Normally CSF pressure is greater than venous pressure. Increases in CSF pressure result in increased absorption, while increases in cerebral venous pressure result in decreased absorption of CSF.[1–7]

THE SPINAL CORD

The spinal cord begins at the foramen magnum and extends to the level of the first or second lumbar vertebra in the adult. The cord is composed of both white and gray matter. The balance of the spinal canal is filled by spinal nerve roots, the meninges, epidural blood vessels, and epidural fat. From the end of the spinal cord to the end of the canal, the nerve roots are collected into a tight bundle of fibers called the *cauda equina.* This name is derived from the appearance of the roots, which resembles a horse's tail. The end of the spinal cord is loosely attached to the end of the spinal canal by the *terminal ligament.*

THE GRAY MATTER

The gray matter serves as the initial processor, much like a telephone switchboard, for incoming sensory signals and final processing of outgoing motor responses. Anatomically, the gray matter is made up of nine laminae and shaped like the letter "H." It is divided in the anterior, lateral, and dorsal horns. In the *anterior horn,* alpha and gamma motor neurons give rise to the nerve fibers that leave via the ventral root to provide motor innervation to skeletal muscle. These connections are provided primarily through intermediate neurons known as cells of Renshaw. They function in an inhibitory capacity to limit excessive activity. Preganglionic neurons of the sympathetic portion of the autonomic nervous system are found in the *lateral horns,* primarily in the thoracolumbar portions of the cord. The *dorsal horn* serves as the gateway for impulses entering via the dorsal roots of the spinal nerves. These fibers carry information from the peripheral nervous system on tactile, temperature, and pain sensations. Intermediate fibers then transmit the impulses to ascending pathways in the spinothalamic tract. The dorsal area of the cord responsible for this comprises laminae II and III and is further identified as the *substantia gelatinosa.*

THE WHITE MATTER

The white matter of the spinal cord is composed of axons of intermediate neurons, including the respective ascending and descending tracts. This area of the spinal cord is divided into sections, similar to those of the gray matter, identified as dorsal, lateral, and ventral columns. Of interest to the anesthesia practitioner are the *spinothalamic tracts* of the dorsal column. These tracts transmit to the brain the impulses responsible for the perception of touch and pain.

THE SPINAL NERVE

There are 31 segments of the spinal cord, and from each segment a pair of spinal nerves arises. Each nerve is composed of efferent motor fibers arising from the anterior and lateral horns and afferent sensory fibers going from the periphery to the dorsal (posterior) horn. Cell bodies of sensory fibers, originating in the spinal ganglia, travel in the dorsal nerve roots, sending branches to both the cord and the periphery. Both the anterior and dorsal nerve roots exit the cord via the intervertebral foramen enclosed in a common dural sheath that extends just past the spinal cord ganglia, where the spinal nerve originates. Following injury and during inflammatory processes, this foramen can become a restricted pathway, resulting in the development of peripheral symptoms of central neural compression.

DERMATOMES AND MYOTOMES

Each spinal nerve provides innervation to a segment of skin designated a dermatome and an area of skeletal muscle known as a myotome. Dermatome maps have been used to determine the level of either spinal cord injury or anesthesia or analgesia provided by regional anesthesia techniques. Although the dermatomes are depicted as being very distinct, there is significant overlap. As many as three dorsal roots must be anesthetized to provide total denervation of a single dermatome. This demonstrates the central interconnection and intermixing of neurons. It is more difficult to determine accurately the segmental innervation of myotomes because individual skeletal muscle groups receive innervation from several anterior nerve roots.

SENSORY PATHWAYS

Sensory signals are transmitted from segments of the body through the spinal nerves into each segment of the spinal cord. The neurons enter the gray matter via the dorsal root. There they synapse and give rise to long fiber tracts that ascend to the brain. The sensory input signals are transmitted by *dorsal column pathways* (dorsal-lemniscal system), *spinocervical tracts,* and *anteriolateral spinothalamic tracts.* The impulses cross to the opposite side in the spinal cord prior to ascending to the thalamus. There is an additional synapse with neurons carrying the sensory stimuli to the cerebral cortex. Nerve fibers from the anteriolateral spinothalamic tracts cross in the anterior commissure and transit to the brain as the ventral and lateral spinothalamic tracts. All sensory input to the cerebral cortex with the exception of input from the olfactory nerves crosses the thalamus. The interaction of spinal (cord) reflexes with peripheral stimuli is apparent in patients with spinal cord injuries.

MOTOR PATHWAYS

There is integration of sensory and motor response within the spinal cord to provide appropriate and immediate motor responses to specific stimuli. The responses occur instantly and may result in either a muscle stretch reflex or a withdrawal reflex in response to a single sensory stimulus. Spinal (cord) reflexes are important in causing emptying of the bladder and rectum. Segmental temperature responses permit localized cutaneous vasodilation or vasoconstriction in response to changes in local skin temperature without the necessity of a global response. As the area of origination of a motor response occurs higher (towards the cortex) in the CNS the more complex the response. The most complex and precise actions originate in the cerebral cortex.

Alpha fibers of the A type arise in the anterior horn of the cord and travel via the anterior root to the skeletal muscle. Within skeletal muscle and tendons, there are muscle spindles and Golgi tendon organs. On an unconscious level, they provide input to the CNS on the stretch, tension, and length of tendons and muscles. During a physical examination, the stretch reflex of the quadriceps femoris and the gastrocnemius muscles can be tested by eliciting the patellar and ankle jerk reflex.

Pathologic lesions in the contralateral cord will result in an exaggerated stretch reflex response. Lesions that result in transection of the brainstem at the level of the pons will result in spasticity. This condition is known as *decerebrate rigidity* and is a result of diffuse facilitation of stretch reflexes. Lesions may also be identified as affecting either upper or lower motor neurons. Lower neurons are in the spinal cord and directly innervate skeletal muscles. *Lesions of the lower motor neurons* are most commonly associated with flaccid paralysis, atrophy of skeletal muscles, and absence of stretch reflex responses. With destruction of *upper motor neurons,* there is spastic paralysis with accentuated stretch reflexes in the absence of skeletal muscle paralysis.

With a painful or noxious stimuli, withdrawal flexor reflexes are most often elicited. This is associated with withdrawal of the stimulated limb and extension of the opposite limb, occurring 0.2 to 0.5 s later (cross-extensor reflex). This action is initiated to push the body away from the object causing the painful stimulus. Because of the need for the signal impulse to pass through several additional neurons, there is a normal time delay in the response. Nociceptive impulses initiated from broken bone edges result in spasm of the surrounding skeletal muscle. Infiltration of local anesthetics at the fracture site may produce relief of symptoms. Peritoneal irritation from peritonitis that results in abdominal muscle spasm is produced by a spinal cord reflex. During abdominal surgery, a similar spasm of the abdominal skeletal muscles occurs from stimulation of the parietal peritoneum and results in extrusion of abdominal contents. This contraction can be attenuated with the use of volatile anesthetics and abolished by regional anesthesia or neuromuscular block drugs.[1–12]

☐ AUTONOMIC NERVOUS SYSTEM

The autonomic nervous system (ANS) is composed of the sympathetic and parasympathetic nervous systems. The ANS is primarily concerned with maintenance of visceral functions and partially responsible for control of blood pressure, gastrointestinal motility and secretion, urinary bladder emptying, and sweating and body temperature. The centers for activation of the ANS are in the hypothalamus, brainstem, and spinal cord. Of the two divisions of the ANS, the *sympathetic nervous system* (SNS) is primarily a global system that, when stimulated, prepares the entire body for "action." The *parasympathetic nervous system* (PSNS) is organ-specific, and its actions will differ depending on which organ system is stimulated. The divisions are considered as physiologic antagonists, so that the actions of each division act to balance the response of the organ system.

THE SYMPATHETIC NERVOUS SYSTEM

The nerve fibers of the SNS arise in the thoracolumbar segments (T1-L2) of the cord. The fibers then pass into the paravertebral sympathetic chain lateral to the spinal cord. From this chain the fibers pass to tissues and organs innervated by the SNS.

The SNS consists of a preganglionic neuron and a postganglionic neuron. The preganglionic neuron's cell body arises in the inter-mediolateral horn of the spinal cord. The neural fibers leave the cord via the anterior root and pass through the white rami into the ganglia. There are 22 pairs of ganglia in a chain along the spinal cord (paravertebral sympathetic chain). The neurons are primarily myelinated, slow-conducting type B fibers. In the ganglia, the preganglionic fibers synapse with the cell body of a postganglionic neuron. In addition, the neuron may not synapse at this level but may pass either cephalad or caudad to synapse with postganglionic neurons (mostly unmyelinated type C fibers) in paravertebral ganglia at other levels in the chain. The postganglionic neuron exits the paravertebral ganglia, traveling to peripheral end organs. Some of the postganglionic neurons return to the spinal nerves via gray rami, traveling with these nerves to provide innervation to vascular smooth muscle, piloerector muscles, and sweat glands. The SNS fibers do not necessarily follow the distribution of the spinal nerve from that segment. Distribution is in part determined by the position of the organ during embryologic development. In the embryo, the position of the heart originates in the neck and the gastrointestinal tract originates in the lower thoracic area.

THE PARASYMPATHETIC NERVOUS SYSTEM

The nerve fibers of the PSNS arise in the posterior fossa and depart the CNS through cranial nerves III, V, VII, IX, and X. Segments of the PSNS also arise from the sacral portion of the spinal cord. Approximately 75% of all PSNS action is mediated through the *vagus* nerve. This nerve supplies innervation to thoracic and abdominal regions of the body. Parasympathetic fibers pass through cranial nerve III to the eye and make up this component of the oculocardiac reflex. Lacrimal, nasal, and submaxillary glands receive PSNS innervation through cranial nerve VII. Parasympathetic innervation to the parotid gland is mediated through cranial nerve IX. The sacral contribution to the PSNS is composed primarily of the second and third sacral nerves. Occasionally, contributions from the first and fourth cranial nerves can be included. They form the sacral plexus on either side of the spinal cord and provide innervation to the distal colon, rectum, bladder, and lower portions of the ureters. In addition, PSNS fibers to the external genitalia transmit impulses that elicit various sexual responses. Unlike the SNS preganglionic neurons, preganglionic fibers of the PSNS originate in the CNS and pass as long fibers to ganglia near the effector organ. Postganglionic neurons are short because of the relationship of the ganglion to the organ of innervation.

NEUROTRANSMITTERS

The propagation of a stimulus along the path of the axon is mediated by ion shifting from extra- to intracellular spaces; however, at the area of the synapse, the mediation is through a chemical compound identified as a *neurotransmitter*. The transmitter is released by the presynaptic neuron into the synaptic cleft. This chemical compound crosses the synaptic cleft and interacts with specific receptors on the postsynaptic neuron. This interaction initiates the process of depolarization in the postsynaptic neuron.

The neurotransmitter of postganglionic fibers of the SNS is *norepinephrine*. These fibers are classified as adrenergic fibers. The parasympathetic postganglionic fibers secrete *acetylcholine* as the neurotransmitter substance. These fibers are identified as cholinergic fibers. Postganglionic sympathetic fibers to sweat glands and to some blood vessels release acetylcholine as the neurotransmitter. The neurotransmitter substance in all preganglionic neurons of both the SNS and the PSNS is acteylcholine. All preganglionic neurons are classified as cholinergic fibers.

Synthesis of norepinephrine is through a series of enzyme-controlled steps that begin in the cytoplasm of the nerve endings and are completed in synaptic vesicles of the postganglionic sympathetic nerve endings. This process begins with the formation of dopamine and then the conversion of the dopamine to norepinephrine by dopamine beta-hydroxylase. Because of the lack of specificity of this process, several medications may enter into the interaction and produce either a weakly active neurotransmitter known as a false transmitter or into an inactive compound that prevents the activation of the receptor site. With a depolarizing action of the cell, norepinephrine is released into the synaptic cleft by the vesicles. To do this, there must be sufficient calcium ions present. Following release, both active and passive mechanisms are responsible for the reuptake or metabolism of norepinephrine. The problem of tachyphylaxis that results when indirect-acting sympathomimetics are used may be a reflection of reduced or depleted stores of neurotransmitter substance.[1–15]

☐ PATHOLOGIC CONDITIONS

NEUROMUSCULAR DISORDERS

Myasthenia Gravis   Myasthenia gravis is a disease process that affects primarily women; however, the incidence in men increases after the age of 40. The patients are differentiated on the basis of symptoms from class 1 to class 4. The disease has an insidious onset and results in fluctuating weakness of the voluntary muscles, a condition exacerbated by exercise and improved by rest. The initial symptom bringing the patient to the clinical practitioner is *diplopia*. Difficulties in swallowing and chewing are also early symptoms. Symptoms can be exacerbated by infection, physical or emotional stress, hyperthyroidism, or drugs such as quinidine, procainamide, and aminoglycoside antibiotics. Medical treatment of myasthenia gravis has been with anticholinesterases since the mid-1930s. The treatment response is variable both between patients and according to time of day. Pyridostigmine can be used effectively because it has fewer side effects than neostigmine. Additional treatment can include the use of immunosuppressants. *Myasthenia gravis* is a disease of the autoimmune system that produces circulating antibodies that effectively reduce the number of available acetylcholine receptors. The disease is primarily a *postsynaptic disorder.* The patient may be slightly resistant to succinylcholine; during recovery, phase II block develops rapidly and recovery is slow. Sensitivity to nondepolarizing neuromuscular blocking drugs has led to the avoidance or minimal use of nondepolarizing muscle relaxants. Traditionally, the use of potent volatile anesthetics has been recommended. Atracurium has been successfully used, with adequate reversal of the muscle relaxant following usage. Neuromuscular monitoring is essential for these patients.

Patients with myasthenia gravis may present with symptoms of either undertreatment with anticholinesterase agents (myasthenic crisis) or overtreatment with anticholinesterase agents (cholinergic crisis). The symptoms include progressive muscle weakness, increased secretions, and bradycardia. Difficulties arise in attempting to differentiate between a cholinergic crisis and overtreatment with anticholinesterase agents. Patients in a myasthenic crisis will have dilated pupils as a result of hypoxia and hypercarbia. The patient with a cholinergic crisis will present with a very constricted pupil as a result of the increased acetylcholine present at the end plates. A differential diagnosis can be further clarified with the administration of 10 mg of edrophonium (Tensilon test). If the patient's muscle strength improves, the possible cause of the muscle weakness is the undertreatment with anticholinesterase agents. If no improvement occurs or the situation worsens, then the probable cause is a cholinergic crisis. This test should not be administered without the means of

supporting ventilation and circulation immediately available.[3–6, 12–13, 16–18]

Muscular Dystrophy   Of the several types of muscular dystrophy, *Duchenne's muscular dystrophy* is the most severe. This is also known as *pseudohypertrophic muscular dystrophy.* A sex-linked recessive trait disorder that is clinically evident in males, it is characterized by a painless degeneration and atrophy of skeletal muscle. Progressive skeletal muscle weakness develops between the ages of 2 and 5 years. Movement limitation is progressive, with restriction of activity and confinement to a wheelchair by age 12. The child may develop axial skeletal muscle imbalance, producing kyphoscoliosis and requiring operative instrumentation for stabilization. Death occurs in the early teen to adult years and may be secondary to *congestive heart failure* or *pneumonia.* While the primary focus has been skeletal muscle degeneration, there is progressive degeneration of cardiac muscle as well. This results in decreased myocardial contractility and mitral regurgitation secondary to papillary muscle dysfunction. With the degeneration of respiratory muscles, there is evidence of restrictive disease patterns upon pulmonary function testing. As the muscle degeneration progresses, an ineffective cough prevents the successful clearance of secretions, resulting in pneumonia and death. Another form of muscular dystrophy, Becker's dystrophy, is similar to Duchenne's. The onset is later in life and progression is considered to be slower. Fascioscapulohumeral dystrophy and limb-girdle dystrophy develop during adulthood. The diseases' severity is significantly less than that of Duchenne's muscular dystrophy.

Management of Anesthesia in
Neuromuscular Disorders

The myocardial dysfunction with Duchenne's muscular dystrophy may potentially result in increased sensitivity to the myocardial depressant effects of potent inhaled anesthetics. Succinylcholine should be *avoided* to prevent the development of massive rhabdomyolysis, hyperkalemia, and cardiac arrest. Patients with Duchenne's muscular dystrophy are susceptible to malignant hyperthermia. There is a longer recovery time from nondepolarizing muscle relaxants. Because of smooth muscle involvement, the resultant hypomotility of the intestinal tract and delayed gastric emptying puts the patient at significant risk of regurgitation and aspiration of gastric acid. This may be further complicated by impaired swallowing mechanisms. There is a higher incidence of pulmonary dysfunction and retention of pulmonary secretions in this group of patients.[3–6, 16, 17]

NEUROLOGICAL DISORDERS

Multiple Sclerosis   Multiple sclerosis (MS) is the most common acquired *nonmyelinating chronic disease* of the CNS. The clinical symptoms are dependent on the sites of demyelination and include visual disturbances, weakness in extremities and parasthesias. The cause is unknown, assumed to be multifactoral, and may be the result of a persistent viral inflammation or an infection that precipitates an autoimmune response. The fundamental lesion is in the white matter of the CNS, although gray matter involvement occurs. Focal edema may result from the inflammation and breakdown of the blood-brain barrier. There are exacerbations of symptoms at unpredictable intervals over a period of several years. There can also be residual symptoms persisting during periods of remission. These residual symptoms may lead to disability. In some individuals, there is improvement of symptoms during pregnancy; however, there may be incidents of exacerbation during the postpartum period. Recovery from an attack probably entails resolution of edema, limited remyelination, and physiologic adaptation. Sensory onset is most commonly transient, with paresthesias in both upper or lower extremities. Early findings include severe sensory loss in the presence of excellent strength and decreased thresholds to two-point discrimination, proprioception, stereognosis, and vibration. Loss of pain and temperature perception may occur initially but infrequently persists. There is no known cure for the demyelination process; however, corticosteroids have been used to promote remission. Their action may be by decreased white matter edema and enhanced neural conduction through partially demyelinated nerve fibers. Diazepam, dantrolene, and baclofen have been used to treat the skeletal muscle spasticity. Patients with MS should avoid excessive fatigue, emotional stress, and hyperthermia. *Temperature control* under anesthesia is a paramount concern, as the demyelinated nerve fibers are extremely sensitive to increased temperature. A temperature increase of as little as 0.5°C may block conduction in demyelinated fibers.

Management of Anesthesia in Multiple Sclerosis

Effective management of anesthesia must include temperature control. Additionally, the symptoms of MS may be exacerbated by anesthesia, particularly regional anesthesia. Patients with MS who receive spinal anesthesia do have an exacerbation of symptoms after surgery. One theory is that the demyelinated areas of the spinal cord might be more sensitive to the effects of local anesthetics, resulting in the extended exacerbations after anesthesia. Epidural and intrathecal medications have been used successfully in the conduct of anesthesia, including the use of narcotics. Increased rates of relapse have been seen following epidural anesthesia and analgesia with bupivacaine in concentrations greater than 0.25%.[3–6, 13, 14, 16, 17]

Seizure Disorders　Seizure disorders are common manifestations of CNS disorders. There is an excessive discharge of large numbers of neurons, with resulting depolarization in a synchronous fashion.

A *grand mal seizure* is a total body response to the central discharge and is normally characterized by tonic-clonic activity. Respiratory activity ceases during the seizure, resulting in hypoxemia and hypercarbia. Normally, the tonic phase may last 20 to 40 s, followed by the clonic phase. In the post-ictal phase, the patient is lethargic and confused. Initial treatment is directed toward maintaining arterial oxygenation and stopping the seizure activity. Diazepam and thiopental are effective drugs for the treatment of acute seizures.

Focal cortical seizures may be sensory or motor, depending on the site of neuronal discharge. They are identified as *jacksonian epilepsy*. There may be no loss of consciousness, although the activity may spread to produce a grand mal seizure.

Petit mal seizures typically occur in children and young adults. They are characterized by brief losses of awareness lasting approximately 30 s, with an immediate return to consciousness. During the seizure, the child may also demonstrate staring, blinking, and rolling of the eyes.

Akinetic seizures occur frequently in children and may result in falling, with a potential for severe head injury. There is a brief, sudden loss of consciousness and inability to maintain postural tone.

Myoclonic seizures are isolated jerks in response to a sensory stimulus. Most often a single muscle group is involved. This type of seizure is frequently associated with degenerative and metabolic brain diseases.

Status epilepticus is a seizure disorder in which the seizure activity continues unabated for 30 min or longer. As the seizure progresses, skeletal muscle activity diminishes and seizure activity may be evident only on the EEG. Respiratory effects of status epilepticus include inhibition of respiratory centers, uncoordinated skeletal muscle activity that impairs ventilation, and abnormal autonomic activity that produces bronchoconstriction. With inadequate airway control and ventilation, the patient is at high risk for the development of hypoxia and hypercarbia. Diazepam and lorazepam have been used in the initial treatment of status epilepticus as has thiopental. The effects of all these medications are short, requiring initiation of therapy with longer-acting medications. Muscle relaxants may be used to secure the airway; however, they should not be used independent of medications to manage the central seizure.

Management of Anesthesia in Seizure Disorders

Normal antiseizure medication should be maintained preoperatively. If the patient will be unable to resume medications immediately postoperatively, parenteral medications should be administered. The potential influence of anticonvulsants on the response to anesthesia drugs must be considered in choosing anesthetic agents and techniques. Choices should preclude the potential to increase seizure activity. Ketamine has been shown to produce seizure activity in patients with known seizure disorders. Avoiding the use of ketamine when alternative medications such as barbiturates, benzodiazepines, and propofol are available should be considered in choosing the anesthetic agents. Propofol is neither an anticonvulsant nor a convulsant drug. There is a *potential pharmacodynamic resistance to nondepolarizing muscle relaxants* in patients being treated with phenytoin and carbamazepine.[3–6, 16, 17, 19, 20]

Parkinson's Disease (Paralysis Agitans)   Parkinson's disease is a *degenerative disease* caused by a loss of dopaminergic fibers and depletion of dopamine in the basal ganglia (Also see Chapter 28.) The depletion of dopamine results in diminished inhibition of the extrapyramidal motor system. The action of acetylcholine is unopposed. The clinical manifestations of the disease include increased spontaneous movements, cogwheel rigidity of the extremities, facial immobility, and rhythmic tremors at rest. These patients may have significant depression, requiring the institution of pharmacologic therapy. Therapeutic interventions are directed at the elevation of central dopamine levels without the development of significant adverse peripheral effects of dopamine. Levodopa, the immediate precursor of dopamine, is clearly the drug of choice for treatment of Parkinson's disease. Levodopa can cross the blood-brain barrier and is converted to dopamine. Peripheral side effects of extended therapy with levodopa include depletion of myocardial norepinephrine stores, peripheral vasoconstriction, and decreased intravascular volume with resultant orthostatic hypotension.

Management of Anesthesia in Parkinson's Disease

The medications used by the patient should be administered on the morning of surgery. Because of the short half-life of levodopa, discontinuing the medication for more than 6 to 12 h can result in severe skeletal muscle rigidity in the postoperative period. This may lead to difficulty in ventilating the patient. Ketamine can potentially produce exaggerated sympathetic responses, with resultant tachycardia and hypertension. Muscle relaxant choices are not influenced by the patient's chronic illness. Potentially hazardous drug interactions can occur with the use of monoamine oxidase (MAO) inhibitors used in the treatment of Parkinson's disease. One such medication is selegiline, an MAO type B inhibitor. Any medication that acts as an antagonist to dopamine, with the result that there is a decrease in the level of the neurotransmitter available, should be avoided. Medications that should be avoided in this group of patients include droperidol, haldoperidol, and other medications of the butyrophenone group.

Autonomic dysfunction is commonly seen in these patients. This can include gastrointestinal dysfunction, manifest as excessive salivation, dysphagia, and esophageal dysfunction. The patient with Parkinson's disease must be considered at *high risk for regurgitation* and potential development of aspiration pneumonitis. The patient is also at high risk for *positional orthostatic hypotension* both from the disease process and the anti-Parkinson medications used in treatment. Such a patient may also develop exaggerated decreases in blood pressure in response to inhaled halogenated anesthetics. Postoperatively, patients with Parkinson's disease are more susceptible to developing confusion and even hallucinations.[3–6, 16, 17, 19–22]

Alzheimer's Disease   This is the most commonly identified cause of dementia in the United States. With increasing life expectancy for both men and women, a larger proportion of the population will be susceptible to this disease. There are more than sixty identified disorders that can result in dementia; however, Alzheimer's disease accounts for 50% to 60% of all reported cases. There is a characteristic deterioration in both intellectual and cognitive ability, leading to an impairment in social function. The diagnosis of Alzheimer's disease is made if the patient exhibits loss of memory and deficits in two or more areas of cognition. Pathologically, there is *cortical atrophy* and the presence of neurofibrillary tangles and neuritic plaques. (Also see Chapter 28.) There is a functional decrease in choline acetyltransferase and a subsequent cholinergic deficit. There is no identified single cause of Alzheimer's disease and no accepted specific therapy. Symptomatic treatment with cholinesterase inhibitors, clonidine, cerebrovascular vasodilators, vitamins, and antidepressants has been attempted with limited success.

Management of Anesthesia in Alzheimer's Disease

No specific complications have been reported following anesthesia for the patient with Alzheimer's disease. The patient is frequently disoriented and uncooperative. Further mental confusion can result from the use of sedative drugs, especially the benzodiazepines. Intravenous anesthesia has been used without problem with these patients; however, an inhaled anesthetic may provide a more rapid and predictable return to the patient's preoperative level of mental function. *Glycopyrrolate* should be used if an anticholinergic agent is required because of the inability of this medication to cross the blood-brain barrier.[3–6, 16, 17, 19–24]

Guillain-Barré Syndrome   This syndrome of *polyradiculoneuritis* (acute idiopathic polyneuritis) develops as either an acute onset of skeletal muscle weakness or paralysis in the legs. The development of paresthesias may precede the development of paralysis. The paralysis is progressive and includes the trunk and arms within several days. As the paralysis progresses cephalad, difficulty in swallowing and impaired ventilation occur. The development and progression occur over 10 to 12 days and recovery is gradual. Acutely, the process may rapidly progress from intact neurologic function to respiratory muscle paralysis within 48 to 72 h. The patient may be able to identify a respiratory or gastrointestinal tract viral illness within 4 weeks of the onset of neurologic symptoms. The nerve demyelination that occurs is felt to be *immunologically mediated,* with a virus serving as an antigen. Ventilatory insufficiency is the most immediate and serious problem. There is autonomic dysfunction in patients with Guillain-Barré syndrome. Wide fluctuations in blood pressure, tachycardia, cardiac dysrhythmias, and cardiac arrest can occur as a result of this dysfunction. Stimulation of the patient may precipitate hypertension, tachycardia, and cardiac dysrhythmias. The use of both alpha- and beta-adrenergic blockade may be required to manage these events.

Management of Anesthesia in Guillain-Barré Syndrome

Compensatory cardiovascular responses may be absent because of loss of autonomic function, with the development of significant hypotension secondary to postural changes, blood loss, or positive airway pressure. Noxious stimuli from laryngoscopy may produce significant increases in heart rate and blood pressure. The use of direct-acting vasopressors or vasodilators rather than indirect acting agents for the control of blood pressure should be considered. *Succinylcholine* should be avoided because of the potential for hyperkalemia following its administration. This risk can potentially extend beyond the recovery period. Nondepolarizing muscle relaxants with minimal cardiovascular effects should be chosen for surgical muscle relaxation. Mechanical ventilation may be required in the immediate postoperative period.[3–6, 16, 17, 19–23]

Autonomic Hyperreflexia/Dysautonomia   Autonomic hyperreflexia is mediation of spinal cord reflexes without further integration of function from higher centers that could potentially inhibit the response. (Also see Chapter 30.) This is a disorder primarily limited to individuals with *spinal cord injuries, especially above the level of T5*. It occurs in approximately 66% to 85% of quadriplegics and high paraplegics. Signs and symptoms are manifest by acute generalized sympathetic hyperactivity. This includes paroxysmal hypertension, bradycardia, and cardiac dysrhythmias that occur in response to stimuli below the level of transection. The most common initiating cause of this problem can be catheterization or bladder irrigation in patients with injuries above T6. Lesions below T5 and above T10 may result in mild elevations of blood pressure with this stimulatory event. All general anesthetics and conduction blocks have been effective in preventing the development of the syndrome. However, spinal and epidural anesthesia may be difficult in this group of patients.[3–6]

☐ CHRONIC PAIN DISORDERS

REFLEX SYMPATHETIC DYSTROPHIES

Reflex sympathetic dystrophy (RSD) develops following another event that may involve injury and damage to tissues, especially in an extremity. It can develop following crush injuries, lacerations, fractures, sprains, and burns. It has been diagnosed following surgery involving the median nerve distribution, including carpal tunnel release and palmar fasciectomy. It may also occur after cerebrovascular accident or myocardial infarction. The patient complains of a burning pain, diffuse tenderness, and pain that occurs with light touch. Both the hand or foot may be common sites, with the pain and hyperalgesia spreading beyond the original site of pain. The additional manifestations will include changes in skin temperature, cyanosis, edema, and hyperhydrosis.

During the early course of the disorder, the skin may be warm and erythematous. At this time there are frequent episodes of severe vasoconstriction. As RSD becomes more of a chronic state, the affected part may remain cool to cold to both perception and touch and the appearance may be pale to cyanotic. Thermograms and vascular scans can be helpful in documenting differences in blood flow between extremities. As the condition further progresses without treatment, dystrophic changes develop. The skin may take on a smooth and glossy appearance. There is demineralization of the bone as well as stiffening and pain in the joint as a result of synovial edema, fibrosis, hyperplasia, and perivascular inflammation.

A selective sympathetic block may be useful in the diagnosis and initial treatment of RSD. With confirmation of the diagnosis, serial blocks of the sympathetic chain in the affected area can provide relief. If there is difficulty in performing the selective sympathetic block, especially in the lumbar region, a lumbar epidural block can be performed. In some patients, continuous epidural blocks have been beneficial. Unlike other "pain" blocks, injections continue until the symptoms are minimal. This may require three to seven injections or more. At the same time, desensitizing techniques should be initiated as well as active range-of-motion exercises. Systemic sympathetic blocking drugs such as prazosin and phenoxybenzamine have been used successfully in the management of RSD. Tricyclic antidepressants and calcium entry blocking agents have also been used.[3–6, 16, 17, 19–23, 25, 26]

POSTHERPETIC/DEAFFERENTATION SYNDROMES

Herpes zoster is a secondary infection related to reactivation of the latent virus in sensory ganglia. It is not a consequence of reinfection with varicella zoster virus (VZV). There is reactivation of latent VZV in the ganglion, transport of the virus down the sensory nerve to the skin, and a concurrent deficiency in immunity. Because of these events, a localized rash develops. In some patients, in particular the immunocompromised, a viremia develops additionally, manifest by widely scattered lesions. The lesions are minute and unilocular vesicles located in the epidermis. Centrally, the ganglion is swollen and hemorrhage can be identified. Maximum degeneration in the posterior nerve root, posterior column, and sensory nerves occurs approximately 2 weeks following the initial dermal eruptions. Development of zoster has been recognized as an early clinical sign of acquired immunodeficiency syndrome (AIDS) in persons at high risk of human immunodeficiency virus (HIV) infection. One of the theories related to the development of pain following the initial outbreak is related to establishing centrally located self-perpetuating loops that develop within the neural synapses.

Herpes zoster presents usually as a unilateral rash that follows the dermatomal distribution of a peripheral nerve. One to three dermatones may be involved. It is most commonly seen in the thoracic area; however, distribution can be identified along the distribution of the facial nerve, neck, and extremities as well. There is pain along the distribution of the nerve during the active phase of the rash; however, the incidence of postherpetic pain begins to increase sharply around the age of 50 years. Zoster involving the trigeminal nerve may also present with symptoms of CNS involvement, including headache, aphasia, and seizures. Contralateral paralysis can develop days to weeks following the onset of trigeminal symptoms and may be related to infection by the virus of the cerebral blood vessels. This is known as *granulomatous angiitis.*

The duration of infection is variable, with the patient no longer being infectious to others after the lesions have dried. The goals of intervention include resolution of the acute problem and minimization of the potential to develop post-herpetic neuralgia. This can include aggressive management with antiviral agents, analgesics, anti-inflammatory agents, antidepressants, vitamin B_{12}, B complex, L-tryptophan, nerve blocks, psychosocial therapy, physical measures, and surgery. Analgesia blocks can be used in the management of the patient. Local anesthetics are injected locally, along the course of the nerve, as a sympathetic block, and in the epidural space. Local anesthetic agents in combination with corticosteroids have been used in the management of the postherpetic neuralgia. However, no intervention has been identified to prevent the development of the neuralgia. The most successful treatment occurs when the intervention is begun within the first 2 weeks after the initial eruptions.[3–6, 16, 17, 19–23, 25, 26]

PHARMACOLOGY

VASOACTIVE AGENTS

All direct-acting vasodilators are considered *cerebral vasodilators.* They abolish autoregulation, thus making CBF passive. These drugs include sodium nitroprusside, nitroglycerin, hydralazine, adenosine, and calcium channel blockers. Cerebral blood flow may go up, go down, or remain the same when these agents are used for the management of blood pressure. Flow becomes dependent on mean arterial pressure. Cerebral blood flow is determined by actual CPP. If the CPP remains high during vasodilator therapy, it is probable that the CBF will increase. If the use of the vasodilating agent results in severe hypotension, the CBF may fall. Cerebral blood flow may be maintained during hypotension as a result of cerebral vasodilation and enhanced flow. With the slow development of hypotension, changes in ICP as a result of changes in cerebral blood volume tend to be blunted. This is related to the compensatory changes in CSF and venous blood volume.[3–5, 9, 19, 20, 23]

Trimethaphan blocks sympathetic ganglia to produce reductions in blood pressure. It also causes pupillary dilation, ileus, and urinary retention. Because of its direct vasodilating properties, its impact on CNS physiology is similar to that of other direct-acting agents. Trimethaphan also impairs cerebral metabolism, with the result that ischemic insults as a result of hypotension are more severe. *Labetalol* and *esmolol* have not been shown to have an effect on CBF.

Alpha$_1$ agonists such as phenylephrine and norepinephrine have little direct effect on the cerebral vasculature. Larger doses may produce a slight decrease in CBF. Alpha$_2$ agonists can produce changes in the CBF independent of changes in the cerebral metabolic rate. Beta agonists have no effect on the cerebral blood flow if the blood-brain barrier is intact. If

it is disrupted, the use of beta agonists will result in an increase in cerebral metabolism and therefore an increase in CBF. *Dopamine* at clinical doses will produce cerebrovasodilation with an increase in CBF.[3–5, 9, 19, 20, 23]

INTRAVENOUS ANESTHETIC AGENTS

All barbiturates in clinical use result in a dose-dependent decrease in cerebral metabolic rate, to a maximum of 50% to 60%. The maximum reduction in metabolism occurs when the EEG becomes isoelectric. Further suppression of metabolism is not possible with barbiturates. Cerebral blood flow is reduced relative to "flow-metabolism coupling." With the induction of anesthesia, metabolism is reduced by approximately 30%. The decreased flow and metabolism are not related to the dose of barbiturate administered. Large decreases can occur with smaller doses and smaller decreases occur with progressively higher doses. The barbiturates *suppress electrical activity* but do nothing to reduce the energy devoted to intrinsic cellular homeostasis. Barbiturates are protective only in *temporary focal ischemia.* Autoregulation will be maintained during barbiturate administration. The hypocapnic response can be blunted by preexisting vasoconstriction induced by barbiturates.

With the use of modest doses of morphine (1 to 3 mg/kg), only slight decreases in cerebral metabolic rate and CBF occur. Autoregulation is normally maintained. Fentanyl produces a dose-dependent reduction in both CBF and cerebral metabolism. Fentanyl, 5 to 15 μg/kg, probably produces a 10% to 30% reduction in both CBF and cerebral metabolism. Higher doses (50 to 100 μg/kg) can result in greater decreases in blood flow and metabolism. Flows may be reduced to about 25 mg/100 g/min. Fentanyl and other synthetic narcotics may possess some mild cerebrovasodilating properties. Autoregulation and carbon dioxide responsiveness are maintained during the administration of fentanyl (in the absence of hypoventilation). The goal of an isoelectric EEG cannot be achieved with fentanyl.

There is a modest reduction in both CBF and cerebral metabolism with the use of benzodiazepines. This may be as great as 20% to 30%. The anesthesia practitioner will be unable to achieve an isoelectric EEG with the use of benzodiazepines. Carbon dioxide responsiveness is maintained with their use as well.

Ketamine produces a marked increase in the cerebral blood flow, with the greatest changes occurring in the limbic system. Intracranial pressure is increased as a reflection of increases in cerebral blood volume. Globally, cerebral metabolism is unchanged; however, regional changes may be present. Ketamine is also capable of producing subcortical seizures. There is an increased resistance to the absorption of CSF by 200%. Carbon dioxide responsiveness is maintained.

Etomidate produces effects similar to those of barbiturates. It can produce an isoelectric EEG. There is no further reduction in CBF, cerebral metabolism, or intracranial pressure following the development of the isoelectric EEG. Prior to the onset of isoelectricity, *spike activity* may be associated with myoclonus. Normal individuals will not exhibit seizure activity; however, small doses may exacerbate seizures foci in predisposed individuals. The hypocapnic response is blunted in a manner similar to that seen with the barbiturates; however, vasodilatory effects of increased carbon dioxide are maintained. The practitioner must also be concerned with the potential for adrenocortical suppression.

Propofol produces effects similar to those of the barbiturates. There is a dose-related change in CBF and cerebral metabolism. Propofol can produce an isoelectric EEG. There may be a significant reduction in the mean arterial blood pressure and thus a significant reduction in cerebral perfusion pressure. High doses of propofol will produce an increase in CBF because of a direct cerebrovasodilatory effect.[3–5, 9,19–21, 23]

INHALED ANESTHETIC AGENTS

Isoflurane is the most commonly used inhalation agent. It produces a dose-related depression in cerebral metabolism. At 2.0 MAC, it will produce an isoelectric EEG with a 50% reduction in cerebral metabolism. There is a dose-related increase in CBF. However, these increases are greater with halothane than with isoflurane. With isoflurane, there are no changes in the cortical flow, while halothane increases cortical flow much more than flow to other areas of the brain. There is a greater increase in flow to the posterior fossa with isoflurane. However, overall CBF is similar with both halothane and isoflurane. Autoregulation is maintained with up to 1.0 MAC of isoflurane. Responsiveness to carbon dioxide is maintained with isoflurane. To prevent increases in intracranial pressure, hyperventilation should be initiated when isoflurane is administered. There is no evidence supporting the premise that isoflurane can protect cerebral tissues from ischemia. Isoflurane has been used to provide controlled hypotension during surgical procedures. There is an increase in the resorption of CSF, but there is no direct impact on production.

Halothane was traditionally presented as a more potent cerebrovasodilator than isoflurane. However, its overall or global vasodilation is not significantly different from that of isoflurane. Halothane *cannot* produce an isoelectric EEG in concentrations used clinically. In animal studies, 6.0 MAC was required to produce an isoelectric EEG. Autoregulation is inhibited at 1.0 MAC. Carbon dioxide responsiveness is maintained at 1.0 MAC. There is a decrease in both the production and resorption of CSF.

Enflurane's effects on CBF and cerebral metabolism is probably similar to those of isoflurane or halothane. At 2.0 MAC, combined with hypocapnia, there is an increased risk of seizures. There is an increase in the production of CSF; however, resorption is inhibited. This may result in increases in ICP over time. Responsiveness to changes in carbon dioxide is maintained.

Nitrous oxide can produce increases in CBF and ICP similar to or greater than that seen with the potent inhalation agents. This could produce negative outcomes in individuals with increased ICP. These increases may be controlled by the concomitant use of intravenous anesthetic agents and hyperventilation.

The inhalation agents cause a reduction in blood flow to the brain as the systemic pressure falls. The *minimum blood flow* required to prevent ipsilateral EEG changes consistent with ischemia in a majority of patients from the potent inhalation agents have been investigated. This is the *critical blood flow* and is identified for halothane as 20 mL/100 g/min, for enflurane as 15 mL/100 g/min, and for isoflurane as 10 mL/100 g/min.

Nitrous oxide also has the potential to increase ICP by increasing the CBF. The response can be blunted by narcotics, barbiturates, and hypocapnia. There is the additional risk of pneumocephalus with the use of nitrous oxide.[3–5, 9, 19, 20, 22, 23]

MUSCLE RELAXANTS

With the nondepolarizing muscle relaxants, there is no significant effect if the heart rate or blood pressure remains unchanged. However, with those medications that cause a release of endogenous histamine, changes can occur in both CBF and ICP. Histamine is a potent cerebrovasodilator. There may be an increase in the intracranial pressure when pancuronium is administered to a patient with nonautoregulating vessels, as are seen with trauma, tumors, and subarachnoid hemorrhage. Finally, *d*-tubocurarine can cause a release of histamine that will result in an increase in ICP.

The depolarizing muscle relaxant succinylcholine can cause an increase in ICP as a result of muscle spindle activation and increased input into the CNS. This will result in further cerebral activation, increased cerebral metabolism, and increased CBF. The increases are transient, and succinylcholine can be used in the neurologic patient if rapid control of the airway is required. Pretreatment with a nondepolarizing muscle relaxant, barbiturates, narcotics, and lidocaine may blunt or prevent the increases seen with succinylcholine. Lidocaine in doses of 1.5 mg/kg administered 3 to 5 min prior to an invasive procedure (such as intubation and suctioning) can help to minimize the changes in intracranial pressure from systemic reactions to these events.[3–5, 9, 19, 20, 23]

DILANTIN (PHENYTOIN)

Phenytoin has been an effective therapeutic medication for seizures since the 1930s. It is similar chemically to barbiturate compounds; however, it does not produce the same level of sedation as the barbiturates. The medication has a long half-life (average 24 h) and can be administered daily. The average daily dose is 250 to 500 mg. Phenytoin is hydroxylated in the liver, conjugated, and then excreted by the kidney. In lower doses, phenytoin exhibits first-order kinetics; but in higher doses, it exhibits zero-order kinetics. Cimetidine can compete for metabolic enzymes, resulting in reduced metabolism of the medication. Phenytoin is highly protein-bound, and drugs such as the antidepressants and oral hyperglycemics compete for binding sites, resulting in increases in the serum dilantin levels. Phenytoin is considered to have a *membrane-stabilizing action*. It acts to alter the movement of sodium, potassium, and calcium at the cellular level as well as membrane potentials and the levels of the neurotransmitters norepinephrine, acetylcholine, and GABA (gamma-aminobutyric acid). There is a block of sustained high-frequency repetitive firing of the action potentials. At higher does, it will interfere with the release of serotonin. Phenytoin has a direct action on the conduction system of the myocardium and can be used effectively as an antidysrhythmic, especially for ventricular dysrhythmias resistant to lidocaine. Patients on long-term therapy with phenytoin may require increased doses of barbiturates. They may be resistant to metocurine, pancurionium, vecuronium, and *d*-tubocurarine. Atracurium has been used successfully without increasing the dosage of the medication.[3–5, 9, 19, 20, 22, 23]

REFERENCES

1. Guyton AC, Hall JE. The nervous system: General principles and sensory physiology. In: *Guyton's Textbook of Medical Physiology*. 9th ed. Philadelphia: Saunders; 1996:565–622.

2. Guyton AC. The nervous system: Motor and integrative neurophysiology. In: *Guyton's Textbook of Medical Physiology*. 9th ed. Philadelphia: Saunders; 1996:685–792.

3. Bendo AA, Kass IS, Hartung J, Cottrell JE. Neurophysiology and neuroanesthesia. In: Barash PG, Cullen, Stoelting, eds. *Clinical Anesthesia*. 2nd ed. Philadelphia: Lippincott; 1992: 871–998.

4. Shapiro HM, Drummond JC. Neurosurgical anesthesia. In: Miller RD, ed. *Anesthesia*, 4th ed. Philadelphia: Lippincott; 1994:1897–1946.

5. Todd MM, Warner DS. Neuroanesthesia: A critical review. In: Rogers MC, Tinker JH, Covino, Longnecker DE, eds. *Principles and Practice of Anesthesiology*. St Louis: Mosby-Year Book; 1993:1599–1648.

6. Kiernan JA. Some functional pathways in the central nervous system. In: Kelly WN, ed. *Textbook of Internal Medicine*. 2nd ed. Philadelphia: Lippincott; 1992:2138–2144.

7. Stoelting RK. Physiology: Central nervous system. In: Stoelting RK, ed. *Pharmacology and Physiology in Anesthesia Practice*. Philadelphia: Lippincott; 1991:612–642.

8. Summer AJ. Structure and function of the peripheral nervous system. In: Kelly WN, ed. *Textbook of Internal Medicine*. 2nd ed. Philadelphia: Lippincott; 1992:2147–2150.

9. Stoelting RK. Physiology: Autonomic nervous system. In: Stoelting RK, ed. *Pharmacology and Physiology in Anesthesia Practice*. Philadelphia: Lippincott; 1991:643–653.

10. Raj PP, Riegler FX. Nerve blocks and other procedures for pain therapy. In: Rogers MC, Tinker JH, Covino, Longnecker DE, eds. *Principles and Practice of Anesthesiology*. St Louis: Mosby-Year Book: 1993:1349–1425.

11. Cousins MJ. Introduction to acute and chronic pain. In: Cousins MJ, Bridenbaugh PO, eds. *Neural Blockade and Pain Management in Clinical Anesthesia*. 2nd ed. Philadelphia: Lippincott; 1988:739–790.

12. Cousins MJ, Dwyer B, Gibb D. Chronic pain and neurolytic neural blockade. In: Cousins MJ, Bridenbaugh PO, eds. *Neural Blockade and Pain Management in Clinical Anesthesia*. 2nd ed. Philadelphia: Lippincott; 1988:1053–1084.

13. Halter JB. Structure and function of the autonomic nervous system. In: Kelly WN, ed. *Textbook of Internal Medicine*. 2nd ed. Philadelphia: Lippincott; 1992:2145–2146.

14. Makatabi M. Basic physiology and pharmacology of the autonomic nervous system. In: Rogers MC, Tinker JH, Covino, Longnecker DE, eds. *Principles and Practice of Anesthesiology*. St Louis: Mosby-Year Book; 1993:1471–1506.

15. Stoelting RK. Physiology: Pain. In: Stoelting RK *Pharmacology and Physiology in Anesthesia Practice*. Philadelphia: Lippincott; 1992:654–660.

16. Ebers CG. Demylenating diseases. In: Kelly WN, ed. *Textbook of Internal Medicine*. 2nd ed. Philadelphia: Lippincott; 1992: 2168–2170.

17. Price DL, Griffin JW, Huffman PN, Cork LC. Neuropathology of toxic degenerative diseases. In: Kelly WN, ed. *Textbook of Internal Medicine*. 2nd ed. Philadelphia: Lippincott; 1992: 2181–2182.

18. Osserman KE, Genkins G. Studies in myasthenia gravis: Review of a twenty-year experience in over 1200 patients. *Mt Sinai J Med*. 1971; 38:497–538.

19. Shelton RC, Ebert MH. Drugs and the central nervous system. In: Wood M, Wood AJJ, eds. *Drugs and Anesthesia: Pharmacology for Anesthesiologists*. 2nd ed. Baltimore: Williams & Wilkins; 1990:571–595.

20. Porter RJ, Meldrum BS. Antiepileptic drugs. In: Katsung B, ed. *Basic and Clinical Pharmacology*. 6th ed. Norwalk, Conn: Appleton & Lange; 1995:361–380.

21. Snow BJ, Peppard RF, Colne DB. Extrapyramidal disorders. In: Kelly WN, ed. *Textbook of Internal Medicine*. 2nd ed. Philadelphia: Lippincott; 1992:2171–2173.

22. Trevor AJ, Way WL. Sedative-hypnotics. In: Katsung B, ed. *Basic and Clinical Pharmacology*. 6th ed. Norwalk, Conn: Appleton & Lange; 1995:333–349.

23. Nicoli RA. Introduction to the pharmacology of CNS drugs. In: Katsung B, ed. *Basic and Clinical Pharmacology*. 6th ed. Norwalk, Conn: Appleton & Lange; 1995:323–332.

24. Bhatt MH, Peppard RF, Colne DB. Chronic dementing diseases. In: Kelly WN, ed. *Textbook of Internal Medicine*. 2nd ed. Philadelphia: Lippincott; 1992:2174–2177.

25. Strichartz GR. Neural physiology and local anesthesia action. In: Cousins MJ, Bridenbaugh PO, eds. *Neural Blockade and Pain Management in Clinical Anesthesia*. 2nd ed. Philadelphia: Lippincott; 1988:25–46.

26. Raj PP. Prognostic and therapeutic local anesthetic blockade. In: Cousins MJ, Bridenbaugh PO, eds. *Neural Blockade and Pain Management in Clinical Anesthesia*. 2nd ed. Philadelphia: Lippincott; 1988:899–934.

☐ QUESTIONS

1. Reductions in cerebral perfusion pressure can occur with closed head injuries when the
   a. Mean arterial pressure is decreased
   b. Intracranial pressure is increased
   c. Carbon dioxide concentration is decreased
   d. Patient is hypovolemic

2. When the cranial vault is open, cerebral perfusion pressure and _____ are equal.
   a. Systolic blood pressure
   b. Diastolic blood pressure
   c. Mean blood pressure
   d. None of the above

3. The use of thiopental in the patient with a space-occupying lesion is preferable because of
   a. The vasodilator effect of the medication
   b. Its role in decreasing cerebral metabolic rate
   c. Its role in decreasing intracranial pressure
   d. All of the above

4. True statements include all **except**:
   a. The parasympathetic postganglionic fibers secrete acetylcholine as the neurotransmitter.
   b. All preganglionic fibers are classified as cholinergic fibers.
   c. Sweat glands receive norepinephrine as the neurotransmitter.
   d. The sympathetic postganglionic fibers secrete norepinephrine as the neurotransmitter.

5. The recommended treatment for hypertension in the patient emerging from general anesthesia following a craniotomy is:
   a. Esmolol
   b. Nitroglycerin
   c. Sodium nitroprusside
   d. Labetalol

6. The critical structure in the cervical spine is
   a. The alanto-axial joint
   b. C1
   c. C2
   d. All of the above

7. The ligaments that prevent displacement of the joint between C1 and C2 are:
   a. Apical
   b. Transverse
   c. Alar
   d. All of the above

8. Patients requiring general anesthesia with a history of _____ should have a cervical neck series prior to the induction of anesthesia.

   a. Down's syndrome
   b. Rheumatoid arthritis
   c. Degenerative joint disease
   d. a and b

9. Procedures used to reduce the mean arterial pressure include:
   a. Antihypertensive therapy
   b. Restricting fluids
   c. Sedation
   d. All of the above

10. Fentanyl _____ μg/kg is administered to achieve the target blood pressure during anesthesia for control of bleeding from a cerebral aneurysm.
    a. 1–4
    b. 5–9
    c. 10–15
    d. 16–19

11. Cerebral edema can be caused by:
    a. Hypertonic saline
    b. Decreased oncotic pressure
    c. Using colloid instead of crystalloid
    d. Hyposmolar solutions

12. Beck's triad includes all *except*
    a. Bradycardia
    b. Distant heart sounds
    c. Hypotension
    d. Jugular distention

13. The nondepolarizing muscle relaxant that has been suggested to increase intracranial pressure in nonautoregulatory vessels is:
    a. Atracurium
    b. Vecuronium
    c. Pancuronium
    d. b and c

14. Autoregulation of cerebral blood flow is relatively constant in the range of _____ torr.
    a. 40–140
    b. 50–150
    c. 60–160
    d. 70–170

15. List the cranial nerve that is active in the oculocardiac reflex.
    a. Trigeminal
    b. Occulomotor
    c. Vagus
    d. a and c

16. The brain has available oxygen stores to provide normal cellular function for _____ sec. following cessation of cerebral blood flow without protective intervention.
  a. 5–10
  b. 11–15
  c. 16–20
  d. No stores are present.

17. The relationship between central venous pressure and absorption of CSF is as follows:
  a. Increased venous pressure decreases absorption.
  b. Decreased venous pressure decreases absorption.
  c. Increased venous pressure increases absorption.
  d. all of the above

18. Secretion of CSF is directly affected by:
  a. Serum osmolality
  b. Intraventricular hydrostatic pressure

  c. Cerebral blood flow
  d. All of the above

19. The _____ produce a dose-dependent decrease in cerebral metabolic rate and are considered to be protective in temporary focal ischemia.
  a. Narcotics
  b. Benzodiazepines
  c. Barbiturates
  d. Agonists-antagonists

20. Autoregulation of cerebral blood flow is maintained with 1.0 MAC of:
  a. Enflurane
  b. Halothane
  c. Isoflurane
  d. None of the above

☐ ANSWERS

1. a	**5.** d	**9.** d	**13.** c	**17.** a
2. c	**6.** d	**10.** c	**14.** b	**18.** d
3. d	**7.** d	**11.** d	**15.** d	**19.** c
4. c	**8.** d	**12.** a	**16.** d	**20.** c

CHAPTER

15

Cardiovascular System

Mary R. Steward

☐ ANATOMY AND PHYSIOLOGY

CARDIAC ANATOMY

The heart is a four-chamber, muscular organ that through a pumping mechanism supplies the body with blood to sustain life. In the adult, the approximate size is 12 cm long, 9 cm wide at the widest point, and 6 cm thick.[1] The weight is 250 to 350 g. Located in the mediastinum within the chest cavity, it is positioned between the lungs and protected structurally by the sternum, ribs, and vertebral column.[1]

The heart is enclosed by a fibroserous membranous sac called the pericardium, which prevents friction when the heart contracts. The fibrous pericardium or the outermost layer is attached to the diaphragm and extends to the great vessels. Beneath this fibrous area is a delicate, thin layer called the serous pericardium. This membrane consists of two layers; the parietal layer, which is fused to the fibrous pericardium, and viseral layer and the epicardium, which is connected to the heart. The pericardial fluid between the two layers lubricates the heart. This fluid is an ultrafiltrate plasma totaling 50 mL.[1]

Beneath the epicardium is the striated muscle portion of the heart, the myocardium. The myocardial striated muscle differs from skeletal muscle in that the cardiac muscle fibers are connected by intercalated disks. Ions that facilitate a change in the action potential, causing depolarization, can diffuse quickly from one cardiac cell to the next. This enables the muscle or syncytium to contract as a unit. There are two syncytiums, the atrial and ventricle.

The endocardium is a connective tissue that lines the innermost layer of the myocardium. This incorporates the papillary muscle and the chordae tendinae. Because the papillary muscle and the chordae tendinae are attached to the cusps of

the interventricular valves, contraction of the muscle prevents eversion of the valves during ventricular systole.[1]

Chambers   The heart has two atria (right and left) and two ventricles (right and left). The atria are separated by the interatrial septum and the ventricles by the interventricular septum.[1]

Right Heart   The right atrium receives deoxygenated blood from the superior vena cava, inferior vena cava, and coronary sinus. Seventy percent of the blood flows from the atrium into the ventricle passively. The other 30% is delivered via an atrial contraction.[1] The tricuspid valve separates the right atrium and right ventricle. Once blood begins to flow through the valve, the papillary muscle relaxes, decreasing the tension on the chordae tendinae and allowing the valve to remain open. As pressure increases in the right ventricle, the papillary muscle contracts, which causes the chordae tendinae to increase the tension. This increased tension inhibits the valve from inverting into the atria, preventing backflow.[1]

The right ventricle will contract, ejecting the deoxygenated blood through the pulmonic valve into the pulmonary artery. The pulmonary valve opens in response to an increase in ventricular pressure; once blood has moved into the pulmonary artery, the volume increases the pressure, causing the valve to close. Blood cannot flow backward through the intact semilunar cusps.

Left Heart   Oxygenated blood flows from the lungs into the left atrium during atrial diastole via the four pulmonary veins. As blood begins to flow through the mitral valve, the papillary muscle relaxes, which decreases the tension in the

251

chordae tendinae. This allows the mitral valve to stay open. Once pressure increases in the left ventricle, the papillary muscle contracts, the chordae tendinae tense, and the valve closes.

During ventricular systole, blood is injected through a semilunar valve, the aortic valve, and into the aorta. The descending aorta supplies the lower extremities and organs; the upper extremities and brain are supplied by the brachiocephalic, the left common carotid, and the left subclavian arteries. These three vessels branch off the aortic arch. At this time during the cardiac cycle the ventricles are contracting and the atria are relaxing, known as ventricle systole. During ventricular diastole the ventricles are relaxing and the atria are contracting.

CORONARY BLOOD FLOW

The heart is supplied with nutrients and oxygen via the coronary arteries (Figure 15–1). The main coronary arteries branch from the base of the aorta and lie directly on the surface of the myocardium, and then go into the smaller arteries.[1] These smaller arteries penetrate into the heart, supplying the heart and conduction system with oxygen.

The *left coronary artery* supplies the anterior and lateral portions of the left ventricle, right bundle branch, left bundle branch, and the anterior and posterior of the mitral papillary muscle. The *circumflex* is a branch off the left coronary artery, which supplies the lateral left ventricle.[2]

The *right coronary artery* supplies the sinoatrial (SA) and the atrioventricular (AV) nodes, posterior interventricular septum, posterior fascicle, left bundle branch, and the interatrial septum.[2] In 80% of the population the right coronary artery is considered dominant, in that it supplies the right ventricle and the posterior portion of the left ventricle. In the other 20% of the population, the left coronary artery is considered dominant.[3]

Deoxygenated blood returns to the heart via the great and small veins, which drain into the coronary sinus and into the right atrium, and the thebesian vein that drains directly through the atrial wall.[3]

Coronary perfusion is intermittent. It is determined by the difference between the aortic and ventricular pressures. When the left ventricle contracts the intramyocardial part of the coronary arteries are occluded. Therefore, left ventricle perfusion occurs during relaxation of the ventricle or diastole. The length of time is also important for perfusion. When comparing a heart rate of 70 versus 90, diastolic time is longer with a slower heart rate, therefore providing more time for the heart to be perfused. Coronary arterial tone also changes blood flow. This could be in response to metabolic demand such as an increase in sympathetic stimulation or hypoxia, which causes a release in adenosine and produces coronary vasodilatation.[3]

CONDUCTION

Neural stimulation (Figure 15–2) of the heart is primarily through the sympathetic and parasympathetic nervous system. The sympathetic fibers originate from cervical ganglions to the cord segments thoracic 1 through 4. The parasympathetic stimulation is through the tenth cranial nerve (the vagus nerve). An increase in sympathetic tone will increase heart rate, whereas an increase in parasympathetic tone will decrease heart rate.[2]

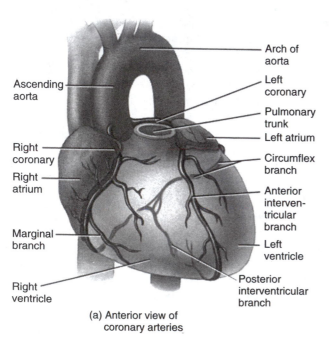

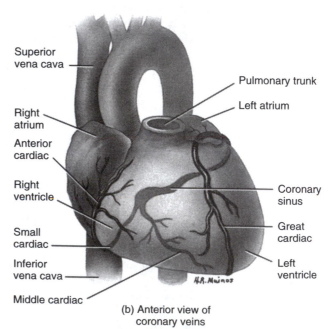

Figure 15–1 Coronary (cardiac) circulation. *A*. Anterior view of arterial distribution *B*. Anterior view of venous drainage. (Reproduced by permission from Tortora and Anagnostakos.[1])

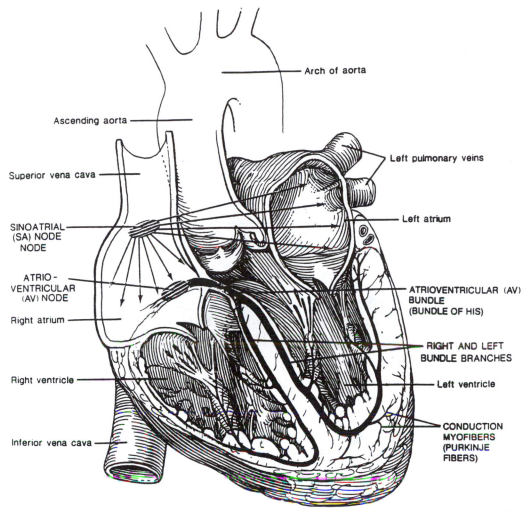

Figure 15-2 Conduction system of the heart. (Reproduced by permission from Tortora and Anagnostakos.[1])

CARDIAC CELL PHYSIOLOGY

Located near the superior vena cava in the right atrium, the SA node initiates an impulse (Figure 15–3). When stimulated, a sudden influx of sodium and a slower influx of calcium causes the resting potential of -85 to -95 mV to reach an action potential of $+20$ mV. After the overshoot potential or spike, the muscle remains depolarized (plateau phase). This plateau is longer in cardiac muscle as compared to skeletal muscle. Once the calcium channels open, the permeability of potassium decreases, thus preventing early recovery. It is the restoration of potassium that returns the SA node to a resting state.[3] During an action potential the cell is unable to be stimulated at a given point. This is the cell's refractory period, during which time it is difficult but not impossible to stimulate the cell. The ventricular refractory period is slightly longer than the atrial period, which facilitates a quicker contraction of the atria compared to the ventricle.[3]

The SA node impulse is rapidly conducted from the right atrium to the left atrium via Bachmann's bundle and to the AV node located in the septal wall of the right atrium, ante-

rior to the coronary sinus and the septal leaflet of the tricuspid valve. The stimulus passes through the AV node to the common bundle of His. These fibers divide into right and left branches, which form the Purkinji fibers. Accessory fibers allow conduction to travel from the SA node to the ventricle without passing through the AV node. These pathways include the Kent fibers that connect the SA node to the right ventricle, the James fibers that conduction bypasses to the bundle of His, and the Mahaim fibers that shunt impulses from the bundle of His to the intraventricular septal myocardium.[6] It takes less than 0.2 second for the SA node stimulus to depolarize the heart.

CARDIAC OXYGEN CONSUMPTION

The myocardium receives 7% of the cardiac output. Normally the myocardium extracts approximately 65% of the oxygen content from the blood.[5] This leaves a narrow margin for the heart to be able to extract more oxygen if needed. Therefore, the heart must be supplied with an adequate amount of blood to meet the demand.

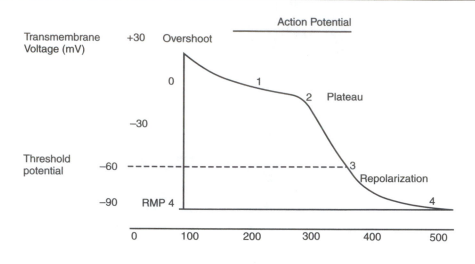

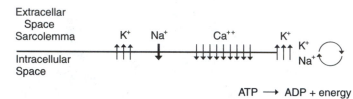

Figure 15–3 Cardiac cell action potential.
Phase 4 Resting membrane potential (RMP) or diastolic repolarization. In this stage the atrial and ventricular permeability of the cells is restored. There is a leakage of Na$^+$ into the cells that will spontaneous depolarize. Potassium moves out of the cell and sodium moves into the cell.
Phase 0 This is the depolarization stage. There is a rapid upstroke due to the fast Na$^+$ channels opening and a decreased permeability to K$^+$. At this point Na$^+$ is moving into the cell.
Phase 1 This is the overshoot stage. There is a rapid repolarization secondary to the inactivation of Na$^+$ channels and increased permeability to K$^+$. K$^+$ is moving out of the cell.
Phase 2 This is the plateau stage. The plateau is due to the activation of slow Ca^{++} channels. Ca^{++} is moving into the cell.
Phase 3 This is the repolarization stage. Ca^{++} channels are inactivated and K$^+$ has an increased permeability. K$^+$ is moving out of the cell.

MYOCARDIAL OXYGEN SUPPLY

Oxygen delivery to the heart is affected by heart rate and diastolic time. It is also affected by coronary perfusion pressure, aortic diastolic blood pressure, and left ventricular end-diastolic pressure (LVEDP). Factors that affect blood delivery are coronary artery diameter and patency, arterial oxygen content, hemoglobin concentration, and viscosity.

MYOCARDIAL OXYGEN DEMAND

The heart's demand for oxygen depends on the basal oxygen requirements, heart rate, wall tension, preload, afterload, and contractility.

MYOCARDIAL OXYGEN SUPPLY–DEMAND BALANCE

Ideally, it is better to have more oxygen than the heart requires to prevent ischemia and infarction. However, it is technically easier to manipulate the demands on the heart versus

the supply. *Tachycardia* is the worst single insult on the heart. This decreases diastolic filling, decreases coronary blood flow, and increases myocardial oxygen consumption. Therefore, slowing heart rate will increase supply and decrease the oxygen consumption. With the use of hemodynamic monitoring, the clinician can select the appropriate medications to decrease wall tension, preload, afterload, and contractility.

HEMODYNAMIC PRESSURES AND PARAMETERS

The necessary hemodynamic measurements for cardiac assessment are presented in Figure 15–4 and Tables 15–1 through 15–10.

NORMAL ELECTROCARDIOGRAM

An electrocardiogram (ECG) is recorded on calibrated paper; the horizontal lines represent time and the vertical lines represent voltage. When measuring the horizontal lines each small box or 1 mm equals 0.04 seconds and the large box or 5 mm

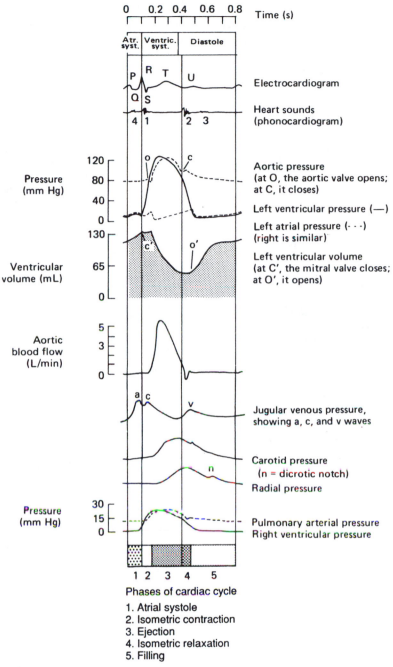

Figure 15-4 Pressures and tracings in the cardiac cycle. (Reproduced by permission from Morgan and Mikhail.[5])

equals 0.20 seconds. For the vertical lines, 1 mm equals 0.1 mV and 5 mm equals 0.5 mV. The components of a normal ECG consist of a P wave, QRS complex, and a T wave. The waves are either inflected or deflected above or below the isoelectric line, which is a straight horizontal line indicating no electrical activity. Any inflection indicates that an electrical impulse is moving toward the positive electrode. A deflection indicates that an electrical impulse is moving away from the negative electrode. In a healthy heart, any electrical activity reflects normal contractility.

Components of an ECG

P wave (normal amplitude < 3 mm)—Represents electrical activity as the right and left atria depolarize.

PR interval (normal 0.12–0.20 second)—Represents the time for the stimulus to leave the SA node and cross junctional tissues, which stimulates the ventricles.

Q wave (normal 0.04 second)—This wave normally does not exist in a healthy heart. It is a negative deflection denoting ventricular depolarization.

Table 15–1
CENTRAL VENOUS PRESSURE (CVP)

Normal: 1–8 mm Hg or 3–8 cm water pressure
Note:　To convert mm Hg to cm H$_2$O multiply mm Hg by 1.34
　　　　(1.34 cm H$_2$O = 1 mm Hg)

Abnormal Wave Forms	Causes
Large a wave	Mitral stenosis, left ventricular failure, tricuspid stenosis, right ventricular hypertrophy from pulmonic stenosis, pulmonary hypertension, pacemaker malfunction
Absent a wave	Atrial fibrillation
Giant v wave	Tricuspid regurgitation, right ventricular ischemia and failure, constrictive pericarditis, cardiac tamponade, papillary muscle ischemia
Absent y descent	Pericardial constriction, cardiac tamponade
Decreased CVP	Hypovolemia, vascular dilation
Increased CVP	Right ventricular failure from right ventricular myocardial infarction or cardiomyopathy; increased pulmonary vascular resistance due to pulmonary edema, hypoxemia, COPD, ARDS, sepsis or shock; mitral stenosis or insufficiency, end-stage left ventricle failure, positive-pressure ventilation

a, atrial contraction
c, ventricular contraction (the tricuspid valve is bulging into the right atrium during ventricular systole)
v, end of ventricular contraction, there is a slow buildup of blood in the atria, while the AV valves are closed
x, end of atrial diastole, there is a decrease in pressure with atrial relaxation
y, isometric relaxation, there is a decrease in atrial pressure as the AV valve opens and the right ventricle fills
ARDS, adult respiratory distress syndrome; COPD, chronic obstructive pulmonary disease

R wave (normal < 13 mm amplitude)—This is a positive inflection denoting ventricular depolarization.
S wave—This is a negative deflection denoting ventricular depolarization.
QRS complex (normal 0.06–0.10 second)—Represents the entire ventricular depolarization.

Table 15–2
RIGHT VENTRICULAR END-SYSTOLIC (RVESP) AND RIGHT VENTRICULAR END-DIASTOLIC (RVEDP) PRESSURES

Normal RVESP: 15–25 mm Hg
Normal RVEDP: 0–8 mm Hg

Abnormal	Causes
Increased RVESP	COPD, ARDS, sepsis, pulmonary edema, hypoxia
Increased RVEDP	Right ventricular failure or cardiomyopathy
Decreased RVEDP	Hypovolemia

ARDS, adult respiratory distress syndrome; COPD, chronic obstructive pulmonary disease; RVEDP, right ventricular end-diastolic pressure; RVESP, right ventricular end-systolic pressure

Table 15–3
PULMONARY ARTERY PRESSURE (PAP)

Normal mean: 10–20 mm Hg; systolic: 15–25 mm Hg; diastolic: 8–15 mm Hg

Abnormal	Causes
Increased PAP systolic	Right ventricular failure, shock, pulmonary edema, COPD, ARDS, cardiac tamponade, hypoxemia, pulmonary hypertension
Increased PAP diastolic	Left ventricular failure, mitral stenosis, pulmonary hypertension, volume overload or AV septal shunt

ARDS, adult respiratory distress syndrome; COPD, chronic obstructive pulmonary disease

T wave (normal rounded)—Represents ventricular repolarization.
ST segment (normal isoelectric)—This symbolizes ventricular repolarization.
QT interval (normal 0.25–.035 second)—Represents ventricular depolarization and repolarization or electrical systole.
U wave—Normally this wave does not exist. It is a positive inflection after the T wave that denotes hypokalemia or hypocalcemia.

PRESSURE/VOLUME LOOPS

Pressure/volume loops express the relationship between intraventricular pressure and left ventricular volume during one cardiac cycle of diastole and systole (Figure 15–5. The loop reflects information regarding the ventricular volume, pressure, compliance, contractility, filling, and ejection. Many cardiac diseases can alter the appearance of the loop. These diseases include valvular disease, ischemia, change in heart rate, and cardiac tamponade.

　　Cardiac medication can also alter the loop. One such medication is phenylephrine, which will increase volume, pressure, and contractility. In an ischemic heart nitroglycerin will decrease the volume and pressure causing a left and down-

Table 15–4
PULMONARY CAPILLARY WEDGE (ARTERY OCCLUSION) PRESSURE (PCWP OR PAOP)

Normal mean: 6–12 mm Hg

Abnormal	Causes
Increased PCWP	Left ventricular failure, pericarditis, mitral valve dysfunction, fluid overload, cardiac tamponade or effusion
Decrease PCWP	Hypovolemia or decrease in afterload

Table 15–5
PULMONARY VASCULAR RESISTANCE (PVR)

$$PVR = \frac{PAP - PCWP}{CO} \times 80$$

Normal: 100–300 dynes/cm/s

Abnormal	Causes
Increased PVR	Pulmonary interstitial pressure, increased blood viscosity, sympathetic stimulation, catecholamines, angiotensin, histamine, serotonin prostaglandin F, hypoxia, hypercarbia, acidemia
Decreased PVR	Pulmonary hypertension, left atrial hypertension, increased pulmonary blood volume, acetylcholine, histamine, bradykinin, prostaglandin-E_1

CO, cardiac output; PAP, pulmonary artery pressure; PCWP, pulmonary capillary wedge pressure

ward shift in the loop; Nipride will also cause a left and downward shift in the loop.

Abnormal Pressure/Volume Loops

Tachycardia
This is characterized by a leftward and downward shift. There is a decrease in pressure, volume, and stroke volume.

Aortic Regurgitation
Acute aortic regurgitation *(volume overload)* is characterized by a rightward shift with an increase of left ventricular end-diastolic volume, increase left ventricular end-systolic volume, and increase in LVEDP. This shows that the ventricle is not compensating. Chronic aortic regurgitation is characterized by a rightward shift with an extreme increase in left ventricular end-diastolic volume, extreme increase in left ventricular end-systolic volume, and mild increase in LVEDP. This reflects that the heart is compensating with an increased compliance.

Aortic Stenosis
Aortic stenosis *(pressure overload)* is characterized by a rightward shift with an increase in pressure. Early aortic stenosis has an increase in left ventricular end-systolic pressure, but the stroke volume is not affected. Moderate aortic

Table 15–6
CORONARY PERFUSION PRESSURE (CPP)

CPP = Diastolic blood pressure − LVEDP

Abnormal	Causes
Decrease	Decreased aortic pressure, increased ventricular end-diastolic pressure, increased heart rate

LVEDP, left ventricular end-diastolic pressure

Table 15–7
EJECTION FRACTION (EF)

$$EF = \frac{EDV - ESV}{EDV}$$

Normal: 55–70%

Abnormal	Causes
Decrease	Severe impairment of ventricular function

EDV, end-diastolic volume; ESV, end-systolic volume

stenosis has an increase in LVEDP, increase in left ventricular end-diastolic volume, but normal ventricular end-systolic volume. Severe aortic stenosis has an extreme increase in left ventricular end-diastolic volume and a decrease stroke volume.

Mitral Regurgitation
Mitral regurgitation *(volume overload)* is characterized by a rightward shift with a decrease in pressure. Acute mitral regurgitation has an increase in LVEDP. In chronic mitral regurgitation there is an increased left ventricular end-diastolic volume and left ventricular end-systolic volume.

Mitral Stenosis
Mitral stenosis *(pressure overload)* is characterized by a leftward shift showing a decrease in volume and amplitude. There is a decrease in left ventricular end-diastolic volume, decrease in left ventricular end-systolic volume, and a decrease in stroke volume.

Cardiac Tamponade
In cardiac tamponade there is a leftward shift with a decrease in amplitude. Stroke volume, left ventricular end-diastolic volume, and left ventricular end-systolic volume are all decreased. In acute cardiac tamponade, each time the heart beats it becomes more restricted. Thus, volume becomes more and more impeded.

VENTRICULAR FUNCTION CURVE

The ventricular function curve or Frank-Starling law of the heart shows the relationship of LVEDP or preload and stroke

Table 15–8
STROKE VOLUME (SV)

$$SV = \frac{CO}{HR} \times 100$$

Normal: 60–90 mL/beat

Abnormal	Causes
Increase	Sympathetic stimulation, positive inotropy, increased preload, reduction of afterload
Decrease	Decreased preload, increased afterload, negative inotropy

CO, cardiac output; HR, heart rate

Table 15-9
CARDIAC OUTPUT (CO)

$CO = SV \times HR$
Normal: 5-6 L/min

Abnormal	Causes
Increased CO	Sepsis, tachycardia, increased blood volume, hyperthyroidism, hyperflow states with hepatic or mesenteric shunting
Decreased CO	Bradycardia, dysrhythmias, decreased blood volume, shock, valvular stenosis, cardiac tamponade, decreased inotropy, hypothermia, increased afterload, restrictive cardiomyopathies

HR, heart rate; SV, stroke volume

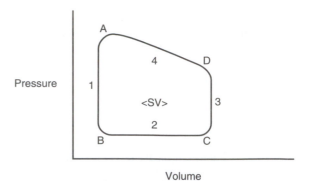

Figure 15-5   Pressure/volume loop.   Phase 1, isovolumetric relaxation (relaxation with filling)   Phase 2, diastolic filling (compliance and preload)   Phase 3, isovolumetric contraction (afterload)   Phase 4, systolic ejection   A, aortic valve closure   B, mitral valve opening   C, mitral valve closure   D, aortic valve opening   A–C represents ventricular systole.   C–A represents ventricular diastole.   Area within the loop represents stroke work index. The width of phase 2 represents stroke volume (SV).

volume. Cardiac muscle is composed of filaments that are able to stretch when the ventricles are filled with blood. When there is an increase in volume and stretch of the cardiac muscle, the force of contraction is stronger. However, this stretch is limited. If the heart is overdistended for a period of time, contractility becomes inadequate, a condition seen in cardiac failure. Factors that influence preload are fiber length, stretch of the filaments, venous return, blood volume, distribution of blood volume, posture, intrathoracic pressure, pericardial pressure, venous tone, cardiac rhythm, and heart rate. Preload can be measured by left ventricular end-diastolic volume, LVEDP, pulmonary capillary wedge pressure, and echocardiograms. As preload increases, the

heart compensates by increasing output. This output is measured by cardiac output, stroke volume, cardiac index, and stroke work index. When the heart begins to fail, cardiac output decreases.

Another factor that affects contractility is wall tension. Afterload is the major contributing factor in wall tension. *Afterload* is the initial resistance that the ventricle must overcome to eject blood across the pulmonic and aortic valves. Afterload of the right ventricle is clinically measured by pulmonary vascular resistance (PVR).

Table 15-10
EQUATIONS FOR ADDITIONAL HEMODYNAMIC PARAMETERS

Parameter	Equation	Normal Value	Comment
Right ventricular stroke work index (RVSWI)	$0.0136 \, (PAP - CVP) \times SI$	5-9 g-m/m^2	
Left ventricular stroke work index (LVSWI)	$0.0136 \, (MAP - PCWP) \times SI$	45-60 g-m/m^2	
Rate pressure product (RPP)	Systolic BP $\times$ HR	>15,000	
Triple index (TI)	Systolic BP $\times$ HR $\times$ PCWP	>180,000	
Stroke index	$\dfrac{SV}{BSA}$	40-60 mL/beat/m^2	
Systemic vascular resistance (SVR)	$\dfrac{(MAP - CVP) \times 80}{CO}$	700-1400 dynes/s/cm	
Cardiac index (CI)	$\dfrac{CO}{BSA}$	2.5-4.0 L/min/m^2	
Diastolic-pressure time index (DPTI)	Coronary perfusion $\times$ diastolic time		Measures left ventricular blood flow
Tension-time index (TTI)	Systolic BP $\times$ systolic time		Measures myocardial O$_2$ demand
	DPTI/TTI	≥ 1 <0.7 associated with subendocardial ischemia	O$_2$ supply-demand balance

BP, blood pressure; BSA, body surface area; CO, cardiac output; CVP, central venous pressure; HR, heart rate; MAP, mean arterial pressure; PAP, pulmonary artery pressure; PCWP, pulmonary capillary wedge pressure; SI, stroke index; SV, stroke volume

PATHOPHYSIOLOGY

ABNORMAL ECG/DYSRHYTHMIAS

When interpreting an ECG, 10 features should be examined:

1. Rhythm—complexes regular or irregular
2. Rate—atrial and ventricular beats per minute
3. P wave—present or absent, relationship to the QRS, size, and shape
4. PR interval—shortened or prolonged
5. QRS complex—size, shape, and polarity
6. QRS interval—shortened or prolonged
7. ST segment—elevated or depressed
8. T wave—size, shape, polarity
9. U wave—follows the T wave, if present
10. QT duration—determine length, shortened or prolonged

ABNORMAL WAVES AND INTERVALS

P Wave   An absent P wave denotes that the atrial stimulus is either nonexistent or the pacing stimulus is coming from a site other than the SA node. An increase in amplitude is a sign of hypertension, cor pulmonale (chronic obstructive pulmonary disease [COPD]), congenital disease, atrial hypertrophy, or AV valve disease. A notched wave is a sign of mitral valve disease.

PR Interval   An interval of less than 0.12 seconds may be a sign of preexcitation syndrome; here the stimulus is initiated from a pacing site other than the SA node. A prolonged interval of greater than 0.20 seconds indicates AV node ischemia or disease. If the intervals vary from beat to beat, a pacing stimulus is coming from various areas and is known as wandering atrial pacing.

QRS Complex   A deep Q wave indicates a past or present myocardial infarction. However, not all myocardial infarctions present with an abnormal Q wave. A prolonged QRS complex may be seen with bundle branch blocks, preexcitation syndromes, ventricular ectopy, hemiblocks, and hyperkalemia. The amplitude of the QRS complex is increased with left ventricular hypertrophy and right ventricular hypertrophy and decreased with heart failure or myocardial infarction.

T Wave   A negative deflection of the T wave indicates myocardial infarction or ischemia. Hyperkalemia causes the T wave to be peaked.

ST Segment   When assessing the ST segment it is important to look for the duration and an elevation or depression in relation to the isoelectric line. Prolongation indicates hypocalcemia. An elevation of more than 1 mm above the isoelectric line may be seen with pericarditis, myocardial infarctions, and aneurysms. Depression of the ST segment can be seen in ischemia, right ventricular hypertrophy, or digitalis toxicity.

U Wave   The presence of a U wave is abnormal and may be seen with hypokalemia or hypocalcemia.

QT Interval   Conditions that cause the QT interval to be prolonged include congestive heart failure, myocardial infarction, hypocalcemia, or myocarditis. A shortened interval is seen in digitalis toxicity, hypercalcemia, or hyperkalemia.

SINUS RHYTHMS

Normal Sinus Rhythm   The arial and ventricular rate of normal sinus rhythm is 60 to 100 beats/min. The rate is regular and the P wave, QRS complex, and T wave are normal.

Sinus Tachycardia   The atrial and ventricular rate is 100 to 150 beats/min. The rate is regular and the P wave, QRS complex, and T wave are normal.

Sinus Bradycardia   The atrial and ventricular rate is less than 60 beats/min. The rate is regular and the P wave, QRS complex, and T wave are normal.

Sinus Dysrhythmia   The atrial and ventricular rate is 80 to 100 beats/min, with a normal P wave, QRS complex, and T wave. However, the PP interval and RR intervals vary. This may be due to the *Herring-Brewer* reflex in which the rate increases with inspiration and decreases with expiration. This is seen in healthy patients, especially athletic men, and does not require treatment.

Sinus Arrest   During sinus arrest no electrical impulse arises from the SA node; the entire complex is absent. The RR intervals vary due to a long pause after the preceding complex. The patient may be asymptomatic. When the pauses become frequent or the patient is symptomatic, treatment with a pacemaker may be necessary.

Sinus Block   During a sinus block the SA node initiates an impulse; however, it is not conducted through the pathway secondary to a block within the SA node. The entire complex is absent. The RR interval is twice the length of the normal complex. This is usually a benign dysrhythmia. However, it may progress to a more serious block that requires treatment.

Sick Sinus Syndrome   This syndrome is characterized by a combination of sinus bradycardia, sinus block, and supraventricular tachydysrhythmias. This is a sign of a failing conduction system. Treatment with a pacemaker is necessary.

ATRIAL DYSRHYTHMIAS

Premature Atrial Contraction   A premature atrial contraction is characterized by a premature P wave that is followed by a normal QRS complex. The RR interval is irregular and the P wave of the ectopic beat may have a different morphology. The reason for this premature P wave is that the stimulus is arising from one or more different atrial foci.

Atrial Tachycardia or Supraventricular Tachycardia   Supraventricular tachycardia (SVT) occurs secondary to an impulse originating *above* the ventricles, within the atrial muscle or AV node. The rate is 150 to 200 beats/min. The PP interval is regular; the RR interval may be irregular and the P wave may be buried within the preceding T wave. This dysrhythmia begins and ends abruptly. Treatment is necessary because the patient is usually symptomatic. A vagal maneuver such as coughing or bearing down or, in a patient under anesthesia, positive-pressure ventilation or endotracheal suctioning, will break the SVT. Pharmacologic intervention may be necessary, using adenosine, β blockers, calcium channel blockers, or digoxin.

Paroxysmal Atrial Tachycardia   During paroxysmal atrial tachycardia the heart rate is 150 to 200 beats/min. It usually begins and ends abruptly and has repeated premature atrial contractions. The PP and PR intervals vary from beat to beat. Patients are usually symptomatic and require treatment, which is the same as for SVT. Overriding pacing may be helpful.

Wandering Atrial Pacemaker   This occurs secondary to the atrial foci originating from various areas within the sinus node and atrial tissue. The PR and RR intervals are irregular.

Atrial Flutter
This a physiologic block within the AV node that does not allow all the atrial impulses to stimulate the AV node. The P waves have the appearance of a sawtooth. Atrial rates are 220 to 300 beats/min. The RR intervals may vary due to the degree of the block. The block is described as the ratio of atrial to ventricular beats.

Atrial Fibrillation   During atrial fibrillation the atrial impulses originate from various foci. The atrial rate is 350 to 500 impulses per minute. Due the rapid atrial activity the P waves are not discernible. Ventricular response varies; thus, RR intervals are irregular. This ectopy does not allow the atrium to contract completely and blood does not flow adequately into the right ventricle. Thus, atrial emboli, known as *mural thrombi*, may occur. Atrial fibrillation can account for as much as a 30% decrease in cardiac output. Treatment depends on the ventricular rate. Rapid rates are treated with digoxin; anticoagulants are used to decrease the formation of mural thrombi.

JUNCTIONAL DYSRHYTHMIAS

Premature Junctional Contractions   The initial impulse in a premature junctional contraction (PJC) comes from within the junctional area. In the premature beat, the P wave may be inverted, absent, or appear before or after the QRS complex. A retrograde PJC occurs when the P wave comes before the QRS complex, secondary to the atria depolarizing before the ventricle. When a P wave occurs after the QRS complex, the ventricles are depolarized before the atria. The impulse is traveling antegrade and then retrograde through the tissue. The RR intervals are irregular secondary to altered conduction.

Junctional Rhythm   In the rhythm the pacemaker originates within the junctional tissue; the rate is 60 to 120 beats/min. Rates of 120 to 200 beats/min are considered junctional tachycardia. The P waves may appear before, during, or after the QRS complex. They may also appear to have an abnormal configuration or are inverted.

VENTRICULAR DYSRHYTHMIAS

Premature Ventricular Contractions   The impulse from the premature ventricular contraction (PVC) is formed in the ventricle, particularly from the bundle of His to the Purkinje fibers. It is characterized by a premature ectopic beat with a wide, bizarre QRS complex and ST-T slopes in the opposite direction of the normal QRS complex. It is usually followed by a compensatory pause. It is benign if fewer than six PVCs occur per minute. Bigeminy is defined as PVCs occurring every other beat. Trigeminy is a PVC occurring every third beat. More than six PVCs per minute can be dangerous especially when three or more occur in a row, which is called ventricular tachycardia. Ventricular tachycardia or ventricular fibrillation may occur if a PVC should hit the T wave. This is lethal and must be treated. Treatment includes medications such as lidocaine, bretylium, and procainamide. Cardioversion or defibrillation may be necessary to convert the rhythm into normal rhythm.

Ventricular Escape Beats   This rhythm is characterized by no P wave and a QRS greater than 0.12 second. When the ventricle does not receive an impulse from the SA or AV node, it will initiate an impulse. When two or more ventricular escape beats occur in a row, it is called idioventricular rhythm. The heart's defense mechanism is to keep beating. However, the ventricular rate is only 20 to 40 beats/min. When rates of 40 to 100 occur, it is known as accelerated idioventricular rhythm. This rhythm must be treated with a pacemaker to sustain cardiac output.

Ventricular Fibrillation   During ventricular fibrillation there is no visible QRS complex. The baseline is erratic and termed as fine or coarse "V Fib," depending on the amplitude of the baseline. This is a lethal dysrhythmia and must be treated with rapid defibrillation and cardiopulmonary resuscitation; epinephrine may be helpful. The underlying cause of the dysrhythmia must be treated.

Ventricular Standstill   In ventricular standstill the P waves are present and the PP intervals are regular. The atrial impulse is unable to stimulate a ventricular impulse; thus, depolarization does not occur. Another name for this lethal rhythm is asystole. Treatment includes cardiopulmonary resuscitation, atropine, and ventricular pacing.

ATRIOVENTRICULAR BLOCKS

First-Degree AV Block   During this block the P wave and QRS complex are normal; however, the PR interval is greater than 0.20 second. This is an incomplete block in which the conduction from the SA node to the AV node is delayed. The patient is asymptomatic and does not require treatment.

Second-Degree AV Block   In this block not all of the atrial impulses are conducted through to the ventricles. The PR interval may be normal, shortened, or prolonged. There are two types of second-degree AV block. *Mobitz I (Wenckebach)* block is characterized by a progressive prolongation of the PR interval until a QRS complex is blocked or "dropped." The RR interval shortens as the PR intervals increase. The rhythm is irregular. In *Mobitz II block* not all of the SA node impulses are conducted through to the AV node. The PP and PR intervals remain constant. It is described as a ratio of number of P waves to every QRS complex (e.g., 2:1, 3:1, etc.).

Third-Degree (Complete) Heart Block   In complete heart block the impulses from the SA node do not reach the AV node. The atrium and ventricle beat at their own intrinsic rates. The PP intervals are regular along with the RR intervals; however, they do not correlate. This is a lethal dysrhythmia that needs immediate treatment, including atropine or pacing or both.

INTRAVENTRICULAR CONDUCTION DEFECTS

Left Bundle Branch Block   During left bundle branch block, the conduction through the bundle branch is blocked on the left side. Conduction is delayed due to the right bundle branch having to stimulate the left ventricle. This is best seen in lead V_1, where the QRS is greater than 0.12 second and the S wave deflects well below the isoelectric line.

Right Bundle Branch Block   In right bundle branch block, conduction through the bundle branch is blocked on the right side. The left side must activate the right side, thus

causing a delay in the impulse. The QRS complex is greater than 0.12 second in V_1 and V_2 with a notched appearance.

Left Anterior Fascicular Block   The anterior fascicle of the left bundle branch is blocked. Therefore, the impulse must conduct through the posterior fascicle and then through the anterior area. This produces a left axis deviation of greater than $-30°$. Leads II, III and aVF show a decrease well below the isoelectric line. Leads I and aVL show a decrease in amplitude in the Q waves and peaked R waves.

Left Posterior Fascicular Block   The posterior fascicle of the left bundle branch is blocked. Therefore, the impulse must conduct through the anterior fascicle and then through the posterior area. This produces a right axis deviation of greater than $+110°$. Leads II, III, and aVF show decreased amplitude in the Q wave and peaked R waves. Lead I shows a decreased amplitude in the R waves and the S waves descend well below the isoelectric line.

Preexcitation Syndrome   During a preexcitation syndrome the impulses from the atria travel through accessory conductive pathways instead of the AV node. It is characterized by a PR interval less than 0.12 second, a wide QRS, and delta waves. It may precipitate paroxysmal atrial tachycardia.

Wolff-Parkinson-White syndrome is a preexcitation dysrhythmia that travels through the bundle of Kent. Treatment may include cardioversion, procainamide HCl, or propranolol (Inderal). For treatment of SVTs in Wolff-Parkinson-White Syndrome, adenosine is helpful in restoring normal sinus rhythm by slowing conduction through the AV node. Verapamil and digoxin may decrease the refractory period in the accessory pathway and should be avoided.

CORONARY ARTERY DISEASE

Coronary artery disease (CAD) occurs when the arteries become partially or totally occluded with artherosclerotic plaque. Cholesterol deposits form on the lining of the artery, causing epithelial damage. Calcifications occur and form artheromas. Once atheromas form, the area becomes thickened with platelets and blood clots. This narrows the lumen of the coronary arteries, hindering blood flow. The myocardium is in danger of ischemia and infarct. Risk factors related to CAD include:

Elevated plasma concentrations of cholesterol, especially low density lipoprotein cholesterol
Cigarette smoking
Hypertension
Diabetes mellitus
Advanced age
Male gender
Family history
Diet

One way to determine if the myocardium is adequately supplied with oxygen is to assess the patient's cardiac reserve through exercise tolerance. When the cardiac demand is increased during exercise, the myocardium supply may be decreased. These patients exhibit signs of dyspnea and angina. If severe, it may lead to myocardial infarction, congestive heart failure, dysrhythmias, and sudden death.

Treatment varies depending on the severity of the CAD. In patients who have identifiable risk factors, treatment is diet control, decreased stress, smoking cessation, and exercise. For progressive disease further treatment such as coronary angioplasty, intracoronary thrombolysis with streptokinase, coronary artery bypass graft surgery, or cardiac transplantation may be warranted.

MYOCARDIAL ISCHEMIA

Myocardial ischemia is caused by an inadequate amount of oxygen being delivered at the myocardial cellular level. Function decreases and LVEDP increases causing an increase in intramyocardial pressure, a decrease in coronary perfusion pressure, and a decrease in blood flow, and leading to an increase in ischemia. It is symptomatically manifested as angina pectoris, which can be vague, mild, or silent. Patients describe this as an extreme, heavy squeezing substernal pain that may radiate to the shoulders, neck, jaw, and arm and is often accompanied by light-headedness, diaphoresis, and nausea. Anginal pain is usually relieved with rest or nitroglycerin. The types of angina pectoris are listed in Table 15–11.

The goal in treating angina is to increase coronary blood supply while decreasing the demand. Intraoperatively ischemia can be detected by changes in the ECG. Typical symptoms are masked under anesthesia with the exception of an awake patient. Medications include nitroglycerin, calcium channel blockers, β-adrenergic antagonists, and oxygen.[6]

Table 15–11
TYPES OF ANGINA PECTORIS

Types	Symptoms
Stable	Pain does not increase in frequency, duration, or severity in months
Unstable	Pain has increased in severity, frequency, and duration; is relieved with rest and medication
Crescendo	Heightening ischemia with impending myocardial infarction
Prinzmetal's	Pain due to coronary spasm, not correlated with exercise, occurs during sleep and rest; treatment with nitroglycerin and calcium channel blockers
Intractable	Increased angina that does not respond to rest or medication; indicates impending myocardial infarction

Table 15–12
CHARACTERISTICS OF TYPES OF MYOCARDIAL INFARCTION

Type/Location	Characteristics
Anterior	Pulmonary edema or cardiogenic shock. Changes in ECG include presence of Q wave, ST elevation, and T wave inversion. Q wave in precordial V leads. ECG changes are seen in leads I, aVL $V_1 - V_2$ with reciprocal changes in leads II, III, and aVF.
Septal	Q wave present in $V_1 - V_3$.
Lateral	ECG changes in lead I and aVL.
Anterolateral	Q wave and inverted T in leads I, II, and $V_4 - V_6$.
Inferior	Right ventricular dysfunction, bradycardia, and AV heart blocks. Q waves present in leads II, III, and aVF and posterior precordial leads, with recipocal changes in leads I, aVL, and anterior precordial leads.
Inferolateral	ECG changes in leads II, III, aVF, $V_5 - V_6$ with reciprocal changes in I and aVL
Anteroseptal	ECG changes in leads $V_1 - V_4$.
Subendocardial	Non-Q wave MI. ST depression with T inversion on epicardial leads. Infarction of the inner third of the myocardium, near the ventricular cavity may lead to decreased ventricular function. This will lead to conduction disorders or papillary muscle dysfunction or both.

MYOCARDIAL INFARCTION

Coronary artery disease may lead to myocardial infarction secondary to occlusion of an epicardial artery. If the muscle fibers are ischemic, death of the tissue can occur within an hour. After the area is infarcted fibrous tissue grows among the fibers. This scarring contracts the size of the infarcted area, preventing aneurysmal effect, a process that takes a few days to occur. Infarction may lead to cardiac failure resulting in decreased cardiac output, pulmonary edema, ventricular fibrillation, and rupture of the infarcted area. The subendocardium is *most* vulnerable to ischemia.

Table 15–12 presents the characteristics of the various areas of infarction.

Assessment of cardiac enzymes further aids diagnosis. Creatine kinase MB appears at 4 to 8 hours, peaks at 16 to 24 hours, and returns to normal at 48 to 72 hours. Lactic dehydrogenase appears at 6 to 24 hours, peaks at 24 to 48 hours, and returns to normal at 72 to 96 hours.

CARDIOGENIC SHOCK

Cardiogenic shock occurs secondary to myocardial infarction with left ventricular involvement. Blood pressure decreases and oliguria develops despite adequate fluid volume. The mean arterial pressure is less than 60 mm Hg and pulmonary wedge pressure is greater than 18 mm Hg. Cardiac index is less than 21 L/min per m². Treatment includes dopamine, dobutamine, or intra-aortic balloon counterpulsation.

HEMORRHAGIC SHOCK

Acute blood loss causes hemorrhagic shock. There is decreased fluid volume, decreased cardiac output, and inadequate tissue perfusion. In early hemorrhage sympathetic stimulation occurs. The patient is tachycardic as blood is being shunted to the heart and brain. Also, arteriolar vasoconstriction decreases renal and splanchnic blood flow, causing a decrease in urinary output. Metabolic lactic acidosis occurs secondary to anaerobic metabolism from shunting of blood to the major organs. Treatment includes whole blood transfusion, crystalloid solutions, vasopressors (to support cerebral and cardiac perfusion), and dopamine (<5 μg/kg per minute) to increase renal blood flow. When including anesthesia, ketamine will support blood pressure and heart rate.

CARDIAC TAMPONADE

Cardiac tamponade occurs secondary to an accumulation of fluid or blood in the pericardial space. Diastolic filling of the heart is impaired secondary to increased intrapericardial pressures, leading to reduced stroke volume and blood pressure. Once this occurs, the sympathetic nervous system is stimulated. Heart rate is increased to maintain cardiac output and peripheral vasoconstriction. Cardiovascular collapse occurs when right ventricular end-diastolic pressure exceeds central venous pressure.

Causes of increased pericardial fluid include chest trauma, postoperation bleeding after cardiac surgery, perforation of the ventricle secondary to insertion of an intracardiac invasive monitor, infection, metastasis from malignant disease, and uremic pericarditis secondary to chronic renal failure. Normally the pericardial space contains 20 to 50 mL pericardial fluid. If the pericardial space fills gradually, the tissue will stretch to tolerate the amount. With acute accumulation, only a small amount can cause cardiac tamponade.

Clinical signs include tachycardia, diaphoresis, compensatory peripheral vasoconstriction, hypotension, elevated venous pressure, distant heart sounds, pulsus paradoxus, Kussmaul's venous sign (an exaggerated distention of neck veins that increases with inspiration), and equalization of central venous and wedge pressures. The heart's silhouette does not change until an accumulation reaches 250 mL. The ECG shows a decrease in voltage of the QRS and T waves with myocardial ischemia. There is also electrical alternans.[6]

Treatment of nontraumatic cardiac tamponade includes percutaneous pericardiocentesis under local anesthesia. If tamponade is due to trauma, pericardiotomy is performed under general anesthesia. However, if the patient is showing signs of decreased cardiac output and hypotension, a pericardiocentesis or pericardial window is performed under local anesthesia. When the patient's cardiac function improves, general anesthesia can be induced. The goal is to maintain *stroke volume*. Anesthesia is started after the area is prepped and surgery is ready to begin. A large-bore intravenous access is needed to administer colloid or crystalloid solutions to keep right atrial pressures above 25 mm Hg; this will help maintain stroke volume by increasing venous return. Induction of anesthesia is with ketamine or benzodiazepines. Avoid positive-pressure ventilation until the chest is open. Avoid blunt coughing on the endotrachial tube, which will increase intrathoracic pressure and impede venous return. Pancuronium is useful as a muscle relaxant secondary to its circulatory effects. Catecholamine infusions may be necessary to maintain cardiac function and blood pressure.[6]

ESSENTIAL HYPERTENSION

The stages of essential hypertension are listed in Table 15−13. Hypertension occurs with the presence of edema and hypertrophy of arteriolar smooth muscle. This decreases the lumen of the blood vessels and impedes blood flow. Blood pressure must increase to maintain a flow rate. When the vessel constricts in response to sympathetic stimulation, the elevation in blood pressure is exaggerated secondary to the already existing narrowed vessel. Blood volume in hypertensive patients is normal to reduced, but there is central redistribution of this volume, presumably as a result of altered tone in capacitance vessels.[6] If untreated, essential hypertension may lead to increased myocardial wall tension, left ventricular hypertrophy, heart failure, myocardial ischemia and infarct, stroke, and congestive heart failure.[6]

VALVULAR HEART DISEASE

Mitral Stenosis Leading to a mechanical obstruction where blood cannot flow into the left ventricle, mitral stenosis is caused by a fusion of the mitral valve leaflets at the commissures secondary to rheumatic carditis. Patients become symptomatic 20 years after the infection when there is

Table 15−13
STAGES OF ESSENTIAL HYPERTENSION

Stage	Characteristics
I Borderline	Systolic >160 mm Hg Diastolic >95 mm Hg
II Sustained diastolic	Diastolic >95 mm Hg with cardiac output normal to slightly decreased
III With major organ involvement	Cerebral hemorrhage, renal dysfunction, congestive heart failure
IV Accelerated	Rapid increased diastolic blood pressure >130 mm Hg with retinopathy
V Malignant	Pressure >200/140 associated with papilledema and encephalopathy

SOURCE: Reproduced by permission from Morgan and Mikhail.[5]

a 50% reduction in the mitral valve orifice. Clinical signs include early diastolic murmur heard at the apex with an audible snap, decreased stroke volume, increased PVR, and left atrial pressure greater than 25 mm Hg. LVEDP and left ventricular volume are normal. Chest x-ray shows a left atrial enlargement. The ECG reveals biphasic P waves and atrial fibrillation. Treatment includes valvuloplasty or valve replacement.[6]

As the disease progresses, dysrhythmias such as atrial fibrillation develop. Pulmonary edema becomes evident secondary to pulmonary pressures that are greater than the oncotic pressure of plasma proteins. Systemic thrombi become a risk secondary to stasis of blood in the distended left atrium and existing atrial fibrillation.

The goal under anesthesia is to maintain a normal heart rate, systemic vascular resistance (SVR), and PVR. When tachycardia exists left ventricular filling is poor and stroke volume and blood pressure are decreased. Prophylactic antibiotics are used to prevent endocarditis. Continue digoxin therapy because decreasing the heart rate allows adequate forward flow of blood. Patients who are taking diuretics should have electrolytes monitored. Those taking anticoagulants need a gradual reduction in prothrombin time until it is 20% normal. Sudden decreases in SVR lead to extreme hypotension. Increasing PVR may cause pulmonary edema, which can be prevented by careful fluid replacement. Factors that increase PVR include arterial hypoxemia, acidosis, α-adrenergic agonists, and nitrous oxide. Therefore, select the anesthetic to avoid increasing the PVR. Trendelenburg position is not well tolerated.

Mitral Regurgitation   In mitral regurgitation left atrial volume overload is secondary to blood flowing back into the left atrium. Causes include acute myocardial infarction leading to papillary muscle dysfunction, endocarditis leading to rupture of the chordae tendinae, progressive mitral valve stenosis, and dilation of the mitral valve secondary to left ventricular hypertrophy.

Clinical signs of mitral regurgitation include systolic murmur heard at the apex, regurgitation fraction greater than 0.6, pulmonary edema, and increased PVR. The ECG shows atrial fibrillation. A pulmonary artery catheter shows *v waves* on the wedge tracing due to backward flow of blood. Treatment is mitral valve replacement.

The anesthetic goal is to maintain a *mild increase* in heart rate, which allows less time for the blood to regurge. SVR should be slightly decreased, which will promote a *forward flow* of blood. In the presence of pulmonary edema secondary to an increased left atrial pressure, giving vasodilating drugs to decrease SVR is effective in increasing cardiac output. Regional anesthesia may cause sudden decreases in SVR, an undesirable event. When administering medications, a dilutional effect occurs secondary to the regurging blood; therefore less drug is needed for the same effect. Vigilant fluid replacement is necessary to maintain preload. Pulmonary artery pressures are useful in assessing cardiac output, left atrial pressure, and PVR. Any increase

in the v wave corresponds with a greater mitral regurgitation.

Mitral Valve Prolapse   Mitral valve abnormalities include redundancy and myxomatous degeneration of the leaflets, dilation of the mitral valve annulus, and elongation and thinning of the chordae tendinae. During systole the leaflets prolapse in the left atrium. Symptoms include an auscultatory click over the apex. A late systolic murmur of regurgitation may be present. This disease occurs in 5% of the population; it is more prevalent in thin, tall people, usually women, associated with high arched palate, pectus excavatum, kyphoscoliosis, hyperextensible joints, and Marfan's syndrome.

Complications include mitral regurgitation, infective endocarditis, ruptured chordae tendinae, transient ischemic attacks, cardiac dysrhythmias, PVCs, AV heart block, ST and T wave changes, and sudden death. Prolapsing of the mitral valve with a backward flow of blood occurs when there is an increased left ventricular emptying. Factors that will increase emptying are increased sympathetic stimulation, reduction in SVR, and upright position. Treatment includes aspirin and dipyridamole (Persantine) to prevent platelet aggregation on the leaflets. β-Adrenergic antagonists are used to prevent preexcitation dysrhythmias and SVT.

The anesthetic goal is to prevent prolapsing of the mitral valve. This is accomplished by blunting sympathetic stimulation, maintaining SVR, and maintaining volume replacement and the heart rate within normal limits. Prophylactic antibiotics are used to prevent endocarditis.

Aortic Stenosis   Forward movement of blood from the left ventricle into the aorta is obstructed by a stenotic aortic valve. There is usually a 30-year latency before the patient becomes symptomatic. Clinical signs include a systolic murmur at the second right interspace, decreased cardiac output, and an increased left ventricular systolic pressure. Once the ventricle wall thickens a concentric hypertrophy will appear on an echocardiogram. The triad of symptoms includes *angina pectoris, dyspnea on exertion,* and *syncope.* Once patients experience congestive heart failure, life expectancy without treatment is less than 5 years. Treatment is percutaneous transluminal valvuloplasty or valve replacement.

Left ventricular filling depends on atrial contraction. Therefore under anesthesia it is crucial to maintain a normal sinus rhythm. Maintaining SVR and intravascular fluid volume is important because any decrease in blood pressure and SVR causes a decrease in stroke volume. General anesthesia is preferred over regional because of the rapid decrease in SVR with regional anesthesia. Any cardiac depressants such as halothane may produce a nodal rhythm that will decrease the atrial kick. Caution should be used with positive-pressure ventilation because an increase in intrathoracic pressure will decrease stroke volume. Bradycardia, SVT, and junctional rhythms must be prevented because they will decrease cardiac output. Prophylactic antibiotics are used to prevent endocarditis.

Aortic Regurgitation Aortic regurgitation is characterized by a decrease in left ventricular stroke volume secondary to blood flowing back into the left ventricle through an incompetent aortic valve. The amount of regurgitation depends on the heart rate and SVR. Chronic aortic regurgitation is secondary to rheumatic fever or persistent systemic hypertension. Acute aortic regurgitation is secondary to infective endocarditis, trauma, or dissection of a thoracic aneurysm. Treatment is aortic valve replacement.

Clinical signs include a diastolic murmur at the second right interspace. Chest x-ray shows left ventricular enlargement. Angina is present secondary to decreased coronary blood flow. The increased myocardial oxygen requirements may result in subendocardial ischemia. Once the left ventricle has hypertrophied, any change in heart rate will result in a decrease in stroke volume because the heart cannot increase contractility.

The anesthetic goal is to maintain *forward flow* of blood, which requires a slight increase in heart rate and a slight decrease in SVR. Fluid volume and contractility must be maintained. Nitrous oxide, opioids, and low concentrations of volatile agents with a nondepolarizing agent are useful for maintenance of anesthesia. Bradycardia and nodal rhythms are undesirable. Pulmonary artery pressure is useful in assessing cardiac output and monitoring preload. Prophylactic antibiotics are used to prevent endocarditis.

CONGESTIVE HEART FAILURE

Heart failure includes CAD, cardiac valve abnormalities, impaired myocardial contractility, and cardiomyopathy. The failure may be right, left, or biventricular. When right-sided failure occurs, symptomatic systemic hypertension is seen. During left-sided failure, pulmonary congestion occurs; this may progress to right-sided failure with hypertension.

In congestive heart failure, stroke volume is decreased secondary to decreased myocardial contractility. Therefore, to increase stroke volume, heart rate needs to be increased. After the heart has been exposed to an increase in cardiac volume and pressure, the ventricle becomes hypertrophied and dilated.

The clinical manifestations of right ventricular failure include dyspnea secondary to interstitial pulmonary edema, orthopnea secondary to shifting of dependent fluid, productive cough with rales, and fatigue. Chest x-ray shows pulmonary venous hypertension and interstitial pulmonary edema. Left ventricular failure has an increased sympathetic activity seen as an increased heart rate and peripheral vasoconstriction.

Treatment includes digitalis to increase myocardial contractility, diuretics, and peripheral vasodilating drugs. Elective surgery should not be performed because of increased morbidity. If emergency surgery is needed, the goal is to maintain cardiac output. An induction agent such as ketamine may be beneficial, while negative inotropes (inhalation agents, pentothal) should be avoided. Maintenance of anesthesia can be supplied with opioids and benzodiazepines. When combining nitrous oxide with opioids and benzodiazepines, cardiac output and blood pressure decrease. Positive-pressure ventilation can be helpful to decrease pulmonary congestion. Regional anesthesia for peripheral surgery is beneficial because it will slightly decrease SVR. Spinal and epidural anesthesia may severely decrease SVR, which will be difficult to control.

IDIOPATHIC HYPERTROPHIC SUBAORTIC STENOSIS

Idiopathic hypertrophic subaortic stenosis (IHSS) is a hypertrophic cardiomyopathy caused by an asymmetrical hypertrophy of the intraventricular septal muscle, which leads to a decrease in stroke volume from the left ventricle. This decrease in flow may also be accentuated by an incompetent mitral valve.[6] Clinical signs of IHSS include syncope, angina pectoris, and congestive heart failure.[6] An ECG may exhibit atrial fibrillation, changes consistent with left ventricle hypertrophy, and the presence of a Q wave.[6] The goal in treating these patients is to decrease the obstruction and increase stroke volume. Factors that will decrease the obstruction include decreasing myocardial contractility with β-adrenergic antagonists and increasing preload and afterload. Factors that will increase the obstruction and impede outflow are increasing myocardial contractility with digitalis, tachycardia, and increasing sympathetic stimulation and decreasing preload and afterload.[6]

The same goals in treating these patients also apply during the administration of anesthetics. Avoiding an increase in sympathetic stimulation is imperative and may be achieved by perioperative sedation and blunting laryngoscopy. The use of β-adrenergic antagonists and volatile anesthetics will decease myocardial contractility. Ketamine should be avoided secondary to it increasing myocardial contractility. Also avoid techniques and medications that will decrease SVR, such as regional anesthesia, curare, and hypovolemia.[6]

ASSOCIATED DRUGS

Sympathomimetics This category includes endogenous catecholamines, synthetic catecholamines, and synthetic non-catecholamines.

Endogenous Catecholamines

Epinephrine is naturally released from the adrenal medulla. At all dosages epinephrine increases myocardial contractility and heart rate, glandular secretions, and metabolic processes in glycogenolysis and lipolysis. At lower doses, vasodilation, broncho dilation and increased cardiac output is seen. This potent α agonist activates β_1 and β_2 when administered subcutaneously or intravenously. The dose for β_2 is 1 to 2 μg/min IV, for β_1 4 μg/min IV, and for α and β effects it is 10 to 20 μg/min IV.

Norepinephrine is an endogenous neurotransmitter released from the postganglionic sympathetic nerve endings. It is a potent α agonist that causes arterial and venous vasoconstriction. The dose for the treatment of hypotension is 4 to 16 μg/min IV.

Dopamine is an endogenous neurotransmitter that increases myocardial contractility, renal blood flow, glomerular filtration rate, urinary output, and sodium excretion. The doses that will affect dopaminergic receptors are 0.5 to 3.0 μg/kg per minute IV; dopaminergic, β_1 and β_2 receptors 3 to 10 μg/kg per min; and alpha receptors, greater than 10 μg/kg per minute IV.

Synthetic Catecholamines

Isoproterenol is a β_1 and β_2 agonist. It is clinically used to bronchodilate, increase heart rate, and decrease PVR. A dose of 1 to 5 μg/min IV will increase heart rate, increase myocardial contractility, increase cardiac automaticity, and decrease SVR secondary to vasodilation.

Dobutamine is a synthetic catecholamine that increases cardiac output and decreases atrial filling. This effect is seen with doses of 2 to 10 μg/kg per minute IV. When doses of more than 10 μg/kg per minute IV are used, tachycardia and cardiac dysrhythmias ensue.

Synthetic Noncatecholamines

Ephedrine is an indirect noncatecholamine that stimulates α-and β-adrenergic receptors. It also stimulates the release of norepinephrine. It is used to treat hypotension particularly in the pregnant patient because uterine blood flow is not altered. It increases cardiac output, systolic and diastolic blood pressure, and heart rate. Doses of 5 to 25 mg IV are given for hypotension. Tachyphylaxis occurs when the second dose is not as effective as the first and is due to blockade of adrenergic receptors. If norepinephrine stores are depleted, ephedrine is ineffective.

Phenylephrine stimulates primary α_1-adrenergic receptors and in small amounts stimulates the release of norepinephrine.[4] Individual doses of 50 to 200 μg IV and a continuous infusion of 20 to 50 μg/min are used to treat hypotension.

Cardiac Glycosides Cardiac glycosides have a direct positive inotropic effect on the heart. They are used to treat cardiac failure, slow ventricular rate as in SVT, paroxysmal atrial tachycardia, atrial fibrillation and atrial flutter; they increase parasympathetic nervous system activity.

Digoxin is a cardiac glycoside; the initial IV dose is up to 10 μg/kg per minute over 30 minutes. The effect is seen in 5 to 30 minutes. The maintenance dose is 0.25 mg daily.

Digitoxin has a greater lipid solubility with 90% to 100% absorption in the gastrointestinal tract. The initial dose is 0.8 to 1.2 mg IV and the maintenance dose is 0.1 mg IV.

Noncatecholamine Nonglyceride Cardiac Inotropes
Calcium is a positive inotrope that increases stroke volume and increases BP. The dose of calcium chloride is 5 to 10 mg/kg IV. Caution should be used when giving it to patients taking digoxin because it may cause dysrhythmias.

Amrinone produces dose-dependent positive inotropic and vasodilating effects. It increases cardiac output and decreases SVR. The dose is 0.5 to 1.5 mg/kg IV; it takes effect within 5 minutes and lasts 2 hours. For a continuous infusion, the dose is 2 to 10 μg/kg/per minute with a maximum dose of 10 mg/kg daily. Adverse side effects include occasional hypotension secondary to vasodilation and *thrombocytopenia* with prolonged therapy.

α-Adrenergic Receptor Antagonist *Phentolamine* is a transient nonselective α-adrenergic antagonist; α_2 blockade decreases norepinephrine release resulting in arterial vasodilation and increased HR. It is used for acute hypertensive emergencies as seen with autonomic hyperreflexia. The dose of 30 to 70 μg/kg IV will produce vasodilation. In addition, phentolamine is used to treat norepinephrine extravasated into skin.

α-Adrenergic Antagonists *Propranolol* is a β_1 and β_2 antagonist. It is used to decrease heart rate and cardiac output and increase peripheral vascular resistance. An adverse effect is increased myocardial oxygen requirements.

Esmolol is a β_1 antagonist with a rapid onset and short action. It is used to decrease heart rate and blood pressure. The initial dose is 10 mg IV, with continuous infusion at 12 mg/min IV.

Combined α- and β-Adrenergic Antagonist *Labetolol* is a selective α_1 and nonselective β_1 and β_2 antagonist used to decrease blood pressure and heart rate. The dose is 0.1 to 0.5 mg/kg IV over 5 minutes with a continuous infusion of 0.1 to 2.0 mg/min.

Peripheral Vasodilators *Nitroprusside* is a direct-acting nonselective peripheral vasodilator that relaxes arterial and venous smooth muscle. It is used to treat hypertensive crisis. The dose for continuous infusion is 0.5 to 2.0 μg/kg per minute not to exceed 8 μg/kg per minute for 1 to 3 hours or 0.5 mg/kg per hour IV. Side effects include metabolic acidosis secondary to cyanide toxicity, decrease in cerebral blood flow, increase in intracoronary steal, and dose-related decreases in platelet aggregation.

Nitroglycerin is an organic nitrate that acts on venous capacitance vessels and relaxes arterial vascular smooth muscle. It is used to decrease myocardial oxygen requirement, relieve angina and pulmonary congestion, decrease preload, decrease SVR thus decreasing afterload, and dilating the coronary arteries. The sublingual dose is 0.3 mg repeated every 5 minutes up to three times or 2% nitroglycerin ointment, 2.5 to 5 cm, which will produce sustained protection for up to 4 hours. A continuous infusion of 0.1 to 7.0 μg/kg/min can be used as prophylaxis against myocardial ischemia.

REFERENCES

1. Tortora GJ, Anagnostakos NP. *Principles of Anatomy and Physiology*. 6th ed. New York: Harper & Row; 1990.
2. Barash PG, Cullen BF, Stoelting RK. *Clinical Anesthesia*. 2nd ed. Philadelphia: JB Lippincott; 1992:989–1020.
3. Guyton AC, Hall JE. *Textbook of Medical Physiology*, 9th ed. Philadelphia: WB Saunders; 1996:107–157.
4. Stoelting RK. *Pharmacology and Physiology in Anesthetic Practice*, 2nd ed. Philadelphia: JB Lippincott; 1991:692–706.
5. Morgan GE, Mikhail MS. *Clinical Anesthesiology*. East Norwalk, Conn: Appleton & Lange; 1992:285–361.
6. Stoelting RK, Dierdorf SF, McCammon RL: *Anesthesia and Co-Existing Disease*. 2nd ed. New York: Churchill Livingstone; 1988:1–54.

☐ QUESTIONS

1. Coronary blood flow is increased in all the following *except:*
   a. Hypoxia
   b. Ventricular relaxation
   c. Decreased heart rate
   d. Ventricular contractility

2. Neural stimulation of the heart is through the:
   a. Sympathetic fibers via the cervical ganglia in the cord segments thoracic 1–4 and parasympathetic via cranial nerve IX
   b. Sympathetic fibers via the cervical ganglia in the cord segments thoracic 1–4 and parasympathetic via cranial nerve X
   c. Sympathetic fibers via the cervical ganglia in the cord segments thoracic 1–8 and parasympathetic via cranial nerve X
   d. Sympathetic fibers via the cord segments thoracic 1–8 and sacral and the parasympathetic cranial nerve X

3. Myocardial oxygen demand may be decreased by:
   a. Tachycardia
   b. Increased afterload
   c. Decreased preload
   d. Increased wall tension

4. In central venous pressure monitoring, an absent a wave is seen in:
   a. Atrial fibrillation
   b. Mitral stenosis
   c. Pulmonary hypertension
   d. Tricuspid stenosis

5. A patient presents with a pulmonary vascular resistance of 500 dynes/cm per second. All of the following may be causes *except:*
   a. Increased blood viscosity
   b. Hypoxia
   c. Pulmonary hypertension
   d. Acidemia

6. A patient presents with a heart rate of 100, blood pressure of 150/90, respiratory rate of 28, temperature of 38°C, central venous pressure 15, pulmonary artery pressure 23/12, wedge 14, and a cardiac output of 6. Calculate the patient's coronary perfusion pressure.
   a. 86 mm Hg
   b. 88 mm Hg
   c. 136 mm Hg
   d. 76 mm Hg

7. Of the following, which are volume overload valvular lesions?
   a. Mitral regurgitation and aortic stenosis
   b. Aortic regurgitation and cardiac tamponade
   c. Aortic regurgitation and mitral regurgitation
   d. Mitral stenosis and aortic regurgitation

8. A shortened QT interval may be seen with:
   a. Hypercalcemia
   b. Hypokalemia
   c. Congestive heart failure
   d. Hypocalcemia

9. Within the pressure/volume loop, where does the mitral valve close?
   a. a
   b. b
   c. c
   d. d

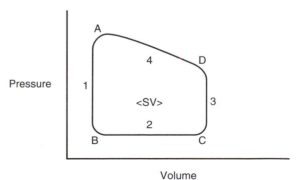

10. The Herring-Breur reflex can be seen in what dysrhythmia?
    a. Sinus arrest
    b. Sinus dysrhythmia
    c. Sick sinus syndrome
    d. Sinus bradycardia

11. Chest pain that is caused by coronary spasm and may be present during rest or sleep is:
    a. Stable angina
    b. Prinzmetal's angina
    c. Unstable angina
    d. Intractable angina

12. You are walking through the postanesthesia care unit and notice asystole on an 81-year-old woman's ECG. The patient is sitting and talking to the nurse. What is your first response?
    a. Administer atropine 1 mg IV
    b. Start cardiopulmonary resuscitation
    c. Defibrillate at 250 joules
    d. Check lead placement

13. What is the triad of symptoms in end-stage aortic stenosis?
    a. Angina, hypertension, and blurred vision
    b. Syncope, angina, and hypertension
    c. Angina, congestive heart failure, and syncope
    d. Hypertension, congestive heart failure, and blurred vision

14. Cardiac tamponade causes a(an):
    a. Increase in pulmonary blood flow
    b. Decrease in stroke volume
    c. Decrease in total peripheral resistance
    d. Increase in coronary perfusion pressure

15. Aortic stenosis can be described as:
    a. Volume overload of the left atrium
    b. Volume overload of the left ventricle
    c. Pressure overload of the left atrium
    d. Pressure overload of the left ventricle

16. High-pitch click followed by a systolic murmur at the apex of the heart is a sign of what valvular abnormality?
    a. Mitral regurgitation
    b. Mitral valve prolapse
    c. Aortic stenosis
    d. Tricuspid regurgitation

17. Epinephrine will do all of the following *except:*
    a. Increase myocardial contractility
    b. Increase heart rate
    c. Inhibit glycogenolysis
    d. Increase glandular secretions

18. Dopamine at doses 0.5 to 3.0 μg/kg per minute will affect what receptors?
    a. Dopaminergic and beta
    b. Alpha
    c. Dopaminergic
    d. Beta 1 and 2

19. Positive inotropic drugs include all *except:*
    a. Norepinephrine
    b. Dobutamine
    c. Calcium
    d. Barbiturates

20. What is present while the cardiac muscle cell is in the resting state?
    a. Sodium ion concentration is greater outside the cell than inside the cell
    b. Potassium ion concentration is greater outside the cell than inside the cell
    c. Unbound calcium is greater inside the cell
    d. The resting membrane potential is -40 to -50 mV

☐ ANSWERS

1.	d	5.	c	9.	c	13.	c	17.	c
2.	b	6.	d	10.	b	14.	b	18.	c
3.	c	7.	c	11.	b	15.	d	19.	d
4.	a	8.	a	12.	d	16.	b	20.	a

Respiratory System

Sherry Ikalowych

The system with which we as anesthetists are most intimately involved and about which we should be the best informed is the respiratory system. Consisting of the lungs and the conduits that lead into the lungs from outside the body, the most important function of the respiratory system is gas exchange. Oxygen enters the lungs via inhalation and is ultimately transported to the mitochondria, where it becomes involved in oxidative phosphorylation and the production of adenosine triphosphate (ATP) (95%). The by-product of the Kreb's cycle, CO_2, is transported back to the lungs, where it is removed from the body via exhalation. The respiratory system performs other functions as well, such as the metabolism of certain drugs, regulation of the temperature of the air entering the respiratory system, filtration of particulate matter and certain toxic substances, serving as a reservoir for the circulation, and converting substances to their active state (i.e., the conversion of angiotensin I to angiotensin II by angiotensin-converting enzyme).

☐ ANATOMY

The respiratory system can be divided into two components, the *conducting zone* and the *respiratory zone*. The conducting region—composed of the nose, nasopharynx, larynx, trachea, bronchi, and bronchioles—ends with the terminal bronchioles. These are collectively known as the conducting airways because their function is to funnel inspired air down to the alveoli. The conducting zone does not participate in gas exchange. Air moves through the conducting zone by bulk flow, propelled by negative intrathoracic pressure, which draws air into it. The respiratory airways consist of the respiratory bronchioles, the alveolar ducts, and the alveoli. This area is where gas exchange occurs. Air moves through

this region by diffusion. The differences in airflow between the two regions account for the phenomenon of the settling of inhaled particles (such as asbestos) in the terminal portion of the conducting zones.

The respiratory system can also be divided into the upper and lower airways. The *upper airway* consists of the nose and the larynx and the *lower airway* of the trachea, lungs, diaphragm, and accessory muscles.

UPPER AIRWAY

When air enters the upper airway, it is composed of approximately 21% oxygen and 79% nitrogen, with virtually no CO_2 or humidification. The main functions of the upper airway are to propel the inhaled air down to the gas exchange areas, to warm and humidify the air, and to remove as much particulate matter and contaminants as possible.

The nose is formed in the fourth week of embryonic life. It is lined with pseudostratified ciliated columnar cells and goblet cells; its cartilage assists in the maintenance of the nose's architecture and in maintaining the patency of the air passages. It also comprises smooth muscle. The olfactory mucosa (the receptors for smell) are located in the roof of the nasal cavities. There are also cavities, or sinuses, connected to the nasal cavities that are air-filled—they are located in the maxillae and in the frontal, ethmoid, and sphenoid bones.

The larynx is located between the trachea and the base of the tongue. It is shaped like a triangle, being more broad and flat at the cephaloid end and more narrow and cylindrical toward the rostral surface, where it joins the trachea. There are *nine cartilages*; three single (the thyroid, cricoid, and epiglottis) and three paired (arytenoids, cuneiforms, and cornicula laryngis). The epiglottis remains of a cartilaginous nature throughout life; but as the larynx ages, the thyroid, cricoid, and arytenoid cartilages, initially hyaline in nature, become ossified. By the time a person reaches the age of 65, these cartilages could be entirely bone. The thyroid cartilage is the most recognizable structure from outside the neck and is also known as the Adam's apple. The space and membrane separating the thyroid cartilage from the cricoid cartilage is known as the cricothyroid membrane. The cricoid cartilage is the only *complete* ring of cartilage in the larynx. The arytenoid cartilages serve as attachments for the vocal cords.

The false cords are thick folds of mucous membrane and ligament attached to the thyroid and arytenoid cartilages—they are not involved in voice generation. The true vocal cords are two thick ligaments covered by a thin layer of mucous membrane that appears whitish yellow; they are usually clearly visible during laryngoscopy. In fact, we use the true vocal cords during laryngoscopy and intubation to identify the tracheal orifice and distinguish the trachea from the esophagus. The approximation of the vocal cords is controlled by certain laryngeal muscles and is innervated by the superior and recurrent branches of the vagus nerve.

LOWER AIRWAY

The trachea is easily identified by the 20 crescent-shaped cartilages anteriorly that are connected by connective tissue heavily laced with elastic fibers. The mucosa is lined by ciliated respiratory epithelium, which propel secretions and foreign particles back up to the nasopharynx.

The trachea ends at a bifurcation known as the *carina*; this is approximately at the level of the fourth or fifth thoracic vertebra. At this level the trachea bifurcates into the left and right mainstem bronchi. The right bronchus is shorter, wider, and straighter than the left bronchus. The bronchi continue to subdivide into smaller bronchi and then into the bronchioles. As mentioned before, each respiratory bronchiole terminates in an alveolar duct, from which the alveolar sacs branch off.

Type I alveolar cells are large, flat cells and line 90% of the alveolar surface—they facilitate gas exchange by minimizing the diffusion surface. Unfortunately for these cells, they are unable to perform mitosis or cellular repair. Therefore, when they are damaged (as they are by a number of agents, including ozone, nitrous oxide, certain chemotherapy agents, and *Pneumocystis carinii*), they lack the ability to regenerate. But when they are damaged as such, there is a proliferation of type II alveolar cells.

There are three primary functions of the *type II* alveolar cells. The first is the transepithelial transport of Na^+ to decrease alveolar fluid. The second is the maintenance of the alveolar epithelium—type II cells have the ability to differentiate into type I alveolar cells if the latter become damaged. And the third function is the synthesis and function of the surface-active material known as *surfactant*. Type II cells in the fetus are mature and capable of producing surfactant by approximately 32 weeks' gestation.

Pulmonary surfactant is secreted into alveolar fluid. It is composed mainly of lipid, with some proteins and carbohy-

drate, and is synthesized shortly after birth in full-term infants. It forms an insoluble film on the surface of the alveolar lining fluid. The purpose of surfactant is to diminish surface tension, which in the alveoli is the molecular force present on the surface of a liquid that makes the surface area exposed to the atmosphere as small as possible. Without surfactant, the surface tension of the alveoli would be so great that the alveoli would collapse. Therefore, surfactant promotes lung expansion with inspiration and prevents lung collapse with expiration. A deficiency or dysfunction in surfactant manifests itself with certain adult lung diseases. It is also seen in premature infants born before the lungs are capable of producing surfactant, leading to respiratory distress syndrome (RDS) in these infants (formerly known as hyaline membrane disease). The development of artificial surfactant (i.e., Exosurf) has been a major therapeutic advancement in the treatment of premature infants with RDS.

The major muscles of ventilation are the diaphragm, the external and internal intercostal muscles, the abdominal wall muscles, and the accessory muscles. The diaphragm, which is innervated by the *phrenic nerve*, is a flat, dome-shaped muscle whose purpose is to temporarily compress the abdominal contents, allowing for a deep, force inspiration. The external intercostal muscles pull the upper ribs outward and the lower ribs upward and outward—a movement that enlarges the thoracic cavity during active inspiration. Just as normal inspiration is an active effort, normal expiration is a passive movement facilitated by the relaxation of muscles that return the thoracic cavity to the preinspiratory size. Forced expiration (as with coughing) occurs due to the work of both the internal intercostal muscles and the abdominal muscles—this is why coughing and deep breathing is so difficult for patients following abdominal or thoracic surgery. The accessory muscles generally come into play only when dyspnea is present—shortening of the scalene and the sternomastoid muscles will raise the first and second ribs and the sternum; this usually appears as a heaving or rocking motion of the neck and shoulders. The use of the accessory muscles during breathing is one of the clinical signs determining whether the patient is having difficulty breathing (nasal flaring is seen only in infants). The patient who depends on the accessory muscles to take in an adequate volume of air will tire quickly due to the considerable amount of energy that must be expended on breathing.

The final component of the ventilatory unit that must be considered is the *pleura*. The visceral layer of the pleura is attached to the lung and its parietal layer to the interior surface of the chest wall. These two layers are held together by a thin film of fluid, and the potential space between the parietal and visceral layers is known as the pleural space. The thin layer of fluid in the pleural space serves as a lubricant, diminishing friction between the two layers as they rub against each other. Numerous lymphatics drain the pleura. The pressure of the fluid in the intrapleural space remains negative at all times due to the difference between the low capillary pressure and the colloid oncotic pressure exerted by the plasma proteins. This negative pressure exceeds the elastic recoil forces of the lung itself, with a net effect of the lung remaining expanded.

Breathing is under both automatic and voluntary control. Ultimate control of ventilation is on the neural level. The pons and the medulla are the areas in the brain involved in respiratory control and are collectively known as the *respiratory center*. This region takes in information from the periphery and integrates it into afferent signals to the respiratory muscles, stimulating inspiration and expiration. Automatic control of ventilation is modulated by input from the chemoreceptors, which are located both centrally and peripherally. The central chemoreceptors are located close to the medulla, near the ninth and tenth cranial nerves, and are surrounded by extracellular fluid. They are sensitive to changes in hydrogen ion (H^+) concentration—increases in hydrogen ion concentration will stimulate breathing, while decreased concentrations will inhibit it. When P_{CO_2} level rise in the circulation, CO_2 will diffuse across the blood-brain barrier from the cerebral vessels (although the blood-brain barrier is relatively impermeable to hydrogen ions and bicarbonate ions, carbon dioxide diffuses easily). The CO_2 will then react with water in the following equilibrium equation:

$$CO_2 + H_2O \rightleftharpoons H_2CO_3 \rightleftharpoons H^+ + HCO_3^-$$

This yields hydrogen ions in amounts depending on the CO_2 levels. If there are high levels of CO_2, the equation moves to the right.

The *peripheral chemoreceptors* are located in the carotid bodies (at the bifurcation of the common carotids) and the aortic bodies (located above and below the aortic arch). These chemoreceptors have a limited role in monitoring CO_2 and pH—their more important function is in the sensing of oxygen concentrations in arterial blood. There is little response from these chemoreceptors as long as the Pa_{O_2} remains above 100 mmHg. When arterial oxygenation falls below 100, the firing rate of the chemoreceptors quickens, stimulating an increase in respiratory rate and depth. In patients with chronically elevated P_{CO_2} levels (such as patients with COPD), the central chemoreceptors become relatively unresponsive because, as a compensatory mechanism, bicarbonate levels in the cerebrospinal fluid become elevated, buffering the increased hydrogen ion concentrations. In these patients the drive to breathe must therefore come from a *decreased P_{O_2}* and is mediated by the peripheral chemoreceptors.

☐ PHYSIOLOGY

In reviewing the physiology of the lung, we must consider several principles that affect the exchange of gases from the alveoli into the bloodstream, the ability of the lung to allow adequate volumes to enter and exit, and principles of both gas flow and the flow of fluid (blood) through a finite vessel. All of these principles must be considered both in the normal lung, with its ability for adequate gas exchange, and in the abnormal respiratory system, whose disease state affects its ability to take in adequate volumes of oxygen and remove CO_2 properly.

DIFFUSION

As discussed previously, air flows through the conducting portion of the respiratory system by bulk flow, propelled by the physical forces of inspiration. Once air reaches the respiratory zone, the cross-sectional area is so large that only diffusion can deliver gases to these areas. The gases under consideration, CO_2 and O_2, are simple molecules that by the physical principles of kinetic movement can freely move within the space of their container. The random kinetic movement of oxygen and carbon dioxide molecules provides the energy with which simple diffusion occurs.

On its most elementary level, diffusion can be defined as the process by which molecules move from an area of higher concentration to one of lower concentration (also known as *equilibrium*). The greater the concentration of a gas, the more pressure it will exert, and the more easily it will diffuse. The cell membranes that compose the blood-gas interface between the alveoli and the capillaries are considered selectively permeable (i.e., they will allow CO_2 and O_2 to pass more readily than H_2O). Diffusion across these membranes follows the principle of simple diffusion: if the concentration of O_2 is higher in the alveoli than in the circulation, O_2 will diffuse across the alveolar capillary membrane from the alveoli into the circulation. Conversely, when the concentration of carbon dioxide in the circulation is higher than in the alveoli, CO_2 will diffuse from the bloodstream into the alveoli.

Fick's law of diffusion states that the amount of gas moving across a membrane is proportional to the area of the tissue but inversely proportional to its thickness. The alveolar membrane is exceedingly thin (> 0.5 μm) and has an area of between 50 and 100 m^2—this makes the lung quite well suited for gas exchange. The principle of equilibrium also applies to the partial pressure of gases in water and tissue. In order for oxygen to be transported to the tissue and CO_2 transported back to the alveoli, these gases must possess the ability to diffuse across both a lipid and a water interface. Each particular gas has a different ability to dissolve into a fluid, this being a constant known as *Henry's law*:

Concentration
    of dissolved gas = pressure $\times$ solubility coefficient

The pressure in this equation is the partial pressure of that particular gas. For example, air has an oxygen concentration of 217, and a pressure at 1 atm of 760 mmHg. Therefore, the partial pressure of oxygen dissolved in room air is approximately 160 mmHg. This refers to the amount of oxygen dissolved in normal arterial blood (not that component carried on the hemoglobin molecule).

Oxygen and carbon dioxide are both highly lipid-soluble. This gives them the ability to cross the cell membrane easily.

Since the alveolus is virtually one layer of cells thick, these gases should be able to cross the alveolar capillary interspace with little difficulty. The limiting factor in diffusion across an alveolus is either the amount of lung water or a thickening or disruption of either the alveolar or the capillary interface.

THE VENTILATION-PERFUSION RELATIONSHIP

If our lungs were perfect, the oxygen content of arterial blood would be equal to the alveolar oxygen concentration. However, since our lungs are not perfect (some being more imperfect than others), we must consider the factors that would increase the alveolar-to-arterial oxygen difference, also known as the *A-a gradient*.

There are essentially four causes of hypoxemia, or low oxygen content in arterial blood. The first is *hypoventilation*—if an inadequate volume of air is inspired, the total lung content of oxygen will ultimately cross into the capillary circulation because the concentration gradient is smaller. There are many causes of hypoventilation, including drugs or alcohol (which suppress the central respiratory drive), postoperative wound splinting, weakness or paralysis of the accessory respiratory muscles. Central causes such as head trauma or pathology lead to increased intracranial pressure. The second cause of hypoxemia is *diffusion abnormalities*. If the alveolar-capillary interface becomes thickened for some reason, according to the Fick equation, the diffusion across this interface will *decrease*. Two major causes of diminished diffusion are an increase in fluid content in the alveoli (as in pulmonary edema) and fibrosis, or a thickening of the alveolar membrane due to injury or infection.

The third cause of hypoxemia is *shunt*, which refers to the blood which would enter the arterial system but bypasses ventilated areas of the lung. Normally, there is a small physiologic shunt in the lungs arising from blood entering from the thebesian veins and the bronchial veins. Shunt becomes significant only in specific cases, as in patients with a congenital heart disease such as atrial septal defects or ventricular septal defects, where a right or left shunt has developed, venous blood mixes with oxygenated blood to dilute the oxygen content of the arterial blood.

And the fourth cause of hypoxemia is mismatching of the *ventilation/perfusion ratio*, or $\dot{V}/\dot{Q}$, ratio. Ventilation and perfusion should be perfectly matched—that is, for every open alveolus containing oxygen, there should be an open capillary passing by to pick up the oxygen and return carbon dioxide for removal. The range of $\dot{V}/\dot{Q}$ in normal patients is approximately 0.8. In patients with pulmonary pathophysiology, the $\dot{V}/\dot{Q}$ would range from near 0, which would represent lungs that are perfused but almost entirely unventilated, to infinite, representing lungs that are ventilated but with varying degrees of diminished perfusion.

When hypoxemia develops, the problem can originate within the alveoli or within the pulmonary circulation. When a patient has a high $\dot{V}/\dot{Q}$, this would indicate a problem with the blood flow through the capillary system that composes the alveolar-capillary gas-exchange units, although on a larger scale the problem could also be in one of the larger pulmonary vessels. With an elevated $\dot{V}/\dot{Q}$, the alveolar ventilation is normal, but there is a diminished blood flow past the alveoli to drop off carbon dioxide and pick up oxygen. This situation is also seen in a patient who is extremely anemic—when the hemoglobin level is very low and the gas-carrying capacity of the blood is depressed, this can also lead to a high $\dot{V}/\dot{Q}$. These patients develop a large alveolar-to-arterial gradient (A-a gradient), which will manifest clinically as a low-end tidal P_{CO_2} and a high P_{CO_2}.

A low $\dot{V}/\dot{Q}$ can be seen as the reverse situation—the pulmonary capillary blood flow is normal but the alveolar ventilation is inadequate. This can be the result of simple hypoventilation but can also be caused by an increase in alveolar fluid (pulmonary edema), obstructive respiratory disease, and a number of other pathologic situations. As the P_{aO_2} drops, the lung will attempt to rectify the problem by constricting blood vessels connected to malfunctioning alveolar units; this will shunt blood flow away from poorly ventilated regions to alveoli with normal ventilation. This mechanism is known as *hypoxic pulmonary vasoconstriction* (HPV), which is used by the lung to rebalance ventilation-to-perfusion matching by redistributing blood flow to areas of the lung that are being well ventilated. A recent study by Morrell et al has shown experimentally that HPV can reduce the shunt fraction up to 50%.

PHYSICAL PROPERTIES OF LUNG FUNCTION

The lungs do not have homogenous blood flow or air movement throughout—regional differences depend not only on $\dot{V}/\dot{Q}$ mismatching but also on patient positioning, voluntary respiratory effort, chest wall compliance, intra-abdominal pressure, etc. Because the lungs have so many elastic fibers within their walls and because of positive pressure within the pleural cavity after inspiration, the lungs will passively return to their pre-inspiratory volume during rest. The lungs are extremely distensible at very low pressures.

The volume of blood that passes through the lungs each minute ($\dot{Q}$) is calculated indirectly using the Fick equation:

$$Q = \frac{V_{O_2}}{Ca_{O_2} - Cv_{O_2}}$$

V_{O_2} is the oxygen consumption per minute, which can be measured by collecting expired gas in a spirometer and measuring its oxygen concentration or by other methods. Once the blood enters the lungs, its regional distribution is unequal and is classically conceptualized by West in his model of the zones of the lung (Fig. 16–1).

If a person stands erect, blood flow increases from the apex to the base. This regional flow difference can be seen as gravity-dependent, because it is essentially due to differences in hydrostatic pressure within and between different blood vessels. When the person changes position and lies supine, the zones change from cephalic-to-rostral and become anterior-to-posterior. When the person lies in the lateral posi-

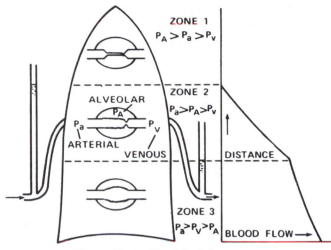

ZONE 1
$P_A > P_a > P_v$

ZONE 2
$P_a > P_A > P_v$

ALVEOLAR
P_A

P_a P_v

ARTERIAL
VENOUS   DISTANCE

ZONE 3
$P_a > P_v > P_A$ BLOOD FLOW →

Figure 16–1   Physiologic lung zones.

tion, the zones change again and become relative to the nondependent ("up") lung and the dependent ("down") lung. Zone 1 is essentially alveolar dead space, because the pulmonary artery pressure (PAP) drops below the alveolar pressure. In the normal lung, the capillaries are not flattened and there is blood flow to this region because PAP is just enough to propel blood up to this zone. There are circumstances under which PAP becomes inadequate to bring blood to this region, such as arterial hypotension and positive-pressure ventilation (increased alveolar pressure). In zone 2, PAP will become higher than alveolar pressure, but venous pressure falls below alveolar pressure, therefore blood flow in this region will be determined by the arterial-to-alveolar gradient. And in zone 3, venous pressure will exceed alveolar pressure, so that flow is determined by the usual difference between arterial and venous pressure.

The elastic forces within the lung are the forces that strive to return the lung to a collapsed state. Forces can be exerted on the lung for expansion, but two major forces (and several others) act to return the lung to its resting or collapsed state. One is the elastic force, and the second is the fluid that lines the alveoli. To better understand how these forces interact, we apply the *LaPlace equation*, which is:

$$P = 2 T/R$$

P is the distending pressure within an alveolus, T is the surface tension of the alveolar fluid, and R is the radius of the alveolus. According to this equation, the pressure necessary to open the alveolus would depend on the size (radius) of the alveolus as well as the surface tension properties of the fluid lining the alveolus. If we assume the surface tension to remain constant, this equation would indicate that the size of the alveolus is inversely proportional to its distending pressure; in other words, the smaller the alveolus, the greater the pressure necessary to distend it. Since in fact all alveoli are different in size, one would assume by this equation that the larger alveoli would distend and the smaller alveoli would remain collapsed. But since this is not the case, there must be

another factor that alters this assumption. That other variable is *surfactant*. By decreasing surface tension even within the small alveoli, the presence of surfactant allows even these small units to expand. But there is a critical volume below which elastic forces will overwhelm these forces that are attempting to keep alveoli open, and the alveoli will collapse. Compliance can be viewed as the opposite of elasticity. *Compliance* is the ability of the alveoli to expand against the forces or pressure resisting such an action. In other words, the higher the compliance, the easier the alveoli are to expand, and an alveolus with low compliance would be able to expand only with much effort (force) applied to it. Compliance can be calculated by the following equation:

$$C = \Delta V/\Delta P$$

where ΔV = change in volume
ΔP = change in pressure

Airway *resistance* can be conceptualized as the opposite of compliance. Resistance is not volume-dependent but rather pressure- and flow-dependent. The following equation helps us to understand the relationship between flow and resistance:

$$R = \Delta P/F$$

where F = flow

The flow of a gas can be seen as the rate at which a gas is displaced, this being influenced by the pressure against which the gas must flow, or the resistance to the molecular movement of the gas. It is also a function of the pressure gradient, or the movement (diffusion) of the gas from an area of higher pressure to one of lower pressure. If the pressure at the latter is high, it will require more force to actively move the gas molecules forward, since the pressure gradient will be low. Conversely, if the pressure of the inward or forward movement of the gas is decreased, the pressure gradient once again is low and gas flow will be diminished.

The resistance to molecular movement is influenced by one other factor, which is laminar versus turbulent flow (Fig. 16–2).

Poiseuille's law applies to *laminar flow*, and states simply that if the driving pressure of a gas is constant, the flow rate will vary with the fourth power of the radius of the airway (r^4). (Also refer to chapter 3.) This indicates that a small decrease in the radius will decrease flow rate drastically and affect gas delivery to the alveoli. Turbulence also influences flow. If molecules of a gas are moving about in a random, chaotic manner, they are very likely to bounce up against the sides of the chamber and even into each other. This disordered or turbulent movement of gas molecules can be a significant cause of a reduction in flow rate. Factors that increase turbulent flow through a conducting system would be tortuous or curving vessels and an increase in particulate matter within the gas stream. Since the upper airway is nor-

bronchiole

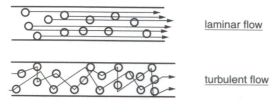

laminar flow

turbulent flow

Figure 16–2 This schematic demonstrates the contrast between laminar and turbulent flow. The top diagram, representing laminar flow shows gas molecules moving through the bronchiole in a smooth, linear manner with little resistance to the molecular movement. The lower diagram represents turbulent flow; molecules of gas are moving about in a random, chaotic manner with molecular flow being hampered by both molecular interaction (gas molecules hitting each other) and by the molecules bouncing off of the sides of the bronchiole.

mally responsible for approximately 50% of the total airway resistance, one can easily understand how any increase in upper airway resistance (such as laryngospasm, obstruction by foreign material, swelling, tumor, etc.) can cause a significant reduction in airflow, both in velocity and amount, as well as an increase in turbulence.

LUNG VOLUMES AND PULMONARY FUNCTION TESTING

As seen from the diagram in Fig. 16–3, the total lung capacity is broken down into several different components that can easily be measured through relatively simple, noninvasive testing. The total lung capacity, or TLC, is the entire volume of air the lung can hold, including the volume that cannot be exhaled (which is the residual volume (RV), or the amount of air that remains in the lungs after a maximum exhalation). The *tidal volume* (V_T) is the amount of air a person can inhale and exhale with a normal breath. The *vital capacity* (VC) is the maximal volume of air that can be exhaled after a normal tidal volume breath. These last two values cannot be

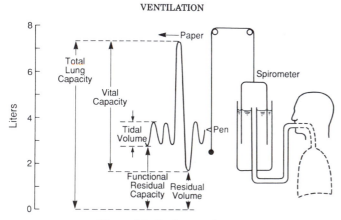

Figure 16–3 Lung volumes.

measured by spirometry but can be evaluated by gas dilution techniques or body plethysmography.

Pulmonary function testing (PFT) is a useful tool in the evaluation of the patient with suspected or confirmed heart and/or lung disease. Frequently it can be difficult to identify patients with lung disease only from subjective and objective history and physical examination. Spirometry is the most widely used noninvasive test to evaluate the nature and degree of airway dysfunction and is used routinely to evaluate air movement during various breathing maneuvers.

It helps to identify preoperative complications in those for whom the risk of surgery would be prohibitive (where the risk of pulmonary morbidity or mortality would outweigh the potential benefits of surgery).

The values that are most useful in the evaluation of a patient's respiratory status would be the *FVC* (forced vital capacity), FEV_1 (forced expiratory volume in 1s), and the *FEV_1/FVC* ratio. A vital capacity of less than 50%, and an FEV_1 of less than 2L (or less than 50% of that predicted for a particular patient) would indicate a patient at risk for postoperative pulmonary complications. Decline in FEV_1 is associated with increased airway responsiveness and is often a predictor for the development of COPD.

Another component, albeit a more invasive test of pulmonary function evaluation, is arterial blood gas measurements. Arterial blood gases are usually drawn via an arterial puncture of the radial or occasionally the femoral artery; the radial artery can easily be palpated via the pulsation along the thumb side of the inner wrist. Arterial blood gases can give us valuable information; disturbances in acid-base balance, whether from respiratory causes or from a metabolic origin, should be identified and corrected in a timely manner in order to avoid further deterioration in patient status. Arterial blood gases (ABGs), depending on the lab and the machine used to calculate the results, will measure several variables; pH, Pa_{CO_2}, Pa_{O_2}, HCO_3 concentration, percent O_2 saturation, and the base excess, and all results are corrected for temperature. Some machines will also measure several electrolytes such as sodium, potassium, and calcium, and many can also measure hematocrit. Because of the importance of this topic, acid-base balance and ABGs will be discussed in further detail.

The pH is defined as the negative log of the hydrogen ion concentration, or

$$pH = -\log [H^+]$$

The hydrogen ions are generated from the chemical reaction of carbon dioxide (the metabolic by-product of cellular metabolism) and water in the following equation:

$$H_2O + CO_2 \rightleftharpoons H_2CO_3 \rightleftharpoons H^+ + HCO_3^-$$

Some of the liberated H^+ ions are bound to hemoglobin. During this process, oxygen is displaced from the hemoglobin because the reduced form of hemoglobin is less acidic than the oxygenated form. This reduced form of hemoglobin in peripheral blood is more receptive to the loading of CO_2 for transport back to the lungs. This phenomenon is referred to as the *Haldane effect*.

Carbonic acid is an important physiologic buffer (others, although more limited, are the orthophosphates and intracellular proteins) whose function is to return a solution to a normal pH. Normal physiologic pH for blood is 7.40, which represents 40 nmol/L of H^+. In humans we accept the range of normal pH as values between 7.35 and 7.45 (approximately). Therefore, a pH of less than 7.35 would indicate too much acid, or acidosis, and a pH of greater than 7.45 would indicate too little H^+, or alkalosis. The pH alone will not be able to identify the source of the increase or decrease in acid load (whether it is of metabolic or respiratory causes). Acute changes in pH (without compensation) can be approximated, as for every change of 1 mmHg in $Paco_2$, there will be a change of 0.01 in the pH—for example, in a patient with respiratory acidosis, if the pH is 7.30, we would expect the $Paco_2$ to be 50 mmHg.

Carbon dioxide is the only form of acid that can be exhaled—most of it is transported dissolved in solution to the lungs or as carbonic acid. It is measured noninvasively by capnography, which analyzes gas concentrations using mass spectrometry or infrared light absorption. The end-tidal Pco_2, which is represented by the plateau on the waveform, approximates $Paco_2$. *In healthy patients, the Pco_2 is about 5 mmHg lower than the actual $Paco_2$.* The kidneys respond to a fall in $Paco_2$ by decreasing its reabsorption and the production of this important buffer. This response takes several days to reach a maximum, however. The $Paco_2$ represents the balance between CO_2 produced on a cellular level and the elimination of CO_2 by the lungs. Normal values for $PAco_2$ lie between 35 and 45 mmHg. If we assume that the metabolic production of CO is constant and there is no rebreathing of CO_2, the $Paco_2$ will indicate (except in specific circumstances such as shivering, increases in body temperature, hyperthyroidism, pheochromocytoma, malignant hyperthermia, and patients receiving IV fluids with a high glucose content) how well the lungs are performing gas exchange. A $Paco_2$ of less than 35 mmHg, or hypocapnea with a normal Ph but without a metabolic explanation is most likely caused by hyperventilation. The etiology of hyperventilation is usually from three causes—anxiety and/or pain, mechanical ventilation, and hypoxemia (via chemoreceptors).

Hypercapnea, on the other hand, is a $Paco_2$ value of greater than 45 mmHg, and the usual explanation for a high $Paco_2$ is hypoventilation. There are also three typical explanations for this condition—they are respiratory depression (commonly seen after administration of narcotics, induction agents, benzodiazepines, and muscle relaxants), increased CO_2 production (such as is seen with malignant hyperpyrexia), and an increased dead space.

$Paco_2$, or arterial oxygen tension, is a measure of the amount of oxygen dissolved in plasma, which determines the percent saturation of hemoglobin. Normal Pao_2 changes with position and age, and it is affected by any pulmonary process that affects gas exchange as well as hypercarbia (because

CO_2 displaces O_2 from the hemoglobin) and systemic changes in O_2 use (such as hypermetabolic states such as hyperthyroidism). Oxygenated and reduced hemoglobin absorbs light of different wavelengths, the values of which have been predetermined. Oxygen saturation is determined by measuring selected wavelengths of light in pulsatile blood using a device known as a pulse oximeter. Pulse oximetry is not a particularly sensitive measure of impaired gas exchange because values are only informative at the steep end of the O_2-hemoglobin dissociation curve. Pao_2 levels equal to or greater than 80 torr will read as a relatively small change in O_2 saturation (97% to 98%). Therefore, according to the curve, oxygen tension can drop to as low as 60 before saturation drops significantly.

Hemoglobin binds with oxygen at the alveolar-capillary interface as the red blood cells in the pulmonary capillaries flow essentially in single file past the alveoli. Normal adult hemoglobin (hemoglobin A) has four binding spots for oxygen and therefore the capacity to carry four oxygen molecules at once. At the tissue level, hemoglobin releases oxygen because the oxygen tension in tissue is low.

The oxygen-hemoglobin dissociation curve represents the relationship between the Po_2 and the amount of hemoglobin that is saturated with oxygen (and therefore the amount of oxygen that will ultimately reach the tissue level). In Fig. 16-4, we see that the curve is steep in the beginning and at approximately a Po_2 of 60 mmHg flattens out considerably. This flat upper portion means that even if the Po_2 of alveolar gas falls, at least to a point, the $HgbO_2$ levels are not

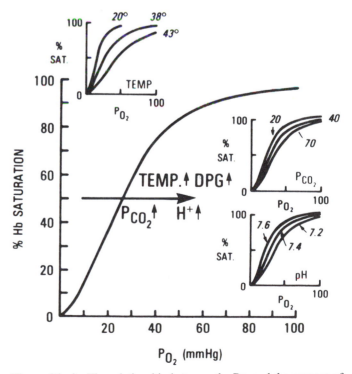

Figure 16-4   The relationship between the Po_2 and the amount of oxygen-saturated hemoglobin is seen with the oxygen-hemoglobin dissociation curve.

affected. But once the P_{O_2} falls below 60 mmHg, O_2 content falls quickly and tissue delivery is compromised. Several factors shift the curve to the left or right—decreased pH and increased P_{CO_2}, temperature, and 2,3-diphosphoglycerate (2, 3-DPG) shift the curve to the right. This facilitates the unloading of oxygen at the tissue level. The same factors but in the opposite direction shift the curve to the left (increase in pH and decrease in temperature, P_{CO_2}, and 2,3-DPG). Although most oxygen is transported on the hemoglobin molecule, a small portion is dissolved in the blood and does contribute slightly to the total oxygen content of blood.

Hypoxemia is a relative term, and values are measured with the F_{IO_2} and several other factors taken into consideration. Strictly speaking, an arterial oxygen saturation of less than 90% is hypoxia; for the normal adult breathing ambient air (with an F_{IO_2} of 21% at 1 atm), the P_{aO_2} should be between 80 and 100. If the patient were breathing supplemental oxygen, we would expect even higher values. The most likely explanation for hypoxemia is hypoventilation, although it can also be caused by absolute shunt (where pulmonary circulation perfuses collapsed or atelectatic alveoli) or a relative shunt as seen with a pulmonary embolus, where blood is shunted through areas of lung were ventilation has not necessarily increased. Whatever the underlying cause of hypoxemia may be, any drop in P_{aO_2} should be addressed appropriately.

In interpreting blood gas results, occasionally a mixed acid-base disturbance will occur, especially if the disease is not purely respiratory or if the patient has more than one metabolic problem. A detailed patient history and physical examination is helpful in interpreting ABG results, especially during an acute episode when the ABG is being drawn (i.e., drug overdose, intractable vomiting, pulmonary embolus). In chronic disease, reabsorption or elimination by the kidney is a compensatory mechanism that takes several days to reach a full effect. On this basis respiratory acidosis or alkalosis as acute (as yet uncompensated) or chronic (partially or nearly compensated) can be classified and will be reflected by the HCO_3 levels that are documented in the ABG results. The therapeutic strategy can then be based on this information and guide treatment accordingly. See Tables 16–1 through 16–4.

Table 16–1
CAUSES OF METABOLIC ACIDOSIS

Normal Anion Gap* (≤ 12 mEq/L)	Increased Anion Gap (>12 mEq/L)
Diarrhea	Lactic acidosis
Retrosigmoidostomy	Starvation
Carbonic anhydrase inhibitors	Diabetic or alcoholic ketoacidosis
Renal tubular acidosis	Methanol, ethylene glycol,
Administration of HCL,	papaldehyde or salicylate
NH3C1, lycine or alginine	ingestion
	Renal insufficiency

*Anion Gap=Serum Na⁻ Serum Cl⁻ Serum HCO_3^-(all in mEq/L)
SOURCE: Reproduced by permission from Selecky PA. *Pulmonary Disease.* 1982

Table 16–2
CAUSES OF METABOLIC ALKALOSIS

Vomiting
Gastric suctioning
Use of diuretics
Hyperaldosteronism
Glucocorticoid administration
Rapid correction of chronic respiratory acidosis
Severe K^+ depletion
Bartter's syndrome
Cushing's syndrome
Villous adenoma of the colon
Volume depletion (contraction of alkalosis)

SOURCE: Reproduced by permission from Selecky PA. *Pulmonary Disease.* 1982

□ PATHOPHYSIOLOGY

Many diverse disease processes ranging from infection to autoimmune or congenital problems to disease caused by environmental contaminants—can affect the lungs. When problems within the respiratory system reach a critical point, gas exchange becomes compromised and oxygen delivery at the cellular level decreases. Respiratory disease is an important part of the overall patient profile and should be a prominent consideration in the anesthetic care plan. A careful evaluation of the patient's subjective symptoms, history, physical examination, laboratory data, electrocardiogram, chest x-ray, review of medications, and, if necessary, pulmonary function tests (PFTs) will be necessary to evaluate the patient with urinary disease, degree of optimization, and risk for surgery and postoperative pulmonary complications. Preoperative evaluation and optimization as such can reduce risk and allow the patient and the anesthetic team to prepare for proper management.

CHRONIC OBSTRUCTIVE PULMONARY DISEASE

Chronic obstructive pulmonary disease (COPD) affects more than 23 million Americans (approximately 1 out of every 10 people) and is the fourth leading cause of death. Patients with severe COPD are at a higher risk for postoperative pulmonary complications such as atelectasis, pneumonia, prolonged postoperative pulmonary complications such as at-

Table 16–3
CAUSES OF RESPIRATORY ACIDOSIS

Increase Wasted Ventilation	Primary alveolar hypoventilation
Severe obstructive lung disease	Obesity
Severe kyphosis	Neuromuscular disease
Severe restrictive lung disease	Myopathy involving respiratory
Bronchospasm	muscles
Normal Wasted Ventilation	Sedative overdose
	General anesthesia

SOURCE: Reproduced by permission from Selecky PA. *Pulmonary Disease.* 1982

Table 16–4
CAUSES OF RESPIRATORY ALKALOSIS

Anxiety, stress	Pneumonia
Fever	Pulmonary embolus
Hypoxemia	Hepatic insufficiency
High altitude	Pregnancy
CNS disease—infection, trauma, tumor	Salicylate intoxication
	Sepsis
CHF	Mechanical ventilation

SOURCE: Reproduced by permission from Selecky PA. *Pulmonary Disease.* 1982

electasis, pneumonia, prolonged postoperative intubation and ventilatory support, and death. Some experts group chronic bronchitis, emphysema, and asthma under the umbrella of COPD, and some classify asthma separately under the heading of reactive airway disease. According to the American Lung Association, 11.4 million Americans suffer from chronic bronchitis, and another 2 million have emphysema; patients frequently present with a mixture of symptoms that blur strict labeling of their disease as emphysema or chronic bronchitis. Both diseases share a common pathophysiology, which is chronic airflow limitation. The major categorical difference lies at the site of disease—for *chronic bronchitis*, the disease is primarily of the airways, and for *emphysema* it is primarily an alveolar disease. Although there are several well-documented contributing factors in the development of COPD (i.e., smoking, environmental air pollution, exposure to respiratory irritants), there has been recent evidence supporting the theory that lytic viral infections could induce chronic lung disease in atopic patients, contributing to the long-term pathogenesis of COPD and asthma.

Chronic Bronchitis Chronic bronchitis is a disease whose hallmark is excessive production of mucus within the conducting airways, which leads to a daily productive cough. This cough is chronic and occurs for at least several months out of the year, especially in the winter. The mucous glands in the large bronchi become hypertrophied, and the number of goblet cells increases (significantly in severe disease). The cilia disappear, and small airways exhibit cellular infiltration, edema of the bronchial walls, and narrowing of the lumens. This sets up the situation where the excessive mucus can become plugged in the small airways, blocking airflow, and leading to a decreased $\dot{V}/\dot{Q}$ and hypoxic pulmonary vasoconstriction (HPV). Hypoxemia and hypocapnea develop, and the patient becomes dyspneic. Chronic hypoxemia stimulates the kidneys to secrete erythropoietin, leading to polycythemia as an attempt to increase oxygen-carrying capacity and delivery.

Severe chronic bronchitics who are chronic CO_2 retainers for many years were thought to have chemoreceptors and respiratory centers that did not respond to increased $Paco_2$ because of chronic exposure. Hypoxemia was thought to be their stimulus to breathe; therefore, if these patients were given supplemental oxygen, theoretically the rise in Pao_2

would lead to a decreased respiratory drive. Recently, studies in patients with COPD in acute respiratory failure indicated that CO_2 drive remained a major determinant of respiratory drive in many of them (Tardiff et al., 1993). But another study (Johnson et al., 1995) concluded that high concentrations of supplemental oxygen decreased FEV in patients with airflow problems, probably relating to the increased density and viscosity of oxygen related to air. Therefore, this aspect of the properties of gas might contribute to the deterioration seen when COPD patients in acute respiratory failure are placed on 100% oxygen. *Therapeutic implications* are to apply to the lowest Fio_2 that would support Pao_2 to acceptable levels.

Cigarette smoking of many packs per year is usually in the patient's history. The patient is typically a stocky male in his 40s or 50s with a plethoric and cyanotic look, leading to the coining of the term "blue bloaters" to describe these patients. Clinically, on auscultation, the patient will have rales, rhonchi, and wheezes. Peripheral edema and jugular vein distention can be present if right ventricular failure occurs. Right ventricular failure, or cor pulmonale, may also cause hepatomegaly. Chest films may show cardiomyopathy, increased pulmonary vascular markings, or frank congestion. These patients use accessory muscles for respiration, increasing their work of breathing. PFTs show a decrease in vital capacity, FEV_1, and FEV_1/FVC ratio, reflecting airway obstruction; increases in residual volume, functional residual capacity, and a possible increase in total lung capacity reflect air trapping. Arterial blood gas abnormalities, such as a low Pao_2 and a high $Paco_2$ can make the patient sleepy and confused or restless and anxious. If their Pao_2 is less than 55, or the O_2 saturation less than 88%, supplemental oxygen is warranted. The pH can be low, but since the condition is chronic the kidney will retain bicarbonate ions and pH will most likely be low normal. They are prone to respiratory tract infections, and their respiratory status is likely to decompensate during these acute episodes. Some sources label the COPD patient with chronic bronchitis as "type B."

Emphysema The "type A," or emphysematous type of COPD, presents a different picture. Unlike the patient with type B or chronic bronchitis, the patient with emphysema does not have much of a cough, and little sputum production—what little sputum is produced is scant and thin. The presenting symptom is usually dyspnea. The pathology of emphysema is a destruction of the alveolar walls and parts of the capillary beds, and the air spaces distal to the conducting airways appear dilated. The small airways can become narrowed, with thin, atrophied walls. There can occasionally be involvement on the large airways. The etiology of emphysema is unknown, although there has been some evidence toward a role of two enzymes, protease and elastase, in the destruction of the elastic tissue in the alveoli. This loss of elastic tissue leads to a loss of elastic recoil. Patients with a genetic deficiency in $\alpha1$-antitrypsin (a single-chain protein synthesized by hepatocytes and macrophages that inhibits certain proteases such as elastase) lack the ability to stop protease enzymes such as elastase from destroying alveolar tissue during acute infections when the polymorphonuclear white cells infiltrate the lung.

Loss of elastic fibers in the lung leads to two problems. The first is overdistended lungs that are unable to return to their resting state or size. The second problem is increased airway resistance due to the narrowing and collapse of small airways, leading to trapping of air in the distal airways. Both of these problems contribute to the overdistension of the lungs. As the lungs continue to distend, the circumference of the chest wall increases, leading to the "barrel chest" appearance that is a cardinal sign of emphysema. The diaphragm is also compressed. Between the loss of elastic recoil, air trapping, chronic use of accessory muscles, and increased respiratory rate, breathing for the emphysematous patient becomes difficult, and these people exert tremendous amounts of energy in their effort to breathe, even at rest. The physical habitus of a person with emphysema becomes thin due to the high caloric expenditure in the work of breathing. Normally, less than 5% of total O_2 consumption is used for the work of breathing. The decreased compliance with emphysema can increase the oxygen necessary to breathe by 50%. This progressively curtails these patients' physical activity, and insidiously, over time, they conserve movement and make lifestyle changes to accommodate the energy necessary simply to breathe. When they breathe, their I/E ratio is very low, and they purse their lips as they exhale, leading to the label "pink puffers."

Chest x-ray shows overinflated lungs with a low, flattened diaphragm, narrowing or obliteration of pulmonary blood vessels, and narrowed mediastinum. The ABGs remain normal unless the person is severely decompensated, because the patient's respiratory rate increases to compensate for the other pathological changes—in fact, the patient can have a respiratory alkalosis with a low Pa_{CO_2} and perhaps a mild decrease in Pa_{O_2}. The emphysema patient as well as the patient with chronic bronchitis is prone to respiratory infections during which the disease can exacerbate and lead to respiratory and/or right heart failure. In addition, there have been studies that indicate that COPD patients have an autonomic nervous system (ANS) dysfunction that leads to a depressed heart rate variability response to sympathetic and vagal stimuli (Volterani, 1994).

The airway changes seen in the COPD patient are not reversible. Therefore, therapy is usually supportive, with a more intensive focus during exacerbations, such as occur with acute infections. Proper nutrition and hydration, expectorants, good health maintenance, and vigilance on the part of the patients and their caretakers are generally the cornerstone of therapy. Patients may be on long-term corticosteroids, and if PFTs have shown a reversible component to their disease, they may be on bronchodilators. If signs of a respiratory infection develop, the patient must be evaluated and placed on an antimicrobial agent expeditiously.

REACTIVE AIRWAY DISEASE

Patients with reactive airways are divided into two groups—those with acute and those with chronically hyperactive airways. Acute airway hypersensitivity is usually seen following a viral upper respiratory infection (URI) and seems to be mediated via *vagally induced* reflex bronchoconstriction. It can last up to *6 weeks* after symptoms of the URI have abated but appears to be blocked by the actions of anticholinergics such as atropine. Airway manipulation appears to be a risk factor for bronchoconstriction in the presence of a viral URI, especially in children. Electively scheduled surgery involving anesthesia is generally delayed several weeks after the symptoms of the URI have disappeared to avoid this potential hazard.

Asthma is a disease of chronic airway hyperactivity. It affects approximately 5% of Americans and is one of the most common chronic diseases seen in children. Many young children (less than 3 years old) have episodes of transient wheezing usually associated with a viral infection; most of these cases showed complete resolution and cessation of episodic wheezing by the age of 6. Martinez et al, in a study published in January 1995, found that children whose wheezing persisted past the age of 6 were likely to be atopic and to have mothers who were asthmatics. Children of mothers who smoke are also more likely to experience wheezing, both transient and persistent. There has been a progressive increase in the prevalence of asthma, and hospitalizations and mortality due to this disease have increased over the past several years. Occupational asthma, either related solely to exposure to respiratory irritants or *IgE-mediated*, is the most prevalent occupational disease in some countries.

Asthma is an overreactivity and hyperresponsiveness of the tracheobronchial conducting zones, leading to the cardinal symptom, which is wheezing. This hyperresponsiveness leads to bronchoconstriction, which narrows the airways to varying degrees. These pathophysiologic changes occur in an episodic manner, but the airways are found to have chronically hypertrophied smooth muscle and hypertrophied mucous glands. Many different events can trigger an asthma attack, including allergies, cold air, exercise, stress, chemical irritants, and upper respiratory infections.

The main diagnostic differentiation between chronic bronchitis and asthma is that asthma responds well to bronchodilator medication (although chronic bronchitis can occasionally respond to some degree). There also tends to be varying degrees of persistent airflow obstruction and morphologic changes between attacks. Obstruction is most common in *medium airways* due to the lack of cartilage support. Between attacks, auscultation of the chest is usually normal, although wheezing can often be elicited with forced expiration. Therefore, it would be important to elicit a history of asthma through patient interview of previous history. An elevated eosinophil count can be present, along with a slight increase in hemoglobin and hematocrit. Chest x-ray may reveal hyperinflated lungs but is otherwise within normal limits.

The ABGs can show a mild respiratory alkalosis, but asthmatics are rarely hypercarbic or hypoxic until their disease is severe or during an attack. A recent study concluded that a reduced chemosensitivity to hypoxia and blunted perception of dyspnea may predispose patients to fatal asthma attacks (Kikuchi et al, 1994).

Patients can infrequently present to the emergency room in status asthmaticus, a condition of continuous wheezing not relieved by the usual therapy. Patients presenting with a "quiet chest" are bronchoconstricted to the point where there is no airflow, presenting a life-threatening emergency. These patients can present exhausted and dehydrated from hours or even a day or two of wheezing and dyspnea. These situations are often too far advanced for nebulized bronchodilator treatments to be effective and require endotrachial intubation and emergency medical therapy.

The usual treatment for asthma is metered-dose bronchodilation by inhaler (especially the beta$_2$-selective agonists), theophyline, steroids, anticholinergics, and cromolyn sodium. Patients with upper respiratory infections and/or who are actively wheezing will usually have elective surgery postponed until their respiratory status is under better control.

RESTRICTIVE DISEASE

Restrictive pulmonary diseases are those in which expansion of the lungs is limited due to either a mechanical defect of the chest wall, increase in intra-abdominal pressure, or neuromuscular disease, causing impedance to lung expansion. A restrictive process can also be caused by disease of the lung itself. In general, the VC is decreased and TLC is decreased. Airflow in large airways is usually preserved, and FEV$_1$/FVC ratio can be *normal*. Small airway obstruction is common with decreased lung compliance, although the airway resistance itself is not always affected. Hypoxemia increases with exertion, and Paco$_2$ is slightly decreased except in severe disease, where it begins to rise. Patients that come for surgery can have restrictive pulmonary problems because of their disease process that is unrelated to the lung itself—these would be conditions such as large abdominal masses, ascites, bowel obstruction, advanced pregnancy or multiple gestations, and surgery involving laparoscopy for gynecologic procedures such as diagnosis of ectopic pregnancy, diagnosis of disease, or tubal ligation. Increases in intra-abdominal pressure have been shown to have a major affect on pulmonary compliance, decreasing it as much as 50% (Obeid et al., 1995).

A broad spectrum of systemic diseases can lead to a restrictive pulmonary picture and is often due to parenchymal lung disease. Diseases that can cause a restrictive lung pattern include sarcoidosis, diffuse interstitial fibrosis, rheumatoid disease, systemic lupus erythmatosus, scleroderma, various collagen vascular disorders, and systemic vasculitic diseases (such as polyarteritis nodosa), polymyositis or dermatomyositis, radiation injury, inhalation lung diseases such as silicosis and asbestosis, talcosis, neurofibromatosis, pectus excavatum, scoliosis, disease induced by certain drugs (especially cancer chemotherapy agents such as methotrexate), and metastatic calcifications or tumor bulk within the chest cavity. In eliciting a history from patients known to have disease that is associated with potential pulmonary problems, follow-up information on lung function is important to determine the degree of lung dysfunction and the respiratory limitations, since restrictive components of these diseases generally are not reversible.

ADULT RESPIRATORY DISTRESS SYNDROME

The term *adult respiratory distress syndrome*, or ARDS, was first used to describe the pathologic pulmonary process noted to afflict trauma patients approximately 24 to 48 h after injury and patients with viral pneumonia and pancreatitis. The same disease process was later described in patients who had undergone major vascular procedures and cardiopulmonary bypass. The series of 12 patients in the study had acute development of tachypnea and diminished pulmonary compliance. The major cause of mortality in these patients was pulmonary failure. When this syndrome was initially studied, the mortality rate was approximately 60%. Almost 20 years later, given the tremendous advancements in critical care medicine, monitoring, and mechanical ventilation, the mortality rate presently approaches 50% (although today, patients succumb to multisystem organ failure instead of respiratory failure per se). ARDS is most recently thought to be not a primary pulmonary process but instead part of a generalized inflammatory reaction to distant tissue trauma.

Several other underlying etiologies such as sepsis, bacterial (as well as viral) pneumonia, aspiration, and massive blood transfusion can all lead to the development of ARDS. *Sepsis* is the most common etiology, and sepsis from nosocomial infection has the highest mortality rate (although the risk of developing ARDS after gastric aspiration is quite high at 30 to 40%). The risk of developing ARDS compounds with increasing numbers of predisposing factors.

ARDS can be divided into four progressive stages, depending on clinical findings, and physiologic and pathologic changes found. In *phase 1*, the only subjective symptom is *dyspnea*. Respiratory alkalosis might be present from tachypnea. At this point, a large number of vasoconstrictive substances have already been released; these mediators initiate various physiologic cascades, neutrophil adherence to the endothelium, and release of oxygen radicals, nitric oxide, and proteases that begin to cause endothelial damage. *Phase 2* generally begins 12 to 24 h after the early symptoms. At this stage lung injury becomes clinically evident, with the patient developing *hypoxemia*, decreased compliance, worsening dyspnea and infiltrates on chest x-ray. Neutrophils infiltrate through the endothelium of capillaries and into the interstitium and alveolar walls, and small thrombi may form in the microvessels. Unlike infant RDS, patients with ARDS will have normal volumes of surfactant, but there is evidence that the surfactant is frequently dysfunctional. The process can resolve at this point if the underlying disease is brought under control. If not, the process will progress to *phase 3*. In phase 3, microemboli or thrombosis of vessels within the microcirculation of the lungs occurs, and hypoxic pulmonary vasoconstriction (HPV) combines with this to *increase dead space ventilation*. At this point, endotracheal intubation and mechanical ventilation become necessary; this in itself can lead to further lung injury due to the potential for barotrauma, oxygen toxicity (via free radical formation), and bacterial colonization of the endotracheal tube (especially with nosocomial organisms such as methicillin resistant Staphylococcus aureus and Pseudomonas). Invasive monitoring is usually initiated at this stage. Characteristically, patients with ARDS will have a high cardiac output, low pulmonary capillary wedge pressure (PCWP), and pulmonary edema; this hemodynamic picture, however, is not exclusive to ARDS and is used only to correlate with the clinical picture for diagnostic purposes. Also, these values can be altered to correlate with the clinical conditions, such as sepsis (which depresses the myocardium, leading to decreased cardiac output) or aggressive fluid resuscitation (increasing fluid pressures).

Other chemical mediators that have been shown to be involved in the progression of ARDS are cytokines such as tumor necrosis factor (TNF) and interleukins-1 and -6 platelet activating factor, macrophage products, free oxygen radicals, proteolytic enzymes, products of arachidonic acid metabolism, and many other substances that have yet to be definitively identified and are derived from neutrophils, macrophages, platelets, and pulmonary endothelium. Activated macrophages, at this stage, can release chemical mediators which perpetuate the pathologic downward spiral without any further influence from the initiating injury.

The final phase, *phase 4*, is similar to phase 3, with the addition of an increased incidence of *lung sepsis* and uncontrolled pulmonary fibrosis caused by an increase in elastic type 1 collagen deposition (under macrophage control). Alveolar edema will usually resolve within 7 to 10 days, but infiltrates on chest x-ray are collagen deposits that preceded fibrosis. The patient will eventually succumb to multisystem organ failure refractory to therapy. Pulmonary edema is a common component of acute respiratory failure and ARDS.

Pulmonary edema is much more complex a process than simple water excess and/or protein crossing microvascular membranes—it involves the interstitium and type I and type II alveolar cells. Changes in the interstitium are an important component in increased membrane permeability.

Intervention is mainly concentrated on determining the underlying disease process and attempting to resolve it. Otherwise the therapeutic goals are mainly supportive—maintenance of acceptable oxygenation and organ perfusion. The patient is placed on a volume-cycled mechanical ventilator on the assist-control mode, with the lowest FiO_2 that still permits adequate arterial blood gas values, with the addition of

positive end-expiratory pressure (PEEP) as necessary and/or as tolerated, or inverse-ratio ventilation. Kacmarek and Venegas (1987) recommend using high respiratory rates (20 to 25 breaths per minute) to compensate for the increased dead space and noncompliant lungs. Other therapeutic measures are fluid restriction (but avoiding hypovolemia by following central filling pressures), exogenous surfactant (still experimental), corticosteroids, antibiotics as indicated, and hemodynamic support.

PULMONARY HYPERTENSION

Pulmonary hypertension is a disease characterized by a progressive increase in pulmonary vascular resistance caused by obliteration or narrowing of resistance in pulmonary arteries. It can be either primary (of unknown etiology) or secondary (caused by various underlying respiratory and/or systemic disorders). Primary pulmonary hypertension is poorly understood and its causes are elusive. There have been recent investigation findings that pulmonary hypertension is associated with an increase in endothelin-1, which is a potent vasoconstrictor and a growth factor for smooth muscle proliferation. Increased expression of endothelin-1, which is produced in the vascular endothelium, is seen in particular in primary pulmonary hypertension and may contribute to the vascular abnormalities (Giaid et al., 1993). There has also been quite a bit of research recently investigating the role of nitric oxide in pulmonary hypertension. Nitric oxide is a known endogenous selective pulmonary vascular vasodilator. A recent study by Giaid and Saleh (1995), found that in primary and secondary pulmonary hypertension there is reduced expression of nitric oxide synthase in the endothelium of pulmonary arteries, correlating with increased vascular resistance in an inversely proportional manner.

The main pathology in pulmonary hypertension is an extensive remodeling of pulmonary vasculature based on a *proliferation* of smooth muscle cells in the tunica media and intima. This thickening reduces the diameter of the resistance vessels, leading to an increase in pulmonary vascular resistance (PVR), increased pulmonary artery pressure (PAP), and increased pressures in the right ventricle, which leads to right ventricular hypertrophy and eventually right ventricular failure. Primary pulmonary hypertension is most frequently seen in young to middle-aged women, and there may be a genetic predisposition to its development, possibly triggered by either drugs or a viral infection. Presenting symptoms are chest pain, exertional dyspnea, and syncope. The high pulmonary vascular tone may actually enhance gas exchange, because frequently when the patients are treated with vasodilator agents or oxygen, $\dot{V}/\dot{Q}$ ratios deteriorate (Augusti, 1993). Secondary pulmonary hypertension is a potential complication of any pulmonary disorder that leads to long-term alveolar hypoxia and arterial hypoxemia. These conditions include severe obstructive lung disease, kyphoscoliosis, neuromuscular diseases, and alveolar hypoventilation syndromes (Vender, 1994). The underlying pathophysiology is the same as in primary pulmonary hypertension, with persistent vasoconstriction and vascular remodeling leading to the narrowing of pulmonary blood vessels. Various therapies have been attempted to treat pulmonary hypertension, including nonselective systemic vasodilators (nitroglycerin, sodium nitroprusside) and inhaled nitric oxide. Severe and irreversible disease would make the patient a candidate for a lung transplant.

TUBERCULOSIS

Tuberculosis is a disease that for a period of time was thought to be well under control in this country. Several decades ago, patients with tuberculosis were sent to institutions or sanitariums, where, under the supervision of medical personnel (to ensure compliance) they were treated with streptomycin. Later, drug therapy was a combination of isoniazid (INH), streptomycin, and aminosalicyclic acid. When, in the 1960s, the trend was to treat tuberculosis patients on an outpatient basis, there was a rise in medication noncompliance, leading to treatment failure and the emergence of drug-resistant bacterial strains. According to an estimate by the World Health Organization, there will be approximately 90 million new cases of tuberculosis between 1990 and 1999; 30 million people are expected to die from tuberculosis-related complications by the year 2000.

Most cases of tuberculosis are caused by the *Mycobacterium tuberculosis* organism, which is transmitted through the respiratory route from person to person. Once the bacterium enters the lung, it grows and induces an inflammatory response in the area, with the proliferation of lymphocytes, macrophages, and connective tissue leading to the formation of a hard nodule around the bacteria called a tubercle. Although the disease process becomes quiescent at this point, the bacteria within the tubercle remain alive (although dormant). After this, a couple of different processes can occur. The tubercle can become a caseous lesion, which can eventually calcify and show up on chest x-ray as a prominent density. Tubercles can also liquefy and form a tuberculous cavity that is filled with air—these cavities are the source of dissemination of infection to new sites, which is known as reactivation. At this stage, the patient becomes infectious once again.

The most common manifestation of pulmonary infection is functional changes such as hyperinflation and restrictive pattern, with increased and occasionally decreased elasticity. Patients can also present with bronchial constriction or fistulas in the small bronchi and can have diminished total lung capacity. There can also be a dysfunction of the thyroid and gonadal axis and occasionally hypoadrenalism.

Typical symptoms of tuberculosis are fever, fatigue, weight loss, and cough, which occasionally produces bloody sputum. Diagnosis is made by chest x-ray, isolation of the organism in sputum culture, and a positive Mantoux or tuberculosis skin test. Therapy is usually chemical, with INH, rifampin, and ethambutal or streptomycin being administered in a combination of at least two drugs at once to avoid drug resistance. Some 10% of the patients today are found to be resistant to INH and/or rifampin. Multiply resistant tuberculosis has recently emerged as a major health problem, with some strains found to be resistant to up to seven drugs (over 90% of these cases were in patients with AIDS), with fatality rates of up to 90%. Surgical resection has even been recommended in selected patients with drug-resistant tuberculosis. Several cases of multidrug-resistant tuberculosis have been reported in physicians and nurses caring for these patients, and the use of submicron molded masks, negative-pressure ventilation of patients' rooms, and ultraviolet light has been advocated by some sources to control nosocomal epidemics (Iseman, 1992). In patients being treated with INH, enflurane should be avoided, as this inhalation agent can enhance defluorination, which may lead to nephrotoxicity.

SMOKING

In 1991, 46.3 million adults (25.7%) in the United States were smoking, and in 1990 approximately 400,000 deaths occurred that were directly related to smoking. According to the Surgeon General's Report, cigarette smoking is the leading cause of pulmonary illness and death in the United States, mainly due to pneumonia, influenza, bronchitis, emphysema, and chronic airway obstruction. These patients can present with subtle changes in their respiratory tracts that can become problematic in the face of stress, such as surgery and general anesthesia. The normal population of mast cells in the human lung is 2%—a higher proportion is found in smokers. Chronic bronchitis results from chronic irritation of the tracheobronchial tree by inhaled irritants, mainly tobacco smoke. Although viral infections lead to similar changes, chronic irritation without infection leads to hypertrophy and hyperplasia of mucus-secreting airway tissue and the appearance of mucus-secreting cells in the distal bronchioli (where they are normally absent). Excessive accumulations of mucus serve as a culture medium for various organisms, particularly *Hemophilus influenzae* and *Streptococcus pneumoniae*. This changes the character of sputum to purulent, leading to inflammation, scarring, and destruction of bronchiolar walls. Even asymptomatic young smokers with normal PFTs were experimentally unable to enhance their rate of mucus clearance by coughing, suggesting changes in mucociliary function (Bennett et al., 1992). There are fewer ciliated cells in smokers, and remaining cilia are abnormal.

Tobacco smoke damages neutrophils, diminishes lysosome activity, and decreases both bronchial surfactant and protease inhibitor. There is an acute increase in airway resistance as the patient is smoking—atropine or beta-$_2$ agonists experimentally attenuate this effect. The smoker also has a transient slight deepening and slowing of respirations. An acute increase in blood pressure and heart rate accompanies cigarette smoking that is associated with an increase in catecholamines; it has been shown experimentally that this is a peripheral effect mediated through adrenal gland stimulation, decreased norepinephrine reuptake, and decreased catecholamine clearance. In fact, it was shown that central sympathetic nervous system activity decreased during smoking, leading to speculation that the central sympathetic drive is inhibited by arterial baroreceptor reflexes (Grassi et al., 1992). Smoking has been shown to cause immediate constriction of proximal and distal epicardial coronary arteries with an increase in coronary resistance vessel tone (Quillen et al., 1993). Further studies done on patients whose only risk factor was smoking showed that during cigarette smoking, there was an increased cardiac output and a fall in pulmonary blood volume; in patients with COPD or pulmonary hypertension there was a transient increase in pulmonary artery pressure but a decrease in pulmonary vascular resistance. Also noted was an increase in neutrophil sequestration in the lungs during smoking (Skwarski et al., 1993).

The incidence of lung cancer, especially *small cell lung cancer*, is increased in smokers. The risk for lung cancer was found to be higher in men than in women relative to the daily intensity of smoking and the number of years of smoking history. Declining ventilatory function associated with persistent symptoms of chronic bronchitis in smokers is also associated with an increased risk of lung cancer. In a recent study, female smokers were found to have 5.34 times greater chance of developing lung cancer than nonsmoking females, and males who smoked had a 4.11 times greater incidence of lung cancer over nonsmoking males (Islam, 1994).

Smokers who quit smoking have a receding incidence of respiratory symptoms such as cough, dyspnea, and sputum production within 3 to 4 months of quitting, while airway conduction, PEF, maximum voluntary ventilation all improve 3 to 6 weeks after smoking cessation. While mucociliary improvement is seen almost immediately, FEV_1 and FVC decreased with age more slowly in ex-smokers than in patients who continued to smoke—the suggestion was that the effects of quitting smoking had a relatively rapid onset and led to a protection against accelerated loss of pulmonary function, even toward some reversal of the effects of smoking (Nemery et al., 1982).

Given that smoking is both a physiologic as well as a psychologic addiction, one should not expect patients to be able to stop smoking preoperatively, especially since smoking is frequently an anxiety-reducing mechanism for these people. If the patients have been hospitalized for a period of time, it is likely they have not smoked because of the hospital's smoke-free environment. Smoking increases the biotransformation of certain drugs via *enzyme induction* by some of the chemicals in tobacco smoke. If the patient is a heavy smoker, up to 15% of the oxygen binding sites on the hemoglobin molecule can be occupied by *carbon monoxide*, decreasing oxygen-carrying capacity. All of the above factors put the smoker at higher risk for postoperative problems, of which the patient should be made aware.

BIBLIOGRAPHY

Aquilina AT, Hall WJ, Douglas RG. Airway reactivity in subjects with viral upper respiratory tract infections: The effects of exercise and cold air. *Am Rev Respir Dis* 1980;122:3–10.

Ashborough DG. Acute respiratory distress in adults. *Lancet* 1967; 2:219–223.

Augusti AG, Rodriguez-Roisin R. Effects of pulmonary hypertension and gas exchange. *Eur Respir J* 1993;6:1371–1377.

Bennett WD, Chapman WF, Gerrity TR. Ineffectiveness of cough for enhancing mucus clearance in asymptomatic smokers. *Chest* 1992;102:412–416.

Boyden EA. *Development of the Lung*. New York: Marcel Dekker; 1977:5–30.

Bullock B, Rosendahl P. *Pathophysiology: Adaptations and Alterations in Function*. 3rd ed. Philadelphia: Lippincott; 1992.

Chan-Yeung M, Malo JL. Occupational asthma. *N Engl J Med* 1995;333:107–112.

Cherniack R. Managing patients who have chronic pulmonary disease. *Anesth Today* 1993; vol 4.

Cigarette smoking-attributable mortality and years of potential life lost—US 1990. *MMWR* 1993;42:645–649.

Cooper PR. *Head Injury*. Baltimore: Williams & Wilkins; 1992: 327–342.

Crapo R. Pulmonary function testing. *N Engl J Med* 1994;331: 25–30.

Crystal R, West J. Development of lung structure. In: *The Lung: Scientific Foundations*. New York: Raven Press; 1991.

Cummings G, Bonsignore G. *Smoking and the Lung*. New York: Plenum Press; 1984.

Dantzer DR. Physiology and pathophysiology of pulmonary gas exchanges. *Hosp Pract* 1986;21:135–157.

De Weese D, Saunders W. *Textbook of Otolaryngology*. St. Louis: Mosby, 1973.

Demling R. Adult respiratory distress syndrome: Current concepts. *New Horizons* 1993;1:371–380.

Ferguson GT, Cherniack R. Management of COPD. *N Engl J Med* 1993;328:1017–1022.

Giaid A, Yanagisawa M, Langleben D, et al. Expression of endothelin-1 in the lungs of patients with pulmonary hypertension. *N Engl J Med* 1993;328:1732–1737.

Goldsberry D, Hurst J. Adult respiratory distress syndrome and sepsis. *New Horizons* 1993;1:324–347.

Gragono AC. *Fundamentals of Acid-Base Balance*. 45th Annual Refresher Course Lectures and Clinical Update Program. American Society of Anesthesiologists, Inc; 1994:154.

Grassi G, Servalle G, Calhoun DA, et al. Cigarette smoking and the adrenergic nervous system. *Clin Exp Hypertens* 1992;14: 251–260.

Gray H. *Gray's Anatomy*. Philadelphia: Running Press; 1974.

Guyton AC. *Medical Physiology*. Philadelphia: Saunders; 1981: 491–502.

Higenbottom T. Pathophysiology of pulmonary hypertension: Role for endothelial dysfunction. *Chest* 1994;105:75–125.

Hodson ME, Geddes DM, eds. *Cystic Fibrosis*. London: Chapman and Hall; 1995:1–13.

Iseman M, Treatment of multidrug-resistant tuberculosis. *N Engl J Med* 1993;329:784–791.

Iseman MD. A leap of faith: What can we do to curtail intrainstitutional transmission of tuberculosis? *Ann Intern Med* 1992;117: 251–253.

Islam SS, Schottenfield D. Declining FEV_1 and chronic productive cough in cigarette smokers: A 25-year prospective study of lung cancer incidence in Michigan. *Cancer Epidemio* 1994;3: 289–298.

Johnson JE, Peacock MD, Hayes JA, et al. Forced expiratory flow is reduced by 100% oxygen in patients with COPD. *South Med J* 1995;88:443–449.

Kacmarek RM, Venegas J. Mechanical ventilatory rates and tidal volumes. *Respir Care* 1987;32:466–478.

Kikuchi Y, Okabe S, Tamura G, et al. Chemosensitivity and perception of dyspnea in patients with a history of near fatal asthma. *N Engl J Med* 1994;330:1329–1334.

Klein EF. *Interpretation of Blood-Gas Measurements*. 43rd Annual Refresher Course Lectures and Clinical Update Program. American Society of Anesthesiologists, Inc; 1992:531.

Kollef MH, Schuster DP. Medical progress: The acute respiratory distress syndrome. *N Engl J Med* 1995;332:27–37.

Leeson CR, Leeson TS, Paparo AA. *Atlas of Histology*. Philadelphia: Saunders; 1985.

Martinez FD, Wright AL, Taussig LM, et al. Asthma and wheezing in the first 6 years of life. *N Engl J Med* 1995;332:133–138.

Massaro D, ed. *Lung Cell Biology*. New York: Marcel Dekker; 1989:487–538.

Morrell NW, Nijran KS, Biggs T, Seed WA. Regional matching of ventilation and perfusion during lobar bronchial occlusion in man. *Clin Sci* 1995;88:179–184.

Murray J. *The Normal Lung*. Philadelphia: Saunders; 1976:95–100.

Murray R, Granner D, Mayes P, Rowell V. *Biochemistry*. Englewood Cliffs, NJ: Prentice-Hall, 1993:15–18.

Nemery B, Moavero NE, Brasseur L, Stanescu DC. Changes in lung function after smoking cessation: An assessment from a cross-sectional survey. *Am Rev Respir Dis* 1982;125:122–124.

Nunn JF. *Applied Respiratory Physiology*. 3rd ed. London: Butterworth; 1987.

Obeid F, Saba A, Fath J, et al. Increases in intraabdominal pressure affects pulmonary compliance. *Arch Surg* 1995;130:544–547.

Oswalt C, Gates G, Fritz M, Holmstrom G. Pulmonary edema as a complication of acute airway obstruction. *JAMA* 1977;238:1833–1835.

Pison U, Obertacke U, Brand M, et al. Altered pulmonary surfactant in uncomplicated and septicemia-complicated courses of acute respiratory failure. *J Trauma* 1990;30:19–26.

Porth C. *Pathophysiology: Concepts of Altered Health States*. Philadelphia: Lippincott; 1990.

Post FA, Soule SG, Willcox, PA, Levitt NS. The spectrum of endocrine dysfunction in active pulmonary tuberculosis. *Clin Endocrinol* 1994;40:367–371.

Prescott L, Harley J, Klein D. Microbiology. William C. Brown, 1990:718–719.

Quillen JF, Rossen JD, Oskarsson HJ, et al. Acute effects of cigarette smoking on the coronary circulation: Constriction of epicardial and resistance vessels. *J Am Coll Cardiol* 1993;22:642–647.

Raviglione M, Snider D, Kochi A. Global epidemiology of tuberculosis. *JAMA* 1995;273:220–226.

Reducing the Health Consequences of Smoking: 25 Years of Progress: A Report of the Surgeon General: Executive Summary. Rockville, MD: Department of Health and Human Services, Publication number (CDC)89–8411, 1989.

Reischman RR. Review of ventilation and perfusion physiology. *Crit Care Nurs* 1988;8:24–26.

Rijcken B, Schouten JP, Xu X, et al. Airway hyperresponsiveness to histamine associated with accelerated decline in FEV_1. *Am J Respir Crit Care Med* 1995;15:1377–1382.

Rubin LJ. Pathology and pathophysiology of primary pulmonary hypertension. *Am J Cardiol* 1995;75:51A–54A.

Russell NJ, Crichton NJ, Emerson PA, Morgan AD. Quantitative assessment of the value of spirometry. *Thorax* 1986;41:360–363.

Shapiro B, Harrison R, Trout C. *Clinical Application of Respiratory Care*. Chicago: Yearbook Medical Publishers; 1979.

Sheeler P, Bianchi D. *Cell and Molecular Biology*. New York: Wiley, 1987;491–502.

Skwarski KM, Gorecka D, Slavinski P, et al. The effects of cigarette smoking on pulmonary hemodynamics. *Chest* 1993;103:1166–1172.

Suchyta MR, Clemmer JP, Elliot CG, et al. The adult respiratory distress syndrome: A report of survival and modifying factors. *Chest* 1992;101:1074–1079.

Swartz M. *Textbook of Physical Diagnosis*. Philadelphia: Saunders; 1994.

Tardif C, Bonmarchand G, Gibon JF, et al. Respiratory response to CO_2 in patients with COPD in acute respiratory failure. *Eur Respir J* 1993;6:611–613.

Tarpy S, Celli B. Long term oxygen therapy. *N Engl J Med* 1995; 333:710–714.

Tobin MJ. *Essentials of Critical Care Medicine*. New York: Churchill Livingstone; 1989:152–156.

Tollinson R. *Clearing the Air: Perspectives on Environmental Tobacco Smoke*. Ashland, MA: Lexington Books; 1988.

Van Golde LMG, Battenburg JJ, Robertson B. The pulmonary surfactant system: Biochemical aspects and functional significance. *Physiol Rev* 1988;68:374.

Vender RL. Chronic hypoxic pulmonary hypertension. *Chest* 1994;106:236–239.

Volterrani M, Scalvini S, Mazzuero G, et al. Decreased heart rate variability in patients with COPD. *Chest* 1994;106:1432–1437.

Walter S. Smoking causes an increase in elastic recoil in the lung, probably caused by inactivation of surfactant. *Ind J Physiol Pharmacol* 1992;36:169–173.

Weinberger SE. Recent advances in pulmonary medicine–Part I. *N Engl J Med* 1993;328:1389–1397.

Weiss KB, Gergen PJ. Changing patterns of asthma hospitalization among children. *JAMA* 1990;264:1688–1692.

West J. *Pulmonary Pathophysiology*. Baltimore: Williams & Wilkins, 1981.

West J. *Respiratory Physiology*. Baltimore: Williams & Wilkins, 1980.

Whitney L. Chronic bronchitis and emphysema: Airing the differences. *Nursing '92* 1992;March:34–41.

Wong D, et al. Factors associated with postoperative pulmonary complications in patients with severe COPD. *Anesth Analg* 1995;80:276–284.

☐ QUESTIONS

1. Carboxyhemoglobin levels decrease within _____ after cessation of smoking.
   a. 24 h
   b. 48 h
   c. 72 h
   d. None of the above

2. The larynx consists of _____ cartilages.
   a. Five
   b. Six
   c. Nine
   d. Ten

3. The cells in the lungs that produce surfactant are the:
   a. Type I alveolar cells
   b. Type II alveolar cells
   c. Type III alveolar cells
   d. Type IV alveolar cells

4. The respiratory center in the brain consists of the:
   a. Cerebral cortex and basal ganglia
   b. Cerebellum and cerebral cortex
   c. Pons and medulla
   d. Medulla and the basal ganglia

5. A major cause of diminished diffusion of gas across the alveoli is:
   a. The thickening of the alveolar membrane due to injury or infection
   b. Hypoventilation
   c. Hyperventilation
   d. Weakness of the accessory muscles

6. A patient with a pulmonary embolus would have a:
   a. High $\dot{V}/\dot{Q}$ ratio
   b. Low $\dot{V}/\dot{Q}$ ratio
   c. High end-tidal P_{CO_2}
   d. None of the above

7. Poiseuille's law applies to:
   a. Compliance versus elasticity
   b. The buffering capacity of the bicarbonate ion system
   c. Gas pressures within a gas tank
   d. Laminar versus turbulent gas flow

8. A decline in the FEV_1 on a pulmonary function test would indicate:
   a. Increased airway responsiveness
   b. Decreased airway responsiveness
   c. Pulmonary embolus
   d. Restrictive pulmonary disease

9. An important physiologic buffer is:
   a. Acetic acid
   b. Phosphoric acid
   c. Carbonic acid
   d. Carbon dioxide

10. The pH reflects the level of _____ in the bloodstream.
    a. Calcium ions
    b. Hydrogen ions
    c. Potassium ions
    d. Sodium ions

11. Patients with chronic hypoxia, such as those with chronic bronchitis, develop polycythemia due to:
    a. The stimulation of erythropoietin from the kidneys
    b. Dehydration
    c. Diminished turnover of red blood cells
    d. Immune deficiency

12. The two enzymes that are thought to play a role in the development of emphysema are:
    a. Collagenase and coagulase
    b. Proteinase and collagenase
    c. Protease and elastase
    d. Protease and collagenase

13. The airways in asthmatics have:
    a. Chronically hypertrophied smooth muscle and hypertrophied mucous glands
    b. Chronically underdeveloped accessory muscles and poor respiratory effort
    c. Poorly developed mucous glands and poor ciliary function
    d. All of the above

14. The most common etiology of ARDS is:
    a. Asthma
    b. Aspiration
    c. Sepsis
    d. Renal failure

15. An endogenous pulmonary vasodilator is:
    a. Oxygen
    b. Halothane
    c. Nitric oxide
    d. Nitrous oxide

16. Closing capacity is:
    a. Related to functional residual capacity (FRC)
    b. The lung volume at which the onset of airway closure occurs
    c. Increased in obesity
    d. All are true.

17. All statements about the respiratory quotient are true *except*:
    a. Under normal circumstances, 5 ml of O_2 is delivered to the tissues in every 100 ml of blood
    b. Under normal circumstances, 4 ml of CO_2 is released into the alveoli for every 100 ml of blood
    c. Will always be 0.8
    d. Refers to the $\dot{V}/\dot{Q}$ ratio within the lungs

18. Pick the correct statement.
    a. The best perfusion and ventilation is in zone 3.
    b. Zone 2 has high venous pressure.
    c. In zone 1, there is very little dead space.
    d. All are true.

19. Pick the false statement. Bronchitis:
    a. Must last at least 3 months within a year to be termed chronic
    b. May occur from infectious or non-infectious causes
    c. Includes abnormal enlargement of the air spaces
    d. Causes the mucous glands in the large bronchi become hypertrophied, leading to excessive mucus production

20. Hypoxic pulmonary vasoconstriction:
    a. Is reduced by inhalational anesthetics
    b. Diverts blood flow from hypoxic to nonhypoxic lung areas
    c. Is reduced by increased intravascular pressure
    d. All are true.

☐ ANSWERS

1. b	**5.** a	**9.** c	**13.** a	**17.** c
2. c	**6.** a	**10.** b	**14.** c	**18.** a
3. b	**7.** d	**11.** a	**15.** c	**19.** c
4. c	**8.** a	**12.** c	**16.** d	**20.** d

CHAPTER
17

Endocrine System

Cynthia K. Rau-Sobotka

Bodily functions are regulated by the nervous system and the endocrine system.[1] The endocrine system influences metabolic cellular activities by means of hormones, chemical substrates secreted by the endocrine gland into the blood for delivery to a distant target site where it exerts its effect. Chemically, hormones are derivatives of amino acids or steroids (gonadal and adrenocortical hormones).[2]

☐ HORMONAL SECRETION AND MECHANISM OF ACTION

Hormone output from most endocrine glands is regulated by a negative feedback system in which increased circulating serum levels of hormone act to reduce its subsequent release from the gland (except in cases of hormone-secreting tumors).[3] Hormones may activate the cyclic adenosine 3′, 5′ monophosphate (cAMP) system of cells (also known as "second messenger"), stimulate genes in the cells to stimulate proteins that initiate cellular activities, or cause protein synthesis in target cells, which act as enzymes or carrier proteins that in turn, activate other cellular functions.[2]

Endocrine diseases are characterized by the deficiency or excess of single or multiple hormones that can have dramatic physiologic and pharmacologic consequences affecting anesthetic management. Understanding endocrine gland pathophysiology is essential for perioperative anesthetic management of the patient with endocrine gland dysfunction. This chapter presents dysfunction of the endocrine organs (pituitary, adrenal, thyroid, parathyroid, pancreas, and reproductive glands) and obesity. A brief review of normal physiology is followed by clinical manifestations and anesthetic considerations of abnormal hormonal activity.

☐ PITUITARY GLAND

The pituitary gland is located in the sella turcica below the base of the brain. Anatomically and functionally, the pituitary is divided into two components: the anterior (adenohypophysis) and the posterior pituitary (neurohypophysis).[4] Pituitary function is under hypothalmic control via vascular connections (hypophyseal portal veins) between the hypothalamus and anterior pituitary and via nerve fibers between the hypothalamus and posterior pituitary.[5] The hypothalamus synthesizes hypothalamic-releasing and -inhibiting factors that are transported to the adenohypophysis by these vascular connections.

ANTERIOR PITUITARY (ADENOHYPOPHYSIS) HORMONES

Under hypothalamic control, the anterior pituitary secretes six hormones: adrenocorticotropic hormone (ACTH), growth hormone (GH), thyroid-stimulating hormone (TSH), follicle-stimulating hormone (FSH), luteinizing hormone (LH), and prolactin.

Adrenocorticotropic Hormone (ACTH)
Physiologic Effects
ACTH is synthesized and stored in the anterior pituitary. It stimulates the adrenal cortex to synthesize and release various corticosteroids (glucocorticoids). Glucocorticoid production, unlike mineralocorticoid production, is dependent on ACTH secretion.[6] Excess ACTH induces adrenal cortex hyperplasia with sustained high output of corticosteroids, whereas, in the absence of ACTH, adrenal cortex atrophy oc-

curs.[3] ACTH elicits adrenal secretion by activating the adenylate cyclase system and cAMP production.[4]

Control of Secretion

Corticotropin secretion is regulated by corticotropin-releasing factor (CRF) from the hypothalamus as well as a negative feedback mechanism dependent on circulating cortisol levels. ACTH and CRF secretion is mainly regulated by cortisol-like steroids, the sleep-wake cycle, and stress.[4] Secretory rates of ACTH and CRF follow a diurnal pattern with maximal activity seen soon after awakening.[3] These diurnal variations are not observed in patients with excessive adrenal cortex activity (i.e., Cushing's disease).[3]

Growth Hormone
Physiologic Effects

Growth hormone is an anabolic hormone that stimulates growth of all body tissues, especially bone and skeletal muscle.[2] GH deficiency in childhood results in short stature, whereas an excess causes gigantism. Acromegaly results from excessive GH in the adult. Specific metabolic effects of GH include increased rate of protein synthesis, increased mobilization of fatty acids, and decreased rate of glucose utilization.[1]

Control of Secretion

Growth hormone secretion is regulated by GH-releasing factor and GH-inhibitory factor (somatostatin), both secreted by the hypothalamus and transported to the anterior pituitary.[3] Hypoglycemia, anxiety, physical exertion, and stress as produced by anesthesia may increase GH secretion.[3]

Thyroid-Stimulating Hormone (Thyrotropin)
Physiologic Effects

Thyrotropin is synthesized and stored in the anterior pituitary. It accelerates all steps involved in thyroid hormone synthesis. TSH effects are elicited through activation of adenylate cyclase and increased formation of cAMP.

Control of Secretion

Thyrotropin-releasing hormone (TRH) produced in the hypothalamus stimulates TSH release; negative feedback of thyroid hormones inhibits it. Sympathetic nervous system stimulation and corticosteroids suppress TSH secretion.[3] An increased TSH level is the most sensitive test for detecting primary hypothyroidism.[5] A low TSH level in a hypothyroid patient indicates pituitary or hypothalamic dysfunction.[4]

Gonadotropins
Physiologic Effects

The two gonadotropins synthesized and released by the adenohypophysis are LH and FSH. FSH stimulates ovarian development or promotes sperm formation in the testes.[1] LH induces ovulation and causes secretion of female sex hormones (estrogen and progesterone) by the ovaries and testosterone by the testes.[1,7]

Control of Secretion

Gonadotropin-releasing hormone produced by the hypothalamus prompts gonadotropin release by the adenohypophysis. In general, gonadal hormones (e.g., estrogen, progesterone, and testosterone) feedback to supress FSH and LH release.[2]

Prolactin
Physiologic Effects

Prolactin, synthesized in the adenohypophysis, promotes mammary gland development and milk production. Suckling increases prolactin secretion. Prolactin-secreting tumors are often accompanied by galactorrhea and, in females, amenorrhea.[3] The most frequent cause of hyperprolactinemia is an anterior pituitary tumor.[7]

Control of Secretion

The hypothalamus secretes both prolactin-releasing hormone and prolactin-inhibiting hormone (dopamine), which increases and decreases prolactin secretion respectively.[2,10]

POSTERIOR PITUITARY (NEUROHYPOPHYSIS) HORMONES

The neurohypophysis is composed of terminal nerve endings of neurons originating in the hypothalamus, which then pass to the posterior pituitary through the pituitary stalk.[3,5] The hypothalamus synthesizes antidiuretic hormone (ADH) and oxytocin. They are stored and released from the posterior pituitary.

Antidiuretic Hormone (Vasopressin, Pitressin)
Physiologic Effects

Vasopressin regulates plasma osmolarity and maintains blood volume. ADH increases water permeability in the collecting ducts causing reabsorption of water, leading to a reduced plasma osmolarity and an increased urine osmolarity (concentrated urine).[7]

Control of Secretion

Vasopressin is released by the posterior pituitary in response to increased blood osmolarity (sensed by osmoreceptors located primarily in the hypothalamus), decreased extracellular volume (hemorrhage or sodium depletion), positive-pressure ventilation, or surgical stimuli.[2-4] The most potent stimulator for ADH secretion is activation of osmoreceptors (increased serum osmolality) in the hypothalamus.[4] Decreased serum osmolarity inhibits ADH release, but the need to restore plasma volume may override osmotic inhibition of ADH.[4] Other actions of ADH include increased blood pressure by constricting vascular smooth muscle (splanchnic, renal, and coronary vascular beds) and hemostasis (increased levels of von Willebrand factor and factor VIII).[4]

Oxytocin
Physiologic Effects

Oxytocin elicits uterine contraction and promotes milk secretion. Natural and synthetic oxytocic drugs (e.g., Pitocin) are used to induce or hasten labor, to stop postpartum bleeding, and to stimulate the milk ejection reflex.[2]

Control of Secretion
As birth nears, uterine and cervical stretching sends afferent impulses to the hypothalamus.[2] The hypothalamus synthesizes oxytocin and triggers its release from the neurohypophysis.

PATHOPHYSIOLOGY OF PITUITARY GLAND AND ANESTHETIC IMPLICATIONS

Acromegaly   Acromegaly is caused by excess GH secretion in the adult, most often from an anterior pituitary adenoma.[4] Excess hypertrophy occurs in connective, skeletal, and soft tissues.

Clinical Manifestations
Manifestations of acromegaly include prognathism (skeletal overgrowth), soft tissue overgrowth (lips, tongue, epiglottis, vocal cords), subglottic narrowing of the trachea, peripheral nerve or artery entrapment, connective tissue overgrowth (recurrent laryngeal nerve paralysis), and glucose intolerance.[7] There is an increased incidence of hypertension, ischemic heart disease, osteoporosis, and osteoarthritis.[5]

Anesthetic Considerations
Airway management of these patients is complicated by distortion of facial and upper airway anatomy. Mask ventilation may be difficult and intubation may be a challenge. If a difficult intubation is anticipated, it is prudent to consider an awake intubation, preferably with a fiberscope, using a smaller endotracheal tube.[5] Serum glucose levels should be monitored. Titrate doses of muscle relaxants and use a nerve stimulator in patients with a history of skeletal muscle weakness. Use of regional anesthesia may be technically difficult or unreliable because of skeletal changes that accompany acromegaly.

Diabetes Insipidus (DI)   Diabetes insipidus (DI) reflects deficient ADH release caused by posterior pituitary destruction (central DI) or failure of the renal tubules to respond to ADH (nephrogenic DI). Patients with nephrogenic DI do not respond to ADH and its analogs (e.g., desmopressin).[4,5] Lesions near the hypothalamus and the pituitary stalk frequently cause DI. Transient DI is commonly seen after head trauma and neurosurgical procedures.[6,7]

Clinical Manifestations
Diabetes insipidus is characterized by polydipsia, polyuria (hypotonic and often > 6 L/day), despite an increased serum osmolarity (hypernatremia), and the absence of hyperglycemia.[6] Hypovolemia and hypernatremia can become life-threatening.

Anesthetic Considerations
Initial management consists of intravenous (IV) hydration if oral intake cannot offset polyuria. Treatment for acute central DI is aqueous IV ADH (100 to 200 mu/h).[4] Desmopressin

(DDAVP) is a longer acting (12 to 24 hours) nasal preparation commonly used.[6] Anesthetic management includes monitoring urine output, serum electrolytes, and osmolarity.

Syndrome of Inappropriate Antidiuretic Hormone (SIADH) Secretion   The inappropriate and excessive secretion of ADH may occur in the presence of diverse pathologic processes, including head injuries, intracranial tumors, pulmonary infections,[10] small-cell carcinoma of the lung, hypothyroidism, adrenal insufficiency, and from drugs such as nicotine, narcotics, clofibrate, chlorpropamide, vincristine, vinblastine, and cyclophosphamide.[4,7] The response theoretically occurs in the majority of patients after surgery.[7] ADH secretion is increased by increased serum osmolality and hypotension. Inappropriate secretion of ADH, without relation to serum osmolality, results in water retention, low output of highly concentrated urine, and dilutional hyponatremia.[10]

Clinical Manifestations
The majority of clinical manifestations associated with SIADH secretion are related to the dilutional hyponatremia and the resulting brain edema.[10] Symptoms may range from weight gain, weakness, lethargy, confusion, and abnormal reflexes to convulsions and coma.[10] Despite fluid retention, peripheral edema and hypertension are rare.[4,10] Monitoring serum and urine sodium and osmolality values supports the diagnosis. SIADH is likely when urine osmolality is higher than serum, and urine sodium is elevated above 20 mEq/L while serum sodium (< 130 mEq/L) and osmolality (< 270 mOsm/L) are decreased.[10] Rapid corrections are not recommended because abrupt reductions in serum sodium concentrations below 110 mEq/L can result in cerebral edema and seizures.[5]

Anesthetic Considerations
The anesthetist must consider the possible presence of renal, cardiac, or liver disease as an etiology for excess body water. Treatment should be directed at the underlying problem. Patients with mild to moderate symptoms of water intoxication usually require only fluid restriction (500 to 1000 mL/d).[10] Patients with acute neurologic symptoms due to hyponatremia may require IV infusion of hypertonic saline (200 to 300 mL of 5% saline) solution.[10] Hyponatremia should be corrected slowly (no faster than 0.5 mEq/L/h) because overly aggressive correction can result in central pontine myelinolysis.[7]

☐ ADRENAL GLAND

The adrenal glands lie at the superior poles of the two kidneys. Each adrenal gland has two functional portions, the medulla and cortex. The adrenal medulla secretes norepinepherine and epinephrine; the adrenal cortex secretes glucocorticoids (e.g., cortisol) and mineralocorticoids (e.g., aldosterone). The adrenal androgens have minimal effects on anesthetic management and will not be discussed further.

ADRENAL MEDULLA

The adrenal medulla is innervated by preganglionic sympathetic fibers that bypass the paravertebral ganglion and pass directly from the spinal cord to the adrenal medulla (analogous to postganglionic neuron).[3] As a specialized part of the sympathetic nervous system (SNS), the adrenal medulla synthesizes and secretes epinephrine (80%) and norepinephrine (20%) in response to SNS stimulation.[4]

Synthesis and Release of Catecholamines The biosynthetic pathway for catecholamines produced in the adrenal medulla involves a series of enzyme controlled steps beginning with tyrosine→DOPA→dopamine→norepinephrine→epinephrine.[7] Cortisol regulates the production of epinephrine. In the medulla, cortisol activates the enzyme phenylethanol-amine N-methyltransferase, necessary for the conversion of norepinephrine to epinephrine.[5] Catechol O-methyltransferase and monamine oxidase provide prompt enzymatic breakdown of catecholamines. Major urinary metabolites of catecholamines are metanephrines and vanillylmandelic acid (VMA). Preganglionic cholinergic acetylcholine release is the triggering event for catecholamine release from the medulla.[3] The catecholamine responses are similar to those produced by direct SNS stimulation.

ADRENAL CORTEX

The adrenal cortex synthesizes three types of hormones classified as glucocorticoids, mineralocorticoids, and androgens (Table 17–1). The two most important corticosteroids are cortisol and aldosterone.

Table 17–1
ENDOGENOUS AND SYNTHETIC CORTICOSTEROIDS

	Glucocorticoid Potency* (Antiinflammatory Effects)	Mineralocorticoid Potency* (Salt-Retaining Effects)	Equivalent Oral or IV Dose* (mg)
Cortisol	1	1	20†
Cortisone	0.8	0.8	25
Prednisolone	4	0.8	5
Prednisone	4	0.8	5
Methylprednisolone	5	0	4
Betamethasone	25	0	0.75
Dexamethasone	25	0	0.75
Triamcinolone	5	0	4
Corticosterone	0.35	15	—
Fludrocortisone	10	125	—
Aldosterone	0	3000	—

* Potencies and equivalent doses are compared with cortisol.
† Assumed daily endogenous cortisol production.
SOURCE: Reproduced by permission from Stoelting and Dierdorf.[5]

Glucocorticoids *Cortisol* is essential for life and has multiple physiologic effects. Metabolic actions include enhanced gluconeogenesis and inhibition of peripheral glucose utilization (elevated blood glucose), protein catabolism, fatty acid mobilization, and anti-inflammatory effects.[3] Cortisol is crucial to the conversion of norepinephrine to epinephrine in the adrenal medulla.[5] About 20 mg cortisol is produced daily in response to ACTH.[4] Cortisol is metabolized by the liver and excreted unchanged by the kidney.

Mineralocorticoids *Aldosterone* is the principal endogenous mineralocorticoid. It is a major regulator of extracellular volume and potassium homeostasis. Aldosterone regulates extracellular fluid volume by promoting renal tubular resorption of sodium and potassium excretion. Aldosterone release is stimulated by the renin–angiotensin system (specifically angiotensin II), hyperkalemia, and ACTH.[4] Hypotension, hypovolemia, congestive heart failure, and surgery result in increased aldosterone levels.[6]

PERIOPERATIVE STEROID REPLACEMENT

The exact dose of corticosteroid or duration of therapy producing pituitary-adrenal axis suppression is unknown. Additionally, it may require as long as 12 months after discontinuation of therapy for recovery of normal pituitary-adrenal axis function.[5] Providing stress steroid coverage poses little risk and because acute adrenal crisis is life-threatening, supplemental steroids are empirically administered to all patients who have received daily steroid therapy for at least 1 week in the year before surgery[4] (see Table 17–1).

A recommended "low-dose" regimen for perioperative corticosteroid supplementation is cortisol (25 mg IV) at induction of anesthesia, followed by a continuous infusion (100 mg IV) over 24 hours.[4,5] Another popular regimen is administration of hydrocortisone 200 to 300 mg/70 kg body weight in divided doses on the day of surgery.[4]

ADRENAL GLAND PATHOPHYSIOLOGY AND ANESTHETIC CONSIDERATIONS

Pheochromocytoma Pheochromocytomas are catecholamine-secreting tumors arising from chromaffin cells of the sympathoadrenal system that accounts for 0.1% of all cases of hypertension.[3] Ninety percent of pheochromocytomas are located in the adrenal medulla, 10% are bilateral, and about 10% are malignant.[8] The tumor most commonly secretes a combination of epinephrine and norepinephrine (percentage of secreted norepinephrine being greater than that of normal gland secretion) and their release is independent of neurogenic control.[4] Pheochromocytoma is diagnosed by confirmation of excessive plasma levels of catecholamines and increased urinary excretion of their metabolites (VMA and metanephrines).[6] Additionally, hypertensive patients without a pheochromocytoma demonstrate decreases in serum catecholamine levels after a single oral clonidine dose (0.3 mg), whereas patients with a tumor demonstrate no decrease.[7] This clonidine suppression test distinguishes the patient with essential hypertension and an elevated catecholamine level from the patient with hypertension due to a pheochromocytoma.[5] Tumor location can be determined by magnetic resonance imaging, computed tomography scan, ultrasound, or scintigraphy.[6] Treatment consists of surgical excision of the tumor.

Clinical Manifestations

The hallmark of pheochromocytoma is paroxysmal or sustained hypertension. The classic triad of diaphoresis, tachycardia, and headache in hypertensive patient is highly suggestive of pheochromocytoma.[7] α_1-Stimulation increases peripheral vascular resistance and arterial blood pressure, which can lead to intravascular volume depletion (increased hematocrit), cerebral hemorrhage, and renal failure.[6] Increased peripheral resistance increases myocardial work and patients are at risk for myocardial ischemia, ventricular hypertrophy, and congestive heart failure.[6] Other symptoms include hyperglycemia (predominant α effect inhibits insulin secretion), mental status changes, hypovolemia-induced orthostatic hypotension, polycythemia, and weight loss.[7] Chronically high levels of circulating catecholamines may produce a cardiomyopathy.[6]

Anesthetic Considerations

Before surgery, α-receptor blockade is usually started with phenoxybenzamine or prazosin, which reduces blood pressure and repletes blood volume (resultant fall in hematocrit).[6] Phenoxybenzamine, an α_1 and α_2 blocker, is most commonly prescribed and patients are maintained on this medication for up to 2 weeks with doses titrated to relieve the signs and symptoms of hypertension.[8] If tachycardia persists, β blockade is started *after* the onset of adequate α blockade. If β receptors are blocked first, unopposed α-mediated vasoconstriction dominates, causing abrupt increases in systemic vascular resistance.[6] A heart depressed by β antagonists in addition to the increased systemic vascular resistance may progress to cardiac failure.

The overall goal is to avoid any drug or event that increases sympathetic outflow, plus the use of invasive monitoring to facilitate early and appropriate intervention of catecholamine-induced changes in cardiovascular status. The α and β antagonists are continued until the day of surgery.[5] Both regional and general anesthesia may be used; however, a disadvantage of regional anesthesia is the resultant sympathectomy compounded by hypotension on tumor excision.[7] Dysrhythmias and severe hypertension may occur with tumor manipulation requiring use of IV nitroprusside (1 to 2 μg/kg), phentolamine (1 to 5 mg IV) or β blockers.[5] With tumor excision, extreme hypotension may follow, requiring volume resuscitation and use of direct-acting vasopressors such as phenylephrine.[4] Recommendations are to avoid the following drugs: halothane, ketamine, vagolytic agents (e.g., anticholinergics, pancuronium), droperidol, and drugs associated with histamine release (e.g., morphine, tubocurarine, and atracurium).[6,7] Because abdominal fasciculations may cause catecholamine release from tumor, the use of succinylcholine is controversial.[6,7]

Hyperaldosteronism   Primary aldosteronism (Conn syndrome) results from intrinsic hypersecretion of aldosterone by the adrenal cortex, which can be due to a unilateral adenoma (aldosteronoma), bilateral hyperplasia, or adrenal gland carcinoma.[3] Secondary hyperaldosteronism is present when increased renin secretion is responsible for excess aldosterone secretion.[4] Measurement of plasma renin activity differentiates the disease as primary (low renin activity) or secondary (high renin activity).[5]

Clinical Manifestations

Mineralocorticoid excess manifestations include hypertension, hypervolemia (due to aldosterone-induced sodium retention), hypokalemia, muscle weakness, and metabolic alkalosis.[5] One should suspect hyperaldosteronism in a patient with diastolic hypertension (100 to 125 mm Hg) and a potassium plasma concentration of less than 3.5 mEq/L.[5] Alkalosis can lower ionized calcium levels leading to tetany.

Anesthetic Considerations

Hypokalemia and hypertension should be treated preoperatively and can be controlled by sodium restriction, potassium supplementation, and the administration of spironolactone (aldosterone antagonist). Hypokalemia may modify responses to nondepolarizing muscle relaxants and can be worsened by hyperventilation.

Hypoaldosteronism   Hyperkalemia despite normal renal function suggests the presence of hypoaldosteronism.[5] Destruction or adrenal gland atrophy results in both mineralocorticoid and glucocorticoid deficiency although unilateral adrenalectomy, protracted heparin therapy, use of angiotensin-converting enzyme inhibitors, and hyporeninemia occasionally cause hypoaldosteronism.[4,5] Hyporeninemic hypoaldosteronism is commonly seen in patients with chronic renal disease or diabetes mellitus.[5] Most patients present with hyperkalemia, metabolic acidosis, and hypotension. Hypoaldosteronism is treated by administration of an exogenous mineralocorticoid (e.g., fludrocortisone) and liberal sodium intake.

Hyperadrenocorticism (Cushing's Disease)   Glucocorticoid excess may be due to overproduction of ACTH by an anterior pituitary adenoma (majority of cases), ectopic ACTH production by a malignant tumor (especially carcinoma of the lungs, kidney, and pancreas), intrinsic adrenal cortex hyperfunction, or exogenous administration of cortisol.[4-6]

Clinical Manifestations

An excess of cortisol results in a syndrome characterized by truncal obesity (redistribution of fat in facial, cervical, and truncal areas), muscle wasting and weakness (protein catabolism), osteoporosis (loss of protein from bone), hypertension, fluid retention, hyperglycemia, hypokalemia, emotional changes, impaired wound healing, susceptibility to infection, and hirsutism.[5] Treatment is adrenalectomy or transphenoidal microadenomectomy.

Anesthetic Considerations

Preoperative preparation should include regulation of hypertension and hyperglycemia and normalization of intravascular fluid volume and electrolytes.[5] Diuresis with the aldosterone antagonist spironolactone mobilizes fluid and helps normalize serum potassium. Preoperative treatment with metyrapone inhibits cortisol synthesis.[5] Careful positioning is essential in the osteopenic patient; preoperative weakness may indicate an increased sensitivity to muscle relaxants. Anesthetic technique or choice of drug is not influenced by the presence of hyperadrenocorticism[4,5] except for the aforementioned. Intraoperative glucocorticoid replacement is recommended for patients undergoing microadenomectomy or bilateral adrenalectomy, which causes a prompt decrease in serum cortisol levels.[5]

Hypoadrenocorticism Primary adrenal insufficiency (Addison's disease) is caused by destruction of the adrenal cortex resulting in a combined glucocorticoid and mineralocorticoid deficiency.[5,9] Secondary adrenal insufficiency results from inadequate ACTH secretion by the pituitary.[4] The most common cause of secondary adrenal insufficiency is exogenous administration of glucocorticoids.[6] Pituitary failure may also result from tumor presence, surgical ablation, radiation therapy, and infection.[4]

Clinical Manifestations

Clinical features of hypoadrenocorticism arise from both a cortisol deficiency (weight loss, hypotension, hypoglycemia, weakness) and an aldosterone deficiency (hypovolemia, hyponatremia, hypotension, hyperkalemia, and metabolic acidosis).[6] Cutaneous hyperpigmentation occurs in most patients with primary adrenal insufficiency due to the compensatory increases in ACTH and β lipoprotein, which stimulates an increase in melanocyte production.[4] Adrenal insufficiency caused by pituitary suppression is not associated with hyperpigmentation or mineralocorticoid deficiency.[4] Acute adrenal insufficiency (*addisonian crisis*) is a medical emergency characterized by circulatory collapse, fever, hypoglycemia, and depressed mentation and can occur in steroid-dependent patients who did not receive stress steroid replacement.[6]

Anesthetic Considerations

Ensure adequate perioperative steroid replacement in patients with a glucocorticoid deficiency (see section on steroid replacement therapy). Avoid etomidate because it suppresses adrenal function.[6]

☐ THYROID GLAND

The thyroid gland is located in the anterior neck, overlying the trachea, just inferior to the larynx. The two principal hormones secreted by the thyroid gland are thyroxine (T_4) and triiodothyronine (T_3), both of which have profound effects on the metabolic rate of the body. T_4 constitutes 95% of hormones released; the remaining 5% is T_3.[7] Peripheral

tissues convert T_4 to T_3, which is three to five times more potent than T_4, has a more rapid onset of effect, and has a shorter half-life (due to less protein binding with T_3).[3] In addition, the thyroid gland also secretes calcitonin, a hormone that causes a reduction in the serum calcium concentration.

SYNTHESIS AND SECRETION OF THYROID HORMONE

Thyroid hormone biosynthesis involves four phases[9] designated as (1) iodide ion trapping (absorbed dietary iodine converted to iodine), (2) oxidation and iodination, (3) hormone storage in thyroid gland as part of thyroglobulin molecule, and (4) proteolysis and release of hormone. All of these steps are regulated by TSH released from the anterior pituitary, which in turn is regulated by a negative feedback system involving thyroid hormone levels and TRH secreted by the hypothalamus. Therefore, disease processes involving the hypothalamus, the anterior pituitary, or the thyroid gland itself may cause thyroid gland dysfunction.

PHYSIOLOGIC EFFECTS

Thyroid hormone produces changes in the speed of biochemical reactions, total body oxygen consumption, and energy production.[4] Although thyroid hormones are important to many aspects of growth and metabolic rate, the anesthetist is most concerned with the cardiac manifestations. These cardiac manifestations of thyroid disease are presumed to be from an alteration in adrenergic receptor physiology as opposed to increase in catecholamine levels.[6,10]

THYROID GLAND PATHOPHYSIOLOGY AND ANESTHETIC CONSIDERATIONS

Hyperthyroidism Hyperthyroidism results from excess secretion of thyroid hormones. The most common etiology is Grave's disease or diffuse toxic goiter (occurs most often in women, ages 20 to 40). Other causes of hyperthyroidism include thyroiditis, TSH-secreting pituitary tumors, Iodine[131] therapy, thyroid adenoma or carcinoma, pregnancy, or overdosage of thyroid replacement hormone.[5,6] Amiodarone, an antiarrhythmic agent, is iodine rich and is a cause of iodine-induced thyrotoxicosis.[5]

Clinical Manifestations

Patients present with weight loss, anxiety, nervousness, heat intolerance, fatigue, muscle weakness, diarrhea, and tremor. A goiter may be noted. Exophthalmus and clubbing of fingers may be seen in patients with Grave's disease. Cardiac features may range from sinus tachycardia, tachydysrhythmias, and increased cardiac output to atrial fibrillation and congestive heart failure.[4,6] Hyperdynamic circulation suggests increased sympathetic activity as well as compensatory attempts to eliminate excess heat. Plasma catecholamine levels are not increased, but β-receptor sensitivity is increased in the hyperthyroid patient.[5] Hyperthyroidism is confirmed by abnormal thyroid function tests, which may include an increased total serum T_4, serum T_3, and free (unbound) T_4.[6] TSH levels are normal or low.

Anesthetic Considerations

Preoperatively, all elective surgery should be deferred until the hyperthyroid patient is rendered euthyroid with medical therapy. Medical treatment includes drugs that inhibit hormone synthesis (propylthiouracil and methimazole), prevent hormone release (e.g., sodium or potassium iodide), or ameliorate the signs of adrenergic overactivity (e.g., propanolol or esmolol).[6] In addition to masking adrenergic overactivity, β antagonists decrease peripheral conversion of T_4 to T_3, but they do not affect thyroid hormone synthesis. Radioactive iodine therapy destroys thyroid cell function but is not recommended in the pregnant patient (may destroy fetal thyroid) and may result in hypothyroidism.[4] Antithyroid and β antagonists should be continued through the morning of surgery.

Preoperative evaluation should include normal thyroid function tests and a recommended resting pulse of less than 85 beats/min.[6] Anxiety may be treated with a benzodiazepine. Avoid anticholinergics (e.g., atropine) because they may interfere with body's normal heat-regulating mechanism and increase heart rate. Evaluation of upper airway for evidence of obstruction from goiter is important.

Intraoperative goals for the hyperthyroid patient include achieving a depth of anesthesia that prevents exaggerated sympathetic response to intubation and surgical stimulation while avoiding drugs that stimulate the sympathetic nervous system (e.g., ketamine, pancuronium, or indirect-acting adrenergic agonists). Thiopental may be the induction agent of choice due to its antithyroid activity at high doses.[4] Hypotension should be treated with direct-acting agents (e.g., phenylephrine). Use of an armored endotracheal tube passed beyond the goiter may prevent kinking and airway obstruction. The incidence of myasthenia gravis is increased in hyperthyroid patients; therefore, muscle relaxants should be titrated carefully. The eyes of patients with Grave's disease should be well protected. Regional anesthesia may be used, but epinepherine-containing solutions should be avoided. Hyperthyroidism does not increase anesthetic requirements (no change in minimum alveolar concentration).[6]

When emergency surgery is necessary before the euthyroid state is achieved, or if perioperatively hyperthyroidism gets out of control, it is recommended to titrate esmolol (IV) 50 to 500 μg/kg[10] or administer propanolol in 0.5-mg IV boluses[4] to restore normal heart rate.

Postoperative Complications of Thyroid Surgery

Postoperative surgical complications of subtotal thyroidectomy include recurrent laryngeal nerve damage, tracheal compression secondary to hematoma or tracheomalacia, and hypoparathyroidism.[6] *Recurrent laryngeal nerve damage* will result in hoarseness (unilateral) or aphonia and stridor (bilateral).[5] Bilateral recurrent laryngeal nerve injury is extremely rare and requires reintubation. Unilateral nerve injury is

more common and often goes unrecognized. Vocal cord function may be evaluated by laryngoscopy immediately after "deep" extubation while the patient is spontaneously breathing. If the vocal cords are nonmoving or assume a midline position, postoperative laryngeal obstruction is likely to occur.[10] *Hematoma formation* may cause airway obstruction due to tracheal compression and tracheal collapse in patients with tracheomalacia. *Hypoparathyroidism* due to inadvertent removal of parathyroid glands will cause hypocalcemia within 24 to 72 hours but may manifest as early as 1 to 3 hours postoperatively.[5] Laryngeal stridor progressing to laryngospasm may be the first suggestion of hypocalcemic tetany.[4] Prompt IV administration of calcium is warranted in this situation.

Thyroid storm (*thyrotoxicosis*) is a life-threatening abrupt exacerbation of hyperthyroidism seen during periods of stress (e.g., infection, surgery, or injury).[4] Manifestations include hyperthermia, tachycardia, anorexia, extreme anxiety, altered consciousness, dehydration, and cardiovasular instability.[5] The onset of thyroid storm associated with surgery is usually 6 to 24 hours after surgery, but may occur intraoperatively, mimicking malignant hyperthermia, pheochromocytoma, or neuroleptic malignant syndrome.[10]

Treatment includes cooling and hydration, IV propanolol or esmolol to maintain heart rate at an acceptable level, administration of antithyroid drugs, blocking release of preformed hormone with iodine, and correction of any precipitating (nonthyroid) cause (e.g., infection).[5,6] Due to coexisting adrenal gland suppression, cortisol (100 to 200 mg every 8 hours) is recommended.[5,6]

Hypothyroidism Hypothyroidism results from inadequate circulating levels of T_3 and T_4, which is estimated to occur in 0.5% to 0.8% of the adult population.[4] The etiology of hypothyroidism is primary, caused by thyroid gland destruction (Hashimoto's thyroiditis, thyroidectomy, radiation therapy, antithyroid medications, iodine deficiency), or secondary caused by failure of the hypothalamic-pituitary axis.[5,6]

Primary failure of the thyroid gland accounts for 95% of all cases of thyroid dysfunction.[4] Hashimoto's thyroiditis (autoimmune disease) is the most common cause of hypothyroidism.[5] The diagnosis of primary hypothyroidism is based on signs and symptoms plus confirmation by a low free T_4 level. An elevated TSH level differentiates primary from secondary hypothyroidism.[6,7] Chronic treatment of hypothyroidism involves exogenous thyroid hormone supplementation.

Clinical Manifestations

Hypothyroidism during the neonatal period can result in cretinism, a condition marked by physical and mental retardation.[7] In the adult, clinical manifestations are usually subtle and include a generalized reduction in metabolic activity resulting in weight gain, cold intolerance, lethargy, muscle fatigue, constipation, and hypoactive reflexes.[4,6] Heart rate, cardiac contractility, and cardiac output are decreased. Peripheral vasoconstriction (cool, dry skin) is characteristic. Cardiac manifestations such as cardiomegaly, pleural effusion, ascites, and peripheral edema may mimic congestive heart failure.[4] There may be adrenal atrophy with decreased cortisol production, dilutional hyponatremia (due to inappropriate ADH secretion), and decreased water excretion.[7]

Myxedema coma is a life-threatening disease resulting from extreme hypothyroidism and is characterized by hypoventilation, hypothermia, hyponatremia, and congestive heart failure.[6] It has been successfully treated with intravenous thyroid hormones.[3]

Anesthetic Considerations

Elective surgery should be deferred in patients with severe hypothyroidism or myxedema coma. Although a euthyroid state is ideal, mild to moderate hypothyroidism does not appear to be an absolute contraindication to surgery.[5] Sedatives should be used cautiously because of an increased sensitivity to depressant drugs. Due to delayed gastric emptying, use of histamine H_2 antagonists is advised. Ketamine is often recommended for induction because hypothyroid patients are more prone to hypotensive effect of anesthetic agents due to decreased cardiac output, blunted baroreceptor reflexes, and hypovolemia.[6] Decreased cardiac output may speed the rate of induction with inhalational agents, but hypothyroidism does not significantly decrease minimum alveolar concentration.[4,5] Acute adrenal insufficiency should be considered if hypotension persists despite treatment with fluids and sympathomimetic drugs.

Other potential problems include hypothermia, prolonged response to muscle relaxants, hypoglycemia, and hyponatremia. Regional anesthesia is an option provided intravascular volume is maintained.[4] Slow drug biotransformation, hypothermia, and respiratory depression in hypothyroid patients may delay recovery from general anesthesia and necessitate prolonged mechanical ventilation.[5,6]

☐ PARATHYROID GLAND

The four parathyroid glands embedded in the posterior aspect of the thyroid gland produce parathyroid hormone (PTH). PTH release is regulated by a negative feedback mechanism dependent on the plasma calcium concentration.[1] Hypocalcemia stimulates PTH release, whereas hypercalcemia suppresses both the synthesis and release of PTH. PTH increases serum calcium concentration by promoting bone resorption, renal calcium resorption, and indirectly enhancing intestinal absorption by its effect on vitamin D metabolism.[4,6] PTH also decreases serum phosphate by increasing renal excretion.[6] The skeleton contains 99% of total body calcium.[6] Of the plasma calcium, 60% is ionized or complexed to organic ions and 40% is protein bound.[6] It is the unbound ionized calcium that is physiologically active and homeostatically regulated.[4]

PARATHYROID PATHOPHYSIOLOGY AND ANESTHETIC CONSIDERATIONS

Hyperparathyroidism   Hyperparathyroidism is present when PTH secretion is increased. Serum calcium levels may be increased, decreased, or unchanged.[5] Causes of *primary* hyperparathyroidism include adenoma, carcinoma, or hyperplasia of the parathyroid gland. *Secondary* hyperparathyroidism is a compensatory response to hypocalcemia produced by diseases such as renal failure or malabsorption syndromes.[4,6] Due to its adaptive rather than autonomous nature, secondary hyperparathyroidism rarely produces hypercalcemia.[4] Ectopic hyperparathyroidism is due to production of PTH or PTH-like substances by a carcinoma.[4,6]

Clinical Manifestations

The majority of clinical manifestations of hyperparathyroidism are caused by hypercalcemia (Table 17–2). Treatment of hyperparathyroidism depends on the cause, but parathyroidectomy is usually preferred.[4]

Anesthetic Considerations

Preoperative preparation should focus on correcting fluid and electrolyte abnormalities. Patients with chronic hypercalcemia should be evaluated for cardiac, renal, and central nervous system abnormalities. Emergency treatment of hypercalcemia is necessary when the serum calcium level exceeds 15 mg/dL (7.5 mEq/L).[4] Lowering the serum calcium level is initially accomplished by hydration (dilutes serum Ca^{++}) and diuresis with IV furosemide, which establishes a sodium diuresis and increases Ca^{++} excretion.[4–6] Other methods of decreasing serum calcium levels include plicamycin (inhibits osteoblastic activity of PTH), glucocorticoids, calcitonin, and dialysis.[4,6] Avoid hypoventilation because acidosis increases ionized calcium. Caution should be used when administering muscle relaxants because of the unpredictable response of the hypercalcemic patient to muscle relaxants and coexisting muscle weakness. Careful positioning of the osteopenic patients prevents pathologic fractures. Postoperative complica-

Table 17–2
EFFECTS OF HYPERPARATHYROIDISM

Organ System	Clinical Manifestations
Cardiovascular	Hypertension, ventricular dysrhythmias, ECG changes (shortened QT interval)*
Renal	Impaired renal concentrating ability, hyperchloremic metabolic acidosis, polyuria, dehydration, polydipsia, renal stones, renal failure
Gastrointestinal	Ileus, nausea and vomiting, peptic ulcer disease, pancreatitis
Musculoskeletal	Muscle weakness, osteoporosis
Neurologic	Mental status changes (delirium, psychosis, coma)

* The QT interval may be prolonged at serum calcium levels > 16 mg/dL.
SOURCE: Reproduced by permission from Morgan GE and Mikhail MS.[6]

tions are similar to those for patients undergoing thyroid surgery.

Hypoparathyroidism Hypoparathyroidism is present when secretion of PTH is deficient or resistance of end-organ tissue to PTH results in hypocalcemia.[4] The most common cause of hypoparathyroidism is the inadvertent removal of the parathyroid glands during thyroid or parathyroid surgery.[10] Other causes include iodine 131 therapy, neck trauma, neoplasia, hemosiderosis, and granulomatous disease.[4,10] Pseudohypoparathyroidism is a congenital disorder in which PTH secretion is intact, but the kidneys are unable to respond to the hormone.[5] Affected patients have hypocalcemia and hyperphosphatemia and are characterized by mental retardation, obesity, short stature, and shortened metacarpals.[4] Severe hypomagnesemia (< 0.8 mEq/L) from any cause can suppress PTH secretion and result in hypocalcemia.[4] Serum calcium, but not ionized calcium, depends on albumin level; therefore, hypoalbuminemia decreases total serum calcium.

Clinical Manifestations

Hypocalcemia (< 8 mg/dL) is responsible for the clinical features of hypoparathyroidism (Table 17–3). Neuromuscular irritability may be evidenced by a positive Chvostek sign, painful twitching of facial muscles following tapping over facial nerve, or Trousseau's sign, carpopedal spasm produced by 3 minutes of limb ischemia using a tourniquet.[7]

Anesthetic Considerations

Calcium and other electrolyte abnormalities should be corrected to bring any symptoms under control before anesthesia and surgery. Emergency treatment of severe symptomatic hypocalcemia is IV administration of calcium gluconate or calcium chloride. Ten milliliters of 10% calcium gluconate contains 93 mg Ca^{++}; 10 mL $CaCl_2$ contains 272 mg Ca^{++}. Calcium, phosphorus, and magnesium levels should be monitored. Hypocalcemia from magnesium depletion should be treated by correcting the magnesium deficit. Phosphorus excess can be treated by elimination of phosphorus from the diet and oral administration of phosphate-binding resins (aluminum hydroxide).[5] Avoid anesthetics that are myocardial depressants in patients with cardiac manifestations of hypocalcemia.[6] Hypocalcemia can be worsened by respiratory alkalosis (hyperventilation) or metabolic alkalosis.

Table 17–3
EFFECTS OF HYPOPARATHYROIDISM

Organ System	Clinical Manifestations
Cardiovascular	Hypotension, congestive heart failure, ECG changes (prolonged QT interval)
Neurologic	Neuromuscular irritability (laryngospasm, inspiratory stridor, tetany, seizures), perioral paresthesia, mental status changes (dementia, depression, psychosis)
Musculoskeletal	Muscle cramps, weakness

SOURCE: Reproduced by permission from Morgan and Mikhail.[6]

☐ PANCREAS

The pancreas (located partially behind the stomach) secretes digestive substances into the duodenum, whereas the islets of Langerhans secrete two important hormones, insulin and glucagon, directly into the blood. The islets of Langerhans are composed of three cells: alpha cells secrete glucagon, beta cells secrete insulin, and delta cells contain secretory granules.[10]

PANCREATIC HORMONES AND FUNCTIONS

Insulin Insulin is a polypeptide anabolic hormone secreted by pancreatic beta cells. Normal daily insulin secretion is 40 to 50 U.[4] Insulin acts through receptor sites on cells. Its release is stimulated by sugars (glucose and fructose), amino acids, gastrointestinal hormones, glucagon, and acetylcholine.[10] Insulin secretion is increased with vagal stimulation, β-adrenergic stimulation, and α-adrenergic blockade.[4] Insulin production continues during fasting periods to prevent catabolism and ketosis. The liver and the kidney metabolize insulin; therefore, prolonged effects may be seen with renal disease.

Important metabolic effects of insulin include increased glucose and potassium entry into muscle and adipose cells; increased synthesis of glycogen, fatty acids, and protein; and decreased gluconeogenesis, glycogenolysis, lipolysis, ketogenesis, and protein catabolism.[6]

Glucagon Glucagon, a polypeptide produced by pancreatic alpha cells, is a potent hyperglycemic agent. Glucagon release is stimulated by hypoglycemia, as well as epinephrine and cortisol, and suppressed by rising glucose levels.[4] Actions of glucagon are opposite to those of insulin. Glucagon stimulates gluconeogenesis and glycogenolysis, increases lipolysis, and enhances amino acid uptake by the liver.[1]

Exogenous Insulin Several types of commercially prepared insulin are available, including pork insulin, beef insulin, and human insulin (Humulin) (Table 17–4). An advantage of human insulin is a decreased risk of developing anti-insulin antibodies. Patients receiving protamine-containing insulin (NPH or protamine zinc insulin) may experience a life-threatening allergic reaction when protamine is administered to antagonize the effects of heparin.[5]

PATHOPHYSIOLOGY OF THE PANCREAS AND ANESTHETIC CONSIDERATIONS

Diabetes Mellitus Diabetes mellitus is a chronic systemic disease caused by a relative or absolute lack of insulin, resulting in inappropriate hyperglycemia. Diagnosis is usually based on a blood glucose level greater than 185 mg/dL present 1 hour after a glucose load.[7] Diabetes is classified as

Table 17–4
COMMERCIALLY AVAILABLE INSULIN PREPARATIONS

	Onset*	Peak effect*	Duration*
Fast-acting			
Regular	30–60 min	2–4 h	5–7 h
Semilente	30–60 min	4–6 h	12–16 h
Intermediate-acting			
Isophane (NPH)	1–2 h	10–20 h	18–24 h
Lente	1–3 h	14–18 h	20–24 h
Long-acting			
Protamine Zinc	4–6 h	16–22 h	25–36 h
Ultralente	4–6 h	24 h	25–36 h

* Approximate

insulin-dependent diabetes mellitus (IDDM or type I) or non–insulin-dependent (NIDDM or type II). Patients with IDDM are often young (juvenile onset), not obese, prone to ketosis, and have very low insulin levels.[6] NIDDM patients (constitute almost 90% of all diabetics), usually experience a gradual onset of the disease later in life, are overweight, not prone to ketosis, have insulin resistance, and are at risk for hyperglycemic hyperosmolar nonketotic (HHNK) coma.[9] Type I patients require insulin to prevent ketoacidosis. Type II patients are treated with diet alone, a hypoglycemic agent, and occasionally insulin. These classifications are only a generalization. A young patient can develop NIDDM and many older adults can develop IDDM.

Secondary causes of diabetes include diseases that alter hormone levels (acromegaly, glucagonoma, Cushing's, pheochromocytoma) or pancreatic damage or destruction.[4]

Clinical Manifestations
Diabetes is manifest as hyperglycemia, glycosuria, and degeneration of small blood vessels. Diabetic patients are subject to many long-term complications that lead to morbidity and premature mortality. Late complications of diabetes include hypertension, coronary artery disease, peripheral and cerebral vascular disease, retinopathy, nephropathy, and peripheral and autonomic neuropathies.[5] Life-threatening, acute complications for diabetics include hypoglycemia, ketoacidosis, and HHNK coma.

In the absence of insulin, the liver converts fatty acids to acetoacetic acid, acetone, and betahydroxybutyrate, leading to *diabetic ketoacidosis*.[7] Manifestations of ketoacidosis include nausea, vomiting, changes in sensorium, dyspnea (compensation for metabolic acidosis), abdominal pain, hyperglycemia (300 to 500 mg/dL), hyperosmolarity, intracellular dehydration, and an osmotic diuresis that leads to profound hypovolemia.[4] Electrolyte abnormalities include hyperkalemia and hyponatremia.[7] The total body potassium content is actually depressed, but it appears elevated due to insufficient insulin to drive it into cells, and acidosis causes movement of potassium out of cells. Treatment consists of correcting the dehydration, hyperglycemia, and total potassium deficit with isotonic fluids, an insulin infusion, and

potassium. Causes for ketoacidosis are stress (e.g., infection, surgery, and trauma), poor patient compliance, or myocardial infarction.[5]

Hypoglycemia in diabetic individuals is the result of excess insulin relative to carbohydrate intake. The brain depends on glucose as an energy source, making it the organ most susceptible to hypoglycemia. If hypoglycemia is not corrected, changes in sensorium may progress from confusion and fainting to convulsions and coma. Many of the systemic manifestations of hypoglycemia result from catecholamine discharge (tachycardia, hypertension, diaphoresis) and may be masked during general anesthesia.[7] Although hypoglycemic symptoms appear at widely differing blood glucose levels and vary from patient to patient, hypoglycemia is generally considered less than 50 mg/dL.[6]

Hyperglycemic, hyperosmolar, nonketotic coma is characterized by plasma hyperosmolarity (> 330 mOsm/L), hyperglycemia (> 600 mg/dL), profound dehydration (hypovolemia), and absence of ketoacidosis (enough available insulin to prevent ketosis).[5] The severe hyperglycemia results in marked osmotic diuresis, which leads to loss of potassium, sodium, and intravascular volume. Severe dehydration may eventually lead to lactic acidosis, renal failure, and predisposition to form intravascular thromboses.[6] The first manifestation of the syndrome can be altered mentation culminating in seizures and coma. Treatment includes fluid resuscitation, small doses of IV regular insulin, and if needed, potassium supplementation.[7] When the glucose level reaches about 300 mg/dL, treatment should progress slowly to prevent cerebral edema. HHNK usually occurs in elderly patients; it is often triggered by infection, trauma, or dehydration and may occur in diabetic (type II) and nondiabetic patients.

Anesthetic Considerations
Preoperative assessment and correction of hyperglycemia, electrolyte abnormalities, and ketoacidosis is important before proceeding with elective surgery. Because perioperative morbidity is related to end-organ damage, a thorough assessment of the cardiovascular, cerebral, and renal systems is essential. Painless myocardial ischemia, orthostatic hypotension, resting tachycardia, lack of heart rate variability, neurogenic bladder, gastroparesis, and impotence may indicate *diabetic neuropathy*.[6] The diabetic patient with evidence of autonomic neuropathy may be at increased risk for aspiration, intraoperative cardiac instability (hypotension requiring vasopressors), and sudden cardiac death.[5,6] Indeed, ischemic heart disease is the most common cause of perioperative morbidity in the diabetic patient.[5] These patients should receive aspiration prophylaxis and a rapid sequence induction if general anesthesia is planned. Invasive monitoring should be considered. Renal involvement manifests as proteinuria and an elevated serum creatinine level. Use strict aseptic technique when placing invasive lines and monitors because diabetic patients have compromised immune systems.

Intraoperative management goals are to prevent hypoglycemia, excessive hyperglycemia, and ketoacidosis. The primary goal is to prevent hypoglycemia by monitoring serum glucose levels and ensuring an adequate supply of ex-

Table 17–5
ORAL HYPOGLYCEMIA DRUGS

	Relative Potency	Duration of Action (h)
First generation		
Tolbutamine	1	6–10
Acetohexamide	2.5	12–18
Tolazamide	5	16–24
Chlorpropamide	6	24–72
Second generation		
Glyburide	150	18–24
Glipizide	100	16–24

SOURCE: Reproduced by permission from Stoelting and Dierdorf.[5]

ogenous glucose. The action of insulin and oral hypoglycemic agents is prolonged in patients with renal disease, making these patients more susceptible to hypoglycemia. It is recommended to maintain a serum glucose level of 120 to 180 mg/dL to avoid hypoglycemia and the deleterious effects of hyperglycemia (hyperosmolarity, osmotic diuresis, electrolyte abnormalities, impaired phagocytic function, and wound healing).[5] Additionally, hyperglycemia may augment the damage caused by cerebral ischemia.[4,6]

The diabetic patient should be scheduled for surgery early in the day. Patients receiving oral hypoglycemics may continue them until the day of surgery, remembering that these drugs have different durations of action (Table 17–5) and may produce hypoglycemia several hours after their administration in the absence of caloric intake. For short procedures in unstressed patients, insulin supplementation may not be needed. Monitor preoperative and postoperative serum glucose levels. Hospital preadmission is probably indicated only for the poorly controlled patient with IDDM.

For patients using insulin, three approaches are used perioperatively. First, the patient receives a fraction (one fourth to one half) of the total morning insulin dose in the form of intermediate acting insulin[4] (see Table 17–4). To lessen the risk of hypoglycemia, the morning glucose should be checked and an IV access established (5% dextrose at 1.5 mL/kg/h) *before* insulin administration.[6] If the patient becomes hypoglycemic (50 to 100 mg/dL), supplemental dextrose can be given. Ten grams of dextrose (50 % dextrose solution) will raise the serum glucose level about 30 to 40 mg/dL in the adult.[6] A second approach is to administer IV regular insulin according to a sliding scale based on frequent serum glucose determinations. One unit of regular insulin usually lowers serum glucose by 25 to 30 mg/dL in the adult.[6] The third approach is to administer a continuous infusion of low-dose insulin at 1 U/h (10 U regular insulin added to 1 L of D_5W and infuse at rate of 1.5 mL/kg/h or 1 unit/h/70 kg).[4,6] If greater flexibility is desired, infuse the D_5W (1 mL/kg/h) and insulin (50 units of regular insulin in 250 mL saline) through separate IV lines.[6] Set the infusion rate, using the following formula: Insulin (U/h)=serum glucose (mg/dL)/150. (*Note:* the denominator should be 100 if the patient is on steroids, markedly obese, or has an infec-

tion.[6,9,10] The key to any management regime is to monitor serum glucose frequently (every 1 to 2 hours) and appreciate patient variability.

Insulinoma   Insulinomas are beta islet cell tumors of the pancreas that produce profound hypoglycemia from the excess release of endogenous insulin. Failure of plasma insulin levels to decrease as blood glucose levels fall is suggestive of an insulinoma.[7] Central nervous system signs and symptoms range from dizziness and clouded sensorium to paresis, seizures, stroke, and coma.[8] Maintenance of a normal blood glucose level is the major challenge during anesthesia for removal of an insulinoma. Because signs and symptoms of hypoglycemia (tachycardia, hypertension, and diaphoresis) may be masked during anesthesia, a glucose infusion should be initiated before induction and continued intraoperatively. Wide fluctuations in blood glucose with tumor manipulation (hypoglycemia) and tumor excision (hyperglycemia) can occur; therefore, blood glucose concentration should be monitored every 15 minutes. An artificial pancreas (Biostar), which continuously analyzes plasma glucose and administers glucose or insulin, has been used for intraoperative management.[7]

☐ REPRODUCTIVE GLANDS

The ovaries, located in the pelvic cavity, release progesterone and estrogen. At puberty, estrogen secretion begins by the ovarian follicles under the influence of FSH. Estrogens stimulate female reproductive system maturation. Progesterone is the principal hormone secreted by the ovaries and it is released in response to high blood levels of LH. Ovulation and normal menses depend on the presence of these ovarian hormones.

The testes, located in the scrotum, produce testosterone, which is responsible for spermatogenesis and external virilization. Gonadal hormone release is regulated by gonadotropins from the hypothalamus (described earlier). Dysfunction of the ovaries or testes has minimal effect on anesthetic management and is not discussed further.

☐ OBESITY

Obesity is the most common nutritional disorder in the United States, affecting about 25% of the population.[11] Generally, obesity is defined as a body weight 20% above the ideal body weight,[10] determined from actuarial tables based on height, sex, and body frame size. Another measure of obesity is the body mass index (BMI), defined as weight (kg) divided by height (m) squared (wt/ht^2).[12] A BMI value of 28 for a man and 27 for a woman corresponds to 20% above the ideal weight.[10,11] A value of 31 is considered a risk for morbid obesity.[10] Also, morbid obesity is twice ideal body weight.[6]

Obese patients are at an increased anesthetic risk because of mechanical and technical difficulties and physiologic changes. Additionally, obesity is associated with many diseases such as hypertension, coronary artery disease, diabetes mellitus, impaired pulmonary function, and gastrointestinal abnormalities that complicate anesthetic management.[11]

CLINICAL MANIFESTATIONS

Morbid obesity has profound physiologic consequences on multiple organ systems. (Figure 17–1). Physiologic changes of respiration include increased oxygen demand, carbon dioxide production, and alveolar ventilation[6] (metabolic rate is proportionate to body weight). Increased pulmonary blood volume and pulmonary artery vasoconstriction due to chronic arterial hypoxemia can lead to pulmonary hypertension and right-sided heart failure.[6]

Obesity is also associated with insulin resistance, an increased incidence of diabetes mellitus, fatty infiltration of the liver, and gastrointestinal pathologies, such as hiatal hernia, poor gastric emptying, gastroesophageal reflux, and increased gastric fluid volume and acidity.

ANESTHETIC CONSIDERATIONS

Preoperatively, premedication with an H_2 antagonist, metoclopramide, or nonparticulate antacids should be considered due to an increased risk of aspiration in the obese patient. Sedatives, hypnotics, and opioids should be used with extreme caution in patients with evidence of preoperative hypoxemia, hypercarbia, or obstructive sleep apnea.[12]

Preoperative cardiopulmonary assessment for morbidly obese patients undergoing major surgery should include a chest radiograph, an electrocardiogram, pulmonary function tests, and a baseline arterial blood gas determination.[6] Particular attention should be directed at any evidence of right or left ventricular failure, hypertension, and coronary artery disease. Monitoring blood pressure may be difficult in the morbidly obese patient; therefore, an arterial catheter may be desirable. Indistinct landmarks and technical difficulties may preclude the use of regional anesthesia. Vital capacity, expiratory reserve volume, and functional residual capacity are decreased because increased abdominal mass limits diaphragmatic excursion, yielding lung volumes suggestive of restrictive lung disease.[11] Chest wall compliance is decreased due to excessive adipose over the thorax, but lung compliance is usually normal.[12] Decreases in lung volumes are exacerbated by the supine and Trendelenberg positions.[6] Arterial oxygen tension is decreased, presumably secondary to ventilation/perfusion abnormalities.[11] Arterial carbon dioxide (CO_2) tension and ventilatory response to CO_2 are usually normal in the obese patient.

Although obese patients are frequently hypoxemic, few are hypercarbic.[6] Obesity hypoventilation syndrome (pickwickian syndrome) is a complication of massive obesity. These patients exhibit somnolence, hypercapnia, alveolar hypoventilation, hypoxemia, pulmonary hypertension, right-sided heart failure, and secondary polycythemia.[10,11] The etiology of this syndrome is unclear, but these patients have a blunted respiratory drive and often have obstructive sleep apnea.[6,11]

The increased oxygen demand present in obese patients results in an increased cardiac workload. Cardiac output and blood volume increase proportionately with rising weight.[12] The increased cardiac output (0.1 L/min/kg of adipose tissue) is due to an increased stroke volume (pulse usually within normal limits) and often results in left ventricular hypertrophy and arterial hypertension.[6] Additionally, particular attention should be given to the airway because these patients may be exceedingly difficult to mask ventilate and intubate. If a difficult intubation is anticipated, an awake intubation with or without a fiberoptic scope is indicated.

Intraoperatively, obese patients should be intubated whenever general anesthesia is administered except for very short procedures. A rapid sequence induction with cricoid pressure minimizes the risk of aspiration. Due to decreased functional residual capacity and increased oxygen consumption, obese patients desaturate rapidly during periods of apnea (induction); therefore adequate denitrogenation of the lungs by breathing 100% oxygen before induction is recommended.[11] Furthermore, controlled ventilation with large tidal volumes and a fraction inspired oxygen greater than 0.5 is recommended.[12] In some morbidly obese patients, the addition of positive end-expiratory pressure may worsen pulmonary hypertension.[6]

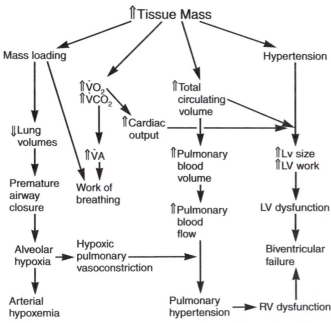

FIGURE 17–1 A schema interrelating the cardiovascular and respiratory abnormalities in morbidly obese patients to the pathophysiologic changes found in such patients. LV, left ventricular; RV, right ventricular; V, ventilation. (Reproduced by permission from Barash P. Clinical Anesthesia, 2nd ed., Lippincott, 1992.)

Obese patients metabolize volatile anesthetics more extensively.[6] Halothane should be avoided because obese patients metabolize the drug by the potentially hepatotoxic reductive pathway.[12] Methoxyflurane and enflurane metabolism is also increased, therefore, increasing the possible risk for fluoride-induced renal toxicity.[12] Decreased functional residual capacity also decreases mixing time for inhaled drugs, accelerating the rate of rise in alveolar concentration for inhaled drugs.

REFERENCES

1. Guyton A. Introduction to endocrine disease. In: Guyton A, ed. *Textbook of Medical Physiology*. 7th ed. Philadelphia: WB Saunders; 1986:876–883.

2. Marieb E. The endocrine system. In: Marieb E, ed. *Human Anatomy and Physiology*. 2nd ed. New York: Benjamin/Cummings Publishing; 1992:540–571.

3. Stoelting R. Endocrine system. In: Stoelting R, ed. *Pharmacology and Physiology in Anesthetic Practice*. Philadelphia: JB Lippincott; 1987:741–759.

4. Graf G, Rosenbaum S. Anesthesia and the endocrine system. In: Barash P, Cullin B, Stoelting R, eds. *Clinical Anesthesia*. 2nd ed. Philadelphia: JB Lippincott; 1992:1237–1265.

5. Stoelting R, Dierdorf S. Endocrine disease. In: Stoelting R, Dierdorf S, eds. *Anesthesia and Co-existing Disease*. 3rd ed. New York: Churchill Livingstone; 1993:339–371.

6. Morgan GE, Mikhail MS. Anesthesia for patients with endocrine disease. In: Morgan GE, Mikhail MS, eds. *Clinical Anesthesiology*. East Norwalk, Conn. Appleton & Lange; 1992:565–576.

7. Stoelting R, Dierdorf S, McCammon R. Endocrine disease. In: Stoelting R, Dierdorf S, McCammon R, eds. *Anesthesia and Co-existing Disease*. 2nd ed. New York: Churchill Livingstone; 1988:473–515.

8. Wall R. Anesthetic challenges in endocrine disease: pheochromocytoma, insulinoma, carcinoid syndrome. *ASA Refresher Course Lectures 146*. Park Ridge, Ill: Society of Anesthesiologists; 1991:1–6.

9. Roizen M. Diseases of the endocrine system. In Katz J, Benumof J, eds. *Anesthesia and Uncommon Diseases*. 3rd ed. Philadelphia: WB Saunders; 1990:245–287.

10. Roizen M. Anesthetic implications of concurrent diseases. In: Miller R, ed. *Anesthesia*. 4th ed. New York: Churchill Livingstone; 1994:903–933.

11. Stoelting R, Dierdorf S. Metabolic and nutritional disorders. In: Stoelting R, Dierdorf S, eds. *Anesthesia and Co-existing Disease*. 3rd ed. New York: Churchill Livingstone; 1993:384–388.

12. Buckley P. Anesthesia and obesity and gastrointestinal disorders. In: Barash P, Cullin B, Stoelting R, eds. *Clinical Anesthesia*. 2nd ed. Philadelphia: Lippincott; 1992:1169–1175.

☐ QUESTIONS

1. A patient with severe untreated hypothyroidism is admitted for emergency appendectomy. A finding consistent with myxedema coma is:
   a. Heat intolerance
   b. Moist skin
   c. Fine hair
   d. Bradycardia

2. All are true of cortisol *except:*
   a. Decreases blood sugar level
   b. Deficiency can lead to cardiovascular collapse
   c. Excess causes hyperglycemia, hypertension, hypokalemia and muscle wasting
   d. Secretion is influenced by ACTH secretion from the pituitary

3. Hyperosmolar coma:
   a. Is usually accompanied by oliguria
   b. Is treated with large doses of insulin
   c. Occurs at osmolar levels greater than 330 mOsm/L
   d. Occurs in the presence of ketosis

4. The time required for a patient to develop adrenal suppression from steroid therapy is:
   a. 1 week
   b. 4 weeks
   c. 6 months
   d. Unknown

5. All are true of inappropriate antidiuretic hormone secretion *except:*
   a. Results in high urine osmolality
   b. Is due to increased secretion of antidiuretic hormone
   c. Results in a low serum sodium
   d. Results in dilute urine

6. Insulin:
   a. Secretion is stimulated by sugars, amino acids, and acetylcholine
   b. Is metabolized solely in the liver
   c. Decreases glucose and potassium uptake into cells
   d. Is secreted by pancreatic alpha cells

7. In diabetes insipidus:
   a. The serum sodium is low
   b. Antidiuretic hormone secretion is deficient
   c. The urine is concentrated
   d. Serum osmolality is low

8. Physiologic changes of obesity include all *except:*
   a. Decreased arterial oxygenation
   b. Decreased functional residual capacity
   c. Decreased ventilatory response to carbon dioxide
   d. Increased carbon dioxide production

9. The patient with pheochromocytoma:
   a. Is usually hypervolemic
   b. Should be treated first with beta antagonists to decrease sympathetic activity
   c. Requires immediate surgical removal of the tumor
   d. Should be treated for 1 to 2 weeks with α blockers

10. All of the following are adrenal cortex hormones *except:*
    a. Epinephrine
    b. Glucocorticoids
    c. Aldosterone
    d. Androgens

11. Treatment for primary hypoadrenocorticism is administration of:
    a. Adrenocorticotropic hormone
    b. Androgens
    c. Cortisol
    d. Spironolactone (aldosterone antagonist)

12. In a patient with pheochromocytoma, one would want to avoid all of the following *except:*
    a. Droperidol
    b. Fluid resuscitation
    c. Anticholinergics
    d. Halothane

13. A patient developed dyspnea 10 hours postthyroidectomy. When obtaining a blood pressure, the nurse noted the patient's blood pressure to be markedly elevated and that the patient's wrist flexed when the blood pressure cuff remained inflated. The cause of the stridor is probably:
    a. Recurrent laryngeal nerve damage
    b. Hematoma formation
    c. Hypocalcemia
    d. Laryngeal edema

14. All are true regarding acromegaly *except:*
    a. Excess growth hormone secretion as an adult
    b. Overgrowth of skeletal and connective tissue

   c. A potential for difficult airway management
   d. Glucose tolerance

15. A patient with rheumatoid arthritis is anesthetized for a hip fracture. She has been on prednisone for 4 months. Perioperatively she suddenly becomes hypotensive. The initial step to be taken is:
    a. Administer hydrocortisone 300 mg IV
    b. Administer a vasopressor (ephedrine)
    c. Establish the cause of the hypotension
    d. Cancel the procedure

16. In hyperparathyroidism the patient may present with all of the following *except:*
    a. A prolonged QT interval
    b. A shortened QT interval
    c. Increased serum calcium
    d. Hypertension

17. The most important goal in the treatment of the diabetic patient undergoing anesthesia is:
    a. Prevent hyperglycemia
    b. Prevent hypoglycemia
    c. Maintain blood sugar 80 to 100 mg/dL
    d. Prevent glycosuria and ketonuria

18. In the patient with hyperaldosteronism, you would expect to see all of the following *except:*
    a. Decreased serum potassium
    b. Hypotension
    c. Muscle weakness
    d. Metabolic alkalosis

19. The adrenal medulla secretes epinephrine and norepinephrine. The percentage of norepinephrine secreted is:
    a. 80%
    b. 20%
    c. 75%
    d. 10%

20. The following hormones are secreted by the anterior pituitary *except:*
    a. Antidiuretic hormone (ADH)
    b. Growth hormone
    c. Adrenocorticotropic hormone (ACTH)
    d. Prolactin

☐ ANSWERS

1. d	**5.** d	**9.** d	**13.** c	**17.** b
2. a	**6.** a	**10.** a	**14.** d	**18.** b
3. c	**7.** b	**11.** c	**15.** c	**19.** b
4. d	**8.** c	**12.** b	**16.** a	**20.** a

CHAPTER

18

The Hepatic System

Celeste G. Villanueva

The many varied and complex functions of the liver are closely related to the workings of virtually every other organ system in the body. The central role of the liver in pharmacokinetics holds tremendous relevance to the choice of drugs utilized in an anesthetic regimen. The formulation of a rational anesthetic plan requires an understanding of the integrated nature of the liver's physiologic functions.

☐ ANATOMY AND PHYSIOLOGY

The largest organ of the body is the liver. In an average adult the organ weighs 1500 g, about 2% of total body weight. The functional units of the liver are lobules. These are cylindrical structures that surround a central vein, which drains into the hepatic vein and into the inferior vena cava. Figure 18–1 illustrates the functional components of the liver lobule. Hepatic cellular plates radiate from the central vein and are surrounded by sinusoids. Blood from branches of both the portal vein and hepatic artery empty into the sinusoids, whose endothelium has large fenestrations, allowing maximal contact of plasma with hepatocytes. Since only one layer of hepatocytes lies between sinusoids, the surface area of hepatocytes exposed to plasma is quite large. Hepatic sinusoids are lined by endothelial cells and *Kupffer cells*, which are macrophages capable of phagocytic activity. The spaces of Disse lie between hepatic cells and the sinusoids; these compartments accommodate the plasma substances that move freely into the space (due to the large fenestrations in the sinusoid endothelium). Terminal lymphatics connect directly with the spaces of Disse, removing excess fluid. Bile canaliculi originate between hepatocytes and drain into terminal bile ducts.

HEPATIC BLOOD FLOW

The liver is the only major organ in the body to receive a dual afferent blood supply. High-pressure saturated blood via the *hepatic artery* makes up 25 to 30% of the total hepatic blood flow (HBF) and low-pressure desaturated blood from the *portal vein* makes up 70 to 75%. Total HBF from these two sources represents 25 to 30% of the cardiac output. An unusual phenomenon exists in the liver: the venous source of blood transports 50 to 60% of the liver's oxygen supply, whereas the arterial source supplies 45 to 50% of the oxygen required. The portal vein contains blood drained from the intestines, pancreas, and the spleen; this, with the arterial blood flow into the liver, is called the splanchnic circulation. Figure 18–2 illustrates the portal circulation.

Control of Hepatic Blood Flow Total HBF is determined by hepatic perfusion pressure (HPP), which is, in turn, determined by mean hepatic artery pressure (MHAP) or mean portal vein pressure (MPVP) minus [hepatic vein pressure (HVP) plus splanchnic vascular resistance (SVR)].

$$HPP = MHAP - (HVP + SVR)$$

Based on this equation, two major causes of decreased HPP are (1) decreased MHAP due to decreased systemic mean arterial pressure, or increased splanchnic vascular resistance, and (2) decreased MPVP due to decreased systemic pressure, or increased HVP.

The presence of an intrinsic autoregulatory mechanism for hepatic arterial flow is controversial. It appears to involve a "reciprocal" relationship between the hepatic artery and the portal vein: a decrease in blood flow through one will result

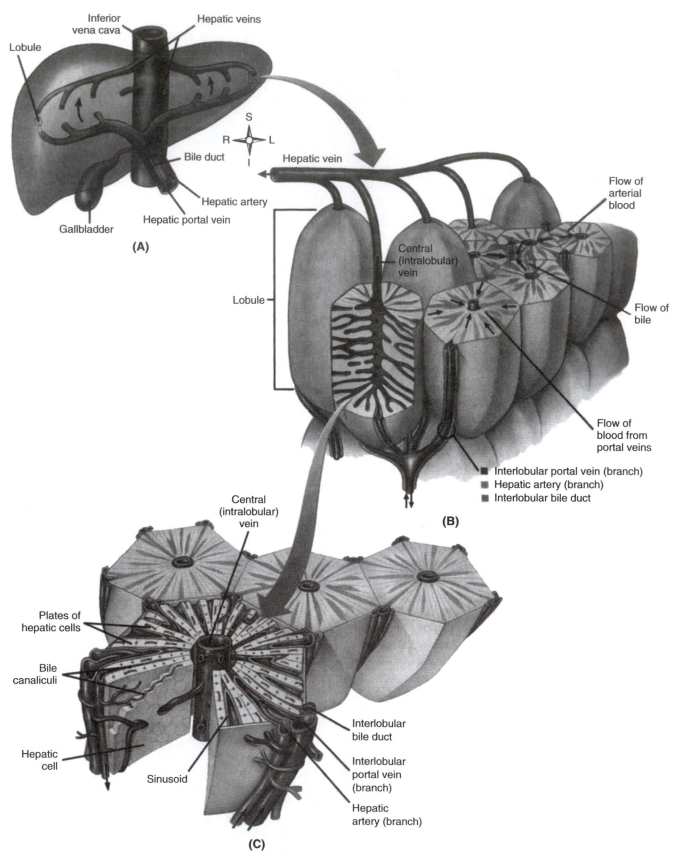

Figure 18–1   Microscopic structure of the liver shows *(A)* the location of liver lobules relative to the overall circulatory scheme of the liver. Enlarged views of several lobules (*B* and *C*) show the vascular scheme of the lobules and the flow of bile from the hepatocytes to the hepatic ducts. (From Thibodeau GA. *Anatomy & Physiology*. 3rd ed. St Louis: Mosby-Year Book; 1996. With permission.)

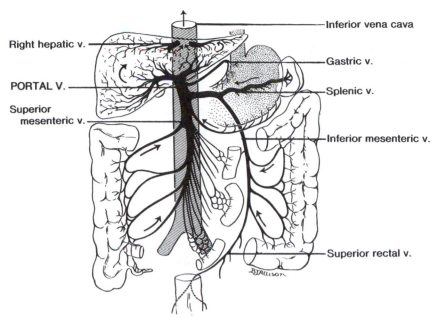

Figure 18–2 Scheme of the portal circulation. (From Moore KL. *Clinically Oriented Anatomy.* 2nd ed. Baltimore: Williams & Wilkins; 1985. With permission.)

in an increase in flow in the other. However, the relatively small contribution of the hepatic artery to total HBF limits the usefulness of this mechanism. Moreover, complete reciprocity is rarely achieved by the portal vein when hepatic artery flow decreases, since portal vein blood flow is limited by low hydrostatic driving pressures and resistance encountered in other parts of the splanchnic circulation. Without a reliable autoregulatory mechanism, the splanchnic viscera are at risk for ischemia in the presence of hypotension or states of increased sympathetic tone. However, the hepatocytes have a mechanism to compensate for the hepatic microcirculation's inability to regulate itself efficiently. They have developed the ability to greatly increase oxygen extraction from sinusoidal blood. This mechanism plays a major role in preserving hepatic integrity during hypoperfused or deoxygenated states.

Sympathetic innervation from T3 to T11 feeds the splanchnic circulation via the splanchnic nerves. In the portal circulation, only *alpha* receptors are found. Diffuse noradrenergic discharge (e.g., in response to a drop in systemic blood pressure) causes a rise in portal pressure, resulting in brisk HBF, which bypasses most of the organ and enters the systemic circulation. Both alpha and beta receptors are present in the hepatic arterial circulation; sympathetic stimulation will cause vasoconstriction of the hepatic artery and mesenteric vessels (which decreases portal inflow), causing a decrease in HBF.

ALTERATIONS IN HEPATIC BLOOD FLOW INDUCED BY ANESTHESIA AND SURGERY

It is clearly established that a reduction in HBF occurs during surgery with either general or regional anesthesia. This reduction can be explained by either the direct or indirect effects of anesthetics or the effects of surgery itself.

Direct Effects of Anesthetics

Inhalation Agents
Portal vein blood flow decreases with a simultaneous increase in hepatic artery blood flow during administration of isoflurane. In contrast, halothane causes a greater decrease in portal vein flow without a concomitant increase in hepatic artery flow. Many studies have demonstrated these findings, indicating that HBF and hepatic oxygen delivery are better preserved with isoflurane. However, even with isoflurane, the increase in hepatic artery flow does not sufficiently compensate for the decrease in portal vein flow. Hence, a reduction of total HBF (of about 25%) is seen with all volatile agents.

Indirect Effects of Anesthetics

Circulatory System
Hepatic blood flow is reduced in proportion to the degree of reduction in cardiac output or mean arterial blood pressure caused by the anesthetic agent. A reduced mean arterial pressure reduces hepatic perfusion pressure, and therefore HBF falls. Decreases in cardiac output stimulate a *reflex sympathetic discharge*, which results in vasoconstriction of the splanchnic vasculature, resulting in decreased HBF.

Assuming an adequate intravascular volume, the reduction in HBF caused by regional anesthetics (both spinal and epidural) is primarily due to the decrease in mean arterial pressure resulting from sympathectomy. Anesthetic levels T7 to T10 lead to a 20% decrease in HBF; levels T2 to T3 can decrease HBF by more than 25%.

Pulmonary System

The effects of ventilation patterns influence HBF primarily due to hemodynamic changes. Mechanical positive-pressure ventilation with high peak inspiratory pressures can significantly reduce venous return and therefore reduce cardiac output. A decrease in venous return not only compromises cardiac output but also increases pressure in the hepatic venous system, which decreases hepatic perfusion pressure, thus lowering HBF. Predictably, the presence of positive end-expiratory pressure potentiates this adverse effect.

Hypoxemia or hypercapnia with acidosis activates a sympathetic discharge and can also reduce HBF.

Surgical Effects on Hepatic Blood Flow Surgical intervention itself adversely affects hepatic flow and function. The *operative site* can more profoundly influence HBF than can anesthetic agents—reductions in HBF occur when surgery is performed near the liver. For example, a cholecystectomy can lower HBF to 50% of normal. In fact, current data strongly suggest that a laparotomy per se causes a decrease in intestinal and liver blood flow. The exact mechanisms for this are not clear; retraction and manipulation of viscera as well as a general stress response involving hormones and other substances (catecholamines, renin-angiotensin, vasopressin) probably have significant roles. The adverse effects of surgery on hepatic function are not usually of clinical consequence except in patients with severe preoperative hepatic disease.

HEPATIC FUNCTIONS

Vascular Functions of the Liver

Reservoir Function

Besides being quite large, the liver is an expandable and compressible organ. The large hepatic veins and the sinusoids are the blood storage components of the liver. Its normal blood volume is 500 mL, or 10% of total blood volume, and it can expand to a capacity of 1 L.

Low resistance to blood flow from the hepatic sinusoids allows large volumes of blood to flow through the portal vein. Furthermore, since the hepatic vein is the liver's outflow tract, changes in hepatic venous pressure alter intrahepatic blood volume. For example, elevation of right atrial pressure—as in congestive heart failure (CHF)—causes back pressure throughout the venous system, forcing the distensible liver to hold excess blood. In contrast, hypovolemia—as in acute hemorrhage—with subsequent reflex sympathetic stimulation will cause vasoconstriction of the hepatic veins and sinusoids, releasing up to 350 mL of blood. Therefore the liver acts as a reservoir, effectively removing excess blood volume from the systemic circulation (sometimes causing hepatic congestion) and supplying extra amounts of blood in states of diminished intravascular blood volume.

Blood Cleansing

The portal vein contains blood from intestinal capillaries, which pick up large amounts of colonic bacteria. The large, highly phagocytic Kupffer cells lining the hepatic sinusoids efficiently remove 99% of the bacteria, plus cellular debris and other particulate matter, from portal blood before they can pass through the sinusoids.

Secretory Function of the Liver

Bile Production and Secretion

Bile, which is composed primarily of bile salts but also contains unconjugated bilirubin, cholesterol, and electrolytes, has two major functions: (1) to emulsify fat particles and (2) to facilitate the absorption of lipids from the intestine. This second function is essential not only to fat metabolism but to the absorption of the fat-soluble vitamins: A, D, E, and K. Vitamin K is necessary for the formation of prothrombin and the coagulation factors VII, IX, and X.

Hepatocytes continually produce bile and secrete it into the bile canaliculi. The canaliculi empty into progressively larger channels to the common bile duct, where the bile empties either into the duodenum or the gallbladder. The gallbladder, which is connected to the common bile duct by the cystic duct, functions as a reservoir for bile. Biliary flow into the duodenum is regulated by the sphincter of *Oddi*.

Between meals, bile is stored in the gallbladder and—via mechanisms involving electrolyte exchange—becomes a concentrated substance. Bile secretion is mediated by cholecystokinin (a hormone released in response to fat and protein ingestion), which stimulates the contraction of the gallbladder; the sphincter of Oddi relaxes as the gallbladder contracts, allowing bile into the duodenum.

Bilirubin Excretion

One of the major end products of hemoglobin degradation is bilirubin. When released into the circulation (free bilirubin), it binds initially to albumin and is transported to the hepatic circulation. Here, the bound bilirubin dissociates from albumin and conjugates with glucuronic acid (conjugated bilirubin). Most of the conjugated bilirubin is excreted into the canaliculi and follows the same pathway as bile. After entering the intestine, it is converted into urobilinogen, which is either excreted in urine or reabsorbed back into the intestine and excreted again by the liver (enterohepatic circulation). Some of the conjugated bilirubin enters the circulation. Unconjugated bilirubin may be neurotoxic and can cause encephalopathy.

When free or conjugated bilirubin accumulates (usually to three times the normal level) in the extracellular fluid space, the skin, sclera, and mucous membranes have a yellowish tint, called *jaundice*. There are two types of jaundice, hemolytic and obstructive. The former is caused by increased destruction of red blood cells and the latter by bile duct obstruction or hepatic cell damage.

Metabolic Functions of the Liver A complete discussion of the metabolic functions of the liver is beyond the scope of this chapter, since they represent some of the more complex and integrated aspects of hepatic physiology. A brief overview of the major roles of the liver in the metabolism of carbohydrates, proteins, and fats is presented, followed by a more extensive review of drug metabolism.

Carbohydrate Metabolism

The liver provides the metabolic machinery for the conversion of several substances into glucose, the body's major energy source. Furthermore, the liver is responsible for *glucose homeostasis*. This involves a dynamic process of constant metabolic activity mediated by hormonal and hepatocellular mechanisms. Important actions of the liver to accomplish the maintenance of normal glucose levels are (1) glycogen storage in the presence of hyperglycemia and (2) glycogenolysis and gluconeogenesis (conversion of amino acids into glucose) during hypoglycemic states. Figure 18–3 summarizes the mechanisms involved in carbohydrate homeostasis.

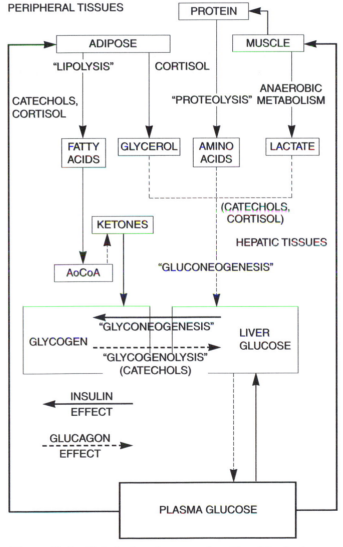

Figure 18–3 Carbohydrate homeostasis achieved by the interaction of the synthetic (anabolic) actions of insulin *(heavy solid arrows)* and the opposing catabolic actions of glucagon *(dashed arrows)*. Major effects of cortisol and catecholamines are also indicated; parentheses indicate actions in concert with insulin or with glucagon. (Adapted from Muravchik S. *The Anesthetic Plan: From Physiologic Principles to Clinical Strategies.* St Louis: Mosby-Year Book; 1991. With permission.)

Protein Metabolism

The role of the liver in protein metabolism is critical to the survival of the human body. The most important aspects of this hepatic function can be summarized as follows: (1) The deamination of amino acids allows these substances to be used in either carbohydrate or fat metabolism. (2) Virtually all plasma proteins including *albumin* and all the *coagulation factors* except factor VIII are of hepatic origin, the most notable exception being the gamma globulins. Albumin is essential for the maintenance of normal plasma oncotic pressure and is the principal protein used for the binding and transport of drugs. The importance of the coagulation factors is obvious. (3) Urea formation aids in the removal of ammonia from body fluids; excessive ammonia in the blood is exceedingly toxic. (4) The interconversion of nonessential amino acids provides substrates for other important metabolic processes.

Fat Metabolism

Principal functions of the liver in fat metabolism are as follows: (1) Beta oxidation of fatty acids and the formation of acetoacetic acid. This process provides a readily available alternative fuel source. (2) The formation of lipoproteins, cholesterol and phospholipids. It is well known that the latter two substances are essential to the synthesis and integrity of most cellular membranes. (3) The conversion of carbohydrates and proteins into fatty acids. This represents yet another way that the liver provides energy sources.

Miscellaneous Metabolic Functions

These include (1) storage of vitamins A, D, and B_{12}; (2) storage of iron; and (3) hormone degradation, notably thyroid hormone, insulin, estrogen, aldosterone, cortisol, glucagon, and antidiuretic hormone (ADH).

Drug Metabolism

Most pharmacologically active compounds are lipid-soluble and are therefore difficult to excrete. Biotransformation of these substances results in more polar, water-soluble, often pharmacologically inactive compounds, which are more easily excreted in bile or urine. *Hepatic biotransformation* reactions are classified as either phase I or phase II. Figure 18–4 summarizes these reaction.

Phase I reactions involve alteration of, addition to, or splitting off of functional groups existing on the active compound. The chemical reactions involved here are oxidation, hydroxylation, and reduction or hydrolysis. Catalyzing phase I reactions are the hepatic microsomal enzymes (mixed oxidase enzymes) located in the smooth endoplasmic reticulum of the liver. *Cytochrome P-450* is a pigmented hemoprotein that appears to play a key role in this enzyme system. Barbiturates and benzodiazepines undergo phase I–type transformation.

The microsomal enzymatic systems of phase I–type reactions have the potential to be enhanced or "induced" by exposure to certain compounds. This means an increase in the production of those enzymes, resulting in increased tolerance to the effect of the drug(s) being metabolized. Some agents commonly known to cause *enzyme induction* are phenobarbi-

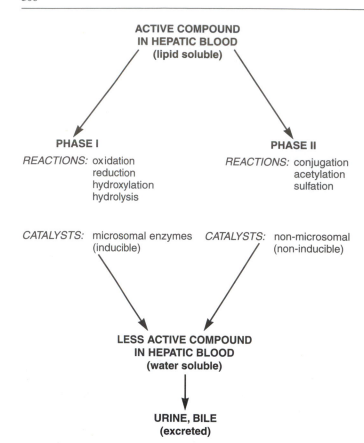

Figure 18–4 Hepatic biotransformation reactions. Most pharmacologic substances undergo sequential biotransformation (phase I, then phase II); endogenous substances (e.g., bilirubin and steroids) undergo phase I only.

tal, tobacco (polycyclic hydrocarbons), rifampin, phenytoin, and (chronic use of) alcohol.

Inhibition of enzyme systems (microsomal or otherwise) results in prolonged duration of drug effects. Some mechanisms for this phenomenon are (1) competitive inhibition, (2) blockade of the enzyme's drug-binding site (e.g., cimetidine blocks the site for meperidine, diazepam, propranolol, and lidocaine), and (3) hepatocellular injury (congestion, toxins, tumor, infections).

Phase II reactions involve conjugation reactions; they may be preceded by phase I reactions. Endogenous substances (e.g., steroids and bilirubin) undergo this type of biotransformation, combining with other substrates (e.g., amino acids, acetate, glucuronic acid, sulfates, methyl groups) to render them more water-soluble. The enzyme systems involved in these reactions are nonmicrosomal and are not capable of being induced. For phase II pathways, maximal metabolic activity is directly influenced by the mass of well-perfused, normal hepatic tissue available.

ANESTHETIC EFFECTS ON HEPATIC FUNCTION

Metabolic Function

Hyperglycemia

Glucose homeostasis is predictably disrupted during general anesthesia. An elevated serum glucose postoperatively is usu-

ally transient, mild, and not associated with ketone production (indicating that insulin levels, at least in nondiabetics, are sufficient and effective). It is generally believed that this alteration in hepatic metabolic function following general anesthesia reflects a nonspecific, stress-related, catecholamine-induced glycogenolysis. Reinforcing this theory is the fact that the blunting of the sympathoadrenal response by high regional anesthesia has been shown to minimize this hyperglycemia.

Drug Metabolism

Halothane may directly inhibit the biotransformation of some drugs (ketamine, warfarin, phenytoin). However, most of the altered pharmacokinetics seen in some drugs after exposure to anesthetics are most likely due to changes in hepatic blood flow.

Secretory Function

Biliary Colic

All opioids can cause spasm of biliary smooth muscle, resulting in increases in intrabiliary pressure, manifest by biliary colic. Narcotics, placed descending in order of likelihood to cause spasm, are fentanyl, morphine, meperidine, butorphanol, and nalbuphine. The actual incidence of sphincter of Oddi spasm is low (3%). The administration of narcotics slowly and in small titrations further decreases the likelihood that this effect will develop. If opioid-induced spasm of the sphincter of Oddi does occur during surgery under a general anesthetic, it may manifest radiographically as a constriction of the common bile duct, and a cholangiogram may be misinterpreted as positive for a common bile duct stone. Glucagon reverses this induced spasm, as do atropine, nitroglycerin, and inhalation agents. Any of these agents can be used to prevent false-positive interpretations of intraoperative cholangiograms.

Postanesthetic Dysfunction A small fraction of patients with no preoperative liver disease demonstrate mild hepatic dysfunction postoperatively (manifest by elevated liver function tests). Making this diagnosis is tricky, since liver function tests are rarely specific and, because of the liver's enormous functional reserves, considerable liver damage must be present before function tests are altered.

The most common cause of postoperative hepatic dysfunction is oxygen deprivation to liver tissue due to hypoxia, hypovolemia, or both. A combination of factors may be responsible, including decreased HBF directly or indirectly related to the anesthesia, the stress response to surgery, or the surgical procedure itself. Not only does surgery in close proximity to the liver reduce HBF, elevations of certain liver enzymes (lactate dehydrogenase and transaminases) often occur. Mild postoperative hepatic dysfunction (in patients with no known preoperative predisposition) is usually self-limiting, requiring no treatment and having no sequelae.

Significant postoperative hepatic dysfunction, evidenced by sustained elevations in liver function tests with clinical symptoms, is usually due to unrecognized preoperative hepatic disease (either unknown chronic hepatitis or acute hepatitis in the incubation phase) or, again, the surgery itself. Postoperative viral hepatitis may be transfusion-related (it usually develops 30 to 70 days posttransfusion). Other explanations for significantly elevated liver function tests postoperatively are sepsis, idiosyncratic drug reactions, and surgical complications.

Hepatic Toxicity Halothane-associated hepatoxicity, or *halothane hepatitis,* is a rare syndrome, but it is associated with a high mortality (50%). First recognized three decades ago, when halothane was introduced for clinical use, it is still the only agent for which hepatic toxicity remains a significant issue. The incidence of halothane hepatitis in adults is 1:10,000 to 30,000. Following a repeat exposure to halothane (up to 28 days after initial exposure), the incidence can be as high as 20%. Prepubertal children seem to have a resistance to this syndrome, with a reported incidence range of 1:80,000 to 200,000. In contrast, the incidence of severe hepatitis due to enflurane or isoflurane is 1:300,000 to 500,000. Studies to date have indicated that the minimal degradation of desflurane correlates with a lack of hepatotoxic effects in humans. Evidence for hepatotoxicity with sevoflurane, which has a greater propensity for degradation, has not yet appeared.

The notion that hepatic injury after exposure to halothane is related to the effects of metabolites formed by biotransformation reactions is not controversial; however, the precise mechanisms have not been clearly elucidated. Some of the clinical manifestations of halothane hepatitis (fever, rash, arthralgia, eosinophilia, and a history of recent exposure to halothane) suggest that an immune-mediated response is involved. Females seem to be more prone to develop the syndrome, and a genetic predisposition may be present. Obesity—with metabolic characteristics of increased microsomal enzyme activity, an enlarged liver mass with high HBF, and therefore enhanced rates of biotransformation—also increases susceptibility.

Since the clinical presentation of halothane hepatitis is similar to that of hepatic disease of many other origins, its diagnosis is one of exclusion. The severity of hepatocellular damage caused by this syndrome varies from mild and asymptomatic to fulminant hepatic necrosis.

☐ HEPATIC PATHOPHYSIOLOGY

ALCOHOLIC LIVER DISEASE

Alcoholic liver disease describes the spectrum of hepatic injury associated with acute and chronic alcoholism. The disease progresses in stages, the final sequelae being cirrhosis and portal hypertension (extensively reviewed under "Cirrhosis," below). The clinical manifestations of disease are frequently absent until, unfortunately, extensive hepatic damage has been done. Furthermore, in cases of subclinical or compensated liver disease, minor stress—and certainly major

stressors such as surgery and anesthesia—can precipitate deterioration of hepatic function.

Pharmacokinetics of Alcohol Alcohol is absorbed by the gastrointestinal tract by simple diffusion and rapidly diffuses throughout the aqueous compartments of the body. Predictably, the blood-brain barrier is quite permeable to alcohol. Only 5 to 15% of the drug is excreted unchanged in urine. Major biotransformation occurs in the liver, which contains all of the enzyme systems necessary for the conversion of alcohol to excretable substances. Other organs may contribute to alcohol metabolism; local degradation in the GI tract results in substantial first-pass metabolism. In fact, variations in the capacity of the gastric mucosa to metabolize alcohol is a major determinant of bioavailability and toxicity. The rate-limiting step in the metabolism of alcohol is intake.

Alcohol and the Liver Alcohol causes fat mobilization from tissue as well as increased hepatic production of fat. Acute alcohol intoxication is probably not associated with excessive increases of fat in the liver; however, prolonged high intake of alcohol results in an accumulation of fat—called alcoholic fatty liver—which represents the first stage of alcoholic liver disease. Hepatomegaly is the clinical manifestation of this stage. Hepatic damage is reversible with cessation of alcohol ingestion.

The product of alcohol metabolism, acetaldehyde, is a toxic substance that binds to proteins, thus inhibiting enzymatic functions. With years of excessive alcohol intake, acetaldehyde causes hepatocyte engorgement with fat, proteins, and water, causing necrosis and fibrosis of hepatic tissue. Thus, alcoholic fatty liver can progress to alcoholic hepatitis (covered in the following section). With continued intake, these pathologic processes become irreversible and cirrhosis ensues.

Chronic alcohol consumption results in induction of the microsomal enzyme systems; however, the effects of enzyme induction are not always predictable and may be outweighed by the severe, alcohol-induced impairment of liver function.

ACUTE HEPATITIS

The term *hepatitis* refers to inflammation of the liver. The disease represents acute hepatocellular injury with a variable amount of cellular necrosis. The most common etiologies are viral, drug-induced, or exposure to a hepatotoxin.

Viral Hepatitis Five types of viral hepatitis have been identified. Hepatitis A (infectious hepatitis) is most common in children in developing countries, but it is frequently seen in adults of the western world. Hepatitis B (serum hepatitis) is the most common form of hepatitis. Hepatitis C (formerly called non-A, non-B hepatitis) is transmitted via blood and blood products. Hepatitis D (delta hepatitis) is found in intravenous drug users who are also carriers of the hepatitis B virus. Hepatitis E (enteric non-A, non-B) is commonly found in underdeveloped countries; its symptoms resemble those of hepatitis A. Other viruses—especially the herpes family, Epstein-Barr, cytomegalovirus, and coxsackieviruses—can also cause hepatitis in addition to their effect on other organs.

The A and E types of hepatitis are transmitted via the oral-fecal route; types B and C are spread via body fluid contact or percutaneously; and hepatitis D, which can only be transmitted to individuals having hepatitis B, spreads percutaneously and via body fluid contact; it can be transmitted orally. Serologic testing is necessary to determine the etiologic viral agent; currently there are tests for the serum markers of hepatitis B and C. Hepatitis D can be detected by the presence of antibody to the virus plus the presence of type B. Testing for hepatitis E is not currently available.

The pathology of viral hepatitis represents a spectrum of hepatocellular damage and disorganization of the normal hepatic lobular architecture. The clinical symptoms reflect the stage and degree to which damage has occurred. A prodromal phase of viral hepatitis is often seen, lasting approximately 1 to 2 weeks. Clinical symptoms are varied and nonspecific: anorexia, nausea and vomiting, fatigue, malaise, arthralgias, myalgias, headache, low-grade fever. Jaundice may or may not follow this phase; if present, it lasts for 2 to 12 weeks, with recovery taking up to 4 months. Resolution of this phase is determined by the normalization of serum transaminase levels. The clinical course of acute hepatitis varies from mild symptomatology to fulminant hepatitis, which is rare. The course of types B and C is usually more prolonged and complicated.

Chronic liver disease develops in about 5 to 10% of cases following hepatitis B and in more than 80% of cases following hepatitis C. (Chronic hepatitis is discussed in the following section.) The degree of chronic disease that is manifest may be mild and slowly progressive or it may be severe, leading rapidly to cirrhosis.

Certain individuals become asymptomatic infectious carriers of the virus, as indicated by the persistence of the hepatitis B surface antigen (HBsAg) in their serum. The current statistics for the known incidence of individuals with hepatitis B or C who are infectious carriers are compelling: there are 3 million carriers of hepatitis B worldwide (1.2 million in the United States) and 3.5 million carriers of hepatitis C in the United States. Infectious carriers of these diseases pose a major health hazard to health providers, especially perioperative service personnel. Universal precautions for avoiding direct contact with blood and secretions are mandatory in the delivery of anesthesia care—gloves, mask, protective eyewear, and needle precautions must be used. A vaccine for hepatitis A is currently under development. Two types of vaccine are available for the prevention of hepatitis B (also, hepatitis B immune globulin may prevent infection after exposure, but it must be given within 48 h to be useful). Hepatitis D is prevented by preventing type B. No vaccine or immune globulin is currently available for hepatitis C or E. Table 18-1 summarizes routes of transmission of viral hepatitis.

Table 18-1
TRANSMISSION OF VIRAL HEPATITIS

	A	B	C	D	E
Food-borne	■				■
Fecal	■				■
Waterborne	■				■
Mollusk-related	■				□
Intrafamilial	■	■	□	■	■
Intrainstitutional	■	■			
Intravenous drug use	□	■	■	■	
Transfusion	◆	■	■	■	
Hemodialysis		■	■	□	
Sexual	□	■	●	■	
Anal/oral sex	■	■			
Oral	■	◆	□	□	■
Household	■	■	□		
Maternal-neonatal		■	●	■	

Key: Confirmed transmission ■; rarely transmitted ◆; suspected □; uncommon ●.
SOURCE: The American Liver Foundation. *Viral Hepatitis: Everbody's Problem.* 1994. With permission.

Drug-Induced Hepatitis This form of acute hepatitis results from direct toxicity of a drug or its metabolites (usually dose-dependent); and/or it may be an idiosyncratic reaction to the drug. Some known hepatotoxic drugs and substances are alcohol, acetaminophen, salicylates, tetracyclines, trichloroethylene, vinyl chloride, carbon tetrachloride, and poisonous mushrooms. Substances known to cause idiosyncratic reactions that lead to acute hepatitis are halothane, phenytoin, sulfonamides, rifampin, and indomethacin. Methyldopa, isoniazid, sodium valproate, and amiodarone can cause both toxic and idiosyncratic reactions, leading to hepatitis. Alcoholic hepatitis is probably the most commonly encountered type of drug-induced hepatitis. The clinical course of this disease resembles that of viral hepatitis.

CHRONIC HEPATITIS

Chronic hepatitis is liver inflammation persistent for more than 6 months. The most common etiology of this disease is prior infection with hepatitis B or C. The presence of chronic hepatitis is determined by elevated serum aminotransferase levels; based on the results of a diagnostic liver biopsy, it has traditionally been classified into three distinct syndromes: chronic persistent hepatitis, chronic lobular hepatitis, and chronic active hepatitis. Although the clinical value of this classification is currently being evaluated, each syndrome is described below.

Chronic persistent hepatitis implies chronic inflammation of portal tracts without inflammatory changes in the rest of the liver lobule. The clinical relevance of this fact is that cirrhosis is characteristically absent; after a course of acute hepatitis, the disease resolves. Chronic lobular hepatitis, a recently described variant of the chronic persistent syndrome, represents similar histologic changes. The difference is that some recurrent exacerbations may occur after an initial course of acute hepatitis, but again, cirrhosis rarely if ever ensues.

Chronic active hepatitis represents inflammation of hepatic tissue as well as damage to the cellular architecture of the lobule. In a significant number of cases, cirrhosis is either evident upon diagnosis or develops eventually. The clinical spectrum of this syndrome ranges from asymptomatic illness to fulminant hepatic failure. Fatigue is common, and jaundice, either persistent or recurrent, is present in the majority of cases. Not uncommonly, symptoms of superimposed acute hepatitis are present—anorexia, malaise, and low-grade fever. Extrahepatic features may also be evident and, in fact, may dominate the clinical picture. Some extrahepatic manifestations of chronic active hepatitis are amenorrhea, arthralgia or arthritis, dermatologic symptoms, pericarditis, anemia, or azotemia. If chronic active hepatitis progresses, the clinical manifestations of cirrhosis will become evident.

The management of chronic active hepatitis involves treatment of extrahepatic manifestations; otherwise, definitive treatment depends on the degree of clinical symptomatology and serologic findings. Patients who are negative for HBsAg are treated with long-term corticosteroid therapy with or without azathioprine.

CIRRHOSIS

Cirrhosis is a generic term comprising all forms of chronic diffuse liver disease. The morphologic definition of this disease includes hepatocyte necrosis, fibrosis of hepatic tissue, and nodular regeneration of the remaining liver tissue. The histologic hallmark of cirrhosis is the extensive disorganization of hepatic lobular structure.

The most common cause of cirrhosis (in the United States) is alcoholic liver disease. Other etiologies include chronic active hepatitis, chronic biliary inflammation or obstruction, chronic right heart failure (cardiac cirrhosis), hemochromatosis, Wilson's disease, and alpha$_1$-antitrypsin deficiency. Regardless of the etiology, the clinical profile of patients with cirrhosis is similar; the following review focuses on alcoholic cirrhosis.

Each morphologic feature of cirrhosis has specific clinical manifestations (Figure 18–5). Hepatocyte necrosis causes a progressive reduction of liver mass, producing jaundice, ascites, and edema, central nervous system (CNS) dysfunction, and cachexia. Fibrosis of hepatic tissue distorts intrahepatic vasculature, causing portal hypertension, with resultant esophageal and gastric varices and splenomegaly. Finally, nodular regeneration leads to distortion of intrahepatic venous and lymphatic systems, which also contributes to portal hypertension and ascites. A generalized derangement of the liver's multiple metabolic and synthetic functions is manifest

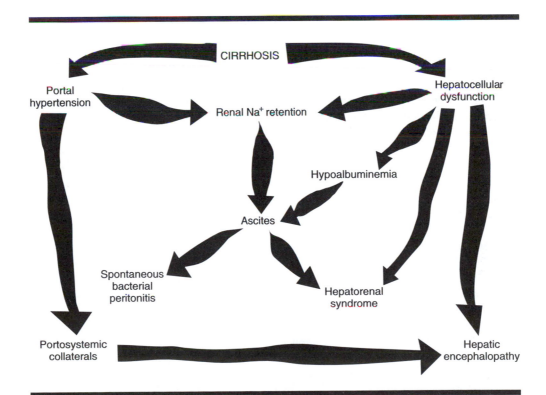

Figure 18–5 Interrelationships between the complications of cirrhosis. (From Wyngaarden JB, ed. *Cecil Textbook of Medicine*. 19th ed. Philadelphia: Saunders; 1992. With permission.)

by multisystem disease, summarized below. It should be noted that clinical signs and symptoms do not necessarily correlate with the severity of hepatic damage. Many patients are asymptomatic until the later stages of the disease.

Gastrointestinal Manifestations Portal hypertension (> 10 mmHg) is a major finding in severe cirrhosis, which leads to the development of venous collaterals in the portal system. The major collateral sites are gastroesophageal (GE), periumbilical, retroperitoneal, and hemorrhoidal. One of the major causes of morbidity and mortality in cirrhosis is massive hemorrhage from GE varices; in addition to depletion of intravascular volume, the increased nitrogenous load due to blood degradation in the intestinal tract leads to encephalopathy.

Cardiovascular Manifestations Systemic cardiovascular function in the presence of portal hypertension is characterized by a number of sequelae. Arteriovenous collaterals and shunting may develop in many organs and tissues, including the lungs, splanchnic organs, skin, and muscles. If myocardial function is maintained, the fall in systemic and pulmonary vascular resistance associated with the opening of shunts between the arterial and venous circulation produces a hyperdynamic state. The arterial blood pressure is low, but the cardiac output is elevated. Total blood volume is increased with decreased viscosity (due to anemia). In the presence of alcoholic cardiomyopathy, this hemodynamic profile may not manifest and a picture of myocardial failure will dominate.

Respiratory Manifestations Hypoxemia in cirrhosis is the result of several factors.

1. Right-to-left shunts due to
   a. $\dot{V}/\dot{Q}$ mismatch (release of endogenous vasodilators— glucagon, ferritin, vasoactive intestinal polypeptides—impairs hypoxic pulmonary vasoconstriction)
   b. Portapulmonary venous communications
   c. Spider angiomas in the lungs
2. Hypoventilation due to ascites (increased closing volumes exceed FRC)
3. Decreased pulmonary diffusion capacity (increased extracellular fluid)
4. Rightward shift of the oxyhemoglobin dissociation curve (increase in 2,3-diphosphoglycerate secondary to anemia)

Hematologic Manifestations Anemia is common and of multifactorial etiology: blood loss (GI bleeds), hemolysis, bone marrow suppression, increased plasma volume, and nutritional deficiencies (vitamin B_{12}). Thrombocytopenia and leukopenia are also common, primarily due to congestive splenomegaly.

Coagulopathies are the direct result of clotting factor deficiencies due to the severely impaired synthetic functions of the liver as well as the inadequate absorption of vitamin K.

The most common deficiency is of factor VII, followed by factors V, X, II (prothrombin), and I (fibrinogen). Enhanced fibrinolysis (due to low clearance of the activators of fibrinolysis) also contributes to abnormal clotting. Fibrin degradation products are not increased, but lower fibrinogen levels may also occur. Specific to alcoholic cirrhosis is alcohol-induced suppression of the function and survival of platelets; this platelet dysfunction also contributes to coagulopathies

Hepatic failure is associated with a substantial decrease in clotting factors, with an increase in the prothrombin time (PT) and partial thromboplastin time (PTT). In fact, changes in the PT usually reflect the extent of liver dysfunction well.

Central Nervous System Manifestations Inadequate hepatocyte function as well as reduced HBF from portacaval shunting leads to insufficient hepatic elimination of waste products (ammonia, methionine metabolites, short-chain fatty acids, and phenols). Hepatic encephalopathy ensues, manifest by alterations in mental status with associated neurologic signs: asterixis, hyperreflexia, or an inverted plantar reflex. Another significant finding specific to hepatic encephalopathy is increased permeability of the blood-brain barrier.

Renal manifestations Renal dysfunction with subsequent electrolyte imbalances is frequently seen in advanced hepatic disease. The clinical manifestations of these imbalances are edema, ascites, and the hepatorenal syndrome.

Inappropriate sodium retention is the primary abnormality in renal function associated with cirrhosis. This results in the accumulation of extracellular fluid with subsequent edema and ascites. The pathogenesis of *ascites* in relation to sodium retention is traditionally explained by two mechanisms, referred to as the "underfilling" and "overflow" theories. Briefly, the underfilling theory proposes that the primary event is a decreased circulating intravascular volume. This event is caused by imbalances of the Starling forces at work in the cirrhotic state (portal hypertension causes increased hydrostatic pressure, and hypoalbuminemia causes a decreased plasma oncotic pressure). Excessive formation of lymph ensues, which seeps out of hepatic tissue due to the distortion of normal lymphatic channels. Eventually lymph accumulates in the peritoneal cavity as ascites, thereby reducing effective circulating plasma volume. Sodium retention then occurs as the result of this relative hypovolemia and secondary hyperaldosteronism. The overflow theory, in contrast, views excessive sodium retention as the primary event, resulting in an increased plasma volume. This, in conjunction with the abnormal Starling forces described above, causes the transudation of fluid out of the splanchic circulation into the peritoneal cavity as ascites. These two theories are not mutually exclusive; a primary defect in sodium retention (outflow theory) may play the major role in early cirrhosis, whereas a decreased effective intravascular volume (underfilling theory) may have the more dominant role in advanced cirrhosis.

Other distortions in renal function that occur with cirrhosis in the presence of ascites are decreased renal perfusion, altered intrarenal hemodynamics, enhanced sodium reabsorption, and an impairment in free water clearance. Hyponatremia is common, with a dilutional etiology. Hypokalemia is also common, attributed to secondary hyperaldosteronism, diuretic therapy, vomiting, or diarrhea.

The most extreme manifestation of the renal dysfunctions just described is seen in the *hepatorenal syndrome,* which usually develops in the classic setting of cirrhosis with portal hypertension and (in particular) ascites of an intractable nature. The pathogenesis of the hepatorenal syndrome is not entirely clear, but renal vasoconstriction, with subsequent decreased renal blood flow, clearly plays a significant role. Clinically, urine output is usually maintained but low (an oliguric state), and the urine sodium concentration is characteristically extremely low. Azotemia is evident.

Hepatorenal syndrome has been closely associated with gastrointestinal bleeds, too vigorous diuretic therapy, sepsis, and major surgery; all of these imply a state of depleted intravascular volume. This points to the wisdom of preventive measures: carefully titrated diuresis for edema and ascites and judicious fluid management. The renal damage caused by the syndrome is extensive and associated with high rates of mortality and morbidity. Treatment is supportive and often unsuccessful without liver transplantation.

☐ ANESTHETIC MANAGEMENT AND CONSIDERATIONS FOR PATIENTS WITH HEPATIC DISEASE

EVALUATION OF HEPATIC FUNCTION

Liver Function Tests Although there are many laboratory tests to measure liver activity, the most common are neither sensitive nor specific. The serum transaminases, for example, are more reflective of hepatocellular structural integrity than hepatic function. Some tests measure the metabolic function of the liver, others the synthetic function. The lack of specificity or sensitivity of liver function tests (LFTs), then, requires that LFTs should always be interpreted in conjunction with other laboratory findings and correlated to the clinical findings. A brief review of the common LFTs follows; the numbers in parentheses represent the range of normal values for each test.

Albumin (3.5 to 5.0 g/dL)

This represents an indirect measurement of the liver's synthetic ability, which may have a predictive value for survival of hepatic disease. The half-life of albumin is from 14 to 21 days; therefore decreased levels may not be evident in acute disease. Values below 2.5 g/dL are indicative of severe hepatic disease. Total body albumin can be elevated in cirrhotic patients with a low serum albumin due to large amounts of albumin in the ascitic fluid.

Other etiologies of hypoalbuminemia are malnutrition (decreased synthesis), nephrotic syndrome, burns, and protein-losing enteropathies (increased losses).

Prothrombin Time (10.9 to 12.8 s)

Normal value ranges actually depend heavily on the controls used. Prothrombin time (PT) is the most important qualitative measure of the hepatic protein synthesis; therefore it is considered to reflect overall liver function. The half-life of prothrombin is 6 h, making this test suitable for assessing hepatic function in acute or chronic disease. The PT does not become elevated until more than 70 to 80% of normal factor activity is absent, therefore a PT prolongation of 3 to 4 s from control reflects a significant reduction in the liver's synthetic function; an increase above 4 s is associated with a poor prognosis in patients with liver disease.

Other etiologies of an elevated PT include vitamin K deficiencies (malnutrition, cystic fibrosis), drugs (coumadin), fibrinolysis, or disseminated intravascular coagulation.

The level of prothrombin indicates the effectiveness of the entire *extrinsic* coagulation pathway. Vitamin K is used to correct this deficiency, which requires at least 24 h to be effective.

Bilirubin

Measurements of bilirubin are differentiated into unconjugated (indirect) bilirubin (0.2 to 0.8 mg/dL), conjugated (direct) bilirubin (0.0 to 0.3 mg/dL), and total bilirubin (≤ 1.1 mg/dL). Intrinsic hepatic disease is implicated when the conjugated (direct) hyperbilirubinemia represents more than 50% of elevations in the total bilirubin. Jaundice usually correlates with a total bilirubin above 3.0 mg/dL.

Transaminases

Aspartate aminotransferase (AST—also known as serum glutamic-oxaloacetic transaminase, or SGOT: 12 to 31 U/L), alanine aminotransferase (ALT—also known as serum glutamate pyruvate transaminase, or SGPT: 10 to 32 U/L). Aspartate aminotransferase is present in the liver as well as the heart, kidneys, and skeletal muscle. ALT is primarily found in the liver. These substances are released in the presence of acute hepatic injury. The magnitude of rise in serum concentration does not always correlate with the severity of the disease, therefore changing levels of the transaminases are not used as consistent predictors of the extent of hepatic disease. Extensive skeletal muscle injury is another etiology of elevated transaminase levels.

Alkaline Phosphatase (90 to 240 U/dL)

Alkaline phosphatase is an enzyme produced primarily by bone but is also made in the liver, small bowel, kidney, and placenta and is excreted into bile. It is released from bile ducts in response to acute injury. Alkaline phosphatase is markedly elevated in obstructive jaundice but not in intrinsic hepatic disease. Other etiologies of elevated alkaline phosphatase are pregnancy and Paget's disease.

Preoperative Assessment

Acute Liver Disease

The need for a preanesthetic evaluation in this context is usually due to acute viral or acute alcoholic hepatitis. Acute alcohol toxicity, with the special challenges it presents to anesthetic management, also falls into this category (see below). In short, any elective surgery should not even be considered until the hepatitis has resolved (in terms of LFTs). Patients with acute hepatitis are at high risk for further deterioration of hepatic function, with progression to hepatic failure and its sequelae (namely, encephalopathy or hepatorenal syndrome).

Surgery should be performed only in emergent situations. Preanesthetic evaluation focuses on the cause and degree of hepatic impairment. The origin of the acute disease can be determined by knowledge of preexisting liver disease or anything that predisposes to it, recent drug exposures, intravenous drug use or excessive alcohol intake, recent blood transfusions, and recent anesthetics. Assessing degree of impairment should be accomplished by an organ systems review. Any degree of mental status change (from subtle alterations in level of consciousness to full-blown encephalopathy) usually indicates severe dysfunction. The cardiovascular system may be in a hyperdynamic state (increased cardiac output due to reduced SVR in the presence of arteriovenous shunting). Hypoxemia may be present due to intrapulmonary shunting; hyperventilation (with subsequent acid/base changes) may be present if ammonia levels are high. Metabolic derangements may be present due to renal involvement. The presence of nausea and vomiting may also potentiate electrolyte imbalance and cause dehydration.

Evaluation of lab tests should include a serum HBsAg, a complete serum electrolyte panel (with blood urea nitrogen and creatinine), LFTs, and a complete blood count. Hypokalemia and metabolic alkalosis are not uncommon and are usually the result of vomiting. Hypoglycemia can be seen due to impaired liver metabolism. The LFTs, which are helpful in evaluating acute disease, are the PT, the transaminases, and alkaline phosphatase—the former because it greatly signifies synthetic function and the latter two because they help make the differential diagnosis of etiology of the hepatitis.

If surgery and anesthesia are absolutely required, dehydration and electrolyte imbalances should be corrected. If a coagulopathy is evident, fresh frozen plasma (immediately effective) and vitamin K (effective within 24 h) can help correct this. Premedication is not usually used so as to avoid precipitating encephalopathy and to minimize drug exposure.

Acute alcohol toxicity greatly complicates anesthetic and surgical management. Intoxicated patients can be obtunded or exhibit inappropriate or combative behavior, making them difficult to assess and manage. They may have ingested or injected other stimulants and/or depressants. Regurgitation and pulmonary aspiration are a high risk. Acute alcohol toxicity lowers MAC and potentiates most anesthetic drug effects; furthermore, the cardiac and respiratory depression caused by anesthetic agents is potentiated. Abnormal laboratory findings may include hypokalemia (if the patient has been vomiting) and hypomagnesemia (seen in chronic alcoholics). Other clinical and lab findings may include those just discussed for acute hepatitis, since acute intoxication may precipitate the move from alcoholic fatty liver disease to acute alcoholic hepatitis.

Alcohol withdrawal during the perioperative period carries a 50% mortality rate. This phenomenon ranges from a relatively minor set of symptoms to delirium tremens, which represents a major withdrawal syndrome. Minor symptoms may appear within a few hours of cessation of drinking and may even start during continued drinking (during which time there has been a significant fall in blood alcohol levels); these symptoms can include anorexia, insomnia, general weakness, tremors, mild disorientation, hallucinations, and convulsions. These symptoms usually peak within 10 to 30 h after drinking has ceased and last approximately 40 to 50 h. *Delirium tremens* (DTs) has an onset of approximately 60 to 80 h after cessation of drinking. True DTs are relatively rare and are characterized by extreme autonomic hyperactivity: tremors, tachycardia, diaphoresis, fever, anxiety, perceptual disorders, hallucinations, and global confusion.

Minor withdrawal should be treated with sedatives, most commonly benzodiazepines. These drugs should be given in amounts sufficient to provide enough sedation to prevent the occurrence of major symptoms. Magnesium may be helpful to treat dysrhythmias secondary to electrolyte imbalance. Beta blockers can be used to attenuate autonomic hyperreactivity, specifically tremors, anxiety, and tachydysrhythmias.

Chronic Liver Disease

(For the purposes of this review, the term *chronic liver disease* assumes some degree of cirrhosis.) Because patients with chronic liver disease have depleted their hepatic functional reserves, they are at great risk to develop hepatic failure. Anesthetic management requires recognition of the multisystem nature of cirrhosis; a preoperative assessment should focus on controlling or preventing its extrahepatic complications.

The *gastrointestinal manifestations* of cirrhosis should be evaluated. A full stomach should be assumed, since gastroesophageal reflux is often present, as is decreased gastric and intestinal motility; the presence of massive ascites especially mandates the usual prophylaxis and precautions for a full stomach. Peptic ulcer disease is not uncommon; therefore information regarding recent gastric bleeding should be elicited. If variceal bleeding has been established (by endoscopy), supportive treatment consists of (1) replacement of blood loss by intravenous fluids and blood products, (2) infusion of vasopressin (high-dose vasopressin may have myocardial ramifications—failure or ischemia); and (3) tamponade with a Sengstaken-Blakemore tube. Bleeding can be stopped with endoscopic sclerosis; if this is not successful or if bleeding recurs, emergency surgery may be required. The type of surgery chosen is usually based on a risk categorization scheme that focuses on hepatic reserve (referred to as Child's classification). Patients with a lower risk score generally undergo shunting procedures; those with high risk scores have ablative surgery, esophageal resection, and gastric devascularization.

Hematologic evaluation is critical. Since anemia is common, the need for preoperative blood transfusions should be balanced against the increased protein breakdown that occurs with excessive blood transfusions—the resultant increase in nitrogen load can precipitate encephalopathy. The decision to transfuse blood preoperatively is often influenced by the presence of coexistent heart disease and the blood loss (which may be exacerbated by increased bleeding tendencies) anticipated with surgery. Coagulation system abnormalities should be evaluated and treated properly before surgery, primarily based on prothrombin (PT) values. A vitamin K (intramuscular) trial for several days may prove helpful in lowering the PT; if this is not successful or if there is no time for normalization of coagulation via vitamin K, then fresh frozen plasma should be used to replenish clotting factors. Thrombocytopenia should also be corrected; ideally the platelet count is brought to over 100,000 per cubic millimeter (each unit of platelets increases the platelet count by 10,000 per cubic millimeter). The use of cryoprecipitate may be necessary for severe coagulopathies.

Fluid and electrolyte balance must also be carefully evaluated, since judicious perioperative fluid management is critical. The preservation of renal function is imperative to avoid the dire circumstances of hepatorenal syndrome. Preoperatively, diuresis for edema and ascites must be accompanied by adequate hydration and must be accomplished slowly (over several days). Initial therapy is bed rest, sodium restriction (< 2 g NaCl per day), and spironolactone. A urine output of approximately 1 mL/kg/h is the goal. Insufficient diuresis is approached with a fluid load of proper volume and composition. The composition of fluid used should be based on serum sodium, potassium, ionized calcium, hematocrit, and glucose; the volume should be titrated against measured filling pressures (via a central venous or pulmonary artery line). Colloid infusions (albumin) are often used to correct acute intravascular fluid deficits. Actual diuretic therapy, when used, is accomplished with either furosemide (0.3 to 2.0 mg/kg), mannitol (1 to 2 g/kg), or both, or renal-dose dopamine (1 to 4 μg/kg/min). The use of low-dose dopamine capitalizes on its renal vasodilatory and antialdosterone effect. These principles of fluid management should be carried into the intraoperative period. The intraoperative effectiveness of mannitol as a means of preventing renal failure has not been conclusively demonstrated.

Common electrolyte findings are hyponatremia (a serum sodium of < 130 mEq/L necessitates water restriction) and hypokalemia, which may require replacement. As a result of impaired hepatic metabolism, hypoglycemia pre- and intraoperatively is a common finding; glucose-containing solutions may be required.

A *pulmonary assessment* should focus on the amount and degree of atelectasis and hypoxemia present. Chest x-rays and arterial blood gases (ABGs) are useful to quantitate this. Significant pulmonary compromise secondary to massive ascites may necessitate a preoperative paracentesis.

The presence of *CNS involvement* should be assessed. Encephalopathy is treated with oral lactulose or neomycin, which decreases the intestinal absorption of ammonia.

INTRAOPERATIVE MONITORING

Routine monitoring is employed, with use of a five-lead electrocardiogram for monitoring of ischemia (e.g., when vasopressin infusions are in use). As always, specific monitoring needs are dictated by the status of the patient and the type of surgery to be done. It is safe to say, however, that patients with symptomatic chronic liver disease warrant close monitoring of the cardiovascular and pulmonary status. Intra-arterial pressure monitoring is often indicated. Beat-to-beat monitoring of rapid blood pressure changes that occur due to excessive bleeding, rapid intercompartmental fluid shifts, and surgical manipulations is invaluable for anesthetic drug and fluid manipulations. Frequent blood sampling for multiple laboratory values is another indication for an intra-arterial line.

Due to the constant seepage of albumin from the liver surface into the peritoneal cavity (part of the process forming ascitic fluid) the evaluation of perioperative intravascular volume shifts and overall fluid balance becomes a more challenging task. Monitoring of central vein or pulmonary artery pressure often aids in the accurate assessment of intravascular volume status and the intelligent management of fluids and transfusions of blood products. Clearly, the decision to place invasive monitoring lines must consider the presence of coagulopathies; treatment of clotting abnormalities may have to precede these procedures, and injudicious attempts at line insertions should be avoided. Frequent monitoring of urine output is also critical to fluid management. These monitoring modes are especially key in the prevention of the hepatorenal syndrome.

Laboratory tests to be followed closely intraoperatively are essentially those used to preoperatively assess the patient (with the exception of some LFTs) and include electrolytes, glucose, ABGs, hematocrit, coagulation panel (PT, PTT, and platelet count).

A peripheral nerve stimulator is also a useful monitor to help titrate doses of muscle relaxants in patients with chronic liver disease, because the effects of muscle relaxants in this population are unpredictable.

ANESTHETIC MANAGEMENT

Anesthesia care required for a patient with significant hepatic dysfunction may be (1) for surgical therapy of the liver disease and its complications or (2) for nonhepatic procedures (e.g., colon resections, cholecystectomy). The first category includes the creation of portasystemic shunts (including transjugular intrahepatic portosystemic shunts (TIPS), transesophageal varix ligations, or injection sclerotherapy of varices.

General Principles   For the most part, the management of patients with acute and chronic liver disease is similar:

1.   The goal of intraoperative management is to preserve existing hepatic function and avoid further hepatic injury.

2. This is accomplished by avoiding substances with potentially adverse effects on hepatic function as well as decreases in hepatic arterial blood flow and oxygen supply.

3. Arterial hypotension as well as a state of reduced cardiac output should be avoided.

4. Increases in splanchnic vascular resistance should be avoided, since the hepatic artery is more heavily relied upon to supply total hepatic blood flow (avoid light anesthesia, hypoxia, hypercarbia).

5. In the absence of a coagulopathy or thrombocytopenia, regional anesthesia is an excellent option for peripheral surgery provided that hypotension is avoided.

6. The preservation of adequate renal blood flow and function is essential to avoid the hepatorenal syndrome.

7. Rapid-sequence induction of anesthesia with cricoid pressure (or awake intubation) is indicated in virtually all patients, since many factors predisposing to regurgitation and pulmonary aspiration exist.

Intravenous Agents   The basic pharmacologic strategy in formulating an anesthetic plan for a patient with liver disease is to assume an unpredictable patient response to anesthetic agents and therefore to avoid using anesthetic agents and adjuvants subject to prolonged effects. Variations in normal drug responses are due to several factors: decreased protein binding, increased volume of distribution, decreased drug metabolism and elimination, and changes in the blood-brain barrier, which increase CNS sensitivity. *Thiopental* undergoes decreased metabolism as well as decreased protein binding; the overall effect is unaltered clearance. Many patients will manifest an increased CNS sensitivity to thiopental; alcoholics tend to show a tolerance for the drug. The *benzodiazepines* are highly protein-bound compounds; a relative overdose of midazolam or diazepam can occur. Furthermore, an increased number of benzodiazepine-specific brain receptors may exist in patients with advanced liver disease, also potentiating a relative overdose. Premedication with anxiolytics is generally avoided or, if these are used, they must be very carefully titrated. Opioids, particularly *fentanyl,* can be used successfully in patients with hepatic disease despite decreased clearance and a prolonged half-life. It has been demonstrated that fentanyl does not decrease hepatic oxygen or blood supply (nor does it decrease hepatic oxygen demand). *Succinylcholine,* despite decreases in plasma cholinesterase activity, has a relatively normal half-life; a prolonged effect does occur when hepatic functional capacity is reduced by 50%. *Mivacurium,* whose duration of action is also inversely related to cholinesterase activity, has demonstrated prolonged effect in patients with liver dysfunction. Due to an expanded extracellular fluid compartment, the volume of distribution for highly ionized drugs such as the *nondepolarizing muscle relaxants* is increased; this means that a higher-than-normal loading dose of the drug may be necessary to accomplish a certain level of relaxation. This holds true for *d-tubocurarine, pancuronium,* and *atracurium* and has recently been demonstrated for *rocuronium.* The volume of distribution for *vecuronium* is not substantially altered; no alteration of initial doses should be expected. Those nondepolarizing muscle relaxants partially relying on hepatic elimination should be associated with a decreased plasma clearance. Therefore smaller-than-normal maintenance doses should be anticipated for curare, pancuronium, and vecuronium. The plasma clearance of rocuronium (in doses up to 0.6 mg/kg) appears to be unaffected by liver disease; therefore the duration of action is unchanged. Titrations of muscle relaxants should always be guided by the use of a peripheral nerve stimulator in the presence of advanced liver disease.

Inhalational Anesthetics   In light of the fact that patients with severe liver disease handle "fixed" intravenous agents in an abnormal and unpredictable fashion, the use of an inhalation-based anesthetic technique seems prudent. *Halothane* should definitely be avoided, since, of all the volatile agents, it is associated with the most prominent decrease in hepatic blood flow and oxygen supply and the highest incidence of moderate postoperative hepatic dysfunction; it is clearly associated with a rare but severe hepatitis. Currently available data indicate that neither *desflurane* nor *sevoflurane* have demonstrated hepatotoxic effects; however, at least for sevoflurane, this has not been reliably confirmed. *Isoflurane* seems to be the inhalation agent of choice provided that adequate cardiac output and arterial pressures are maintained. *Nitrous oxide per se* is not contraindicated in patients with liver disease; it has not been associated with anesthesia-related hepatic complications. However, in advanced liver disease, the imperative to maximize oxygen delivery to hepatic tissue may preclude the use of nitrous oxide.

Fluid Management   As mentioned under "Preoperative Assessment" above, fluid management of the patient with significant chronic liver disease includes low-salt solutions. In the intraoperative phase, sodium restriction is still key, but the preservation of intravascular volume and maintenance of urine output become the main priorities. Colloids often become the solutions of choice; they are particularly effective in preventing profound hypotension and renal hypoperfusion after the drainage of massive ascites.

The principles of intraoperative blood product transfusion in patients with liver disease follow those cited previously for preoperative preparation. Intraoperatively, excessive bleeding is due not only to coagulopathies but also to venous engorgement from portal hypertension and the presence of adhesions from prior surgeries. Clearly, in the intraoperative phase, one should be prepared with adequate blood products and sufficient intravenous access to accommodate transfusion needs. Large-bore intravenous access along with pressurized, rapid-infusion fluid warmers should be employed. Whole blood, when available, may be preferable to packed red blood cells, since replacement of clotting factors is also necessary. Calcium binding by the citrate preservative used in blood products can result in clinically significant hypocalcemia (ionized calcium), especially when liver disease exists, since citrate metabolism is primarily hepatic. When massive blood transfusions are given, calcium replacement should be anticipated to counteract the negative inotropic effect of hypocalcemia.

SURGICAL PROCEDURES INVOLVING THE LIVER

HEPATIC RESECTION

Preoperative Considerations Hepatic resections are performed on patients with primary hepatic neoplasms, metastatic tumors from the gastrointestinal tract, or injuries due to trauma, with resultant necrosis of hepatic tissue. Liver function may be entirely normal in these patients, or they may exhibit the range of hepatocellular dysfunction described in the previous sections of this chapter. Hepatocellular carcinoma is commonly seen in males above 50 years of age and is associated with chronic, active hepatitis B with resultant cirrhosis.

Tumors may surround major vascular structures, impeding their flow. It is important to gain information regarding the tumor size and the extent of involvement (if any) of vascular structures in order to be adequately prepared for major intraoperative blood and fluid losses.

Surgical Considerations Most major resections can be performed via a transabdominal approach, although in some cases a thoracoabdominal approach is used. During lobar resections, the corresponding hepatic artery, portal vein, and bile duct are isolated and ligated; if possible, the major hepatic vein of the involved lobe is ligated at its entry into the vena cava. Control of bleeding and the achievement of adequate hemostasis is a major focus of the surgical technique.

Intraoperative Considerations Regardless of the patient's preoperative liver function, the potential for massive blood loss during hepatic resections should be a major focus

in the formulation of an anesthetic plan. (Obviously, a cirrhotic patient with coagulopathies presents an even greater challenge in this regard.) Massive blood transfusions may be required; therefore adequate amounts of appropriate blood products must be immediately available. (One possible guideline is 2 units FFP plus 6 units PLT per 10 units PRBCs). Adequate venous access with large-bore intravenous catheters is critical. Fluid and blood warmers are essential, and high-pressure rapid-transfusion devices should be considered; if the patient's condition does not include cancer, blood salvage devices can be utilized.

The placement of invasive monitoring lines depends on the patient's overall medical status and provider preference. With the distinct potential for major blood loss, placement of an intra-arterial pressure line for close blood pressure monitoring and frequent blood sampling would seem advantageous. If the extent of the resection is not known prior to exploration of the abdomen, appropriate additional catheters and monitoring lines should be established prior to the actual start of resection.

General endotracheal anesthesia is utilized with or without an epidural catheter for postoperative analgesia. If the site of resection is known beforehand, the placement of a left double-lumen endotracheal tube may improve surgical exposure. The choice of induction agents depends heavily on the patient's preoperative status and whether or not the procedure is emergent. Maintenance techniques should focus on avoiding hypotension (due to its deleterious effects on remaining hepatic tissue). Following major hepatic resections accompanied by massive transfusion of blood and fluid, postoperative mechanical ventilation should be seriously considered. However, because of its detrimental effects on hepatic blood flow, prolonged positive-pressure ventilation should be avoided, especially in light of the well-established fact that patients with normal liver function preoperatively may have significant postoperative impairment of liver function due to loss of liver mass, surgical trauma, or sustained hepatic hypoperfusion.

BIBLIOGRAPHY

Eger EI. New inhaled anesthetics. In: Feeley TW, Royston D, eds. *International Anesthesiology Clinics: New Drugs in Anesthesia.* Vol 33, no 1. Boston: Little, Brown; 1995:61–80.

Faust RJ, ed. *Anesthesiology Review.* 2nd ed. New York: Churchill Livingstone; 1994:73–77, 100–101, 187–189, 521–524.

Fiamengo SA. Alcoholism. In: Yao FF, Artusio JF: *Anesthesiology: Problem-Oriented Patient Management.* 3rd ed. Philadelphia: Lippincott; 1993:693–707.

Ganong WF, ed. *Review of Medical Physiology.* 17th ed. Norwalk, Conn: Appleton & Lange; 1995:458–463, 568–569.

Gelman S. Anesthesia for the patient with liver disease. In: Barash PG, ed: *ASA Refresher Courses in Anesthesiology.* Vol 20. Philadelphia: Lippincott; 1992:85–98.

Guyton AG. *Textbook of Medical Physiology.* 8th ed. Philadelphia: Saunders; 1991:771–776.

Higuchi H, Sumikura H. Renal function in patients with high serum fluoride concentrations after prolonged sevoflurane anesthesia. *Anesthesiology* 1995; 83:449–458.

Isselbacher KJ, Braunwald E, eds. *Harrison's Principles of Internal Medicine.* 13th ed. New York: McGraw-Hill; 1994:1458–1478, 1478–1483, 1483–1495.

Jaffe RA, Samuels SI, eds. *Anesthesiologist's Manual of Surgical Procedures.* New York: Raven Press; 1994:361–365.

Miller RD, ed. *Anesthesia.* 3rd ed. New York: Churchill Livingstone; 1990:585–600, 1809–1828.

Muravchik S. *The Anesthetic Plan: From Physiologic Principles* to *Clinical Strategies*. St Louis: Mosby-Year Book; 1991: 250–285.

Morgan GE, Mikhail MS. *Clinical Anesthesiology*. Norwalk, Conn: Appleton & Lange; 1992:544–554, 555–564.

Stoelting RK. *Pharmacology & Physiology in Anesthetic Practice*. 2nd ed. Philadelphia: Lippincott; 1991:782–794.

Stoelting RK, Dierdorf SF. *Anesthesia and Co-Existing Disease*. 2nd ed. New York: Churchill Livingstone; 1988:355–392.

☐ QUESTIONS

1. Blood flow to the liver:
   a. Is made up of a dual afferent supply: the hepatic artery and the splanchnic artery
   b. Is supplied by the hepatic artery (75% of total hepatic blood flow) and the portal vein (25% of total hepatic blood flow)
   c. Is decreased with sympathetic stimulation
   d. Is closely autoregulated during surgery and anesthesia via a dopaminergic mechanism

2. The functions of the liver include all of the following *except:*
   a. Biotransformation of pharmacologically active compounds
   b. The production of gamma globulins and factor VIII
   c. To act as a reservoir for blood
   d. To produce and secrete bile

3. The liver synthesizes albumin, the major serum protein. Which statement is true of albumin?
   a. Synthesis of albumin in the adult is higher than that in the neonate.
   b. Hypoalbuminemia increases the free fraction of protein-bound drugs, enhancing drug sensitivity.
   c. Serum albumin represents an indirect measure of the liver's synthetic ability; since the half-life of albumin is 14 to 21 h, it is an accurate measure of acute liver disease.
   d. Serum albumin represents an indirect measure of the liver's synthetic ability; since the half-life of albumin is 14 to 21 days, an elevated level (>5.0 g/dL) indicates the presence of chronic liver disease.

4. The liver plays a key role in glucose homeostasis; all of the following mechanisms are involved in this function *except:*
   a. Glycogen storage and gluconeogenesis
   b. Glucagon synthesis
   c. Glyconeogenesis (insulin-mediated)
   d. Synthesis of glucose from galactose

5. Which of the following statements is true for phase I reactions of hepatic biotransformation?
   a. They involve conjugation reactions and are catalyzed by noninducible enzymes.
   b. They involve conjugation and autooxidation reactions.
   c. They involve the oxidation, reduction, or hydrolysis of compounds and are catalyzed by the hepatic microsomal enzymes, which are inducible.
   d. They are catalyzed by the cytochrome P-450 system of enzymes, resulting in compounds that are less polar than their parent compounds and that are water-insoluble.

6. A 42-year-old man is scheduled for a septorhinoplasty. A preanesthetic evaluation reveals that he is more than likely in the early stages of acute viral hepatitis. Which statement is true regarding considerations for his anesthetic care?
   a. Patients with acute viral hepatitis should never undergo general anesthesia.
   b. The patient is not an acceptable candidate for elective surgery since he is at high risk for exacerbating his hepatic dysfunction.
   c. The patient is an acceptable candidate for general anesthesia since he is in the early stages of acute hepatitis and otherwise healthy.
   d. Patients with acute viral hepatitis can undergo general anesthesia as long as the inhalation agents are avoided.

7. The cirrhotic patient with portal hypertension and ascites:
   a. Usually has elevated total body albumin with an associated hyperalbuminemia
   b. Will manifest high hepatic artery pressures but low portal vein pressures
   c. May demonstrate a hyperdynamic cardiovascular state if myocardial function is maintained
   d. Should be aggressively diuresed to alleviate the severe cardiorespiratory effects of ascites

8. The hepatorenal syndrome:
   a. Represents a compensatory mechanism by the liver to increase renal blood flow during periods of renal hypoperfusion
   b. Represents a minor degree of renal impairment and is usually reversible with moderate fluid restriction and loop diuretics
   c. Manifests as oliguric renal failure in the severely cirrhotic patient
   d. Can be avoided in the cirrhotic patient by active diuresis of ascites and edema

9. All of the following statements are true about coagulopathies in severe hepatic failure *except:*
   a. They are the direct result of severely impaired synthetic functions of the liver.

   b. They are the result of inadequate absorption of vitamin K.
   c. All of the coagulation factors (except factor VIII) are deficient.
   d. Vitamin K therapy is not helpful.

10. Which of the following statements is true regarding the anesthetic management of a patient with severe hepatic disease?
   a. Deliberate hypotensive techniques work well to minimize intraoperative bleeding, especially when coagulopathies are present.
   b. All anesthetic agents should essentially be given in one half the usual doses in order to avoid prolonged drug effects.
   c. Regional anesthesia should always be avoided, since hypotension will decrease hepatic perfusion pressures.
   d. The volume of distribution of highly ionized drugs is increased, therefore higher-than-normal loading doses of nondepolarizing muscle relaxants may need to be given to accomplish adequate relaxation.

11. All of the following are true regarding the effects of anesthesia and surgery on hepatic blood flow (HBF) *except* which one?
   a. A reduction in HBF occurs with general and regional anesthetics; this is due to both the direct and indirect effects of anesthetics.
   b. Surgical intervention itself (e.g., an exploratory laparotomy) has not been demonstrated to have any effect on HBF.
   c. Mechanical positive pressure ventilation affects HBF primarily through hemodynamic changes.
   d. A subarachnoid block to a T2 level can significantly decrease HBF.

12. Jaundice:
   a. Is either hemolytic or obstructive in etiology
   b. Usually occurs when total serum bilirubin exceeds 0.5 mg/dL
   c. Is the result of elevated serum unconjugated bilirubin and not of elevated conjugated bilirubin
   d. Is the result of elevated serum conjugated bilirubin and not of elevated serum unconjugated bilirubin

13. What are some of the risk factors associated with halothane hepatitis?
   a. Obesity, male gender, and family history of cirrhotic liver disease
   b. Obesity, female gender, and family history of immune disorders
   c. Obesity, male gender, genetic predisposition, and prior exposure to halothane
   d. Obesity, female gender, genetic predisposition, and prior exposure to halothane

14. Which liver function tests assess hepatic synthetic function?
   a. PTT, albumin
   b. PT, albumin
   c. Albumin, ALP
   d. Albumin, AST, ALT

15. Which of the following is true for cirrhosis of the liver?
   a. Cirrhosis of the liver is synonymous with end-stage liver failure.
   b. Clinical signs and symptoms directly correlate with the extent and severity of hepatocyte damage.
   c. The pathogenesis of alcoholic cirrhosis differs from that of cardiac cirrhosis.
   d. The morphologic definition of cirrhosis includes hepatocyte necrosis, fibrosis of hepatic tissue, and nodular regeneration of the remaining liver tissue.

16. All of the following statements regarding alcohol withdrawal during the perioperative period are true *except* that it:
   a. Includes the possibility of delirium tremens with an onset of approximately 60–80 hours post cessation of drinking.
   b. Is excluded as a possibility if the patient has not had a seizure within 24 h after cessation of drinking.
   c. Is associated with a 50% mortality rate.
   d. Is not predictive of hepatic dysfunction postoperatively.

17. Fluid and electrolyte management of a cirrhotic patient includes all of the following *except:*
   a. An initial period of bed rest, sodium restriction, and spironolactone
   b. Diuresis for edema and ascites, accompanied by adequate hydration
   c. Primarily glucose-rich crystalloids, since colloids are contraindicated
   d. Diuresis with furosemide and/or mannitol, or renal dose dopamine

18. Hepatorenal syndrome differs from acute tubular necrosis (ATN):
   a. Since ATN is caused by renal tubular injury from ischemic or toxic injury and hepatorenal syndrome involves impaired glomerular filtration due to decreased RBF
   b. Since ATN is manifest by an elevated serum creatinine and oliguria and the hepatorenal syndrome is characterized by high-output renal failure
   c. In that ATN may respond to drug therapy (e.g., diuretics, dopamine) and is often reversible. Hepatorenal syndrome is not often responsive to drug therapy and is only reversible through normalization of hepatic function
   d. **a.** and **c.** are correct

19. Acute hepatitis:
    a. Can be either drug-induced or viral in etiology
    b. Involves acute hepatocellular injury with a variable amount of cellular necrosis
    c. Represents a strong contraindication for anesthesia
    d. All are correct

20. Anesthetic management in patients with acute and chronic liver disease:

a. Is similar in that the goal of intraoperative management is to preserve existing hepatic function and avoid further hepatic injury
b. Avoids thiopental, since this can be hepatotoxic
c. Is similar in that the plasma half-life of all drugs is shortened significantly
d. Includes slow, controlled induction sequences to prevent myocardial strain

☐ ANSWERS

1. c	5. c	9. d	13. d	17. c
2. b	6. c	10. d	14. b	18. d
3. b	7. c	11. b	15. d	19. d
4. b	8. c	12. a	16. b	20. a

The Renal System

Celeste G. Villanueva

An understanding of renal physiology is essential to the proper management of anesthetic care, since a patient's renal function greatly influences decisions made regarding pharmacologic choices and dosages, fluid management, and therapies involving electrolytes and acid-base adjustments.

☐ ANATOMY AND PHYSIOLOGY

The kidneys are paired retroperitoneal organs situated on either side of the vertebral column. The upper pole of each kidney lies opposite T12 and the lower pole opposite L3. They derive their sensory innervation from levels T12-L2. Each kidney is divided into a cortical (outer) and medullary (inner) region.

NEPHRON

The nephron is the functional unit of the kidney, being capable of forming urine; therefore an explanation of the workings of a single nephron essentially constitutes a description of the entire kidney's function. There are approximately 1.2 million nephrons in each kidney. Each nephron's basic function is to clear the blood plasma of unwanted metabolic end products and excess amounts of substances normally found in blood plasma.

The glomerulus is the portion of the nephron designed to form an ultrafiltrate of blood. The filtered fluid is passed along a tortuous tubule made up of distinct segments, each containing a specific type of epithelial cell along its lumen. The type of cell implements the functional role of that particular segment. These roles are either to secrete solutes into or reabsorb solutes out of the tubule, modifying the composition of the ultrafiltrate. Urine, the end product of the nephron, is then drained into the renal pelvis and into a single ureter.

The nephron is usually divided into the following anatomic and functional components: (1) the glomerulus, (2) the peritubular capillaries and vasa recta, (3) the proximal convoluted tubule, (4) the loop of Henle, (5) the distal renal tubule, (6) the collecting tubule, and (7) the juxtaglomerular apparatus. Figure 19–1 illustrates the functional nephron.

Cortical nephrons are those whose glomeruli lie close to the outer surface of the kidney and whose loops of Henle are very short. Juxtamedullary nephrons have glomeruli that lie close to the medulla. Their loops of Henle are characteristically long and dip deep into the medullary region. The distinction of nephrons according to regions of the kidney is important, relating to the nephron is ability to form a maximally concentrated urine.

The Glomerulus The glomerulus is essentially a convoluted capillary network. It is encased in Bowman's capsule, which is actually the blind, expanded end of a renal tubule deeply invaginated by the glomerular capillaries. Blood flow to the glomerular capillaries is supplied by the *afferent arteriole* and channeled away by the *efferent arteriole*. The efferent arteriole offers considerable resistance to blood flow, making the glomerular capillary network a high-pressure system. The multilayered interface between the endothelial cells of the glomerular capillaries and the epithelial cells of Bowman's capsule forms a highly efficient, size-selective, and charge-selective filter, allowing the passage of water, low-molecular-weight substances, and cations from glomerular capillary blood. For all practical purposes, the composition of the ultrafiltrate formed in the glomerulus is the same as plasma, differing primarily in the lack of red blood cells and any significant amount of proteins.

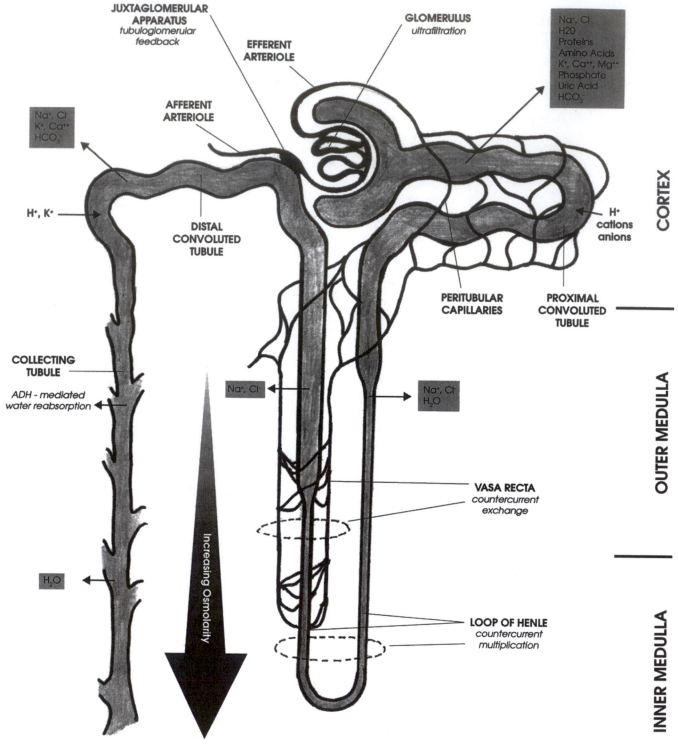

Figure 19–1.   Functional structure of the nephron.

Peritubular Capillaries and Vasa Recta   Each nephron has a peritubular capillary network that emanates from its efferent arteriole and surrounds cortical nephron segments. These low-pressure capillary beds are extremely porous and reabsorb vast amounts of fluids and solutes that flow from the tubules to interstitial spaces. Peritubular capillaries empty into the arcuate vein, which empties into the renal vein, which returns "cleansed" ultrafiltrate to the systemic circulation.

Juxtamedullary nephrons are surrounded not only by a peritubular capillary network but also by the vasa recta, a network of blood vessels that descend deep into the medulla and surround the lower portions of the long loops of Henle. The vasa recta have a key role in the countercurrent mechanism of urine concentration.

The Proximal Tubule   The primary function of the proximal tubule is sodium reabsorption via active transport of sodium (fueled by sodium-potassium-stimulated ATPase). Sodium reabsorption is coupled with reabsorption of phosphate, glucose, and amino acids (via carrier proteins and sodium cotransport). The absorption of cations (potassium, calcium, and magnesium) occurs as a result of the net loss of intracellular positive charges due to Na^+ K^+-ATPase activity. Chloride reabsorption occurs passively via a concentration gradient.

The proximal tubule is highly permeable to water. Because of the concentration gradient of solutes formed by the reabsorption processes just described, osmosis of water occurs from the tubular lumen to the peritubular capillaries so rapidly that the osmolar concentration of the solutes on either side of the tubule border is similar (isotonic). Some 65 to 75% of the glomerular ultrafiltrate is reabsorbed in the proximal tubule.

Active secretion of hydrogen ions (H^+) occurs in the proximal tubule, which, in turn, allows for the reabsorption of the most of the bicarbonate ions (HCO_3^-) in the glomerular ultrafiltrate. Other substances that are actively secreted from the ultrafiltrate by the proximal tubule are organic cations (creatinine, cimetidine, quinidine) and organic anions (urate, keto acids, penicillins, cephalosporins, diuretics, salicyclates, most x-ray contrast dyes).

The Loop of the Henle   The remaining 25 to 35% of the glomerular ultrafiltrate drains into the thin descending limb of the loop of Henle which is as permeable to water as the proximal tubule, though not as metabolically active. Its primary function is to passively reabsorb water via an osmotic gradient, and solutes (sodium, chloride, potassium, calcium, and magnesium) via a concentration gradient.

Once the loop makes a "U" turn, it is called the *ascending loop of Henle,* which is divided into two functionally distinct segments: the thin and thick limbs. The thin ascending limb is not as water-permeable as its descending counterpart, but it shares the latter's functional role of water and solute reabsorption. Throughout the loop of Henle, approximately 15% of the glomerular filtrate is reabsorbed.

In the thick ascending limb, active transport of chloride to the interstitium creates a slightly positive charge within the tubule. Sodium diffuses out of the tubule via an electrical gradient and then is actively transported into the interstitium and reabsorbed. Coupled to this process is potassium and chloride reabsorption, while calcium and magnesium are also reabsorbed in large amounts in this segment of the tubule.

An important characteristic of the thick ascending limb is its total impermeability to water. As a result, tubular fluid draining out of the loop of Henle is hypotonic and the interstitium surrounding the loop is hypertonic. The establishment around the loop of Henle of a hypertonic medullary interstitium in association with tubular filtrate—which is hypertonic at the base of the loop and hypotonic upon leaving the loop—is the essence of the countercurrent multiplier mechanism.

The Distal Tubule   After passing through the loop of Henle, 10 to 20% of the ultrafiltrate is left to enter the distal tubule. This portion of the nephron is divided into (1) the early segment, which contains the juxtaglomerular apparatus (discussed below), (2) the diluting segment, and (3) the late distal tubule.

The epithelial cells in the diluting segment are similar to those in the proximal tubule, and sodium reabsorption occurs by essentially the same mechanism. However, in great contrast to the proximal tubule, the diluting segment of the distal tubule is virtually impermeable to water. Hence, as the name implies, the diluting segment delivers a very dilute filtrate to the late distal tubule. The late distal tubule (also called the connecting segment) is a site for aldosterone-mediated sodium reabsorption. The water permeability of this portion varies, regulated by antidiuretic hormone (ADH). Another important function of the distal tubule is the absorption of parathyroid hormone and (vitamin D–mediated) calcium reabsorption.

Collecting Tubule   In this portion of the nephron, the glomerular ultrafiltrate, which at this point is called urine, becomes either highly concentrated or highly dilute, highly acidic or highly basic. The two functional divisions of this segment are (1) the cortical collecting tubule and (2) the inner medullary collecting duct.

The cortical collecting tubule is the principal site of aldosterone-mediated sodium reabsorption, which is coupled to chloride reabsorption, hydrogen ion secretion, or potassium secretion (which is also aldosterone-mediated). Water permeability in this segment is also determined by ADH activity.

The inner medullary collecting duct is the principal site of ADH action in the nephron, providing the nephron with the ability to either dilute or concentrate urine (see "Renal Functions," below). The medullary portions of the collecting ducts of all the nephrons in one kidney eventually join together, emptying urine into the renal pelvis.

Both segments of the collecting tubule are capable of hydrogen ion secretion. This occurs via an ATPase driven pump mechanism, where a hydrogen ion is secreted and a bicarbonate ion is reabsorbed, making the collecting tubules a major site for the control of acid/base balance.

The Role of Urea

Urea is the most abundant of metabolic waste products that must be eliminated by the kidneys. The process by which it becomes highly concentrated for excretion in the urine simultaneously plays an important role in the establishment of a hypertonic medullary interstitium.

The lumens of the loop of Henle and distal tubule are quite impermeable to urea; the result is a high concentration of urea flowing into the collecting tubules. The cortical collecting tubule remains virtually impermeable to urea, whereas the urea permeability in the inner medullary collecting tubule varies with the presence of ADH (increased ADH causes increased urea permeability). Therefore, in the presence of ADH, water reabsorption is increased, further increasing urea concentration within the tubules. Urea, which is now able to flow freely into the interstitium, does so according to a concentration gradient, increasing the tonicity of the medullary interstitium.

The Juxtaglomerular Apparatus   The juxtaglomerular apparatus (JGA) is the portion of each nephron where specialized cells in the afferent arteriole (juxtaglomerular or JG cells) come in contact with a histologically distinct segment of the early distal tubule (the *macula densa*). The JG cells produce and release *renin* in response to decreased blood pressure, renal ischemia, or sympathetic stimulation. Renin is the hormone that mediates the formation of angiotensin II, a potent vasoconstrictor that plays a major role in some of the processes regulating renal blood flow and the glomerular filtration rate. Table 19–1 outlines and summarizes the functional divisions of the nephron.

Table 19–1
SUMMARY OF NEPHRON SEGMENTS AND THEIR FUNCTIONS

Nephron Segment	Function
Glomerulus	Ultrafiltration of blood
Peritubular capillaries	Reabsorption of solutes from interstitium
Vasa recta	Countercurrent exchanger

Proximal tubule	Reabsorption
	  Sodium, chloride, glucose, protein, amino acids, potassium, calcium, magnesium, phosphate, uric acid, urea, bicarbonate
	Secretion
	  Hydrogen ions, organic anions, cations
	Ammonia production

Loop of Henle	Reabsorption Sodium, chloride, water, potassium, calcium, magnesium Countercurrent multiplier

Distal tubule	Reabsorption
	  Sodium, chloride, water, potassium, calcium, bicarbonate
	Secretion
	  Hydrogen ion, potassium, calcium

Collecting tubule	Reabsorption
	  Sodium, chloride, water, potassium, calcium, bicarbonate
	Secretion
	  Hydrogen ion, potassium
	Ammonia production

Juxtaglomerular apparatus	Renin secretion Tubuloglomerular feedback

RENAL BLOOD FLOW

In a resting state, 20 to 25% of the cardiac output (1.2 to 1.3 L/min) perfuses both kidneys. Relative to total body mass, this is an enormous amount of blood perfusing an organ. The rate of urine formation is 1 mL/min, indicating the high metabolic energy requirement for urine production. In the kidneys, O_2 consumption (18 mL/min) is determined by the renal blood flow (RBF); the inverse is true in all other body organs. Normal RBF far exceeds metabolic demands. This high rate of the flow is essential to the process of urine formation and renal function in general.

There are regional differences in RBF. Blood flow in terms of milliliters of blood per gram of tissue per minute is greatest in the cortex. The rate of perfusion gradually decreases from the outer to the inner medulla and slows to a downright sluggish drip in the innermost regions of the kidney. This difference in blood flow has relevance to the countercurrent exchange mechanism of the vasa recta.

Glomerular Filtration Rate   The amount of glomerular filtrate formed per minute in both kidneys is considered the glomerular filtration rate (GFR). The average GFR is 125 mL/min, which translates to 180 L of glomerular filtrate formed per day. The kidneys filter in 1 day a volume of fluid equivalent to 4 times the total body water, 15 times the ECF, and 60 times the plasma volume. Approximately 99% of the ultrafiltrate that passes through each nephron is reabsorbed back into the systemic circulation, making the average amount of urine formed per day between 1 to 2 L.

Regulation of RBF and GFR   The regulatory mechanisms that influence both RBF and GFR are complex and interrelated. The following represents a summary of the major regulatory systems at play.

Autoregulation of RBF
Renal blood flow remains constant within a range of arterial pressures (60 to 180 mmHg) due to an autoregulatory phenomenon. The mechanisms involve local metabolic factors (O_2, CO_2, and pH) and a contractile response of the afferent arteriole smooth musculature to stretch. Higher arterial pressures stimulate vasoconstriction of the afferent arteriole, causing less blood to flow into the glomerulus. Lower arterial pressure cause vasodilation of the afferent arteriole, allowing more blood to flow into the glomerulus. Autoregulation of RBF is intrinsic; however, it is not sustained in the presence of persistent (approximately 10 min) changes in arterial pressure. Outside the range of autoregulatory limits, RBF and GFR become pressure-dependent. When mean arterial pressures fall below 40 to 50 mmHg, the GFR falls essentially to zero.

Autoregulation of GFR
The autoregulation of the GFR exerts a long-term and far more profound effect on the urine output—a 5% change in the GFR in either direction results in significant increases or decreases in the urine output. This process occurs in the JGA

and is effective within approximately the same range of arterial blood pressures in which RBF autoregulation occurs (60 to 160 mmHg).

Two feedback mechanisms work in concert to accomplish the precise degree of GFR regulation; together, they are referred to as *tubuloglomerular feedback:* (1) an afferent arteriolar vasodilator feedback and (2) an efferent arteriolar vasoconstrictor feedback. A low GFR causes overreabsorption of chloride in the distal tubule and therefore a decreased chloride concentration in the macula densa. This causes afferent arteriolar dilatation, which increases blood flow into the glomerulus, resulting in a rise of the GFR back to normal. A low chloride ion concentration in the macula densa also stimulates renin to be released from the JG cells of the JGA, which causes the formation of angiotensin II. There is a vasoconstrictive effect of angiotensin II, especially on the efferent arteriole. This increased resistance to glomerular outflow causes increased blood pressure in the glomerular capillaries, resulting in an increase in the GFR back to normal. (This is thought to be the explanation for the renal failure that develops in patients with poor renal perfusion who are using ACE inhibitors). Part of this GFR-preserving mechanism involves angiotensin induced prostaglandin synthesis, which causes renal vasodilation and tempers the vasoconstrictive effects of angiotensin II. *(Which is why NSAIDs, which inhibit prostaglandin synthesis, can adversely affect GFR.)* Figure 19-2 illustrates the relationship between the autoregulation of RBF and GFR. Figure 19–3 illustrates the mechanism of GFR autoregulation.

Sympathetic Stimulation

The renal vasculature and tubular segments are richly innervated by sympathetic outflow tracts from the T4 to the L1 levels of the spinal cord. Sympathetic stimulation of the kidneys, as occurs with the rise in catecholamines associated with surgical stress or the administration of exogenous catecholamines, causes constriction of the renal vessels in general, with a preferential constriction of the afferent arteriole. This decreases both RBF and GFR. Sympathetic stimulation of the renal nerves also causes increased renin secretion, which triggers the efferent arteriole part of the tubu-

loglomerular feedback system, thereby counteracting a GFR decrease. Varying intensities of sympathetic stimulation appear to result in graded degrees of renin-angiotensin–mediated effects on GFR. That is, the amount of renin secreted in response to lower levels of sympathetic stimulation permits a normal GFR (despite a decrease in RBF), whereas the significantly higher renin levels in response to excessive sympathetic stimulation result in a greatly decreased RBF and GFR.

Sympathetic stimulation can cause redistribution of RBF to the medulla (which means greater flow to the juxtamedullary nephrons); the overall significance of this response to the regulation of GFR is controversial.

Cardiac Output

Cardiac output directly affects RBF and GFR in a parallel fashion. The increased perfusion pressures caused by a raised cardiac output increase glomerular flow and therefore GFR.

ANESTHESIA-INDUCED ALTERATIONS IN RENAL BLOOD FLOW

The effects of anesthesia on renal flow and function are usually described in terms of being direct or indirect, the latter generally considered as having the more profound influence.

Indirect Effects

Circulatory System

Virtually all of the inhalation and intravenous agents used to deliver a general anesthetic decrease arterial blood pressure, either due to myocardial depression or decreased systemic vascular resistance. Below the blood pressure limits of RBF and GFR autoregulation, these agents can produce a dose-dependent reduction in RBF, GFR, urinary flow, and sodium excretion. The sympathetic blockade with resultant hypotension caused by subarachnoid and epidural anesthetics can also cause reductions in renal function, the magnitude of the reduction paralleling the degree of sympathetic blockade. It has been determined that the reduction in renal function is less marked in regional anesthetics.

Sympathetic Nervous System

Sympathetic stimulation occurs during anesthesia (of any type) in the perioperative period in response to a variety of circumstances: intense surgical simulation, tissue trauma, light anesthesia, or as a compensatory response to anesthesia-induced hypotension. Renal sympathetic activity generates a powerful endocrine response (discussed in the following section). Sustained and intense sympathetic activity tends to decrease RBF and GFR—and therefore urine output—due to a vasoconstricted renal vasculature.

Endocrine System

The hormonal changes that occur during anesthesia greatly influence renal flow and function and represent a complex interplay of the circulatory and neuronal effects just discussed. Again, the stressful events that evoke the release of the hormones are painful surgical stimulation, circulatory depres-

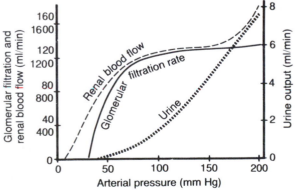

Figure 19–2. Autoregulation of glomerular filtration rate and renal blood flow. (From Guyton AC. *Textbook of Medical Physiology.* 8th ed. Philadelphia: Saunders; 1991. With permission.)

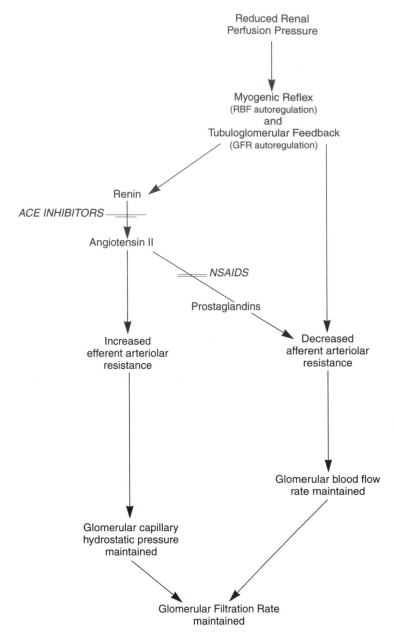

Figure 19–3.   Mechanism of GFR autoregulation.

sion resulting from anesthetic agents, hypovolemia or hemorrhage, hypoxia, or acid/base derangements. Levels of ADH, catecholamines (epinephrine and norepinephrine), renin, angiotensin II, and aldosterone are all *increased* during anesthesia. The catecholamines and angiotensin II decrease RBF (remember, GFR is maintained, despite a decrease in RBF, within autoregulatory limits) and ADH causes decreased urine volume. Aldosterone promotes sodium retention and subsequent expansion of the extracellular fluid compartment. The water-retentive effect of ADH may dominate here, causing a tendency toward a decreased serum sodium after anesthesia. The combined effect of ADH and aldosterone may be partly responsible for postoperative fluid retention.

It is important to emphasize that the indirect effects of anesthesia on renal function have clearly been demonstrated to be transient, *reversible* phenomena. Furthermore, the adverse effects on renal function can be attenuated or abolished by adequate *preoperative hydration* and the maintenance of an adequate intravascular volume and blood pressure during the perioperative period.

Direct Effects

Inhalation Agents

The worrisome adverse renal effect of the volatile anesthetics is nephrotoxicity induced by the release of a metabolic end product, the inorganic fluoride ion (F^-). Fluoride elimination is dependent on GFR; therefore individuals with compromised renal function are predisposed to this problem. Fluoride-induced nephrotoxicity, manifest by high-output renal failure, was a major problem with methoxyflurane. Halothane, isoflurane, and desflurane do not release enough fluoride as metabolic end products to pose a risk of nephrotoxicity.

Enflurane and sevoflurane are considered by some to present a theoretical risk. Prolonged enflurane administration—9.6 minimum alveolar concentration (MAC) hours or more—can lead to significantly high fluoride levels, but this degree of exposure is rare; still, the use of enflurane in the presence of renal impairment is not often recommended. The risk of nephrotoxicity with the use of sevoflurane remains, to date, controversial. The focus of the debate is sevoflurane's in vivo instability (producing Fl^-) and in vitro instability (producing compound A, also nephrotoxic). In sufficient doses and for sufficiently long periods of exposure, sevoflurane may cause injury to renal tubules. In healthy patients without renal disease, this has not been clinically significant; however, further studies are under way to establish the safety of sevoflurane in patients with preexisting renal disease.

In terms of the direct effects on RBF, halothane decreases renal vascular resistance and perfusion pressures proportionally, therefore it does not directly decrease RBF. Enflurane has been shown to decreases RBF. At 1 MAC, isoflurane minimally alters RBF and significantly decreases renal vascular resistance; however, with increased anesthetic depth, RBF is decreased due to the greater indirect effect of decreased perfusion pressure.

Studies indicate that halothane has no direct effect on the autoregulation of RBF (there are no data for isoflurane or desflurane).

Intravenous Agents

The direct effects on renal function of narcotics and barbiturates, when used alone, have been demonstrated to be nonexistent or of minor importance. Two drugs have been found to preserve normal renal function: ketamine maintains renal function in the context of hemorrhagic hypovolemia and droperidol (an alpha-adrenergic antagonist) prevents the sympathetic-induced redistribution of renal blood flow, which tends to decrease GFR.

RENAL FUNCTIONS

Excretion of Metabolic End Products   The process and mechanisms by which urine is formed from glomerular filtrate was outlined in the previous section as the functional role of the each segment of the nephron was described. The kidney has mechanisms to either dilute or concentrate urine.

Urine dilution is mediated by ADH in the late distal tubules and the collecting ducts. Decreased levels of ADH decrease water permeability; therefore less water is reabsorbed, resulting in dilute urine. Conversely, increased levels of ADH increase permeability to water, causing increased water reabsorption into blood and hence a less dilute urine.

Urine concentration is accomplished via the *countercurrent system*. This is dependent on (1) the establishment of a hypertonic medullary interstitium via the countercurrent multiplier mechanism of the loop of Henle; (2) the sluggish blood flow in the vasa recta, which minimizes the amount of solutes removed from the interstitium; and (3) the countercurrent exchange mechanism of the vasa recta. The parallel streams of flow in opposing directions (the two arms of the U tube) enable fluid and solutes to exchange freely and rapidly, making it possible for very high concentrations of solute to be maintained at the tip of the U tube with negligible washout of solute.

The excretion of concentrated urine occurs in the presence of high levels of ADH, which cause the collecting ducts to become highly permeable to water. The water is pulled by osmosis (toward the hypertonic medullary interstitium) out of the collecting duct, leaving highly concentrated urine in the duct to drain into the renal pelvis. Figure 19–4 illustrates the countercurrent system.

Regulation of the Volume and Composition of Body Fluids   The kidneys control (1) blood volume, (2) the volume of the extracellular fluid (ECF), (3) osmolarity of the body fluids, and (4) plasma ion concentrations.

Blood volume is controlled via a simple feedback loop. An increased blood volume increases cardiac output, which increases arterial blood pressure. Renal blood flow and GFR are eventually increased by the increased blood pressure, which increases urine output, thereby decreasing blood volume. The control of the ECF volume, not surprisingly, occurs simultaneously to blood volume control. What varies is the relative ratio of the ECF to blood volume; the ECF compartment serves as a reservoir for excess fluid that is not contained in the blood circulation.

The control of body fluid osmolarity by the kidney is me-

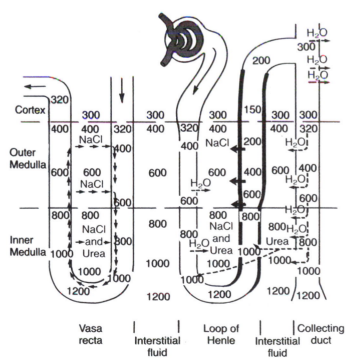

Figure 19–4.   The countercurrent mechanism of urine concentration. The loop of Henle functions as a countercurrent multiplier and the vasa recta as a countercurrent exchanger. Numerical values are in milliosmoles per liter. (From Guyton AC. *Textbook of Medical Physiology*. 8th ed. Philadelphia: Saunders; 1991. With permission.)

diated by *osmo-sodium receptor–ADH feedback.* Osmo-sodium receptors (in the anterior hypothalamus) detect the sodium concentration of the ECF and stimulate the release of ADH (from the posterior pituitary). The greater the sodium concentration (the higher the ECF osmolarity), the greater the rate of ADH secretion. Water reabsorption then increases, thus diluting the sodium concentration and bringing the ECF osmolarity back toward normal.

The kidneys regulate the plasma concentration of potassium, sodium, calcium, phosphate, and magnesium; potassium and sodium control are mediated by aldosterone, which promotes potassium secretion and sodium reabsorption. Long-term control of calcium is mediated by parathyroid hormone, whose secretion is stimulated by low calcium plasma concentrations and whose action is to enhance calcium reabsorption in the renal tubules. Phosphate reabsorption in the renal tubules is mediated by an overflow mechanism, whereby any amount in excess of the renal tubules' transport maximum for the ion is excreted. The mechanism for magnesium control is not well understood.

Acid-Base Regulation   The kidneys help regulate plasma hydrogen ion concentration by either acidification or alkalinization of the urine. The proximal renal tubule normally secretes hydrogen ions in exchange for bicarbonate ion filtration. In an acidotic state, hydrogen ion secretion exceeds bicarbonate ion filtration, causing excess hydrogen ion to be excreted in the urine; the converse is true in an alkalotic state. Higher CO_2 levels stimulate more rapid secretion of hydrogen ion; lower CO_2 levels decrease the secretion rate.

The renal regulatory mechanisms for acid-base balance have a slow onset (hours) but are complete—that is, these mechanisms are capable of neutralizing virtually every excess acid or alkali in body fluids.

Hormone Production   In addition to renin, which has already been discussed, the kidneys produce erythropoietin and 1,25-dihydroxycholecalciferol. Erythropoietin stimulates hemoglobin synthesis and the production and release of red blood cells from the bone marrow. The primary stimulus for erythropoietin secretion is hypoxia; other factors that facilitate its secretion are the alkalosis of high altitudes, catecholamines, and adenosine.

1,25-dihydroxycholecalciferol (calcitriol) is a steroid whose primary function is to facilitate Ca^+ reabsorption from the intestines and the kidneys.

□ RENAL PATHOPHYSIOLOGY

ACUTE RENAL FAILURE

Acute renal failure (ARF) refers to the rapid deterioration of renal function, which is not immediately reversible by altering extrarenal factors. The hallmark of ARF is azotemia (re-tention of nitrogenous waste products). *Prerenal* azotemia is the result of hypoperfusion of the kidneys and is most often due to decreased perfusion pressures and/or renal vasoconstriction. Correcting intravascular volume, improving cardiac function and blood pressure, and decreasing renal vascular resistance can reverse this process. *Postrenal* azotemia is due to obstruction of the urinary tract, with flow from both kidneys interrupted. Rapid recognition of obstruction and its subsequent relief reverses this azotemia. If untreated, both prerenal and postrenal azotemia can progress to ARF. *Renal* azotemia is caused by intrinsic renal disease, renal ischemia, or nephrotoxic agents and can rapidly progress to ARF. *Acute tubular necrosis* (ATN) is the term used when AFR is the result of ischemia or toxins. Causes of ARF are listed in Table 19–2. The vast majority of cases of ARF are the result of trauma or surgery.

Identifying patients and procedures at high risk for developing ARF in the perioperative setting is important. Age (> 50 years) is a factor, since renal reserve falls progressively with age; cardiac or hepatic failure (associated with abnormal renal hemodynamics); cardiac surgery and abdominal aortic surgery (aortic cross-clamping); obstructive jaundice; septic shock; obstetric problems (postpartum hemorrhage, amniotic fluid embolism, and toxemia); crush injury (rhabdomyolysis and myoglobinuria); prolonged immobilization; and malignant hyperthermia are the major risk factors.

Acute renal failure represents a spectrum of renal dysfunction, with classifications based on the rate of urine formation and the quality of urine produced. It can be oliguric (urinary volume < 400 mL/day), nonoliguric (> 400 mL/day), or anuric (< 100 mL/day). The tubular concentrating ability of the kidneys varies with the type of ARF (prerenal, renal, postrenal) and is reflected in a variety of renal function tests (see "Evaluation of Renal Function," below). Because treatment for the different types of ARF varies, it is critical that the proper differential diagnosis of ARF be made.

Management of ARF can be divided into preventive and therapeutic approaches. Preventive measures are discussed under "Anesthetic Management," below. Treatment of established ARF involves primarily supportive care, with fluid, sodium, potassium, and protein restriction. Dialysis (peritoneal or hemodialysis), and, more recently, continuous arteriovenous hemodialysis (CAVHD) is employed to treat or prevent the uremic complications of ARF.

The clinical course of ARF is variable since, in most scenarios, ARF is one of many organ system dysfunctions. The morbidity and mortality of this disease is high, with sepsis being the most common cause of death.

CHRONIC RENAL FAILURE

The progressive and irreversible loss of nephron function and decline in GFR over at least a 3- to 6-month course is considered chronic renal failure (CRF). The most common causes

Table 19–2
CAUSES OF ACUTE RENAL FAILURE

Location of Primary Disorder	Clinical Examples
Prerenal	
Absolute decrease in effective blood volume	Hemorrhage, skin losses (burns, sweating), gastrointestinal losses (diarrhea, vomiting), renal losses (diuretics, glycosuria), fluid pooling (peritonitis, burns)
Relative decrease in blood volume (ineffective arterial volume)	Congestive heart failure, dysrhythmias, sepsis, anaphylaxis, liver failure
Arterial occlusion	Bilateral thromboembolism, thromboembolism of solitary kidney, aortic or renal artery aneurysm
Postrenal	
Ureteral obstruction	Bilateral or solitary kidney (calculi, neoplasm, clot, retroperitoneal fibrosis, iatrogenic)
Ureteral obstruction	Prostatitis
Venous occlusion	Bilateral or solitary kidney (renal vein thrombosis, neoplasm, iatrogenic)
Intrarenal	
Vascular	Vasculitis, malignant hypertension, vasopressors, eclampsia, microangiopathy, hyperviscosity states, nonsteroidal anti-inflammatory drugs, hypercalcemia, iodinated radiocontrast agents
Glomerulus	Acute glomerulonephritis
Tubular injury	
Ischemia	Profound hypotension, postrenal transplant, vasopressors, microvascular constriction
Intratubular pigments	Hemoglobinuria, myoglobinuria
Intratubular proteins	Myeloma
Intratubular crystals	Uric acid, oxalate, sulfonamides, phenazopyridine hydrochloride
Tubulointerstitial	Interstitial nephritis due to drugs, infection, radiation
Nephrotoxins	Antibiotics (gentamicin, kanamycin, neomycin, amikacin, tobramycin, streptomycin, cephaloridine, amphotericin B; metals (mercury, bismuth, uranium, arsenic, silver, cadmium, iron, antimony); solvents (carbon tetrachloride, glycol, tetrachlorethylene); iodinated contrast agents; streptozotocin, cisplatin

SOURCE: Wyngaarden JB, ed. *Cecil Textbook of Medicine.* 19th ed. Philadelphia: Saunders; 1992. With permission.

of CRF are hypertension, nephrosclerosis, diabetic nephropathy, chronic glomerulonephritis, pyelonephritis, and polycystic kidney disease. Stages of CRF are determined by the percentage of functioning nephrons: (1) decreased renal reserve (40%), (2) renal insufficiency (10 to 40%) and (3) uremia (10%). The *uremic syndrome* involves dialysis-dependent renal failure with widespread organ system involvement.

The manifestations of CRF represent multi–organ system dysfunction and are summarized in Table 19–3. The major derangements are discussed.

Table 19–3
THE UREMIC SYNDROME

1. Electrolyte disorders
   a. Potassium: hyperkalemia, total body depletion
   b. Sodium: salt-losing nephropathy, sodium retention
   c. Acidosis: metabolic acidosis with high "anion gap," type IV renal tubular acidosis (hyporeninemic hypoaldosteronism)
   d. Calcium: tendency toward hypocalcemia—phosphate retention and secondary hyperparathyroidism, with vitamin D deficiency
   e. Phosphate: hyperphosphatemia contributes to disorders of calcium metabolism
   f. Magnesium: accumulation due to excessive intake
   g. Aluminum: accumulation due to excessive intake
2. Cardiovascular abnormalities
   a. Accelerated atherosclerosis
   b. Hypertension
   c. Pericarditis
   d. Myocardial dysfunction
3. Hematologic abnormalities
   a. Anemia: erythropoietin deficiency, iron deficiency
   b. Leukocyte dysfunction: infection
   c. Hemorrhagic diathesis: defective platelet function
4. Gastrointestinal disorders
   a. Anorexia, nausea, vomiting, gastroparesis
   b. Gastrointestinal bleeding
   c. Disorders of taste
5. Renal osteodystrophy
   a. Osteomalacia
   b. Osteitis fibrosa (secondary hyperparathyroidism)
   c. Osteosclerosis
   d. Osteoporosis
6. Neurologic abnormalities
   a. Central nervous system: insomnia, fatigue, psychological symptoms, asterixis
   b. Peripheral neuropathy: stocking-glove sensory neuropathy
7. Myopathy: especially of proximal muscles
8. Impaired carbohydrate tolerance: peripheral resistance to insulin, hypoglycemia
9. Endocrine and metabolic disorders
   a. Glucose intolerance: insulin resistance, insulin degradation, hypoglycemia
   b. Other endocrine disorders: fertility, sterility
   c. Hypothermia
10. Hyperuricemia: clinical gout is rare; pseudogout occurs
11. Pruritus, soft tissue calcification, uremic frost

SOURCE: Wyngaarden JB. *Cecil Textbook of Medicine.* 19th ed. Philadelphia: Saunders; 1992. With permission.

Metabolic Manifestations Multiple electrolyte and metabolic abnormalities occur, including metabolic acidosis, hyperkalemia, hyperphosphatemia, hypermagnesemia, hyperuricemia, hypocalcemia, and hypoalbuminemia. The metabolic acidosis results from a high anion gap, due to decreased excretion of nonvolatile acids. Acidemia increases the proportion of drugs existing in the nonionized, unbound state, which increases their availability to effector sites. Water retention can result in hyponatremia, and sodium retention can cause ECF overload. Hyperkalemia is a potentially lethal abnormality due to its myocardial ramifications, especially since it can be exacerbated by factors commonly present in the perioperative period: tissue trauma, hemolysis, acidosis, infection, blood transfusions.

Cardiovascular Manifestations Systemic arterial hypertension is caused by abnormal renin-angiotensin activity and sodium retention. Tendencies toward fluid overload, anemia, and left ventricular hypertrophy in addition to hypertension result in a predisposition for congestive heart failure and pulmonary edema. Coronary artery disease is not uncommon in CRF (primarily due to hypertriglyceridemia), nor are dysrhythmias and conduction blocks, which are usually due to the metabolic abnormalities. Uremic cardiomyopathy and pericarditis as well as pleural or pericardial effusions also occur. Postdialysis hypovolemia is also an indirect result of CRF.

Hematologic Manifestations Anemia, an ubiquitous finding in CRF, is due to decreased erythropoietin, decreased survival of red blood cell's (RBC), and increased tendencies to bleed. Compensation for the resulting decreased O_2-carrying capacity is an increased cardiac output, decreased blood viscosity, and increased 2,3-diphosphoglycerate. The metabolic acidosis of CRF favors a right shift in the oxyhemoglobin dissociation curve, which promotes an easier release of oxygen from hemoglobin to the tissues, aiding in the patient's tolerance of the anemia.

Coagulopathy is primarily due to decreased platelet adhesiveness and is contributed to by coexisting liver disease or postdialysis heparinization. Impaired leukocyte function is also common; it causes a very high susceptibility to infection and sepsis.

Neurologic Manifestations Autonomic neuropathy is common in CRF, which alters the normal hemodynamic responses to changes in blood pressure and intravascular volume. Delayed gastric emptying also results (gastroparesis), with the subsequent predisposition to pulmonary aspiration. Peripheral neuropathies, especially of the distal extremities, are common. Other neurologic manifestations are related to degrees of encephalopathy.

☐ ANESTHETIC MANAGEMENT AND CONSIDERATIONS FOR PATIENTS WITH RENAL DISEASE

EVALUATION OF RENAL FUNCTION

The anesthetic care of patients with any degree of renal dysfunction, regardless of its etiology, is based upon the status of their preoperative renal function. The basic parameters for measuring renal function and guidelines for the preoperative assessment of the patient with renal disease is reviewed below.

Renal Function Tests

Urine

Urinalysis (UA) is the most common and useful noninvasive diagnostic test. The information gained from a routine UA includes pH, specific gravity, urinary sediment, and quantitative detection of glucose, protein, and blood. Urinary pH is not diagnostic; however, in conjunction with a serum pH and HCO_3, it is useful in evaluating renal tubular acidification function. Specific gravity reflects urine osmolality, which relates to renal tubular concentrating ability. Dipstick glucose elevations can indicate a tubular defect, decreased tubular reabsorption capacity, or hyperglycemia. Abnormalities in dipstick urine protein levels are more accurately assessed with 24-h urine collections. Hematuria (by dipstick or microscopic analysis) can signify inflammation, infection, trauma, stones, coagulopathy, or bleeding due to tumor. Microscopic analysis of urinary sediment can show casts, which indicate disease at the nephron level, or crystals, which are more indicative of metabolic problems.

Creatinine Clearance

Creatinine, an end product of muscle metabolism, is excreted solely by the kidneys. Its excretion is mainly determined by the GFR, hence creatinine clearance (Ccr) is the index used to estimate GFR. *Creatinine clearance is defined as the volume of plasma totally cleared of creatinine by the kidney per unit time and is expressed in terms of milliliters per minute.* Measurements of Ccr are usually determined over 24 h; however, 2-h collections are accurate. Correlations of Ccr to renal function are as follows: mild renal impairment (40 to 60 mL/min), moderate renal dysfunction, usually with symptoms (25 to 60 mL/min), and overt renal failure (< 25 mL/min).

Serum Creatinine

Creatinine production, as mentioned previously, is proportionate to muscle mass. It is excreted solely by the proximal tubules of the kidneys. Certain drugs (e.g., cimetidine) block creatinine secretion and increase serum creatinine without affecting GFR; large meat meals also increase serum creatinine without affecting GFR. Other nonrenal variables may be responsible for creatinine elevation, therefore serum creatinine is not considered a sensitive measure of changing renal function.

However, serum creatinine is still commonly utilized as an indicator of renal function, its value being inversely related to GFR. Normal serum creatinine is 0.8 to 1.3 mg/dL in men and 0.6 to 1.0 mg/dL in women.

Blood Urea Nitrogen

Renal handling of blood urea nitrogen (BUN) is complex; its serum levels are directly related to protein catabolism, which is not always consistent. The BUN is not used as a reliable indicator of GFR.

Tubular Function Tests

Tubular function tests reflect the kidney's ability to perform its usual homeostatic functions. These tests include (1) urinary sodium, which reflects volume status (< 20 mEq/L suggests volume depletion) and (2) fractional excretion of sodium (F_ENa), which is reflective of renal tubular Na reabsorption ($< 1\%$ suggests normo- or hypovolemia, whereas $> 1\%$ indicates tubular damage). Renal function tests are summarized in Table 19–4.

Preoperative Assessment

Acute Renal Failure

Most patients with ARF or who are developing ARF and require surgery and anesthesia are critically ill. Their renal dysfunction is usually due to prolonged shock, sepsis, or trauma and/or is associated with a major postoperative complication.

In cases of impending ARF, a thorough renal evaluation can lead to a timely recognition of the disease and implementation of strategies to either reverse the ARF immediately or at least prevent further reductions in renal function. A review of the patient's recent daily urine outputs in correlation with the laboratory indices of renal function can aid in this assessment. For patients with established ARF, an evaluation should be made of the efficacy of recent dialysis treatments to ensure as optimal a metabolic and hemodynamic status as possible.

Chronic Renal Failure

The focus of a preoperative evaluation should be the optimization of the patient's medical condition. The degree of renal impairment, which is reflected in the frequency of dialysis, should be ascertained and the date of the latest dialysis known. Any correction or reversal of uremic abnormalities that is possible should be done.

A careful evaluation of the cardiopulmonary status should be made, including indications of either fluid overload or hypovolemia (usually postdialysis). Exercise tolerance, recent blood pressure ranges, changes in weight, and chest x-ray findings are helpful with this. The electrocardiogram (ECG) should be checked for signs of hyperkalemia and hypocalcemia as well as ischemia or rhythm disturbances. An echocardiogram may be indicated for patients exhibiting symptoms of a pericardial effusion.

Table 19–4
RENAL FUNCTION TESTS

Test	Normal Value	Calculation	Interpretation
Serum creatinine	0.6–1.5 mg/dL (60–130 mmol/L)		Increases as GFR decreases
Urine creatinine (Ucr)	15–25 mg/kg body weight/day (0.13/0.22 mmol/kg/day)		Elevated in prerenal azotemia; decreased in parenchymal renal failure
Serum sodium (SNa)	135–145 mEq/L (135–145 mmol/L)		Decreased with chronic renal failure
Urine sodium (UNa)	Variable		Decreased with dehydration; increased with salt loading and renal failure
Serum osmolality (SOsm)	285–295 mOsm/kg H_2O (285–295 mmol/kg)		Decreased with renal failure; increased with dehydration
Urine osmolality (UOsm)	Variable		Decreased with renal failure; increased with dehydration
Urine flow rate (V) function	1 mL/min		Poor indication of renal function; varies with H_2O intake
Creatinine clearance (Ccr)	110–150 mL/min 105–132 mL/min or 104–125 mL/min 1.73 m²BSA	Ccr = Ucr/Ser × V	Decreased with decreased GFR; increased with volume load or high creatinine load
Free water clearance (CH_2O)	− 25 to − 100 mL/day	CH_2O = V (1−UOsm/SOsm)	Increased to positive with renal failure or volume loading; decreased with dehydration
Fractional excretion of sodium (F_ENa)	$< 1\%$	$F_E Na = \dfrac{UNa \times SCr}{UCr \times SNa} \times 100\%$	Increased with parenchymal renal failure

m²BSA = body surface area expressed in meters²; Ucr/Ser = urine to serum ratio of creatinine; V = urinary flow rate; V = urinary flow rate, UOsm/SOsm = urine to serum osmolar ratio; UNa = urine sodium, SCr = serum creatinine, UCr = urine creatinine, SNa = serum sodium.
SOURCE: Grande CM. *Textbook of Trauma, Anesthesia, and Critical Care.* St Louis: Mosby; 1993. With permission.

Arterial blood gases are helpful for checking acid base balance as well as for hypoxemia. A moderate metabolic acidosis is frequently present. Other preoperative laboratory values of importance include electrolytes, albumin, hemoglobin, platelet count, and a coagulation panel. Since multiple perioperative events are capable of raising potassium levels, serum potassium values higher than 5.5 to 6.0 mEq/L should warrant a postponement of elective surgery until normalization of potassium can be accomplished with dialysis. If emergency surgery is required, hyperkalemia may be treated with glucose/insulin and hyperventilation. Anemia will be a predictable finding; hematocrits of 15 to 25% are usually tolerated well. Therefore low hematocrits are not treated with RBC transfusions unless the anemia is severe and/or in association with severe coronary artery disease or if significant intraoperative blood loss is expected. Platelet counts are often low; however, the primary problem is usually platelet dysfunction. Hemodialysis (by eliminating the compounds that cause platelet dysfunction) usually restores adequate platelet function.

INTRAOPERATIVE MONITORING

The patient's general medical condition and the surgical procedure dictate any monitoring requirements beyond what is currently considered standard. Patients with ARF typically come to the operating room with indwelling invasive monitoring lines because their critical status entails several indications for aggressive hemodynamic monitoring. For both ARF and CRF patients undergoing surgeries associated with significant blood loss and fluid shifts, the need for accurate monitoring of intravascular volume may call for intra-arterial, central venous, and pulmonary artery lines. Frequent analysis of electrolytes and hematocrit values may also be an indication for placement of an intra-arterial line.

Close monitoring of urine output in patients with ARF or impending ARF is critical (recognizing that urine output is not always reflective of adequate renal function). Use of a peripheral nerve stimulator allows for titration of muscle relaxants according to an individual's response, since drug effects are unpredictable in patients with renal disease. During the placement of monitors and the positioning of patients, care should be taken with the extremities where dialysis access devices or sites are located.

ANESTHETIC MANAGEMENT

General Principles   (1) Utilize a technique and drugs that will maintain maximally available RBF and GFR, especially during those phases of anesthesia where hypotension is likely (postinduction, no surgical stimulation, major and rapid blood loss). (2) Minimize the exposure of the kidneys to nephrotoxins (see Table 19–5). (Principles 1 and 2 pertain to patients with ARF). (3) Although most drugs that are used to provide anesthesia are converted to inactive metabolites in the liver and do not depend on renal function to ter-

Table 19–5
NEPHROTOXIC AGENTS

Agent	Remarks
Antibiotics	
Gentamycin	Reduce dose or increase interval
Tobramycin	during renal failure
Amikacin	Monitor blood levels to guide dose or interval
Cephaltohin	Prolong interval in renal failure
Cephalexin	
Semisynthetic penicillins	
Rifampin	Monitor blood levels to guide
Vancomycin	dosage intervals
Amphotericin B	
Analgesics and anti-inflammatory drugs	
Heroin	
Phenacetin	Cyclooxygenase inhibitors impair
Phenylbutazone	vasodilator prostaglandin
Indomethacin	synthesis and autoregulation
Ketorolac	
Anesthetics	
Methoxyflurane	
Radiocontrast agents	Forced diuresis protective to kidney
Angiotensin-converting enzyme inhibitors	Avoid in combination with nonsteroidal antiinflammatory drugs
Organic solvents	
Diesel fuel	
Glue (sniffed)	
Biologic substances	
Hemoglobin	Alkalinize urine and forced diuresis
Myoglobin	

SOURCE: Grande CM. *Textbook of Trauma, Anesthesia, and Critical Care.* St Louis: Mosby-Year Book; 1993.

minate their action, a modification of dosages for certain drugs should be made to prevent accumulation of those drugs or their active metabolites. (4) The pharmacologic actions of drugs may be altered as a result of the systemic effects of azotemia (e.g., decreased protein binding, greater brain penetration due to changes in the blood-brain barrier). (5) Prophylaxis for pulmonary aspiration should be considered (for CRF patients with delayed gastric emptying), especially when nausea, vomiting, and GI bleeding are present. (6) Spontaneous ventilation under anesthesia can result in respiratory acidosis, which can potentially exacerbate preexisting acidemia; therefore, controlled ventilation may be preferable. (7) Avoid respiratory alkalosis, since it favors a left shift of the oxyhemoglobin dissociation curve; this shift is not tolerated well in anemic states, it exacerbates hypocalcemia and may reduce cerebral blood flow. (8) The duration of local anesthetics used in regional techniques may be decreased by as much as 40% due to acidosis and increases in cardiac output.

Intravenous Agents   Decreased protein binding of *barbiturates* and *etomidate* enhances their pharmacologic effects, therefore doses should be reduced and titrated to effect;

their pharmacokinetics (as well as that of *propofol*) are unchanged by renal disease. Some of the active hepatic metabolites of *ketamine* are excreted by the kidney, so accumulation might occur. The hypertensive effect of ketamine may exacerbate the hypertension seen in renal disease.

Benzodiazepines are also less protein-bound; therefore an increased sensitivity results. The active metabolites of *diazepam* in particular may accumulate. The effects, pharmacokinetics, and elimination of *fentanyl, sufentanil,* and *alfentanil* are unchanged by renal function. The active metabolites of *morphine* and *meperidine* do accumulate and have been shown to prolong respiratory depression. Accumulation of a metabolite of meperidine (normeperidine) can cause seizures.

Opioid agonists-antagonists (butorphanol, nalbuphine, and buprenorphine) pharmacokinetics are unchanged. *Anticholinergic agents* (atropine and glycopyrrolate) have active metabolites that depend on renal excretion, therefore accumulation is a theoretical risk; in the usual doses this is not a problem. *Droperidol* metabolites may accumulate after large doses, but small doses (< 2.5 mg) can be used in the presence of renal disease. *Metoclopramide* will accumulate, since it is partly excreted in the urine. *Ondansetron* undergoes extensive hepatic degradation, making accumulation less likely.

Succinylcholine may be used safely in the absence of hyperkalemia (> 5 mEq/L). Dialysis lowers serum cholinesterase levels, potentially prolonging the effect of succinylcholine. Since it is degraded in plasma by ester hydrolysis and Hofmann elimination, the pharmacologic profile of *atracurium* is unchanged by renal disease. *Mivacurium* is minimally dependent on renal excretion (metabolized by plasma cholinesterase) and can be safely used. Some 10% to 20% of *vecuronium* is dependent on renal elimination and its action is only slightly prolonged in patients with renal disease. The fact that vecuronium is devoid of cardiovascular side effects makes it a safe choice for the hemodynamically unstable patient. *Curare, pancuronium, pipecuronium,* and *doxacurium* have a definite prolonged effect, since these drugs are primarily eliminated in the urine. The anticholinesterase agents (*edrophonium, neostigmine,* and *pyridostigmine*) also depend primarily on renal excretion; therefore their actions are prolonged, usually more so than those of the nondepolarizing muscle relaxants.

Inhalational Agents Since the halogenated volatile agents do not depend at all on renal function for elimination and do not seem to have a direct effect on autoregulation of RBF, they are safe choices for patients with renal disease. Furthermore, if adequate arterial pressure and cardiac output are maintained during the delivery of an inhalation-based anesthetic, the renal autoregulatory mechanisms will maintain an adequate GFR.

With the exception of *methoxyflurane* and *enflurane* (which, with prolonged exposure, could be nephrotoxic), any of the volatile agents (*isoflurane, halothane, desflurane*) can be used with low risk for toxicity. The use of *sevoflurane* is controversial. *Nitrous oxide* is not contraindicated in renal disease; however, the patient's degree of anemia and the associated decrease in oxygen-carrying capacity may call for the use of high inspired oxygen concentrations.

The volatile agents provide a steady, titratable depth of anesthesia and are useful in controlling intraoperative hypertension and reducing the dose of muscle relaxants necessary for adequate surgical exposure. The blood-gas partition coefficients for the inhalation agents are decreased by 15% to 25% in the presence of severe anemia; therefore the rate of induction and emergence from general anesthesia may be increased.

Fluid Management In situations of prerenal azotemia that have the potential to progress to ARF, fluid therapy is the mainstay of prevention of further decrease in renal function. Adequate intravascular volume should be maintained to restore RBF and GFR. In some instances it is possible to convert oliguric ARF to nonoliguric ARF (which holds a better prognosis) by using diuretics or dopamine in conjunction with adequate intravascular volume replacement. Mannitol is effective in increasing GFR and provides a flushing effect (for toxin washout), furosemide is useful in maintaining urinary output. Renal dose dopamine (1 to 3 µg/kg/min) improves GFR by improving RBF (specifically, intracortical redistribution of blood flow).

Patients with established ARF undergoing surgical procedures with minimal blood and insensible fluid losses require careful replacement of the insensible losses. Procedures associated with major fluid losses or shifts require replacement with isotonic crystalloids, colloids, or both. There is justifiable concern with fluid overload; however, the risk:benefit ratio must be weighed in terms of the consequences of fluid overload (which is treatable) versus the consequences of a worsening renal failure.

Patients with CRF require very judicious replacement of intraoperative fluid and blood losses. Lactated Ringer's solution (4 mEq K^+/mL) is best avoided, especially when large volume replacements are a potential. Dextrose-containing solutions should also be avoided due to the predisposition to glucose intolerance.

Anesthesia for Placement of Arteriovenous Access Perhaps the most common type of surgical procedure performed on patients with CRF is the creation of vascular access in an upper extremity for the purpose of hemodialysis. Access is usually in the form of a subcutaneous arteriovenous (AV) fistula using a variety of combinations of upper extremity veins and arteries. In the absence of suitable veins, prosthetic grafts are placed. Patients with CRF who undergo hemodialysis frequently return to the operating room for thrombectomies (not uncommonly, clots form in the vascular access site) or revision/replacement of their fistulas/grafts. Typically, these are ASA III and IV patients requiring the full range of anesthetic considerations just reviewed.

The anesthetic techniques used for this type of procedure are monitored anesthesia care, upper extremity blocks, or general anesthesia. Local anesthetic infiltration with monitored anesthesia care is usually sufficient for the initial creation of a vascular access, simple declotting, or revision procedures. Upper extremity blocks are also used (in the absence of a coagulopathy), especially when multiple revisions have been attempted and more extensive vascular invasion is anticipated. General anesthesia may be required for those patients in whom local anesthesia is insufficient or for whom regional anesthesia is either contraindicated or unsuccessful.

SURGICAL PROCEDURES INVOLVING THE KIDNEY

NEPHRECTOMY

Preoperative Considerations   Nephrectomies are classified as simple, partial, or radical. Simple nephrectomies are performed for benign conditions on patients who span the age and illness spectrum. Partial nephrectomies are indicated for benign tumors, small renal cell carcinomas, or anatomic abnormalities; the patient population also encompasses a wide range of age and physical status. Radical nephrectomies are performed for malignancies. The highest incidence of urologic cancers occurs in elderly males; furthermore, there are possible associations of renal carcinoma with cigarette smoking. For these reasons, the coexistence of coronary artery disease and chronic obstructive pulmonary disease is not uncommon. Hypertensive disease (of renal origin) may also be present. Impaired renal function may be the result of advanced age or due to postrenal causes if urinary tract obstruction is present.

Surgical Considerations   The procedure involves ligation of the renal artery and vein, and removal of the kidney, adrenal and surrounding fat, and fascia. Although most tumors are confined to the kidney, tumor extension into the inferior vena cava, hepatic vein, or right atrium does occur, greatly increasing the risk for a pulmonary embolus. If the tumor involves the renal vein and/or the inferior vena cava (IVC), the IVC may be clamped. If a large atrial thrombus occurs, cardiopulmonary bypass may be required.

The surgical incision is either thoracoabdominal (large tumor with a thrombus present), transabdominal, or flank, with the latter two being the most common. The flank incision necessitates a modified lateral decubitus position with marked flexion and elevation of the kidney rest to produce optimal exposure of the kidney. This position is notorious for producing hypotension due to compression of the great vessels, pooling of blood in the lower extremities, and reduced venous return from the upper body.

The proximity of the surgical site to the diaphragm results in the risk of a pneumothorax if the pleura is inadvertently entered. If a thoracoabdominal incision is used, chest tubes are routinely placed.

Intraoperative Considerations   General endotracheal anesthesia is usually recommended for nephrectomies. Regional anesthesia (spinal or epidural) is theoretically possible; however, the procedure can be lengthy and the extreme positioning (for flank incisions) would lead to patient discomfort and ventilatory difficulty. General anesthesia in combination with a spinal or epidural offers the advantages of decreased general anesthetic requirements and an excellent route for postoperative analgesia.

The choice of technique and pharmacologic agents should be dictated by the patient's coexistent medical problems. Similarly, the use of invasive monitoring is dependent upon the patient's preoperative status. The hypotension that occurs with the placement of the patient in the lateral position can be minimized by volume loading, careful titration of anesthetic depth, and gradual assumption of the position. The usual precautions taken for injuries associated with the lateral position should be taken (See also Chapter 10.) Close monitoring of the intravascular volume and blood loss (which can be rapid and large) is essential and may necessitate the placement of an intra-arterial pressure monitor. Urine output, monitored frequently, should be correlated to the phase of the surgical procedure, as the urinary flow may be interrupted during the operation. Vigilance for signs and symptoms of a pneumothorax should be maintained; a postoperative chest x-ray should be taken to exclude the presence of this complication.

RADICAL NEPHRECTOMY FOR WILMS' TUMOR

Preoperative Considerations   Nephroblastoma (Wilms' tumor) is the second most common solid abdominal tumor of childhood. This malignancy occurs in otherwise healthy children less than 4 years of age (one third of those affected are less than 1 year old). Bilateral nephroblastomas occur in 3% to 10% of patients. Common clinical findings in these patients are anemia, disturbances in micturition, and GI symptoms (vomiting, constipation, or diarrhea). Hypertension (sometimes severe enough to cause encephalopathy or CHF) may occur due to renin secretion by the tumor or secondary renin secretion from compression of the renal vasculature by the tumor.

Extrarenal tumor extension of nephroblastomas is not uncommon; invasion into the renal vein occurs in as many as 40% of cases, the IVC in less than 10%, and the right atrium in less than 1%. A thorough preoperative evaluation of the extent of tumor involvement is essential to optimal surgical and anesthetic management of patients undergoing a Wilms' tumor resection. A cardiac evaluation includes ultrasonography or computed tomography to reveal large vessel involvement and an echocardiogram to rule out right atrial involvement as well as to evaluate the ventricular function. In addition to a complete cardiac assessment, the presence of renal, hepatic (dysfunction due to mass effect or vascular obstruction), and pulmonary (lungs are the most common site of metastasis) involvement should be revealed. Some children with Wilms' tumors are treated with prenephrectomy radiation and/or chemotherapy; hence the type, dose, and secondary effects of the radiation or chemotherapeutic agents must be considered. (See also Chapter 32.)

Infants and children undergoing this procedure will be in varying states of health, depending on the stage of the tumor upon diagnosis. Prior to the initiation of anesthesia, severe anemia should be corrected (usually to a hemoglobin of 10 g/dL^{-1}), as well as electrolyte and acid/base derangements. Adequate prehydration must be accomplished, especially in cases of severe preoperative hypertension with a resulting contracted intravascular volume.

Surgical Considerations   The intent of the operation is to explore the abdomen for actual tumor involvement, and if operable, to do a radical nephrectomy. Extensive tumor involvement may necessitate radical en bloc resections. The patient is placed supine; a transverse incision that can be extended to the flank is used. Because the tumors are large and frequently involve major vessels, extreme preparedness for thoracic extension of the procedure and massive blood loss is critical. When IVC and/or right atrial involvement is known or suspected, preparations for utilizing cardiopulmonary bypass (CPB) must be accomplished. That is, access to the great vessels for CPB via a median sternotomy is accomplished prior to manipulation of the tumor.

Intraoperative Considerations   General endotracheal anesthesia with an intravenous induction is indicated, using techniques that take into consideration the patient's cardiac reserve. Where there is a large abdominal mass, a modified rapid-sequence induction is recommended and continuous stomach decompression maintained. Because of the potential for interrupted IVC blood flow, large-bore intravenous access via the upper extremities or the external jugular vein is preferred. Monitoring includes intra-arterial and central venous (placed with extreme caution to avoid disruption of tumor thrombus) pressure as well as continuous urine output. Intraoperative complications to anticipate and prepare for are hypotension (due to massive blood loss or IVC obstruction), pulmonary embolus (due to tumor embolism), hypertension (due to tumor or adrenal manipulation), hypothermia (extensive open abdominal exposure of long duration), and hypoventilation (large abdominal retractors and packing). Especially in cases with extrarenal extension of the tumor, a coordinated effort involving pediatric and cardiac surgeons and the anesthesia providers is essential in the management of Wilms' tumor resections.

BIBLIOGRAPHY

Brenner BM ed. *Brenner & Rector's The Kidney.* 5th ed, vol 1. Philadelphia: Saunders; 1996.

Brown BR. Anesthetic management of the patient with abnormal liver function. In: *44th Annual Refresher Course Lectures and Clinical Update Program.*: American Society of Anesthesiologists; 1993–chap 241:1–6.

Caldwell JE. New skeletal muscle relaxants. In: Feeley TW, Royston D, eds. *International Anesthesiology Clinics: New Drugs in Anesthesia.* Vol 33, no 1. Boston: Little, Brown, 1995:39–60.

Faust RJ. ed. *Anesthesiology Review.* 2nd ed. New York: Churchill Livingstone, 1994:79–81, 98–99, 515–516.

Ganong WF, ed. *Review of Medical Physiology.* 17th ed. Norwalk, Conn: Appleton & Lange; 1995—chap 24:418–422; chap 38:641–669; chap 39:670–677.

Green DM. The diagnosis and management of Wilms' tumor. In: *The Pediatric Clinics of North America: Symposium on Pediatric Oncology.* Vol 32, no 3. Philadelphia: Saunders, 1985:735–750.

Green DM, Finkelstein JZ, et al: Remaining problems in the treatment of patients with Wilms' tumor. In: Horowitz ME, Pizzo PA, eds. *The Pediatric Clinics of North America: Solid Tumors in Children.* Vol 38, no 2. Philadelphia: Saunders, 1991:475–488.

Gregory G, ed. *Pediatric Anesthesia.* Vol 2, 2nd ed. New York: Churchill Livingstone, 1989:1012–1013, 1028–1029.

Guyton AC, *Textbook of Medical Physiology.* 8th ed. Philadelphia: Saunders; 1991:286–295; 298–307; 308–318; 320–328; 330–342.

Jaffe RA, Samuels SI, eds. *Anesthesiologist's Manual of Surgical Procedures.* New York: Raven Press, 1994:262–267, 559–564.

Mazze RI. Renal effects of sevoflurane. *Anesthesiology.* 1995; 83:443–445.

Mehernoor FW, White PF. New antiemetic drugs. In: Feeley TW, Royston D, eds. *International Anesthesiology Clinics: New Drugs in Anesthesia.* Vol 33, no 1. Boston: Little, Brown; 1995:1–20.

Miller RD, ed. *Anesthesia.* 3rd ed. New York: Churchill Livingstone, 1990:601–619, 1791–1808.

Muravchik S. *The Anesthetic Plan: From Physiologic Principles to Clinical Strategies.* St Louis: Mosby-Year Book; 1991:286–324.

Morgan GE, Mikhail MS. *Clinical Anesthesiology.* Norwalk, Conn: Appleton & Lange, 1992:509–522, 523–533.

Przybylol HJ, Stevenson GW. Anesthetic management of children with intracardiac extension of abdominal tumors. *Anesth Analg* 1994; 78:172–175.

Sladen RN. Perioperative renal protection. In: *44th Annual Refresher Course Lectures and Clinical Update Program.* American Society of Anesthesiologists; 1993:1–7.

Stene JK. Acute renal failure. In Grande CM, ed. *Textbook of Trauma Anesthesia and Critical Care.* St Louis: Mosby-Year Book; 1993:856–864.

Stene JK. Trauma patients with acute and chronic renal failure. In: Grande CM, ed. *Textbook of Trauma Anesthesia and Critical Care.* St Louis: Mosby-Year Book; 1993:737–743.

Stoelting RK. *Pharmacology & Physiology in Anesthetic Practice.* 2nd ed. Philadelphia: Lippincott; 1991:769–781.

Stoelting RK, Dierdorf SF. *Anesthesia and Co-Existing Disease.* 2nd ed. New York: Churchill Livingstone; 1988:409–443, 864–866.

Waugaman W, ed. *Principles and Practice of Nurse Anesthesia.* Norwalk, Conn: Appleton & Lange; 1988:309–319.

Yao FS. Kidney transplant. In: Yao FS, Artusio JF. *Anesthesiology Problem-Oriented Patient Management.* 3rd ed. Philadelphia: Lippincott; 1993:446–464.

☐ QUESTIONS

1. Which of the following is true about the nephron?
   a. The glomerular capillary network is a high-pressure system.
   b. The primary function of the proximal tubule is sodium reabsorption.
   c. The distal tubule is impermeable to water.
   d. All are correct.

2. In relation to anesthesia-induced changes in renal blood flow, which of the following is true?
   a. Surgical stimulation, light anesthesia, or hypotension may cause a decrease in RBF, GFR, and urine output.
   b. Catecholamines and angiotensin II increase RBF.
   c. Levels of ADH are increased during general anesthesia and may cause an increase in urine output.
   d. All inhalational anesthetics have the inorganic fluoride ion as a metabolite and are therefore potentially nephrotoxic.

3. Acute renal failure:
   a. Causes the retention of nitrogenous waste products
   b. Is either prerenal, renal, or postrenal in origin
   c. Can occur as the result of a crush injury of the lower extremity
   d. All are correct.

4. Chronic renal failure results in several metabolic and electrolyte disturbances, including:
   a. Decreased pH, decreased K^+, decreased phosphate, increased Mg^{++}, increased Ca^{++}
   b. Decreased pH, increased K^+, decreased phosphate, increased Mg^{++}, decreased Ca^{++}, decreased albumin, increased uric acid
   c. Increased pH, increased K^+, increased phosphate, increased Mg^{++}, decreased Ca^{++}
   d. Decreased pH, increased K^+, increased phosphate, increased Mg^{++}, increased uric acid, decreased Ca^{++}, decreased albumin

5. Treatment of hyperkalemia includes all except:
   a. Hyperventilation
   b. Use of lactated Ringer's solution for all intravenous maintenance therapy
   c. Insulin/glucose therapy
   d. Dialysis

6. The renal function test that most effectively assesses glomerular filtration is:
   a. Free water clearance
   b. Fractional excretion of sodium
   c. Urine-to-plasma creatinine ratios
   d. Creatinine clearance

7. A 64-year-old male with a history of IDDM, HTN, and chronic renal insufficiency is scheduled for an emergency exploratory laparotomy for an obstruction of the small bowel. His preop Cr is 2.1. Anesthesia management for this patient includes all of the following except:
   a. Prophylactic use of renal dose dopamine as early as possible
   b. Maintenance of an adequate intravascular volume
   c. Avoidance of NSAIDs and aminoglycosides
   d. Maintenance of arterial pressure within the autoregulatory range of RBF and GFR

8. Clinical manifestations associated with chronic renal failure include all of the following except:
   a. Hypertension
   b. Anemia
   c. Thrombocytopenia
   d. Increased gastric emptying time

9. All of the following statements regarding acid base regulation are true except:
   a. The proximal tubule normally secretes H^+ in exchange for HCO_3^- filtration.
   b. In an acidotic state, the urine pH decreases.
   c. The regulatory mechanism for acid-base balance has a rapid onset.
   d. Elevated CO_2 levels stimulate more rapid secretion of H^+.

10. NSAIDs are contraindicated in patients with renal disease because:
    a. They are protein bound.
    b. They are metabolized by the kidney.
    c. Prostaglandin inhibitors decrease intrinsic renal vasodilitation, thereby decreasing RBF and GFR.
    d. They undergo phase II biotransformation.

11. Renal blood flow:
    a. Is hampered by prostaglandins
    b. Represents 40% of cardiac output
    c. Is autoregulated over a arterial pressure range of 60 to 80 mmHg
    d. Is not influenced by neural factors
    e. Is autoregulated by tubuloglomerular feedback

12. The term countercurrent system refers to:
    a. A hepatic mechanism for blood cleansing involving Kupffer cells in the sinusoids
    b. A renal process involving the macula densa and the vasa recta, which concentrates urine
    c. The renal mechanism by which the proximal and distal tubules create a hypertonic medullary interstitium

   d. The renal mechanism involving the loop of Henle and the vasa recta to create and maintain a hypertonic medullary interstitium

   e. The renal mechanism by which the loop of Henle creates a hypertonic cortical interstitium and the vasa recta maintain this hypertonicity due to its brisk flow

13. A patient's azotemia is thought to be prerenal in origin. You would expect:

   a. That this condition is irreversible, therefore hemodialysis should be anticipated

   b. An oliguric state with a decreased 24-h creatinine clearance, with normal urinary sediment

   c. A dilute urine with a higher-than-normal amount of casts seen in microscopic analysis

   d. An anuric state with an increased 24-h creatinine clearance

   e. A normal urine output of high osmolality

14. Antidiuretic hormone (ADH) is required in the formation of concentrated urine because:

   a. It decreases the active transport of sodium in the proximal and distal tubules.

   b. It is released in response to increased stretch of the atrial baroreceptors.

   c. It increases the permeability of the distal convoluted tubule to water.

   d. It decreases the permeability of the proximal convoluted tubule to sodium.

   e. Its release from the hypothalamus is stimulated by the osmoreceptors in the posterior pituitary gland.

15. Acid-base regulation in the kidneys is primarily accomplished in the renal tubules by:

   a. Reabsorption of chloride in the loop of Henle

   b. Excretion of phosphates in the proximal tubule

   c. Reabsorption of bicarbonate

   d. Secretion of urea

   e. An ADH-mediated increase in water reabsorption

16. Which of the following statements is true regarding the regulation of the glomerular filtration rate (GFR)?

   a. It is primarily influenced by the intracapsular hydrostatic pressure.

   b. Autoregulation of GFR is accomplished via simultaneous effects on the afferent and efferent arterioles.

   c. Autoregulation of GFR occurs in direct response to ADH levels.

   d. Regulation of GFR depends primarily on the plasma colloid oncotic pressure in the glomerulus.

   e. Autoregulation of GFR is not mediated by the juxtaglomerular apparatus.

17. A 48-year-old man with end-stage renal disease has been on hemodialysis for 8 years. He is scheduled for a revision of his AV fistula. Preoperative laboratory tests

indicate a hemoglobin of 7 g/100 mL. Which of the following statements is true regarding anemia in patients with chronic renal failure (CRF)?

   a. Hemoglobin concentrations of 5 to 7 g/100 mL are unusual, even for CRF patients; therefore surgery should be postponed until the etiology of the anemia can be determined.

   b. The primary cause of anemia in CRF is iron deficiency due to frequent sampling and blood loss in hemodialysis coils.

   c. Chronic anemia is not uncommon in CRF. Compensatory findings for low hemoglobin concentrations include an increased cardiac output, increased levels of 2,3 DPG, and a right shift of the oxygen dissociation curve.

   d. The acidemia of CRF causes a left shift of the oxygen dissociation curve, with resultant easy release of oxygen from hemoglobin to tissue, thereby compensating for anemia.

   e. Hemoglobin concentrations of 5 to 7 g/100 mL are not uncommon in CRF patients, necessitating frequent blood transfusions, especially prior to surgery.

18. A 56-year-old female with a known history of CRF is scheduled for emergency surgery, which requires general anesthesia. It is not known when she last had hemodialysis. Anesthetic considerations for induction of general anesthesia include:

   a. Rapid sequence induction, with succinylcholine as the best choice of muscle relaxant for facilitating tracheal intubation

   b. Rapid-sequence induction, with succinylcholine contraindicated, since decreased pseudocholinesterase levels (found in CRF) will greatly prolong its effect

   c. An awake fiberoptic intubation, since depolarizing muscle relaxants are contraindicated in CRF patients

   d. Rapid-sequence induction; a serum potassium level, if known prior to induction, will help determine if succinylcholine can be safely used

   e. Checking the ECG tracing in lead V for hyperkalemic changes prior to initiating a rapid-sequence induction with succinylcholine

19. Which statement best reflects the direct effect of halogenated inhalation anesthetics on renal function?

   a. All of the currently available volatile anesthetics are metabolized in the body to a significant degree; therefore they should be considered nephrotoxic.

   b. Isoflurane undergoes minimal biotransformation; therefore it presents a minimal risk for nephrotoxicity.

   c. Nephrotoxicity due to an inhalation anesthetic is the result of the decrease in GFR caused by the product of biotransformation, the inorganic fluoride ion.

   d. The use of halogenated inhalation agents in conjunction with nitrous oxide is not recommended in delivering a general anesthetic to patients with pre-existing renal disease.

e. The direct effects of the inhalation agents on the kidney more profoundly affect renal function than do the indirect effects of inhalation agents.

20. Choose the statement that most accurately reflects the use of nondepolarizing muscle relaxants in patients with chronic renal failure.

a. Atracurium and mivacurium are the preferred muscle relaxants due to their metabolism by enzymatic ester hydrolysis and nonenzymatic alkaline hydrolysis (Hofmann elimination).

b. Mivacurium is the short-acting muscle relaxant of choice since its use does not affect intracellular potassium and it is metabolized by Hofmann elimination.

c. Vecuronium is primarily excreted in the liver, but since 10 to 20% of the drug is excreted by the kidneys, it cannot be used without risk of nephrotoxicity.

d. The elimination half-life of atracurium is unchanged in patients with CRF, and the elimination half-life of vecuronium is prolonged.

e. Hypermagnesemia may accompany CRF, which shortens the duration of nondepolarizing muscle relaxants.

☐ ANSWERS

1.	d	5.	b	9.	c	13.	b	17.	c
2.	a	6.	d	10.	c	14.	c	18.	d
3.	d	7.	a	11.	c	15.	c	19.	b
4.	d	8.	c	12.	d	16.	b	20.	d

CHAPTER
20

Hematology

Rita Weiss

☐ RED BLOOD CELLS (ERYTHROCYTES)

ANATOMY AND PHYSIOLOGY

One of the largest organs in the body, the bone marrow, is the primary site of erythrocyte of red blood cell (RBC) production. The RBCs originate as nucleated cells and in the process of maturation the nucleus is extruded (Fig. 20–1). The erythroblastic island is the anatomic unit of erythropoiesis in the normal adult.[1] The process of *erythropoiesis* is the production of a constant number of RBCs needed to maintain homeostasis. The life span of the mature RBC is approximately 120 days. The cell circulates as a deformable biconcave disk and is eventually removed from the circulation by the spleen. The spleen will sequester RBCs that are senescent or have structural alterations. Aberrations in the morphology can be produced by changes in the cell membrane such as cytoskeleton abnormalities, alterations in the lipid bilayer, and decreased concentration of adenosine triphosphate (ATP). Table 20–1 lists the normal components of blood.

The function of the RBC is the transportation of oxygen and carbon dioxide. The RBC membrane is bilaminar. Cytoskeletal proteins below this membrane play a crucial role in maintaining the stability of the membrane and the shape of the RBC. Alteration of the membrane structure by deficiencies of spectrin, phospholipid, or cholesterol will shorten the life span of the cell. This semipermeable membrane allows water and anions, HCO^{-3} and Cl^-, to enter the cell and excludes the movement of cations such as Na^+ and K^+. The energy necessary to maintain the RBC membrane is derived almost exclusively from the Embden-Meyerhof anaerobic

pathway. As the RBC ages, the anaerobic pathway becomes less efficient, causing the membrane to be deformed and removed from the circulation by the spleen. The protein hemoglobin is degraded into its components and recycled.

The earliest RBC contains a nucleus composed of DNA. As the cells mature, extrusion of the nucleus occurs and it is during this developmental stage that the majority of the hemoglobin is made. At the time of birth, the major hemoglobin production is hemoglobin F, accounting for up to 85% of the total hemoglobin.[2] The level of hemoglobin F is inversely proportional to gestational age and unaffected by environment and oxygen tension that occurs at birth.[3] The affinity for oxygen is *greater* in hemoglobin F than in hemoglobin A, facilitating the transfer of oxygen from mother to fetus. The oxygen tension at which the hemoglobin of cord blood is 50% saturated is 6 to 8 mm Hg lower than that of adult blood. Hemoglobin F will decrease as the infant matures and by 4 to 6 months will have attained approximately 40% to 50% of hemoglobin A. In the adult, hemoglobin A comprises 95% of the total hemoglobin, the remainder of which is the minor hemoglobins A_2 and F. Amino acid sequence defines the primary structure of globin so that any alteration in the position can affect stability and function of the molecule and impair its ability to bind oxygen. Oxygen is bound to the protein hemoglobin during its course through the pulmonary circulation, becoming almost fully saturated (1.34 mL O_2/g hemoglobin) and is then released during perfusion through the capillary beds. This exchange of gases (oxygen for the metabolic end product, carbon dioxide) is necessary for tissue and organ survival. This process is known as *respiratory movement*. The affinity of hemoglobin for oxygen is modified by three intracellular cofactors: hydrogen ion, carbon dioxide, and 2,3-diphosphoglycerate (2,3-DPG). Increasing the concentration of each of these can cause a shift to the

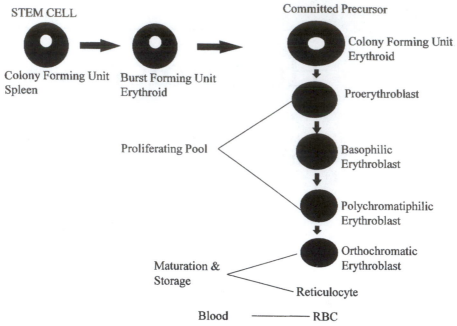

Figure 20–1 Red blood cell maturation

Table 20–1
CELLULAR COMPONENTS OF THE BLOOD

Cell	Structural Characteristics	Normal Amounts in Circulating Blood	Function	Life Span
Erythrocyte (red blood cell)	Nonnucleated cytoplasmic disk containing hemoglobin	4.2–6.2 million/mm³	Gas transport to and from tissue cells and lungs	80–120 days
Leukocyte (white blood cell)	Nucleated cell	5000–10,000/mm³	Bodily defense mechanisms	See below
Lymphocyte	Mononuclear immunocyte	25–33% of leukocyte count (leukocyte has differential)	Humoral and cell-mediated immunity	Days or years depending on type
Monocyte and macrophage	Large mononuclear phagocyte	3–7% of leukocyte differential	Phagocytosis; mononuclear phagocyte system	Months or years
Eosinophil	Segmented polymorphonuclear granulocyte	1–4% of leukocyte differential	Phagocytosis, antibody-mediated defense against parasites, allergic reactions, associated with Hodgkin's disease, recovery phase of infection	Unknown
Neutrophil	Segmented polymorphonuclear granulocyte	57–67% of leukocyte differential	Phagocytosis, particularly during early phase of inflammation	4 d
Basophil	Segmented polymorphonuclear granulocyte	0–0.75% of leukocyte differential	Unknown, but associated with allergic reactions and mechanical irritation	Unknown
Platelet	Irregularly shaped cytoplasmic fragment (not a cell)	140,000–340,000/mm³	Hemostasis following vascular injury; normal coagulation and clot formation/retraction	8–11 d

SOURCE: Reproduced by permission from McCance KL, Huether SE, eds. *Pathophysiology: The Biologic Basis for Disease in Adults and Children.* CV Mosby; 1990:755.

right in the oxygen dissociation curve decreasing oxygen affinity. Changes in the oxygen affinity with pH is known as the Bohr effect[4,5] exemplified by the equation:[6]

$$Deoxy\ Hb \rightleftharpoons Oxy\ Hb + H^+$$

The exchange of oxygen and carbon dioxide in the lungs and tissues is a function of this effect. As oxygen is bound to hemoglobin in the lungs, carbon dioxide is released. This raises the pH, resulting in a shift to the left of the affinity curve. This carbon dioxide elimination promotes carbon dioxide pick up on the tissue level and is known as *Haldane effect*. In contrast, the acidic environment of the tissues due to the increased concentration of carbon dioxide enhances oxygen delivery to the tissues. This is known as the *Bohr effect*. The oxygen affinity of hemoglobin is expressed in terms of P_{50}, the oxygen tension at which hemoglobin is half-saturated. The value of the P_{50} is taken from the midpoint of the oxygen dissociation curve and does not reflect the shape of the curve. As the affinity for oxygen increases, the P_{50} becomes smaller or shifted to the left. Conversely, for high P_{50} values there is a lower affinity of oxygen for hemoglobin and a shift to the right (Fig. 20–2). When hemoglobin unloads oxygen, the resulting conformation of the deoxyhemoglobin molecule is known as the tense (T) form, which has a lower affinity for oxygen.[7] When hemoglobin loads oxygen and becomes oxyhemoglobin, 2,3-DPG is expelled in the relaxed (R) form. This molecule has a greater affinity for oxygen.

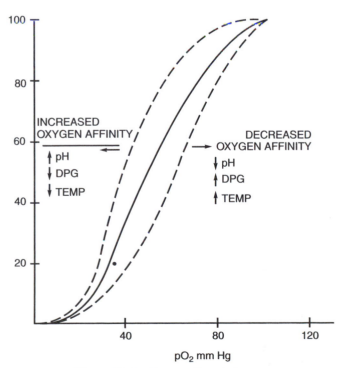

Figure 20–2   Oxygen dissociation curve

ABNORMALITIES

Anemia   *Anemia* is defined as a hemoglobin concentration below normal for age, gender, and altitude of residence. This results in the reduced oxygen-carrying capacity of hemoglobin and tissue hypoxia. Factors that can cause this condition are blood loss, excessive RBC destruction, or abnormal RBC production (Table 20–2).

Typically, iron deficiency anemia in the adult (mean corpuscular volume [MCV] < 80 fL) is the result of gastrointestinal blood loss or menometrorrhagia. Clinically, the degree of the patient's symptoms depends on the level of hemoglobin and the chronicity of the underlying conditions. To compensate for this form of chronic anemia, the oxygen dissociation curve shifts to the right due to an increase in the concentration of 2,3-DPG. However, because of a reduction of the arterial oxygen saturation, the cardiac output increases, leading to tachycardia at rest.

The most common cause for macrocytosis (MCV > 100 fL) is megaloblastic anemia. The deficiency of vitamin B_{12}, folic acid, or both is the primary cause for this condition. Inherited or drug-induced impairment of DNA synthesis can also cause an elevated MCV. In addition to anemia, patients may present with peripheral neuropathy, hepatosplenomegaly, and icterus.

Normocytic anemias present with a MCV in the range of 81 to 99 fL. The increased or decreased production of erythrocytes can help to define the clinical entities. The anemias of chronic disease including chronic renal insufficiency are in this general category. *Erythropoietin* is a glycoprotein produced by the kidney, which functions as the physiologic stimulus for RBC production. The decreased effect of erythropoietin associated with renal disease accounts for the anemia commonly seen. Erythropoietin can also be stimulated by hypoxia. With the advent of recombinant erythropoietin as an exogenous stimulus to RBC production, the transfusion requirement associated with the chronic anemias can be significantly reduced. In surgical candidates who wish to have autologous donations or in patients whose religious beliefs prohibit blood product transfusion, this hormone replacement can be given preoperatively to boost the RBC count. Although most erythropoietin supplements currently employed are administered subcutaneously, it must be noted that currently available intravenous forms of recombinant erythropoietin contain 2.5 mg of human albumin.[8]

Hemoglobinopathies   *Hemoglobinopathy* refers to a genetic disorder in which the hemoglobin is structurally abnormal or one of the hemoglobin chains has an altered rate of production. *Sickle cell anemia* is a hemoglobinopathy inherited as a homozygous autosomal recessive trait. As the hemoglobin is deoxygenated, the RBC becomes sickled. Hemoglobin S molecules have a tendency to bind to one another at the oxygen release sites increasing viscosity and causing stasis of blood flow. The hallmarks of this disease are chronic anemia, bone and joint pain, frequent infection, and vaso-

Table 20–2
MORPHOLOGIC CLASSIFICATION OF ANEMIAS

Morphology and Cause of Reduced Oxygen-Carrying Capacity of Blood	Name and Mechanism of Anemic Condition	Primary Cause of Associated Disorder
Macrocytic-normochromic anemia: large, abnormally shaped erythrocytes but normal hemoglobin concentrations	Pernicious anemia: lack of vitamin B_{12} (cobalamin) for erythropoiesis; abnormal DNA and RNA synthesis in the erythroblast; premature cell death	Congenital or acquired deficiency of intrinsic factor (IF); genetic disorder of DNA synthesis
	Folate-deficiency anemia: lack of folate for erythropoiesis; premature cell death	Dietary folate deficiency
Microcytic hypochromic anemia: small, abnormally shaped erythrocytes and reduced hemoglobin concentration	Iron-deficiency anemia: lack of iron for hemoglobin production; insufficient hemoglobin	Chronic blood loss; dietary iron deficiency, disruption of iron metabolism or iron cycle
	Sideroblastic anemia: dysfunctional iron uptake by erythroblasts and defective porphyrin and heme synthesis	Congenital dysfunction of iron metabolism in erythroblasts, acquired dysfunction of iron metabolism as a result of drugs or toxins
	Thalassemia: impaired synthesis of α or β chain of hemoglobin A; phagocytosis of abnormal erythroblasts in the marrow	Congenital genetic defect of globin synthesis
Normocytic-normochromic anemia: destruction or depletion of normal erythroblasts or mature erythrocytes	Aplasic anemia: insufficient erythropoiesis	Depressed stem cell proliferation resulting in bone marrow aplasia
	Posthemorrhagic anemia: blood loss	Acute or chronic hemorrhage that stimulates increased erythropoiesis, which eventually depletes body iron
	Hemolytic anemia: premature destruction (lysis) of mature erythrocytes in the circulation	Any condition that increases fragility of erythrocytes
	Sickle cell anemia: abnormal hemoglobin synthesis, abnormal cell shape with susceptibility to damage, lysis, and phagocytosis	Congenital dysfunction of hemoglobin synthesis
	Anemia of chronic disease: abnormally increased demand for new erythrocytes	Chronic infection or inflammation; malignancy

Source: Reproduced by permission from McCance KL, Huether SE, eds. *Pathophysiology: The Biologic Basis for Disease in Adults and Children.* CV Mosby; 1990:785.

occlusive events leading to obstruction of the microcirculation by the altered RBC morphology (sickle cell). In addition, this destruction decreases the RBC normal life span from 120 to 12 days. The chronic anemia associated with this condition causes an increase in cardiac output and subsequent cardiac enlargement. Congestive heart failure may develop as a result of myocardial hemosiderosis from multiple transfusions. There is a notable decrease in the pulmonary vital capacity and oxygen saturation as a result of infarcted pulmonary tissue caused by the shunting of blood in the lungs. This can further lead to pulmonary hypertension when sludging occurs in the small pulmonary arteries. Acute episodes of *sickle cell crisis* can be precipitated by numerous conditions including hypoxemia, hypothermia, acidosis, infection, and dehydration. The partial pressure of oxygen when decreased below its normal value favors the formation of sickle cells. This condition is fostered by acidosis. Hypothermia causes vasoconstriction leading to impairment of blood flow and deoxygenation of hemoglobin S. The same mechanism accounts for the effects of dehydration.

Anesthetic Management
Meticulous monitoring of these patients is crucial to avoid these complications. In particular oxygen saturation monitoring is important. Because oversedation may lead to hypoventilation and acidosis, it should be avoided. Patients with sickle cell disease must be well hydrated and hypothermia aggressively prevented. Supplemental oxygen should be administered intraoperatively as well as postoperatively. Preoperative transfusions may be indicated. The carrier state for sickle cell disease is sickle cell trait (presence of hemoglobins A and S), which is the most benign form of the sickling disorders. Sickle cell trait, however, produces no significant clinical manifestation and does not require special anesthetic considerations.

Thalassemia   The thalassemias result from decreased or absent globin chain synthesis. The degree and severity of clinical manifestations depend on which of the globin chains is affected. A decrease or absence of α chain production is widely seen throughout Africa, Mediterranean countries,

Southeast Asia, and parts of India and Pakistan. The absence of one or two genes for the production of the α chains does not have significant clinical manifestations. However, a three-gene deletion known as hemoglobin H disease results in a mild to moderate form of α thalassemia that may require transfusion. A four-gene deletion of the α chain is incompatible with life (*hydrops fetalis*). In the most severe form of viable thalassemia, *Cooley's anemia*, there is a complete absence of β chain production (β^0) resulting in no normal adult hemoglobin A formation. In Cooley's anemia, the predominant hemoglobin is hemoglobin F with an increased amount of the minor hemoglobin, A_2.

Anesthetic Management

In addition to severe anemia, this disease is characterized by cephalofacial deformities, hepatomegaly, splenomegaly, and spinal cord compression. Chronic anemia leads to repeated transfusions, thereby causing hemosiderosis and end-organ failure of the heart, lung, and kidney. These physical manifestations of the disorder pose a challenge to the anesthesia provider. The overgrowth of the maxilla can make intubation technically difficult. The hepatomegaly leads to impaired synthesis of clotting factors, increasing the risk of operative bleeding. The massive transfusion requirement and subsequent myocardial hemosiderosis predisposes to congestive heart failure and dysrhythmias. Splenomegaly can lead to thrombocytopenia as well as leukopenia.

Polycythemia or Erythrocytosis The term *polycythemia* or *erythrocytosis* refers to the increase in the concentration of RBC and may not be associated with an increase in the RBC mass. In the condition of relative or pseudoerythrocytosis, the concentration of the RBC is greater than normal by loss of blood plasma and not an actual increase in the RBC number. This arises when there is loss of bodily fluids or decreased fluid intake; this may occur transiently as a result of burns, diabetic acidosis, or shock. Chronic relative erythrocytosis (Gaisböck's syndrome or stress erythrocytosis) occurs, in general, in middle-aged men with a long history of hypertension, obesity, or excessive smoking. Absolute erythrocytosis is a true increase in the number of RBCs in the circulation leading to an increase in blood volume as well. At high altitudes, there is decreased atmospheric oxygen pressure, which can cause fatigue, headache, dizziness, nausea, and vomiting if the ascent is too rapid. The compensatory mechanism involves erythropoietin, produced in the kidney. Anoxia or insufficient oxygen supply to the tissues results in erythropoietin stimulation and the resultant increased RBC production. Acclimatization usually involves an increase in 2,3-DPG resulting in a shift to the right of the oxygen dissociation curve and better oxygen delivery to the tissues.

A second cause of erythrocytosis can be seen in some patients with chronic pulmonary disease in whom oxygenation of the circulating blood through the lungs is inadequate. Congenital heart defects such as right-to-left shunt also result in an increase in the size of the RBC mass as a result of low oxygen tension from shunting of unoxygenated blood through the lungs. In obese patients in whom there is an inadequate ventilatory drive (Pickwickians), cyanosis, hypercapnia, and right-sided heart failure may develop. If the affinity for oxygen is increased, as occurs in certain atypical hemoglobinopathies, there may be a tendency to develop erythrocytosis. High RBC mass can lead to the clinical symptoms of headache, dizziness, and visual defects.

Anesthetic Management

Before elective surgery hematocrit levels should be reduced to normal levels by phlebotomy. With emergency surgery crystalloids or colloids should be infused intravenously to decrease hyperviscosity. Without these measures increased blood viscosity may lead to a more frequent occurrence of hemorrhage or thrombosis. When these symptoms occur associated with leukocytosis, thrombocytosis, and splenomegaly, a diagnosis of *Polycythemia vera* must be considered, especially in older Jewish men. Total RBC volume is increased but the arterial oxygen saturation may be normal. After many years of proliferative activity, some patients develop a "spent" phase characterized by marrow fibrosis and a need for transfusion.

☐ WHITE BLOOD CELLS (LEUKOCYTES)

The white blood cell (WBC) series (see Table 20–1) refers to five distinct groups of cells: the granulocytes (neutrophils, basophils, and eosinophils), lymphocytes, and monocytes. The special function of each type of leukocyte depends on the production of chemical substances stored in the cells. Leukocytes have an important role in the body's defense mechanisms and in the immune response.

GRANULOCYTES

Neutrophils Neutrophils are the most common circulating leukocyte. Maturation of the bone marrow precursor cells into the granulocyte-macrophage cell series depends on the glycoproteins called *colony-stimulating factors* (CSF). Granulocyte-macrophage colony-stimulating factor (GM-CSF) is produced by activated T lymphocytes and stimulates the growth and differentiation of the granulocytes and macrophage precursor cells. Granulocyte colony stimulating factor (G–CSF) is a more specific stimulator and activator of neutrophil production and function.

The bone marrow is the site of production and maturation of the neutrophils before their release into the blood and tissues. The length of stay in the marrow before release is 6 to 10 days. The total neutrophil blood pool consists of circulating cells and those adherent to the endothelium of small vessels (marginated neutrophil pool), which can readily enter the circulation at times of exercise or stress. Ether anesthesia can produce an increase in the number of leukocytes. Once the neutrophils enter the tissues, however, they do not reenter the blood.

The primary function of the mature circulating neutrophil is host defense. The neutrophils are well suited for this phagocytic role by their specialized cytoplasmic granules and plasma membranes. Neutrophils are attracted to sites of infection or inflammation by chemotactic factors creating a chemical gradient that directs neutrophil migration toward the source of the chemotactic factor. *Opsonization* is the process whereby microorganisms are "coated" by plasma antibodies and complement. Neutrophils then ingest an opsonized microorganism by surrounding it with pseudopodia that fuse and enclose the microbe within an intracellular vesicle (phagosome). The various cytoplasmic granules of the neutrophil fuse with this vesicle and by a process of degranulation, discharge their contents to help in the digestive process. The metabolites produced together with material discharged into the phagosome by the granules kill ingested microbes. The interaction of immune complexes and complement can promote neutrophil activity including leakage or secretion of extracellular granular proteins and toxic metabolic products into the surrounding tissue contributing to tissue injury and autoimmune inflammatory reactions. These can have deleterious effects on the neutrophil as well as the endothelium.

Basophils   The basophil represents the least common granulocyte in the human circulation. It contains proteoglycans and is the primary source of heparin and histamine in human blood. The clinical manifestations present in immediate hypersensitivity reactions are due to the release of the products from within the basophil and its kindred present in tissues, the mast call. Several anesthetic agents are notable for causing histamine release (Table 20–3).

These anesthetics should be administered with caution or avoided altogether in patients with known sensitivities. Histamine is an autocoid capable of exerting profound effects on the cardiovascular system (vasodilatation), airways (bronchoconstriction), and gastrointestinal system via gastric H^+ secretion. Because of its molecular size, histamine will not readily cross the blood–brain barrier.

Table 20–3
ANESTHETICS AND RELATED DRUGS NOTABLE FOR ANTIHISTAMINE RELEASE

morphine
atracurium
curare
para-aminobenzoic ester agents
penicillin
vancomycin
protamine
thiamylal
thiopental
methylmethacrylate
colloid volume expanders

Eosinophils   The mature eosinophil constitutes about 2% of the leukocytes in blood and bone marrow and participates in phagocytosis and killing of protozoa as well as allergic and inflammatory reactions. Eosinophils preferentially reside in the skin, lung, and gastrointestinal tract.

Abnormalities

Neutrophilia
The condition of *neutrophilia* is characterized by the increased numbers of peripheral blood neutrophils. The five mechanisms of action primarily responsible for this are:

Increased production
Mobilization from the marrow maturation storage pool
Demargination
Decreased egress from the circulating pool
Extramedullary hematopoiesis

The major causes of neutrophilic leukocytosis are:

Infection (primarily bacterial)
Inflammation (collagen vascular diseases)
Tissue damage or necrosis (surgery)
Metabolic disorders (ketoacidosis)
Drugs and hormones (epinephrine and glucocorticoids)
Malignant neoplasms (leukemia)
Physiologic conditions (severe stress)
Hereditary conditions
Miscellaneous causes such as acute hemorrhage or hemolysis

Neutropenia
Patients with profound granulocytopenia are at risk for serious infectious complications. Some drugs, especially chemotherapeutic agents, are marrow suppressive and result in decreased numbers of neutrophils. In contrast, the neutropenia found in one fourth of the African-American population is not associated with increased risk of infection. Chronic idiopathic neutropenia and neutropenia in association with immune disorders are more infrequent causes

Leukemias
Acute Myelogenous Leukemia
Acute myelogenous leukemia (AML) is the most frequent form of acute leukemia in adults, arising from a single pluripotential hematopoietic stem cell. The incidence of AML is approximately 2/100,000 with higher male preponderance. Hereditary factors (Down's syndrome) and environmental (radiation or benzene exposure) have been cited as etiologic factors. Several tumors, especially Hodgkin's disease, lymphomas, myeloma, and ovarian and breast carcinomas are associated with the occurrence of secondary AML.[9,10]

The most frequent presenting complaints of patients with AML are fatigue, infection, and bleeding. Anemia, ecchymoses, and organomegaly may be present. In hyperleukocytic leukemia, the excessive WBC count can cause blood flow stasis leading to stupor or coma, retinal engorgement, papilledema, and respiratory distress. The mainstay of treatment has been chemotherapy with an anthracycline and cytosine arabinoside. Occasionally more immediate measures such as leukopheresis are necessary to prevent injury to the endothelium leading to hemorrhage, respiratory compromise, and coronary occlusion.

The cure rate is usually between 10% and 30% depending on age, preexisting myelodysplastic or myeloproliferative disorder, and cytogenetic factors. The intensive chemotherapy required to treat this disease is associated with a wide range of complications. Granulocytopenias predispose to increased risk of infection and are the primary cause of morbidity along with symptomatic anemia and thrombocytopenia requiring blood product support. The anthracyclines can lead to cardiac toxicity, reduced ejection fraction, and subsequent heart failure. Extramedullary leukemic cell infiltrates can cause superior vena cava obstruction, cranial nerve palsy, or other neurologic symptoms. In appropriate younger patients, marrow transplantation has improved long-term survival.

Chronic Myelogenous Leukemia

Chronic myelogenous leukemia (CML) is a clonal disorder of a pluripotential stem cell that gives rise to lymphocytes, leukocytes, erythrocytes, and platelets. The incidence increases with age and accounts for about 25% of adult leukemias. Clinically, the disease has three distinct phases. The *chronic phase* may present asymptomatically as an abnormal blood count or with fevers, splenomegaly, and bleeding. Although variable, usually within 3 years, the patient may complain of bone pain; progressive hepatosplenomegaly is noted and the patient develops more marked anemia and thrombocytopenia. The *accelerated phase* typically leads to the *blast phase* within 3 to 6 months. The development of AML is generally refractory to standard induction chemotherapy. Bone marrow transplantation in the chronic phase of this disorder offers an opportunity to change the natural history of this disease.

LYMPHOCYTES

The function of the immune system is to protect the body from damage by various microorganisms. The monocytes, macrophages, and neutrophils function as phagocytes by taking up foreign material and breaking it down. Eosinophils, basophils, mast cells, and platelets function as the accessory cells in the immune response process. Lymphocytes are the controlling cell of the immune response and are comprised of two main cell types, T cells and B cells.

T cells are responsible for *cell-mediated immunity*. They develop in the thymus where they acquire a specific surface receptor molecule, the antigen receptor. Each of the several subtypes of T cells has a different function. T-helper cells are lymphocytes that help B cells to produce antibody. These T cells express CD_4 surface antigen and comprise about 65% of the blood T cells. They also work with cytotoxic T cells and release lymphokines, which can activate macrophages. In this capacity, they function as T-inducer cells. The cytotoxic T cells are lymphocytes that can destroy target cells

that have abnormal or altered membranes. The suppressor T cell regulates the action of the lymphocytes and expresses the surface antigen CD_8. They make up 25% to 35% of the peripheral T cells. These cells act to control the specific interaction between antigens, T cells, and B cells so that the magnitude of the immune response is regulated.

B cells are the mediators of *humoral immunity* and are primarily derived from the bone marrow. They are usually under control of specific regulatory T cells and differentiate into the mature plasma cell. Immunoglobulins are glycoproteins or antigen-specific antibodies produced by B lymphocytes or plasma cells. Their primary function is to bind antigens.

Immunoglobulin G (IgG) constitutes approximately 80% of the immunoglobulin in adult plasma and is the only one to cross the placental barrier to provide passive immunity to the newborn. The four major subclasses are designated IgG_1, IgG_2, IgG_3, and IgG_4. The average half-life of the IgG molecule is 21 days. About 13% of the immunoglobulins is immunoglobulin A (IgA) with a half-life of 6 days. These secretory immunoglobulins are the principle antibody in saliva, tears and the fluids of the gastrointestinal, respiratory, and urinary tracts. Immunoglobulin M (IgM) comprises about 6% of total immunoglobulin and is referred to as a macroglobulin because of its large molecular weight. IgM also has a half-life of 6 days. Less than 1% of the plasma immunoglobulin is expressed as immunoglobulin D (IgD). Immunoglobulin E (IgE), the reaginic antibody, is present in even lower amounts except in patients with parasitic infections or atopic children. In allergic patients, the antigen–antibody binding of IgE induces the release of histamine, serotonin, leukotrienes, and eosinophilic chemotactic factor.

Abnormalities
Acute Lymphoblastic Leukemia

Acute lymphoblastic leukemia (ALL) is the most common malignant disease of children. Typically, the patient may present insidiously or with symptoms related to the bone marrow replacement by immature lymphoblasts. Weakness, fatigue, pallor, infection, or bleeding may be present. ALL is classified into three subdivisions based on cell size, population, and characteristics of the nucleus and cytoplasm. In the adult, the disease is associated with a much poorer prognosis. Although ALL is treated with chemotherapeutic drugs, radiation therapy and intrathecal drugs are also used because the central nervous system (CNS) and testes may be sanctuaries for leukemic cell infiltrates. The incidence of infection and need for blood product support are the same as in AML. In patients treated at a young age or in long-term survivors, late complications such as learning disorders or leukoencephalopathy may develop.

Chronic Lymphocytic Leukemia

Chronic lymphocytic leukemia (CLL) is characterized by proliferation of B-cell lymphocytes usually in the adult population over the age of 50. The indications for treatment for CLL include disease-related symptoms such as fever, autoimmune hemolytic anemia or thrombocytopenia, massive organomegaly or lymphadenopathy, and bacterial infections. The latter is due primarily to the development of hypogammaglobulinemia causing impaired immunity. There is also an associated increased risk in second malignancies such as melanoma, multiple myeloma, and colorectal or lung carcinoma.

General Considerations

Care for the leukemic patient involves multisystem compromise secondary to the disease process or from the actual treatment of the disease (radiation and chemotherapy). (See Chap. 32).

Immunodeficiency Disorders Primary immunodeficiencies are genetically determined disorders that cause increased susceptibility to infection in affected individuals. These involve defects in the T or B lymphocyte or the phagocytic or complement system. Over 70 disorders have been described of which the antibody deficiencies may comprise up to 50% and the T-lymphocyte or cellular immunodeficiencies about 30%. Most of these disorders have their onset in childhood. Because of the X-linked nature of many of these disorders, 70% of primary immunodeficiencies occur in males.[11, 12] The major clinical manifestation of these disorders is susceptibility to and frequency of infections. Recurrent respiratory infections are common as well as gastrointestinal symptoms such as diarrhea and malabsorption. Infections with major gram-positive organisms frequently indicate a deficiency in antibody opsonization or complement activation. Cellular immunodeficiency usually results in viral or fungal infections such as oral thrush. Recurrent gram-negative infections are potential signs of a phagocytic deficiency.

Secondary immunodeficiencies are a result of illness or condition that causes an impaired immune response. Patients are predisposed to the subsequent development of lymphoid malignancies. This is clearly seen in the increased risk of high-grade non-Hodgkin's lymphoma and primary lymphoma of the brain seen in patients infected with human immunodeficiency virus (HIV). If there is clonal proliferation of B lymphocytes leading to increased levels of IgM or IgA, a hyperviscosity syndrome may be present with resultant CNS symptoms. These monoclonal proteins may also impair hemostasis by interfering with the function of platelets or coagulation proteins.

General Considerations

In general, patients with immunodeficiency should not be given live vaccines. Good nutrition and dental health is to be encouraged as well as prompt or prophylactic antibiotic usage. For patients presenting for surgical procedures good sterile technique is requisite. These patients are likely to be on extensive antibiotic and coagulation therapy. In addition to those with congenital immunodeficiencies, patients receiving chemotherapy for malignant conditions or immunosuppressive therapy for collagen vascular disease or transplantation constitute a population of comprised hosts with increased susceptibility to infection. Breakdown of the mucosa of the respiratory or gastrointestinal system provides a portal of entry for infectious organisms. Granulocytopenia, usually as a result of cytotoxic chemotherapy, is a major risk for bacterial and fungal infections especially when the granulocyte count is below 1000 μL. Impaired humoral immunity in patients with multiple myeloma and CLL accounts for the increased infections with encapsulated organisms.

Patients with T-cell immunodeficiency may require irradiated blood products to reduce the risk of possible graft-versus-host disease. Gamma globulin injection is also an effective replacement therapy for most forms of antibody deficiency with the notable exception of IgA-deficient patients. This primary immunodeficient condition may occur in as many as 1 in 600 persons. Usually these patients are asymptomatic. Transfusion of plasma or gamma globulin should be avoided because this can result in the production of anti-IgA antibodies leading to possible anaphylactic reactions when blood products are administered.

☐ PLATELETS

The platelet is a fragmented cell derived from the megakaryocyte in the bone marrow. The morphology of the platelet reflects its physiologic role in the process of hemostasis. It possesses a unique quality to adhere to foreign surfaces forming aggregates in response to such stimuli as thrombin, adenosine diphosphate, and catecholamine. For the platelet to function normally, certain factors must be present including adequate numbers of platelets, structurally normal platelets, membrane-responsive receptors, and normal numbers and contents of storage granules. At any one time, 80% of the platelets are in the circulation; the remaining 20% are in the spleen with a free interchange between the two compartments. The normal life span of the platelet is 10 days. Platelets adhere to damaged endothelium to form the platelet plug and promote thrombin production. The first phase of adhesion requires the presence of von Willebrand's factor and fibrinogen. The second phase, platelet aggregation, is the release reaction involving extrusion of the contents of the granules and is induced by thrombin. The control mechanism for this process is the concentration of cyclic adenosine 3'5'-monophosphate (AMP). Aggregation of the platelet at the site of injury provides the surface for procoagulant activity and the formation of the hemostatic plug.

Disorders of the platelets are either qualitative or quantitative. The common clinical findings of both are petechiae, purpura, or mucosal bleeding. Qualitative platelet disorders can be divided into thrombocytopenias or thrombocytoses. *Thrombocytopenia* is generally considered when the platelet count is less than 100,000/mm³. Acquired platelet production defects can be caused by a wide variety of conditions including marrow infiltrative diseases, drug-induced suppression, aplastic anemia, cyclic thrombocytopenia, and renal failure. Decreased platelet numbers can also be caused by increased consumption or destruction of platelets, such as that in the hemolytic uremic syndromes or thrombotic thrombocytopenic purpura (TTP). Commonly encountered is the thrombocytopenia caused by hypersplenism secondary to a number of different etiologies. Thrombocytosis is generally a benign process associated with an asymptomatic increase in the number of platelets. This can be the result of infection, malignancy, or collagen vascular disorders. Primary thrombocythemia, however, is a malignant process of uncontrolled platelet production with a clinical course characterized by splenomegaly, hemorrhage, or thrombosis.

Functional platelet defects may be hereditary. Acquired platelet defects affecting platelet function and documented by abnormal platelet aggregation studies may be caused by the myeloproliferative syndromes, uremia, or malignant paraproteinemias. The most common acquired cause of platelet dysfunction is the effect of medications such as aspirin, anti-inflammatory drugs, antibiotics, and anesthetics.

Evaluation of platelet function should begin with a platelet count. An accurate history of easy bruising or bleeding should be part of the initial screening process. Further assessment of platelet function can be made with platelet aggregation studies that include the platelet response to various agonists such as collagen, thrombin, epinephrine, and arachidonic acid. The bleeding time test can also be used; however, this procedure is invasive and often inaccurate because of variables in technique.

☐ CLOTTING AND HEMOSTASIS

The transformation of blood from a liquid to gel state is a complex process whose end result is the cessation of blood flow or hemostasis (Table 20–4). Impairment of this process occurs as a result of:

Decreased synthesis of clotting factors
Production of abnormal molecules that interfere with the coagulation pathways
Loss or consumption of the coagulation factors
Inactivation of these factors by inhibitors or antibodies[15 (p 365)]

Abnormal clotting can also occur as a result of vitamin K deficiency, liver disease, hemorrhage, or a consumptive coagulopathy such as disseminated intravascular coagulation (DIC), induction of anticoagulant therapy, and treatment with various drugs.

Fibrinogen is a large glycoprotein produced in the liver; it participates in the final stages of coagulation. The interaction of fibrinogen with the enzyme thrombin yields a network of insoluble strands called fibrin.[13(p 277)] Afibrinogenemia, a rare inherited autosomal recessive trait, can cause profuse bleeding after slight trauma and delay in wound healing. Initial symptoms include bleeding from the umbilical cord. Other symptoms can include intracranial bleeding, epistaxis, gastrointestinal bleeding, and menorrhagia. Hemathrosis is uncommon in this disorder. Mild to moderate thrombocytopenia can occur but platelet counts are rarely less than $100,000/\mu L$.[14,15] Treatment for this disorder includes cryoprecipitate, fresh-frozen plasma (FFP), and whole blood transfusions if profuse bleeding has occurred. Dysfibrinogenemia is a qualitative defect that can be either inherited, mostly as an autosomal dominant trait, or acquired due to some underlying disease, most often liver disease. Alterations in this structure can lead to defects in fibrin formation and, therefore, affect the clotting process.

Prothrombin is synthesized in the liver and is the most abundant of the vitamin K-dependent blood clotting

Table 20–4
SOURCE OF CLOTTING FACTORS—MINIMUM LEVELS NECESSARY FOR HEMOSTASIS AND TREATMENT

Clotting Factors		Substance	Source	Minimal Level for Surgical Hemostasis (% of Normal)	Clinical Syndrome Caused by Deficiency	Treatment
I	Fibrinogen	Plasma protein	Liver	50–100	Yes	Cryoprecipitate
II	Prothrombin[a]	Plasma protein	Liver	20–40	Yes	Plasma
III	Thromboplastin	Lipoprotein and phospholipid	Released from damaged tissues		No	
IV	Calcium	Ion in plasma	Diet and bones		No	
V	Proaccelerin	Plasma protein	Liver	5–20	Yes	Fresh or frozen plasma
VII	Proconvertin[a]	Plasma protein	Liver	10–20	Yes	Plasma
VIII	Antihemophilic factor	Plasma protein	Subunit by endothelium	30	Yes	Cryoprecipitate, plasma
IX	Christmas factor[a]	Plasma protein	Liver	20–25	Yes	Plasma or II, VII, IX, X concentrate
X	Stuart-Prower factor[a]	Plasma protein	Liver and plasma	10–20	Yes	Plasma
XI	Plasma thromboplastin antecedent	Plasma protein	Possibly liver	20–30	Mild	Plasma
XII	Hageman factor	Plasma protein	Liver and plasma	0	No	Plasma
XIII	Fibrin-stabilizing factor	Plasma protein	Liver, platelets, plasma	1–3	Yes	Plasma

[a] Denotes dependency on vitamin K for synthesis

proteins.[16] Deficiencies of prothrombin delay generation of thrombin thus contributing to hemorrhagic symptoms.

The initiation of the coagulation pathways in vivo begins with the extrinsic system involving components of the vascular and blood elements. The predominant plasma protein of the extrinsic system is factor VII, a vitamin K-dependent protein. Factor VII deficiency is a rare inherited autosomal recessive trait[17,18] clinically presenting with deep muscle hematomas, joint hemorrhage, epistaxis, and menorrhagia. Factor VII deficiency can be acquired with liver disease, warfarin therapy, or vitamin K deficiency and, therefore, treatment modalities include FFP, prothrombin complex concentrates, and vitamin K.

Factor VIII circulates as a complex of von Willebrand factor (FVIII: vWF) and the procoagulant, factor VIII (FVIII:C).[19] *Hemophilia A* is the most common hereditary coagulation disorder and is carried on the X chromosome. The defect is not an absence of factor VIII complex, but rather a molecular defect or absence of its procoagulant portion (FVIII:C)[20] Hemarthrosis is a primary symptom involving knees, elbows, ankles, shoulders, hips, and wrists. Other symptoms include hematuria, intracranial bleeding, hematomas, and unexplained spontaneous hemorrhage. Levels of 30% of normal activity is the ideal therapeutic level for maintaining hemostasis.

von Willebrand's disease (vWD) differs from classical hemophilia A in three important ways: autosomal inheritance rather than sex-linked, consistently prolonged bleeding times, and mucocutaneous bleeding rather than hemarthroses and deep muscle hemorrhage. The bleeding is due to the inability of platelets to adhere to the subendothelial surface following injury to the blood vessel.[21,22] vWF is an acute phase reactant and will increase during times of stress, pregnancy, or after surgery. This makes the diagnosis or evaluation of patients suspected of having this disorder difficult. Concentrates of factor VIII, cryoprecipitate, and vWF have been used to treat vWD. The use of commercial factor VIII concentrates is not useful because they lack the high molecular weight multimers of vWF. Desmopressin (DDAVP) is a synthetic vasopressin used to treat patients with diabetes insipidus. It also causes both the vWF and FVIII:C to rise and can be used to treat patients before dental work or surgery and after bleeding episodes, avoiding the risk of exposure to blood products. In type IIb, DDAVP can cause thrombocytopenia and is, therefore, contraindicated.

Factor IX deficiency, hemophilia B or *Christmas factor*, is a sex-linked recessive bleeding disorder. Acquired deficiency states can be seen in patients with liver disease, vitamin K deficiency, and those on oral anticoagulant therapy. The most serious complication in patients with hemophilia B is the formation of antibodies to factor IX.

Deficiency of factor X may occur at any age with the most severe hemorrhagic symptoms occurring in the very young. Clinical symptoms range from easy bruising, epistaxis, gastrointestinal bleeding, or menorrhagia in mildly affected patients to hemarthrosis, CNS hemorrhage, and severe postopertive bleeding in the most severely affected patients.

Acquired factor X deficiencies usually coincide with other vitamin K-dependent factor disorders.

Factor XI is a plasma glycoprotein that participates in the intrinsic coagulation pathway.[17] Factor XI deficiency, once known as Rosenthal syndrome or hemophilia C, is seen predominately in the Ashkenazi Jewish population and is inherited as an autosomal recessive trait. Factor XI is the only factor of the contact system where a deficiency may lead to a bleeding diathesis. Levels of factor XI may fluctuate with time and bleeding episodes vary in response to a variety of surgical procedures.[23] Levels of less than 15% factor activity are considered severely deficient and result in postoperative bleeding unless corrected with the use of FFP.

The deficiency of factor XII, Hageman trait, is inherited in an autosomal recessive fashion. This disorder is not associated with clinical bleeding or hemorrhage. There may, however, be an increased incidence of thrombotic events such as myocardial infarction or thromboembolism.

Circulating anticoagulants are acquired inhibitors of the coagulation mechanism. Nonspecific inhibitors such as lupus anticoagulants have been associated with thrombosis, fetal wastage, and thrombocytopenia. They occur spontaneously or associated with autoimmune diseases such as systemic lupus erythematosus, acquired immunodeficiency syndrome (AIDS), infectious diseases (bacterial, viral, protozoal), antibiotic and other drug exposure, strokes, spontaneous abortions, and lymphoproliferative disorders. Patients possessing lupus-like anticoagulants present in the laboratory with a prolonged activated partial thromboplastin time (aPTT) and normal prothrombin time (PT).

When assessing the preoperative patient for increased bleeding potential, the platelet count, PT, and aPTT must be evaluated, in addition to asking the patient about a history of bleeding problems. Care must be taken in the collection of the specimen from a nonheparinized line. If any results are suspicious, a bleeding time, which is the best indication of platelet function, may be necessary.

☐ COMPLICATIONS OF TRANSFUSION THERAPY

There is a significant risk that transfusion of blood and blood products may result in the patient's death. Assessing adverse reactions may be more complicated in the anesthetized patient, which accounts for about 50% of the transfusions given.[24,25] Reactions can be classified into two categories: immediate and delayed. Immediate transfusion reactions begin within minutes to hours and may be nonspecific. In the anesthetized patient, generalized oozing secondary to DIC or unexplained shock may be the clinical manifestations. The bleeding diathesis requires restitution with cryoprecipitate, platelet concentrates, and FFP.

Hemolytic reactions may be due to intravascular breakdown resulting from an ABO incompatibility or extravascular destruction. Clinically, the patient may develop fever, low back pain, or chest tightness at which time the transfusion should be stopped immediately. Blood and urine samples should be submitted for evidence of hemolysis and the specimen retyped for confirmation of the initial crossmatch. Institution of lifesaving measures should not be withheld until laboratory results are available. To avoid acute tubular necrosis, renal blood flow must be maintained with intravenous fluids, mannitol, or diuretics. *Febrile reactions* may be due to a hemolytic reaction or sensitivity to WBC or platelet antigens. The latter may be confused with a true hemolytic reaction and can be prevented if leukocyte-poor blood or filtration is used during transfusion. Noncardiogenic pulmonary edema with acute respiratory distress, chills, fever, and tachycardia may be induced by the reaction to leukocyte and platelet antigens and usually responds to supportive measures. *Allergic reactions* may be caused by sensitivity to plasma proteins or other agents transferred from donor to recipient and result in pruritus, urticaria, or, in severe cases, anaphylaxis. In an *anaphylactic reaction*, an antigen attaches to a "sensitized" cell via IgE antibodies formed during a prior antigen exposure. This union of antigen–antibody on the cell membranes of mast cells and basophils leads to release of vasoactive substances such as histamine, leukotrienes, and prostaglandins. Clinically, symptoms develop quickly and are characterized by bronchospasm, laryngeal edema, hypotension, and hypovolemia secondary to increased capillary permeability. Depending on the severity, antihistamines or epinephrine may be needed. Anaphylaxis may also result when IgA present in plasma of transfused blood reacts with the anti-IgA in IgA-deficient patients. Rarer complications associated with transfusion of blood or blood products are congestive heart failure due to circulatory overload, air embolism, bleeding from dilution of coagulation factors with large volumes of transfused blood, and shock due to bacterial contamination.

Delayed transfusion reactions can occur days or weeks after transfusion. Jaundice can develop as a result of delayed hemolytic reaction with the subsequent onset of a positive direct antiglobulin reaction or Coombs' test. Posttransfusion purpura is the thrombocytopenia that occurs within 1 week of transfusion. Hepatitis B, hepatitis C (non-A non-B), cytomegalovirus, malaria, and HIV are infectious diseases transmissible by transfusion. Other complications include iron overload or hemosiderosis, graft-versus-host disease, and alloimmunization.

☐ HUMAN IMMUNODEFICIENCY VIRUS (ACQUIRED IMMUNODEFICIENCY SYNDROME)

The constellation of HIV diseases is characterized by predisposition to opportunistic infections and malignancies. HIV-associated diseases are caused by the action of retroviruses. Unique to all retroviruses is a DNA polymerase, reverse transcriptase, which permits the virus to encode the RNA message into double-stranded DNA. These "infected" DNA strands integrate into the host DNA. Transmission of this virus has been documented through sexual contact, parenterally, or by transplacental route.

One of the first manifestations of HIV infection is the increased susceptibility to opportunistic infections as a result of the decline in circulating CD_4 lymphocytes and a reversal of the CD_4/CD_8 lymphocyte ratio.[26] The decrease is progressive and correlates with the risk of AIDS-defining opportunistic infections.

The stages of disease can be classified into primary infection, which may be associated with a transient mononucleosis-like syndrome; an asymptomatic period of varying length; illness associated with one or several features, namely, weight loss, periods of fever, diarrhea, lymphadenopathy, and dermatitis (a constellation termed AIDS-related complex or ARC); and finally AIDS-defining illness with opportunistic infections, malignancies, or dementia.[6(p 976)]

Several hematologic complications are associated with HIV infection including impaired hematopoiesis, immune-mediated cytopenias, and coagulopathies. The frequency and severity of these problems correlate with the severity of the disease complex. Approximately 15% of asymptomatic HIV-infected subjects have mild anemia.[27] The pathogenesis of the anemia includes anemia of chronic disease due to infection or inflammation, defective erythropoiesis, drug-induced myelosuppression, autoimmune hemolytic disease, and neoplasia. Granulocytopenia, with or without lymphopenia, occurs in approximately 8% of asymptomatic HIV carriers. The pathogenesis is usually multifactorial, including the myelosuppressive effect of the drugs used to treat AIDS. The overall incidence of thrombocytopenia increases with disease progression. Immune mechanisms are responsible for premature platelet destruction. Although corticosteroids induce a transient increase in platelet count, there is an increased risk of compromising the immune status even further. Splenectomy or intravenous gamma globulin are useful alternate therapies. A prolonged aPTT and normal PT can also be noted.

With advanced disease, patients with AIDS are at an increased risk of opportunistic infections and the development of neoplastic diseases, the most common being Kaposi's sarcoma. Those who acquire the virus by sexual contact seem to be at increased risk. The treatment is usually palliative and may require radiation therapy, chemotherapy, or cryotherapy. AIDS is also associated with an increase in malignant lymphomas.

☐ OTHER HEMOSTATIC DEFECTS

In most surgical procedures requiring extracorporeal circuits, a mild defect in hemostasis is induced. In addition, these patients may already have preexisting defects in their clotting ability secondary to the underlying disease process necessitating the surgery. To minimize the operative risk, a detailed patient history, physical examination, and laboratory evaluation for potential bleeding problems is essential.

Many vascular defects are associated with significant hemorrhagic diatheses and present with petechiae, purpura, ecchymoses, and telangiectasia.[28,29(p 44)] The most common disorders include hereditary hemorrhagic telangiectasia, malignant paraprotein disorders, collagen vascular disorders, and aspirin ingestion.

Surgical bleeding usually does not occur if the platelet count is over 100,000/mm[3]. The most common causes of thrombocytopenia in surgical patients are drug induced with aspirin, antibiotics, and diuretics as the leading offenders. Infection, liver disease, malignancy, and immune thrombocytopenic purpura are also included in the more common etiologies. Qualitative defects in platelet function can also account for operative hemorrhage. Conditions most commonly associated with chronic or subacute underlying DIC processes in patients who are candidates for prosthetic devices or general surgical procedures are septicemia, disseminated solid malignancy, crush injuries, tissue necrosis, burns, selected liver and biliary diseases, and obstetric accidents including amniotic fluid embolism, placental abruption, toxemia, and the retained fetus syndrome.[29–32]

Early studies in cardiopulmonary bypass documented significant thrombocytopenia and the degree of platelet reduction was related to time on bypass and more pronounced with perfusions lasting longer than 60 minutes.[33] Platelet function impairment occurs in all patients and is usually the result of prior ingestion of warfarin-type drugs, cyanotic heart disease, hypothermic perfusions, and preoperative ingestion of drugs known to interfere with platelet function. Clearly, the distinction between operative bleeding secondary to technique or impairment of the hemostatic mechanism is essential for correct management.

The most common defects that may occur with prosthetic devices are a frank coagulation factor and platelet consumption with subsequent thrombocytopenia and resultant hemorrhage; partial platelet degranulation with subsequent defective platelet function and resultant hemorrhage; in cases of oxygenation or dialysis membranes, fibrin–platelet deposition will render the exchange ineffective and provide a focus for thromboembolus; and micro- or macrothromboemboli of platelets or fibrin may give rise to serious clinical vaso-occlusive problems. The use of anticoagulants, including warfarin-type drugs, heparin, and platelet-suppressive agents, tends to normalize thrombotic and thromboembolic complications with prosthetic devices.[29(p 233),34] These complications are also linked to the use of arterial and venous catheters and the intra-aortic balloon pump used for unstable cardiac status, cardiogenic shock, low output, or dysrhythmias.

REFERENCES

1. Bessis M. *Living Blood Cells and Their Ultrastructure.* New York: Springer-Verlag; 1973.
2. Oski FA, Nainam JL. *Hematologic Problems in the newborn.* 3rd ed. Philadelphia: WB Saunders; 1982.
3. Bard H. Postnatal fetal and adult hemoglobin synthesis in early preterm infants. *J Clin Invest.* 1973; 52:1789.
4. Astrup P. Red-cell pH and oxygen affinity of hemoglobin. *N Engl J Med.* 1970; 283:202.
5. Riggs A. Functional properties of hemoglobin. *Physiol Rev.* 1965; 45:619.
6. William WJ, Beutler E, Erslev AJ, Lichtman MA. *Hematology.* 4th ed. New York: McGraw-Hill; 1990:382, 976.
7. Harmening DM. *Clinical Hematology and Fundamentals of Hemostasis.* Philadelphia: FA Davis; 1992:12.
8. Hansell, D. *Clinical Anesthesia Procedures of the Massachusetts General Hospital.* 4th ed. Boston: Little, Brown; 1993:525.
9. Coltman C Jr. Treatment related leukemias. In: Bloomfield CD, ed. *Adult Leukemias.* The Hague: Marinus Nijhoff, 1982:62.
10. Koeffler HP, Rowley JD. Therapy related acute nonlymphocytic leukemia. In: Wiernik PH, Canellos GP, Dutcher JP, Kyle RA eds. *Neoplastic Diseases of the Blood.* New York; Churchill Livingstone; 1985:357.
11. Hayakawa H, Iwata T, Yata J, Kobayashi N. Primary immunodeficiency syndrome in Japan. I. Overview of a nationwide survey on primary immunodeficiency syndrome. *J Clin Immunol* 1981; 1:31–39
12. Medical Research Council Working Party. Hypogammaglobulinemia in the United Kingdom. *Lancet* 1969; 1:163.
13. Rock G. Defects of plasma clotting factors. In: Pittiglio DH, Sacher RA, eds. *Clinical Hematology and Fundamentals of Hemostasis.* Philadelphia: FA Davis; 1987: 277, 365.
14. Bommer W, Kunzer W, Schroer H. Kongenitale Afinrinogename. Teil I. *Ann Paediatr* 1963; 200:46.
15. Gralnick HR, Connaghan DG. In: Williams WJ, Beutler E, Ersler AJ, Lichtman MA, eds. *Hematology.* 5th ed. New York: McGraw-Hill, 1994:1441.
16. Davie EW, Fujikawa K, Kisiel W. The coagulation cascade: Initiation, maintenance and regulation. *Biochemistry.* 1991; 30: 10363–10370.
17. Hall CA, Rapaport SI, Ames SB, DeGroot JA. A clinical and family study of hereditary proconvertin (factor VII). *Am J Med.* 1964; 37:172.
18. Dische FE, Benfield V. Congenital factor VII deficiency: haematological and genetic aspects. *Acta Haematol.* 1959; 21:257.
19. Tuddenham EGD, Lane RS, Rotblat F, et al. Response to infusion of proelectrolyte fractionated human factor VIII concentrates in human hemophilia A and von Willebrand disease. *Br J Haematol.* 1982; 52:259.
20. Hoyer LW, Rick ME. Implications of immunological methods for measuring antihemophilic factor (factor VIII). *Ann N Y Acad Sci.* 1975; 240:97.
21. Coller BS. Von Willebrand's disease. In: Ratnoff OD, Farbes CD, eds. *Disorders of Hemostasis.* Orlando, Fla: Grune & Stratton; 1984:241.
22. Holmber L, Nelson IM. Von Willebrand's disease. In: *Clinics in Hematology: Coagulation Disorders.* Philadelphia: WB Saunders; 1985:461.
23. DeLa Cadena RA, Wachtfogel YT, Colman RW. Contact activa-

tion pathway: Inflammation and coagulation. In: Colman RW, Hirsh J, Marder VJ, Salzman EW, eds. *Hemostasis and Thrombosis: Basic Principles and Clinical Practice*. 3rd ed. Philadelphia: JB Lippincott; 1994:230.

24. Stehling LC, Ellison N, Faust RJ, et al: A survey of transfusion practices among anesthesiologists. *Vox Sang*. 1987; 52:60.
25. Van Dijk PM, Kleine JW. The transfusion reaction in anaesthesiological practice. *Acta Anaesthesiol Belg*. 1976; 4:274.
26. Zunich KM, Lane HC. Immunologic abnormalities in HIV infection. *Hematol Oncol Clin North Am* 1991; 5:215.
27. Zon LI, Groopman JE. Hematologic manifestations of the human immune deficiency virus (HIV). *Semin Hematol* 1988; 25:208.
28. Bick RL. Vascular disorders associated with thrombo-hemorrhagic phenomenon. *Semin Thromb Hemost* 1979; 5:167.
29. Bick RL. Vascular disorders associated with thrombo-hemorrhagic phenomenon. In: Bick RL, *Disorders of Hemostasis and Thrombosis. Principles of Clinical Practice*. New York: Thieme; 1985; 44, 157, 223.
30. Bick RL. Disseminated intravascular coagulation and related syndromes: Etiology, pathophysiology, diagnosis and management. *Am J Hematol* 1978; 5:265.
31. Bick RL. Disseminated intravascular coagulation and related syndromes: A clinical review. *Semin Thromb Hemost*. 1988;14:299.
32. Bick RL. Disseminated intravascular coagulation. In: Abe T, Yamanaka M, eds. *Disseminated Intravascular Coagulation*. Boca Raton, Fla: CRC Press, 1983:31.
33. Kevy SV, Glickman RM, Bernhard WF, et al: The pathogenesis and control of the hemorrhagic defect in open heart surgery. *Surg Gynecol Obstet*. 1966; 123:313–318.
34. Bick RL. Alterations of hemostasis associated with surgery, cardiopulmonary bypass surgery and prosthetic devices. In: Ratnoff OD, Forbes CD, eds: *Disorders of Hemostasis*. 2nd ed. Philadelphia: WB Saunders, 1989:379.

☐ QUESTIONS

1. Major causes of neutrophilic leukocytosis are:
   a. Ketoacidosis
   b. Bacterial infection
   c. Surgery
   d. All of the above

2. Which of the following statements regarding delayed transfusion reactions are correct?
   a. It can occur days or weeks after transfusion.
   b. Transmission of infectious diseases including hepatitis, cytomegalovirus, and human immunodeficiency virus can occur.
   c. Graft-versus-host disease can occur.
   d. All are true.

3. A patient requiring an emergency exploratory laparotomy presents with a prothrombin time/partial thromboplastin time of 12.6/25.2, a platelet count of 250,000 and a bleeding time of 12 minutes. The best treatment would be
   a. Infusion of 6 units of platelets intraoperatively
   b. Administration of desmopressin (DDAVP)
   c. Infusion of fresh-frozen plasma
   d. Repeat laboratory studies preoperatively

4. Which of the following statements about thrombocytopenia is *incorrect*?
   a. Surgical bleed may occur with platelet count less than 75,000.
   b. At any time, two thirds of the platelets are in circulation, the remaining one third in the spleen.
   c. Normal platelet count is 150,000 to 450,000/μL.
   d. One unit of platelet concentrate will increase the platelet count 5000 to 10,000 mm.[3]

5. Administration of fresh-frozen plasma replaces which factors:
   a. V
   b. III
   c. VIII
   d. V and VIII

6. All of the following cause sickling of the red blood cells *except:*
   a. Hypothermia
   b. Increased 2,3-DPG
   c. Respiratory alkalosis
   d. Dehydration

7. Which of the following statements about von Willebrand's disease is (are) *true?*
   a. Autosomal versus sex-linked trait
   b. Perioperative treatment includes infusion of cryoprecipitate.
   c. Bleeding is due to an inability of the platelets to adhere.
   d. All of the above

8. A 57-year-old man with Cooley's anemia (β thalassemia) presents with a suspected ruptured appendix. All statements are true *except:*
   a. Potential overgrowth of the maxilla can make airway management and intubation difficult.
   b. This patient is considered a "full stomach" related to chronic hepatomegaly.
   c. Spinal cord compression may be present.
   d. Chronic splenomegaly can cause thrombocytopenia and leukopenia.

9. Factor IX deficiency is a sex-linked recessive bleeding disorder also known as Christmas factor. True or false?
   a. True
   b. False

10. Intraoperatively you are administering 1 U packed red cells to a 36-year-old woman undergoing an acoustic neuroma resection who is otherwise healthy. Twenty minutes after hanging the blood you notice the patient's

temperature has risen 1.7°. Otherwise no other changes are noted. Correct management would include:
a. Send the remaining blood to the blood bank.
b. Remove existing filter from blood tubing.
c. Initiate diuretic therapy.
d. Slow transfusion rate down.

11. Choose the one *correct* statement:
a. Immunoglobulins are antigen-specific antibodies produced by T lymphocytes.
b. IgA is the only immunoglobulin to cross the placenta for passive immunity to the newborn.
c. IgE induces the release of histamine, serotonin, leukotrienes, and eosinophilic chemotactic factor in the allergic patient.
d. IgD is principally found in saliva, tears and fluids of the gastrointestinal, respiratory, and urinary tracts.

12. A 55-year-old man is scheduled for insertion of Hickman catheter prior to treatment for lung carcinoma. On physical examination he is found to be anemic with adenopathy and organomegaly. The most likely coexisting disease is:
a. Chronic myelogenous leukemia
b. Acute lymphoblastic leukemia
c. Chronic lymphocytic leukemia
d. Neutrophilia

13. Once entering into circulation, platelets survive approximately:
a. 5 days
b. 10 days
c. 30 days
d. 120 days

14. A 32-year-old woman is scheduled for open reduction, internal fixation of the left ankle. She has sickle cell disease and has been hospitalized in the past for sickle cell crisis. Major anesthetic concerns include all *except:*
a. Meticulous attention to all sterile techniques during invasive procedures to diminish risk of infection
b. Avoidance of tourniquet
c. Prompt treatment of febrile episodes with a cooling blanket
d. Careful attention to adequate hydration and blood loss replacement

15. Which of the following statements about primary immunodeficiency disorders is *incorrect?*
a. Most have onset in childhood.
b. Affects females more than males

c. Increased susceptibility to infection
d. Genetically determined disorder

16. Which of the following statements about anemia are *correct?*
a. Aplastic anemia is due to bone marrow damage as with radiation therapy.
b. Pernicious anemia is caused by poorly absorbed B_{12}, folic acid, or intrinsic factor causing red blood cells to fail to mature. This leads to compensating oversized and irregularly shaped hemoglobin.
c. When exposed to low concentrations of oxygen, hemoglobin S sickles in shape forming crystals that can damage cell membranes.
d. Hereditary spherocytosis is a disease in which the erythrocyte count may be normal. But the red cell is more spherical in shape than the normal biconcave disk. Membrane fragility and splenic sequestration can lead to hemolytic anemia.
e. All are correct.

17. The affinity of hemoglobin for O_2 is altered by H^+, CO_2 and 2,3-DPG. Increasing P_{CO_2} and decreasing O_2 concentration is known as the:
a. Joules-Thompson effect
b. Haldane effect
c. Bohr effect
d. Oxyhemoglobin dissociation curve

18. A 35-year-old man has a preoperative test result of prothrombin time 12.5 and partial thromboplastin time 42.0. He has no history of bleeding. The most appropriate initial presurgical evaluation should include which of the following:
a. Repeat laboratory tests.
b. Proceed with surgery.
c. Transfuse 2 U fresh-frozen plasma.
d. Infuse 10 U fresh-frozen plasma platelet concentrate.

19. All of the following are manifestations of human immunodeficiency virus *except:*
a. Hypogammaglobulinemia
b. Decreased CD_4 lymphocytes
c. Delayed or absent hypersensitivity skin reactions
d. Increased susceptibility to opportunistic infection

20. By what mechanism does coumadin work?
a. Prolonging prothrombin time
b. Inhibiting platelet adhesion
c. Inhibiting vitamin K-dependent factors (II, VII, IX, and X)
d. a and c

☐ ANSWERS

1.	d	**5.**	d	**9.**	a	**13.**	b	**17.**	c
2.	d	**6.**	c	**10.**	d	**14.**	c	**18.**	a
3.	b	**7.**	d	**11.**	c	**15.**	b	**19.**	a
4.	b	**8.**	b	**12.**	c	**16.**	e	**20.**	d

SIX

Anesthetic Considerations for the Surgical Patient

CHAPTER

21

Cardiothoracic Anesthesia

John C. Kastor

Cardiothoracic and vascular anesthesia is a large area to cover within the confines of one chapter. Whole books have been written about each area covered here, and I encourage all anesthetists to use these books for a more in-depth look at this subject. It is assumed that the anesthetist has a working knowledge of the physiology and pharmacology connected with these systems. This chapter is designed to be a quick reference guide.

☐ CARDIAC PROCEDURES

OPEN HEART SURGERY

Anesthetic considerations for cardiac surgery should include hemodynamic goals, surgical requirements, choice of anesthetic drugs and techniques, monitoring, and cardiopulmonary bypass (CPB). Ideally, a normal, angina-free, hemodynamic state should be maintained during the surgery. Optimal oxygen supply–demand balance is achieved when the heart is beating slowly and is small and well perfused. This will allow for *maximum end-diastolic time*, which is the time that the coronary arteries receive their blood supply, and will allow for adequate coronary artery perfusion pressure.

Surgical requirements include length of time of surgery, time of extubation, need for muscle relaxation, and need for increased inspired oxygen fraction (FIO$_2$). The choice of anesthetic techniques is left up to the practitioner, and no one technique has been shown to be superior to another. The most common technique is a narcotic-oxygen technique, but it can be used in conjunction with inhalation agents. A regional anesthetic may be used to help with postoperative pain management. A high-dose narcotic-oxygen technique has the advantage of producing less myocardial depression while maintaining a stable heart rate during stimulating events such as intubation, placement of monitoring lines, surgical stimulation, and when relaxants such as pancuronium are used. *Narcotics* also suppress the normal stress reactions such as the release of antidiuretic hormone, growth hormone, and endogenous epinephrine or norepinephrine. If early extubation is anticipated careful titration of narcotic and relaxant should be used. Awareness with a narcotic-oxygen technique has been reported, but the incidence seems to be small. The use of Versed or other amnesic drugs helps prevent this problem.

General anesthesia with volatile anesthetics, such as isoflurane, has the advantage of reversing myocardial depression quickly and easily while providing reliable suppression of untoward sympathetic responses and awareness. The disadvantages include lowering of blood pressure, lack of postoperative analgesia, and coronary steal. *Coronary steal* is theoretically caused by decreasing the pressure in the coronary vasculature and thus stealing blood from small collaterals that may be feeding an area blocked in its main blood supply. The use of *nitrous oxide* is controversial. Most institutions avoid its use to reduce the possibility of enlarging air bubbles.

Monitoring Monitoring should include electrocardiography (ECG) with leads II and V$_5$, two sources of temperature (nasal, esophageal, Swan-Ganz, rectal or bladder), direct invasive arterial pressure and possibly a pulmonary artery catheter, central venous pressure (CVP) catheter, and transesophageal echocardiography (TEE). All but the TEE and temperature probes should be inserted before induction with the patient sedated and supplemental oxygen administered. Monitoring of ST segment trend analysis is useful for recognition of *ischemia*. Pulse oximetry provides information about rate as well as oxygen saturation. Use of a noninvasive blood pressure cuff is necessary until an arterial line is connected.

Preparation   Venous access may be through two large-bore peripheral intravenous sites, or if peripheral access is limited, then double cannulation of the internal jugular vein is the most common practice. If prominent, the external jugular may be used. The right radial artery should be used whenever compromise of the left subclavian artery may occur, as in retracting for exposure of the *left internal mammary artery*. This may cause damping of the arterial tracing. The left radial artery should be used whenever compromise of the *innominate artery* may occur. A femoral artery may be used if radial or brachial arteries cannot be cannulated. The internal jugular is the most common site for placement of a pulmonary artery catheter, and a side port can be used for intravenous introduction of vasoactive drugs. Preinduction measurements of arterial pressure, pulmonary artery pressure, pulmonary capillary wedge pressure (PCWP), CVP, and cardiac output should be obtained for baseline measurements.

All drugs should be made ready and clearly labeled. Vasoactive drugs that may be used include phenylephrine, $CaCl_2$, nitroglycerin, epinephrine, Neo-Synephrine, dopamine, dobutamine, and amrinone. Initial heparin dosage for preparation for CPB is 300 to 400 U/kg and should be drawn up prior to starting anesthesia should it become necessary to go on CPB emergently. Anesthetic drugs should be ready and selected using hemodynamic effects, duration of action, and cost as primary considerations.

Anesthesia Considerations   On arrival to the operating room, any drug infusions being given to the patient should be continued until the initiation of CPB. Induction should be slow and controlled, with 100% oxygen given. Airway control must be maintained without the use of excess positive pressure during inspiration or exhalation. Induction agents should be given according to the patient's hemodynamic status. Intubation can cause a sympathetic discharge with hypertension and tachycardia. The use of deeper anesthesia, liberal narcotics, intravenous lidocaine, or nitroglycerin, 2–4 $\mu g/kg$, may be necessary to avoid this response. After the endotracheal tube has been secured and bilateral breath sounds determined, a TEE probe may be inserted through the mouth and into the esophagus. A complete evaluation of the heart should include checking for mitral and aortic valve regurgitation, aortic calcification, and generalized wall motion. For coronary artery bypass graft surgery (CABG), the best view to use with the TEE probe is the *short axis view* of the left ventricle (Fig. 21–1) and is accomplished by placing the probe into the stomach and bringing the tip up facing the diaphragm. This will allow the anesthetist to view the wall motion, thickness of the wall, and size of the ventricle. Ischemia can be seen in this view if the motion of the wall changes. *Temperature probes* should be inserted in the nasal pharyngeal area, showing brain temperature, and in the bladder with a temperature-tipped bladder catheter. These will

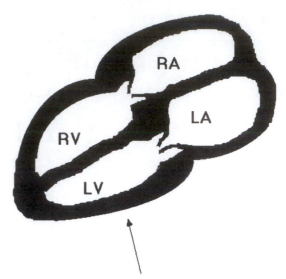

Figure 21–1   Short axis view of the left ventricle.

show more accurately when reheating of the patient has been successful.

Arterial blood gases, after a period of mechanical ventilation, should be obtained as well as blood glucose, electrolytes, and a baseline activated clotting time (ACT). From induction until time of CPB, the anesthetic goal is to ensure minimal hemodynamic alteration and a smooth transition. Stimuli that can cause hypertension and tachycardia such as skin incision, sternal splitting, spreading the sternum with a retractor, opening and suturing the pericardium, and manipulating the aorta should be anticipated and anesthesia adjusted accordingly. Ventilation should be discontinued and the lungs deflated during *sternal splitting* to prevent an accidental pneumothorax.

Coronary Artery Bypass Graft   Coronary artery bypass graft is the most common surgical procedure done on the heart today. This is done primarily for occlusive coronary artery disease (CAD) that cannot be treated medically with coronary angioplasty. In this surgery, autologous veins and internal mammary arteries can be used to bypass areas in the coronary artery circulation where blockage has occurred. These patients usually present with one or more other problems in addition to occluded coronary arteries. It is common to see diabetes, renal failure, hypertension, vascular disease, and pulmonary disease in these patients.

Cardiopulmonary Bypass Preparation   Heparin is a large mucopolysaccharide that prevents blood clotting by accelerating the formation of antithrombin III, which, in turn, forms a complex with activated thrombin. This neutral complex leads to anticoagulation.

Heparin is given when requested by the surgeon, and an ACT should be obtained 3 to 5 minutes after the dose is administered. Blood should be aspirated before and after the dose of heparin has been given to make sure that the venous line has not infiltrated before or during the injection of heparin. The goal is for an ACT of 480 seconds or higher, and if not reached, then additional heparin is given. A rare resistance to heparin anticoagulation may be secondary to *antithrombin III deficiency*. If the initial heparin dose does not cause a significant rise in the ACT, and an additional dose does not bring the ACT up to 480 seconds or more, then antithrombin III deficiency should be considered, and fresh-frozen plasma (FFP), usually 1 to 2 U, should be given. The ACT should be repeated, and additional heparin given if necessary.

Once the surgeon has secured arterial and venous cannulation, then the patient will be placed on CPB. When complete CPB has been achieved, the anesthetist should:

1. pull the pulmonary artery catheter back about 5 cm to avoid its becoming permanently wedged during manipulation of the heart,
2. stop all intravenous solutions,
3. discontinue mechanical ventilation and apply about 1 L oxygen to the breathing circuit,
4. empty the urine collection bag so that the urinary output can be measured while on CPB, and
5. discontinue all anesthetic and other drugs being given to the patient.

They will be administered by the perfusionist through the CPB pump. The left ventricle size is observed with the TEE monitor for signs of filling and the perfusionist notified if filling occurs.

While the patient is on bypass, preparations for coming off of bypass can begin. The pacemaker generator batteries are inserted, and parameters programmed in for both arterial and ventricular lead testing. All medications that will be necessary after bypass must be prepared. If cardioplegia is used during bypass, temperature leads will have to be connected to monitor the temperature of the heart. Doppler lines may need to be connected to test the flow of blood through coronary bypass grafts.

Cardiopulmonary Bypass During CPB the heart and lungs are replaced by a pump and oxygenator which provide a nonpulsating blood flow and allow for systemic hypothermia. The patient is anticoagulated and hemodiluted.

Abnormal blood-gas and blood-plastic interfaces are formed, which damage blood cells and denature blood proteins. The normal filtering function of the lungs is lost and organ damage and dysfunction can occur. Suction devices to evacuate fluids and blood from the surgical site are attached to the pump and oxygenator. A schematic diagram of the CPB circuit is shown in Fig. 21–2.

Venous drainage is usually accomplished by a single cannula inserted into the right atrium, although a second cannula may be inserted into the inferior vena cava. The blood then flows by gravity to a reservoir that helps to buffer fluctuations in venous return. The reservoir has a built-in oxygenator in which the blood is oxygenated and carbon dioxide is removed. A heat exchanger attached to the reservoir allows cooling and rewarming of the blood. Next a microfilter and

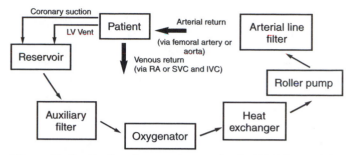

Figure 21–2 Cardiopulmonary bypass circuit. LV, left ventricle; RA, right atrium; SVC, superior vena cava; IVC, inferior vena cava. (Reproduced by permission from Thomson.[1])

bubble trap are inserted into the arterial line to prevent particulate and gas embolism. A manometer is used to monitor pressure in the arterial return line. The *arterial cannula* is usually placed into the aorta, but it can be placed into the femoral artery, if the surgeon is working on the ascending or descending thoracic aorta.

In addition to the primary circuit, there are several auxiliary circuits. Cardiotomy suctions are connected to the pump, which bring free blood, air, and particulate matter from the surgical field. This must undergo settling and microfiltration in a separate reservoir before being fed into the main reservoir for oxygenation. A ventricular vent catheter may also be inserted into the left ventricle to prevent overdistention and damage. If cardioplegia solution is used, an additional circuit is needed with the heat exchanger. A typical *cardioplegia solution* consists of potassium, 30 mmol/L; sodium, 109 mmol/L; chloride, 114 mmol/L; calcium, 1 mmol/L; bicarbonate, 27 mmol/L; glucose, 28 mmol/L; and mannitol, 54 mmol/L.

Membrane oxygenators are the most commonly used and consist of a semipermeable membrane, which allows gas exchange across the membrane, separating the blood from the gases. Gas microembolism, a problem found when using a bubble-through oxygenator, usually does not occur with the membrane oxygenator. The blood-plastic interfaces formed during perfusion can cause blood damage, but it is thought that the membrane quickly becomes coated with a thin layer of denatured blood protein, resulting in blood damage. Membrane oxygenators can be used for long periods of time with fewer complications to the patient. Prior to bypass, the pumps are primed with 1500 to 2500 mL normal saline. Priming with this amount of normal saline leads to a desired intraoperative hematocrit in the low twenties.

Hypothermia Deliberate hypothermia of 20° to 28°F is accomplished in the reservoir to reduce metabolism during bypass. A reduced metabolism will allow vital organs to better tolerate the insult of bypass for a longer period of time. It also decreases the flow requirements while on bypass, reducing the total physiologic insult. Another advantage of hypothermia is the prolonged period of cardiac arrest that patients can tolerate without causing brain and cellular damage. Many changes occur with hypothermia and CBP; therefore, it is important to check electrolytes, glucose, hematocrits, pH, and ACT intraoperatively and adjust accordingly. The perfusionist will draw samples of blood from the reservoir at prescribed intervals to run checks on all of these parameters. If intermittent cross-clamping of the aorta is used by the surgeon during CABG surgery, cardioplegia solution is not used.

Rewarming the patient is started at the surgeon's request. Adequate rewarming to 37°C can be monitored from the bladder or rectal probe.

When the patient is coming off CPB, the anesthetist should have vasoactive and inotropic drugs ready to administer. *Protamine*, 1 mg/100 U heparin, should be administered slowly to reverse the anticoagulation of the heparin by neutralization, thus forming an inactive complex. If protamine is given too rapidly, a *type I (anaphylactic)* reaction can result. This is manifested by systemic hypotension due to peripheral vasodilation and pulmonary hypertension and may be caused by the release of histamine, leukotrienes, or other endogenous vasoactive substances that cause vasodilation.[2] Although antihistamines can attenuate this reaction, slow administration works equally well. After the protamine is administered, wait 3 to 5 minutes and then check an ACT to determine if the ACT is back to preoperative levels.

Post-CPB

As the patient is taken off of bypass intravenous fluids are restarted; the pulmonary artery catheter is advanced to a position that allows a PCWP reading; cardiac output is obtained; anesthetic agents are given; and ECG and TEE monitors are observed for signs of ischemia, dysrhythmias, and left ventricular wall function. Usually, the patient's intravascular volume will be low and must be increased with crystalloids, packed cells, and plasma expanders. A blood scavenging system can be used to process blood lost from the operative site and returned to the patient. From the reservoir the perfusionist can return volume to the patient, before the arterial cannula is discontinued. At this time electrolytes and arterial blood gases must be measured and corrected, pacemaker leads tested, and generators set to three times above thresholds obtained.

If myocardial ischemia and cardiogenic shock are present, the use of an intra-aortic balloon pump (IABP) may be necessary. A misnomer, the IABP actually augments coronary blood flow and reduces impedance to ventricular ejection. The *IABP* consists of a catheter with an elongated balloon at the end that is inflated and deflated in a synchronized fashion with the heartbeat. It can receive its stimulus from an ECG or from an arterial pressure line. The length of the balloon is measured by laying the balloon on the patient's chest at the angle of Louis and measuring down to the femoral artery. It is then inserted into the femoral artery and advanced up into the central aorta and then into the correct position in the proximal segment of the descending aorta.

Coexisting Disease
DIABETES

Up to 22% of patients presenting for CABG have diabetes. Surgical stress, hypothermia, and epinephrine infusion can contribute to a resistance to insulin. Cardioplegia is high in dextrose and can exacerbate this situation. Intraoperative blood sugar levels should be monitored and controlled with insulin, preferably with an infusion technique.

RENAL DISEASE

Renal failure can occur after CABG and is thought to be a result of inadequate renal profusion.[3] Patients with renal impairment may require diuretics or low-dose dopamine to maintain adequate urine output. Intraoperatively, adequate circulating volume, cardiac output, and urine flow must be maintained.

HYPERTENSION

Preoperatively, hypertension should be controlled, otherwise left ventricular hypertrophy and congestive heart failure (CHF) are increased risks. Careful monitoring of left ventricular function with PCWP and short axis view TEE is necessary.

VASCULAR DISEASE

Vascular disease can be present in patients presenting for CABG. Peripheral vascular disease can be of importance in placement of arterial catheters. A history of transient ischemic attacks (TIAs), stroke, or carotid bruits will need to be evaluated for carotid stenosis. If carotid stenosis is documented, simultaneous CABG and carotid endarterectomy may be planned.

PULMONARY DISEASE

Pulmonary function should be optimized at time of surgery. Pulmonary function tests will provide clinical information for evaluating the ease and timing of extubation postoperatively. There is a predictive value in the results of these tests and the patient's ability to breath for himself or herself.

COAGULOPATHIES

These patients may have received an intravenous thrombolytic drug (e.g., tissue plasminogen activator) within the past 24 hours and can be expected to develop a coagulopathy after CPB. This coagulopathy will not respond to the reversal of the heparin given before CPB, and may require FFP, cryoprecipitate, or an antifibrinolytic agent such as aminocaproic acid (Amicar) to reverse the affects of the intravenous thrombolytic drugs.[4] Patients with unstable angina may be kept on intravenous heparin until the time of surgery, necessitating a baseline ACT before the administration of heparin CPB.

VALVULAR PROCEDURES

The mortality rate for patients undergoing valvular procedures on the heart remains in the third to tenth percentile. Statistical improvement should be the goal for all concerned with the perioperative care of these patients. The most common valvular procedures on the heart involve the aortic and mitral valves (Table 21–1).

Table 21–1
ANESTHETIC GOALS FOR MANAGEMENT OF VALVULAR LESIONS

	Heart Rate	Contractility	Afterload	Preload
Aortic Stenosis	Normal or slightly decreased	Normal	Maintain normal	Increase
Aortic Regurgitation	Normal or slightly elevated	Normal or slightly increased	Decrease	Normal/ Elevated
Mitral Stenosis	Normal or slightly decreased	Normal	Normal or slightly decreased	Increase
Mitral Regurgitation	Normal or slightly elevated	Normal	Decrease	Normal/ Elevated

Aortic Valvular Disease   Conditions of the aortic valve include congenital or acquired *aortic stenosis*. If congenital, it can be either unicuspid, bicuspid, or tricuspid, with bicuspid the most common, occurring in more than 50% of patients. Aortic insufficiency occurs in 90% of patients with unicuspid disease.[5] With acquired aortic stenosis, calcification of the leaflets of the valve is the most common, and the stenosis increases with age. The patient is usually asymptomatic for a period of years (as long as 50 or more). *Angina*, *syncope*, and *CHF* are the most common symptoms. Patients may be treated medically for a period of time, but the more severe the symptoms, the more an invasive procedure is indicated. The stenotic valve causes an obstruction during LV ejection resulting in a decreased cardiac output and LV hypertropy. Failure can occur and oxygen demand will increase due to the increased workload of the heart. Patients with aortic stenosis and angina may have underlying CAD.

Diagnosis is made by symptoms, cardiac catheterization, and echocardiography, both transthoracic and transesophageal. A cardiac catheterization will help rule out the possibility of underlying CAD.

Aortic insufficiency may be acquired or congenital. If congenital, it is usually associated with other cardiac anomalies and rarely occurs as a single lesion. Rheumatic heart disease and endocarditis are the most common causes of acquired aortic insufficiency. The history is one of a long asymptomatic period as the left ventricle progressively enlarges, and CHF and angina occur. Treatment is valve replacement. Diagnosis is made on the basis of symptoms. An echocardiogram will show valvular regurgitation and an enlarged left ventricle. Severity is best measured by cardiac catheterization.

Idiopathic hypertropic subaortic stenosis (IHSS) is a thickening of the myocardium below the aortic valve that can lead to partial outflow obstruction of the left ventricle. This is usually caused by a autosomal dominant genetic defect.[6] Patients may present with nonspecific symptoms such as chest pain, palpitations, dyspnea, and syncope. Findings are consistent with left ventricular outflow obstruction, which usually occurs in older patients. IHSS is usually treated medically, and surgery is reserved for patients who do not respond to medical treatment. β blockers and verapamil have been used for medical treatment. Surgical management is myotomy-myomectomy through a transaortic approach. For patients presenting with IHSS, *halothane,* which decreases contractility of the ventricle due to myocardium depression, is preferred. Preload and afterload must be maintained with volume replacement and phenylephrine. Heart rate should be maintained at preoperative levels with β blockade and verapamil as needed.

Anesthetic Management
When presenting for noncardiac surgery, either regional or general anesthesia may be used. Monitoring will be determined by existing symptoms and the type of surgery the patient is undergoing. Monitoring of these patients should consist of an ECG with a continuous display of a modified V_5 lead because the hypertrophied left ventricle is prone to ischemia. Direct arterial monitoring is probably indicated for these patients even for relative minor surgery. Filling pressures via a Swan-Ganz pulmonary artery catheter should be monitored whenever significant volume shifts are anticipated. This will indicate the left ventricular filling pressure and alert to the possibility of left ventricular failure. Also, the pulmonary artery catheter allows an accurate core temperature reading, sampling of mixed venous oxygen content, and a reliable cardiac output index.

If using regional anesthesia, a "solid" block is desired and use of sedation is essential. Spinal anesthesia usually produces a better quality of both motor and sensory anesthesia than does epidural anesthesia. Medication should be chosen to allow for an adequate length of time to accommodate the proposed surgery. A sufficient volume of anesthetic drug should be used to provide for an adequate level of anesthesia. If epidural anesthesia is chosen, it is desirable to achieve both a motor and sensory block. Anxiety, which can increase the workload of the heart, is not well tolerated.

For patients with aortic insufficiency, all techniques for general anesthesia are acceptable; however, a narcotic technique is desired. This helps avoid significant myocardial depression and control tachycardia. The muscle relaxant should be devoid of cardiac effects. If using Sufenta, pancuronium may be used for its sympathomimetic properties to counter the potential for bradycardia, nodal rhythm, heart block, and transient sinus arrest. Avoid increases in afterload and keep the intravascular volume stable. Early treatment of hypotension is essential regardless of it etiology. Tachydysrhythmias of any origin require equally aggressive treatment because of associated increase in myocardial oxygen demand. Appropriate drug therapies include edrophonium, adenosine, esmolol, or verapamil. Bradycardias should be treated immediately with atropine or other vagal blocking agents.

Mitral Valvular Disease Mitral valvular disease is usually either mitral stenosis or mitral regurgitation. Rheumatic fever is the most common cause for *mitral stenosis* and occurs in women more than men. Symptoms usually occur in the fourth or fifth decades of life with acute onset of CHF and paroxysmal attacks of atrial fibrillation. Ventricular underloading causes pulmonary hypertension and leads to pulmonary edema. Again, cardiac catheterization and echocardiography as well as patient symptoms confirm the diagnosis.

Mitral regurgitation (MR) occurs due to a disease of the valve leaflets, the papillary muscles, or chordae tendineae. Rheumatic disease is the most common cause of leaflet disease, though it can also be caused by bacterial endocarditis and acute myocardial infarction. Mitral valve prolapse is a common valvular anomaly affecting 5% to 8% of the population. About 15% of these patients will develop varying severity of MR. Papillary muscle dysfunction is usually caused by ischemia. The history includes lassitude and easy fatigability. Diagnosis is the same as for mitral stenosis.

Anesthetic Management

Goals for noncardiac surgery anesthetic management should include maintaining appropriately full volume, and avoiding exacerbation of preexisting pulmonary hypertension. *Bradycardia* must be avoided with MR as this causes increased LV volume, diminished forward cardiac output, and increased regurgitation. Supplemental oxygen should always accompany preoperative medication. Minimal monitoring should include ECG, noninvasive blood pressure (arterial) monitoring, and oxygen saturation. A pulmonary artery catheter should be used to measure PCWP when major volume shifts are expected.

Either regional or general anesthesia may be used. The *Trendelenberg* position increases the work of breathing and should be avoided. Oxygen-narcotic techniques for general anesthesia are best for patients with pulmonary hypertension. Nitrous oxide is rarely used in these patients due to conflicting data regarding this drug's potential *pulmonary vasoconstrictive* properties. Hypercarbia, hypoxia, and all anesthetics that cause increased PVR should be avoided. Muscle relaxants that avoid cardiovascular side effects are preferred. After all other causes of tachycardia have been corrected (light anesthesia, hypercarbia, hypoxia, etc.) β blockers are desirable. Hypotension is best corrected with volume and vasoconstrictors should be avoided. Dopamine, epinephrine, and dobutamine are appropriate treatment for hypotension unrelated to volume depletion. Cardiac output and blood pressure are increased without excessive increases in heart rate. Finally, any increase in systemic vascular resistance (SVR) will worsen chronic mitral regurgitation. Therefore, afterload reduction may be desirable.

Aortic Operations Operations on the aorta may include operations on the aortic arch, the ascending aorta, and the descending thoracic aorta. Aortic aneurysms are classified according to their etiology. Degenerative aneurysms occur from weakening of the medial layer, which allows a ballooning out of the aortic walls. Two classifications of this type of aneurysm are: (1) atherosclerotic aneurysms in which the process starts in the intima and then proceeds to the media and (2) Marfan's syndrome, which is a dominant inherited disorder of the connective tissue that may lead to abnormalities in the aortic media.

Aortic dissections are caused by an intimal tear that progresses to a separation of layers of the aortic wall, creating a false lumen that runs parallel to the true lumen. This tear usually occurs in the ascending aorta. Complications of dissections are rupture, cardiac tamponade, aortic insufficiency, and obstruction of the true lumina of aortic branches, including the coronary arteries, leading to ischemia of the organs supplied by those branches involved.

A major anesthetic concern with aortic arch procedures is providing cerebral protection. The technique of choice today is deep hypothermic circulatory arrest using CPB with femoral artery cannulization. The temperature needed to produce an isoelectric electroencephalogram (EEG) is approximately 18°C. The period of circulatory arrest, in which there is no cerebral complication, is approximately 45 minutes at 18°C and 1 hour at 15°C.[7] The best estimate of the brain temperature is measured in the *nasopharyngeal* area.

Complications

If a shunt is not used during the cross-clamping period, an inevitable complication of thoracic aorta surgery is hypertension. The proximal end of the aorta is the site for hypertension. Nitroprusside should be started slowly before aortic cross-clamping. Nitroglycerin might be necessary in some cases. Unclamping can lead to a sudden lowering of the systemic vascular resistance, accumulation of metabolites or endogenous vasoactive substances, and cardiac depression due to ischemia.

The surgeon should notify the anesthesia team as unclamping approaches, to allow discontinuation of vasodilator drugs and infusion of adequate volume to counter the hypotension that occurs. Vasopressors may be necessary until an adequate volume is established. Acidosis should be anticipated, and a sodium bicarbonate infusion can be given during cross-clamping. If hypotension persists, reclamping may be necessary until the problem is resolved.

At this point, unclamping can be reattempted. When needed, a scavengering system to recycle major blood loss should be used. Volume replacement is with crystalloids, plasma, and red blood cells according to hematocrit levels and the intraoperative coagulation studies. Hypothermia and the administration of mannitol before CPB provide renal protection.

Over half the complications that lead to perioperative mortality are cardiac in nature. Not surprisingly, there is a direct correlation between aortic aneurysm and presence of CAD. Unfortunately, a cardiac evaluation may be difficult due to significant arterial disease in this population.

The most feared major complication of thoracic aortic surgery is paraplegia from spinal cord ischemia. During aortic cross-clamping, arteries that supply the spinal cord can be compromised. Cross-clamping for more than 30 minutes increases the incidence of paraplegia. Acute dissections have a higher incidence of paraplegia than other forms of aneurysms.

In addition to shunting and CPB with hypothermia, somatosensory evoked potentials should be monitored during cross-clamping to identify important intercostal arteries that will need to be anastomosed to the aortic graft. Barbiturates and corticosteroids may offer further spinal cord and cerebral protection with prolonged cross-clamping time. Other measures of protection include cerebrospinal fluid drainage via a subdural catheter and injection of papaverine into the subdural space to dilate the anterior spinal artery.

CONGENITAL HEART ANOMALIES

Congenital heart defects occur in approximately 8 of 1000 live births and may be discovered soon after birth, in infancy, or later in childhood. Congenital heart diseases are structural in nature and may lead to CHF, cyanosis, or both. The categories of pediatric heart disease are shown in Table 21–2. Classification of the disease depends on the type of lesion.

Special anesthetic concerns include altered inhalation and intravenous induction, avoidance of crying which may exacerbate cyanosis, and a thorough understanding of the pathophysiology of each anomaly. Some of the more common anomalies are ventricular septal defect, atrial septal defect, and tetralogy of Fallot. Further classification places lesions into three categories: lesions that cause outflow obstruction, lesions that cause right-to-left shunts, and lesions that cause left-to-right shunts. The presence of a shunt can lead to chamber pressure overload or chamber volume overload. In addition, there may be mixed lesions that improve or worsen the primary defect. In some cases, survival from one defect may depend on the presence of a secondary lesion (pulmonary atresia with a ventricular septal defect). Cyanotic congenital defects, which allow unoxygenated blood to enter the systemic arterial circulation, require early surgical intervention. Emergency shunting procedures are done immediately, with major defect corrections done at a later age.

Ventricular Septal Defect Ventricular septal defect is the most common congenital defect. There is a left-to-right shunting of the blood in the ventricles. Consequently, the left ventricle will enlarge as it takes on the work of pumping blood to the systemic vasculature system and the pulmonary system, through the septal defect. Pulmonary blood flow is increased. Once CHF develops, surgical intervention is indicated to close the septal defect and prevent irreversible pulmonary hypertension. The pharmacokinetics of the inhaled and intravenous agents are not appreciably altered. Antibiotic prophylaxis against bacterial endocarditis is necessary in the presence of VSD.

Atrial Septal Defect Atrial septal defect is of special concern to the anesthetist. Because of the possibility of air embolism, the utmost vigilance must be given to avoiding the entrainment of any air into the intravenous line. Anesthetics and events that lead to an increase in SVR should be avoided because this worsens the existing shunt. Although the right ventricle may dilate, these children do well and right-sided failure is unlikely. A left-to-right shunt can speed the alveolar equilibration of inhaled anesthetic and would thus increase the speed of induction. The opposite is true of intravenous drugs because recirculation prolongs induction tine.

Transposition of the Great Vessels and Tetralogy of Fallot Tetralogy of Fallot has four components: right ventricular outlet obstruction (pulmonary stenosis), right ventricular hypertrophy, ventricular septal defect, and overriding aorta. With transposition of the great vessels, the aorta arises from the right ventricle, and the pulmonary artery arises from the left ventricle. Surgical intervention is indicated with both of these defects. A primary anesthetic goal is to maintain a *sufficient pulmonary blood flow* to maintain acceptable oxygen content when oxygenated pulmonary venous blood returns to the heart and mixes with systemic venous blood. Because intraoperative maintenance of SVR and pulmonary blood flow is crucial, all agents that will compromise this goal must be avoided. Pharmacologic agents to avoid include those that release histamine, volatile anesthetics, and ganglionic and alpha-adrenergic blockers. Pancuronium can be safely used to maintain blood pressure, SVR, HR, and cardiac output. Ketamine, either intramuscularly or intravenously, is useful in maintaining pulmonary blood flow.[9] Phenylephrine can be used to help maintain peripheral resistance.

Table 21–2
CLASSIFICATION OF CONGENITAL HEART DISEASE

1. Pressure overload on the right or left ventricle
   Aortic stenosis
   Pulmonary stenosis
   Coarctation of the aorta
   Hypoplastic left heart syndrome
2. Volume overload on the ventricle or atrium
   Ventricular septal defect
   Patent ductus arteriosus
   Endocardial cushion defects
   Atrial septal defect
3. Cyanosis due to obstruction of pulmonary blood flow
   Tetralogy of Fallot
   Pulmonary atresia
   Tricuspid atresia
4. Cyanosis due to a common mixing chamber
   Total anomalous pulmonary venous return
   Truncus arteriosus
   Double-outlet right ventricle
   Single ventricle
5. Cyanosis due to separation of the systemic and pulmonary circulations
   Transposition of the great vessels

SOURCE: Reproduced by permission from Rothstein.[8]

CONDUCTION DISEASES

Conduction disease may require electrical stimulation of the heart or correction of aberrant electrical conditions with defibrillation. Indications for the placement of permanent pacemakers are: (1) complete heart block with symptomatic bradycardia, or CHF, (2) asystole persisting more than 3 seconds, (3) suppression of ventricular dysrhythmias, (4) persistent and symptomatic second-degree atrioventricular block when it results in symptomatic bradycardia, (5) sick sinus syndrome, and (6) chronic bifascicular or trifascicular block. These can occur in CAD, valvular heart disease, and calcification of the conduction system.

Pacemaker Insertion   The pacemakers leads are usually inserted transvenously under local or monitored anesthesia care. A subclavian vein is usually cannulated to allow the placement of the leads. The leads are placed under fluoroscopy, and a generator is then implanted in the subcutaneous tissues. The leads can be ventricular, or atrial and ventricular that allow synchronized atrial and ventricular stimulation to occur. Atrial and ventricular leads are used when the "atrial kick" that helps fill the ventricles is needed. During cardiac surgery, electrodes are placed directly into the heart muscle and then attached to an external generator.

Anesthetic Considerations
Sedation is usually accomplished with narcotics and Versed. Monitoring requirements for placement of transvenous leads are a good ECG pattern without interference and a pulse oximeter with plethysmography to see perfusion of each complex. This is particularly important if the ECG becomes unreadable.

Premature ventricular contractions may occur when the intracardiac leads are placed. Lidocaine may be indicated if they become too numerous.

After the generator has been connected to the leads and placed into its "pouch" in the subcutaneous tissue of the chest, the anesthetist should watch the ECG to make sure that the generator is functioning properly, that is, sensing and stimulating properly. If a pacemaker spike is seen with no response from the heart, check for lead placement or generator malfunction. If a pacemaker should fail during surgery, placing a magnet over the generator will change from a sensing to an asynchronous (fixed) mode.

Complications
Electrocautery can reprogram programmable pacemakers by simulating the electromagnetic code for reprogramming. If this should occur, placing a magnet over the generator will put it into the fixed mode and then it can be reprogrammed later.

Pacemaker leads have been known to puncture the ventricle where myocardial infarction is present. This can lead to cardiac tamponade. Surgery may be necessary to correct the puncture site.

Automatic Implantable Cardioverter Defibrillator Insertion   Automatic implantable cardioverter defibrillators (AICDs) have been developed to treat cardiac dysrhythmias with accessory pathways, both right and left sided. The device requires the transvenous placement of leads, one for sensing the heart rate, one for sensing the morphology of the QRS complex, and one for delivering the shocks. The last two functions are usually handled by one lead. The generator needs to sense eight beats of the abnormal dysrhythmia to be activated, and then it delays for 2.5 seconds to make sure that the dysrhythmia is still present before delivering a shock. The first shock is usually 30 joules, and if the dysrhythmia is still present, it will shock again for five shocks. The automatic implantable cardioverter defibrillator generator and leads are also capable of pacing if the need arises.

Anesthetic Considerations
Monitoring should be appropriate to each patient and the surgical risk. Anesthetic considerations should be the same as for any patient coming to surgery for transvenous placement of leads. These patients will have been on antidysrhythmic drugs, and most of these should have been discontinued. One drug, amiodarone, will probably be continued due to its long half-life, but amiodarone therapy can lead to both myocardial and pulmonary complications. Because amiodarone in the presence of vasodilators and myocardial depressants can lead to refractory bradycardia and profound hypotension, the proper selection of intraoperative anesthetic agents is crucial. After the generator has been connected, the dysrhythmia is produced to make sure the generator is sensing and functioning well and how effective pharmacological intervention is.

When caring for the patient with an AICD during noncardic surgery, the implanted device should be deactivated immediately before surgery (when electrocautery will be used) and then reactivated in the OR or recovery room. Intraoperatively, anesthetic management is unchanged; however, external defibrillation pads should be available and applied transcutaneously.

☐ VASCULAR PROCEDURES

AORTIC ANEURYSMS

Vascular procedures for aortic aneurysm are either infrarenal or suprarenal. *Renal failure* is a major complication of aortic procedures. This is related to prolonged surgery involving extensive tissue manipulation, substantial fluid loss into the third space, and potentially massive blood loss. If the aneurysm involves the renal arteries or above, frank ischemia to the kidneys or altered renal hemodynamics due to cross-clamping of the aorta may occur. Patients who develop acute renal failure postoperatively have a high mortality rate, as high as 78% in one report.[10]

Treatment includes prevention of hypotension and maintenance of proper intravascular volume. Mannitol may be used before cross-clamping to help preserve renal function in the presence of hypovolemia. It is critical to maintain a urine output of at least 0.5 mL/kg intraoperatively.

Patients with aortic aneurysms have a high incidence of CAD, and they should have a thorough cardiac work-up before surgery. The patient may need to have CABG before the aortic aneurysm is resected.

Cross-clamping the aorta does not affect cardiac output or heart rate, but it can increase mean arterial pressure (MAP) by 40%. The arterial pressure below the clamp decreases about 15%, myocardial wall tension increases, and coronary blood flow increases by about 40%.[11,12] Nitroprusside may be used to help lower the MAP after cross-clamping occurs, but it will also lower coronary blood flow.

Before the clamp is released, vasodilating drugs should be discontinued, cystolloid solutions infused, and inhalation agents reduced to low concentrations. The surgeon should release the clamp slowly to allow for homeostatic mechanisms to maintain the blood pressure within acceptable limits. Hypotension after cross-clamp release is usually due to low SVR in the lower body and buildup of vasodilating metabolites during the ischemic cross-clamp period. Treatment consists of a vasoactive drug such as phenylephrine and fluid infusion. The blood from the lower extremities will be very acidotic, and pH must be checked after release.

Spinal cord ischemia risk after abdominal aortic surgery is about 0.25%. Postoperatively, spinal cord complications are more common in cases of ruptured aneurysms.[13] The patients present with an anterior spinal artery syndrome with loss of motor function and pinprick sensation, but they have vibration and proprioception. The spinal cord receives its blood supply from the vertebral arteries and from the thoracic and abdominal aorta. One anterior and two posterior arteries descend along the cord. Intercostal arteries supply blood to the anterior and posterior arteries in the upper thoracic area; in the lower thoracic and lumbar cord, the anterior spinal artery is supplied by the thoracolumbar artery of Adamkiewicz. This artery has a variable origin from the aorta, arising between T-5 and L-2. It may be damaged during surgical dissection or occluded by cross-clamping.[13]

Aortic Artery Emergencies If patients present with a ruptured abdominal aortic aneurysm or dissecting aortic aneurysm, the mortality rate is high. These patients require immediate surgery to control the bleeding and replace the area of the aorta involved with the aneurysm. Speed is essential and several large-bore venous access lines should be placed before induction. These patients may have cardiopulmonary resuscitation in progress when they arrive in the operating room, and a standard induction may not be possible. If ruptured, the retroperitoneal space will fill with blood and, if intact, can tamponade the ruptured aneurysm until an incision is made into the space. Hypotension is a major problem facing the anesthetist, and drugs that would exaggerate this

problem should be avoided. Ketamine may be a good induction drug because it stimulates the sympathetic nervous system, which will help increase the blood pressure. A muscle relaxant may be all the anesthetist has time to give to allow the surgery to begin. Vasoactive drugs should be started, and vascular volume replaced with hetastarch preparations, plasmanate, and crystalloid solutions. Type-specific blood products should be given when not enough time exists to cross-match blood products. Blood scavenger systems should be used and the blood returned to the patient. ECG, blood pressure, and oxygen saturation should be monitored. Once bleeding is controlled, and the vascular volume is being addressed, then arterial lines, central pulmonary catheter, and central venous access can be inserted. Dysrhythmias causing hypotension should be diagnosed and corrected. Infusions should include vasoactive drugs, inotropic drugs, nitroglycerin, and lidocaine. A "renal" dose of dopamine, 2 μg/kg/min, should be started. The pH and electrolytes should be checked and adjusted if metabolic acidosis is present. Kidney function is monitored by urinary output and specific gravity.

CAROTID ENDARTERECTOMY

Carotid endarterectomies are done on patients who have a 75% occlusion of the carotid artery and have symptoms such as TIAs, carotid bruits, or stroke. Some centers feel that a carotid endarterectomy is a prophylactic procedure and should be done on asymptomatic patients with 75% occlusion. Mortality and morbidity following carotid surgery is reported to be from 5% to 6% depending on absence of symptoms.[14] Because there is a correlation between carotid disease and CAD, ischemic heart muscle is the major cause of mortality and morbidity. CABG and carotid endarterectomies are often done at the same time or in staged procedures. Cerebrovascular accidents are common with this surgery.

These patients may appear healthy; however, after a careful history and examination, disease can usually be found. The anesthetist should obtain a complete cardiac work-up and antihypertensive medication history, including the half-life of all drugs. Blood pressure can be labile during surgery and cardiac complications are not uncommon. Other diseases, such as diabetes, should be well controlled. If chronic obstructive pulmonary disease is severe, pulmonary function tests should be obtained. Hyperventilation should be *avoided* in these patients because it may lead to cerebral ischemia.

Monitoring should include an ECG with a V_5 lead and ST segment analysis, oxygen saturation, and direct intra-arterial measurement of the blood pressure. It is usually not necessary for a pulmonary artery catheter, but some practitioners prefer to have a central venous access for administration of vasoactive drugs and inotropes. Cerebral protection may be either mechanical or pharmacologic. Table 21–3 lists the types of protection that can be used to help reduce the incident of cerebral injury. Surgeons have the option of using a shunt to bypass the area of stenosis while performing the en-

Table 21–3
CEREBRAL PROTECTION

Mechanical
   Shunts
Pharmacologic
   Barbiturates
   Hypothermia
   Isoflurane
   Calcium channel blockers
      Nimodipine
      Lidoflazine
      Flunarazene
   Benzodiazepines
   Etomidate
   Iron chelators (deferoxamine)
   Enzymes (catalase, superoxide dismutase)
   Naloxone
   Acetazolamide

SOURCE: Reproduced by permission from Youngberg and Gold.[15]

darterectomy, or clamping the artery above the lesion, opening the artery, performing the endarterectomy, and then suturing the artery and releasing the clamp. Many will monitor the EEG and use a shunt if changes occur, for shunting is associated with a fixed percentage of embolism. The surgeon should inactivate the pressor receptors at the carotid bifurcation to keep from causing stimulation and a vagal response of bradycardia. This is usually accomplished by applying topical local anesthesia on the bifurcation or injecting lidocaine into the pressor receptors. EEGs may be monitored during surgery to observe for signs of reduced cerebral blood flow.

Anesthetic Choice The use of either regional or general anesthesia depends on the skill of the anesthesia provider and the wishes of the surgeon and patient. When using a general anesthesia technique, keep in mind that early evaluation of the patient is desired by the surgeon. Hypotension is avoided by using low concentrations of inhaled agents, intravenous fluids, and injection of lidocaine into the carotid sinus. MAP is maintained at 10% to 20% *above normal* with the cautious use of vasopressors when the carotid is cross-clamped and after release of the clamp. This will help the surgeon recognize any leaking around the sutures in the artery. If hypertension is encountered, inhaled agents, narcotics, nitroglycerin, nitroprusside, labatelol, or esmolol can be used. The use of vasodilating infusions may be necessary at this time until the underlying cause of hypertension is corrected. The incidence of hypertension is highest at the termination of anesthesia when the vasodilating effect of the inhaled agent is no longer present and the patient is awakening and may be anxious and have pain. Postoperative evaluation of the patient should include movement of all extremities, strength of hand grasp bilaterally, ability to protrude the tongue in the midline, (hypoglossal nerve) and facial symmetry when smiling (facial nerve). Persistent hoarseness may indicate recurrent laryngeal nerve trauma.

Complications The most common life-threatening emergencies postoperatively are acute carotid occlusion and carotid artery hemorrhage. It is important to maintain postoperative MAP at preoperative levels. Vasoactive drugs such as phenylephrine and nitroprusside should be in an infusion form and kept with the patient in both the postanesthesia care unit (PACU) and the ICU. If TIAs should occur in the postoperative period, as would be the case with carotid occlusion, then raising the MAP, heparinization, and return to the operating room for angiography and possibly redoing endarterectomy are indicated. Carotid artery hemorrhage is diagnosed by swelling in the neck and can result in life-threatening airway obstruction. Reintubation is necessary for airway control and for return to the operating room for arterial repair. Fiberoptic bronchoscopy equipment should be available if needed emergently. The treatment is immediate opening of the wound to relieve the pressure on the airway and direct pressure to the carotid artery proximal to the area of surgery.

LOWER ARTERIAL SURGERY

Patients who present for lower revascularization often have multiple systemic disease and limited organ reserves. Once these patients have been brought to their optimal condition for surgery, the choice of anesthetic technique continues to be controversial. Most of these patients have occlusive disease in their peripheral arterial system due to athrosclerosis. Common revascularization procedures are aortofemoral bypass graft for disease in the iliac arteries, femoral-popliteal bypass graft, femoral-tibial bypass graft, and popliteal-tibial bypass graft. Patients may present with acute ischemic attacks due to thromboembolism. Emergency surgery is indicated to relieve the thrombus and allow the return of blood flow to the affected extremity. This can usually be done under monitored anesthesia care with local anesthesia and sedation.

Arteriosclerotic heart disease is prevalent with peripheral vascular disease. Therefore, a complete cardiac work-up is essential. Many of these patients will also have hypertension, chronic obstructive pulmonary disease (COPD), and diabetes. Each disease, and its severity, will have an effect on the anesthetic plan.

MONITORING Basic monitoring should consist of a dual-channel ECG with a V_5 lead to detect ischemia, and lead II for early detection of cardiac dysrhythmias, plus an ST segment analysis to help with detection of ischemia. Oxygen saturation, end-tidal carbon dioxide monitoring, and temperature monitoring are included. Measures to keep the patient normothermic, such as fluid warmers, heated humidifiers for the breathing circuit, and heating blankets like Bair Huggers, should be used. Maintaining body temperature is important with these patients during surgery. Allowing body temperature to decrease during surgery can cause the arteries to vasoconstrict and impede the flow of blood in the newly revascularized arteries. This can lead to clot formation and vasospasm and make it difficult to ascertain the success of the procedure. Measures to maintain normothermia should be carried over into the PACU and ICU. Hourly measurement of urine output helps in monitoring vascular volume. Although noninvasive blood pressure monitoring can be used, invasive arterial catheterization is more accurate and will allow frequent monitoring of ventilation with blood gas sampling. An Allen test may be performed before intra-arterial cannulization to make sure that both arteries supplying the hand are patent. This test is easily performed, but is somewhat controversial in its ability to tell if the ulnar artery is patent.

Anesthesia Choice Anesthetic choice will depend on the procedure to be done. An embolectomy is usually performed under monitored anesthesia care with the surgeon administering local anesthesia and the anesthetist sedating the patient with narcotics and benzodiazepines.

Revascularization procedures involving grafts from the aortic arch to the upper extremities will require general anesthesia. If a patient has already been anticoagulated, then regional anesthesia is contraindicated. For lower extremity procedures, regional or general anesthesia may be used. The usual regional techniques for this are continuous epidural anesthesia/analgesia or subarachnoid block. The advantages of regional anesthesia are hemodynamic stability and a smoother intraoperative and postoperative course. Cardiac benefits include less myocardial ischemia with a regional technique.[16] Regional techniques may help with the surgical outcome by causing a sympathetic block leading to reduced vascular tone and producing decreased vascular resistance.

Despite the advantages of regional anesthesia, the sympathetic block from regional anesthesia may be detrimental for patients with hypertension, significant CAD, or hypotension. For patients with COPD or other pulmonary problems, regional anesthesia may not be as safe as once believed. When considering using a regional block on someone who is going to be anticoagulated, it is generally thought that if you follow three guidelines it is acceptable to do a regional on these patients: (1) the patients were properly selected without preexisting coagulation abnormalities (i.e., no history of leukemia, hemophilia, blood dyscrasias, thrombocytopenia, or preoperative anticoagulation therapy); (2) if the regional technique was traumatic or yielded a bloody tap, the patient's surgery was canceled and rescheduled for general anesthesia the following day; and (3) anticoagulation with heparin was closely monitored to keep the activated clotting time approximately twice the baseline value.[17]

☐ PULMONARY SYSTEM PROCEDURES

Rigid bronchoscopy is usually indicated for the removal of foreign bodies from the tracheobronchial tree. Moderate or massive hemoptysis is also an indication for rigid bronchoscopy. It is the procedure of choice for granulation tissue

or tumor blocking the airway, and one can obtain very large biopsy specimen through this scope. When using the rigid scope, ventilation must be accomplished either through the scope, in a side port using jet ventilation, or by a small endotracheal tube.

For surgical procedures, the flexible fiberscope can be manipulated into the periphery of the lungs for better visualization of bronchial lesions. For the anesthetist, the flexible scope can aid in intubations. See Chapter 24 for further discussion on bronchoscopies.

MEDIASTINOSCOPY

Mediastinoscopy provides access to mediastinal lymph nodes in the presence of carcinoma of the lungs and mediastinal tumors. Absolute contraindications are: (1) anterior mediastinal tumors, (2) inoperable tumor, (3) previous recurrent laryngeal nerve injury, (4) extremely debilitated condition, (5) ascending aortic aneurysm, and (6) previous mediastinoscopy. Relative contraindications include thoracic inlet obstruction and the presence of a superior vena cava syndrome.

The surgical approach is usually through a suprasternal incision, and general anesthesia with muscle relaxation is indicated. Because pneumothorax is a potential complication, nitrous oxide should be avoided. The innominate artery can be compressed by the scope; therefore, the right radial or carotid pulses should be monitored and the surgeon made aware if compression occurs. This can be done with a right radial catheter or pulse oximetry reading. Because compression will alter flow to the right arm, a blood pressure cuff should be placed on the left side for an accurate pressure indicator. Hemorrhage should be anticipated, and at least two large-bore intravenous catheters should be started. Preoperatively, blood should be typed and crossmatched. Masses in the mediastinum can compress the trachea and collapse has been reported. *Mediastinal lymphadenopathy leading to tracheal collapse when muscle relaxants are given is an important indication for awake fiberoptic intubation.*

THORACOSCOPY

Thoracoscopy is indicated for pleural effusions and lesions of the lung and pleura. It is also used for the introduction of chemical agents for pleurodesis for recurrent pneumothorax. This can be done either under local anesthesia or with a general anesthetic. If done under local anesthesia, heavy sedation may be necessary. When general anesthesia is used, a double-lumen endobronchial tube is used for lung isolation and deflation.

INTRATHORACIC PROCEDURES

Anesthesia for open lung procedures that require a full thoracotomy, such as wedge resection, lobectomy, or pneumonectomy, are a challenge for the anesthetist. Preoperative evaluation is extremely important. Hemodynamic status, pulmonary status, and other underlying medical problems must be evaluated to provide the safest anesthesia and postoperative course possible. Pulmonary function testing will be necessary to plan for optimal postoperative extubation. If the forced expired volume in 1 second is abnormal, then a *split lung test* should be obtained.

Anesthesia affects lung volumes by reducing the functional residual capacity (FRC) of the lungs by an increase in lung elastic recoil and a decrease in chest recoil.[18,19] This is important because airway closure and absorption atelectasis may occur when the closing capacity exceeds the end-expiratory lung volume. The decrease in FRC produces an increase in airway resistance. Patients having lung surgery are at risk for increased airway resistance. Excess pulmonary mucus, blood, and tumor cell production are present and will worsen the situation. Many have COPD, asthma, or other lung diseases that can alter airway caliber and reactivity.

Anesthetics affect airway resistance in different ways. Halothane appears to produce direct smooth muscle bronchomotor relaxation. Isoflurane has some bronchodilation effects and may be preferred over halothane because it does not cause myocardial depression. Intravenous drugs that can cause histamine release and bronchoconstriction should be avoided. Deep anesthesia will protect against reflex bronchospasm.

One-lung ventilation has become popular for intrathoracic procedures on the lungs. However, hypoxemia with PaO_2 of less than 70 mm Hg has been reported to occur in 15% to 25% of cases.[20] Ventilation/perfusion mismatch has an effect on PaO_2, and shunting is particularly prominent during one-lung ventilation. Hypoxic pulmonary vasoconstriction (HPV) occurs as blood is shunted away from areas of atelectasis. This can be restored after lung expansion has occurred if

100% oxygen is used. If nitrous oxide is used, low concentrations should be used because a higher than normal FIO_2 is sometimes necessary in these patients. Because 100% FIO_2 can cause absorption atelectasis, it should be used only after positive end-expiratory pressure to the dependent lung and continuous positive airway pressure to the nondependent lung have been first tried.

Selection of anesthetic agents requires consideration of the multiple, sometimes conflicting effects of drugs. Table 21–4[21] lists some drugs used in anesthesia and their desirable and undesirable properties related to their use for lung surgery. Drug effects, underlying diseases, position of the patient during surgery, and effects of the surgery all must be considered when planning the anesthetic approach to each patient. No single agent or technique is always recommended. Clinical judgment and past experience of the anesthetist are factors in the selection and use of anesthetics for intrathoracic surgery.

Esophageal procedures through an intrathoracic approach have similar anesthetic considerations as for lung surgery. The esophagus lies in close proximity to the major vessels of the chest, the aorta and vena cava, and to the heart. Major hemorrhage is a risk, and placement of at least two large-bore intravenous catheters is appropriate. In addition, typed and crossmatched blood should be available. During heart and lung manipulation, cardiac dysrhythmias are not uncommon. Along with the routine monitoring, intra-arterial catheterization is indicated for pressure monitoring and arterial sampling. Central venous access is required for fluid replacement, delivery of medications, and CVP monitoring. If cardiac status requires, a pulmonary artery catheter may be needed.

Awake intubation, or rapid sequence induction with cricoid pressure, should be used for patients at high risk for

Table 21–4
PROPERTIES OF ANESTHETICS

Anesthetic	Desirable	Undesirable
Volatile	Permits use of high FIO_2	Inhibits HPV
	Bronchodilation	Myocardial depression
	Diminishes airway reflexes	
	Readily eliminated	
Narcotics	Do not inhibit HPV	Not general anesthetics
	No myocardial depression when used alone	May depress ventilation in immediate postoperative period
	Provide postoperative analgesia	
Nitrous oxide	Readily eliminated	Reduces FIO_2
	Probably no effect on HPV	
Ketamine	Diminishes airway irritability	Myocardial ischemia
	Does not inhibit HPV	Emergence delirium
	Cardiovascular stability during hypovolemia	
Thiopental	Does not inhibit HPV	Minor potential for histamine release and bronchospasm
Muscle relaxants	Facilitate mechanical ventilation	Potential for postoperative weakness
	Enhance surgical exposure	Possible histamine release and bronchospasm
	Minimize doses of general anesthetics	Need for use of reversal agent
Cholinesterase inhibitors	Reverse neuromuscular blockade	May produce acetylcholine-mediated bronchospasm

HPV, hypoxic pulmonary vasoconstriction.
Source: Reproduced by permission from Siegel and Brodsky.[21]

aspiration. Awake fiberoptic intubation may be indicated in some circumstances. For lower esophageal surgery through a thoracoabdominal incision, a regular endotracheal tube will suffice. If a thoracotomy incision is necessary, then a double-lumen endobronchial tube should be used for surgical exposure. Some investigators recommend the use of a right-sided endobronchial tube for right thoracotomies and a left-sided one for left thoracotomies. Some advocate the use of a left-sided tube for either sided thoracotomies.[22]

If bowel is present, the use of nitrous oxide is contraindicated because it will cross into the bowel by diffusion. In one-lung ventilation, which requires high concentrations of inspired oxygen, nitrous oxide is also contraindicated.

ENDOBRONCHIAL INTUBATION

Endobronchial (one-lung) intubation is used for thoracic surgery and in the management of critically ill patients requiring differential lung ventilation such as pulmonary lavage. The technique allows selective one lung ventilation. The collapsed lung will experience distal parenchymal collapse. Table 21–5 lists the indications for one-lung anesthesia. Many techniques may be used for one-lung ventilation, such as bronchial blockers, single-lumen endobronchial tubes, and double-lumen endobronchial tubes. The use of left-sided double-lumen endobronchial tubes offers distinct advantages over the bronchial blockers and single-lumen tubes. For example, once in place, selective ventilation and suctioning are possible in either lung.

With the double-lumen endobronchial tube, one lumen is long enough to reach into one of the mainstem bronchi and has an occlusion cuff near the tip of the lumen. The other lumen is shorter, larger, and fits in the distal trachea. It too, has an occlusion cuff near its tip, however, proximal to the take-off of the endobronchial lumen. The two lumens have dual connectors at the proximal end with capped ports that allow passage of a flexible fiberoptic bronchoscope, position checking, and passage of a suction catheter into each lumen. These connectors are then fit to a Y piece,

Table 21–5
INDICATIONS FOR ONE-LUNG ANESTHESIA

Control of secretions
  Abscess
  Bronchiectasis
  Hemoptysis
Airway control
  Bronchopleural fistula
    Chronic
    Acute
  Sleeve resection
Quiet surgical field/improved exposure
Teaching

SOURCE: Reproduced by permission from Wilson.[23]

which connects to the breathing circuit. Two pilot tubes connect to the two occlusion cuffs. A stylet is inserted into the bronchial lumen giving the lumen a curve for intubation.

Placement of a Double-Lumen Endobronchial Tube
After induction and muscle relaxation, a laryngoscopy is performed and the tube is held with the curve facing anteriorly. After passing the endobronchial and tracheal lumens past the cords, the entire tube is rotated either right or left, depending on whether it is a right- or left-sided tube. The stylet is removed and the entire tube is then advanced until resistance is met with the carina. At this time, the tracheal occlusion cuff may be inflated, and both lumens connected to the breathing circuit with the Y connector. Preliminary placement is ascertained by bilateral breath sounds and chest movement.

Next, it is absolutely necessary to check that the endobronchial lumen is placed into the proper bronchus and that the tracheal lumen is sitting away from the carina. A flexible fiberoptic bronchoscope is inserted through the port on top of the connector of the tracheal lumen and is passed, under vision, down the tracheal lumen until the carina and take off of the nonintubated bronchus are visible. The bronchial lumen should be seen going into the selected bronchus. While watching the endobronchial lumen, its occlusion cuff is inflated. The cuff should be visualized as it inflates and fills the space between the wall of the tube and the bronchus. Next, the fiberscope is inserted into the other bronchus to check for a clear take-off view of the bronchioles to the various lobes of the lung. If a right-sided endobronchial tube is used, it is necessary to use the flexible fiberoptic bronchoscope in both lumens to check distance from the carina and the tip of the tracheal lumen. Next, the endobronchial lumen is checked for right mainstem bronchus placement to make sure that the opening to the upper lobe of the lung has not been blocked by the endobronchial lumen. There is an opening on the side of the endobronchial lumen, as well as on the end, that should be placed over the opening to the upper lobe. The fiberscope can confirm that this side opening is over the opening to the upper lobe, and the tip of the scope can be flexed to look directly at the openings to make sure they line up.

For lung isolation, the cuff on the endobronchial tube must be inflated for a seal, then a clamp is placed across the proximal end of the endobronchial lumen occluding it entirely; this will isolate that lung. If the lung is to be deflated, the clamp is placed proximal to the connector of the endobronchial lumen, but distal to the Y connector. Next the port on the connector that allows the passage of the fiberscope or suction catheter is opened, which will allow the lung to deflate and still be isolated. To isolate and allow deflation of the other lung, both cuffs are inflated to seal, and then the tracheal lumen is clamped with a clamp placed proximal to the connector on the tracheal lumen, but distal to the Y connector; the port on the connector on the tracheal lumen is opened.

Complications Complications of using the double-lumen endobronchial tubes are trauma, malposition, and hypoxemia. Direct laryngeal trauma, such as arytenoid dislocation, can occur due to the size and bulk of these tubes. Laceration and rupture of the trachea has been reported.[24] This can be diagnosed by the presence of a large leak with mediastinal and subcutaneous air. If this occurs, the tip of the tube may be seen in the surgical field and prompt repair of the tear is indicated.

Malposition causing impaired gas exchange may occur at any time. Once the tube is positioned and checked, it should be secured. If there is any doubt about its placement during the procedure, check again with the fiberscope. Inappropriate tube size may partially occlude the mainstem bronchus.

Because one-lung ventilation has risks that can lead to systemic hypoxemia, it is imperative to optimize dependent lung ventilation. Appropriate inspired oxygen tension, rate, and tidal volume should be used. An anesthetic technique should be used to allow the use of near 100% oxygen. This will help bring the PaO_2 up to acceptable levels and cause vasodilation in the dependent lung, thus helping the dependent lung accept some of the circulatory shift from the nondependent, hypoxic, pulmonary vasoconstricted lung.

Less than 10 mL/kg tidal volume may result in atelectasis in the dependent lung. Yet larger tidal volumes might cause high airway pressures, and thus increased vascular resistance. If a tidal volume 10 mL/kg produces high airway pressure, the tidal volume should be lowered until a desired airway pressure is obtained. Dependent lung positive end-expiratory pressure should initially be avoided because of the possibility of developing dependent lung vascular resistance.[25]

Respiratory rate should be increased by about 20%. The goal is to keep a $PaCO_2$ of about 40 mm Hg. Minute ventilation will remain constant, but there will be ventilation/perfusion mismatch. Frequent arterial blood gases should be sampled and oxygen saturation should be monitored. Adjustments can be made according to the PaO_2, $PaCO_2$, pH, and oxygen saturation. Table 21–6 offers a plan to obtain

Table 21–6
OVERALL ONE-LUNG VENTILATION PLAN

1.	Maintain two-lung ventilation until pleura is opened	
2.	Dependent lung	$FIO_2 = 1.0$ $TV = 8–10$ ml/kg $RR =$ So that $PaCO_2 = 40$ mm Hg $PEEP = 0–5$ mm Hg
3.	If severe hypoxemia occurs	(a) Check position of double-lumen tube with fiberoptic bronchoscopy (b) Check hemodynamic status (c) Nondependent lung CPAP (d) Dependent lung PEEP (e) Two-lung ventilation (f) Clamp pulmonary artery as soon as possible (for pneumonectomy)

CPAP, continuous positive airway pressure; FIO_2, inspired oxygen concentration; PEEP, positive end-expiratory pressure; RR, respiratory rate; TV, tidal volume.
SOURCE: Reproduced by permission from Benumof.[26]

satisfactory arterial oxygenation during one-lung ventilation.

☐ SUMMARY

Cardiothoracic and vascular anesthesia requires anesthetists to use their skills to their fullest. The diseases of the heart, vasculature, and lungs make preoperative assessment of all organ systems mandatory and intraoperative management difficult. The anesthetist is required to have a complete understanding of the pathophysiology and pharmacology and the relationship between the anesthetic drugs and diseases. Invasive monitoring techniques are used more routinely than for any other patients. The postoperative period is also a challenge. What happens to these patients in the intraoperative period will affect the outcome of the procedure and the patient's course in the postoperative period.

REFERENCES

1. Thomson IR. Technical aspects of cardiopulmonary bypass. In: *Manual of Cardiac Anesthesia*. 2nd ed. New York: Churchill Livingstone 1993:479–499.
2. Spiess BD, Chang S-PB. Intraoperative coagulation disorders. In: *Manual of Cardiac Anesthesia*. 2nd ed. 1993:517–552.
3. Hilberman M, Myers BD, Carrie BJ, et al. Acute renal failure following cardiac surgery. *J Thorac Cardiovasc Surg*. 1979; 77: 880–888.
4. Aprile AE, Palmer TJ. The intraoperative use of Amicar to reduce bleeding associated with open heart surgery. *Journal of the American Association of Nurse Anesthetists*. 1995; 63.
5. Jackson JM. Valvular heart disease. In: *Manual of Cardiac Anesthesia*. 2nd ed. New York: Churchill Livingstone 1993: 81–127.
6. Hejtmancik JF, Brink PA, Towbin J, et al. Localization of gene for familial hypertrophic cardiomyopathy to chromosome 14q1 in a diverse US population. *Circulation*. 1991;83: 1592–1597.
7. Kouchoukos NT, Wareing TH, Izumoto H, et al. Elective hypothermic cardiopulmonary bypass and circulatory arrest for spinal cord protection during operations on the thoraco-abdominal aorta. *J Thorac Cardiovasc Surg*. 1990; 99:659–664.
8. Rothstein, P. Congenital heart disease. In: *Manual of Cardiac Anesthesia*. New York: Churchill Livingstone 1993:197–243.

9. Vaughan RW, Stephen MD. Ketamine for corrective cardiac surgery in children. *South Med J*. 1973; 66:1226–1230.
10. Gornick CC Jr, Kjellstrand CM. Acute renal failure complicating aortic aneurysm surgery. *Nephron*. 1983; 35:145–157.
11. Roberts AJ, Nora JD, Hughes WA, et al. Cardiac and renal responses to cross-clamping of the descending thoracic aorta. *J Thorac Cardiovasc Surg*. 1983; 86:732–741.
12. Livesay JJ, Cooley DA, Ventemiglia RA, et al. Surgical experience in descending thoracic aneurysmectomy with and without adjuncts to avoid ischemia. *Ann Thorac Surg*. 1985;39: 37–46.
13. Kwitka G, Kidney SA, Nugent M. Thoracic and abdominal aortic aneurysm resections. In: *Vascular Anesthesia*. New York: Churchill Livingstone; 1991:389.
14. Fode NC, Sundt TM Jr, Robertson JT, et al. Multicenter retrospective review of results and complications of carotid endarterectomy in 1981. *Stroke*. 1986; 17:370–376.
15. Youngberg JA, Gold MD. Carotid artery surgery: Perioperative anesthetic considerations. In: *Vascular Anesthesia*. New York: Churchill Livingstone; 1991:351.
16. Reiz S, Balfors E, Sorensen MB, et al. Coronary hemodynamic effects of general anesthesia and surgery. Modification by epidural analgesia in patients with ischemic heart disease. *Regional Anesth*. 1982;7(suppl):S8.
17. Rao TLK, El-Etr AA. Anticoagulation following placement of epidural and subarachnoid catheters: an evaluation of neurologic sequelae. *Anesthesiology*. 1981; 85:618–620.
18. Hewlett AM, Hulands GH, Nunn JF, Heath JR. Functional residual capacity during anesthesia: II. Spontaneous respiration. *Br J Anaesth*. 1974; 46:486–495.
19. Don HF, Wahba M, Cuadrado L, Kelkar K. The effects of anesthesia and 100 percent oxygen on the functional residual capacity of the lungs. *Anesthesiology*. 1970; 32:521–529.
20. Kerr JH, Smith AC, Prys-Roberts C, et al. Observations during endobronchial anesthesia. II: oxygenation. *Br J Anaesth*. 1974; 46:84–92.
21. Siegel LC, Brodsky JB. Choice of anesthetic agents for intrathoracic surgery. In: *Thoracic Anesthesia*. 2nd ed. New York: Churchill Livingstone; 1991:347–370
22. Aitkenhead AR. Anesthesia for esophageal surgery. In: Gothard JW, ed. *Thoracic Anesthesia*. London: Bailliere-Tindall; 1987:181–206.
23. Wilson RS. Endobronchial intubation. In: *Thoracic Anesthesia*. 2nd ed. 1991:371–388.
24. Wagner DL, Gammage GW, Wong ML. Tracheal rupture following the insertion of a disposable double-lumen endotracheal tube. *Anesthesiology*. 1985; 63:698–700.
25. Kerr JH. Physiological aspects of one-lung (endobronchial) anesthesia. *Int Anesthesiol Clin*. 1972; 10:61–78.
26. Benumof JL. Conventional and differential lung management of one-lung ventilation. In: *Anesthesia for Thoracic Surgery*. Philadelphia: WB Saunders; 1987:chap 11.

☐ QUESTIONS

1. During cardiopulmonary bypass surgery the ideal temperature range for induced hypothermia is 14° to 24°C. True or False?
   a. True
   b. False

2. Cyanotic heart diseases caused by right-to-left intracardiac shunt include:
   a. Pulmonary atresia
   b. Tricuspid atresia
   c. Tetralogy of Fallot
   d. All of the above

3. All are true of amrinone *except*:
   a. Increases contractility
   b. Vasodilates (decreases afterload)
   c. Decreases calcium uptake by the sarcoplasmic reticulum
   d. Phosphodiesterase inhibitor

4. All may contribute to hypotension once the cross-clamp is removed from the aorta *except*:
   a. Lactic acid release causing myocardial depression
   b. Relative hypovolemia
   c. Sudden increase in systemic vascular resistance with unclamping of the aorta
   d. Release of endogenous vasoactive substances

5. Which agent is the best choice in the anesthetic management of the patient with tetralogy of Fallot?
   a. Isoflurane
   b. Pancuronium
   c. Hydralazine
   d. *d*-Tubocurarine

6. After what amount of time is there increased risk of spinal cord damage with cross-clamping the aorta?
   a. 30 minutes
   b. 40 minutes
   c. 60 minutes
   d. 90 minutes

7. Methods of spinal cord protection prior to aortic cross clamping include all *except*:
   a. Corticosteroids
   b. Somatosensory evoked potential monitoring
   c. Hypothermia
   d. Inject papavarine into the aortic aneurysm

8. True statements regarding protamine include all *except*:
   a. A positively charged alkaline protamine combines with a negatively charged acid heparin to form an inactive complex devoid of anticoagulant activity.
   b. Anaphylactic or anaphylactoid reactions are rare.
   c. Hemodynamic instability with rapid administration is probably caused by histamine and leukotriene release.
   d. Pretreatment with antihistamines may attenuate pulmonary hypertension induced by protamine administration.

9. During total bypass perfusion, mean arterial pressure should be maintained between:
   a. 25 and 50 mm Hg
   b. 40 and 90 mm Hg
   c. 100 and 120 mm Hg
   d. 120 and 150 mm Hg

10. Intraoperative considerations for pacemaker insertion include:
    a. Electrocautery can reprogram pacemakers.
    b. Succinylcholine can produce pacemaker standstill when pacemaker is in sensing mode.
    c. Etomidate should be avoided because of potential for myoclonus in about one third of patients during induction.
    d. All of the above

11. Absolute contraindications to mediastinoscopy include all except:
    a. Ascending aortic aneurysm
    b. Thoracic inlet obstruction
    c. Previous mediastinoscopy
    d. None of the above

12. Which is not an acceptable intraoperative anesthetic intervention in the patient with idiopathic hypertropic aortic stenosis?
    a. Inderal
    b. Calcium chloride
    c. Halothane
    d. 1000 mL bolus of 0.9 normal saline

13. True statements include:
    a. A properly inserted endobronchial tube ensures that the right mainstem bronchus will be blocked by the endobronchial lumen.
    b. Optimal tidal volumes during one-lung anesthesia are 15 mL/kg.
    c. Complications of endobronchial intubation include arytenoid dislocation, tracheal tear and hypoxia with malposition.
    d. None of the above

14. Which statement is true regarding cardiopulmonary bypass?
    a. The bypass machine allows perfusion through a pulsatile blood flow throughout the body.
    b. Damaged blood cells are a normal consequence of CPB as abnormal blood-gas and blood-plastic interfaces are formed.
    c. During CPB the patient must remain hemoconcentrated and anticoagulated.
    d. All statements are false.

15. A patient presents for a mediastinoscopy. Which statement is correct regarding intraoperative monitoring?
    a. The blood pressure cuff should be on the right arm and pulse oximetry on the left.
    b. The blood pressure cuff should be on the left arm and pulse oximetry on the right.
    c. The blood pressure cuff should be on the left arm and pulse oximetry on the left.
    d. The blood pressure cuff should be on the right arm and pulse oximetry on the right.

16. Which statement is false regarding the anesthetic management of patients with tetralogy of Fallot?
    a. Increased pulmonary vascular resistance will worsen shunt.
    b. Ketamine should never be used for an induction agent.
    c. With tetralogy of Fallot, pulmonary blood flow is reduced.
    d. A decrease in systemic vascular resistance should be avoided.

17. The best way to prevent hypotension associated with removal of cross-clamp is volume infusion prior to release. True or False?
    a. True
    b. False

18. True statements include:
    a. Hypothermia during revascularization surgery may lead to arterial vasoconstriction.
    b. Hypotension due to a sympathetic block during regional anesthesia may be beneficial in the patient undergoing an aortofemoral bypass graft.
    c. The best anesthetic choice for an emergency thrombectomy is a general anesthetic with rapid sequence intubation.
    d. All statements are false.

19. Indications for one-lung anesthesia include all of the following except:
    a. Airway control
    b. Improved surgical exposure
    c. Improved ventilation/perfusion ratio
    d. Control of secretions

20. Right-to-left intracardiac or intrapulmonary shunt:
    a. Speeds induction with an inhaled anesthetic
    b. Slows induction with an inhaled anesthetic
    c. Will never have a significant effect
    d. Slows induction with an intravenous anesthetic

☐ ANSWERS

1. b	**5.** b	**9.** b	**13.** c	**17.** a
2. d	**6.** a	**10.** d	**14.** b	**18.** a
3. c	**7.** d	**11.** b	**15.** b	**19.** c
4. c	**8.** b	**12.** b	**16.** b	**20.** b

CHAPTER 22

Neuroanesthesia

Wayne E. Ellis

☐ PATHOLOGIC CONDITIONS

The anesthesia practitioner is confronted with several dilemmas with the neurosurgical patient; however, most common situations can be grouped into areas of trauma, intracranial bleeding, or space-occupying lesions. Each area has some specific concerns for the practitioner that moderate the care administered during the anesthetic to improve positive outcomes.

TRAUMA

The incidence of head trauma in the United States is tremendous. The average figure is 200/100,000 trauma incidents per year. Each year, 500,000 people sustain severe head trauma with approximately 50,000 dying before they reach definitive medical treatment facilities. Head injuries account for approximately one third of all the trauma deaths in the United States. Fifty percent of head trauma incidents are as the result of motor vehicle accidents. As many as 50% of patients with head trauma will have other associated injuries that predispose the individual to hypotension, hypoxia, and anemia. Closed head trauma accounts for approximately 82% of all patients and the remaining 18% are related to penetrating head injuries.[1-6]

HEMATOMAS

Bleeding into the intracranial vault as a result of trauma can produce symptoms of increased intracranial pressure (ICP) and if untreated will result in the patient's death. The majority of surgery after trauma to the patient is to evacuate a cerebral hematoma.

Subdural Hematoma   There are three classifications of subdural hematomas. In an *acute* subdural hematoma, the symptoms present within 24 hours of incident. With a *subacute* subdural hematoma, the symptoms may be delayed from 24 hours to 10 days following injury. The *chronic* subdural hematoma may present with symptoms developing 10 days or longer after injury. The most common cause of a subdural hematoma is rupture of arachnoid veins. Clinical signs and symptoms are variable and are a result of both location and size of the hematoma. They include signs of increased ICP and midline shift from the hematoma's displacement of tissues.

Epidural Hematoma   This hematoma results from separation of the dura from the skull with the tearing of meningeal veins. The resulting hematoma causes further separation of the dura and additional vascular injury. The most common presenting symptoms include a loss of consciousness with the injury, a return to consciousness, and progressively increasing severity of headache over several hours. In the untreated patient, this can lead to further neurologic deterioration, unconsciousness, and death. Surgical intervention is required to drain the hematoma and control continued bleeding. About one third of the patients do not lose consciousness. Another one third of the patients do not regain consciousness following injury.

Intracerebral Hematoma   Intracerebral hematoma following intracranial injury may occur in approximately 20% to 25% of all patients with severe head trauma. Symptoms vary and depend on the location of the injury, size of the hematoma, and potential for continued bleeding. For most intracerebral hematomas, surgery is not required. The symptoms may develop late, presenting as late at 10 to 14 days after the injury. Neurologic status deteriorates rapidly after an initial period of improvement. Medical treatment is focused on reducing ICP; surgical intervention is directed at evacuation of the hematoma.

Anesthesia Management The initial management of the patient must include establishing the airway and ensuring responsiveness of the cardiovascular system. Reinitiating oxygenation and adequate circulation must be of the highest priority before concern for the patient's neurologic status. If the patient is having seizures, they must be aggressively and rapidly treated. All patients must be considered to have a *full stomach* after the trauma incident. Following most head injuries, patients should be evaluated for stability of the cervical spine as indicated. If the stability of the cervical spine cannot be confirmed, *in-line stabilization* should be maintained during all movement of the patient and airway manipulations. Succinylcholine may be used to secure the airway if clinically necessary. In the presence of an unstable cervical spine, the fiberoptic bronchoscope may be used to obtain access to the trachea.

Resuscitation of the patient should include returning the intravascular volume to near normal. There is no advantage in using either colloid or crystalloid in the resuscitation period. *Cerebral edema* is not associated with oncotic pressure but with changes in osmolality. Hyposmolar solutions should be avoided in this patient population. Glucose solutions should also be avoided. Hyperglycemia is associated with poor outcomes. Evaluation of the blood sugar should be initiated before glucose infusions are started to ensure that treatment of hypoglycemia is the only reason for use of the solution.

Following the establishment of adequate ventilation, oxygenation, and circulation, the patient's neurologic status can be evaluated. The Glasgow Coma Scale can be used to evaluate the severity of the injury and to assign a prognosis to the patient. This evaluation cannot be accomplished if the patient is either hypoxic or hypotensive. The evaluation should be conducted 6 hours post-injury to permit the effects of drugs used to have dissipated. All causes of alteration in mental status must be evaluated in the patient. Diagnostic tests include radiographic examination of the neck, cervical spine, and skull; computed tomography (CT) scan; and possibly magnetic resonance imaging (MRI). To manage increased ICP, the head of the bed should be elevated to ensure increased venous drainage from the cranial vault. Temporarily, the carbon dioxide level can be lowered to between 25 and 30 mmHg to reduce cerebral blood flow and decrease cerebral blood volume. It may be necessary to paralyze and sedate the patient to permit the management of the airway and ventilation. Mannitol 0.5 to 1.0g/kg is administered to minimize cerebral edema. This is especially indicated if signs of herniation occur. Mannitol 1.0 g/kg will result in a reduction of total brain water of approximately 90 mL while increasing serum osmolality by 18 osm/L. Lasix (furosemide) causes an isosmotic contraction of the extracerebral extracellular space. This results in a decrease in cerebral blood volume, cere-

brospinal fluid (CSF), and sodium transport within the brain. The effects on ICP with Lasix are less than those seen with mannitol.

When providing care for the patient with head trauma, the practitioner must be concerned about the potential for both primary injury and secondary injury. A primary injury is related to the tissue damage that occurs at the time of insult. Secondary injury refers to the injury that results from microvascular or biochemical alterations initiated by the primary insult. Systemic causes of secondary injury include arterial hypotension, hypoxia, anemia, hypoglycemia, hyperthermia, hypertension, osmotic imbalance, coagulopathy, and sepsis. Intracranial events that contribute to secondary injury include subdural and epidural hematomas, contusions, intracerebral hematomas, increased ICP, edema, cerebral vasospasm, cerebral hyperemia, and post-traumatic epilepsy.

Several interventions have been proposed to assist in minimizing secondary injury. Methylprednisolone inhibits lipid peroxidation of cell membranes. No improvements in outcome in head trauma occur; however, improvement in neurologic scores has been demonstrated if methylprednisolone is given within 8 hours of spinal cord injury. The loading dose is 30 mg/kg followed by 5.4 mg/kg/h for the next 23 hours. Tirilizad is a synthetic 21-aminosteroid that prevents lipid peroxidation. This medication lacks the glucocorticoid and mineralocorticoid activities of methylprednisolone. The hypotension that develops after administration may contribute to increased negative outcomes in head trauma patients. *N*-methyl-D-aspartate receptor antagonist and polyethylene glycol-superofide dimutase are antioxidants and free radical scavengers that may have some benefit in the management of secondary injury after head trauma.

Depending on the severity of the injury and type of trauma the patient may be either conscious or unconscious. If unconscious, procedures should be undertaken to secure the airway immediately and initiate hyperventilation. The anesthesia practitioner should assume that the ICP is elevated and select agents and techniques that will minimize the risks of further increases in ICP.

All of the potent inhalation agents have the potential to increase ICP because of cerebral vasodilation leading to increased cerebral blood flow. The development of mild hypocapnea through hyperventilation will reduce this effect. *Hyperventilation* should be initiated before the use of halothane and can be initiated at the same time as isoflurane inhalation is begun. *All of the inhalation agents uncouple the relationship between cerebral blood flow and cerebral oxygen consumption/metabolic rate in a dose-dependent fashion.*

Emergence should proceed slowly using the same concerns and cautions initiated during induction. Airway and control of the blood pressure should be the principle concerns during emergence. If drugs are required for the control of blood pressure, labetolol and hydralazine can be administered. Coughing and straining on the endotracheal tube should be avoided. Both events will result in increased ICP. Lidocaine 1.5 mg/kg can be administered before emergence to assist the patient in tolerating the endotracheal tube. Consideration of the patient's ability to adequately ventilate and protect the airway should guide the practitioner in the decision to keep the patient intubated and ventilated.

Following completion of the surgical intervention, the patient should be evaluated and monitored carefully for the next 12 to 72 hours. There is the potential for developing cerebral edema in the postoperative period. The head of the bed should remain elevated, coughing and bucking should be avoided, and neurologic evaluation continued. Sedation or muscle relaxation should be continued as indicated to provide ventilation and oxygenation while preserving normal systolic, diastolic, and mean arterial blood pressures. Aggressive treatment of seizures, systemic hypertension, and hyperthermia must be initiated to prevent further secondary injury.[1-10]

SPACE-OCCUPYING LESIONS

One of the primary concerns with space-occupying lesions is the potential for increased ICP and the resulting decrease in cerebral perfusion pressure (CPP). This can ultimately result in ischemic changes to other regions of the brain from decreased perfusion, anaerobic metabolism, and buildup of toxic products of metabolism. With increased brain volume, there is increased difficulty in performing the surgical procedure, as well as increased mortality. If the patient is alert and oriented, and displays a normal level of consciousness, there is less potential for problems relating to increased ICP.

The anesthesia practitioner may become involved in the management of this patient from the beginning of a work-up to provide assistance with CT scan and MRI or to provide anesthesia for the definitive surgical procedure. In developing a care plan for this patient, the initial decision concerns premedication. Benzodiazepines have no direct cerebrovascular effects and do not product significant hypercarbia unless doses are administered that render the patient unconscious. Opioids should not be used to provide relief of headache pain in this patient. The potential for respiratory depression may be enhanced by increased ICP. Anticonvulsants and antihypertensive agents should be kept current. It is more harmful to the patient and creates a more difficult sequence of events during induction if the anesthesia practitioner must also manage either a seizure or hypertensive crisis.

The patient should be transported to the operating room in the head-up position. Thirty degrees of Fowler's position will facilitate increased venous drainage and provide a match between CPP and gravity. The choice of monitoring the patient should be based on the patient's preoperative condition and the amount and type of preoperative sedation used.

The selection of monitors for the surgical procedure should include all standard monitors recommended for general anesthesia, including electrocardiogram (ECG) noninvasive blood pressure monitoring, pulse oximetry, and monitoring of heart sounds, respiration, and temperature. An arterial cannula should be inserted to monitor beat to beat, the systolic blood pressure and the mean arterial pressure (MAP).

The indwelling catheter will also provide the anesthetist with the ability to assess arterial blood gases, monitoring changes in carbon dioxide content and pH directly. A Foley catheter should be inserted to monitor urine output and thus intravascular fluid status. Additionally, in suprasellar lesions and midbrain tumors, the catheter can be an aid in the differential diagnosis of diabetes insipidus. Central venous pressure (CVP) monitoring should be considered when the patient is in the sitting position; for aneurysm surgery; when a large blood loss is anticipated; and with vascular lesions, olfactory groove meningiomas, sphenoid wing procedures, and basilar brain tumors.

Induction of general anesthesia can be initiated with most medications and techniques in clinical practice. In midline lesions and hydrocephalus, an inhalation induction with halothane should be avoided. Ketamine should be avoided in most patients with central nervous system (CNS) lesions. Dramatic changes in the ICP can result from the use of ketamine for induction. In the combative patient and those suffering from either mental retardation or mental illness, the benefits of a rapid induction from a single intramuscular injection may be greater than the risks. Thiopental is the most commonly used induction agent. The advantages of rapid action, cerebral vasodilation, decreased cerebral metabolic rate, and decreased ICP support this choice. When hemodynamic stability is a concern during induction, etomidate may be the chosen induction agent.

In choosing a muscle relaxant, the quality of the airway must be evaluated. If a rapid sequence induction with immediate securing of the airway is required, succinylcholine may be used. ICP is transiently increased. This can be reduced by the use of narcotics, benzodiazepines, or pretreatment with a nondepolarizing muscle relaxant. In choosing a nondepolarizing muscle relaxant for intubation and maintenance of relaxation during the procedure, medications that cause histamine release should be avoided. Both rocuronium (0.8 to 1.2 mg/kg) and vecuronium (0.1 to 0.2 mg/kg) can provide sufficient relaxation to secure the airway rapidly. When using the longer-acting muscle relaxants, the ability to secure the airway safely must be paramount during decision making.

During anesthesia, volatile anesthetic agents without hyperventilation increase cerebral blood flow and thus can increase ICP and cerebral blood volume. The intravenous barbiturates and narcotics can reduce cerebral blood flow with a resulting decrease in ICP. Nitrous oxide will cause an increase in cerebral blood flow and ICP. Propofol has been used successfully with the additional benefit of reduced postoperative nausea and vomiting. With the current focus on cost reductions, the cheapest anesthesia combination is thiopental, vecuronium, fentanyl, oxygen, and nitrous oxide. Induction can be obtained with fentanyl 10 μg/kg with a continuous infusion of 2 μg/kg/h during maintenance.

Emergence should proceed slowly with the same concerns and cautions initiated during induction. Concern for the airway and control of the blood pressure should be maintained. If pharmacologic agents are required for the control of blood pressure, labetolol and hydralazine can be administered.

Coughing and straining on the endotracheal tube should be avoided. Both events will increase the ICP. Lidocaine 1.5 mg/kg should be administered before emergence to assist the patient in tolerating the endotracheal tube. Consideration of the patient's ability to adequately ventilate and protect the airway should guide the practitioner in the decision to keep the patient intubated and ventilated. The practitioner must establish goals for emergence and recovery. The blood pressure should be maintained within the range of "normal" for the patient as demonstrated by preoperative nonstress baseline readings. The patient should be awake and follow instructions within 30 minutes of termination of the anesthetic. If these do not occur, the patient should be evaluated to determine if other deficits exist.[4-11]

CEREBRAL ANEURYSM

Cerebral aneurysm has a population incidence of 1% per year. Only about 1% of the patients will develop symptoms following rupture of the aneurysm. The incidence is described as 1:10,000 people per year. Approximately 30,000 individuals in the United States and Canada have aneurysmal subarachnoid hemorrhage (SAH) per year. Of this group, approximately one third die immediately or in the first few hours after rupture. Kassel and colleagues reviewed data on 2922 patients and found that approximately 30% of all patients are functional survivors. The incidence of SAH increases with age. There is a higher incidence of rupture in women compared with men. African-Americans are at higher risk than Caucasians. There is an increased risk of SAH for smokers compared with nonsmokers. Hypertension may be a predisposing factor in the U.S. population.

The patient with an SAH will have a sudden escape of arterial blood into the subarachnoid space. This causes an initial increase in the ICP toward the systemic diastolic pressure. Global ischemia may develop from reductions in CPP and decreased available oxygen supplies. In the patients admitted to the hospital, the ICP gradually declines, resulting in an improvement in cerebral perfusion. This process may take approximately 15 minutes. Cerebral function will gradually improve as perfusion and oxygenation to the brain are restored. The clinical symptoms may include the abrupt onset of a severe headache in 85% to 95% of patients. There will be an alteration in the level of consciousness including loss of consciousness. Approximately 20% of all patients will develop seizures. The patient will complain of nausea and vomiting. In 25% to 50% of patients, a premonitory headache may have developed in preceding weeks that could be connected to a minor hemorrhage or "leak" from the aneurysm. Meningeal irritation from blood may produce signs that are similar to the presentation of meningitis including nucal rigidity and photophobia. Specific neurologic signs will depend on the size of the hematoma, the specific area of injury, the duration of decreased cerebral blood flow, and the presence of vasospasm. The increased ICP can result from edema that is a secondary development of the direct injury.[4-10]

Diagnosis is made by an evaluation of the patient's symptoms in conjunction with the use of CT scans, which will provide clues to the location and magnitude of the bleeding. Additional information on the size of the ventricles may provide practitioners with information on the possibility of hydrocephalus. In approximately 15% to 20% of patients, no detectable site of bleeding can be identified. In 5% to 34% of patients, multiple aneurysms are present. In approximately 90% of patients the aneurysm is contained within the anterior circulation. Lumbar puncture will reveal xanthochroma for several days after the initial bleeding. The procedure can place the patient at risk for herniation.

Complications *Rebleeding* is one of the most serious of complications with a 60% to 70% fatality rate for patients who rebleed. The highest risk of rebleeding is in the first 14 days following the initial bleeding event. In an effort to prevent rebleeding, increases in MAP and decreases in ICP should be avoided. Procedures initiated to prevent these problems include reduction in systemic blood pressure, fluid restriction to the point of dehydration, and sedation. The surgeon's goal will be to operate as soon as possible. All of the procedures used to control ICP and MAP have an impact on the induction and management of anesthesia.

Another serious complication is the development of cerebral vasospasm. *Cerebral vasospasm* is the delayed narrowing of large capacitance arteries at the base of the brain after SAH. It is often associated with evidence of diminished perfusion in the territory distal to the injury in the affected vessel. Evidence of vasospasm will appear on radiographic studies in 50% of patients; however, 30% to 35% of patients will present with clinical symptoms. Cerebral vasospasm occurs approximately 3 to 5 days following the initial bleeding. Maximum narrowing will occur in 5 to 14 days with a gradual resolution of the problem. Approximately 20% of patients with vasospasm will die or develop symptoms of a stroke despite therapeutic interventions. In patients with cerebral vasospasm, decreases in MAP should be avoided. It is necessary to initiate therapeutic measures to ensure relaxation of the smooth muscle of vessel walls. Nimodipine, a calcium entry blocker, is one medication currently used for this purpose. In an effort to maintain the MAP, vasopressors may be used as well as hypervolemic hemodilution.

Acute hydrocephalus has been identified in 20% to 30% of all patients following SAH. The etiology is usually obstruction from intraventricular blood following the hemorrhage. If the level of consciousness is deteriorating, a ventriculostomy is usually performed. There is a potential for an increased rate of bleeding following ventriculostomy. Approximately 50% to 80% of patients will have an improvement in symptoms after the procedure.

Brain edema and *seizures* are potential complications of SAH. Direct insult and injury to the tissues, prolonged periods of either global or localized ischemia, and the presence of hematoma may be the basis of the brain edema. Dexamethasone (Decadron) is frequently administered to the patients; however, evidence clearly demonstrating effectiveness of this therapy is not available. Seizures develop because of focal injury. The potential for rebleeding increases during seizures. To prevent seizures, anticonvulsant medications are routinely ordered. Once the therapeutic blood level is established this medication should not be withheld.

Following SAH, 50% to 80% of patients will have *abnormal ECGs.* ST-T wave changes are most frequently seen in these patients. The changes are similar to changes seen with myocardial infarction. Prolongation of the QT, P wave changes, U waves, and dysrhythmias may also be seen. The posterior hypothalamus may alter autonomic control of the cardiac repolarization process, which is neurogenic and not cardiogenic. Norepinephrine is released from the adrenal medulla and sympathetic efferents. Ischemic changes in the subendocardium can occur either through direct toxicity of norepinephrine or acute increases in afterload. If myocardial ischemia or infarction is suspected, then induced hypotension should be avoided.

Hyponatremia is seen in 10% to 34% of patients, developing several days after the hemorrhage. Clinical manifestations include impaired consciousness, asterixis, muscle weakness, seizures, and coma. With cerebral salt-wasting syndrome, atrial natriuretic factor is elevated and this results in volume contraction and high urine sodium concentration. Hypovolemia should be avoided in these patients. The use of isotonic solutions for maintenance of fluid status is suggested.

Anesthesia Management The goals for the management of anesthesia are to prevent rupture of the aneurysm, facilitate surgical exposure, minimize intraoperative neurologic injury, and facilitate a rapid stable recovery to permit early neurologic evaluation. Marked increases in the MAP and decreases in ICP must be avoided. This patient should not be hyperventilated and CSF must not be drained. To facilitate surgical exposure, the patient must be positioned with the head up, hyperventilated, and CSF drained once the bone flap is opened. To minimize neurologic injury, the brain must be relaxed to facilitate placement of retractors and improve the possibilities of securing the aneurysm. Hyperventilation and low airway pressure can be used to facilitate the decrease in brain volume, if vasospasm is present, or if the patient is of a poor clinical grade.

The choice of premedication should be based on clinical indications. If the patient is anxious, then monitored sedation may be required during transport of the patient and placement of invasive monitors. In this patient, the insertion of the indwelling arterial line should precede induction of anesthesia. The establishment of a CVP monitor before induction may assist in the determination of volume status. Rebleeding during induction is of low risk and seems to be related to uncontrolled hypertensive events during induction, intubation, or painful manipulations. Opioids, β-blockers, and lidocaine may be used to minimize the responses to these interventions and reduce the potential for increased transmural pressure. This will result in reductions in CPP, causing focal and global deficits, especially in patients who have impaired autoregulation and vasospasm. Brief periods of decreased CPP

are less detrimental than sudden increases in transmural pressure.

During the maintenance of anesthesia, the goal is to maintain hemodynamic stability while avoiding marked hypertensive responses to painful stimuli including burr holes and insertion of pins.

Emergence should be rapid and controlled. If pharmacologic agents are required for the control of blood pressure, labetolol and hydralazine can be administered. Coughing and straining on the endotracheal tube should be avoided; both will increase the ICP. Lidocaine 1.5 mg/kg should be administered before emergence to assist the patient in tolerating the endotracheal tube. Consideration of the patient's ability to adequately ventilate and protect the airway should guide the practitioner in the decision to keep the patient intubated and ventilated. The blood pressure should be maintained within the range of "normal" for the patient as demonstrated by preoperative nonstress baseline readings. The patient should be awake and follow instructions within 30 minutes of termination of the anesthetic. If these do not occur, evaluation of the patient should be made to determine if other deficits exist.[4–14]

☐ NEUROSURGIC PROCEDURES IN THE SITTING POSITION

Posterior fossa craniotomies are accomplished in either the sitting position or in the prone position. The choice of the sitting position has been favored in the past because of the exposure of the brain stem. The change of surgical position from sitting to prone has occurred because of the higher incidence of air embolism in the sitting position. Studies have identified the potential problem of air embolus formation in the sitting position. This physiologic problem can occur in all positions; however, the anesthesia practitioner is less likely to monitor for an air embolism in other positions. Doppler monitoring is used to identify the infusion of air into the vascular space. Black and colleagues identified that 30% to 25% of patients will experience hypotension during the surgical procedure. Less respiratory compromise occurs in the sitting position when compared with the prone position.[11]

Shapiro and coworkers compared the incidence of deterioration of cranial nerve function between the sitting and prone position and found that there was a 10% increased incidence in the prone position.[5,6,11] Approximately 65% of patients whose surgery is performed in the sitting position have little to no change in cranial nerve function. Concern is related to injury of cranial nerves involved in airway function (IX, X, XI) from surgical traction, compression of blood supply, or surgical excision. No monitors are available that adequately monitor the function of these nerves; however, if there are more than two or three events during the surgery that result in either hemodynamic or respiratory symptoms such as hypertension, tachycardia, bradycardia, or inspiratory effort, the patient remains intubated until awake. These symptoms may reflect injury to the brain stem or nerves from surgical traction or excisions of tissue.[4,5,7]

Standard monitors are used for a craniotomy in the sitting position. In addition, a central venous catheter should be inserted. The catheter should have multiple openings, which should be at the tip to facilitate removal of air from the *right atrium*. An indwelling arterial catheter can be used to monitor beat-to-beat variability in arterial pressure, monitor changes in MAP, calculate CPP, and facilitate the measurement of arterial blood gases. Monitoring of CVP is not an accurate means of measuring venous sinus pressure.

One of the concerns during anesthesia with the cranial vault open is the entrainment of air. Several procedures have been attempted to decrease the potential for entrainment of air including increasing the CVP and positive end-respiratory pressure (PEEP). Increasing CVP does not consistently decrease the potential for air entrainment. The catheter should be placed at the junction of the superior vena cava and the right atrium. PEEP has been used to minimize the amount of air entrainment; however, the success of this technique also depends on the venous sinus pressure. Neck compression and increasing intra-abdominal pressure have been suggested.[4-12]

☐ TRANSSPHENOIDAL APPROACH

The transsphenoidal approach is used to gain access to tumors of the pituitary gland or other tumors in the area of the sella turcica. The patient may be in either the supine position or with the head of the bed elevated 10° to 15°. The major concerns with this approach are related to the airway. Because both the anesthesia practitioner and the surgeon will have mutual concern for the airway, minimizing the potential for emergent problems is preeminent. Securing of the endotracheal tube to the lower jaw and teeth by wiring the tube to the central incisors can provide additional security. The potential for bone fragments and blood to enter the pharynx can be minimized with the insertion of a throat pack. Maintaining an orogastric tube during the procedure may be beneficial in maintaining an empty stomach; however, the tube may act as a wick for secretions, blood, and irrigating solutions to enter the hypopharynx even with a throat pack in place.

Tumors of the sella turcica or suprasellar region rarely have accompanying increased ICP. Maneuvers to reduce ICP may provide additional difficulty to the surgeon. When the brain size is reduced, the pituitary gland retracts from the base of the sella turcica and "floats" upward into the cranial vault. Some neurosurgeons may request that the patient be ventilated to maintain a slight hypercarbia. This causes the increased blood volume in the cranial vault to force the pituitary gland into the seat of the sella turcica.

Another concern for the anesthesia practitioner is the location of the internal carotid to the sella turcica. The internal carotid artery is slightly lateral to the sella turcica. Surgical procedures for tumors that extend beyond the borders of the sella turcica can potentially injure the vessels. This will result in severe hemorrhage and increase the incidence of fatality with this procedure.[4-6]

☐ GENERAL ANESTHESIA MANAGEMENT IN NEUROANESTHESIA

Before the administration of general anesthesia, the neurologic status of the patient should be completely evaluated. This should include an evaluation of the patient's level of consciousness and response to environmental stimuli including orientation to time, place, and person. The airway should be carefully evaluated to determine the anesthesia practitioner's ability to secure the airway. Hypoxia and increased stimulus from airway manipulation may be causes of increased ICP.

For elective surgical procedures, the patient may require sedation if anxious, before arrival in the operating room. Low doses of benzodiazepines, such as midazolam up to 0.05 mg/kg, may be used. Benzodiazepines that can limit anxiety and have limited ability to cause respiratory depression and hypercapnia should be chosen.

Preinduction monitoring should include noninvasive blood pressure, ECG, pulse oximetry, end-tidal carbon dioxide, precordial pulse, and temperature monitoring. Close monitoring of the arterial pressure requires the establishment of an arterial line prior to induction. Assessment of volume status is crucial; therefore, a central venous catheter should be inserted before beginning the surgical procedure. If the patient is to be placed in the sitting position, the accurate placement of a multiorifice catheter in the right ventricle is necessary. If air is entrained during the surgical procedure, the patient should be turned *right side up* and head lowered so that the air can be trapped in the lower portion of the right ventricle. Proper placement should be assessed with the Doppler device in place. Placement of the catheter in the antecubital vessel will minimize the potential for collapse of the lung with subclavian puncture or restriction of cerebral drainage from cannulation of a jugular vein. During the establishment of invasive monitoring devices, the patient's blood pressure should be monitored carefully and measures taken to prevent increased systolic blood pressure. The anesthesia practitioner should begin to preoxygenate the patient during this time also.

The goal of induction should be to avoid uncontrolled rises in the blood pressure while securing the airway. Thiopental 4.0 mg/kg should be administered for induction of anesthesia following prehydration with 5 to 10 mL/kg of normal saline. This will minimize the potential for precipitous hypotension. Prior to the administration of the muscle relaxant, complete assessment of the airway should be accomplished. If there are any doubts regarding the ability to secure the airway, other procedures should be instituted first to secure the airway. The patient should be totally relaxed with a muscle relaxant before manipulation of the airway. The patient's relaxation status should be monitored with a peripheral nerve stimulator. The choice of muscle relaxant depends on the status of the airway, the potential for a full stomach, and the potential for aspiration. Rocuronium 0.8 to 1.2 mg/kg can provide adequate muscle relaxation within 60 to 75 seconds. Rocuronium in doses above 1.2 mg/kg can result in slight tachycardia. Other muscle relaxants such as vecuronium and metubine can be used safely. Muscle relaxants that potentially release histamine on administration should be avoided. Succinylcholine 1.5 mg/kg can be administered safely; however, the short duration of the muscle relaxation after administration will require additional nondepolarizing muscle relaxant before the patient is positioned. Concerns for changing blood pressure can be controlled with the administration of fentanyl 10 μg/kg, lidocaine 1.5 mg/kg, or esmolol 0.5 mg/kg.

Hyperventilation should begin as soon as the endotracheal tube is in place (unless otherwise indicated, i.e., tumors of the sella turcica or cerebral aneurysm). The ventilator settings should be adjusted to maintain the end-tidal carbon dioxide level in the mid-20 mm Hg range. Baseline arterial carbon dioxide levels can be determined to establish that the arterial carbon dioxide level is approximately 25 mm Hg.

Following induction and initiation of hyperventilation, 10 to 15 μg/kg fentanyl is titrated intravenously over 5 to 10 minutes. Isoflurane can be used to maintain the systolic blood pressure at the levels identified prior to induction. The patient must have sufficient anesthetic to prevent hypertensive responses to stimuli. Both narcotics and volatile anesthetic agents cause cerebral vasodilation and increase cerebral blood flow. This causes an increase in cerebral volume. Initiation of hyperventilation and reduction of carbon dioxide levels cause vasoconstriction and may minimize the effects of both the narcotics and inhalation agents.

During maintenance of anesthesia, the goal is to provide a quiet surgical field, decreased brain volume, and maintenance of cerebral oxygen requirements. Analgesia is maintained with fentanyl 2 μg/kg/h via either a continuous infusion or intermittent bolus administration. Muscle relaxation should be maintained during the procedure. If the surgical procedure will last longer than 3 hours, vecuronium can replace rocuronium. If the procedure is to be less than 3 hours, either muscle relaxant will provide sufficient relaxation for the procedure. One twitch on the train-of-four monitor should be maintained.

The blood pressure should be controlled to minimize rises in systolic blood pressure without significantly lowering the MAP. Nitrous oxide can be added to the anesthetic technique if the ICP is not significantly elevated. Once the dura is open, the ICP is essentially zero. Following opening of the dura, techniques should be used to provide the surgeon with optimal brain tissue compliance. Mannitol may be required at this time and if significant results are not obtained it may be necessary to drain CSF via a lumbar drain.

Systemic blood pressure should be reduced but the MAP should not be lowered below normal levels of autoregulation. MAP should be maintained between 60 and 70 mm Hg during the surgical procedure. If there is a high risk of cerebral vasospasm, a mean of 50 to 60 mm Hg may be too low to ensure adequate CPP. Nitroprusside, nitroglycerin, and β blockers (esmolol) may be required to maintain systemic pressures. Thiopental may be used to provide electroencephalographic burst suppression during the surgical procedure especially if the procedure is an aneurysm clipping. Thiopental should be administered in 100- to 200-mg increments every 5 minutes as tolerated by the arterial pressure. To achieve burst suppression, the dose of thiopental may be up to 20 mg/kg over 30 minutes.

Hypothermia may be protective in this patient. Temperature ranges of 30° to 34°C provide decreased cerebral oxygen consumption. However, it may be difficult to rewarm the patient at the end of the procedure.

During emergence and the initial period following surgery, the goal is to maintain oxygenation and perfusion of cerebral tissues and control systolic blood pressure. Slow withdrawal of inhalation agents and opioids provides a gentle emergence. The continuous infusion of opioids should be discontinued at the termination of the procedure. The inhalation agent should be discontinued when security of the airway is returned to the anesthesia practitioner. The same care provided to the patient during induction should be continued during emergence. Because one of the goals of this portion of the anesthetic is to provide an awake patient as soon as possible to evaluate the neurologic status, additional sedative medications should be administered only as a last choice.[4-11]

REFERENCES

1. Caplan LM, Miller SM, Trundorf H. Trauma overview. In: Caplan LM, Miller SM, Trundorf H, eds. *Trauma Anesthesia and Intensive Care*. Philadelphia: JB Lippincott; 1991:3–29.

2. Miller SM. Management of central nervous system injuries. In: Caplan LM, Miller SM, Trundorf H, eds. *Trauma Anesthesia and Intensive Care*. Philadelphia: JB Lippincott; 1991: 321–351.

3. Markison RE, Trunkey DD. Establishment of care priorities. In: Caplan LM, Miller SM, Trundorf H, eds. *Trauma Anesthesia and Intensive Care*. Philadelphia: JB Lippincott; 1991:29–42.

4. Bendo AA, Kass IS, Hartung J, Cottrell JE. Neurophysiology and neuroanesthesia. In: Barash PG, Cullen BF, Stoelting RK, eds. *Clinical Anesthesia*. 2nd ed. Philadelphia: JB Lippincott; 1992:871–998.

5. Shapiro HM, Drummond JC. Neurosurgical anesthesia. In: Miller RD, ed. *Anesthesia*. 4th ed. Philadelphia: JB Lippincott; 1994:1897–1946.

6. Todd MM, Warner DS. Neuroanesthesia: a critical review. In: Rogers MC, Tinker JH, Covino, and Longnecker DE, eds. *Principles and Practice of Anesthesiology*. St. Louis: Mosby-Yearbook, 1993:1599–1648.

7. Nicoli RA. Introduction to the pharmacology of CNS drugs. In:

Katsung B, ed. *Basic and Clinical Pharmacology*. 6th ed. East Norwalk, Conn: Appleton & Lange; 1995:323–332.

8. Trevor AJ, Way WL. Sedative-hypnotics. In: Katsung B, ed. *Basic and Clinical Pharmacology*. 6th ed. East Norwalk, Conn: Appleton & Lange; 1995:333–349.

9. Porter RJ, Meldrum BS. Antiepileptic drugs. In: Katsung B, ed. *Basic and Clinical Pharmacology*. 6th ed. East Norwalk, Conn: Appleton & Lange; 1995:361–380.

10. Shelton RC, Ebert MH. Drugs and the central nervous system. In: Wood M, Wood AJJ, eds. *Drugs and Anesthesia: Pharmacology for Anesthesiologists*. 2nd ed. Baltimore: Williams & Wilkins; 1990:571–595.

11. Black S, Ockert DB, Oliver WK, Cucchiara RF. Outcome following posterior fossa craniectomy in patients in sitting or horizontal positions. *Anesthesiology*. 1988;69:49–56.

12. Hibino H, Matsuura M. Cerebral venous sinus pressure in seated dogs: impact of PEEP, central venous compression, and abdominal compression. *Anesthesiology*. 1985;63:184–189.

13. Kassel NF, Torner JC, Jance JA, et al: The International Cooperative Study on the Timing of Aneurysm Surgery: part 2. Surgical results. *J Neurosurg*. 1990;73:37–47.

14. Haley EC, Kassell NF, Torner JC, et al. The International Cooperative Study on the Timing of Aneurysm Surgery: the North American experience. *Stroke*. 1992;23:205–214.

☐ QUESTIONS

1. A 58-year-old woman scheduled for a frontal craniotomy for a possible cystic lesion is complaining of a severe mid-frontal headache radiating to the occipital area and "fuzzy" vision. She has asked for medication for the headache. What agents would you avoid in providing her analgesia?
   a. Benzodiazepines
   b. Agonist-antagonists
   c. Opioids
   d. None of the above

2.–4. Match the technique with a desired outcome:
   2. ⎯⎯ Isoflurane-nitrous   a. Decreased nausea
   3. ⎯⎯ Fentanyl-nitrous   b. Intracranial pressure <20
   4. ⎯⎯ Propofol-fentanyl   c. Faster wake-up

5. A primary reason for decreasing sitting position craniotomies has been:
   a. That other positions provide better surgical exposure
   b. Concern about the increased incidence of air embolus
   c. The difficulty in preserving blood pressure during surgery
   d. None of the above

6. Postanesthesia deterioration of cranial nerve function is ⎯⎯⎯⎯⎯⎯⎯⎯ in the sitting position when compared to patients whose surgical procedure is accomplished in the prone position.
   a. Less
   b. More
   c. The same
   d. Not a factor

7. To monitor the cerebral perfusion pressure during craniotomy, the a-line should be zeroed at the level of the:
   a. Mandible
   b. Heart, calculating the CPF mathematically
   c. Incision
   d. The ear lobe

8. When the patient's central venous pressure is maintained at a high level, there is a significant decrease in the potential for entrainment of air. True or false?
   a. True
   b. False

9. A central venous pressure catheter that is inserted for the purpose of removing air if it is entrained into the central circulation should be:
   a. Placed at the junction of the right atrium and superior vena cava
   b. A multiorifice catheter
   c. In the subclavian vein
   d. a and b

10. Anesthetics that increase ICP include all *expect*:
   a. Ketamine
   b. Enflurane
   c. Droperidol
   d. N_2O

11. Ketamine is considered an acceptable induction agent in patients with a space-occupying lesion when the patient suffers from
   a. Guillaine Barré syndrome
   b. COPD
   c. Mental retardation
   d. Multipe sclerosis

12. Postoperative complications associated with subarachnoid hemorrhage (SAH) repair include:
   a. Hyponatremia
   b. Rebleeding
   c. Cerebral vasospasm
   d. All of the above

13. Epidural hematomas result from a rapid arterial bleed into the dural space. True or false?
   a. True
   b. False

14. In the presence of facial trauma, patients with suspected basilar skull fractures should obtain airway control via:
    a. Nasal endotracheal tube
    b. Oral endotracheal tube
    c. Cricothyrotomy
    d. Controlled tracheotomy

15. One of the cardinal signs of a ruptured cerebral aneurysm is a complaint of the abrupt onset of a "severe headache" followed by an alteration or loss of consciousness in most patients. True or false?
    a. True
    b. False

16. In an effort to reduce or prevent cerebral vascular vasospasm, the practitioner can:
    a. Avoid decreases in mean arterial pressure
    b. Inhibit fibrinolysis
    c. Relax cerebral arteries
    d. All of the above

17. For airway management of a head trauma patient one must consider:
    a. All trauma patients are considered to have a full stomach
    b. The need to rule out cervical spine fracture
    c. In-line stabilization of the head alone with a rapid sequence induction
    d. All of the above

18. A 81-year-old woman is undergoing a craniotomy in the sitting position. Suddenly the patient becomes hypotensive and air is heard on the precordial Doppler. All are appropriate actions expect.
    a. Discontinue the N_2O
    b. Hyperventilate to a $ETCO_2$ of 20
    c. Aspirate fluid from the central venous catheter
    d. Flood the surgical field with normal saline

19. After which surgical procedure might you want the patient to remain intubated postoperatively?
    a. Cerebral aneurysm clipping
    b. Ventriculostomy
    c. Craniotomy for astrocytoma of the posterior fossa
    d. All of the above

20. Elevation in intracranial pressure is controlled by:
    a. Placing the patient in the Trendelenberg position
    b. Allowing the patient to hypoventilate
    c. Maintaining the systolic blood pressure at greater than 160 mm Hg
    d. Preventing seizures from occurring

☐ ANSWERS

1.	c	5.	b	9.	d	13.	b	17.	d
2.	b	6.	a	10.	c	14.	b	18.	b
3.	c	7.	d	11.	c	15.	a	19.	c
4.	a	8.	b	12.	d	16.	d	20.	d

CHAPTER
23

Anesthesia for Abdominal and Genitourologic Surgery

Laura Baker

☐ ABDOMINAL PROCEDURES AND ANESTHETIC MANAGEMENT

A thorough preoperative evaluation is necessary to provide a safe anesthetic to a patient for whom an intra-abdominal procedure is planned. This includes knowledge of gastrointestinal disease and its affect on other systems. Assessment of perioperative fluid status, any metabolic or hematologic derangements, and history of previous abdominal surgery, radiation therapy, infection, or steroid use is also necessary. The anesthetic technique is then determined by factors relating to the patient, the operation, the anesthesia provider, and the surgeon.

HERNIA REPAIRS

A field block in combination with intravenous sedation is a common method of providing anesthesia for a hernia repair. General or regional anesthesia are alternative techniques. A sensory level of T-4 to T-6 is required if a regional technique is used.

A field block often consists of a mixture of lidocaine and bupivacaine. This solution is injected at the external and internal oblique muscles to block the ilioguinal and iliohypogastric nerves. Subcutaneous infiltration and local injections in the area of the spermatic cord and internal ring are also required. During a field block, it is important to avoid epinephrine because its use may be associated with ischemia of the base of the penis or spermatic cord. Rare complications of this procedure include hematoma formation and motor blockade of the femoral nerve.

ABDOMINOPERINEAL RESECTION

The presence of malignant lesions or inflammatory disease of the lower sigmoid colon, rectum, or anus may require an abdominoperineal resection. The principal disorders comprising inflammatory bowel disease are Crohn's disease and ulcerative colitis.

Inflammatory lesions are located primarily in the mucosa and submucosa of the colon in ulcerative colitis. The mucosa is friable with a tendency to bleed easily. As a result, patients typically present with bloody diarrhea and abdominal pain.

Fulminant colitis, present in 5% of patients, is a severe form of ulcerative colitis that can be complicated by toxic megacolon or perforation. Predominant symptoms include multiple bouts of bloody diarrhea and weight loss over several weeks. Patients may be pale, febrile, and tachycardic with postural changes in blood pressure. Abdominal guarding, distention, and absent bowel sounds are common. Laboratory results may reveal the presence of a low hematocrit, hypokalemia, hypoalbuminemia, blood urea nitrogen (BUN) elevation, and leukocytosis. Initial treatment consists of immediate fluid resuscitation, steroids, cultures, and a radiograph to rule out the presence of free air in the peritoneal cavity. Systemic steroids are the mainstay of therapy. The administration of steroids may be continued for a duration of 1 to 2 weeks. An NPO status is also maintained on these patients, allowing the bowel to rest. Total parenteral nutrition may be necessary. Broad-spectrum antibiotics and cyclosporine may be initiated if symptoms do not improve or ulcerative colitis is severe. Surgery is indicated if the patient shows no response to the above measures.

Skip lesions or the presence of normal tissue alternating

with areas of inflammation characterize Crohn's disease. Lesions involve all the layers of the bowel wall, mesenteries, and associated lymph nodes. Right lower quadrant abdominal pain, bloodless diarrhea, fever, fatigue, weight loss, and the presence of anal fissures, fistulas, or perirectal abscesses are common. These patients may be at risk for macrocytic anemia, cholelithiasis, and renal calculi. Fulminant colitis and toxic megacolon may also occur in patients with Crohn's disease. However, this syndrome is less common than in patients with ulcerative colitis. The presence of bowel obstruction, abscess formation, perforation, and possible hemorrhage may require emergent surgery in patients with Crohn's disease.

SMALL-BOWEL OBSTRUCTION

Patients with bowel obstructions commonly present with nausea, vomiting, and abdominal distention. The mortality rate is 1% in previously healthy patients and higher in compromised patients.

When an obstruction occurs in the small bowel, a segment of intestine proximal to the obstruction distends with gas and fluid. Small-bowel secretion increases and absorption decreases. Blood supply can be compromised as the bowel dilates, leaving these patients at risk for bowel necrosis, perforation, bacteremia, and septicemia. Because of the risk of bowel necrosis and perforation, an urgent operation is necessary.

LARGE-BOWEL OBSTRUCTION

Large-bowel obstruction is determined by the activity of the ileocecal valve. If the ileocecal valve is competent in a patient with large-bowel obstruction, the large bowel will show dilation, which may impair blood supply. The patient may be at risk for bowel necrosis and perforation. If the ileocecal valve is not competent the contents of the large bowel will reflux into the small bowel and cause vomiting. Obstruction in the large bowel usually occurs more slowly than small-bowel obstruction. However, severe fluid and electrolyte abnormalities, as in patients with small-bowel obstructions, can still occur.

Factors that influence the management of anesthesia include control of the airway and fluid and electrolyte balance. A rapid sequence induction with cricoid pressure is essential in a patient with a full stomach. The risk of aspiration may also be diminished by the judicious use of sodium citrate, ranitidine or famotidine, metoclopramide, and nasogastric tube insertion. Primary goals during maintenance of anesthesia include appropriate fluid management, exposure of the surgical field, and measures to ensure normothermia. Fluid replacement should be based on clinical and laboratory data.

Fluid loss from surgical bleeding, sequestration, evaporation, and nasogastric and ascitic drainage must be considered. Serial measurements of the hematocrit, electrolytes, and BUN must be obtained. Exposure of the surgical field is facilitated by the use of potent inhalational agents and non-

depolarizing muscle relaxants. *Avoid* N_2O because its use may cause expansion of the air spaces within the bowel, leading to possible bowel ischemia or surgical difficulty during closure. During emergence, *neostigmine* should be used with caution because the drug increases bowel motility and may cause anastomic disruption.

PANCREATITIS

The majority of cases of pancreatitis result from excessive alcohol intake or the presence of gallstones. Blunt abdominal trauma, penetrating peptic ulcer, hypercalcemia, hyperlipidemia, or genetic predisposition are less frequent causes. Pancreatitis may also occur idiopathically.

Activated pancreatic enzymes are released into the gland and surrounding tissues causing inflammation. In addition, bacterial endotoxin, pancreatic protease, and other active agents are released into the systemic circulation. Pancreatic protease and endotoxin, in turn, activate the complement system. Complement system activation causes release of substances that exert local toxic effects on pulmonary epithelium, resulting in increases in permeability. This is also thought to occur in other organs.

The most common symptom is epigastric pain that can radiate to the back. Diffuse abdominal tenderness and rebound, nausea, vomiting, and fever may also occur. If pancreatitis is severe, symptoms of profound dehydration appear, including tachycardia and postural hypotension. Pleural effusions may be present, especially on the left. Hemorrhagic pancreatitis may be indicated in 1% to 2% of patients by Turner's or Cullen's sign. Turner's sign is a bluish discoloration in the flank; Cullen's sign is a bluish discoloration in the umbilical area. These two signs are caused by retroperitoneal dissection of blood.

An elevation in serum lipase concentration may appear early in the attack of pancreatitis. However, diagnosis is usually based on an elevation in serum and urinary amylase levels. Liver function tests are generally normal. The hematocrit may be elevated or decreased from dehydration or blood loss. In severe pancreatitis, hypocalcemia may be present.

Early identification of patients at risk for complications and aggressive treatment may decrease the mortality rate. Treatment includes fluid resuscitation, close attention to electrolytes (especially sodium, potassium, magnesium and calcium), use of nasogastric tubes, total parenteral nutrition, and opioids for analgesia. Supplemental oxygen should be administered if the Pao_2 level is below 70. Severe pancreatitis may be complicated by acute respiratory distress syndrome, myocardial depression, renal insufficiency, and gastric stress ulceration. A patient experiencing complications or signs and symptoms of shock will probably require time in an intensive care unit, intubation, and placement of an arterial line and Swan-Ganz catheter.

Surgical management of the patient is necessary if a pancreatic abscess develops. An abscess is usually fatal unless it is drained surgically. Broad-spectrum antibiotics are also prescribed. However, the condition is severe and diagnosis is difficult, resulting in a mortality rate of about 20%.

GASTROINTESTINAL BLEEDING

Surgery for control of gastrointestinal bleeding is required in 10% to 20% of patients. The majority of patients cease bleeding within 24 to 48 hours with conservative medical management.

These patients, if brought to the operating room, are frequently hypovolemic. Significant blood loss has occurred when a decrease of 10 to 20 mm Hg in the systolic blood pressure is associated with a concurrent increase in the heart rate of 10 to 20 beats/min when the patient changes from a supine to a sitting position. Laboratory data may reveal hemoconcentration, reflected by a normal hematocrit and an elevation in the BUN, which occurs from increased nitrogen absorption in the small intestine.

If hypotension is prolonged because of massive gastrointestinal bleeding, liver necrosis, mesenteric insufficiency, acute renal failure, and myocardial ischemia can occur.

SPLENECTOMY

The most common indication for a splenectomy is trauma from a motor vehicle accident. Patients may present in severe hypovolemic shock or have minimal to absent signs and symptoms. The majority of patients have generalized abdominal pain, most severe in the left upper quadrant. Referred pain to the left shoulder or cervical region, nausea and vomiting may also occur. Laparotomy is indicated in approximately 75% of patients. Splenectomy may also be performed for staging of Hodgkin's lymphoma or treatment of idiopathic thrombocytopenic purpura. Splenectomy may be associated with a large loss of blood. Large-bore intravenous lines and general anesthesia are necessary.

LAPAROSCOPIC PROCEDURES

Cholecystectomy   Biliary tract disease is present in approximately 15 to 20 million adults. Obstruction of the biliary tract by gallstones usually causes acute cholecystitis. These patients present with abrupt onset of severe epigastric pain that radiates to the right upper abdomen and increases with inspiration (known as the Murphy sign). Patients may have a fever, mild leukocytosis, and elevations in plasma bilirubin, alkaline phosphatase, and amylase levels. Jaundice will be present if the cystic duct is completely obstructed by gallstones.

The first laparoscopic cholecystectomy was reported by a French surgeon in 1987. Advantages of laparoscopic surgery include a shorter hospital stay, faster recovery, less postoperative pain, and a smaller incision. A pneumoperitoneum is created for this surgery by inserting a Veress needle through a small infraumbilical incision. Carbon dioxide is then insufflated until an intra-abdominal pressure of 12 to 15 mm Hg has been reached. The surgical field is visualized with a video laparoscopic camera and monitor. Additional incisions are made for instruments used to dissect the gallbladder. For further discussion on gallbladder please see Chapter 18.

A surgeon will often request a reverse Trendelenberg position with a left lateral tilt to provide exposure of the surgical field. Further exposure is facilitated by the use of a nasogastric tube and Foley catheter to decompress the stomach and bladder, respectively. General anesthesia with controlled ventilation is preferred. Controlled ventilation prevents hypercarbia that may result from absorption of CO_2 from the peritoneal cavity, mechanical impairment of the diaphragm by the pneumoperitoneum, and depression of ventilation by anesthetics.

To maintain normocarbia during laparoscopic procedures, it may be necessary to increase the minute volume by 20% to 30%. Laparoscopic surgery is also associated with changes in the patient's cardiovascular status. An increase in the mean arterial pressure may represent an elevation in afterload. A decline in the cardiac index then occurs. These changes probably represent a combination of events including the effects of general anesthesia and impedance of venous return caused by the reverse Trendelenberg position and insufflation of CO_2. This scenario may put patients with cardiovascular disease at risk for ischemia during laparoscopic cholecystectomies. This problem may be accentuated if tachycardia occurs. Conversion to an open cholecystectomy may be necessary.

Complications during a laparoscopic cholecystectomy include possible injury to biliary structures, bowel perforation, and possible cardiovascular collapse from laceration of an intra-abdominal blood vessel or venous air embolism. A gas embolism should be immediately suspected if hypotension and acute pulmonary edema occur. The insufflation of gas should be terminated immediately. Subcutaneous emphysema may occur if the Veress needle does not penetrate into the peritoneum before the insufflation of gas. If subcutaneous emphysema occurs a chest x-ray should be obtained to rule out the possibility of pneumothorax or pneumomediastinum caused by the gas entering the thorax through weakened areas in the diaphragm. Vasovagal reflex or bradycardia may result from the manipulation of intra-abdominal structures or massive distention of the peritoneal cavity. Conversion to an open cholecystectomy may be necessary if difficulty in identification and mobilization of the cystic duct or bleeding occur.

Appendectomy   A diagnostic laparoscopy may be done in a patient presenting with acute appendicitis. This procedure may prevent an unnecessary laparotomy from being done, especially in women. If a patient has a perforated appendix, a laparotomy is the surgical technique of choice.

Pheochromocytoma   A pheochromocytoma is a catecholamine-secreting tumor usually found in the adrenal medulla. Characteristic signs and symptoms include paroxysmal hypertension, tachycardia, diaphoresis, headache, tremors, and palpitations. α_1-Mediated suppression of insulin release may result in hyperglycemia. Catecholamine-induced cardiomyopathy and congestive heart failure can also occur.

A computed tomography (CT) scan is extremely accurate in diagnosing pheochromocytoma. Laboratory determinations of urinary catecholamines and their metabolites are useful but require rigid dietary and drug restrictions by patients. Oral clonidine may be useful in distinguishing patients with essential hypertension from patients with hypertension secondary to pheochromocytoma. In patients with essential hypertension, oral clonidine suppresses catecholamine secretion but does not do so in patients with pheochromocytoma.

Preoperative preparation of the patient includes use of α antagonists. Adequate α blockade prevents vasoconstriction caused by catecholamines released by the tumor and lowers the blood pressure. Dysrhythmias can be controlled with β blockade once α blockade has been initiated. The patient should never receive β blockers before instituting α antagonists because β blockers are negative inotropes and in these patients the depressed heart would be unable to maintain a cardiac output against an elevated systemic vascular resistance caused by the huge catecholamine release by the pheochromocytoma. If cardiomyopathy is suspected, an echocardiogram to evaluate left ventricular function and a chest x-ray to determine possible presence of congestive heart failure may be necessary. A hematocrit over 45 percent may indicate a contracted blood volume. Preoperative fluid may be required. A baseline glucose level should be obtained. During surgical excision of a pheochromocytoma, a nephrectomy may be required; therefore, renal function must be assessed before surgery. Finally, a multiple endocrine neoplasia and hyperparathyroidism may be present if the patient is hypercalcemic.

Intubation of the trachea, tumor manipulation, and the period of time after ligation of the tumor's venous drainage are intraoperative periods of danger for these patients. Anxiolytics should be given preoperatively. Gentle transfer of the patient to the operating room table prevents any undue strain that could cause catecholamine release. A large-bore intravenous line, arterial line, electrocardiogram monitor, temperature probe, urinary catheter, and central venous line are essential for safe anesthetic management. If cardiomyopathy is suspected, a Swan-Ganz catheter is also necessary.

The anesthetic induction should be deep, combining the use of sodium thiopental, isoflurane, and lidocaine. Nipride should be immediately available. Cardiac dysrhythmias can be treated with lidocaine or esmolol. Vecuronium is the preferred choice for muscle relaxation because of its lack of histamine release or vagolytic effects. Avoid *droperidol* because it may enhance catecholamine release by occupying presynaptic dopaminergic receptors on chromaffin cells, which normally inhibit the release of catecholamines.

Hypotension from an immediate decline in circulating catecholamine, profound depth of anesthesia, and hypovolemia may occur after the tumor is removed. At this point, anesthetic management will consist of decreasing the concentration of isoflurane, fluid resuscitation, and possible blood pressure support with phenylephrine or norepinephrine.

Hypoglycemia, hypertension, and hypotension are possible postoperative complications. Hypoxia, hypercarbia, urinary retention, or an undiagnosed pheochromocytoma may cause hypertension. Necessary measures may include: controlled ventilation, bladder catheterization, and pharmacological control of blood pressure. Hypotension is rare. If hypotension occurs, it is treated with volume administration. If, however, hypotension is acute, it may indicate intra-abdominal bleeding, necessitating reoperation. Further management must include use of glucose-containing solutions once the tumor is removed. This decreases the potential for profound hypoglycemia, which may cause loss of consciousness and respiratory arrest. In the first 24 hours, frequent glucose determinations are required. Also see Chapter 17.

CARCINOID SYNDROME

Carcinoid tumors, present in 5% to 7% of the general population, are frequently small with multiple sites. The most common site is the *gastrointestinal tract*. Fifty percent of the tumors occur in the appendix, 25% in the ileum, and 20% in the rectum. Tumors may also occur in the bronchi. More than 20 mediators have now been associated with carcinoid syndrome. Kallikreins, serotonin, and prostaglandins are some of the vasoactive substances released. When the output of the vasoactive substances exceeds the ability of the liver to inactivate them, carcinoid syndrome occurs.

Carcinoid syndrome develops in 5% of patients with carcinoid tumors. It is usually associated with metastasis of ileal carcinoid tumors and multiple systems may be affected. Ninety percent of patients have flushing of the face and upper body, 75% have diarrhea, 33% have right-sided heart disease, and 20% will experience wheezing and bronchoconstriction. Premature atrial contractions or supraventricular dysrhythmias are also possible. Diagnosis is based on signs and symptoms and elevation of urinary 5-hydroxyindoleacetic concentrations.

Surgery may be necessary for ligation of a hepatic artery, resection of a carcinoid tumor, relief of bowel obstruction, or tricuspid or pulmonary valve replacement. A life-threatening carcinoid crisis with cardiovascular collapse, hypotension, tachycardia, or hypertension can be precipitated by stress, induction of anesthesia, surgical manipulation, or even by prepping the abdominal wall before surgery. Current medications should be continued preoperatively. Somatostatin (antiserotonin) analogues such as octreotide, which prevents release of ectopic hormones, can be given preoperatively. Somatostatin analogues should also be available for immediate intraoperative administration. Avoid succinylcholine, ketamine, and drugs that release histamine. Succinylcholine can cause fasciculations, pressure on the tumor, and hormone release. The use of ketamine, which stimulates the sympathetic nervous system, may be associated with the release of kallikreins. It is also important to avoid hypotension, hypercapnia, and hypothermia which can cause release of endogenous catecholamines. Hypotension must be treated with fluid in patients with carcinoid syndrome, because catecholamine use may also precipitate mediator release and impair resuscitation. Finally, sedation is associated with increased levels of serotonin and anesthetic requirements may be decreased in these patients.

GENITOUROLOGIC PROCEDURES AND ANESTHETIC MANAGEMENT

A large percentage of patients in whom genitourologic surgery is necessary are elderly. Preoperative preparation must consider concominant disease, functional decline in most organ systems, and consequent loss of reserve. Elderly patients require extra care when moving and positioning, are more susceptible to hypothermia, and have a diminished requirement for most anesthetics. Anesthetic agents should be titrated slowly, remembering that elderly patients have a prolonged circulation time. Regional techniques of anesthesia may be superior to the administration of general anesthesia in many genitourologic procedures. Postoperative mental impairment may be reduced by use of a regional technique if minimal sedation is required. The awake patient is often able to describe early signs and symptoms of complications during a transurethral resection of the prostate (TURP). Finally, regional techniques are associated with a significant decrease in blood loss and reduction in the incidence of thromboembolic events during radical prostatectomies and radical cystectomies.

CYSTOSCOPY

These procedures are frequently done on an outpatient basis. Indications for cystoscopy are removal of a bladder tumor, treatment of uretheral strictures, or retrograde catheterization. Cystoscopy may also be performed for diagnostic studies including diagnosis of prostatic hypertrophy.

The administration of anesthesia is determined by the amount of stimulation encountered during these procedures. Minor cystologic procedures may only require local anesthesia using 2% lidocaine jelly with or without monitored anesthesia care. If dilation of the urethra or bladder distention is performed, a regional technique with a T-10 sensory level or general anesthesia is necessary. Instrumentation of the ureters, done during a retrograde catheterization, requires a regional technique with a sensory level of T-6 or the administration of general anesthesia.

TRANSURETHRAL RESECTION OF THE PROSTATE

Benign prostatic hypertrophy, prostate cancer, and bladder contracture can cause bladder neck obstruction. TURP is the most common operation performed for treatment of bladder obstruction. A resectoscope is used to perform this procedure; 1.5% glycine or Cytal and a mixture of 2.7% sorbitol and .5% mannitol are used to distend the bladder, provide vi-

Table 23–1
COMPLICATIONS ASSOCIATED WITH TURP

Complication	Signs/Symptoms
Hemorrhage	Hypotension, tachycardia, sweating, pallor
Perforation of urinary bladder	Abdominal or shoulder pain, nausea, vomiting, abdominal rigidity
Intravascular absorption of irrigating fluid	Hypervolemia, pulmonary edema, congestive heart failure, hypertension, widened pulse pressure, slowing of heart rate, dyspnea, cyanosis, cerebral edema, restlessness, headache, nausea vomiting, confusion, coma, seizures,
Hypothermia	
Bacteremia	Sudden unexplained cardiovascular collapse

sualization, and disperse the electrical current from a wire loop used to resect tissue and coagulate blood vessels. *Complications* include hemorrhage, perforation of the urinary bladder, intravascular absorption of irrigating fluid, hypothermia, and bacteremia. Signs and symptoms associated with complications during this procedure are listed in Table 23–1.

The TURP syndrome is caused by intravascular absorption of irrigating fluid. Central nervous system symptoms are usually seen when the sodium level is *below 120 mEq/L*. At a sodium level of 115 mEq/L, ST segment elevation, T wave inversion, widening of the QRS, bradycardia, and ventricular ectopic beats can occur. Ventricular tachycardia, ventricular fibrillation, generalized seizures, and respiratory arrest are possible if the sodium level falls below 100 mEq/L. The height of the fluid column, the duration of the procedure, size of openings in the venous sinuses, and amount of bladder distention used all influence the amount of fluid absorbed.

A spinal anesthetic to a T-10 sensory level is generally preferred in these patients. The awake patient can be helpful to the anesthesia provider in detecting early signs and symptoms of possible complications. If the awake patient describes a change in sensorium, this may indicate dilutional hyponatremia or ammonia intoxication. Immediate recognition of the TURP syndrome is essential. An early sign of excess fluid absorption may be indicated by progressive increases in arterial or central venous or pulmonary capillary wedge pressures. If TURP syndrome occurs the surgery must be stopped as soon as possible. An arterial blood sample should be sent to determine the arterial blood gas and sodium levels. Treatment should consist of fluid restriction and furosemide administration if symptoms are mild. Hypertonic saline may be required for severe symptomatology.

Intraperitoneal perforation is another possible complication during a TURP procedure. If intraperitoneal perforation occurs, the conscious patient may complain of abdominal pain. Irritation of the diaphragm will cause additional referred pain to the shoulder. Aggressive therapy is not required for small perforations. Insertion of uretheral catheters allow the kidneys to excrete the intraperitoneal fluid. Suprapubic drainage or surgical exploration may be necessary for larger perforations.

RADICAL PROSTATECTOMY

If a prostate is greater than 100 g, an open prostatectomy is usually performed. This can be done using a suprapubic, retropubic, or perineal approach. The patient is at risk for deep-vein thrombosis and pulmonary embolism following major abdominal surgery. Results from a recent study suggested early ambulation, use of compression stockings, and continuous epidural patient-controlled analgesia may prevent such complications. The use of epidural anesthesia may also decrease intraoperative blood loss and postoperative pain in patients requiring this procedure.

RADICAL CYSTECTOMY

A radical cystectomy is the removal of the bladder and creation of an ileal conduit for patients with bladder cancer. Preoperatively, these patients often receive radiation therapy, which may make surgical dissection difficult. If nutritional deficiencies exist, hyperalimentation therapy may be initiated. Patients may also be dehydrated as a result of extensive preoperative bowel preps. If regional techniques are used, these patients must be hydrated before instituting anesthesia.

During a radical cystectomy the anesthesia provider loses the ability to measure the urine output once the ureters are disconnected. Routine monitors, large-bore intravenous lines and an arterial line are necessary. A central venous catheter to monitor intravascular volume status must also be inserted. Additional anesthetic management goals must consider the prolonged length of surgery and ability to maintain normothermia.

NEPHRECTOMY

A lateral decubitus position and elevation of a kidney rest are used in patients requiring this procedure. The great vessels are compressed, blood pools in the lower extremities, and venous return is reduced from the upper portion of the body as a result of this position. Volume loading and careful turning of the patient can minimize potential hypotension. For further discussion, see Chapter 19.

RENAL TRANSPLANT

Nine thousand renal transplants are performed each year. Ten percent of these patients have end-stage renal disease. Major problems encountered in patients with renal failure include hypertension and cardiac failure, anemia, hyperkalemia, coagulopathy, and decreased resistance to infection. If the patient's current medical regime includes the use of corticosteroids, these should be given preoperatively to avoid adrenal insufficiency. Hemodialysis within 24 hours before surgery may optimize outcome.

These patients are at risk for a full stomach. If the potassium level is normal, succinylcholine and cricoid pressure are used to secure the airway. Atacurium or vecuronium, which do not rely on renal excretion, should be used for maintenance. A central venous pressure catheter may be used to guide fluid replacement.

When the vascular clamps are released from the common iliac vessels, blood returning to the systemic circulation will be high in potassium and acid metabolites. Hypotension and cardiac arrest are possible but rare. Renal perfusion is promoted once circulation is restored to the allograft and lower extremities. This may be achieved by the use of temporary dopamine infusions, mannitol, bolus administration of crystalloid, or reduction in the depth of anesthesia to obtain a high-normal blood pressure.

Cyclosporine is given for immunosuppression. However, rejection can still occur. Hyperthermia, disseminated intravascular coagulation, and deterioration of the urine output are delayed signs of rejection.

☐ GYNECOLOGIC PROCEDURES AND ANESTHETIC MANAGEMENT

A woman may undergo gynecologic surgery for diagnostic or therapeutic purposes. She may present with abnormal bleeding, suspected neoplasm, or infertility problems. Repair of weakened anatomic structures may also be performed. The preanesthetic evaluation must consider any disease process the patient may be presenting with as a reason for the surgery, the presence of coexisting disease, history of previous surgery, and possible previous chemotherapy.

An intra-abdominal, transabdominal, transvaginal, or perineal surgical approach may be used for gynecologic surgery. Hysterectomy, oophorectomy, cystectomy, salpingectomy, myomectomy, and debulking procedure are done using an intra-abdominal approach. A Pfannensteil or transverse incision is frequently used to provide access for the surgeon and a cosmetically pleasing result for the patient. If the patient is obese or the surgeon requires a wider exposure, a vertical incision may be used. Because a vertical incision intrudes on the upper abdomen, respiratory compromise may occur postoperatively. Many factors influence the choice of anesthetic, including: the difficulty of the dissection, tumor size if present, degree of exposure, positioning of the patient, duration of the surgery, and blood loss. If wide exposure or steep Trendelenburg position is required, a regional anesthetic is usually insufficient and general anesthesia is used.

A patient with a ruptured ectopic pregnancy is at risk for pulmonary aspiration and is potentially hemodynamically compromised because of massive bleeding into the peritoneal cavity. A safe, rapid sequence anesthetic induction with cricoid pressure and rapid fluid resuscitation are also necessary in these patients.

A transabdominal approach using a laparoscope may be used for myomectomies, removal of ectopic pregnancies, and laparoscopic vaginal hysterectomies. A laparoscopic tubal ligation is a common procedure.

Dilation and curettage, hysteroscopy, cone biopsy, and vaginal hysterectomy are transvaginal procedures. A dilation and curettage is usually a brief procedure. Local anesthesia with sedation is a common technique. General or regional anesthesia may be alternative methods. *Cervical dilation* is the most painful stimulus during a dilation and curettage. A dilation and curettage and hysteroscopy may often be included in the same procedure.

Intrauterine irrigating solutions used during the hysteroscopy can cause hemodilution, volume expansion, pulmonary edema, and possible coagulopathy. An epidural or spinal anesthetic allows the patient to remain awake, which can aid in early detection of signs and symptoms of volume expansion. A woman requiring a vaginal hysterectomy usually has some loss of pelvic support and a pelvic suspension can be done simultaneously. Vasopressin or epinephrine may be injected into the cervix before a cone biopsy to decrease the blood loss from this highly vascularized area.

In the perineal area laser fulgurations of vulvar neoplasms, papillomas, drainage of Bartholin's gland abscesses, vulvar biopsies, and vulvectomies can be done using regional, general, or local anesthesia. Intact viral DNA has been detected in plumes when a carbon dioxide laser is used to treat papillomas and warts. Operating room personnel should be protected from laser plumes by holding the smoke evacuator 2 inches away from the tissue being vaporized. *Herpetic whitlow* is an infection of the digits that may be transmitted to health care personnel as tissue is being vaporized.

ASSISTED REPRODUCTIVE TECHNIQUES

In vitro fertilization refers to oocytes or primitive ova that are fertilized with spermatozoa and incubated in culture media. These procedures are usually done on healthy outpatients. Propofol is an ideal agent associated with little postoperative nausea and vomiting and sedation. However, in a recent study the use of isoflurane and nitrous oxide was associated with a higher percentage of pregnancies with evidence of viable fetal cardiac activity, or evidence of a fetal heart rate over 100 in comparison to the use of propofol and nitrous oxide for anesthesia maintenance (Anesthesiology. 1995; 82(2):352–358). Further investigation continues.

Planning an anesthetic begins with the preoperative evaluation. The anesthetist selects an anesthetic based on several considerations—the presence of coexisting disease, requirements for the proposed operative procedure, age, and preference of the patient. Often more than one technique is possible and the appropriate technique is selected based on the unique needs of the patient.

BIBLIOGRAPHY

Agin C. Anesthesia for transurethral prostate surgery. *Int Anesth Clin.* 1993; 31(1):25–46.

Baker CC, Huynh T. Acute pancreatitis surgical management. *Crit Care Clin.* 1995; 11(2):311–321.

Barash PG, Cullen BF, Stoelting RK. *Clinical Anesthesia.* 2nd ed. Philadelphia: JB Lippincott; 1992.

Cunningham AJ. Laparoscopic surgery—anesthetic implications. *Surg Endos.* 1994; 8(11):1272–1284.

Deutsh, S. Anesthesia for Urologic Surgery. *ASA Refresher Courses in Anesthesiology.* 1992; Volume 20:77–83.

Hastings GE, Weber RJ. Inflammatory bowel disease. Part I: clinical features and diagnosis. *Am Fam Physician.* 1993; 47(3): 598–628.

Lantz PE, Smith JD. Fatal carbon dioxide embolism complicating attempted laparoscopic cholecystectomy—case report and literature review. *J Forensic Sci.* 1994; 39(6):1468–1480.

Pulleritis J, Ein S, Williamson J. Anaesthesia for phaeochromocytoma. *Can J Anaesth.* 1988; 35(5):526–534.

Roy RC, Carter RF, Wright PD. Somatostatin, anaesthesia and the carcinoid syndrome. *Anaesthesia.* 1987; 42(6):627–632.

Sevarino FB. Anesthesia for gynecology. *Postgraduate Assembly in Anesthesiology.* 1993.

Shir Y, Frank SM, Brendler CB, et al. Postoperative morbidity is similar in patients anesthetized with epidural and general anesthesia for radical prostatectomy. *Urology.* 1994; 44(2):232–236.

Shir Y, Raja SN, Frank SM. The effect of epidural versus general anesthesia on postoperative pain and analgesic requirements in patients undergoing radical prostatectomy. *Anesthesiology.* 1994; 80(1):49–56.

Shir Y, Raja SN, Frank SM, et al. Intraoperative blood loss during radical retropublic prostatectomy: epidural versus general anesthesia. *Urology.* 1995; 45(6):993–999.

Stoelting RK. *Pharmacology and Physiology in Anesthetic Practice,* 2nd ed. Philadelphia: JB Lippincott; 1991.

Stoetlting RK, Dierdorf SF, McCammon RL. *Anesthesia and Co-Existing Disease.* 3rd ed. New York: Churchill Livingstone; 1993.

Vincent RD, Syrop CH, Van Voorhis BJ, et al. An evaluation of the effect of anesthetic technique on reproductive success after laparoscopic pronuclear stage transfer. *Anesthesiology.* 1995; 82(2):352–358.

Wahba RW, Beique F, Kleiman SJ. Cardiop;ulmonary function and laparoscopic cholescystectomy. *Can J Anaesth.* 1995; 42(1):51–63.

Wall RT III. Anesthetic challenge in the patient with endocrine disease: pheochromocytoma, insulinoma, carcinoid syndrome. *ASA Refresher Course Lectures #143,* 1993.

Way LN. *Current Surgical Diagnosis and Treatment.* 9th ed. East Norwalk, Conn: Appleton & Lange: 1991.

☐ QUESTIONS

1. CO_2 is the distending gas of choice during creation of a pneumoperitoneum because it can be resorbed more readily than other gases. True or False?
   a. True
   b. False

2. Hypercalcemia is a complication of pancreatitis. True or False?
   a. True
   b. False

3. Which of the following statements is false?
   a. Carcinoid tumors may be scattered throughout the body, but primarily reside in the gastrointestinal tract and bronchi.
   b. Classic signs and symptoms of carcinoid syndrome include light-headedness, dizziness, clouded sensorium, paresis, seizures, possible stroke, and coma; signs and symptoms usually occur 5 hours after food intake.
   c. The overproduction of serotonin is the hallmark of carcinoid syndrome although over 20 mediators have been identified.
   d. Hepatic artery occlusion may be done to devascularize a carcinoid tumor but does not provide long-term control.

4. The patient with carcinoid syndrome may be receiving which of the following medications?
   1. Lasix
   2. Salbutamol
   3. Diazoxide
   4. Loperamide
      Choose one answer:
      a. 3
      b. 1,2,4
      c. 1,4
      d. All of the above

5. What agent or agents antagonize opioid-induced spasm of the sphincter of Oddi?
   1. Naloxone
   2. Glucagon
   3. Nalbuphine
   4. Insulin
      Choose one answer:
      a. 1
      b. 1,2,3
      c. 1,3,4
      d. 4

6. Where are pheochromocytomas located?
   a. Crypts of Langerhans
   b. Neural crest

   c. Chromaffin tissue
   d. Submucosa of the colon

7. Which α_1-blocking agent is preferred in the preoperative treatment of pheochromocytoma?
   a. Prazosin
   b. Labetolol
   c. Phenoxybenzamine
   d. Propanolol

8. An adequate sensory level for a transurethral resection of the prostate must be:
   a. T-4
   b. T-6
   c. T-10
   d. T-12

9. What are the metabolites of the catecholamines?
   1. Metanephrine
   2. Dopamine
   3. Normetanephrine
   4. Vanillymandelic acid
      Choose one answer:
      a. 1,3
      b. 2,4
      c. 1,3,4
      d. 1,2,3

10. When do plasma catecholamine levels return to normal after surgery for pheochromocytoma?
    a. 24 hours
    b. 5–7 days
    c. 7–10 days
    d. 30 days

11. List potential side effects of phenoxybenzamine:
    1. Postural hypotension
    2. Gastrointestinal irritation
    3. Mydriasis
    4. Reflex tachycardia
       Choose one answer:
       a. 1,4
       b. 1,3
       c. 2,3,4
       d. 1,2,4

12. What is the predominant catecholamine secreted in pheochromocytomas?
    a. Epinephrine
    b. Norepinephrine

13. What is the dose of nitroprusside?
    a. 1–2 μg/kg
    b. 2–5 μg/kg

c. 5–10 μg/kg
d. 10–20 μg/kg

14. When would you suspect cyanide toxicity during a Nipride infusion?
1. Patient is unresponsive to Nipride despite increases in dose
2. Decrease in oxygen consumption
3. Metabolic alkalosis
4. Dose greater than 8 μg/kg
Choose one answer:
a. 1,2,3
b. 1,4
c. 2,4
d. 2,3,4

15. What is the treatment for cyanide toxicity?
a. Sodium thiosulfate
b. Sodium nitrate
c. Both sodium thiosulfate and sodium nitrate

16. A patient experiences transient blindness during a transurethral resection of the prostate. What can you attribute this to?
a. Hyponatremia
b. Hyperammonemia
c. Glycine toxicity
d. Hyperoxaluria

17. When irrigating fluids are used, what is the rate of fluid absorption per minute?
a. 10 mL/min
b. 20 mL/min
c. 50 mL/min
d. 150 mL/min

18. Irrigating fluids used during a transurethral resection of the prostate must be:
a. Hypotonic
b. An electrolyte solution
c. Isotonic
d. Distilled water

19. Inflammatory bowel disease may also be associated with peripheral and axial arthritis, iritis, and urolithiasis. True or False?
a. True
b. False

20. A 32-year-old woman presents with lower abdominal pain that was colicky and is now steady. She is pale, cold, and clammy. Her pulse is 120 and her blood pressure is 85/40. Laboratory results reveal a hematocrit of 23 and a moderate leukocytosis. She has missed one menstrual period but now has mild vaginal bleeding. She is complaining of shoulder pain. What is your diagnosis?
a. Fulminant colitis
b. Acute appendicitis
c. Tubal pregnancy

ANSWERS

1. a
2. b
3. b
4. b
5. b
6. c
7. c
8. c
9. c
10. c
11. d
12. b
13. a
14. b
15. c
16. c
17. b
18. c
19. a
20. c

24

Anesthesia for Eye, Head, and Neck Surgery

Colleen T. Ober
Laura Wild McIntosh

The intricate nature of eye, head, and neck pathology and anesthetic interplay requires a well planned and thought out anesthetic management. To balance the surgical, anatomic, and anesthetic concerns, the anesthetist should have a thorough knowledge of the anatomic structures, the effects of anesthetics involved, and related drug interactions. In addition, the degree of possible perioperative compromise should be fully understood.

This chapter reviews the basic anatomy and physiology, the common surgical procedures, and the general anesthetic management and considerations of patients presenting for eye, head, and neck surgery.

☐ ANESTHESIA FOR EYE SURGERY

ANATOMY AND PHYSIOLOGY OF THE EYE

Structures The eyeball normally functions as a closed unit generating and maintaining its own pressures. The anterior transparent surface of the eye is the cornea. The anterior chamber is a space located between the cornea and iris. Its shape is maintained partially by the aqueous humor, which is formed at a rate of 2 to 3 μL each minute.[1] The aqueous humor is formed by the ciliary body and is secreted by the ciliary processes, which lie behind the iris. The canal of Schlemm, actually a circumferential blood vein normally filled with aqueous humor, provides an exit pathway for the aqueous out of the eye into the extraocular veins. Behind the anterior chamber is the iris, a pigmented collection of circular and radially oriented muscle fibers that constrict and relax. The pupil is the opening at the center of the iris. As light enters the pupil it falls on the lens. The lens is a transparent biconvex body between the posterior chamber and the vitreous body that refracts the light to focus the image that falls on the retina. Between the lens and the retina is the vitreous humor, a more gelatinous and less free-flowing substance than the aqueous humor. Behind this is the retina, the posterior inner surface of the eyeball. As light falls on this region, cones and rods are excited and light impulses are translated into neural impulses that are then passed along the optic nerve to be interpreted by the brain. Encircling the posterior surface of the eyeball and contiguous with the corneal surface is the sclera. This is the tough white covering that protects the eye and provides an external sheath for the optic nerve and maintains the shape (Fig. 24–1). The eyeball is encased within a bony framework consisting of the frontal, zygomatic, greater wing of sphenoid, maxilla, palatine, lacrimal, and ethmoid bones of the skull.

Innervation Despite the size, the eyeball is a highly innervated and sensitive organ, receiving both sympathetic and parasympathetic innervation. The sympathetic stimulation causes mydriasis (pupillary dilation); parasympathetic stimulation causes miosis (pupillary constriction). Sympathetic innervation originates with an impulse in the intermediolateral horn cells in the spinal cord, then passes to the superior cervical ganglion, to the postganglionic neurons and finally to the iris. There is weak sympathetic innervation to the ciliary muscle.[1] The parasympathetic innervation of the eyeball is via the oculomotor nerve (cranial nerve III). The oculomotor nerve passes to the ciliary ganglion where the presynaptic nerves synapse with the postsynaptic nerves. From here these fibers travel through the ciliary nerves to the eyeball where the ciliary muscle and the sphincter of the iris become excited.

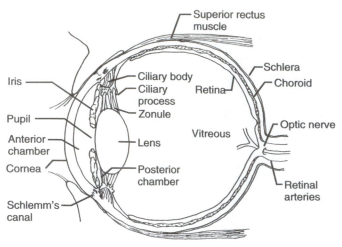

Figure 24-1   Structures of the eye.

Musculature   Movement of the eyeball within the orbit occurs through the concerted work of six extraocular muscles: medial and lateral rectus muscles, superior and inferior rectus muscles and the superior and inferior obliques (Fig. 24-2). These muscles are innervated by cranial nerves III (oculomotor), IV (trochlear), and VI (abducens).

ANESTHETIC MANAGEMENT AND CONSIDERATIONS

Monitoring   Whether under general anesthesia or local sedation with a regional anesthetic, standard monitoring is necessary. Because surgical procedures on the eye have mini-

mal systemic implications, it is unusual to need invasive monitoring. Predictably, the patient is out of view and the airway is unaccessible, which necessitates a stringent plan of care to ensure an uncompromised airway. Oversedation should be avoided because this may compromise airway patency and lead to excessive $Paco_2$. The presence of hypercarbia is thought to augment the incidence and severity of the oculocardiac reflex in either local or general anesthesia. Precordial stethoscope and oxygen saturation (Sao_2) monitoring provide ongoing status of adequate ventilation and oxygenation. End-tidal CO_2 ($ETCO_2$) monitoring in the sedated patient can warn of hypercarbia and in the general anesthetic may help in the differential diagnosis of malignant hyperthermia. During general anesthesia the endotracheal tube should be well secured to avoid accidental extubation, tube kinks, and disconnects. For this purpose, anode or oral Rae® tubes may be used.

Blood pressure is continually monitored. Often ophthalmic patients represent the ASA classification status 2 or 3 because advanced age makes systemic diseases more prevalent. Although chronic hypertension is somewhat tolerated in this population, acute episodes can lead to extrusion of ocular contents in the open eye. Persistent hypotension can lead to retinal hypoperfusion and ischemia.

Standard monitoring of the electrocardiogram (ECG) serves as a critical indicator of dysrhythmias, which may occur during ophthalmic procedures secondary to the delicate interplay of ocular innervation, surgical manipulation, and anesthetic presence. The alert practitioner will recognize and immediately treat any perioperative dysrhythmias.

Retrobulbar and Peribulbar Block

Technique
The retrobulbar block (Fig. 24-3) is performed by injecting 5 to 7 mL of a 50:50 mixture of 2% lidocaine and 0.75% bupivicaine solution containing 1:200,000 epinephrine into the muscle conus behind the globe in the area of the ciliary nerve and ganglion. The needle is positioned inferiorly as local is injected. A separate injection to the facial nerve prevents squeezing motion by providing a motor blockade of the orbicularis oculi muscle.[2]

Complications
Regional blockade of the eyeball can lead to a oculocardiac reflex resulting in hemodynamic instability. For this reason the patient must be fully monitored at this time. A rare but potential complication is a subarachnoid injection in which supportive or resuscitative care is needed.[3] Also rare but possible is the diffusion of local anesthetic into the optic nerve sheath causing brief unconsciousness and apnea for approximately 15 minutes. Although there is a period of unconsciousness, the patient usually remains hemodynamically stable with an adequate pulse rate and blood pressure.[2] *The most common complication of a block is hemorrhage.*[4] A final complication of the retrobulbar and peribulbar block is a rise in the intraocular pressure (IOP). For this reason a regional block is contraindicated in the penetrating and open eye injury.

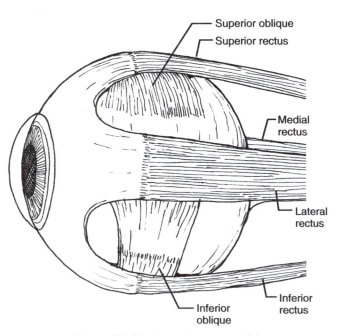

Figure 24-2   Extrinsic muscles of the eye.

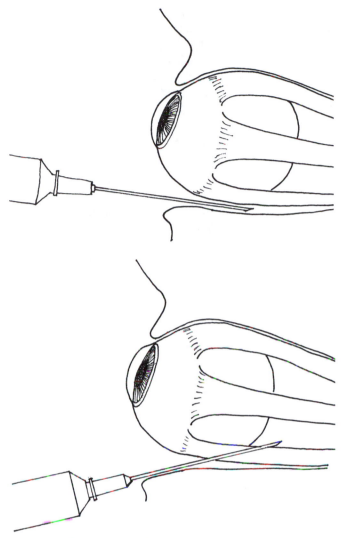

Figure 24–3 Administration of retrobulbar block. Patient looks supranasally as a 23- to 25-gauge needle is advanced 1.5 cm along the inferior aspect of the eye. The needle is then redirected upward approximately 30° and slightly medially until it passes into the muscular cone of the eye.

Sedation

Sedation is usually necessary before performing a local block. Both propofol and thiopental offer rapid onset with a quick wake-up, usually before the surgeon has returned from scrubbing. Timing should allow for prolonged sedation onset and duration in the elderly patient, related to a generalized slowing in circulation time and metabolism. In the awake sedated patient coughing, straining, and patient movement must be prevented intraoperatively. At all times equipment and drugs for general anesthesia should be available in the event an immediate need for a general anesthetic arises.

General Anesthesia When planning for a general anesthetic, avoiding a detrimental increase in IOP should be a major concern. Only agents that do not increase IOP should be used. Once the globe is opened, succinylcholine as either a bolus or infusion should be avoided.[5] Situations that raise the IOP, such as hypercarbia or prolonged hypertension, must

be prevented. Intravenous lidocaine 1 mg/kg will attenuate straining and coughing during intubation and extubation. Postoperative straining due to nausea and vomiting may be diminished by premedication with an antiemetic.

Oculocardiac reflex The oculocardiac reflex is mediated through the *trigeminal afferent* and *vagal efferent* pathways. Stimulation of this reflex can result in sinus bradycardia, junctional rhythm, ectopic atrial rhythm, atrioventricular blockade, wandering pacemaker, idioventricular rhythm, ventricular bigeminy, multifocal premature ventricular contractions, ventricular tachycardia, fibrillation, and asystole. However, bradycardia is most commonly seen. Pressure on the globe and traction on the medial rectus muscle is the most common cause and generally lessens with subsequent stimulation. The best treatment is to alert the surgeon to cease pressure or pulling. If this is unsuccessful atropine 0.007 mg/kg intravenously will work. Alternatively, the surgeon may supplement the block, thereby eliminating the afferent pathway in this reflex.

Intraocular Pressure The average IOP is 15 mm Hg with a range of 12 to 20 mm Hg.[1] It is maintained by a resistance of aqueous humor outflow through the trabeculae network to the canal of Schlemm. A pathologic increase in IOP is greater than 25 mm Hg. Intraoperative management should attempt to avoid increases in IOP at all times. A significant increase in IOP may cause extrusion of ocular contents in the open globe, leading to permanent damage and blindness.

Anesthetic-Induced Alterations in Intraocular Pressure

INDUCTION AGENTS

Thiopental, propofol, and etomidate will lower IOP. Because ketamine is believed to raise IOP and is known to cause blepharospasm, blood pressure elevations, vomiting, and nystagmus, it would seem prudent to avoid it altogether in ophthalmic procedures.

MAINTENANCE AGENTS

Inhaled anesthetics will all lower IOP. However, if any of these agents are used in the spontaneously breathing patient, a dose-dependent hypoventilation and hypercarbia may be seen, which would then lead to an increased IOP. Likewise, hyperventilation will decrease IOP.

MUSCLE RELAXANTS

All nondepolarizing muscle relaxants will predictably lower IOP. For this reason nondepolarizers offer an attractive intubating option. Unfortunately these agents have a longer onset and duration, making them a less than ideal rapid sequence induction choice. In addition, because onset predictability and twitch correlation are less likely than with succinylcholine, bucking and coughing during laryngoscopy and intubation may occur. The use of lidocaine 1 mg/kg before both intubation and extubation will reliably attenuate a rise in IOP. Succinylcholine will raise the IOP by 5 to 10 mm Hg for 5 to 10 minutes.[6] For this reason succinylcholine has always had a questionable, albeit controversial role in ophthalmic care. However, to place this increase into perspective, it is necessary to know that a normal blink will raise IOP by 10 to 15 mm Hg and forceful eyelid closure by more than 70 mm Hg.[7]

Glaucoma   Glaucoma is caused by the outflow obstruction of aqueous humor. It is characterized by an increase in IOP that jeopardizes blood flow to the optic nerve leading to neuronal insufficiency and subsequent blindness. Glaucoma remains a major cause of blindness in the United States. Eyedrops used to treat glaucoma do so by altering IOP, either by decreasing secretion or increasing outflow of aqueous humor.

Nitrous Oxide Use   Because nitrous oxide will diffuse into any space or potential space, it should not be used for 5 days after injection of an air bubble and 10 days after sulfur hexafluoride injection. This information may need to be elicited either from the previous operative report or from a consult with the surgeon.[6] Nitrous oxide should be discontinued 15 minutes before injection of gas bubble during surgical procedures on the retina.

Related Drug Interactions

Echothiopate
Echothiopate is the only organophosphorus anticholinesterase agent with any clinical use. This long-acting miotic causes a fall in IOP, primarily by lowering the resistance to the outflow of aqueous humor.[8] Because it is an irreversible agent, plasma cholinesterase activity will be depressed for 4 to 6 weeks after discontinuation. A prolonged action with succinylcholine can be anticipated and the use of a twitch monitor should be standard. In addition, a delay in metabolism of ester local anesthetics should be expected.[4]

β Blockers   β Blockers are used in the ophthalmic patient to reduce the production of aqueous humor. Certain systemic side effects are caused by this class of drugs. Timolol is a nonselective β-adrenergic antagonist. Side effects include bradycardia, congestive heart failure (CHF) in susceptible patients, and bronchospasm in the presence of obstructive airway diseases. Betaxolol is β_1 specific and is less likely to cause bronchospasm. However, it is contraindicated in patients with a history of CHF, sinus bradycardia, and certain heart blocks.

Pilocarpine Hydrochloride   Pilocarpine is a parasympathomimetic agent. When given, this miotic drug reduces IOP in the presence of glaucoma. Side effects from this drug are minimal.

Phenylephrine   Phenylephrine eyedrops are used as mydriatics (pupillary dilation) and may cause hypertension. A 2.5% solution is less likely to cause hypertension than a 10% solution.[2]

Acetazolamide   Acetazolamide (Diamox) is a carbonic anhydrase inhibitor that reduces the secretion of aqueous hu-

mor. It can be given orally or intravenously. Chronic use can lead to metabolic acidosis from renal excretion of bicarbonate ions and potassium. Hypokalemia and hyponatremia may also occur. It should be avoided in patients with sulfonamide allergies. Serious side effects related to Stevens-Johnson syndrome, fulminant hepatic necrosis, agranulocytosis, and aplastic anemia have been reported.[9]

SURGICAL PROCEDURES

Open Globe Injuries and Foreign Body Removal   This scenario provides a conflict of interest for the anesthetic care plan. First it is necessary to determine the last oral intake. More than likely these patients will be considered to have full stomachs. Although a retrobulbar block with an open globe or penetrating eye injury, and full stomach is ideal, it is nevertheless contraindicated because it will increase the IOP. Therefore one must balance aspiration precautions against further damage to the eye that may be caused by succinylcholine administration and intubation. Although some advocate a rapid sequence intubation with the use of a nondepolarizing muscle relaxant,[5] a rapid sequence intubation with succinylcholine has proven to be just as safe, and safer when the airway is questionable.[7] Also crucial to a successful repair is a quiet field, necessary to prevent extrusion of ocular contents, which could lead to permanent blindness. Movement, straining, and coughing must be avoided to prevent further injury.

Scleral Buckling   This procedure is one treatment for a detached retina. A band is surgically placed circumferentially around the posterior surface of the sclera to repair a tear in the retina. If not corrected, the vitreous protrudes through the tear resulting in a loss of vision. The anesthetic management will require a reduction in the IOP. General anesthesia may be indicated for a lengthy procedure. Nitrous oxide must be discontinued before air or sulfur hexafluoride is injected.

Cataract Extraction   Cataracts are formed by denaturization of the lens proteins, which then coagulate and form an opacity that impairs vision. Treatment is the surgical removal of the entire lens and usually an implantation of an artificial lens for return of visual acuity. Often a cataract extraction is performed in an ambulatory surgical setting under retro- or peribulbar block with sedation and standard monitoring. However, this requires an alert, cooperative patient. General anesthesia is indicated if the patient is unable to tolerate an awake procedure, for example, senility, coughing, inability to lie flat, or claustrophobia. The typical patient presenting for cataract extraction is elderly with multiple health problems; diabetes, coronary artery disease, CHF, chronic obstructive pulmonary disease (COPD), and hypertension. Intravenous fluids should be carefully monitored. Common medications seen with this population are digoxin, furosemide (Lasix), and antihypertensive agents. Cardiovascular side effects of these drugs may be compounded by ophthalmic medications such as β blockers.

☐ ANESTHESIA FOR EAR SURGERY

ANATOMY AND PHYSIOLOGY

Structures The ear receives sound and transmits it to the central nervous system (CNS) to be deciphered and interpreted.[1] The tympanic membrane, or the eardrum, separates the outer ear from the middle ear. Within the inner ear is the cochlea, the major sensory organ for hearing. In addition to hearing, the vestibular apparatus within the inner ear is the organ of equilibrium.

Innervation The acoustic nerve (cranial nerve III) is responsible for hearing and balance. Disorders associated with this nerve include endolymphatic hydrops (Ménière's disease) and vestibular neuronitis. Vestibular neuronitis is a benign irritation of the eighth cranial nerve and manifests as vertigo, vomiting, and gait disturbances without hearing loss.[10] When these presenting symptoms are seen in addition to hearing loss, Ménière's disease should be suspected. Treatment is surgical resection of the vestibular nerve, if bed rest and benzodiazepines are ineffective.[10] Another benign growth on the eighth cranial nerve is an acoustic neuroma. Successful tumor excision is curative.

ANESTHETIC MANAGEMENT AND CONSIDERATIONS

Monitoring Any surgical procedure on the ear will mean that the patient is out of view and the airway will become inaccessible once surgery begins. Extra precautions should be taken to secure the airway. Endotracheal tubes should be well fitted to avoid accidental extubation, tube kinks, and disconnects. Anode or oral Rae® tubes may be used for this purpose.

Nitrous Oxide Because nitrous oxide is 34 times more soluble than nitrogen,[11] it is capable of diffusing into and expanding the middle ear, causing pressure elevations and possible tympanic membrane rupture. This may manifest as bright red blood in the ear channel. Normally, passive opening of the eustachian tube in a ball-valve fashion will relieve pressure of the middle ear in excess of 200 to 350 mm H_2O into the nasopharynx. In the presence of narrowed eustachian tubes secondary to inflammation, infection, or scar tissue after an adenoidectomy, the inability to relieve the middle ear pressure passively under general anesthesia can lead to rupture.[12]

Facial Nerve Function Ear surgery will often require monitoring of cranial nerve VII (the facial nerve) function during dissection around this area. Intubation should be performed with a short-acting agent such as succinylcholine or mivacurium (Mivacron). Anesthetic depth can be maintained with inhalational agents.

Nausea Any inner ear manipulation can cause postoperative nausea, vomiting, and vertigo. To attenuate this problem droperidol may be administered perioperatively.

SURGICAL PROCEDURES

Bilateral Myringotomy and Tubes Most often, this procedure is done on the infant or toddler. (See Chap. 25 for pediatric anesthetic management.) Because of the brevity involved in draining the ears and inserting tubes, a mask anesthetic is all that is needed. Positioning of the child requires the anesthetist to be both in control of the airway at all times and free of the surgical approach. Depending on the child's history and the length of surgery, intravenous access may be necessary. This is one case where inserting an intravenous line may very well double the time spent in the operating room. Postoperative pain requirements are minimal if at all.

Mastoidectomy/Tympanoplasty This procedure will require general anesthesia for a quiet field. Muscle relaxants should be avoided to monitor facial nerve function.[13] If used, a peripheral nerve stimulator should ensure neuromuscular function of 10% to 20%.[11] Intraoperative nitrous oxide should be avoided altogether or limited to 50% until 5 minutes before tympanic membrane graft placement at which point it should be discontinued. This should be discussed with the surgeon. Administration of antiemetics is essential.

Parotidectomy For lesions of the parotid gland, the main trunk of the seventh cranial nerve is identified, exposed, and dissected along the external surface of the nerve.[14] For this reason muscle relaxation should not be used. As stated earlier, a secured airway must be established because of intraoperative inaccessibiltiy. Depending on the pathology, this procedure may progress to a radical neck dissection. (Refer to section on radical neck dissection in this chapter.)

Acoustic Neuroma These benign neurofibromas of the eighth cranial nerve arise within the internal auditory meatus of the ear. Extensive nerve resection is required and electromyographic (EMG) monitoring is used to preserve facial nerve function. Anesthetic agents do not appreciably alter EMG monitoring except that neuromuscular blocking agents should be avoided.[15]

☐ ANESTHESIA FOR OROPHARYNGEAL AND NECK SURGERY

ANATOMY AND PHYSIOLOGY OF THE NOSE, OROPHARYNX, UPPER AIRWAY, AND NECK

Structures/Innervation The nose and oropharynx are part of the conduction system of breathing. Clear opening of these passages allows for air to enter the body and gas exchange to occur. Any anomalies can greatly impede gas flow and ultimately compromise respiration. Distinct functions of the nose include warming, humidifying, and filtering air.

The nasal cavity consists of the paranasal sinuses; the maxillary, ethmoid, frontoethmoid and sphenoid sinuses are air-filled cavities with mucosal lining. Other structures include the nasal septum, the choanae, or turbinates, and the pharyngeal wall. The blood supply to the nose is via the *internal mammary* branch of the external carotid.

The pharynx runs midline from behind the nasal passages to the larynx. The carotid sheath and its structures (internal jugular, common and internal carotids, and vagus nerve) are located in the neck lateral to the pharynx.[16] The pharynx is divided into three parts: the nasopharynx, oropharynx, and the laryngeal pharynx. Also located in the pharynx near the base of the tongue are the palatine tonsils and other lymphoid structures. The nasopharynx communicates with the pharynx by way of the choanae. The most prominent structure in the oropharynx is the tongue. The tongue is the most frequent cause of upper airway obstruction because both the genioglossis and styloglossis muscles are relaxed under anesthesia. The sensory innervation to the base of the tongue and the pharynx is supplied by the *glossopharyngeal nerve.*

The larynx is a box-shaped structure located from C-4 to C-6. The larynx connects to the trachea and is the entrance into the respiratory tract. The larynx consists of nine cartilages, three paired cartilages and three single cartilages. The single cartilages include the thyroid, cricoid, and epiglottis. The cricoid cartilage is the only one that is a complete ring. Therefore, when pressure is applied, the back of the cricoid cartilage occludes the esophagus and prevents gastric contents from passing into the oropharynx. The cricoid cartilage is the narrowest part of the airway in a child. The epiglottis is a leaf-shaped cartilage that inserts between the two plates of the thyroid. The three paired cartilages are the arytenoid, corniculate, and cuneiform.

The true vocal cords are white ligamentous structures attached to the thyroid cartilage anteriorly and to the artenoid cartilage posteriorly. The space between the vocal cords is the glottic opening. The glottis is the narrowest part of the airway in adults.

There are three types of laryngeal muscles: the *abductors,* which externally rotate and open the cords; the *adductors,* which close the glottis; and a third set that tense and relax the vocal cords. The *cricothyroids* are responsible for vocal cord tension and the motor innervation for these muscles is provided by the *superior laryngeal nerve.* The *thyroarytenoid* muscles relax the vocal cords.

Innervation of the larynx is provided by branches of the glossopharyngeal and the vagus nerve. Sensory innervation to the epiglottis and mucous membranes of the larynx are provided by the *superior laryngeal nerve* branch of the vagus. Sensory innervation to the vocal cords and the upper trachea is provided by the *recurrent laryngeal nerve* branch of the vagus.[17] It is imperative to fully understand the sensory and motor innervation to the upper airway before performing regional anesthetic blocks.

The anesthetist must also be familiar with the structures of the neck and their close proximity to the operative area. The facial, trigeminal, glossopharyngeal, and recurrent laryngeal nerves can be easily damaged during head and neck surgery. In addition, blood supply from the internal carotid, common carotid, and internal and external jugular may be impaired by accidental ligation with potential for severe hemorrhage from accidental transection of these vessels.

ANESTHETIC MANAGEMENT AND CONCERNS

Monitoring Adequate monitoring for all head and neck procedures is crucial whether performed under local anesthetic blocks or general anesthesia. Routine monitoring equipment should include an ECG, pulse oximetry, $ETCO_2$, noninvasive blood pressure cuff, temperature probe, and possibly an arterial line. An ECG is necessary to detect potential dysrhythmias from either local anesthetic toxicity or from manipulation of the vagus nerve during radical neck dissection. Dysrhythmias may indicate inadequate anesthesia and inadequate ventilation. Pulse oximetry is necessary to ensure adequate ventilation before and after induction. Many clients with head and neck masses may have existing alterations in oxygenation related to airway obstruction. Intraoperatively, lack of access to the airway requires not only pulse oximetry but $ETCO_2$ monitoring capabilities. It is also helpful to monitor peak airway pressures in the ventilated patient. Endotracheal tubes are easily kinked and displaced from manipulation of the head and neck. Studies have indicated that the endotracheal tube moves inward approximately 5 mm with *neck flexion* and outward 6 mm with *neck extension.*[18] Movement of the endotracheal tube can lead to potential endobronchial intubation (notice an increase in peak airway pressure) or accidental extubation.

Use of an arterial line is helpful when there is a requirement for frequent arterial blood gas sampling such as during prolonged rigid bronchoscopy where use of alternate modes of ventilation does not allow for $ETCO_2$ monitoring, or if the patient's preoperative cardiopulmonary status necessitates careful blood pressure monitoring or postoperative ventilation.

Because there is usually no significant blood loss or major fluid shift, central venous monitoring is not necessary for routine head and neck cases. Central pressure monitoring may be considered in patients with severe cardiac disease. However, line placement may be difficult because of previous head and neck radiation or surgery, and the monitoring line may interfere with surgical access.

A peripheral nerve stimulator is necessary when using muscle relaxants.

Key Points for Anesthetic Management Versatile airway management skills and ventilation techniques are required for providing anesthesia for head and neck surgery. Deep planes of anesthesia are needed to blunt cardiovascular and airway flexes, yet brief procedures often require rapid emergence.

The anesthetist must be prepared with nasal and oropharyngeal airways; a variety of endotracheal tubes in different sizes should be available, including anode, armor, cuffed and uncuffed, and laser-proof. A fiberoptic bronchoscope, a jet ventilator, and a proficient head and neck surgeon should be ready in case an emergency surgical airway is required.

A large-bore intravenous line should be inserted for potential fluid resuscitation because of the proximity of major vascular structures. Prolonged procedures, tonsillectomies, and some nasal operations may be associated with more significant blood loss. Vigilant monitoring of intake and output (if urinary drainage catheter is in place) is important. Note blood on lap pads, pharyngeal packs, and in suction canisters. Occult blood can be swallowed or hidden in the drapes.

The choice of anesthetic technique is determined by type of procedure, patient and surgeon preference, and underlying airway pathology. If a general anesthetic is chosen, discuss with the surgeon preference for oral versus nasal intubation and the most desirable endotracheal tube. Once this decision is made assess the patient to determine the most efficacious means for tracheal intubation. Can a standard intravenous induction proceed safely or does the patient require an awake fiberoptic intubation? Extra precautions must be taken to ensure a secure airway intraoperatively.

Physical Assessment Physical assessment should include detecting the presence of possible airway obstruction. Airway compromise can be demonstrated by wheezing, increased work of breathing, and stridor. Inspiratory stridor during quiet breathing suggests airway stenosis, with an airway diameter of less than 4 cm.[19] Before sedating any patient with potential airway compromise it is advisable to be familiar with indirect laryngoscope reports, as well as a posteroanterior and lateral neck x-ray, chest x-ray, and computed tomography (CT) scan reports. Pulmonary function tests may be required for patients with significant COPD or upper airway obstruction from tumor impingement. The flow–volume loop is most significant for diagnosing upper airway obstruction. Alterations in the flow–volume loop curve will vary depending on whether the lesion is fixed or variable, and if variable, whether lesions are intrathoracic or extrathoracic.[20]

Patients with advanced age, coexisting cardiac disease, prior chemotherapy, or symptoms of cor pulmonale should have a preoperative echocardiogram.

Regional Anesthesia for Head and Neck Surgery
Topical Instillation
Cocaine, lidocaine and benzocaine spray are frequently used topical anesthetics for head and neck surgery. Cocaine is a local ester anesthetic that is readily absorbed from mucosal membranes. *Cocaine* blocks the reuptake of norepinephrine and epinephrine at adrenergic nerve endings thereby producing vasoconstriction, which decreases blood loss, making it a desirable topical anesthetic in nasal and oropharyngeal surgery. Cocaine is for topical use only. The absorption of cocaine is enhanced by inflammation of the vascular nasal mucosa and should be instilled over 10 to 15 minutes to avoid systemic toxicity. Cocaine toxicity will occur when topical doses exceed *3 mg/kg*.[21]

The versatility of lidocaine makes it the most popular local anesthetic in use today. Lidocaine is used plain or with epinephrine for local nerve blocks to facilitate head and neck surgery. The *maximum* injected dose of lidocaine plain is 4 mg/kg, and up to 7 mg/kg with epinephrine. Lidocaine-soaked pledgets can be inserted into each pyriform sinus, producing anesthesia of the internal laryngeal nerve.[22] Lidocaine can be sprayed directly onto the tongue, both valleculae, the epiglottis, and vocal cords to provide adequate oropharyngeal anesthesia for endoscopic procedures. Lidocaine may also be instilled to the suction port to anesthetize the recurrent laryngeal nerve or given intravenously (dose of 1.5 mg/kg) to suppress the cough[23] reflex during flexible bronchoscopy.

Hurricaine® and Cetacaine® sprays are commonly used for topical anesthesia of the oropharynx and upper airway. Both these solutions contain benzocaine, which, like prilocaine, can produce *methemoglobinemia*. Doses of benzocaine of 15 to 25 mg/kg can cause detectable levels of methemoglobin.[24]

Methemoglobinemia will give the patient a cyanotic appearance and decrease the oxygen-carrying capacity in the blood with diminished pulse oximetry values. Treatment of methemoglobinemia is with methylene blue 1 to 2 mg/kg of body weight.

Superior Laryngeal Nerve Block
A superior laryngeal block is performed to provide sensory anesthesia to the mucosa of the base of the tongue, larynx, laryngeal surface of the epiglottis, and part of the posterior larynx (Fig. 24–4).

With the patient lying supine, head extended, the hyoid and superior portion of the thyroid cartilage are identified. A 23-gauge needle is introduced laterally and directed at the greater cornu of the hyoid, while slight retraction of the skin and carotid sheath is held posteriorly. After contact with the bone is made, the needle is carefully walked off caudad until it slips off the hyoid and through the thyrohyoid membrane (a "pop" will be felt).[25] Once in the membrane, carefully aspirate for blood or air and then inject 2.5 mL of 1% lidocaine solution. This should be repeated on the opposite side. The thyrohyoid membrane may be entered by identifying the superior cornu of the thyroid cartilage and walking the needle superiorly off the thyroid cartilage until the membrane is felt.

Complications include systemic local anesthesia toxicity and possible aspiration from loss of upper airway reflexes.

Transcricoid Puncture
A direct transcricoid puncture provides anesthesia to the upper and lower airways. The cricothyroid membrane is identified and a small skin wheal of local anesthetic is injected. With a 5-mL syringe, a 25-gauge needle is inserted through the cricothyroid membrane. Aspiration of air confirms adequate positioning in the trachea; then 2 to 4 mL of 2% lidocaine is injected as the patient inspires. Patient coughing will usually confirm a successful block and will spread the local anesthetic along the airway. Contraindications include an en-

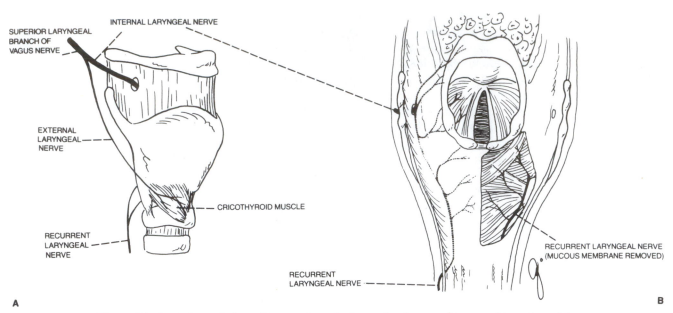

Figure 24–4   *A.* Lateral view of larynx show the internal and external laryngeal branches of the superior laryngeal branch of the vagus nerve. *B.* The distribution of the terminal branches of the internal and recurrent laryngeal nerves. The larynx is viewed from above and posteriorly.

larged thyroid, tracheal mass, deviated trachea, and coagulopathies. Complications are local anesthesia toxicity, hematoma at injection site, local infection, broken needles, and subcutaneous emphysema.[26]

Local Anesthetic Complications

Because systemic toxicity from local anesthetics is possible after both regional blockade and topical application, standard monitoring in addition to intravenous access should be established before the induction of regional blockade. Oxygen and emergency airway equipment should be available. Local anesthetics readily cross the blood–brain barrier and the first signs of toxicity will be CNS alterations such as tinnitus, dizziness, perioral numbness, restlessness, slurred speech, and muscle twitching. Tonic-clonic seizures may rapidly ensue following the start of muscle twitching.[27] Treatment of local anesthetic toxicity is with oxygen and hyperventilation. Diazepam and thiopental should be readily available to suppress anesthetic-induced seizures.

Adjunct Drugs for Head and Neck Surgery

Anticholinergics

Premedication with anticholinergics helps to diminish vagal tone, decrease secretions, and increase bronchodilation. Glycopyrrolate, a quarternary ammonium compound, does not cross the blood–brain barrier and may be a better choice in outpatient surgery because of lack of sedative effects. Antisialagogue effects are equal with atropine and glycopyrrolate.[28]

Corticosteroids

Glucocorticoids such as prednisolone and dexamethasone (0.1 to 0.2 mg/kg intravenously) may be given perioperatively to reduce anticipated laryngeal edema especially after laser operations in the upper airway.

Postoperative Complications   Common postoperative complications seen with head and neck surgery include airway edema, bleeding, upper airway obstruction, postobstruction pulmonary edema, and an increased incidence of laryngeal spasm. Upper airway obstruction may be caused by retained pharyngeal packs, soft tissue obstruction, tumor, debris from laser surgery, incomplete muscle relaxant reversal, or recurrent laryngeal nerve damage. If upper airway obstruction is from the tongue or relaxed soft tissue, a nasal airway may be inserted in the semiconscious patient.

Initial treatment of laryngeal spasm is with forward jaw thrust and application of positive airway pressure via mask with 100% oxygen. If laryngeal spasm continues, succinylcholine 0.15 to 0.3 mg/kg intravenously should be given.

☐ NASAL, SINUS, AND COSMETIC SURGERIES

SURGICAL PROCEDURES

Common nasal procedures include closed reductions of fractures, nasal polypectomy, submucosal resection, rhinoplasty, and Caldwell-Luc and nasal endoscopic sinus surgery. These are commonly done on an outpatient basis and may be done under local anesthesia with sedation.

Nasal and Sinus Surgery   Nasal procedures such as rhinoplasty, polypectomies, and closed reductions can be performed under local anesthesia. Anesthetic considerations should include potential local anesthetic toxicity, airway obstruction, sharing the field with the surgeon, and potential bleeding. If general anesthesia is used, a topical vasoconstrictor such as epinephrine is also used to decrease bleeding.

These patients should be extubated awake after thorough oropharyngeal suctioning.

Sinus surgery is most frequently performed to drain sinuses, excise inflamed and excess tissue, and diagnose tumors or other intranasal obstruction. Most operations are performed on the maxillary and ethmoid sinuses. The maxillary sinus is the most common site of infection and inflammation.[29] Surgery of the frontoethmoid or sphenoid sinuses are associated with an increase in potential intracranial complications. General anesthesia is usually required for radical antrostomy or Caldwell-Luc operations. These operations may be performed for chronic maxillary sinusitis, diagnosis of suspected tumors, or treatment of an oral antral fistula.

Anesthetic considerations for sinus surgery include adequate assessment of preoperative airway obstruction because chronic congestion may obliterate nasal passage openings. Blood loss from the highly vascular nasal mucosa should be anticipated. A vasoconstrictor such as epinephrine is frequently used under general anesthesia. Cocaine for anesthesia and vasoconstriction may also be used. It should be noted that injecting epinephrine in addition to cocaine does not further increase vasoconstriction. General anesthesia is associated with increased blood loss over regional anesthesia even when epinephrine is injected. This may be related to the vasodilatory properties of the inhalation agents. Studies have indicated that general anesthesia with propofol maintenance may be associated with less blood loss than with an inhalation maintenance.[30] A cuffed endotracheal tube and posterior pharyngeal packing should be used to avoid aspiration of blood. Keep a count of the throat packs and document on your record. Antiemetics should be given perioperatively.

Endoscopic sinus surgery is performed with the assistance of a rigid magnifying scope with a fiberoptic light source. Local anesthesia with sedation is the anesthetic of choice. The same considerations for other sinus surgeries apply. Postoperative intercerebral hematoma from accidental introduction of the endoscope into the cribriform plate is possible.

Table 24–1 lists other complications of sinus surgery.

☐ TONSILLECTOMY AND ADENOIDECTOMY

The patient presenting for tonsillectomy and adenoidectomy will very likely have increased airway obstruction and poten-

Table 24–1
COMPLICATIONS OF SINUS SURGERY

- Bleeding—keep head of bed elevated 15°
- Postoperative nausea and vomiting
- Air embolism
- Cerebral hematoma
- Cerebral spinal fluid leaks
- Infection
- Local anesthetic toxicity

Table 24–2
INDICATIONS FOR TONSILLECTOMY

- Recurrent tonsillitis (4–7 acute episodes in one season to 5 episodes per year for 2 years)
- Peritonsillar abscess
- Acute airway obstruction
- Recurrent tonsillitis associated with cardiac valvular disease or otitis media
- Obstruction that produces cor pulmonale
- Sleep apnea
- Hearing loss
- Dysphagia, difficulty eating

tial systemic involvement from recurrent illness or from congenital anomalies.

ANATOMY

Adenoids are a large mass of lymphoid tissue located on the posterior wall of the nasopharynx. Hyperplasia of adenoid tissue results in otitis media. The tonsils are paired masses of lymphoid tissue located on the lateral walls of the oropharynx. Surgery is required when tonsilar hyperplasia produces obstruction or if there is chronic recurrent tonsillitis (Table 24–2).

SURGERY

Surgery involves entering the oropharynx and curetting the enlarged tonsillar and adenoid tissue. The surgeon will control bleeding with cautery or with the use of potassium titanyl phosphorus (KTP) laser. Usual blood loss is 4 mL/kg, although much of it may go unnoticed as it passes into the patient's stomach. The average mortality from tonsillectomy is 0.003% with hemorrhage and airway obstruction being the leading causes of morbidity and mortality.[31]

Preoperative Evaluation Preoperatively the patient should be evaluated for degree of airway obstruction, history of sleep apnea, and CHF. Most children will not present for tonsillectomy until tonsillar hyperplasia results in airway obstruction of 50% to 75%.[32] Children with craniofacial anomalies such as those with trisomy 21, acromegaly, micrognathia, and retrognathia will demonstrate airway obstruction with a lesser degree of tonsillary hyperplasia. Carefully assess the airway and potential for difficult intubation. A history of sleep apnea suggests airway obstruction as well as potential pulmonary hypertension. *Pulmonary hypertension* is present in 3% of children presenting for surgery and these patients may exhibit signs and symptoms of CHF. A thorough physical examination for presence of rales, pedal edema, jugular vein distention, and hepatomegaly should be performed.

Preoperative Testing
Routine preoperative testing should include a complete blood count and urinalysis. More extensive testing such as elec-

trolytes, bleeding time and prothrombin time/partial thromboplastin time (PT/PTT) may be necessary in the patient with a history of sleep apnea or potential bleeding dyscrasias.

Contraindications

Surgery should not proceed if there is evidence of infection, increased bleeding time, bleeding diathesis, or anemia. If the patient has an elevated PT/PTT and surgery cannot be delayed, blood should be available and platelets should be transfused in the preoperative period.

Anesthetic Considerations   Reliable intravenous access is necessary for potential large hidden blood loss. Routine monitoring is required for all patients. The ECG should be monitored for alterations in heart rate. Light anesthesia, hypoxia, hyperthermia, and hypovolemia may all produce dysrhythmias. A precordial stethoscope is necessary to listen to breath sounds during and after induction. The endotracheal tube must be well secured to prevent accidental disconnects or extubation.

Premedication

The routine use of premedication in anesthesia has been questioned. However, in the pediatric population, premedication will help the patient separate from parents and alleviate anxiety. Oral midazolam 50 to 75 µg/kg in children is an excellent anxiolytic and it may have some postoperative antiemetic effect.[33] The use of a narcotic may also provide sedation as well as postoperative analgesia. *Do not premedicate with a history of sleep apnea.*

Induction

In adults or older children an intravenous induction with propofol or thiopental and muscle relaxant may be desirable. Intravenous inductions are associated with a rapid loss of consciousness and of the airway; therefore, in patients with airway obstruction, a cautious inhalation induction maintaining spontaneous respirations is the best choice to avoid the potential of total airway occlusion. Use of an endotracheal tube (flexibend or Rae®) is necessary to ensure adequate ventilation and to prevent aspiration of excised tissue and blood. Uncuffed tubes should fit snuggly with an air leak at 25 cm. Pharyngeal packs may be used by the surgeon to prevent blood in the stomach. Laryngeal mask airways have been used for tonsillectomy without evidence of aspiration of blood.[34]

Maintenance

Maintenance of anesthesia can be with inhalation or intravenous agents. Nitrous oxide-narcotic techniques have been associated with an increase in postoperative nausea and vomiting and may delay emergence. New inhalation agents with low blood solubility such as desflurane and sevoflurane provide for rapid induction and emergence. Sevoflurane is especially advantageous for inhalation inductions with less incidence of laryngeal spasm.[35] However, sevoflurane is associated with the production of inorganic fluoride and the production of compound A, which theoretically may preclude nephrotoxicity.[36] Desflurane is not associated with organ toxicity, but cannot be used as an induction agent because of the high incidence of laryngeal spasm.[37]

Emergence

It is important that protective reflexes are intact before extubation to avoid airway obstruction and aspiration. The stomach should be emptied and the oropharynx thoroughly suctioned before the patient is awakened. Deep extubation may avoid coughing and straining on the endotracheal tube, which may precipitate bleeding. Extubation in the "tonsil position" (lateral, slight Trendelenberg, and head down) allows for pooled secretions to drain away from the trachea.

Postoperative Considerations   In the postoperative period small doses of narcotic or acetominophen can be used for analgesia. The use of ketorolac has been associated with increased blood loss in tonsillectomy patients.[38]

The most common complications include laryngeal spasm, airway obstruction from edema, retained tissue or retained pharyngeal packs, nausea and vomiting, and bleeding. The most insidious complication after tonsillectomy is bleeding. Most significant bleeding occurs in the first 9 hours after surgery and up to 10 days postoperatively (late bleeding is often associated with infection). Increased swallowing, tachycardia, and orthostatic blood pressure changes noted in the postanesthesia care unit may be indicative of bleeding. If bleeding is suspected the initial course of action is hydration with balanced salt solutions. Initially, packing the area may stop the bleeding. If reoperation is needed, blood should be available. Continue to hydrate, and place pressure on the ipsilateral carotid artery to slow bleeding. *Rapid sequence induction* or awake fiberoptic intubation is performed after adequately emptying of the stomach with a nasogastric tube.

RETROPHARYNGEAL MASS/LUDWIG'S ANGINA

Retropharyngeal and peritonsillar abscesses are common in childhood. Peritonsillar abscess can cause severe pain, trismus, and respiratory obstruction. Peritonsillar abscess is usually a complication following streptococcal tonsillitis. Treatment of choice for both retropharyngeal and peritonsillar abscess is systemic antibiotics (penicillin) and surgical incision and drainage if necessary. Anesthetic management includes cautious assessment of potential airway obstruction and avoidance of accidental rupture of mass when intubating the patient.

Ludwig's angina is a rapidly progressing cellulitis of the submandibular and sublingual spaces including the anterior neck and the floor of the mouth. Streptococcus is the causative pathogen. On physical assessment these patients will demonstrate fever, elevation of the tongue with protrusion, shortness of breath, possible stridor, and an inability to swallow. Airway compromise from rapidly progressing edema heralds eminent danger. Emergent control of the airway followed by surgical incision and drainage is necessary. Airway control with tracheostomy under local anesthesia is considered safest. However, some suggest that tracheostomy may not be absolutely indicated and that awake fiberoptic bronchoscopy can provide a secure airway.[39] Extubation or decannulation is safe only when edema has resolved.

DENTAL EXTRACTIONS

Dental extractions are not usually performed on healthy patients in the operating room. Therefore, the anesthetist can assume that this patient has some systemic or congenital disease (such as cerebral palsy or trisomy 21). Induction of general anesthesia with either intravenous drugs or volatile agents is possible. A nasal endotracheal tube is preferably on the opposite side of where the surgeon will be working. Nasal vasoconstriction and adequate lubrication may decrease nasopharyngeal trauma. Patients with trisomy 21 may have difficult mask airways from small oropharynx, enlarged tonsils, and large tongues. In addition, coexisting cardiac disease is present in 40% of these patients.[40] Patients with cerebral palsy have an increased incidence of gastric reflux.[41]

☐ ANESTHESIA FOR LASER SURGERY

Lasers are frequently used in head and neck surgery in conjunction with microlaryngoscopy or during fiberoptic or rigid bronchoscopy to debulk tumors. The carbon dioxide laser is most commonly used in head and neck surgery. Benefits include surgical precision and less thermal damage to surrounding tissues. The neodymium: yttrium-aluminum-garnet (Nd:YAG) laser has deepest penetration and is used for debulking of tumors. (For further discussion on laser considerations, see Chap. 1.)

☐ MICROLARYNGOSCOPY

Microlaryngoscopy is performed for diagnosis and excision of upper airway lesions or polyps, or for voice augmentation procedures. Some of these cases may entail the use of a laser.

PREOPERATIVE ASSESSMENT

Preoperative laboratory tests should be performed based on extent of planned operation and present medical history of each patient. Preoperatively the patient should be examined for any signs of airway obstruction. Knowledge of the location and size of the mass is important. Ask the surgeon about the findings on indirect laryngoscopy, chest x-ray, and CT scan. Depending on the pathology, local or general anesthesia can be used. If general anesthesia is required appropriate tube size and placement should be discussed with the surgeon. In addition, the anesthetist must be familiar with alternate modes of ventilation and the surgical time frame.

ANESTHETIC MANAGEMENT

Microlaryngoscopy is a brief, highly stimulating surgery. Local anesthesia using regional and topical anesthesia (see beginning of chapter for description of techniques) is usually reserved for small biopsies, polyps, and voice augmentation procedures. Voice augmentation procedures are usually performed in patients with preexisting vocal cord damage. The surgeon will use a Teflon injection or small stents to alter vocal cord function. The key is light sedation. Small doses of narcotic and midazolam will suffice. If the patient is unable to phonate on the surgeon's request, the success of the surgery may be compromised.

Goals of general anesthesia include safe airway management, control of sympathetic nervous system response to laryngoscopy, immobility of vocal cords, and protection from aspiration. It is likely these patients have upper airway tumors or enlarged polyps that may produce a ball-valve effect and make mask ventilation and intubation difficult. In the absence of airway obstruction, general anesthesia can be safely induced with intravenous agents. Proceed with intubation cautiously to avoid accidental removal of the tumor. Most frequently the anesthetist will intubate the trachea with a small flexible endotracheal tube with an internal diameter of 5.0 to 6.0 mm. The tube should be placed and secured on the left side of the patient's mouth. Check peak airway pressures and ensure adequate ventilation before turning the table for surgical exposure.

Five percent of microlaryngoscopy procedures involve the posterior commisure or lower third of the vocal cords. The placement of an endotracheal tube (even a small one) can create technical difficulty for the surgeon and alternate modes of ventilation with a hand-held jet ventilator or high-frequency positive-pressure ventilation may be required. Subglottic jet ventilation using a small 3.0-mm tube below the glottis has also been described.[42]

Maintenance of anesthesia with short-acting inhalation and intravenous agents is preferred. Vocal cord paralysis is required for optimal surgical exposure. This can be achieved with the use of succinylcholine drip or by using a short-acting nondepolarizing muscle relaxant. Plan for immediate reversal and monitor twitch status accordingly. Narcotics are helpful to blunt sympathetic nervous system response; however, these patients should be wide awake at the end of the operation. The use of esmolol or labetalol to blunt cardiac reflexes, especially in patients with a history of cardiovascular disease, may be prudent. If jet or high-frequency ventilation is used, total intravenous anesthesia is desirable to prevent environmental contamination.

Emergence from anesthesia should include adequate oropharyngeal suctioning, humidified oxygen, and observation in the postanesthesia care unit for signs of postextubation croup or laryngeal spasm. Racemic epinephrine or steroids may be added to decrease airway edema.

☐ FIBEROPTIC BRONCHOSCOPY

Fiberoptic bronchoscopy is useful for diagnostic purposes of airway biopsies and cultures and for performing therapeutic measures such as bronchopulmonary lavage for recurrent pneumonia or small foreign body removal. The flexibility of the bronchoscope allows for greater patient comfort, less damage to dentition, less need for neck extension, and better visualization of right upper bronchus.

ANESTHETIC MANAGEMENT

Fiberoptic bronchoscopy can be comfortably performed under local anesthesia with superior laryngeal nerve and transcricoid anesthesia. In addition, local anesthetic instilled through the suction port of the bronchoscope will anesthetize the carina. Sedation with propofol is an excellent choice with either a continuous drip or intermittant boluses. Propofol provides equivalent sedation when compared to midazolam with faster awakening,[43] which is important with these brief procedures. Small doses of narcotic (alfentanil or fentanyl) will be helpful to blunt cough reflex. Fiberoptic bronchoscopy diminishes PaO_2 by 20 mm Hg, which may last for up to 4 hours.[44] Therefore, oxygen should be administered via nasal cannula throughout the perioperative period.

General Anesthesia   Premedication with atropine or glycopyrrolate is beneficial before bronchoscopy. Intravenous induction is acceptable in the absence of airway obstruction. The trachea is intubated with a large endotracheal tube (usually 8.0 for women and 9.0 for men) for passing of the fiberoptic scope. The choice of muscle relaxation will depend on the duration of the procedure. Frequently, diagnostic bronchoscopy under general anesthesia is followed by mediastinoscopy, thorascopy, or thoracotomy and the use of a longer-acting muscle relaxant would be acceptable. During bronchoscopy, the anesthetist will have one hand ventilating the patient and the other hand on the endotracheal tube to prevent movement. Fiberoptic bronchoscopy increases peak airway pressures when the scope is advanced through the endotracheal tube. The decreased cross-sectional area across the tube leads to a positive end-expiratory pressure effect, which may cause barotrauma.

COMPLICATIONS

Complications during fiberoptic bronchoscopy include hypercarbia, hypoxemia, barotrauma, cardiac dysrhythmias, mediastinal emphysema, and pneumothorax. Postoperative chest x-ray should be attained after bronchoscopy to rule out complications.

☐ RIGID BRONCHOSCOPY

Rigid bronchoscopy is performed for excision of tracheal masses, debulking of airway tumors, removal of large and distal foreign bodies, placement of tracheal stents, and control of pulmonary hemorrhage.

ANESTHETIC MANAGEMENT

General anesthesia is the best choice for patients presenting for rigid bronchoscopy. Premedication with an antisialagogue will decrease secretions, allowing for better visualization of airway structures. Preoperative sedation should be used judiciously with consideration of patient's existing cardiopulmonary status and the presence of airway obstruction from tumors or other foreign bodies. Good positioning is vital to assist the surgeon with visualization. The patient will be supine with the head extended at the very top of the operating room table. The use of a roll under the patient's shoulders will aid in extension. Immediately after induction the patient will be turned toward the surgeon. The anesthetist must work closely with the surgeon to ensure adequate ventilation of the patient during the operation.

Inhalation induction should be performed for foreign body aspiration or when there is evidence of airway obstruction from tracheal or mediastinal masses. In the absence of airway obstruction an intravenous induction is acceptable. Again, choice of maintenance anesthetic agent and muscle relaxant will depend on the length of procedure and mode of ventilation. After induction ensure adequate airway before turning the patient over to the surgeon.

MODES OF VENTILATION

Ventilation during rigid bronchoscopy can be a challenge. A rigid bronchoscope with a side arm attachment allows for positive-pressure ventilation and administration of volatile agents. The pharynx should be packed to prevent air and inhalation agent from contaminating the environment. Unfortunately, during prolonged operations the use of intermittant ventilation leads to unacceptable increase in $PaCO_2$ and hypoxia.

Jet Ventilation   The use of jet ventilation with rigid bronchoscopy was initially presented by Sanders in 1966.[45] The jet ventilator delivers pulses of oxygen at a pressure of 50 psi. This high positive pressure at the proximal end of the bronchoscope produces negative pressure at the other end and entrains room air (Venturi effect). The tidal volume and peak airway pressure delivered to the patient is the sum of the delivered pressure to the jet ventilator, the diameter and size of the bronchoscope, and the lung compliance of the patient.[46] The advantage is that you can adequately ventilate the patient without the need of an endotracheal tube. Patients with poor compliance, bulbous emphysema, or obesity are not good candidates for jet ventilation.

Complications of jet ventilation include pneumothorax, mediastinal air, tension pneumothorax, subcutaneous emphysema, hypoxemia, hypercarbia, awareness, and gastric distention.

High-Frequency Positive-Pressure Ventilation   High-frequency positive-pressure ventilation uses a ventilator that provides lung insufflation with a tidal volume of 100 to 150 mL at a frequency of 60 times per minute. Advantages include no room air entrainment and the ability to set the forced inspired oxygen (FIO_2) according to the patient's needs.[47]

FOREIGN BODY ASPIRATION

Aspiration of foreign objects occurs most frequently in the pediatric population and it is one of the leading causes of fatal injuries in children under age 4. The most frequent site of foreign body aspiration is the right bronchus. Wheezing is the presenting sign in 65% to 75% of patients with foreign body aspiration. Other signs and symptoms include choking, coughing, tachycardia, aphonia, and cyanosis. Visualization of foreign objects with chest x-ray may not be possible; however, hyperinflation of the obstructed lung and distal atelectasis to the foreign body may be noted on radiographic examination.

Anesthetic Management The anesthetic management will depend on the location of the airway obstruction. If the obstruction is located at the level of the larynx, a simple laryngoscopy with Macgill forceps should allow for easy removal of the offending object. If the foreign body is located in the distal larynx or the trachea, the patient should be taken to the operating room immediately and an inhalation induction performed, maintaining spontaneous respiration. *Do not assist respiration* because this may move the object and further compromise ventilation.

The surgeon will remove foreign bodies usually with a rigid bronchoscope; fiberoptic bronchoscopes are useful for small foreign objects in proximal airways. Supportive measures include the use of humidified oxygen, racemic epinephrine, bronchodilators, and steroids.

COMPLICATIONS OF RIGID BRONCHOSCOPY

Damage to dentition, gums and upper lips can be avoided by the use of a mouth guard. Other complications are tracheal tears from the introduction of the bronchoscope and vagal stimulation from the extreme head extension. Complications related to ventilation include hypoxemia, hypercarbia, barotrauma, mediastinal emphysema, and dysrhythmias. Table 24–3 compares fiberoptic and rigid bronchoscopy.

☐ RADICAL NECK DISSECTION

Much of the anesthetic management guidelines on this topic have been covered at the beginning of this chapter and in Chapter 32 under cancer surgery. Special considerations for a radical neck dissection concern vagal stimulation from the surgeon working in proximity to the carotid sinus. The development of prolonged QT intervals seen especially during right radical neck dissection may occur from manipulation of the *right stellate ganglion*. The alteration in rhythm with this prolonged QT interval can quickly progress to ventricular tachycardia.[48] Small doses of local anesthetic injected near the carotid sinus may block vagal reflexes.

Venous air embolism can occur during radical neck dissection from open neck veins during surgery and head-up position. Careful monitoring of end-tidal nitrogen and carbon dioxide is necessary. Treat air embolism immediately (see Chap. 31 for anesthetic complications and management).

Table 24–3
A COMPARISON OF FIBEROPTIC AND RIGID BRONCHOSCOPY

Fiberoptic Bronchoscopy	Rigid Bronchoscopy
Increased patient comfort	Better control of hemorrhage
Easily performed under regional anesthesia	Best performed under general anesthesia
Less damage to teeth	Greater damage to teeth and gums
Greater visualization of upper lobe	Better visualization down to the carina
Removal of small foreign objects	Used to remove large foreign objects
No hyperextension of neck necessary	Greater incidence of vagal responses from severe head neck extension requied for procedure
Repositioning of endotracheal and required endobronchial tubes	Alternate modes of ventilation Including jet ventilation, periods of apnea and HFPPV
Good for bronchopulmonary lavage	Good for vascular tumors
Diagnosis of lung masses	Endobronchial resections

COMPLICATIONS

Hypoxia, PEEP effect, cardiac dysrhymias mediastinal emphysema, pneumothorax	Hemorrhage, bronchospasm, tracheal or bronchial perforation, subglottic edema, barotrauma, hypercarbia, hypoxia, cardiac dysrhythmias

HFPPV, high-frequency positive-pressure ventilation; PEEP, positive end-expiratory ventilation

☐ TRACHEOSTOMY

Tracheostomy is usually performed in debilitated patients who have been intubated for a prolonged period of time or for patients undergoing extensive head and neck procedures. Ideally the patient will already be intubated. Tracheostomy as a primary surgical airway for the trauma patient or acute arrest patient is usually performed under local anesthesia. Often transport of the patient from the intensive care unit to the operating room with all vasoactive medication and intravenous lines intact will be the greatest challenge. For a general anesthetic, induction is with intravenous agents such as thiopental or etomidate, (depending on patient status,) narcotics, and a neuromuscular blocking agent. The patient should be maintained on 100% oxygen with an inhalation agent before the tracheostomy tube is in place. Once the surgeon has established exposure, the anesthetist will be asked to slowly remove the endotracheal tube, without completely removing it until the tracheostomy cannula is in place and adequate chest expansion and $ETCO_2$ waveform is confirmed.

Complications of tracheostomy include tube displacement, pneumothorax, and hemorrhage. A chest x-ray should confirm placement after surgery.

REFERENCES

1. Guyton AC, Hall JE. *Textbook of Medical Physiology,* 9th ed. Philadelphia: WB Saunders, 1996:623–635.
2. Acquadro M. Anesthesia in head, and neck surgery. In: Davison JK, Eckhardt WF III, Perese DA, eds. *Clinical Anesthesia Procedures of the Massachusetts General Hospital.* Boston: Little, Brown; 1993:390–412.
3. Tatum PA, Defalque RJ. Subarachnoid injection during retrobulbar block: a case report. *American Association of Nurse Anesthetists Journal.* 1994; 49–52.
4. McGoldrick KE. Anesthesia and the eye. In: Barash PG, Cullen BF, Stoelting RK, eds. *Clinical Anesthesia.* 2nd ed. Philadelphia; JB Lippincott; 1994:1095–1113.
5. Smith RB. Open globe. In: Bready LL, Smith RB, eds. *Decision Making in Anesthesiology.* 2nd ed. St. Louis: CV Mosby; 1992:320–321.
6. Morgan GE, Mikhail MS. *Clinical Anesthesiology.* East Norwalk, Conn: Appleton & Lange; 1992:583–591.
7. McGoldrick KE. The open globe: is an alternative to succinylcholine necessary? *J Clin Anesth.* 1993; 5:1–4.
8. Taylor P. Anticholinesterase agents. In: Gilman AG, Rall TW, Nies AS, Taylor P, eds. *The Pharmacological Basis of Therapeutics.* 8th ed. New York: Pergamon Press; 1990:131–149.
9. Olin BR, ed. *Drug Facts and Comparisons.* Loose leaf drug information service. St. Louis: A Wolters Kluwer Company; 1996:139a, 285e.
10. Stoelting RK, Dierdorf SF, McCammon RL, eds. *Anesthesia and Co-existing disease.* 2nd ed. New York: Churchill Livingstone; 1988:263–354.
11. Stoelting RK, Miller RD. *Basics of Anesthesia,* 2nd ed. New York: Churchill Livingstone; 1989:357–368.
12. Ohryn M. Tympanic membrane rupture following general anesthesia with nitrous oxide: a case report. *American Association of Nurse Anesthetists Journal.* 1995; 63:42–44.
13. Dutton RP, Goldstein AD. *The Anesthesiologist's Guide to the OR: Prepped.* Boston: Little, Brown; 1995:81.
14. Schwartz SI, Shires TG, Spencer FC, Husser WC, eds. *Principles of Surgery.* 5th ed. New York: McGraw-Hill; 1991:222–239
15. Black S, Cucchiara RF. Neurological monitoring. In: Miller RD, ed. *Anesthesia.* 3rd ed. New York: Churchill Livingstone; 1990:1185–1207.
16. Feinstein R, Owens WD. Anesthesia for ENT. In: Barash P, Cullen F, Stoelting R, eds. *Clinical Anesthesia.* Philadelphia: JB Lippincott: 1989.
17. Stoelting RK. Lungs. In: *Pharmacology and Physiology in Anesthetic Practice.* 2nd ed. Philadelphia, PA.: JB Lippincott; 1991:720.
18. Yap SJ, Morris RW, Pybus DA. Alterations in endotracheal tube position during general anesthesia. *Anaesth Intensive Care* 1994; 22:586–588.
19. Reed AP, Kaplan JA. Upper airway diagnostic procedures—laryngoscopy, bronchoscopy. In: *Clinical Cases in Anesthesia.* New York: Churchill Livingstone; 1989:41–48.
20. Beyer-Young P, Wilson RS. Anesthetic management for tracheal resection and reconstruction. *J Cardiothorac Vasc Anesthesia.* 1988; 2:821–835.
21. McGoldrick KE. Otorhinolaryngolic surgery. In: *Ambulatory Anesthesia.* Baltimore: Williams & Wilkins; 1994:420.
22. Curling PE. Anesthesia for thoracic diagnostic procedures. In: Kaplan JA, ed. *Thoracic Anesthesia.* New York: Churchill Livingstone;1983:322.
23. Poulton TJ, James FM. Cough suppression by lidocaine. *Anesthesiology.* 1979; 50:470–472.
24. Ellis FD, Seiler JG, Palmore MM. Methemoglobinemia: a complication after fiberoptic orotracheal intubation with benzocaine spray. *J Bone Joint Surg.* 1995; 77 (6):937–939.
25. Gotta AW, Sullivan CA. Anaesthesia of the upper airway using topical anaesthetic and superior laryngeal nerve block. *Br J Anaesth.* 1981; 53:1055–1057.
26. Curling, p 323.
27. Stoelting, R. Local anesthetics. In: *Pharmacology and Physiology in Anesthetic Practice.* 2nd ed. Philadelphia: JB Lippincott; 1991:159.
28. Gronnebech H, Johansson G, Sedebol M, Valentin N. Glycopyrrolate vs. atropine during anaesthesia for laryngoscopy and bronchoscopy. *Acta Anaesthesiol Scand.* 1993; 37:454–457.
29. McGoldrick KE. Otorhinolaryngolic surgery. In: *Ambulatory Anesthesiology.* Baltimore; Williams & Wilkins; 1994:485.
30. Blackwell K, Ross DA, Kapur P, Calcaterra TC. Propofol for endoscopic sinus surgery. *Am J Otolaryngol.* 1993; 14(4): 262–266.
31. Reed A, Kaplan J. Tonsillectomy. In *Clinical Cases in Anesthesia.* New York: Churchill Livingstone:1989:33–40.
32. Montgomery JN, Watson CB, Mackie AM. Anesthesia for tonsillectomy and adenoidectomy. *Otolaryngological Clinics of North America.* May 1987; 20(2):335
33. Splinter WM, et al. Midazolam reduces vomiting after tonsillectomy in children. *Can J Anaesth.* 1993; 40:1171–1177.
34. Webster AC, Morley-Forster PK, Dain S, Ganapthy S, Ruby R, Cook, MJ. Anaesthesia for adenotonsillectomy: a comparison between tracheal intubation and the armoured laryngeal mask airway. *Can J Anaesth.* 1993; 40:1171–1177.
35. Lerman J. Sevoflurane in pediatric anesthesia. *Anesth Anal.* 1995; 81:S4–10.
36. Malan TP. Sevoflurane and renal function. *Anesth Analg.* 1995; 81:S39–45.
37. Suprane (desflurane): prescribing information. Anaquest Inc., Liberty Corner, NJ.
38. Rusy LM, Houch CS, Sullivan LJ, et al. A double-blind evaluation of ketorolac tromethamine versus acetaminophen in pediatric tonsillectomy: analgesia and bleeding. *Anesth Analg.* 1995; 80:226–229.
39. Hart BT. Tracheotomy for Ludwig's angina. *Oral Surg Oral Med Oral Pathol.* 1994; 78:414–415. Letter.
40. Stoelting RK, Dierdorf SF., & McCammon RL. Pediatric patients. In *Anesthesia and Co-existing Disease* 2nd ed. New York: Churchill-Livingstone; 1988:842.
41. Ibid., p 837.
42. Hudsaker DH. Anesthesia for microlaryngeal surgery: the case for subglottic jet ventilation. *Laryngoscope.* 1994; 104:1–30.
43. Clarkson K, Power CK, O'Connell F, Pathmakanthan S, Burke CK. A comparative evaluation of propofol and midazolam as sedative agents in fiberoptic bronchoscopy. *Chest.* 1993; 104:1029–1031.
44. Curling, p 325.
45. Sanders RD. Two ventilating attachments for bronchoscopes. *Del Med J.* 1967; 39:170–175, 192..
46. Sosis MB. Venturi jet ventilation of the lungs. *Problems in Anesthesia.* 1993; 7:239–246.
47. Borg U, Eriksson I, Sjostrand U. High-frequency positive-pressure ventilation (HFPPV): a review based upon its use during bronchoscopy and laryngoscopy and microlaryngeal surgery under general anesthesia. *Anesth Analg.* 1980; 59:594–601.
48. Otteni JC, Pottecher T, Bonner G, Flesch H, Diebolt JR. Prolongation of the Q-T interval and sudden cardiac arrest following right radical neck dissection. *Anesthesiology.* 1983; 59: 358–361.

☐ QUESTIONS

1. Which of the following may cause a decrease in intraocular pressure?
   a. Ketamine, N_2O
   b. Curare, fentanyl
   c. Hypoventilation, retrobulbar injection
   d. Halothane, hyperventilation

2. The oculocardiac reflex may cause all of the following *except:*
   a. Cardiac arrest
   b. Increased intensity with subsequent stimulation
   c. Ventricular fibrillation
   d. Nodal rhythm

3. A 26-year-old woman is scheduled for parotidectomy. The best anesthetic management for this patient includes:
   a. GETA with 0.4% Forane, O_2 35%/N_2O 65%, vecuronium
   b. Facial nerve block with IV sedation
   c. GETA with propofol infusion, O_2 100%, vecuronium
   d. GETA with propofol infusion, O_2 30%, N_2O 70%

4. The surgeon is about to instill the sulfur hexafluoride bubble prior to the completion of a scleral buckling. Appropriate actions include:
   a. Deepening the anesthetic
   b. Turning off of the N_2O for the remainder of the case
   c. Administer atropine 0.2 mg IV
   d. Check the patient's airway pressures

5. The cranial nerve(s) responsible for movement of the eyeball is (are)
   a. CN III (oculomotor nerve)
   b. CN IV (trochlear nerve)
   c. CN VI (abducens nerve)
   d. All of the above

6. The efferent limb of the oculocardiac reflex is which nerve?
   a. Facial
   b. Trigeminal
   c. Vagus
   d. Optic

7. A 75-year-old woman presents for an emergency retinal reattachment. Medications include omeprazole, Vasotec, and timolol and echothiophate. Rapid sequence induction and intubation proceed uneventfully. Fifteen minutes later you notice that twitches have not yet returned. The most likely cause is:
   a. Decreased circulation time related to advanced age

   b. Homozygous atypical plasma cholinesterase
   c. Side effect of echothiophate therapy
   d. Side effect of timolol therapy

8. An 8-year-old child is scheduled for a tympanoplasty. The child has had multiple, yet uneventful anesthetics for chronic ear infections. True statements include all *except:*
   a. Because N_2O is 34 times more soluble than nitrogen, it should be avoided to prevent rapid absorption into the middle ear.
   b. Droperidol after induction may decrease postoperative nausea and vomiting induced by middle ear manipulation.
   c. Halothane is the volatile agent of choice when the surgeon informs you epinephrine will be used to produce vasoconstriction.
   d. Use of muscle relaxants may be contraindicated.

9. The primary cranial nerve responsible for equilibrium is:
   a. CN IV (trochlear nerve)
   b. CN V (trigeminal nerve)
   c. CN VII (facial nerve)
   d. CN VIII (acoustic nerve)

10. During a 7-hour abdominoplasty on a 42-year-old woman, you suddenly notice bright red blood present in the patient's external auditory canal. Anesthesia is being maintained with 0.8% Forane, 40% O_2, and 60% N_2O. A likely cause for the blood is:
    a. Intracerebral hemorrhage
    b. Tympanic membrane rupture
    c. Early stage disseminated intravascular coagulation
    d. None of the above

11. A 32-year-old woman presents for nasal endoscopy for recurrent sinusitis. Preoperative vital signs are blood pressure 110/70, heart rate 84, respiratory rate 20, SaO_2 99% on room air. Four percent cocaine pledgets (1.5 mL total volume) are inserted into the pyriform sinus. Midazolam 2 mg with 200 μg alfentanil is given intravenously for sedation. On introduction of the endoscope, the patient's vital signs are 160/100, heart rate 130, SaO_2 98% and the patient is agitated. The most likely cause of the changes in vital signs is
    a. Local anesthetic toxicity
    b. Hypoxemia
    c. Insufficient regional anesthesia and intravenous sedation
    d. Penetration of the endoscope into the cribiform palate

12. The internal laryngeal nerve can be blocked by:
   a. Superior laryngeal nerve block with injection of 2 mL lidocaine
   b. Transcricoid puncture with injection of 4 mL 4% lidocaine
   c. Insertion of lidocaine soaked pledgets into the pryiform sinus
   d. a and c

13. The muscles responsible for opening the vocal cords are:
   a. The abductors, which externally rotate and open the vocal cords
   b. The adductors, which internally rotate and open the vocal cords
   c. The cricothyroid, which tenses and opens the vocal cords
   d. The epiglottis, which relaxes to open the vocal cords

14. Indications for tonsillectomy include all of the following *except:*
   a. Recurrent tonsillitis with five episodes in two consecutive years
   b. Tonsil obstruction that causes sleep apnea
   c. Otitis media
   d. Tonsil obstruction that leads to dysphagia and difficulty eating

15. Michael is a 3-year-old 16-kg boy who is in the postoperative care unit 3 hours after a tonsillectomy/adenoidectomy with bilateral myringotomy and tubes. He is restless and vital signs are: pressure 80/40, heart rate 135, respiratory rate 28, SaO$_2$ 97% on room air. His hemoglobin is 9.7 mg/dL. He has been vomiting bloody emesis for the last 20 minutes. Reexploration of the operative site is planned. Anesthetic intervention for this patient would include:
   a. Hydrate with balanced salt solutions, order a type and crossmatch and proceed with an inhalational induction.
   b. Hydrate with balanced salt solutions, send type and crossmatch, hold pressure on the contralateral carotid, and proceed with an intravenous induction.
   c. Send type and crossmatch stat, place pharyngeal packing, and hold reexploration for 2 hours while the patient is observed.
   d. Hydrate with balanced salt solutions. Send type and crossmatch, hold pressure on the ipsilateral carotid and perform a rapid sequence induction.

16. Anesthetic management for a patient with Ludwig's angina would include:
   a. Immediate tracheostomy under local anesthesia
   b. Rapid sequence intravenous induction with cricoid pressure
   c. Start a nitroglycerine drip prior to intravenous induction with high-dose narcotics and etomidate
   d. Inhalation induction, direct laryngoscopy, and maintenance with a volatile agent and spontaneous ventilation.

17. Complications of jet ventilation include all of the following *except:*
   a. Barotrauma
   b. Hemorrhage
   c. Subcutaneous emphysema
   d. Hypoxia

18. When comparing flexible bronchoscopy to rigid bronchoscopy, the advantage of rigid bronchoscopy is
   a. Convenient and well accepted by patients when using regional anesthesia
   b. Better control of pulmonary hemorrhage
   c. Better visualization of the upper lobe bronchus
   d. Easier ventilation, with either mechanical ventilation or spontaneous ventilation

19. A 4-year-old, 18-kg patient presents to the emergency department with shortness of breath, wheezing, and tachycardia. She has a history of environmental allergies. Her mother states, "She was just fine playing with her marbles while I was driving." Treatment should include:
   a. Start humidified oxygen, β agonist via hand-held nebulizer, and begin an aminophylline infusion.
   b. Start humidified oxygen, racemic epinephrine, throat cultures, go to the operating room stat, and proceed with an inhalational induction.
   c. Start humidified oxygen. Send patient directly to the operation room and proceed with an inhalational induction maintaining spontaneous respirations. Rigid bronchoscopy performed by surgeon.
   d. Start humidified oxygen. Send patient directly to the operation room. Proceed with a rapid sequence induction and flexible bronchoscopy.

20. During a right radical neck dissection the patient's heart rate drops to 40 immediately followed by ventricular tachycardia. Vital signs are blood pressure 58/35, heart rate over 180, SaO$_2$ 96% on 100% FIO$_2$, end-tidal CO$_2$ is 26. The precipitating cause of this event is:
   a. Vagal stimulation from working near the carotid baroreceptors
   b. Pulmonary air embolism
   c. Sympathetic stimulation from light anesthesia
   d. Stimulation of the right stellate ganglia, which produces a prolonged QT syndrome that progresses to ventricular tachycardia

☐ ANSWERS

1. d	**5.** d	**9.** d	**13.** a	**17.** b
2. b	**6.** c	**10.** b	**14.** c	**18.** b
3. d	**7.** c	**11.** c	**15.** d	**19.** c
4. b	**8.** c	**12.** d	**16.** a	**20.** d

CHAPTER
25

Pediatric Anesthesia

Linda Downs

The purpose of this chapter is to provide a basic review of the principles and practice required to deliver anesthesia care to the pediatric patient. The significant differences between the infant, pediatric, and adult patient must be considered when making decisions about delivering anesthesia care.

☐ ANATOMY AND PHYSIOLOGY

AIRWAY

The pediatric airway can be more difficult to manage than the adult because of anatomic differences; however, this difficulty can be overcome with relative experience. Neonates have small nares, a large tongue, small mandibles, small oral cavities, and an airway that easily obstructs.[1] Obstruction occurs due to a short neck and the chin meeting the chest at the level of the second rib[2] (Figure 25–1).

ANATOMIC DIFFERENCES (Table 25–1)

The epiglottis of the infant is stiff, longer, narrower, and U shaped.[3]

The laryngeal reflex is strong. Apnea, bradycardia, and laryngospasm are common. Laryngospasms can be triggered by water, foreign bodies, noxious gases, and airway manipulation.[2]

Infants are obligatory nasal breathers until the age of 3 months.[4]

BODY SURFACE AREA

Body surface area (BSA) closely parallels variation in basal metabolic rate. Newborns have large BSA compared to

their weight. A normal newborn is 3 kg, which is one ninth the adult size in BSA, is about one third the length of an adult and is about one twentieth the adult size in weight. Large BSA/weight ratio accounts for differences in fluids, calories, heat, and drug requirements.[2]

METABOLIC RATE

The metabolic rate is greatly increased in infants.

Caloric needs:
Term infant	30 kcal/m^2/h
2 years	50 kcal/m^2/h
Adult	35–40 kcal/m^2/h

Because the infant has a large BSA/weight ratio, the caloric requirements are extremely high.[2]

RELATIVE SIZE AND PROPORTION

Significant differences that affect anesthetic management exist between the child and adult. The neck is extremely weak and cannot support the weight of the head. The chest is relatively small in relation to the protuberant abdomen and the abdominal muscles are weak. The arms and legs are poorly developed, which leads to difficulty in positioning.[2]

CENTRAL AND AUTONOMIC NERVOUS SYSTEM

The brain of a neonate weighs one tenth of the body weight as compared to one fiftieth in the adult. The brain grows rapidly, doubling by 6 months and tripling by 1 year. At birth one fourth of neuronal cells are present and cells in the cortex and brain stem are completely developed by 1

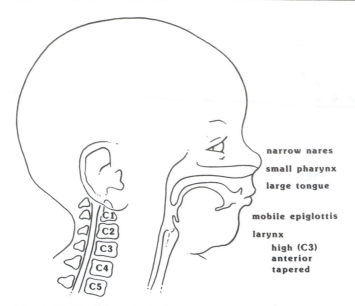

narrow nares

small pharynx

large tongue

mobile epiglottis

larynx

high (C3)
anterior
tapered

Figure 25–1 Schematic depiction of the anatomic characteristics of the neonate, which may influence the ease of intubation of the trachea during direct laryngoscopy. (Reproduced by permission from Stoelting and Dierdorf.[6])

year. Myelinization is complete by 3 years. The spinal cord at birth extends to L-3 and by 1 year it reaches its permanent position of L-1.[2]

The autonomic nervous system is relatively developed at birth. The parasympathetic system is fully functional at birth. However, the sympathetic system is not fully developed until 4 to 6 months of age.[2] This accounts for the parasympathetic system predominance at birth. Bradycardia is easily induced by vagal stimulation or hypoxia. Procedures that may induce bradycardia are laryngoscopy, intubation, crying with Valsalva, and placement of esophageal stethoscope or rectal temperature probe.[2]

RESPIRATORY SYSTEM

At term the lungs are still maturing. Adult-type alveoli are just forming. Alevolar ventilation is doubled in neonates to meet the increased demand for oxygen. This increase in alveolar ventilation is achieved by an increase in respiratory rate.[5]

Table 25–1
ANATOMIC DIFFERENCES BETWEEN CHILDREN AND ADULTS

Structure	Infants	3-year-old	Puberty/Adult
Epiglottis	midline C-1	C-3	C-4
Glottis	midline C-3	C-4–5	C-5
Cricoid	superior C-4	mid C-5	C-6
Vocal cords	angled	angled	perpendicular
Narrowest point	cricoid	cricoid	larynx

Table 25–2
MEAN PULMONARY FUNCTION VALUES

	Neonate (3 kg)	Adult (70 kg)
Oxygen consumption (ml·kg^{-1}·min^{-1})	6.4	3.5
Alveolar ventilation (ml·kg^{-1}·min^{-1})	130	60
Carbon dioxide production (ml·kg^{-1}·min^{-1})	6	3
Tidal volume (ml·kg^{-1})	6	6
Breathing frequency (min)	35	15
Vital capacity (ml·kg^{-1})	35	70
Functional residual capacity (ml·kg^{-1})	30	35
Tracheal length (cm)	5.5	12
PaO$_2$ (F$_I$O$_2$ 0.21, mmHg)	65–85	85–95
PaCO$_2$ (mmHg)	30–36	36–44
pH	7.34–7.40	7.36–7.44

SOURCE: Reproduced by permission from Stoelting and Dierdorf.[6]

Differences in respiratory parameters in the infant include (Table 25–2):

1. Lower functional residual capacity, which limits oxygen reserve
2. Lower closing volumes
3. Lower lung compliance, secondary to small alveoli
4. Greater chest wall compliance due to the cartilaginous chest wall, rather than the fixed rib cage of the adult
5. Oxygen requirements of 6 mL/kg as compared to 3 mL/kg for the adult
6. Carbon dioxide production doubled[4]

Tidal volume and dead space per kilogram remain constant. Peak inspiratory pressures, 15 to 20 cm H$_2$O, required for adequate ventilation are also the same for both child and adult.[4] Hypoxia and hypercarbia in the infant will depress respirations rather than stimulate them as in the adult. This is related to immaturity of the central nervous system control of ventilation.[6] Immaturity of the muscles of respiration cause fatigue, which leads to airway obstruction and hypoxia.[7]

CARDIOVASCULAR SYSTEM

During the first minute of life the infant must change from fetal circulation to adult circulation. The foramen ovale closes secondary to increased systemic vascular resistance (SVR) and a decrease in pulmonary vascular resistance (PVR). Anatomic closure is within 4 to 10 days; however, there is probe patency of this structure in 50% of 5-year-old children and 25% of all adults.[6,8] The ductus venosus closes by constriction due to increased oxygen levels. The ductus arteriosus may remain open for 10 to 15 hours with permanent closure in 2 to 3 weeks.[6] Closure occurs in the presence of increased levels of oxygen, decreased prostaglandin levels, and normal acid–base balance. The pulmonary vascular bed is reactive to hypoxia, acidosis, and hypothermia, which leads to an increase in PVR and a condition known as persistent fetal circulation.[7]

Cardiac output is 30% to 60% increased in neonates to meet the increased oxygen demand. The average cardiac output is 200 mL/kg/min, which decreases with age to 100 mL/kg/min by adolescence. Cardiac index of 2.5 to 4.2 L/min/m^2 varies little with age. Stroke volume in the newborn is 4 mL/beat.[8] Cardiac output determinants are contractility, heat rate, preload and afterload. The major determinant of cardiac output in the pediatric patient, up to age 2 years, is heart rate. Changes in preload have little effect on cardiac output due to fewer sarcomeres and less contractile mass in the infants' ventricles.[8] Therefore, the pediatric ventricle is relatively stiff and cardiac output is greatly dependent on heart rate. Infants have decreased catecholamine stores and blunted response to exogenous catecholamines.[4] Normal sinus rhythm predominates; however, sinus dysrhythmias occur frequently and are benign.[8]

FLUID AND ELECTROLYTE METABOLISM

Maturation of the kidney continues for 6 months after full term. Nephrons are completely formed at 36 weeks' gestation. Glomerular filtration is lower in the neonate because of high renal vascular resistance. The full-term infant can conserve sodium but the preterm infant cannot. The preterm infant has prolonged glomerulotubular imbalance resulting in sodium wastage and hyponatremia.[2] Concentrating ability is limited at birth. Glomerular filtration rate is increased two to three times in the first 3 months. Extracellular fluid is approximately 40% of body weight in the newborn compared to 20% in the adult. An increased metabolic rate results in an accelerated turnover of extracellular fluid.[5] A decrease in blood pressure without an increase in heart rate is the hallmark of intravascular depletion in the neonate.

Fluid maintenance:

0–10 kg	4 mL/kg/h
10–20 kg	2 mL/kg/h
>20 kg	1 mL/kg/h

For example, a 15-kg child requires 4 times 10 = 40 + 2 times 5 = 10 total = 50 mL/h[4]

Choice of fluids:
Maintenance should be with D$_5$W$\frac{1}{4}$NS.
Replacement/deficit should be with Ringer's lactate.

Replacement fluid includes third-space loss, blood loss and loss from fever, if present. Third-space loss may be estimated at 2 mL/h for atraumatic surgery, 4 mL/h for moderate surgery, and 6 to 10 mL/h for extensive surgery.[5] Water loss from fever can be as much as 12% per degree.

Blood volume:

Premature	100 mL/kg
Full term	85–90 mL/kg
Infant	80 mL/kg
Adult	65–70 mL/kg[4]

Hematocrit:

Full term	55%
3 months	30%
6 months	35%

Decrease at 3 months is caused by decreased erythropoietin production, shorter red blood cell survival time, and an increase in plasma volume.

Coagulation tests in the neonate are abnormal. Vitamin K-dependent factors (II, VII, IX, X) are low, which leads to an increase in prothrombin time (PT) and partial thromboplastin time (PTT). Despite laboratory values coagulation in the neonate is normal.[6]

TEMPERATURE REGULATION

Infants do not shiver; they regulate temperature through nonshivering thermogenesis by metabolism of brown fat. Brown fat accounts for 2% to 6% of total body weight and is found in six areas: between the scapulae, in small masses around blood vessels, in the neck and axilla, mediastinally, around internal mammary vessels, and around the adrenal glands. Nonshivering thermogenesis is mediated by the sympathetic nervous system. Cold stress leads to increased norepinephrine production and brown fat metabolism. Shivering thermogenesis slowly takes over by 1 year of age.[9]

Heat loss is by four mechanisms: conduction, radiation, convection, and evaporation. Radiation accounts for the greatest amount of heat loss due to the large BSA/volume ratio. Radiant heat loss is decreased in a warm room.

Prevention of hypothermia is a must for the pediatric patient because it leads to: increased oxygen demand, increased PVR, increased SVR, and right-to-left shunting. Hypothermia can be avoided by:

Heating operating room to 80° to 85°
Using radiant heater during induction, insertion of catheters, and emergence
Setting warming blankets at 40°C
Covering the head—40% loss
Warming fluids via hot line for IVs and irrigation fluids
Humidifying gases—minimizes convective and evaporative losses from the respiratory tract.[9]

Intraoperative temperature monitoring is an American Society of Anesthesiologists (ASA) standard for all children. Nasal pharyngeal probes can cause nosebleeds in children with large adenoids. Esophageal probes that are placed properly in the distal third of the esophagus are the best monitor of the intubated patient. However, it must be kept in mind that an inaccurately positioned probe will produce a false reading. Axillary temperatures are unreliable and accuracy of skin probes varies with placement.[9]

NEUROMUSCULAR JUNCTION

Immaturity of the neuromuscular junction (NMJ) and a decreased amount of pseudocholinesterase activity exists in the neonate.[2] Maturation of the NMJ occurs by 2 months of age.[16]

Because of a larger volume of distribution compared to the adult, higher doses of succinylcholine per kilogram are required. Children are more prone to cardiac dysrhythmias, myoglobinemia, and malignant hyperthermia after succinylcholine administration. Bradycardia can be prevented by pretreatment with atropine. Infants do not fasciculate; therefore, pretreatment is not required. The response of nondepolarizing agents is variable. The immature NMJ tends to increase sensitivity, whereas the increase in extracellular fluid dilutes the concentration. Duration of action may be prolonged in neonates if the drug depends on liver metabolism.[4]

FETAL HEMOGLOBIN

Hemoglobin F is the predominant type of hemoglobin in the fetus. Neonates have 60% to 90% hemoglobin F. By 6 months of age hemoglobin A/hemoglobin F is equal.[10] Hemoglobin F has a decreased concentration of 2,3-diphosphoglycerate and results in a leftward shift of the oxyhemoglobin dissociation curve. This makes the hemoglobin have a high affinity for oxygen, which enables the oxygen transfer from placenta to the fetus. Normal umbilical vein Po_2 is 28 mm Hg with a saturation of 80%. Hemoglobin A would have a saturation of only 50% at this level. The P_{50} of hemoglobin F is 19 compared to 26 for hemoglobin A. After birth hemoglobin F impairs release of oxygen to the tissues.[10] The decreased release of oxygen to tissues is offset by the increased oxygen delivery secondary to the increase in hemoglobin concentration. By 4 months of age the oxyhemoglobin dissociation curve is approximately the same as for the adult.[6]

☐ PATHOPHYSIOLOGY

AIRWAY

Children may have congenital or acquired conditions that make airway management a challenge.

Asthma   Asthma is the most common respiratory disease in children. Asthma presents as either extrinsic or intrinsic. Extrinsic is also called allergic and is the most common type; intrinsic is exercise or cold induced.

All types of asthma are associated with increased IgE levels. The child with asthma carries a high risk of intraoperative bronchospasm.

Preoperatively the anesthesia care provider should:

1.   Inquire as to what factors trigger an episode.
2.   Ask when the last episode occurred—elective surgery should be postponed for 4 to 6 weeks.
3.   Assess for upper respiratory infection (URI)—in an asthmatic child URI is associated with an increased risk of bronchospasm; elective surgery should be postponed for 4 to 6 weeks after the URI is resolved.

4.   Inquire if steroids are used; a stress dose may be required.
5.   If the child is on theophylline, determine if a therapeutic level is obtained.

Preoperatively on the day of surgery:

1.   Bronchodilators should be administered.
2.   Theophylline, β_2 agonists (albuterol, metaproterenol), or steroids should be administered before induction.

During induction, manipulation of the airway and light anesthesia can precipitate bronchospasm. If at all possible avoid endotracheal intubation. If a secured airway is necessary, adequate depth of anesthesia must be obtained before intubation. If wheezing occurs intraoperatively measures must be taken to prevent deterioration.

1.   Increase fraction inspired oxygen (Fio_2)
2.   Deepen anesthetic—all inhalation agents are bronchodilators.
3.   Administer muscle relaxants; this prevents exaggerated expiratory efforts that increase lower airway obstruction.
4.   Lidocaine 1 mg/kg intravenously (IV)
5.   Aerosol β_2 agonists
6.   If wheezing continues, an aminophylline drip, 1 mg/kg/ h, may be instituted after a loading dose of 6 mg/kg over 20 minutes. If aminophylline is started, the halothane should be discontinued to prevent dysrhythmias. Isoflurane and enflurane are not dysrhythmogenic.

Two techniques for emergence of the asthmatic patient are acceptable. The choice will depend on the type of procedure.

1.   Awake extubation—the patient is fully awake and breathing spontaneously. Lidocaine 1 mg/kg or a small dose of narcotic will reduce irritation from the endotracheal tube. Administration of aerosol β_2 agonist is helpful.
2.   Deep extubation—the patient is extubated while still deeply anesthetized with inhalation agent and allowed to emerge without stimulus of the endotracheal tube. This technique is not recommended for tonsillectomy or any other procedure on the upper airway.[11]

Bronchopulmonary Dysplagia   Bronchopulmonary dysplagia (BPD) is a chronic pulmonary disorder in children with a history of respiratory distress syndrome (RDS). Precipitating factors include a need for prolonged high Fio_2 and positive-pressure ventilation. The degree of BPD correlates with the degree of RDS. Pulmonary dysfunction is greatest during the first year of life with a slow resolution occurring with increasing age. This improvement is due to proliferation of alveolar saccules, which occurs rapidly in infancy and early childhood. Newborns have 30 million as compared to 300 million in the adult.[6]

Characteristics include:

1. Increased airway reactivity and resistance
2. Decreased pulmonary compliance
3. Ventilation/perfusion (V/Q) mismatch
4. Decreased arterial oxygenation
5. Tachypnea[5,6]

Oxygen consumption is increased by 25%, in the patient with BPD, due to increased work of breathing.[6]

Management of anesthesia includes:

1. Intubation
2. Increased F_{IO_2}
3. Mechanical ventilation
4. Deep plane of anesthesia before intubation of trachea[6]

Pierre Robin Syndrome   Pierre Robin syndrome is a congenital syndrome with the following characteristics:

1. Micrognathia
2. Glossoptosis (posterior displacement of the tongue)
3. Cleft palate
4. Associated congenital heart disease[6,12]

Acute upper airway obstruction occurs in the neonate or infant. This obstruction may require the tongue to be sutured down and forward. These infants require awake intubation due to the difficulty of intubation.[12]

Epiglottitis and Croup   Epiglottitis is a bacterial infection from *Haemophilus influenzae* type B. It can be fatal if not treated expediently and properly. Edema of supraglottic tissues obstructs the airway (Table 25–3).

The child presents to the operating room in a sitting position, drooling, tongue protruding, hypoxic, lethargic, and with a high fever.[4,6]

Induction and maintenance of anesthesia is with a volatile agent, usually halothane and oxygen. Before induction the room and personnel should be prepared for an emergency cricothyrotomy or tracheostomy. Induction is started with the child in a sitting position and once drowsy the child is placed supine and assisted ventilation is required. Adequate depth of anesthesia is a must. The endotracheal tube size may be one to two sizes smaller than expected for the age. After successful intubation, a direct laryngoscopy is performed to confirm the diagnosis. The child will remain intubated for 48 to 96 hours, until the edema has resolved. Extubation is performed in the operating room after the temperature is normal, neutrophil count is decreased, and clinical signs of decreased airway edema are present.[6]

Croup is a viral infection. Treatment usually does not require an anesthetic. Patients with a history of croup have hyperreactive airways. This should be considered in patients presenting to the operating room for other procedures.[5,6]

Postintubation Laryngeal Edema   Incidence of this is highest in children aged 1 to 4 and occurrence is within 3 hours of extubation.[6]

Causes include:

1. Manipulation of the airway—especially repeated attempts
2. Tight fitting endotracheal tube

Table 25–3
CLINICAL FEATURES OF EPIGLOTTITIS (SUPRAGLOTTITIS) AND LARYNGOTRACHEOBRONCHITIS

	Epiglottitis	Laryngotracheobronchitis
Age group affected	2–6 y	≤2 y
Incidence	Accounts for 5% of children with stridor	Accounts for about 80% of children with stridor
Etiologic agent	Bacterial *(Haemophilus influenzae)*	Viral
Onset	Rapid over 24 h	Gradual over 24–72 h
Signs and symptoms	Inspiratory stridor	Inspiratory stridor
	Pharyngitis	Croupy cough
	Drooling	Rhinorrhea
	Fever (often >39°C)	Fever (rarely >39°C)
	Lethargic to restless	
	Insists on sitting up and leaning forward	
	Tachypnea	
	Cyanosis	
Laboratory	Neutrophilia	Lymphocytosis
Lateral radiograph of the neck	Swollen epiglottis	Narrowing of the subglottic area
Treatment	Oxygen	Oxygen
	Urgent intubation of the trachea or tracheostomy during general anesthesia	Aerosolized racemic epinephrine
	Fluids	Humidity
	Antibiotics	Fluids
	Corticosteroids(?)	Corticosteroids
		Intubation of the trachea for severe airway obstruction

SOURCE: Reproduced by permission from Stoelting and Dierdorf.[6]

4. Change in patient's position after intubation
5. Coexisting URI
6. Head and neck procedures

Prevention consists of inserting a tube ensuring an audible air leak at 15–25 cm H_2O.

Treatment consists of racemic epinephrine inhalation treatment of 0.05 mL/kg (maximum 0.5 mL) racemic in 2 mL saline. The usefulness of dexamethasone, 0.1 to 0.2 mg/kg IV, remains questionable. Rarely is reintubation or tracheostomy needed.[6,10]

Tracheoesophageal Fistula Tracheoesophageal fistula (TEF) is a congenital malformation of the trachea and esophagus. There are five different types of TEF (Figure 25–2); 20% of patients have coexisting cardiac anomalies and 30% to 40% are premature.

Diagnosis is made when a catheter cannot be placed into the stomach or when the newborn becomes cyanotic and coughs with feedings. Aspiration is common.[5,6]

Treatment consists of decompression of the upper pouch and surgical correction. The infant should remain in a sitting position until surgical intervention is possible to prevent aspiration. Surgery consists of ligation of the defect and primary anastomosis of the esophagus. If this is not possible, due to a short esophagus, a gastrostomy and esophagotomy are performed until the infant is able to have the final procedure. The final procedure consists of a colon interposition done at about 2 years of age.[6,13]

Intubation is usually accomplished awake to prevent further aspiration.[4,6,7] Proper endotracheal tube placement is crucial; the tip should be above the carina but below the fistula. Accidental right mainstem intubation leads to drastic desaturation.[6] Fiberoptic intubation is not necessary in these patients, but it may be helpful in confirming tube placement.[6] Surgery is done in the left lateral position. A precordial stethoscope should be placed in the dependent axilla to detect mainstem obstruction during retraction.[4] Avoid high airway pressures, which lead to gastric distension; if the patient has a gastrostomy tube in place open it to air or place in a jar of water.[6,7]

Postoperative complications include gastroesophageal reflux, aspiration, anastomosis leakage, tracheomalacia, and esophageal strictures.[4,6,7]

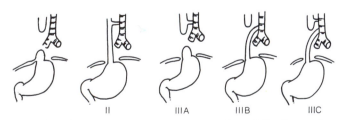

Figure 25–2 The five types of tracheoesophageal fistula are classified as I, II, IIIA, IIIB, and IIIC, depending on the anatomic characteristics of the trachea and esophagus. A blind upper esophageal pouch and a fistula connecting the stomach to the trachea (IIIB) is the most common type of tracheoesophageal fistula. (Reproduced by permission from Stoelting and Dierdorf.[6])

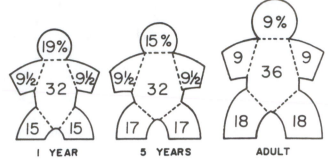

Figure 25–3 In determining the percentage of body surface area involved by thermal injury, one must consider the age of the patient. (Reproduced by permission from Stoelting and Dierdorf.[6])

BURNS

The severity of a burn depends on the BSA involved and the thickness of the burn (Figure 25–3). Partial thickness burns involve the superficial dermis and usually heal without a skin graft. Full thickness burns require skin grafts. Mortality increases with the severity of the burn.[6,14]

Pathophysiologic responses to burns include:

1. Decrease in cardiac output is initially due to a low molecular weight myocardial depressant factor and then to acute hypovolemia. Cardiac output increases after the first 24 hours due to a hyperdynamic state. Blood pressure and heart rate increase while cardiac output is two times normal. Pulmonary edema is rare during first few days but may occur when fluid is being reabsorbed into the intravascular volume.[6]

2. Hypertension is present in 30% of children in the postburn period and is usually transient. It may be due to an increase in catecholamine levels. Treatment may be required with hydralazine or nitroprusside.

3. Decreased intravascular volume is usually proportionate to the depth and extent of the burn. There is a large amount of third spacing due to increased osmotic pressure. Increased permeability is greatest at the burn site but exists throughout the body. Severe hypoglycemia occurs. Loss of fluid from evaporation averages approximately 4 mL/kg, based on percentage of BSA burned. A child weighing 40 kg with 50% burns will require 8000 mL fluid in the first 24 hours. Administer two thirds of the fluid in the first 8 hours. Capillary integrity is restored by the second day; fluid and plasma losses are decreased. Colloid solutions are administered on the second day.[6,14]

4. Airway edema is severe with thermal or chemical injury. Hoarseness, stridor, and tachypnea require immediate intubation to prevent complete obstruction.[6]

5. Smoke inhalation leads to a chemical pneumonitis. Treatment includes warm humidified air, positive-pressure ventilation with positive end-expiratory pressure if Pa_{O_2} is less than 60 mm Hg on room air.[6]

6. Carbon monoxide inhalation is the most immediate cause of death. Carbon monoxide has 200 times the

affinity for hemoglobin as does oxygen. Patients present with pink cheeks and low oxygen saturations. Carboxyhemoglobin levels should be determined and treatment should be with 100% oxygen by mask or endotracheal tube.[15,16]

7. Circumferential burns restrict the thorax, as healing begins, and escharotomy may be required.[6]

8. Metabolism increases in proportion to the percent burned and the patient becomes hypermetabolic until the burn is healed. There is an increase in catecholamine levels, hyperthermia, increased catabolism, increased oxygen consumption, tachypnea, increased heart rate, and increased carbon dioxide production.[6,15,16]

9. Ileus is almost always seen with thermal injury, requiring the insertion of a nasogastric tube. Acute ulceration of the stomach known as Curling's ulcer is a life-threatening complication. Duodenal ulcer occurs two times more frequently in children than adults. Treatment is with antacids and H_2 antagonists.[6]

10. Decreased renal blood flow and glomerular filtration rate occur due to the decrease in cardiac output, decreased intracellular volume, and increase in catecholamine levels. Decreased renal blood flow leads to an increase in renin–angiotensin effect. There is a loss of potassium, calcium, and magnesium with a retention of sodium and water. Aggressive fluid resuscitation increases both renal blood flow and glomerular filtration rates. Urine output should be maintained at a minimum of 1 mL/kg/h.[6]

11. The potassium level initially increases due to necrosis and hemolysis, and then is followed by a decrease due to renal losses. Cardiac dysrhythmias may occur.[6]

12. Endocrine responses include an increase in corticotropin, antidiuretic hormone, renin, angiotensin, aldosterone, glucagon, and catecholamines. An increase in catecholamines, especially norepinephrine, causes intense vasoconstriction of skin and splanchnic vessels. Ischemia of the gastrointestinal tract may result. Plasma glucose increases result from increases in catecholamines.[6]

13. Blood viscosity increases and the increase in factors V and VIII continues for several weeks. This may lead to disseminated intravascular coagulation.[6]

14. An altered immune response is demonstrated in burn patients. Infections are common in the burn, the eschar, the lungs, and the intestinal tract. Strict aseptic technique must be maintained at all times.[6]

Anesthetic management includes:

1. Intubation is imperative if any airway damage has been assessed. Edema develops quickly.

2. A nasogastric tube is needed.

3. Monitoring and IV access may be limited; needle electrodes may be necessary. An arterial line for blood drawing and blood pressure monitoring may also be required.[6,14]

4. Warming devices are crucial because thermoregulation is totally obliterated. Increased ambient temperature and warmed airway gases, IV fluids, and irrigation fluids are imperative intraoperative measures.[14]

5. Blood loss, especially during removal of eschar, can be 2% to 3% of blood volume for every 1% BSA to be excised. Transfuse early. Assess blood loss by arterial line, central venous pressures, and urine output.[14]

6. Drug responses are altered in the burned patient. All drugs must be given IV to prevent poor absorption. IV and inhaled drugs may have an exaggerated effect due to increased blood flow to vessel-rich groups. Inhaled drugs during the first 24 hours after the burn when the cardiac output is decreased may further depress the heart. Ketamine or narcotics may be the drugs of choice.[14] Albumin levels are low; therefore, requirements of protein-bound drugs (pentothal, benzodiazepams) are reduced. Ketamine can be used in reduced dosages of 0.25 to 0.50 mg/kg. If the patient is severely hypovolemic and sympathetic tone is high, ketamine acts as a myocardial depressant. While the patient is hypermetabolic, oxygen consumption, glucose consumption, and carbon dioxide production are markedly increased. Adequate oxygenation and ventilation should be maintained.[14]

7. After burn injury a denervation occurs and postjunctional acetylcholine receptors increase. This leads to hyperkalemia if succinylcholine is administered. Controversy exists over when this occurs after the injury—it can be as little as 24 hours after burn up to 50 days after injury. The safest action is to avoid succinylcholine completely.[6,14] Resistance to nondepolarizing agents occurs when greater than 30% BSA is burned. This is due to extrajunctional cholinergic receptors or an altered affinity of cholinergic receptors for acetylcholine.

8. Choice of agent depends on the procedure being done. Again, ketamine is a good choice for dressing changes because it offers some postoperative analgesia. Halothane is favored for inhalation because it maintains spontaneous respirations and a high level of oxygen may be administered. It is best to avoid nitrous oxide due to the high oxygen consumption.[6,14]

DOWN'S SYNDROME—TRISOMY 21

Characteristics of these children include flat faces with oblique palpebral fissures, simian crease, dysplastic middle phalanx of the fifth finger, and fat pad at the back of the neck. The upper airway is chronically obstructed due to a narrow nasopharynx, large tonsils and adenoids, and hypertrophy of the tongue. The incidence of accompanying congenital heart disease is 40%. Endocardial cushion defect is the most commonly seen associated cardiac anomaly. These children may also present with ventricular septal defect, tetrology of Fallot, patent ductus arteriosus, or atrial septal defect.[6,17] There is a high incidence of cataracts and strabismus as well as otitis media. Asymptomatic dislocation of the atlas on the axis is present in 20%. Care must be taken when manipulating the head and neck for intubation.[6,17]

A small dose of ketamine may be needed to facilitate induction of anesthesia. The airway may be difficult to maintain once the patient is asleep because of the facial and oral characteristics, but intubation is usually not difficult. If the patient has no heart disease, either an inhalation or narcotic technique can be used.[6] Meticulous avoidance of air bubbles in the IV lines is important because many of these patients have a right-to-left shunt.[4]

Postoperatively these patients are more prone to stridor and upper airway obstruction. They should be fully awake before extubation and should be closely observed in the postanesthesia care unit (PACU). If airway edema is suspected, a racemic epinephrine treatment may be given to reduce the edema.[17]

PHARMACOLOGY

Pharmacologic responses differ in the child and the adult. The minimal alveolar concentration (MAC) is lower in the neonate and preterm infants require even less volatile agent, in direct proportion to their age. A 32-week neonate would require less than a 34-week neonate. MAC increases until 2 to 3 months of age and then it declines to that of the adult except for a short period of time during puberty when it again rises.[4,5] There is a rapid induction and emergence in infants due to rapid uptake of anesthetics. This is due to high alveolar ventilation, low functional residual capacity (FRC), and a large vessel-rich group in infants.[4] Blood pressure in infants and neonates is more sensitive to volatile anesthetics because of their inability to compensate for vasodilatation. They are unable to increase the heart rate or vasoconstrict blood vessels.[4]

The neonate has decreased hepatic and renal clearance, which can prolong the duration of action of some drugs. Drugs such as theophylline, phenytoin (Dilantin), and diazepam (Valium) have a decreased clearance in the neonate, which increases by 5 to 6 months. Protein binding is decreased in infants leading to increased drug availability and greater drug effect.[6]

BARBITURATES AND OPIOIDS

The cytochrome P-450 pathway is mature at 1 month of age. Neonates have an immature blood–brain barrier and decreased ability to metabolize drugs, which may be responsible for toxic effects of barbiturates.[4] The elimination half-life of pentothal is shorter than in the adult due to increased blood flow and a rapid clearance.[18] Neonates require lower dosages for induction but by the age of 5 to 15 the requirement increases.[6]

Neonates and infants are more resistant to ketamine and require higher doses. The dose of ketamine required to prevent movement is four times greater in infants younger than 6 months than in 6-year-old children. Studies have shown there is little metabolism of ketamine in the newborn. The high doses required in the infant will lead to respiratory depression and apnea. Ketamine should be avoided in the child with hydrocephalus due to the increase in intracranial pressure that it causes. Ketamine also raises pulmonary artery pressure and should be avoided in children with congenital heart disease.[10,18]

Fentanyl and sufentanyl appear to be safe and cause no hemodynamic changes in the neonate or the preterm infant.[6] Morphine sulfate should be used with caution in the neonate due to decreased conjugation and impaired renal function, which decreases the rate of clearance.[18] In the infant meperidine (Demerol) has a half-life that is about twice that of the adult. Neonates excrete 25% to 40% of meperidine within 48 hours.[18]

Neonates and infants have a larger volume of distribution than the adult, which results in the need for a higher dose of succinylcholine (2 mg/kg IV, 4 mg/kg IM). Succinylcholine produces small changes in intragastric pressures in children. It does cause more bradycardia in children and pretreatment with atropine is required. Infants are more sensitive to nondepolarizing agents; however, the dose per kilogram is calculated the same as for the adult due to the larger volume of distribution.[5,6]

Duration of muscle relaxants is variable in the infant and child. Atracurium, which does not depend on hepatic transformation, has a shorter duration of action in infants, whereas the duration of vecuronium may be increased due to immaturity of the hepatic system.[4,6]

Antagonism of a neuromuscular blockade is reliable and may require a smaller dose of anticholinesterase drug than the adult; however, it is not necessary in clinical practice to alter the dose.[4–6]

ANESTHESIA PROCEDURES

PYLORIC STENOSIS

Pyloric stenosis occurs in 1 of 500 births with 95% of cases occurring in boys.[19] It is predominate in first-born boys with a strong family history.[6]

There is a thickening of the smooth muscle around the pyloris with edema of surrounding mucosa.[20] The infant presents with projectile vomiting between the second to sixth week of life. An olive-sized mass is palpable at the site.[19]

Pyloric stenosis is a medical emergency and surgery should not proceed until medically treated. Infants present with hypokalemic, hypochloremic metabolic alkalosis with a compensatory respiratory acidosis.[6]

Fluid and electrolyte replacement usually requires 12 to 48 hours depending on degree of imbalance. Before surgical intervention the infant should have normal skin turgor, sodium level greater than 130 mEq/L, potassium level greater than 3 mEq/L, chloride level greater than 85 mEq/L, and a urine output of 1 to 2 mL/kg/h.[21] Fluid resuscitation should be with a balanced salt solution with potassium added after the infant voids. Maintenance fluid should be with $D_5W\frac{1}{2}NS$. When the infant is medically stable a pyloromyotomy may be performed.[19]

These infants are considered to have a full stomach and are at great risk for aspiration pneumonitis. The nasogastric tube should be suctioned prior to induction. An awake intubation is preferred but a rapid sequence intubation with the Sellick maneuver is acceptable.[6] Muscle relaxation can be provided by atracurium or Mivacron.[21]

Postoperatively, respiratory depression may be noted due to cerebrospinal fluid alkalosis, preoperative electrolyte imbalance, and intraoperative hyperventilation. Extubation should be delayed until the infant is fully awake and vigorous.[6] Hypoglycemia may occur 2 to 3 hours postoperatively due to cessation of glucose infusion and depletion of glycogen stores.[6,20]

TONSILLECTOMY AND ADENOIDECTOMY

Patients requiring tonsillectomy and adenoidectomy have hypertrophy of lymphoid tissues.[4] Usually patients presenting for this procedure are children or young adults who have developed obstructive sleep apnea due to relaxed pharyngeal muscles and obstruction of the airway by the enlarged tissues. If left untreated, pulmonary hypertension or cor pulmonale results from chronic obstruction and hypoxia.[22]

If the PT, PTT, and platelet count are abnormal the surgery should be postponed until they are normalized.[4] Sedatives or hypnotics should be avoided to prevent respiratory depression and further hypoxia. An antisialagogue may be given preoperatively to decrease oralpharyngeal secretions.[22] A reinforced endotracheal tube or oral Rae tube should be used to prevent endotracheal tube obstruction caused by the mouth gag. Blood loss is difficult to estimate. The child should be given adequate amounts of crystalloid fluids. Extubation should not be performed unless the child is fully awake and able to protect the airway. Careful suctioning of the stomach and posterior pharynx should be done before extubation to decrease the risk of laryngospasm. Transport the patient in the tonsil position, lateral, head down, to the PACU.[22] This position facilitates drainage of any blood or secretions that may be in the posterior pharynx.

Sleep apnea may continue into the postoperative period due to a central component. Monitoring in the PACU is of utmost importance. The most common postoperative complication is bleeding, which presents with frequent swallowing, restlessness, pallor, tachycardia, and hypotension. If reoperation is necessary, the child must be fluid resuscitated before return to the operating room. Intubation must be either awake or rapid sequence with the Sellick maneuver.[22] Ketamine may be the drug of choice due to intravascular fluid depletion. Bleeding may occur within the first 6 hours or between postoperative days 5 to 10 when the eschar falls off and leaves an exposed tonsillar bed.[22]

CLEFT PALATE/CLEFT LIP

Both lip and palate clefts occur in 1/1000 births; cleft palate alone occurs in 1/2500 births. These children may have associated anomalies including congenital heart disease. Infants with cleft palate or lip have difficulty feeding and are prone to aspiration pneumonitis. They are also prone to otitis media.[6]

Cleft lips are usually repaired at 2 to 3 months of age and cleft palate at approximately 18 months of age.

Induction of anesthesia depends on the degree of airway obstruction. In the child with no other anomalies a standard IV induction is possible but in a child with other anomalies, such as Pierre Robin syndrome, an inhalation induction while maintaining spontaneous respirations may be required.[6] Intubation may be difficult if the laryngoscope blade slips into the cleft. Packing the cleft may facilitate intubation.[6] Airway obstruction may occur after induction due to relaxed pharyngeal muscles and a large tongue. An awake intubation may be necessary. Intubation should be with an oral Rae tube to prevent kinking by the mouth gag.[6] Maintenance is with a volatile agent and muscle relaxation.[23] All air bubbles should be carefully removed from IVs due to the incidence of associated cardiac anomalies. Extubation must only be done when the patient is fully awake.[6]

Postoperatively, airway obstruction may be due to edema of the tongue from the mouth gag, mucosal swelling, subglottic edema, flap edema, or posterior displacement of the tongue.[23] Respiratory difficulty may also be caused by blocked nasal passages and because infants are obligatory nasal breathers they must adjust to oral breathing.[23] A decrease in the anterior-posterior oropharyngeal distance may also lead to hypoxia and apnea.[23] A suture may be placed through the tongue and taped to the cheek. If airway obstruction occurs, the tongue can be displaced forward.[6] Because of copious secretions and blood, these children are prone to laryngospasm after extubation. Treatment must be readily available in the PACU.[24]

DIAPHRAGMATIC HERNIA

Incomplete closure of the diaphragm causes herniation of bowel into the thorax that results in a hypoplastic lung on the affected side.[6] It becomes apparent soon after birth that a diaphragmatic hernia exists. The infant presents with a scaphoid abdomen, bowel sounds in the chest (usually on the left), barrel chest, and significant hypoxia. Chest radiography reveals bowel in the thoracic cage. Persistent fetal circulation is common due to hypoxia, acidosis, and an increase in pulmonary vascular resistance. Other anomalies associated with diaphragmatic hernia are congenital heart disease and malrotation of the bowel.[6,25]

The stomach must be decompressed immediately to decrease distention of bowel, which further hinders lung function. When ventilation becomes necessary, an awake intubation is required. Do not exceed 25 cm peak airway pressure during ventilation, which may cause a tension pneumothorax of the functioning lung.[6,25]

Awake intubation is mandatory. Ventilation should be done with low peak airway pressures and high rates. A respiratory rate of 50 to 100 is appropriate. Avoid nitrous oxide, which increases the free air in the bowel within the thoracic cage, making ventilation difficult. Monitor the infant with all standard monitors plus an arterial line and Foley catheter. Narcotic technique is a good choice because the infant will require postoperative ventilation. Do not attempt to reinflate the hypoplastic lung following the reduction of the hernia because this may lead to a pneumothorax on the contralateral side. Signs and symptoms of a pneumothorax on the contralateral side include rapid desaturation and bradycardia leading to sudden cardiac arrest. If the abdominal closure is tight secondary to a small abdominal cavity, the result will be increased peak airway pressures, decreased functional residual capacity, and compression of the inferior vena cava.[6] IV access of the lower extremities should be avoided because venous return will be decreased if the inferior vena cava becomes compressed.[26] Postoperatively, extracorporeal membrane oxygenation may be required if the lung tissue is severely hypoplastic.[26] The prognosis for these infants remains poor, even with early surgical intervention. Death usually occurs due to hypoplasia of lung tissue and persistent fetal circulation.[6]

OMPHALOCELE AND GASTROSCHISIS

These anomalies appear similar; however, there are important differences between them.

The incidence of omphalocele is 1/6000 to 10,000 births, with a male predominance; the incidence of gastroschisis is 1/30,000, with no sexual predominance.[26]

An omphalocele results from failure of part or all of the intestine to return to the abdominal cavity at approximately the tenth week of gestation. Gastroschisis results from the interruption of the omphalomesenteric artery with resultant dissolution of the layers of the abdominal wall.[21]

An omphalocele is midline and has a covering of amnion, whereas a gastroschisis has no amnion covering and is usually right-sided lateral in position.

There is a 75% incidence of associated congenital anomalies in patients with an omphalocele. Commonly seen anomalies are cardiac anomalies, trisomy 21, and Beckwith syndrome, which consists of organomegaly, macroglossia, and hypoglycemia. Epigastric omphaloceles are associated with cardiac and lung anomalies, whereas hypogastric omphaloceles are associated with extrophy of the bladder and other genitourinary disorders. Gastroschisis is rarely associated with any other anomalies.[27]

The incidence of preterm delivery is higher with gastroschisis than in those with an omphalocele.[6,21,26] Preoperative preparation of the child with either an omphalocele or a gastroschisis includes the prevention of infection and minimization of heat and fluid loss. Exposed viscera should be covered with moist dressings and a plastic bag to prevent evaporative fluid and heat loss. A nasogastric tube should be passed to decompress the stomach and prevent aspiration.

Fluid resuscitation should begin immediately at 6 to 12 mL/kg/h.[6] The infant with gastroschisis has a greater fluid loss due to the fact that there is no hernia sac covering the viscera.[21] Hypovolemia leads to hemoconcentration and metabolic acidosis. Plasma albumin and colloid oncotic pressure are decreased. Albumin replacement should be given at the rate of 25% of the replacement fluids. Sodium bicarbonate should be given slowly to correct the metabolic acidosis. Urine output of 1 to 2 mL/kg/h indicates adequate hydration.[6]

The goal of surgery is to close the defect; however, a primary closure is not always possible. When the defect is large, closure may lead to vascular insufficiency to the bowel and lower extremities, compression of the inferior vena cava and respiratory insufficiency.[6,21] A Silastic silo is used to cover defects that cannot be closed primarily. The abdominal contents are wrapped in a Dacron-Silastic bag and suspended above the infant and the contents are slowly returned to the abdomen over a period of a few days.[6,21]

Awake intubation is needed after nasogastric suctioning and preoxygenation. Anesthetic technique may be either narcotic or volatile agent or a combination. Nitrous oxide should be avoided to prevent further distention of the bowel. Muscle relaxation must be maintained; however, it must be closely monitored because excessive relaxation may give an inaccurate assessment of the primary closure. Airway pressures must be monitored to detect changes in pulmonary compliance, especially during abdominal closure.[6,21] Heat loss in the operating room should be prevented by keeping the room warm, using airway humidifiers, using warming blankets, and warming all fluids.[26]

Postoperatively, monitoring of blood gases, fluids, and electrolytes is essential. Postoperative ventilation is usually required for 24 to 48 hours. Complications include hypertension and edema of extremities. Hypertension is caused by increased abdominal pressure with resultant decreased circulation to the kidney causing renin release. Third-space fluid shifts continue for 3 to 4 days. Fluid management should be guided by central venous pressures and urine output.[21,26]

STRABISMUS REPAIR

Strabismus is caused by weakened extraocular muscles. Strabismus is the most common pediatric ocular surgery. Anesthetic concerns include increased incidence of oculocardiac reflex, postoperative nausea and vomiting, and malignant hyperthermia.[28] The use of succinylcholine remains controversial because patients with strabismus are believed to have an increased predisposition to malignant hyperthermia.[29]

Oculocardiac reflex manifests as bradycardia in response to:

1. Traction on the rectus muscles especially the median
2. Direct pressure on the globe
3. Administration of a retrobulbar block
4. Ocular trauma
5. Ocular pain

6. Ocular manipulation[29]
7. Pain, hypoxia, or increased carbon dioxide
8. Retrobulbar hemorrhage[29,30]

The afferent pathway is via the trigeminal nerve and the efferent pathway is via the vagus nerve causing the bradycardia. Other dysrhythmias may be noted such as premature ventricular contractions, junctional rhythm, atrioventricular block, wandering pacemaker, ventricular tachycardia, and asystole. Pediatric patients have a higher incidence of oculocardiac reflex due to an increased vagal tone. Preoperative atropine or glycopyrrolate may decrease the incidence of the reflex. If the oculocardiac reflex occurs:

1. Inform the surgeon to stop retraction and manipulation.
2. Increase the depth of anesthesia.

The heart rate should increase within 20 seconds. The oculocardiac reflex will fatigue with constant manipulation; however, if it continues IV atropine (0.007 mg/kg) or glycopyrrolate (0.004–0.008 mg/kg IV) should be administered.

Succinylcholine causes bradycardia in the pediatric population; because this same population is prone to the oculocardiac reflex (OCR), it is best to avoid succinylcholine if possible. Succinylcholine also interferes with the forced duction test the surgeon performs to determine if the strabismus is secondary to a paretic muscle or a restrictive force that prevents eye movement. The use of succinylcholine is contraindicated within 20 minutes of performing the test. Succinylcholine is also associated with a fourfold increase of myoglobinemia in the strabismus patient.[29]

Incidence of postoperative nausea and vomiting is increased in patients with strabismus repair. Prophylactic administration of droperidol (0.075 mg/kg) at induction decreases the incidence from 85% to 10%.[30]

Intubation should be facilitated by a nondepolarizing muscle relaxant. Monitoring for the OCR is of utmost importance. Should bradycardia develop follow the steps outlined above. Temperature should be monitored. Droperidol should be administered at induction to prevent nausea and vomiting.[31] Emergence should be smooth; measures should be taken to prevent bucking, such as deep extubation or administration of lidocaine or narcotic.[31]

☐ NEONATAL RESUSCITATION

The neonate must be assessed immediately after birth to identify and intervene if the infant is depressed. The neonate may be depressed due to trauma, placental insufficiency, drugs given to the mother, or congenital anomalies. Breathing should begin by 30 seconds and be sustained by 90 seconds. If this does not occur, the neonate is considered severely depressed.[32]

The Apgar score was developed by Dr. Virginia Apgar to identify depressed infants who required resuscitation. It is based on five vital signs:

1. Heart rate
2. Respiratory effort
3. Muscle tone
4. Reflex irritability
5. Color

Scores are taken at 1 and 5 minutes of life.[32] The amount of resuscitation depends on the Apgar score at 1 minute. Apgar scores of 8 to 10 require only gentle stimulation such as drying, flicking the foot, or rubbing the back. Scores of 5 to 7 need a moderate amount of stimulation with oxygen given by insufflation. Scores of 3 to 4 require temporary assisted positive-pressure ventilation with a mask and bag. An Apgar score of 0 to 2 requires immediate intubation; chest compressions may be required. Indications for ventilation are persistent apnea, heart rate less than 100, and sustained central cyanosis with 100% oxygen. Ventilation should be at a rate of 40/min. Initial breaths may require up to 40 cm H_2O but should be kept less than 30 cm H_2O after initial inflation. If after 1 minute the infant is spontaneously breathing then ventilation can be stopped. If the heart rate remains below 60, immediate intubation and chest compressions are required at a rate of 120/min. Use a 2.5 to 3.0 uncuffed endotracheal tube and a Miller 00 or 0 blade.

Vascular access must be obtained, the umbilical vein being the easiest. Volume resuscitation should be initiated if the blood pressure is low, there is a faint pulse with an adequate heart rate, or a poor response to resuscitation. Fluid should either be Ringer's lactate or packed cells at the rate of 10 mL/kg.[32–34]

MECONIUM ASPIRATION

If meconium-stained fluid is noted, the anesthetist must be ready to treat a depressed infant. Meconium is thick material that will lead to hypoxia, atelectasis, pneumothorax, and persistent fetal circulation if not removed from the trachea. Treatment consists of suctioning the trachea before the first breath. Suctioning without ventilation should continue until the return is clear. Ventilation will only advance the meconium into the alveoli and obstruct them.[32,35]

DRUGS

Epinephrine: 0.1–0.3 mL/kg of 1:10,000 for asystole or heart rate of less than 80 during chest compressions and ventilation. May be administered IV or endotracheal.[34,35]

Calcium: 30 mg/kg CaCl or 100 mg/kg calcium gluconate if magnesium toxicity is suspected.[34]

Naloxone: 0.01 mg/kg if the cause of respiratory depression is believed to be due to maternal narcotic dose. Do not give to infants of addicted mothers.[32,34,36]

Glucose: 4 mL/kg of 10% solution for documented hypoglycemia. Hyperglycemia may worsen hypoxic neurologic deficits.[34]

Sodium bicarbonate: 2 mEq/kg should be given only if a metabolic acidosis is present. It must be administered slowly (1 mEq/kg/min) to prevent cerebral hemorrhage due to hyperosmolarity and fragile cerebral vessels.[34]

For more complete information, see Table 25–4.

☐ ANESTHETIC EQUIPMENT

Pediatric patients may require different equipment than the adult patient because of the difference in their size and lung compliancy.

BREATHING SYSTEMS (Table 25–5)

Semiopen systems include a gas reservoir bag, use of a unidirectional valve, or high fresh gas flow rates to prevent rebreathing of carbon dioxide. Advantages of these systems are that they are lightweight, portable, easy to clean, and offer low resistance to breathing. Assisted or controlled ventilation is possible. A unidirectional valve directs fresh gas flow to the patient and exhaled gases out of the system. The disadvantage of the valve is that it increases the resistance to breathing. High fresh gas flows are needed when there is no unidirectional valve to prevent rebreathing of exhaled gases.

The Mapleson systems are used for pediatric patients under 10 kg in weight. The differences of these systems is the placement of the overflow valve (Figure 25–4).

In *Mapleson A*, the overflow valve is near the patient and the fresh gas flow is located at the end of the corrugated tubing. This system is the most efficient for the spontaneously breathing patient.

In *Mapleson B*, fresh gas flow is just distal to the overflow valve located near the patient. This design is less efficient during spontaneous ventilation than the Mapleson A. A fresh gas flow of two times the patient's minute ventilation is required to prevent rebreathing.

Mapleson C, is the same as Mapleson B with a shorter expiratory limb. Fresh gas flow should be two times the patient's minute ventilation. This may be used with either spontaneous or controlled ventilation.

Mapleson D resembles Mapleson A except the location of the fresh gas flow and the overflow valve are reversed. Fresh gas flow placed near the patient results in efficient carbon dioxide removal with any type of ventilation. Fresh gas flow must be two times the patient's minute ventilation.[37–39]

The *Bain system* is the most common system used for pediatric patients. Its advantage is the decreased resistance to breathing. The primary sources of resistance to breathing are the endotracheal tube, valves, and the carbon dioxide absorber.[40] It is a modification of the Mapleson D system. The fresh gas flow enters through a narrow tube within the corrugated expiratory limb, creating a countercurrent type mechanism. This results in the rewarming of inspiratory gases, better humidification due to partial rebreathing, and the ability to scavenge exhaled gases. During controlled ventilation a fresh gas flows of 70 mL/kg is required; however, during

Table 25–4
PEDIATRIC DRUG DOSAGES

Drug	Comment	Dosage
Aminophylline	Loading dose administered over 20 minutes	5 mg/kg
	Maintenance dose (therapeutic level: 10–20 µg/mL)	0.5–0.9 mg/kg/h
Atropine	IV or IM	0.01–0.02 mg/kg
Bretylium	Loading dose	5 mg/kg
Cardioversion		0.2–1 J/kg
Chloral hydrate	Oral administration	50–100 mg/kg
Dantrolene	Initial dose (10 mg/kg maximum)	2.5 mg/kg
Defibrillation	First attempt	2 J/kg
	Subsequent attempts	4 J/kg
Dextrose	$D_{25}W$ or $D_{50}W$	0.5–1 g/kg
Diazepam	Sedation	0.1 mg/kg
Digoxin	Three divided doses over 24 h	0.02–0.04 mg/kg
Dopamine	Infusion	2–20 µg/kg/min
Droperidol		0.01–0.05 mg/kg
Edrophonium	Depends on degree of paralysis	0.5–1 mg/kg
Ephedrine		0.1 mg/kg
Epinephrine	Bolus	0.01 mg/kg
	Infusion	0.1–1.0 µg/kg/min
Furosemide		0.2–1 mg/kg
Insulin	Infusion	0.02–0.1 units/kg/h
Isoproterenol	Infusion	0.1–1 µg/kg/min
Ketamine	Induction (IV)	1–2 mg/kg
	(IM)	5–10 mg/kg
Lidocaine	Loading	1 mg/kg
	Maintenance	20–50 µg/kg/min
Mannitol		0.25–1 g/kg
Meperidine	Pain relief (IV)	0.02–0.05 mg/kg
	Premedication (IM)	1 mg/kg
Methohexital	Induction (IV)	1–2 mg/kg
	(per rectum)	25–30 mg/kg
Metoclopramide		0.1 mg/kg
Morphine	Pain relief (IV)	0.02–0.05 mg/kg
	Premedication (IM)	0.1 mg/kg
Naloxone		0.01 mg/kg
Neostigmine	Depends on degree of paralysis	35–70 µg/kg
Nitroprusside	Infusion	0.5–8 µg/kg/min
Norepinephrine	Infusion	0.1–1 µg/kg/min
Pentobarbital	Premedication (IM)	4–6 mg/kg
Phenylephrine		1–2 µg/kg
Propranolol		0.01 mg/kg
Prostaglandin E_1	Infusion	0.1 µg/kg/min
Sodium bicarbonate		1–2 meq/kg
Succinylcholine	Intubation (IV)	1–2 mg/kg
	(IM)	4–6 mg/kg
Thiopental	Induction (IV)	3–6 mg/kg
	(per rectum)	25–30 mg/kg
Verapamil		0.1–0.3 mg/kg

* Dosages are for intravenous administration if not otherwise specified.
Source: Reproduced by permission from Morgan & Mikhail.[4]

spontaneous breathing the fresh gas flow must be increased to 100 to 300 mL/kg to prevent rebreathing.[40]

Advantages of the Bain system are there is less equipment to interfere with the surgical field, less likelihood of kinking the endotracheal tube due to its light weight, and the ability

Table 25–5
CLASSIFICATION OF ANESTHETIC BREATHING SYSTEMS

System	Gas Reservoir Bag	Rebreathing of Exhaled Gases	Chemical Neutralization of Carbon Dioxide	Unidirectional Valves	Fresh Gas Inflow Rate*
Open					
Insufflation	No	No	No	None	Unknown
Open drop	No	No	No	None	Unknown
Semiopen					
Mapleson A, B, C, D	Yes	No†	No	One	High
Bain	Yes	No†	No	One	High
Mapleson E	No	No†	No	None	High
Mapleson F (Jackson-Rees)	Yes	No†	No	One	High
Semiclosed					
Circle	Yes	Partial	Yes	Three	Moderate
Closed	Yes	Total	Yes	Three	Low

* High, greater than 6 L/min; moderate, 3–6 L/min; low, 0.3–0.5 L/min.
† No rebreathing of exhaled gases only when fresh gas inflow is adequate.
SOURCE: Reproduced by permission from Stoelting & Miller.[5]

to mount the circuit on the anesthesia machine and allow for scavenging of exhaled gases.[38]

Complications associated with the Bain system are increased resistance to breathing, rebreathing due to unrecognized disconnection of the inner tube, and absence of fresh gas flow due to unrecognized kinking of the inner tube.[40]

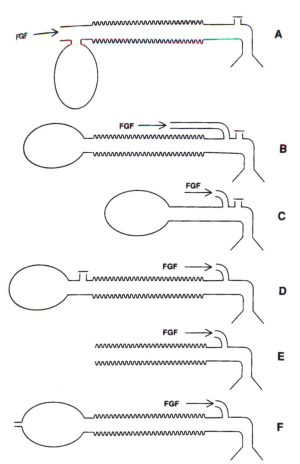

Figure 25–4 Anesthetic breathing systems classified as semiopen Mapleson A through F. (Reproduced by permission from Stoelting and Miller.[5])

Semiclosed systems are commonly used for both pediatric and adult patients. They provide for partial rebreathing and contain a system for neutralizing carbon dioxide. Advantages are conservation of some heat and moisture and lower fresh gas flows that can reduce the amount of inhalation agent used. Disadvantages of this system are increased resistance to breathing due to unidirectional valves and the carbon dioxide cannisters, less portability, and increased risk of malfunction.[37]

The circle system is the most common semiclosed breathing system. Components of this are:

1. Unidirectional inspiratory and expiratory valves
2. Inspiratory and expiratory corrugated tubing
3. Carbon dioxide cannister
4. Gas reservoir bag
5. Adjustable pressure-limiting valve
6. Airway pressure gauge
7. Oxygen analyzer
8. Scavenger system[41]

Pediatric circle systems must be designed to minimize dead space and resistance to breathing. They use short, narrow caliber hoses and smaller carbon dioxide absorbers.

ANESTHESIA MASKS

A mask increases dead space, which becomes a concern if the patient is not going to be intubated. The Randel-Baker mask decreases dead space, is molded to conform to many faces, and is low profile making procedures like probe and irrigation possible. Masks should be clear for better observation of the face for color and secretions.[40]

AIRWAYS

Oral and nasal airways are important to open an obstructed airway. The insertion of an oral airway must be done when the level of anesthesia is deep enough that the airway does not precipitate a laryngospasm. Nasal airways are usually better tolerated than the oral airway. An endotracheal tube may be used as a nasal airway if none is available. The length should be measured from the tip of the nose to the base of the ear.[40]

ENDOTRACHEAL TUBES

Endotracheal tubes decrease dead space of the natural extrathoracic airway. The endotracheal tube dramatically increases resistance to breathing. This is governed by the Hagen-Poiseuille law, which states that during laminar flow resistance is proportional to the length of the tube and inversely proportional to the fourth power of the radius.

Mucosal damage may occur due to an endotracheal tube that is too large for the trachea. In pediatric patients 1 mm of edema may narrow the airway by 33%, yet in an adult the same amount of edema narrows the airway only 3% to 9%.

The size of an endotracheal tube may be estimated; however, once inserted the presence of a leak must be assessed. It is best to have a leak at 20 to 25 cm H_2O.

Recommended sizes are:

< 1000 g	2.5
> 1000 g	3.0
neonate to 3 months	3.0
3–9 months	3.5
9–18 months	4.0
> 2 y	$\dfrac{age\ (y + 16)}{4}$

Cuffed tubes should not be used until the age of 8. A cuff will increase the outer diameter of the tube by 0.5 mm.

Rae tubes are frequently used for cases such as ear-nose-throat where it is necessary to have the tube curve away from the surgical field. These tubes are available with either oral or nasal bends in them.[40]

The length of the tube can be estimated at three times the internal diameter. The tube should be secured at the lip at this length. For example, a 4.0 endotracheal tube should be secured at 12 cm at the lip.

It should be kept in mind that flexion or extension of the neck will move the endotracheal tube 1.5 cm. This is important in cases such as tonsillectomy or thyroidectomy where the neck is hyperextended to perform the procedure.

LARYNGOSCOPE BLADES

The most common blade is the straight Miller blade, which makes intubation of the infant easier due to the cephalad larynx. For older children either a Miller or a Mac blade may be used. Many other available blades are modifications of the Miller blade.[40]

REFERENCES

1. Loftness SL. Pediatric anesthesia. In: Waugaman WR, Rigor B, Katz L, Bradshaw H, Garde J, eds. *Principles and Practice of Nurse Anesthesia.* East Norwalk, Conn: Appleton & Lange; 1988:401–409.
2. Motoyama EK. Special considerations of pediatric anesthesia. In: Motoyama EK, ed. *Smith's Anesthesia for Infants and Children.* 5th ed. St. Louis: CV Mosby; 1990:7–9.
3. Stoelting LC. Management of the airway. In: Barash PG, Cullen BF, Stoelting RK, eds. *Clinical Anesthesia.* 2nd ed. Philadelphia: JB Lippincott; 1992:686.
4. Morgan GE, Mikhail MS. Pediatric anesthesia. In: Morgan GE, Mikhail MS, eds. *Clinical Anesthesiology.* East Norwalk, Conn: Appleton & Lange; 1992:630–642.
5. Stoelting RK, Miller RD. Pediatrics. In: Stoelting RK, Miller RD, eds. *Basics of Anesthesia.* 3rd ed. New York: Churchill Livingstone, 1994:381–392.
6. Stoelting RK, Dierdorf SF. Diseases common to the pediatric patient. In: Stoelting RK, Dierdorf SF, eds. *Anesthesia and Co-Existing Disease.* 3rd ed. New York: Churchill Livingstone; 1993:579–627.
7. Berry FA. Neonatal anesthesia. In: Barash PG, Cullen BF, Stoelting RK, eds. *Clinical Anesthesia.* 2nd ed. Philadelphia: JB Lippincott; 1992:1308–1325.
8. Schieber RA. Cardiovascular physiology in infants and children. In: Motoyama EK, ed. *Smith's Anesthesia for Infants and Children.* 5th ed. St. Louis: CV Mosby; 1990:84–86.
9. Davis PJ. Temperature regulation in infants and children. In: Motoyama EK, ed. *Smith's Anesthesia for Infants and Children.* 5th ed. St. Louis: CV Mosby; 1990:146–156.
10. Cook DR. Pediatric anesthesia. In: Barash PG, Cullen BF, Stoelting RK, eds. *Clinical Anesthesia.* 2nd ed. Philadelphia: JB Lippincott; 1992:1335–1347.
11. Spear RM, Deshpande JK, Davis PJ. Systemic disorders in pediatric anesthesia. In: Motoyama EK, ed. *Smith's Anesthesia for Infants and Children.* 5th ed. St. Louis: CV Mosby; 1990:781–785.
12. Spear RM, Deshpande JK, Davis PJ. Anesthesia for general, urologic, and plastic surgery: In: Motoyama EK, ed. *Smith's Anesthesia for Infants and Children.* 5th ed. St. Louis: CV Mosby; 1990:603–606.
13. Bikhazi GB, Davis PJ. Anesthesia for neonates and premature infants. In: Motoyama EK, ed. *Smith's Anesthesia for Infants and Children.* 5th ed. St. Louis: CV Mosby; 1990:441–453.
14. Creasman M, Bradshaw M. Update for nurse anesthetists—anesthetic considerations for the burn patient. *AANA J.* 1995; 63:257–265.
15. Morgan GE, Mikhail MS. Anesthesia for the trauma patient. In: Morgan GE, Mikhail MS, eds. *Clinical Anesthesiology.* East Norwalk, Conn: Appleton & Lange; 1992:596–598.
16. Priano LL. Trauma and burns. In: Barash PG, Cullen BF, Stoelting RK, eds. *Clinical Anesthesia.* 2nd ed. Philadelphia: JB Lippincott; 1992:1421–1422.

17. Stensrud PE, VATER association and trisomy-21. In: Faust RJ, ed. *Anesthesiology Review*. 2nd ed. New York: Churchill Livingstone; 1994:438–439.

18. Cook DR, Davis PJ. Pharmacology of pediatric anesthesia. In: Motoyama EK, ed. *Smith's Anesthesia for Infants and Children*. 5th ed. St. Louis: CV Mosby; 1990:157–191.

19. Spear RM, Deshpande JK, Davis PJ. Anesthesia for general, urologic, and plastic surgery. In: Motoyama EK, ed. *Smith's Anesthesia for Infants and Children*. 5th ed. St. Louis: CV Mosby; 1990:592.

20. Friedhoff RJ. Pyloric stenosis. In: Faust RJ, ed. *Anesthesiology Review*. 2nd ed. New York: Churchill Livingstone; 1994;436–437.

21. Berry FA. Neonatal anesthesia. In: Barash PG, Cullen BF, Stoelting RK, eds. *Clinical Anesthesia*. 2nd ed. Philadelphia: JB Lippincott; 1992:1322–1329.

22. Feinstein R, Owens WD. Anesthesia for ear, nose and throat surgery. In: Barash PG, Cullen BF, Stoelting RK, eds. *Clinical Anesthesia*. 2nd ed. Philadelphia: JB Lippincott; 1992: 1118–1120.

23. Spear RM, Deshpande JK, Davis PJ. Anesthesia for general, urologic, and plastic surgery. In: Motoyama EK, ed. *Smith's Anesthesia for Infants and Children*. 5th ed. St. Louis: CV Mosby; 1990:607–609.

24. Wallender WH. Congenital pediatric airway problems. In: Faust RJ, ed. *Anesthesiology Review*. 2nd ed. New York: Churchill Livingstone; 1994:416–417.

25. Wallender WH. Congenital diaphragmatic hernia. In: Faust RJ, ed. *Anesthesiology Review*. 2nd ed. New York: Churchill Livingstone; 1994:429–431.

26. Bikhazi GB, Davis PJ. Anesthesia for neonates and premature infants. In: Motoyama EK, ed. *Smith's Anesthesia for Infants and Children*. 5th ed. St. Louis: CV Mosby; 1990:441–452.

27. Binegar WG. Other neonatal emergencies: tracheoesophageal fistual, omphalocele. In: Faust RJ, ed. *Anesthesiology Review*. 2nd ed. New York: Churchill Livingstone; 1994:432–433.

28. Stoelting RK, Miller RD. Ophthalmology and otolaryngology. In Stoelting RK, Miller RD, eds. *Basics of Anesthesia*. 3rd ed. New York: Churchill Livingstone; 1994:345–346.

29. Christopherson TJ. Succinylcholine and strabismus surgery. In: Faust RJ, ed. *Anesthesiology Review*. 2nd ed. New York: Churchill Livingstone; 1994:535–538.

30. McGoldrick KE. Anesthesia for ophthalmic surgery. In: Motoyama EK, ed. *Smith's Anesthesia for Infants and Children*. 5th ed. St. Louis: CV Mosby; 1990:633.

31. McGoldrick KE. Anesthesia and the eye. In: Barash PG, Cullen BE, Stoelting RK, eds. *Clinical Anesthesia*. 2nd ed. Philadelphia: JB Lippincott; 1992:1107–1109.

32. Cohen SE. Evaluation of the neonate, resuscitation of the newborn. In: Shnider SM, Levinson G, eds. *Anesthesia for Obstetrics*. 2nd ed. Baltimore: Williams & Wilkins;1 984; 489–520.

33. Stoelting RK, Miller RD. Obstetrics. In: Stoelting RK, Miller RD, eds. *Basics of Anesthesia*. 3rd ed. New York: Churchill Livingstone; 1994:376–378.

34. Morgan GE, Mikhail MS. Obstetric anesthesia. In: Morgan GE, Mikhail MS, eds. *Clinical Anesthesiology*. East Norwalk, Conn: Appleton & Lange; 1992:626–627.

35. Lockwood SA. Meconium aspiration. In Faust, RJ, ed. *Anesthesiology Review*. 2nd ed. New York: Churchill Livingstone; 1994:427.

36. Woodworth GE. Neonatal resuscitation. In Faust RJ, ed. *Anesthesiology Review*. 2nd ed. New York: Churchill Livingstone; 1994:468–469.

37. Stoelting RK, Miller RD. Anesthesia systems. In Stoelting RK, Miller RD, eds. *Basics of Anesthesia*. 3rd ed. New York: Churchill Livingstone; 1994:133–138.

38. Reed KS. Pediatric breathing circuits. In: Faust RJ, ed. *Anesthesiology Review*. 2nd ed. New York: Churchill Livingstone; 1994:444–446.

39. Andrews JJ. Anesthesia systems. In: Barash PG, Cullen BF, Stoelting RK, eds. *Clinical Anesthesia*. 2nd ed. Philadelphia: JB Lippincott; 1992:653–657.

40. Steven JM, Cohen DE. Anesthesia equipment and monitoring. In: Motoyama EK, ed. *Smith's Anesthesia for Infants and Children*. 5th ed. St. Louis: CV Mosby; 1990:218–232.

41. Morgan GE, Mikhail MS. Breathing systems. In: Morgan GE, Mikhail MS, eds. *Clinical Anesthesiology*. East Norwalk, Conn: Appleton & Lange; 1992:23–31.

☐ QUESTIONS

1. In the term infant which one of the following is correct regarding respiratory parameters?
   a. Decreased FRC, increased closing volume, increased oxygen requirements, decreased carbon dioxide production
   b. Increased FRC, increased closing volume, decreased oxygen requirements, increased carbon dioxide production
   c. Decreased FRC, decreased closing volume, increased oxygen requirements, increased carbon dioxide production
   d. Increased FRC, increased closing volume, decreased oxygen requirement, decreased carbon dioxide production

2. The mechanism that causes the greatest amount of heat loss in the operating room:
   a. Evaporation
   b. Radiation
   c. Convection
   d. Conduction

3. The major determinate of cardiac output in the infant is:
   a. Preload
   b. Afterload
   c. Heart rate
   d. Contractility

4. The Bain system is a modification of which other system?
   a. Mapleson A
   b. Mapleson B
   c. Mapleson C
   d. Mapleson D

5. The amount of fluid required in the first 24 hours after a 15-kg patient sustains 50% burns of the body is:
   a. 1000 mL
   b. 1200 mL
   c. 1500 mL
   d. 3000 mL

6. An awake intubation *may* be required in all of the following *except?*
   a. Pyloric stenosis
   b. Diaphragmatic hernia
   c. Cleft palate
   d. Down's syndrome

7. The incidence of accompanying congenital anomalies is highest with:
   a. Omphalocele
   b. Gastroschisis
   c. Diaphragmatic hernia
   d. Cleft palate

8. All the following are true about the oculocardiac reflex *except?*
   a. More common in the adult than the pediatric patient
   b. May be caused by traction on the rectus muscle
   c. May be caused by hemorrhage
   d. Mediated afferently by the trigeminal nerve and efferently by the vagus nerve

9. A neonate is born with meconium staining; the proper action is to:
   a. Suction oralpharynx and stimulate
   b. Intubate, suction, intubate, suction until clear then stimulate to breathe
   c. Ambu with 100% oxygen
   d. Stimulate to cough

10. The infant's spinal cord ends at what level?
    a. L-1
    b. L-2
    c. L-3
    d. L-4

11. A patient who is returning to the operating room due to a tonsillar bleed after tonsillectomy and adenoidectomy should have the following induction?
    a. Inhalation with halothane
    b. Ketamine, succinylcholine, Sellick maneuver, intubate
    c. Diprivan, Norcuron, ventilate, intubate
    d. Ketamine, Pavulon, ventilate, intubate

12. Which is the *incorrect* management of a 4-year-old patient presenting with epiglottitis?
    a. Mask induction with halothane
    b. Maintain in sitting position.
    c. Have a tracheostomy set and an ENT surgeon available
    d. Intubate in the emergency room

13. The proper placement of an endotracheal tube in the patient with a tracheoesophageal fistula is:

a. Right mainstem bronchus
b. Above the carina but below the fistula
c. Above the carina and above the fistula
d. Left mainstem bronchus

14. Fetal hemoglobin has a P_{50} that is:
    a. Higher than the adult value
    b. 26
    c. 19
    d. 50

15. Which of the following is true about croup?
    a. It is viral.
    b. It is bacterial.
    c. It is a surgical emergency.
    d. It is caused by *Haemophilus* B.

16. Which is true about succinylcholine?
    a. It may be used on burn patients on the tenth day postburn.
    b. It causes bradycardia more in the adult patient than the pediatric patient.
    c. It is contraindicated for the patient with an acute AP.
    d. It interferes with the forced duction test in patients with strabismus.

17. A patient with a diaphragmatic hernia presents to the operating room; all of the following are correct *except:*
    a. Decompress the stomach with a nasogastric tube
    b. Awake intubation
    c. Inflate the affected lung after the repair has been done
    d. Avoid N_2O during the procedure

18. Minimal alveolar concentration is lowest in which group of patients?
    a. Adolescents
    b. 29-week preterm infants
    c. Full-term infants
    d. Toddlers

19. The amount of succinylcholine needed for the pediatric patient is:
    a. The same as for an adult
    b. Less than for an adult
    c. Two times the adult dose
    d. Four times the adult dose

20. The patient with a pyloric stenosis will present to the hospital with projectile vomiting and which of the following electrolyte abnormalities?
    a. Hyperchloremic, hypokalemic, metabolic acidosis
    b. Hyperchloremic, hyperkalemic, metabolic alkalosis
    c. Hypokalemic, hypochloremic, metabolic alkalosis
    d. Hypokalemic, hypochloremic, metabolic acidosis

☐ ANSWERS

1.	c	**5.**	d	**9.**	b	**13.**	b	**17.**	c
2.	b	**6.**	d	**10.**	c	**14.**	c	**18.**	b
3.	c	**7.**	a	**11.**	b	**15.**	a	**19.**	c
4.	d	**8.**	a	**12.**	d	**16.**	d	**20.**	c

CHAPTER
26

Obstetric Anesthesia

Joan Fox

☐ ANATOMY AND PHYSIOLOGY

Pregnancy produces many physiologic changes in every maternal organ system. These changes alter the normal response to anesthesia, creating unique challenges in the anesthesia management of the obstetric patient. The anesthetist is caring for two patients—the mother and the fetus.

AIRWAY AND RESPIRATORY CHANGES

The changes in airway physiology of the parturient are of primary concern for the anesthetist. Vascular engorgement of the respiratory mucosa may predispose to difficult anatomic visualization during laryngoscopy. Small endotracheal tubes are used because trauma, obstruction, and bleeding can occur during instrumentation and intubation.

The physiologic respiratory changes during pregnancy include an increase in oxygen consumption and minute ventilation, up to 50%. This leads to rapid induction in these patients. Tidal volume and respiratory rate also increase. Anatomic and physiologic changes during pregnancy lead to alterations in pulmonary function, ventilation, and gas exchange.[1] Because of an elevation of the diaphragm by the gravid uterus, functional residual capacity is decreased by 15% to 20%, leading to an increased shunt fraction and less oxygen reserve. Airway closure exists in 30% of parturients during tidal ventilation. These factors can lead to a rapid decrease in PaO_2 during induction, despite preoxygenation.[2]

CARDIOVASCULAR CHANGES

The cardiovascular system is continuously and progressively stressed during pregnancy. Cardiovascular components are increased to meet the heightened demands of maternal and fetal metabolism. During the first trimester, cardiac output is increased approximately 30% to 40%. An additional slight increase occurs during the second trimester. The greatest increase (up to 50%) in cardiac output is seen during labor and immediately after delivery. This increase in cardiac output is due to a 15% increase in heart rate and a 30% increase in stroke volume. Blood pressure is not increased during normal pregnancy because of a 21% decrease in systemic vascular resistance and a 34% decrease in pulmonary vascular resistance.[3] A decrease in systemic vascular resistance is observed with a lower systolic blood pressure and a greater diastolic blood pressure in the second trimester. Cardiac output does not return to normal until approximately 2 weeks after delivery.[1]

In the supine position, the gravid uterus compresses the aorta and inferior vena cava, obstructing venous return to the heart. This creates a decrease in cardiac output, usually seen around the 28th week of pregnancy. Ten percent to 15% of women become hypotensive and diaphoretic when placed in the supine position, developing supine hypotensive syndrome. A decrease in uterine blood flow may result in fetal asphyxia.

Aortocaval compression is a significant but preventable cause of fetal distress. The combination of hypotension, increased uterine venous pressure, and decreased uterine blood flow can produce fetal distress. This can be easily prevented by placing a wedge 15° under the right hip of the supine parturient at 28 weeks or longer gestation. This maneuver causes left uterine displacement, greatly improving uterine arterial perfusion and increasing oxygen delivery to the fetus. If hypotension is not restored in 1 to 2 minutes after left uterine displacement, ephedrine, which preserves uterine blood flow, should be administered in 5- to 10-mg increments. Systolic blood pressure should be maintained at or above 100 mm Hg.

GASTROINTESTINAL TRACT

Anatomic and hormonal changes during pregnancy place the parturient at high risk for esophageal regurgitation and pulmonary aspiration. The upward displacement of the stomach by the uterus causes increased intragastric pressure and incompetence of the gastroesophageal sphincter. *Progesterone* inhibits gastric motility and food absorption, leading to decreased gastric emptying. Gastric emptying time is also prolonged by labor, apprehension, and pain. Pulmonary aspiration of gastric contents with a pH of 2.5 or less, in a quantity greater than 0.4 mL/kg is associated with the development of *Mendelson's syndrome.*[4] Mendelson's syndrome is characterized by an increase in aveolar-arterial oxygen gradient, bronchospasm, and pulmonary edema, which eventually can lead to adult respiratory distress syndrome. Gastric pH can be rapidly elevated above 2.5 with the oral administration of 30 mL of a clear, nonparticulate, antacid such as sodium citrate. This effect can last for an hour or more in most parturients.[4] The H_2 blockers are reliable in raising pH and lowering gastric volume, but they require 60 to 90 minutes for optimal effect. In an emergency induction of general anesthesia, their protection against aspiration is limited.

INTRAVASCULAR BLOOD VOLUME

At term, maternal blood volume has increased by 1000 to 1500 mL (approximately 85 to 90 mL/kg). This increased blood volume allows women to easily tolerate the blood loss associated with delivery. The average blood loss of a normal vaginal delivery is 400 to 600 mL. The blood loss is approximately doubled with the delivery of twins. The average cesarean section blood loss is 800 to 1000 mL. The dilutional anemia of pregnancy is caused by an increase in plasma volume coupled with an increase in red cell mass. Hemoglobin levels average between 10 and 12 g/dL and hematocrit levels between 30 and 36 mL/dL. The reduction of hemoglobin is offset by the increase in cardiac output. In terms of tissue oxygen delivery, this shifts the hemoglobin dissociation curve to the *right*. A rightward shift lowers oxygen affinity. This displaces oxygen from hemoglobin, making more oxygen available to the tissues. The pregnant woman becomes hypercoagulable as gestation progresses, related to an increase in the clotting factor substrate. This physiologic mechanism is needed to avoid excessive maternal blood loss at delivery.[3]

CENTRAL NERVOUS SYSTEM

The physiologic changes of the central nervous system (CNS) during pregnancy have an effect on the anesthetic requirement for parturients. Progesterone, which rises to a level 20 times normal at term, has a *sedative* effect on the mother, decreasing anesthetic needs. The minimum aveolar

concentration (MAC) requirement for inhalation agents progressively decreases during pregnancy (halothane by 25% and isoflurane up to 40%). A surge in β-endorphin levels may also decrease MAC.[1]

Intrathecal and epidural local anesthetic requirements are also decreased. The enhanced sensitivity to local anesthetics is related to the engorgement of the epidural venous plexus. This engorgement decreases the volume of subarachnoid and epidural spaces. Other factors include the increased sensitivity of nerve fibers or enhanced diffusion of local anesthetics to membrane receptor sites.

The pregnant patient has an altered metabolism of protein, carbohydrates, and fat in favor of fetal growth and development. This alteration increases the overall basal metabolic rate of the parturient.

UTERINE BLOOD FLOW

Uterine blood flow increases throughout pregnancy and at term is approximately 700 mL/min. This represents 10% of the cardiac output. About 80% of the uterine blood flow passes through the intervillous space. The remainder mostly supplies the myometrium. Autoregulation is absent during pregnancy because the uterine vasculature is maximally dilated. *Uterine blood flow equals the uterine artery pressure minus the uterine venous pressure divided by uterine vascular resistance.*[5]

Three major factors are responsible for a decrease in uterine blood flow during pregnancy:

1. Hypotension (caused by aortocaval compression, hypovolemia, or sympathetic blockade)
2. Vasoconstriction (stress-induced release of catecholamines)
3. Uterine contractions (hypertonic contractions or Pitocin infusions compromise blood flow)[1]

INNERVATION

Uterine contractions and cervical dilation are the two components responsible for pain in the first stage of labor. Pain impulses travel along the visceral afferent fibers via the sympathetic nerves to the spinal cord where they enter at T-10 to L-1. Stretching of the perineum, caused by the beginning of fetal descent, produces the pain that occurs in the second stage of labor. The pudendal nerve provides sensory innervation of the perineum through segments S-2 to S-4.

☐ PATHOPHYSIOLOGY

PRE-ECLAMPSIA

Pre-eclampsia is a characterized by hypertension, proteinuria, and edema and is referred to as toxemia of pregnancy. Symptoms of pre-eclampsia or pregnancy-induced hypertension usually appear after the 20th week of pregnancy and usually resolve within 48 hours of delivery of the fetus. If grand mal convulsions accompany this hypertensive disorder, the condition is known as eclampsia.

Although the cause is still unclear, many authors suggest that pre-eclampsia is related to an immunologic rejection of fetal tissue causing placental vasculitis and ischemia. Miller discusses that the cause of pre-eclampsia is thought to be related to decreased placental perfusion. This results in an increased production of renin, angiotension, aldosterone, and thromboplastin and the placental imbalance of the prostaglandins prostacycline and thromboxane.[5] This alteration in prostaglandin metabolism causes vasoconstriction and intravascular volume depletion despite the retention of sodium and water, resulting in generalized edema. Severe pregnancy-induced hypertension significantly increases both maternal and fetal mortality and morbidity. Endothelial damage increases platelet adherence, which may lead to coagulopathies or disseminated intravascular coagulation (DIC). An elevation of liver enzymes is one of the hallmarks of the *HELLP* (hemolysis, elevated liver enzymes, low platelet count) *syndrome*. This syndrome has been described in pre-eclampsia usually occurring before 36 weeks' gestation.[3] Symptoms of worsening pre-eclampsia include CNS manifestations such as headache, visual disturbances, or seizures, as well as hepatic capsular distention that manifests as epigastric pain. The disease can progress rapidly with the development of liver and renal failure. The most common causes of death are pulmonary edema and cerebral hemorrhage.[1] The best treatment of pre-eclampsia is prompt delivery of the fetus. Management goals include:

1. Prevention of seizure
2. Reduction of blood pressure
3. Improvement of uteroplacental perfusion

Magnesium sulfate is used to treat the signs and symptoms of pre-eclampsia: hyperreflexia, convulsions, and irritability of the CNS. MgSO4 reduces the *presynaptic* release of acetylcholine, which decreases the hyperactivity at the neuromuscular junction. The therapeutic range is 4 to 6 mg/L. MgSO4 may cause skeletal muscle weakness, respiratory depression, and cardiac arrest. Patients receiving MgSO4 are more sensitive to depolarizing and nondepolarizing muscle relaxants. Intravenous calcium chloride or gluconate may counteract the adverse effects of MgSO4 in the newborn and the mother.[6] The treatment of seizures seen in the eclamptic patient consists of oxygenation, ventilation, and intravenous administration of 50 to 150 mg thiopental. Diazepam is not used because it readily crosses the placenta to cause neonatal depression (hypotonia, hypothermia, and decreased respirations).

Ideally, patients with severe eclampsia should have a central venous pressure or pulmonary artery catheter placed for fluid management. The patient should be well hydrated before the use of epidural, caudal, or spinal anesthesia.

The use of regional anesthesia for the patient with pre-eclampsia or eclampsia is controversial. Some authors believe that regional anesthesia may further compromise uteroplacental circulation secondary to the sympathetic block and maternal hypotension. Still other clinicians recommend epidural anesthesia for a cesarean section in the pre-eclampic patient who is volume repleated and has normal clotting factors. A continuous epidural is thought to control blood pressure and pain and to increase renal and uterine perfusion. To avoid the risk of epidural hematoma, coagulation studies should be performed prior to the block. A platelet count should be above 100,000/mm3 before a regional block is performed. Coagulopathies (platelet counts less than 100,000/mm3) are managed with the transfusion of platelets, fresh-frozen plasma, and cryoprecipitate, as needed. Platelet counts of 35,000/mm3 are consistent with cerebral hemorrhage and even death.

General anesthesia may be necessary for emergency cesarean section in the event of fetal distress. Soft-tissue edema, periglottic swelling, and systemic and pulmonary hypertension are all factors that may increase the patient's risks under anesthesia.

PLACENTA PREVIA

The major cause of maternal mortality is hemorrhage. Placental previa is painless, bright red bleeding after the seventh month of pregnancy. Placenta previa occurs when the placenta is implanted at or very near to the cervical os. The placenta prematurely separates from the myometrium during cervical dilation. The anesthetist should be prepared with a double setup for both general or regional anesthesia in the case of an emergency cesarean section when the diagnosis of placenta previa is being made. Profound maternal hemorrhagic shock can result from placental bleeding. If the diagnosis of placenta previa is confirmed, and the patient is actively bleeding, an emergency cesarean section under general anesthesia is performed immediately.[3] If the patient is hypotensive, intravenous ketamine (0.75 mg/kg) can be used for induction. Blood volume and fluid balance must be restored prior to induction. If the diagnosis of placenta previa is confirmed and the patient is not bleeding, cesarean section is still performed at this time, but regional anesthesia can be used if no evidence of hypovolemia is present.

ABRUPTIO PLACENTA

Abruptio placenta is seen as dark red, painful vaginal bleeding and is caused by the premature separation of the placenta before birth. Ths is the most common cause of DIC in pregnancy. Consumption of coagulation factors and activation of the fibrinolytic system occur frequently and should be treated with colloids (fresh-frozen plasma, and cryoprecipitate). The anesthetist must be prepared for an emergency cesarean section with major bleeding. Regional anesthesia is contraindicated for patients in hypovolemic shock or with severe coagulation abnormalities.

UTERINE RUPTURE

Uterine rupture is uncommon (1/3000 deliveries) but can occur during labor from:

1. Dehiscense of a scar from a previous cesarean section, extensive myomectomy or uterine reconstruction
2. Intrauterine manipulation (forceps)
3. Spontaneous rupture after prolonged labor in patients with hypertonic contractions[1]

Uterine rupture presents as either frank hemorrhage or as hypotension with occult bleeding in the abdomen. Severe abdominal pain and cessation of fetal heart tones are also observed. Treatment requires volume resuscitation and immediate laparotomy under general anesthesia.[1]

AMNIOTIC FLUID EMBOLISM

Amniotic fluid embolism occurs in 1/20,000 to 30,000 deliveries and in most cases is fatal. Ten percent of maternal deaths result from amniotic fluid embolism. The pathology involves a tear through the amnion or chorion. This opens uterine or endocervical veins at a pressure sufficient to force fluid into the venous circulation. Major manifestations are pulmonary embolism, DIC, and uterine atony.[2] Diagnosis is established by fetal elements in maternal circulation (autopsy). It is clinically suggested by respiratory distress, shock, hemorrhage from DIC, and coma. Pulmonary edema, cyanosis, altered mental status, and seizures may be present. Treatment is directed at aggressive cardiopulmonary resuscitation and delivery of the fetus.[2]

INVERTED UTERUS

The reported incidence of inverted uterus is approximately 1/1700 deliveries.[7] The inverted uterus actually turns inside out so the placenta surface appears on the outside. Inversion may be partial with the fundus inverted inside the lower uterine segment, or complete with the uterus turned inside out protruding from the vagina. Inversion produces profuse continuous postpartum bleeding.

Treatment of uterine inversion consists of immediate reduction of the inversion with restoration of intravascular volume. Continued firm pressure against the fundus from inside the uterus is necessary for reduction; uterine relaxation may be required for this manipulation. If the uterus has become tightly contracted on itself, general anesthesia with a volatile agent (usually halothane) may be required. However, a patient who has been bleeding from an inverted uterus may be so hypovolemic despite vigorous resuscitation that a high concentration of halothane may be unwise, leading to profound vasodilation and hypotension. Halothane concentrations above 1.6% reversibly relax the uterus and block the response to oxytocin infusion. Forane also produces uterine relaxation, but to a lesser extent, as compared to halothane. *Nitroglycerin* administered intravenously as a bolus in doses from 50 to 150 μg provides successful uterine relaxation for removal of retained placenta, breech extraction, and replacement of an inverted uterus.[8]

☐ PHARMACOLOGY

INHALATION AGENTS

The MAC requirement progressively decreases by as much as 40% during pregnancy. When general anesthesia is required, 50% O_2 and N_2O is generally administered with 1.0% enflurane, 0.75% isoflurane, or 0.5% halothane to prevent maternal recall. Volatile inhalation anesthetics decrease blood pressure and consequently decrease uteroplacental blood flow. However, in concentrations less than 1 MAC, effects are generally minor.

INTRAVENOUS AGENTS

Nearly all narcotics, analgesics, and sedatives cross the placenta and have an effect on the fetus. Fetal depression limits the use of these agents to early stages of labor.

Meperidine is the most commonly used narcotic. It can be given in doses of 12.5 to 25 mg intravenously. Maximum maternal and fetal respiratory depression is seen in 10 to 20 minutes. Meperidine is administered 4 hours prior to delivery because fetal levels are the *highest* 2 to 3 hours after the mother receives the drug.

Fentanyl 1 μg/kg provides prompt pain relief without severe neonatal depression. *Ketamine* provides adequate analgesia in 2 to 5 minutes without neonatal depression. (Fetal depression can be seen with doses as small as 1 mg/kg.) *Diazepam* is no longer used in labor because of its potential for profound neonatal depression. The anesthetic properties of benzodiazepines are undesirable for labor and delivery for women who want to remember their delivery.

Nondepolarizing muscle relaxants can be safely used in general anesthesia because of their low lipid solubility and increased molecular weight. These properties prevent the drug from crossing the placenta and paralyzing the fetus.

Succinylcholine can be safely used for intubation and general anesthesia for cesarean section. A prolonged block may be related to a normal decrease in plasma cholinesterase during pregnancy. *Sodium pentathol,* less than 4 mg/kg, crosses the placenta but can be safely used in general anesthesia. *Promethazine* (Phenergan) provides sedation and reduces anxiety and incidence of nausea. It does not attenuate neonatal depression when combined with meperidine. *Naloxone* 0.01 mg/kg intravenously or intramuscularly may be administered to the newborn to reverse opioid depression. It should not be given to neonates whose mothers are addicted to narcotics.

REGIONAL AGENTS

Local anesthetic requirements in the obstetric patient are lowered by 30% to 50% of the normal dose. Regional techniques using the epidural or intrathecal route are the most popular methods of pain relief during labor and delivery. Traditionally, regional anesthesia is believed to prolong labor if administered too early. Studies show that epidural or spinal anesthesia up to T-10 has little effect on labor once the patient is in the active phase.

The best time to initiate the block in primiparas in when the cervix is dilated *5 to 6 cm* because this does not appear to alter the course of labor. The proper time to initiate regional anesthesia in multiparas is at cervical dilation of *3 to 4 cm*.[9]

α AND β AGONISTS/ANTAGONISTS

Uterine muscle has both α and β receptors. α-Receptor stimulation causes uterine contraction; β_2-receptor stimulation produces relaxation. *Phenylephrine* is an α-adrenergic agent that can cause uterine arterial constriction and even tetanic uterine contractions. *Ephedrine* stimulates both α and β receptors but is β predominant. It increases blood pressure by vasoconstriction, but its major action is from cardiac stimulation. Peripheral and uterine blood flow increases. Ephedrine maintains uterine perfusion, and it is the drug of choice for obstetric anesthesia.

TOCOLYTICS

Terbutaline and ritodrine are selective β_2 agonists, used to inhibit preterm labor and produce myometrial inhibition, bronchodilation, and vasodilation. The undesirable effects include tachycardia, hypotension, and restlessness. In general, tocolytics are used for fetal and gestational ages between 20 and 36 weeks, cervical dilation less than 4 cm, and cervical effacement less than 80%.

OXYTONICS

The primary use of oxytonics is to stimulate uterine contraction, to augment labor, or to control postpartum bleeding and uterine atony. The most frequently used drugs include oxytocin, which originates from the posterior pituitary, or Pitocin, a synthetic version of the hormone. Oxytocin acts on uterine smooth muscle to stimulate both frequency and force of contractions. It decreases systolic and diastolic blood pressure and causes tachycardia. An antidiuretic effect can be seen in high doses, leading to water intoxication, cerebral edema, and convulsions.[2]

☐ ANESTHESIA TECHNIQUES

GENERAL ANESTHESIA

Because of the risk of pulmonary aspiration and failed intubation, general anesthesia is indicated only when an emergency delivery is necessary (Table 26–1) or if the mother refuses regional anesthesia. Indications for general anesthesia include fetal distress during the second stage, tetanic uterine contractions, breech extraction, version and extraction, manual removal of retained placenta, and replacement of inverted uterus.[1] In the event of a general anesthetic, excessive hyperventilation should be avoided because this misadventure leads to a reduction in uterine and umbilical blood flow, in addition to an increased affinity of oxygen to maternal hemoglobin and less placental transfer. Risks and benefits of general anesthesia are listed in Table 26–2.

REGIONAL ANESTHESIA

Regional techniques using an epidural catheter or intrathecal route combined with local anesthetics and narcotics are the

---

Table 26–1
GENERAL ANESTHESIA TECHNIQUE FOR EMERGENCY DELIVERY

1. Place wedge under the right hip for left uterine displacement.
2. Preoxygenate for 3–5 min with 100% O_2.
3. Defasciculation with curare or nondepolarizer not necessary (most pregnant patients do not fasciculate).
4. Administer 500–1000 mL of a nonglucose balanced salt solution via a large-bore IV.
5. Rapid sequence induction. Cricoid pressure (once abdomen has been prepped and draped and surgeons are ready). Induction proceeds with 4 mg/kg IV thiopental followed immediately by 1.5 mg/kg IV Anectine.
6. Laryngoscopy and intubation performed using 6–7 mm endotracheal tube. (Have a plan for handling unexpected difficult intubation.)
7. After successful intubation, bilateral breath sounds confirmed, 1–2 MAC of any inhalation agent. O_2 50% with N_2O (if oxygenating well).
8. If skeletal muscle relation necessary, atracurium, vecuronium, or Anectine drip may be used.
9. Potent inhalation agents are discontinued once the umbilical cord has been clamped (may cause uterine atony) or decrease to 0.5 MAC.
10. Oxytocin infusion started, 20–40 U/L.
11. Skeletal muscle relaxants reversed. Patient extubated when awake and meets extubation criteria.

Table 26–2
GENERAL ANESTHESIA RISKS AND BENEFITS

Risks	Benefits
1. Maternal aspiration and inability to intubate the trachea remain the major causes of maternal morbidity and mortality.	1. Rapid induction
2. Fetal depression from sedation	2. Control over airway
3. Maternal hyperventilation, leading to fetal hypoxemia and acidoses	3. Less hypotension than regional

SOURCE: Reproduced by permission from Wadlington.[2]

most popular for effective management of pain during labor and delivery.[1] Continuous lumbar epidural anesthesia is the most versatile technique because it can be used for anesthesia in the first stage of labor (pain relief), vaginal delivery, or cesarean section if necessary. Pain in the first stage requires T-10 to L-1 sensory level (1.2 mL of local anesthetic per dermatone). A cesarean section requires a T-4 sensory level block.

Single-shot epidural, spinal, or caudal anesthesia is appropriate in the second stage of labor to initiate pain relief just prior to vaginal delivery. Administration of 5 to 10 mL of the original local anesthetic through the epidural catheter can extend analgesia to the sacral segments, S-2 to S-4, during the second stage of labor.

CAUDAL

This form of epidural analgesia has become less popular for use during labor. It requires 15 to 20 mL local anesthetic to reach the T-10 level. This technique blocks the sacral spinal cord segments. It can inhibit proper rotation of the fetal head in the second stage. Caudal epidural anesthesia is technically more difficult to perform with many anatomic variations in the sacral vertebrae. Is is especially difficult to locate in obese patients.[7]

☐ ANESTHESIA PROCEDURES

CESAREAN DELIVERY

Cesarean section can be performed under general or regional anesthesia. No one anesthetic technique causes fetal hypoxia/acidosis as does uterine incision to delivery time greater than 90 seconds (Tables 26–3 and 26–4).

NORMAL, SPONTANEOUS VAGINAL DELIVERY

Systemic drugs administered during labor are generally used in the first and second stages of labor. Sedative tranquilizers are used, either alone or in combination with a narcotic during the first stage of labor. Narcotics are used to relieve pain during the first and second stages of labor. In the past, ketamine was used in small doses as an analgesic during the second stage of labor. However, the use of ketamine is now discouraged because of its hallucinogenic effects on the mother.

Table 26–3
INDICATIONS FOR CESAREAN DELIVERY

1. Fetal distress
2. Regional anesthesia contraindicated
3. Need for uterine relaxation
4. Massive bleeding, uterine rupture, etc.

Table 26–4
REGIONAL ANESTHESIA FOR CESAREAN SECTION

1. Less neonatal exposure to drugs
2. Decreased pulmonary aspiration
3. Less need for systemic pain medications
4. Awake mother can bond with baby
5. Epidural catheter for postoperative pain relief (cesarean section requires T-4 sensory level)

Barbituates have lost their popularity because of their prolonged depressant effects on the neonate.

Regional Anesthesia for Normal Vaginal Delivery Regional blocks for labor and vaginal delivery are the most commonly used techniques for analgesia. Regional blocks provide pain relief while allowing the parturient to be awake to experience the delivery. Regional anesthesia is less likely to produce drug-induced depression in the fetus or aspiration pneumonitis in the mother. The most common forms of regional anesthesia for normal vaginal delivery are spinal, lumbar epidural, caudal, paracervical, pudendal, and local perineal infiltration.

Paracervical Block
This is usually performed by the obstetrician to provide analgesia during the first stage of labor. Local anesthetic is injected via the submucosa into the fornix of the vagina lateral to the cervix. This technique should anesthetize all the viceral sensory nerve fibers from the uterus, cervix, and upper fibers. The somatic sensory nerve fibers are not blocked.

The major disadvantage of the paracervical block is the high incidence of fetal bradycardia that occurs after the block. This bradycardia is associated with fetal acidosis, decreased oxygenation, and an increased likelihood of neonatal depression. Bradycardia may be related to decreased uterine blood flow caused by constriction of the uterine artery and high levels of local anesthetics in fetal blood.[5]

Pudendal Nerve Blocks
These blocks are most often given by obstetricians to provide perineal anesthesia during the second stage of labor. A block of S-2 to S-4 nerves is useful during delivery in combination with other techniques.

Spinal Anesthesia
Because of the profound motor paralysis that it induces, spinal anesthesia (Table 26–5) is limited to delivery. Lidocaine 5% using 30 to 50 mg is injected with the patient in the sitting position, often called a saddle block. Postdural puncture headache is believed to be caused by a leak of cerebrospinal fluid (CSF) through a puncture in the dura from the spinal needle. The size of the needle used is thought to affect the leakage of CSF from the needle hole. This is especially true in younger women, who are at a greater risk for postdural puncture headache for this reason. A 26-gauge spinal

Table 26–5
SPINAL ANESTHESIA

Techniques for spinal anesthesia (saddle block). Initiate just prior to delivery:
1. Fluid bolus 500–1000 mL
2. Patient sitting or left lateral decubitus
3. 25-, 26-, or 22-gauge Whitacre needle decreases likelihood of postdural puncture headache
4. Hyperbaric tetracaine 3–4 mg or lidocaine 20–40 mg, for perineal anesthesia
5. T-10 sensory level

SOURCE: Reproduced by permission from Morgan and Mikhail.[1]

needle is recommended to decrease the incidence of postdural puncture headache in these patients.

Epidural Anesthesia

Segmental epidural anesthesia (Table 26–6) uses a catheter in the lumbar epidural space, which provides pain relief at T-10 to L-1. This can be extended to S-2 to S-4 to provide analgesia during delivery. The epidural catheter has become the most common method of providing anesthesia for normal vaginal delivery. The most frequent complication of spinal and epidural anesthesia is maternal hypotension (systolic blood pressure less than 100 mm Hg or 20% decrease). Hypotension can be avoided with prehydration using 500 to 1000 mL of balanced salt solution and left uterine displacement to prevent aortocaval compression.

NONOBSTETRIC PROCEDURES

Pregnant women undergoing nonobstetric procedures require special anesthetic management to avoid injury to the fetus. The basic management goals are:

Table 26–6
REGIONAL ANESTHESIA TECHNIQUE

Epidural activation:
1. IV administration of H_2-receptor antagonist or 30 mL sodium citrate
2. Administer 1000–1500 mL IV bolus lactated Ringer's (15–20 mL/kg via large-bore IV)
3. Epidural space identified L-2–L-3 or L-3–L-4 in sitting position. (If supine, maintain left lateral decubitus.)
4. Give 3–4 mL test dose of local anesthetic 1.5% lidocaine with 1:200,000 epinephrine. (Local anesthetic choices vary. Barash recommends lidocaine 45 mg with 15 μg epinephrine.)
5. Observe for signs of intravascular injection (60 s) or intrathecal injection (3–5 min).
6. After 3–5 min if signs of intravascular or intrathecal injection are absent, may give additional 10–15 mL of local anesthetic (rate 5 mL every 30 s).
7. Lay patient supine with left uterine displacement and in slight Trendelenburg. Monitor blood pressure every 1–3 min for first 15 min, then 5 min thereafter.[9]
8. Ensure proper room setup for general anesthesia and that resuscitative drugs and equipment are available.

1. Avoidance of teratogenic drugs
2. Avoidance of fetal asphyxia
3. Prevention of preterm labor

In the first 2 weeks of life, teratogens have either lethal or no effect. The third through the eighth weeks are the most critical period. Drug exposure can lead to major developmental abnormalities. After the eighth week organogenesis is complete and organ growth occurs. Exposure to anesthetics should be kept to a minimum.[1]

Intrauterine fetal asphyxia is avoided by maintaining maternal Pao_2 and $PaCo_2$ at normal levels. As maternal Pao_2 increases, fetal Pao_2 also increases. Severe maternal hyperventilation may cause a decrease in umbilical and uterine blood flow and fetal oxygenation.

Although studies suggest that anesthesia during pregnancy is associated with preterm labor, no one agent or technique has been associated with a higher incidence of premature delivery.[5] Nearly 1% to 2% of all pregnant patients require surgery during pregnancy. Abdominal procedures are the most commonly performed (appendectomy 1/1500 pregnancies, cholecystectomy 1/2000 to 10,000 pregnancies).[1] Elective surgery should be deferred until at least 6 weeks after delivery. Urgent surgery should be deferred until the second or third trimester.

If emergency surgery is necessary, it should be performed under regional block if possible. Premedication should be minimized. If general anesthesia is necessary, all considerations for maternal safety should be implemented (prevention of aspiration and aortocaval compression). Ideally, after 16 weeks' gestation, fetal heart rate should be monitored continually during surgery. Administration of benzodiazepines is discouraged during the first trimester because of the association between diazepam and congenital abnormalities seen in laboratory animals. There was some controversy in the literature regarding the use of N_2O during the first trimester. N_2O inhibits maternal and fetal *methionine synthase*. Methionine synthase is a vitamin B_{12}-containing enzyme involved in folate metabolism and DNA synthesis. This inhibition of methionine synthase was thought to be the primary mechanism for the reproductive abnormalities seen in rats, but no evidence in humans has been noted. Due to this fact, 50% N_2O can be safely administered without teratogenic effects.[5]

Postpartum Tubal Ligation   If desired, postpartum tubal ligation can be performed immediately after delivery, when general or continuous epidural anesthesia is administered for cesarean section. If a continuous epidural catheter is administered for vaginal delivery, it can be left in place up to 48 hours for subsequent tubal ligation. This delay allows for a period of elective fasting. A sensory level of T-4 to T-5 is required for analgesia. Lidocaine 2% can be administered to reactivate the epidural, with a volume up to 20 mL. If the patient has not had anesthesia for delivery, either regional or general anesthesia can be used for sterilization. Regional anesthesia is preferred in this setting due to the risks of pulmonary aspiration associated with general anesthesia. If general anesthesia is used, a minimum of 8 hours of fasting is recommended. Patients are premedicated with histamine blockers (H_2) or clear antacids. Rapid sequence induction with cricoid pressure is mandatory. The patient should only be extubated when completely awake.

Circlage Treatment of an incompetent cervix (cervical cirlage) requires general anesthesia with rapid sequence induction or local anesthesia with intravenous sedation early in pregnancy. Spinal and epidural anesthesia has also been used with success. Teratogenic drugs are avoided. Usually Demerol is the narcotic of choice. Maternal and fetal safety is maintained continuously.

☐ MATERNAL FETAL CIRCULATION

The fetus depends on the placenta for gas exchange, nutrition, and water elimination. Maternal and fetal tissues form the placenta, and its blood supply is derived from both the mother and the fetus. The placenta is composed of fetal tissues that lie in maternal vascular spaces. This enables the fetal capillaries within the villi to exchange substances within the maternal blood. Medications administered to the mother enter the fetal circulation primarily by passive diffusion. Most drugs in anesthesia have a low molecular weight (less

Table 26–7
PLACENTAL TRANSFER OF DRUGS

Contributed by:
1. Molecular weight
2. Nonionized drug
3. Lipid-soluble drug

than 500), are partially nonionized at physiologic pH, have a high lipid solubility, and are partially nonprotein bound in maternal blood. This means that almost all drugs used to produce anesthesia, analgesia, or sedation will rapidly cross the placenta[5] (Table 26–7).

Lipid-soluble drugs such as thiopental diffuse rapidly. Neuromuscular blocking drugs, such as all the muscle relaxants, are highly ionized and have a low lipid solubility. This makes transfer across the placenta difficult. Drugs that are highly protein bound such as bupivacaine also diffuse poorly across the placenta.[5] As more of the drug exists in the free, nonionized form at physiologic pH, it becomes more diffusable across the placenta. Factors tending to increase maternal drug concentration are high total doses, use of slowly metabolized drugs, and administration of drugs into highly vascular areas. Once the drug crosses the placenta, the effects on the fetus depend on drug uptake, distribution, metabolism, and elimination in the fetus.[5]

REFERENCES

1. Morgan, GE, Mikhail MS. *Clinical Anesthesiology.* East Norwalk, Conn: Appleton & Lange; 1992:611–629.
2. Wadlington, JS. Anesthesia for obstetrics and gynecology. In: *Clinical Anesthesia Procedures for the Massachusetts General Hospital.* Boston: Little, Brown; 1993:457–475.
3. Snider SM, Levinson G. *Anesthesia for Obstetrics.* Baltimore: Williams & Wilkins; 1993: 385–390.
4. Dripps, RD, Eckenhoff JE, Vandam LD, eds. *Introduction to Anesthesia.* Philadelphia: WB Saunders; 1992:333–348.
5. Miller RD. *Anesthesia.* New York: Churchill Livingstone; 1992:1829–1874.
6. Sandor, JJ. Anesthesia for the pre-eclamptic patient. In: Faust R, ed. *Anesthesia Review.* 2nd ed. New York: Churchill Livingstone; 1994:447–449.
7. James FM, Wheeler SN, Dewan DM. *Obstetric Anesthesia: The Complicated Patient.* Philadelphia: FA Davis; 1988.
8. Pan PH. Crisis management in obstetrical emergencies. *Anesthesia Today.* 1995;6(4):10–14.
9. Barash PG, Cullen BF, Stoelting RK, eds. *Clinical Anesthesia.* Philadelphia: JB Lppincott; 1992:1267–1305.
10. Koff HD. Placenta previa. In: Yao FS, Artusio JF, eds. *Anesthesiology.* 3rd ed. Philadelphia: JB Lippincott; 1993:477–492.
11. Rosinia FA. Determining the criteria for selecting general versus regional anesthesia for obstetric patients. *Anesthesia Today.* 1995;6(4):1–4.
12. Stoelting, RK, Dierdorf SF, McCammon RL. *Anesthesia and Co-Existing Disease.* New York: Churchill Livingstone; 1988:807–804.

☐ QUESTIONS

1. Respiratory changes seen in pregnancy are:
   a. Increased O_2 consumption, decreased minute ventilation, increased respiratory rate
   b. Increased tidal volume, decreased functional residual capacity, increased respiratory rate
   c. Increased minute ventilation, decreased O_2 consumption, increased functional residual capacity
   d. Decreased O_2 consumption, increased minute ventilation, increased respiratory rate

2. The oxyhemoglobin curve is shifted to the _____ in the pregnant patient.
   a. Right
   b. Left

c. Not shifted at all
d. None of the above

3. Dilutional anemia from pregnancy is caused by:
   a. Increased plasma volume, decreased red blood cell mass
   b. Increased plasma volume, increased red blood cell mass
   c. Decreased plasma volume, decreased red blood cell mass
   d. None of the above

4. Pain in the first stage of labor is innervated through:
   a. the pudendal nerve
   b. the sacral plexus
   c. T-10 to L-1
   d. S-2 to S-4

5. Placenta previa best presents as:
   a. Painless bright red bleeding
   b. Painful bright red bleeding
   c. Painless dark red bleeding
   d. Painful dark red bleeding

6. Uterine blood flow equals:
   a. Uterine vascular resistance minus uterine artery pressure divided by venous pressure
   b. Uterine arterial pressure minus uterine venous pressure divided by uterine vascular resistance

7. Inverted uterus is best reversed and treated under general anesthesia with:
   a. Halothane 1.6% and fluid resuscitation
   b. Halothane 0.5%
   c. Ethrane 0.75%
   d. Ethrane 1.14%

8. The anesthetic requirement in pregnancy is:
   a. Decreased inhalation agents, increased local anesthetic, and decreased IV sedatives
   b. Increased inhalation agents, decreased local anesthetic, and increased IV sedatives
   c. Increased inhalation agents, increased local anesthetic, and decreased IV sedatives
   d. Decreased inhalation agents, decreased local anesthetic, and decreased IV sedatives

9. In a pre-eclamptic patient with blood pressure 180/110, heart rate 100, respiratory rate 30, the best anesthetic plan with a bleeding time under 6 minutes is:
   a. General anesthesia rapid sequence induction with ketamine 1 mg/kg
   b. Continuous epidural anesthesia 0.75% bupivicaine total 20 mL
   c. General anesthesia rapid sequence induction with pentathol 3 to 5 mg/kg, balanced salt solution
   d. One-shot spinal 5% lidocaine 20 mL

10. A pre-eclamptic patient has just exhibited a grand mal seizure. The best treatment is:
    a. Valium 10 mg to control convulsion
    b. Magnesium sulfate 20 mEq/L
    c. Anectine 100 mg
    d. Pentathol 50 to 150 mL

11. A patient becomes dyspneic, hypotensive, cyanotic, and clammy after insertion of epidural catheter during a uterine contraction. The most likely cause is:
    a. Intravascular injection of local anesthetic
    b. Cerebral toxicity from local anesthetic
    c. Amniotic fluid embolism
    d. Placenta abruptio

12. After supporting the patient with oxygen and fluids, she suddenly experiences cardiac collapse. You should:
    a. Aggressively resuscitate the mother and prepare for stat cesarean section of fetus
    b. Do nothing because mortality rate is approximately 86% for the mother
    c. Give phenylephrine 100 mg to increase blood pressure
    d. Give Narcan to reverse respiratory depression

13. Uterine rupture can be caused by:
    a. Dehiscence of scar
    b. Forceps delivery
    c. Tetanic uterine contractions from Pitocin
    d. All of the above

14. The greatest risk under general anesthesia during pregnancy is:
    a. Difficult intubation
    b. Pulmonary aspiration
    c. Placenta transfer of drugs to fetus
    d. All of the above

15. Spinal anesthesia for normal vaginal delivery is limited to:
    a. The first stage of labor
    b. Immediately prior to delivery
    c. In the active stage
    d. In the latent stage

16. Pregnancy-induced hypertension causes which hormonal changes?
    a. Increased prostacycline, increase thromboxane, decrease renin
    b. Increased renin, increase angiotension, decrease thromboxane
    c. Decreased renin, decrease prostacycline, increase thromboxane
    d. None of the above

17. Absolute contraindications of regional anesthesia include:

a. Patient refusal
b. Active bleeding
c. Coagulopathy
d. All of the above

18. What are the maternal cardiovascular changes of pregnancy?
    a. Increased heart rate, increased stroke volume, increased blood pressure
    b. Decreased diastolic blood pressure, decreased stroke volume
    c. Decreased vascular resistance, increased blood pressure, increased vascular resistance
    d. Increased red blood cell volume, increased stroke volume, decreased vascular resistance

19. Your patient presents with dark red vaginal bleeding and disseminated intravascular coagulation. Anesthesia management for delivery of fetus includes:
    a. Epidural anesthesia for cesarean section
    b. Normal vaginal delivery
    c. Rapid sequence induction with ketamine 0.75 mg/kg
    d. Mask induction with 1.5% halothane

20. Maternal hypotension is treated by:
    a. Ephedrine 5-mg increments IV
    b. Phenylephrine 40 mg IV
    c. Left uterine displacement
    d. Both a and c

☐ ANSWERS

1. b	5. a	9. c	13. d	17. d
2. a	6. b	10. d	14. d	18. d
3. b	7. a	11. c	15. b	19. c
4. c	8. d	12. a	16. b	20. d

Orthopedic Anesthesia

Charles R. Barton
Minnette Beeson

The practice of orthopedic care has changed dramatically in the last several years due to factors that range from prevention or effective early treatment of chronic diseases to improvement of materials through space age technology. Today the incidence of orthopedic problems related to poliomyelities is rare because that disease is nearly eliminated. Likewise, rickets and scurvy, tuberculosis, chronic osteomyelitis, and septic arthritis are often prevented or treated effectively to reduce the necessity of surgery. Improved screening and use of early nonsurgical or simpler surgical treatment of congenital problems such as clubfoot, hip dysplasia, and idiopathic scoliosis often improve patient outcomes without major surgical interventions.

Former joint reconstruction, when available, required custom-made prosthetic components and had a high mortality rate. Today a wide variety of joint replacement systems are available for the shoulder, fingers, hip, and knee. They are standardized and well fitting and increase the quality of life for thousands of patients. Internal and external fixation devices have become extremely sophisticated, now composed of stronger, more resilient materials. Intramedullary rodding devices enable a patient to ambulate within 24 hours of surgery, drastically reducing the incidence of thrombophlebitis and its subsequent morbidity.

Vast improvements have been made in video technology and imaging. When used in conjunction with pressure-sensitive irrigation systems, they allow ideal joint visualization and operative conditions. Sophisticated intratrocar oscillating drills and operative instrumentation permit closed procedures previously requiring an open joint. These advances have reduced recovery time, prolonged bone and joint function, and minimized pain.

Many subspecialties within the field of orthopedics have developed. Today there are specialists for hip surgery, shoulder surgery, foot surgery, and cancer and bone tumor treatment. Often physicians specialize in revision of reconstructive surgery. Sports medicine has become a science of its own[1] and more information than ever before has been compiled about the mechanism of bone and joint healing.

Not all of the changes seen have been positive. Orthopedic injuries have increased in variety and scope due to high-speed motor vehicular and industrial accidents and as the result of armed assaults. Repetitive motion injuries are seen frequently in industrial and computer-related activities.

With the innovations seen in orthopedic surgery over the last several years, provision of appropriate anesthesia drugs and techniques has become more challenging. The anesthetist must be familiar with a wide variety of orthopedic-related procedures and techniques. This chapter highlights the anesthetic considerations that need to be addressed for many of these procedures.

☐ ANESTHETIC CONSIDERATIONS

COEXISTING DISEASES

The advanced technology and enhancement of technique available to the healthy and medically compromised patient have created a challenge for the anesthesia care provider. The degree and occurrence of complications likely during the perioperative period has been altered. The anesthesia care provider must consider not only the inherent pitfalls of the patient's orthopedic injury and surgical procedure, but also the associated medical conditions.

It is now possible to provide orthopedic care to a population of patients previously ineligible due to the associated risks. Many systemic alterations are likely to exist in this extended patient population. Cardiac disease has been reported as high as 60% in the elderly surgical patient[2] and is among many systemic alterations anesthesia care providers are likely to encounter. Elderly patients frequently have some degree of hypertension and atherosclerosis with associated end-organ disease. Patients taking antihypertensive agents often present in a relatively dehydrated state. Many age-related pulmonary changes occur. Other alterations associated with the aging process that are of concern to the anesthesia care provider include inevitable decreases in organ function and altered responses to drugs.[4]

Many patients requiring fracture reduction have sustained injury as a result of a fall or trauma, and associated injury or causative factors must be diagnosed and treated. Many patients may be taking chronic anti-inflammatory agents that may alter their body's ability to achieve hemostasis. Chronic steroid therapy may suppress adrenal cortical function and alter their ability to respond to stress.

Common Related Musculoskeletal Disorders
Osteoarthritis and Rheumatoid Arthritis
Patients requiring orthopedic surgery frequently have degenerative or rheumatic joint disease. Arthritis is a general term used to describe inflammation of the joints. However, two distinctly different processes cause joint degeneration and loss of function.

OSTEOARTHRITIS
Osteoarthritis affects the articular cartilage, with minimal inflammatory reaction. Progressive degeneration of cartilage leads to changes in subchondral bone and joint structure. Diagnostic components include stiffness and pain with movement and relief with rest. Stiffness usually resides with joint motion. The disease is differentiated from rheumatoid arthritis by bony enlargements or Heberden's nodes in the distal interphalangeal joints (this joint is spared in rheumatoid arthritis). Joint trauma, advanced age, and heredity increase the incidence.[4] One to several joints may be affected, but knee and hip involvement are the most common. Degenerative disease of vertebral bodies and intervertebral disks, especially the middle to lower cervical spine and lower lumbar area, is likely in advanced cases as is the incidence of herniated nucleus pulposus and compression of nerve roots.[5]

Suggested therapy includes heat and anti-inflammatory drugs for the relief of pain. In the advanced stages of the disease, reconstructive joint surgery may be necessary.

RHEUMATOID ARTHRITIS
Rheumatoid arthritis is a chronic inflammatory disease of unknown etiology. It has been speculated that it is a disease of viral origin.[6] It has also been speculated that its onset could possibly be triggered in a susceptible host by a cellular immune response.[7] In some patients, onset of the disease may coincide with trauma, surgical procedures, childbirth, or exposure to temperature extremes. The disease can affect several symmetric joints and its onset and subsequent progression may be acute or gradual, marked with remissions and exacerbations. The terminal interphalangeal joints are spared (distinguishes from osteoarthritis); the proximal interphalangeal joints develop Bouchard's nodes.[4] Other diagnostic criteria, although nonspecific, include the presence of anti-immunoglobin antibody (also positive in systemic lupus erythematosus, pulmonary fibrosis, and viral hepatitis).

Because rheumatoid arthritis is an *autoimmune disease*, it has other systemic consequences. Patients can develop vasculitis from immune complex deposition on the wall of small vessels, which may manifest as myocardial, cerebral, or gastrointestinal ischemia. The pericardial lining may thicken, or pericardial effusions can develop. Pulmonary tissue fibrosis can lead to the development of pulmonary nodules, interstitial inflammation, and plural effusions. Other systemic concerns are a mild anemia that could be aggravated by an anti-inflammatory regime and a 10% incidence of keratoconjunctivitis.[3] Treatment includes analgesics, anti-inflammatories, and immunosuppressives. Long-term therapy of any one of these medications has the potential for significant side effects. Antimalarial drugs may be added when nonsteroidals are not effective. Surgical interventions such as synovectomy and joint replacement surgery may be indicated with progressive disease states.

Rheumatoid involvement of the cervical spine is common, causing pain and limitation of motion for the patient. *Subluxation* of C-1 and C-2 (atlas-axis) is possible with head and neck manipulation, and in extreme cases can cause a separation of the atlanto-odontoid articulation. Arthritic involvement of the temporomandibular joint may lead to marked limitations in mouth opening, causing airway management concerns. Acute or chronic cricoarytenoid arthritis can limit the abduction and adduction of the vocal cords and could increase the degree of difficulty during intubation.

The need for preoperative cervical spine radiographs in patients with rheumatoid disease is controversial. One study was conducted that suggested they were unnecessary due to a lack of effect on subsequent anesthetic management. The investigators did not perform procedures that required hyperextension of the neck. Their investigation revealed a 5.5% incidence of unsuspected C-1 to C-2 subluxations in asymptomatic patients with rheumatoid disease before elective surgery.[7]

Muscular Dystrophies
Muscular dystrophy is characterized by painless degeneration and atrophy of skeletal muscle. The disease increases the permeability of muscle membranes, and plasma kinase levels are markedly increased early in the course of the disease.[3]

At least five forms of the disease are recognized, each with unique onset and clinical manifestations. The most common form, pseudohypertrophic, or *Duchenne's*, is associated with many conditions likely to seriously affect a patient's perioperative course. In this progressive disorder, fatty infiltration of muscle tissue leads to cardiac muscle degeneration. Electrocardiographic (ECG) changes and mitral regurgitation are likely. Volatile agents must be used with caution due to increased myocardial sensitivity to their depressing effects.

Narcotics must be used judiciously due to potential respiratory depressing effects. With disease progression, respiratory insufficiency ensues and, eventually, development of kyphoscoliosis and restrictive airway disease are manifest. Pulmonary reserves will be lost, and 30% of the related deaths are due to decreased respiratory function.[3]

There is an exaggerated serum potassium elevation with succinylcholine administration due to the increased permeability of skeletal muscle membranes. Response to nondepolarizing agents is usually normal, although the degree of blockade may be difficult to assess because of uneven muscle wasting. Along with the underlying state of weakness, even a slight prolongation could have serious consequences.[3]

Duchenne's dystrophy is also associated with an increased risk for *malignant hyperthermia* during the anesthetic course. Dantrolene must be readily available. Other anesthetic concerns are an increased risk for aspiration because of gastrointestinal hypomotility. Therefore, full stomach precautions should be taken.[3] See also Chap. 14.

Scleroderma

Scleroderma manifests as a progressive inflammation and fibrosis of skin, viscera, and vasculature. The process affects cardiac muscle, coronary vessels, and the cardiac conduction system. Vascular tone is altered, and it may be difficult to anticipate vascular response. Systemic hypertension is common due to arterial vasoconstriction and may be difficult to control. Significant hypotension may ensue with volatile anesthetic agents after induction. Arterial line insertion may be difficult and cause arterial thrombosis. Warming measures should be instituted, including warming the operating room, to avoid vasoconstriction due to hypothermia. Pulmonary involvement manifests as pulmonary hypertension. Pulmonary interstitial fibrosis results in decreased compliance and arterial hypoxemia.[3]

Typically the skin is tight and shiny. The patient's mouth usually narrows and mandibular motion may be limited. Fiberoptic laryngoscopy may be indicated for intubation. Excess bleeding may occur with traumatic intubation.

There are other anesthetic considerations. The disease process affects the gastrointestinal tract, leading to dysphagia and reflux of gastric acid. Preoperative treatment with H^+ blockers and nonparticulate antacids is indicated. Because of accelerated hypertension, patients are prone to corneal abrasions and peripheral or cranial neuropathies. *Renal failure* is the most common cause of death, and a significant degree of renal insufficiency may be present early in the disease.[3]

PREOPERATIVE ASSESSMENT

Because of the many associated musculoskeletal disease processes, preoperative clinical assessment of the orthopedic patient is essential. The choice of anesthetic technique may be determined by eliciting a detailed, accurate patient history and assessing the patient's current condition. Areas of special concern for all surgical candidates include assessment of the cervical spine, mobility of the temporomandibular joint, and potential for arthritic laryngeal changes for airway management. The patient's cardiovascular status should be assessed

for pre-existing dysrhythmias, hypertension, coronary artery disease, and chronic obstructive pulmonary disease.

Other concurrent drug therapy that must be considered, in addition to those previously mentioned, include cardiac inotropic and antidysrhythmics and antihypertensive agents. The preoperative studies usually recommended for most orthopedic procedures include hemoglobin and hematocrit. If the patient is taking antihypertensives or diuretics, an electrolyte panel is indicated because serum potassium and hydration status may be altered. If significant blood loss or fluid volume changes are anticipated, baseline laboratory values may be helpful. Urinalysis will help diagnose preoperative urinary tract infections. If an underlying infective process is identified, sometimes surgery will be deferred. Coagulation profiles, platelet count, and bleeding times can be helpful diagnostic indicators when anti-inflammatory agents are taken chronically. Preoperative chest x-rays and ECGs and other evaluative cardiovascular and pulmonary studies may be indicated with advancing disease states.

MONITORING

Vital sign monitoring should be tailored to the patient's history, state of health, and surgical procedure. Routine monitoring includes ECG, noninvasive blood pressure, core temperature, oxygen saturation, capnography, and agent analysis. The insertion of a Foley catheter and measurement of urine output can help assess the volume status, renal function, and the presence of hemoglobinuria often seen in hemolytic blood transfusion reactions.

Invasive monitoring helps guide intraoperative management in the patient with known or anticipated volume status changes and those at risk for embolus, prolonged procedures, and when deliberate hypotensive technique is used. Continuous blood pressure monitoring with an arterial catheter is indicated when the potential for massive blood loss exists, when the accuracy of noninvasive blood pressure monitoring is unreliable, with the coexistence of cardiovascular disease, and when frequent arterial blood gas analysis will help manage the care of the patient intraoperatively. A central venous catheter may be an adjunct to assess volume status and guide volume replacement and as a means to aspirate an air embolus when this is a risk. The need for pulmonary artery catheterization is indicated when severe cardiovascular disease is present, such as left ventricular dysfunction, or a guide to volume replacement when massive quantities of blood are lost, or when the patient would be physiologically sensitive to blood and fluid replacement.

POSITIONING

Position-related injury increases in patients with coexisting disease states because their tissues and body systems have less resistance to the compromises surgical positioning imposes. These disease processes need to be identified and managed intraoperatively because the compromised regional blood flow may lead to increased risk of ischemia and subsequent neurovascular damage.

Many conditions in patients undergoing orthopedic procedures and anesthesia alter their compensatory mechanisms. Osteoarthritis, rheumatoid arthritis, systemic lupus erythematosus, polymyositis, dermatomyositis, scleroderma, muscular dystrophies, diabetes mellitus, cachexia, and obesity may limit the patient's ability to move muscles and joints normally or to maintain normal vascularity. All present challenges for uncomplicated intraoperative positioning (see Chap. 10).

STERILE TECHNIQUE

Strict adherence to sterile technique is of vital importance in orthopedic surgery because contamination could lead to bone destruction, sepsis, and death. Bacteria may be introduced through the patients' skin, oropharyngeal bacteria, cross contamination from other patients, bacteria from lint or dust particles, as well as airborne bacteria from the head and neck of operating room personnel.[8]

PROPHYLACTIC ANTIBIOTICS

Parenteral prophylactic antibiotics are used routinely in clean and uncontaminated orthopedic procedures because so many studies have shown a reduced infection rate with their use. Cefazolin is a first-generation cephalosporin and the antibiotic of choice primarily because of its coverage against staphylococci. Antibiotics should be given preoperatively, on induction of anesthesia, or at least 10 minutes before inflation of a tourniquet. Based on evidence in the current literature, 24 hours of postoperative coverage appears to be adequate[9] unless the wound is contaminated with soil or human bite, in which case extended coverage may be necessary.

LAMINAR AIR FLOW

Laminar air flow is used at some institutions to minimize the risk of infection from cross contamination. This type of ventilation is able to filter airborne particles. The standard air exchange within an operating room ranges from 12 to 15 exchanges an hour. A laminar air flow system can provide up to 500 air exchanges per hour.[8] Its major disadvantages include noise, increased drying of operative field, and decreasing body temperature due to convective losses.

WARMING MEASURES

Optimal physiologic functioning is maintained at a normal body temperature. Patients lose heat from a variety of mechanisms. Heat lost through *radiation* is the primary preoperative mechanism of heat loss. All areas of the patient's body not essential for surgery and anesthesia should be kept covered, including the head. *Evaporative* heat loss occurs through large surgical incisions and by skin damaged burns. *Convective* heat loss occurs as air circulates across uncovered body parts during surgery. Ambient room temperatures should be maintained. Heat is lost from *conduction* if any body part is in direct proximity with cooler surfaces on the table or equipment.

Hypothermia has numerous adverse physiologic effects including impaired hemostasis, impaired leukocyte function, reduced cardiac output, and decreased stress hormone release. It is important to avoid hypothermia by warming blood, fluids, and gases. The *most effective* means of warming a patient is by a forced air warming blanket placed over the patient. Many different types of surface warming devices are available for intraoperative use.

BLOOD TRANSFUSION

It is generally accepted that a safe minimum of a hematocrit of 25% and hemoglobin of 8 g/dL in previously healthy patients, a hemoglobin of 6 g/dL in well compensated chronic anemic patients, and a hemoglobin of 10 g/dL in patients who are unable or in whom it would be undesirable to increase their cardiac outputs to compensate for anemia. But the current philosophy on the need for transfusion therapy is based on the patient's hemodynamic and physiologic parameters, not on a target minimum hematocrit and hemoglobin level.

If the potential for significant intraoperative blood loss is a concern, the patient can be prepared in several ways. In anticipation of transfusion, a patient may predeposit 2 to 3 U whole blood 1 to 2 weeks before surgery. A second option is to donate 1 to 2 U immediately before surgery that is replaced with colloids or crystalloids. This autologous blood may be reinfused at the end of the procedure or earlier if necessary.

Intra- and postoperative salvage is possible with the use of a "cell saver" unit that selectively collects, filters, and centrifuges red blood cells for readministration. If blood loss is unanticipated or the patient is unable to predeposit or receive salvaged blood due to a contaminative or infective process, homologous transfusion is an option. Typed and crossmatched blood is always preferred, but universal donor blood is always an option in an emergency. Patients should be typed and screened, at the very least, for any procedure with a remote possibility of blood loss, and typed and crossmatched if transfusion is anticipated.

TOURNIQUET

Pressure and Timing　A pneumatic cuff or tourniquet is used to minimize blood loss from the operative site. Its disadvantages include sustained compression to tissues, nerves, and blood vessels that may be problematic if used for extended periods of time. Although safe limits are unknown, recommended ranges vary from 1 to 4 hours. Damage caused by transient ischemia usually resolves within 1 to 24 hours.

Other disadvantages include intraoperative reaction to sustained tourniquet pressure. After 45 minutes the awake patient may complain of dull aching pain, even when regional analgesia is otherwise adequate, or the patient under a general anesthetic may exhibit elevations of blood pressure and heart rate due to sustained tourniquet pressure.

Hemodynamic Changes When the cuff is rapidly deflated, the patient can experience transient metabolic acidosis, washout of K^+, and elevation of $PaCO_2$[8] that could cause a transient vasovagal reaction or hypotensive episode.

Sickle Cell The use of a tourniquet should be avoided in patients with sickle cell disease or trait. Tourniquet inflation produces vascular occlusion and localized hypoxemia that initiates structural changes in the red blood cell that produce sickling. These sickled red blood cells are not able to carry oxygen to tissues and can obstruct small arterioles when the tourniquet is deflated. These effects are not reversed by increasing systemic oxygen delivery.[10]

HYPOTENSIVE TECHNIQUE

Hypotensive technique is an option often used when the risk of operative blood loss is great. It is most often used during extensive spinal fusions with instrumentation and hip surgery. It combines the use of volatile anesthetics and peripheral vasodilators to maintain the mean blood pressure 20% below mean blood pressure in hypertensive patients and up to 60% below mean blood pressure in normotensive patients and, therefore, reduces blood loss.[8] One of the major disadvantages is a potential for uncontrolled hypotension after methylmethacrylate application.

METHYLMETHACRYLATE

Methylmethacrylate is a self-polymerizing, space-filling mortar used to transmit compressive loads from bone to prosthesis.[11] It helps achieve fixation by entering both the bone surface and the deliberate irregularities placed in the prosthesis. It is a cementing substance, not a glue. Its use is often associated with hypotension caused by *decreases in systemic vascular resistance* and *direct myocardial depression*. There are many explanations offered for this effect, including systemic absorption of a volatile monomer released,[12] or effect from emboli forced into the circulation as the prosthesis is inserted into an open medullary channel,[13] or from the effects of heating bone marrow and blood and subsequent release of thrombotic and vasoactive substances,[14] and from the hydrolysis of the methylmethacrylate to methacrylate acid.[15] The hypotensive effect may appear within 30 to 60 seconds after insertion of the cement, or up to 10 minutes after the prosthesis is inserted, and may be treated with vasopressors. Hypotension usually terminates spontaneously in less than 5 minutes.[16a] Because the onset and duration of hypotensive episodes vary, all of the postulated mechanisms probably play a role in one patient or another.[16a] These adverse systemic responses are augmented by volatile inhalation agents, and they should be used with caution immediately before, during, and after methylmethacrylate administration. It

would seem prudent to accommodate a slight increase in the patient's blood pressure 5 to 10 minutes before cement application. Hypoxemia, presumably as a result of fat and marrow emboli, has been reported. This can be prevented by maximizing alveolar oxygen tension before prosthesis insertion.[16a] In extreme cases, cardiovascular collapse may occur.

Reactions to methylmethacrylate have been reported and are more common with subsequent exposure and affect patients undergoing their second joint replacement surgery and those undergoing revision of the same joint.[16b]

☐ ANESTHETIC CONSIDERATIONS FOR PROCEDURES OF THE SPINE

The most common procedures of the spine include operations for herniated intervertebral disks, including laminectomy, microdiskectomy, and chemonucleolysis; and spinal fusions for scoliosis, vertebral fractures, or spinal instability.[16a] After induction, the sitting-prone position using an Andrew's frame is often used for the majority of procedures necessitating a posterior surgical approach (see Chap. 10). Procedures necessitating a high anterior approach, such as cervical diskectomy or fusion, are usually performed in the supine position using head tongs and a counterweight system. A sitting position may be used for some posterior cervical laminectomies. Thoracoabdominal procedures of the lower spine are performed with the patient in the supine position. Combined anteroposterior surgeries may require intraoperative repositioning and need careful preoperative planning to facilitate safe and coordinated patient care. Anesthetic concerns include the potential for airway compromise and complications related to unstable cervical spine.

LAMINECTOMY/DISKECTOMY

Microlumbar diskectomy is safe and cost effective when performed as an outpatient procedure. It produces immediate improvement and allows early return to regular activities.[17]

Chymopapain In the 1980s chymopapain was commonly used to treat herniated disk in a procedure known as chemonucleolysis. Due to a 1% incidence of anaphylactic reactions occurring in individuals receiving this treatment, the procedure is now largely discontinued and therefore is mostly of historical interest.[18] Chymopapain is a proteolytic enzyme that is obtained from the tropical tree *Carica papaya* that was first isolated in 1941 by Jansen and Balls.[19] Dr. L. Smith, an orthopedic surgeon, began experiments in 1959 to treat herniated disks.[20] This technique involves the injection of chymopapain into the nucleus pulposus. Subsequently this proteolytic enzyme causes digestion of that part of the disks, relieving compression of the adjacent nerve root.[21]

Chymopapain is actually a form of papaya latex, which may explain its potential of causing anaphylactic reactions in a manner that is similar to that seen with the latex derived from rubber trees. The precise mechanism of action of chymopapain on an intervertebral disk is not known. It has been postulated that the rapid hydrolysis of intradiskal protein-mucopolysaccharide complexes following chymopapain injection might release substances into the bloodstream capable of triggering an acute anaphylactic reaction.[22] These substances alone, the chymopapain alone, or a combination of these substances may be the basis of anaphylactic reactions in susceptible individuals. A retrospective study demonstrates that the signs and symptoms of anaphylaxis occur very rapidly following injection of chymopapain.[23] Of 164 cases of anaphylaxis following chymopapain injection, 54% of signs occurred within 5 minutes, 30% within 10 minutes, and 10% within 20 minutes. The use of skin testing has been proposed as useful in selecting candidates for this procedure, but unfortunately there can be a significant percentage of false-positive and false-negative results.[24] The preparation for patients undergoing any procedure that may precipitate an anaphylactic reaction to agents such as chymopapain or latex derived from rubber trees has been described.[25]

SPINAL FUSION/INSTRUMENTATION

Scoliosis Scoliosis is a deformity of the thoracolumbar spine and rib cage caused by lateral deviation and rotation of the vertebral bodies. The disease can be congenital or progressive. With a 40° deformity, respiratory compromise develops as a result of one hemithorax being compressed toward residual volume, and the other being expanded toward total lung capacity. When the angle of deformity exceeds 65°, decreasing lung volumes and mechanical impairments lead to severe restrictive changes. This increases physiologic shunting and dead space altering ventilation perfusion ratios, causing decreases in Pa_{O_2}, increases in Pa_{CO_2}, and increases in the work of breathing.[16a] Patients exposed to chronic hypercapnia do not respond normally to further increases in Pa_{CO_2} and will hypoventilate when inhaling a high inspired oxygen concentration.[16a] Pulmonary vascular resistance is elevated, leading to right ventricular hypertrophy and cor pulmonale.[16a]

Preoperative pulmonary function testing and arterial blood gas analysis can help determine the severity of the impairment.[16a] Right ventricular hypertrophy is caused by increased pulmonary vascular resistance. ECG findings will often reflect the presence of cor pulmonale. Pulmonology and cardiology consultation may be beneficial in the preparation of the patient with scoliosis for surgery.

The advent of Harrington instrumentation helped correct the severity and progression of these spinal deformities. Today, patients with scoliosis are now operated on as a matter of routine. Many instrumentation setups are available and offer the advantage of speed, versatility, and convenience. The procedure can be accomplished in one or two stages combined with anteroposterior spinal fusions. If an anterior approach is used, anesthesia care providers can expect an increase in operative time, blood loss, and postoperative length of stay. Complications increase with those individuals over 40 years of age or with coexisting diseases.

Monitoring and Intraoperative Wake-up

An intraoperative wake-up test is used by some surgeons to assess the (anterior cord) *motor function* after instrumentation has been placed. In anticipation of this test, inform the patient of the plan and explain what will be asked. The patient should be reassured there will be no pain experienced and that uncontrolled patient movement during this procedure can be hazardous. The anesthesia care provider must carefully assess the patient's baseline motor and sensory function of both upper and lower extremities because preoperative deficits may be present.

A 40- to 60-minute advanced notice of the test by the surgeon is ideal. During this time, neuromuscular blockade can be allowed to diminish, if the patient's condition permits, while monitoring the train-of-four response on a peripheral nerve stimulator. The nondepolarizing muscular blockade may also be reversed at the appropriate time. Inhalation agents can be decreased, and narcotics should be titrated to provide some analgesia, but not fully depress respiratory efforts. Narcotics can also be reversed if necessary. As signs of lightening are observed, request a hand squeeze. If present, elicit bilateral foot movement and assess the degree of patient compliance and resulting motor ability. Anesthesia may be reinduced with thiopental (1 mg/kg) and increased concentrations of inhalation agents. Potential complications include dislodgment of spinal instrumentation or accidental extubation with uncontrolled patient movement and air embolus.

Gokel and colleagues reported on the use of fentanyl-propofol and alfentanil-propofol as a method of providing the wake-up test in 60 patients undergoing spinal surgery.[26] The technique involves induction of anesthesia with either fentanyl 2 μg/kg or alfentanil 20 μg/kg intravenously, along with propofol 1 to 2 mg/kg intravenously and vecuronium for relaxation and 33% to 40% O_2 and nitrous oxide. The patients are maintained with continuous fentanyl (2 to 3 μg/kg/h) by infusion or alfentanil (50 to 60 μg/kg/h) by infusion and propofol 2 to 3 mg/kg/h. If required, opioid boluses are administered and, generally, further doses of neuromuscular blocking agents are not required if adequate anesthetic depth can be achieved. When the wake-up period is required the propofol infusion and nitrous oxide are discontinued while the opioid infusion and controlled ventilation are continued with 100% O_2. The patient is awakened with verbal stimulus and asked to move both feet and toes. At the end of the wake-up test, propofol 1 mg/kg is given as an intravenous bolus. Anesthesia is maintained with both opioid and propofol infusion along with nitrous oxide. This technique provided extremely rapid awakening in a calm manner without a cumulative effect. The patients responded to the request to open their eyes in 4.3 ± 2.2 minutes in the fentanyl group and 4.1 ± 2.9 minutes in the alfentanil group. The time to neurologic examination was 6.2 ± 2.1 minutes and 5.8 ± 2.1 minutes for the fentanyl and alfentanil groups, respectively. An alternative wake-up technique can be accomplished with midazolam and opioids along with nitrous oxide and neuromuscular blocking agents. If needed, flumazenil could be used to reverse the benzodiazepine effect during the wake-up test period.

Monitoring of the spinal cord can also be accomplished through somatosensory and motor evoked potentials when relieving a cord compression or to correct a spinal deformity.[27]

ANESTHETIC CONSIDERATIONS FOR PROCEDURES OF THE UPPER EXTREMITY

SHOULDER SURGERY

Shoulder procedures may be done in the lateral decubitus or "lawn-chair" position. Anesthetic choices include regional blockade or general anesthesia. Shorter procedures such as examinations and manipulations under anesthesia may be best accomplished under a general anesthetic. Generally, succinylcholine is used for the short and intense relaxation that is needed for shoulder manipulation in patients with capsular adhesions that are often referred to as "frozen shoulder." Although major shoulder procedures can be performed under regional anesthesia, they are also generally done under general anesthesia. Regional anesthesia requires either a supraclavicular block or a paravertebral block along with supplemental blocks. Patient acceptance tends to be low and a high degree of familiarity with these types of blocks is generally not found among most anesthesia providers. General anesthesia techniques are supplemented with moderately higher doses of narcotics to help in postanesthesia pain control (i.e., 3 to 5 µg/kg fentanyl). During wound closure, local infiltration of the surgical field with long-acting local anesthetics (e.g., bupivicaine) will help significantly for immediate postoperative pain management. General anesthetic considerations include protection of the endotracheal tube, airway circuit, and appropriate head support due to the close proximity of the airway and surgical site.

Arthroscopy and Arthroplasty Up until this past decade, shoulder surgery has been done via an open method. Today, because of advancing technology, many shoulder procedures are performed through an arthroscope. Its advantages include minimal incisions, decreased postoperative morbidity, and potentially faster rehabilitation.[28] Shoulder arthroscopy has been beneficial in the diagnosis of rotator cuff tears, subacromial impingement, glenohumeral instability, secondary inflammation, calcific deposits, and arthritis. Shoulder arthroscopy has also been beneficial in the treatment of resistant frozen shoulder.[29]

OPEN REDUCTION AND INTERNAL FIXATION OF THE ARM, ELBOW, AND WRIST

Fractures of the arm, elbow, and wrist that cannot be treated adequately with closed reduction require open reduction and internal fixation (ORIF). The goal is to provide stable anatomic reduction and can be accomplished with a variety of plates, screws, and wires.

There are many anesthetic choices for procedures on the upper extremity. However, the choice may be limited by the necessity of a bone graft that is usually obtained from the iliac crest to facilitate reduction and could increase risk of surgical blood loss.

Complications associated with wrist fractures include infection (if the fracture is open), compartment syndrome, and neurologic and occasionally vascular compromise. Open fractures are considered urgent because debridement and irrigation are needed within 8 hours of the injury. In this instance, full stomach precautions should be instituted. A fasciotomy may be indicated at the time of surgery, and the wound would remain open with splint applied. The incidence of vascular compromise is higher with severe crush or high-energy injuries and is a surgical emergency. If possible, vascularity must be immediately restored. Broad-spectrum antibiotic coverage is indicated in open fractures.

CARPAL TUNNEL RELEASE

Compression of the median nerve at the wrist results in carpal tunnel syndrome. Pain, paresthesia, and loss of motor function (primarily inability to oppose the thumb and little finger) that are associated can be improved by transection of the transverse carpal ligament through either an open palmar or an endoscopic approach. The procedure may be performed under local or intravenous regional anesthesia if the procedure will take under an hour, or axillary blockade. Bleeding may be controlled with the use of a pneumatic tourniquet placed on the upper arm or, if a local infiltration technique is used, adrenaline may be added to the local anesthetic agent.[30]

UPPER EXTREMITY BLOCKS

Brachial Plexus Brachial plexus blocks can be used for operative procedures of the neck, arm, and shoulder. The nerves of the brachial plexus can be blocked anywhere along their course from the emergence from the intervertebral foramina and entrance into the sheath between the anterior and middle scalene muscles until they terminate in the specific nerves of the hands. Several approaches are used—the interscalene, supraclavicular, or axillary techniques. Like other regional anesthetic techniques, blockade of the brachial plexus or more distal sites usually provides the patient with the advantage of avoiding a general anesthetic and its associated side effects and potential complications.

The brachial plexus supplies all of the motor and most of the sensory innervation to the upper extremity. The remaining areas and the skin over the shoulder are supplied by the descending branches of the cervical plexus (C-3 to C-4), and the posterior medial aspect of the arm extending nearly to the elbow is supplied by the intercostal brachial branch of T-2.[28]

Supraclavicular Block The supraclavicular block targets the brachial plexus at the level where it is most compactly arranged. The needle insertion point is directly superior to the clavicle. A low volume of fluid is injected, and in experienced hands a quick onset is obtained. The supraclavicular (or paraclavicular) approach is used for procedures of the upper arm and hand. Because this procedure is done so close to the apex of the lung, one of the most serious complications is the development of a pneumothorax and toxic reactions secondary to increased blood levels of local anesthetic drugs. Nerve damage and neuritis have been reported with this block. Due to the location and nature of this technique the *phrenic nerve* is unilaterally anesthetized in 40% to 60% of the patients, and the incidence of *Horner's syndrome* is 70% to 90% with injected volumes of greater than 50 mL.[31]

Interscalene Block The interscalene block is effective for operations of the upper arm and shoulder. It is not as effective for surgeries of the forearm and hand because the ulnar area is not always blocked. Often, the skin over the shoulder (C-3 to C-4) and the medial aspect of the upper arm (T-2) will need to be infiltrated with additional local anesthetic for adequate sensory blockade. The needle is inserted more superiorly than the supraclavicular approach, in a plane between two scalene muscles, also called the paravertebral or interscalene space. Therefore, the risk of pneumothorax is decreased. However, inadvertent epidural or spinal anesthesia has been reported. The vertebral artery is in close proximity to the needle insertion point, and there is a risk of intravascular injection of local anesthetics. *Phrenic nerve* blockade is an inevitable consequence, and subsequent hemidiaphragmatic paralysis may not be tolerated well in patients with preexisting respiratory alterations. The vagus, recurrent laryngeal, and branches of the cervical sympathetic nerves are sometimes blocked, in which case the patient will need to be reassured that this is a common side effect and normally does not pose a serious medical problem.[31]

Axillary Block An axillary block is the most effective regional technique for procedures of the forearm and hand. With this approach the musculocutaneous nerve is the most difficult to block, and infiltration of local anesthetic into the coracobrachialis muscle is often necessary to augment analgesia.[31]

Bier Block Intravenous regional anesthesia is a safe and cost-effective outpatient anesthetic for upper extremity fracture treatment in children[32] and adults. A continuous intravenous line is started to keep the vein open on the nonoperative extremity. A 22-gauge indwelling intravenous catheter and heparin lock are placed in the operative extremity as distal as possible in the arm so as not to interfere with the operative site. Forty to 50 mL preservative-free 0.5% lidocaine is injected into an exsanguinated extremity. Approximately 1 hour of adequate analgesia will be provided before tourniquet pain becomes severe. A double-cuff tourniquet may be used to help minimize the discomfort. The proximal cuff would be inflated during the local anesthetic administration, then the distal cuff inflated, then proximal deflated after distal cuff inflation is confirmed.

The most serious complication related to intravenous regional blocks is systemic local anesthetic toxicity. Toxic reactions have occurred after abrupt tourniquet deflation early in the procedure. Signs and symptoms of *toxicity* include tinnitus, dizziness, blurred vision, seizure activity, decreasing heart rate, and decreasing blood pressure. For procedures less than 40 minutes, the tourniquet should be deflated briefly ($<$ 10 seconds), then reinflated while observing the patient for signs of toxicity for 60 to 90 seconds before final deflation.

Other complications associated with intravenous regional block include inadequate block and thrombophlebitis.

☐ ANESTHETIC CONSIDERATIONS FOR PROCEDURES OF THE HIP, FEMUR, AND KNEE

As with upper extremity fractures and dislocations, injuries that compromise vascular or neurologic integrity are surgical emergencies and must be reduced immediately. Patients with fractures of the pelvis and femur must be monitored closely for signs and symptoms of hemorrhage because blood loss may be much greater than evident from superficial inspection. Hip fractures are common in the elderly, and anesthetic care should focus on optimizing physiologic reserve and effects of age-related diseases. Traction may be instituted for initial treatment of hip fractures, but most require ORIF to facilitate proper healing and function.[33]

Anesthetic management should be based on the patient's condition. Many patients are candidates for regional and combined regional techniques. Options include peripheral nerve block (i.e., femoral and sciatic nerves); subarachnoid blocks using hypobaric (operative side up) or hyperbaric (operative side down) techniques; epidural anesthesia, alone or in combination with general anesthesia; and general anesthesia.[33]

RECONSTRUCTIVE SURGERY

Most patients requiring reconstructive surgery are geriatric patients with coexisting rheumatic or degenerative or congenital joint alterations. Most are receiving chronic steroid therapy and large doses of nonsteroid anti-inflammatory medications. Therefore, thorough preoperative clinical assessment is mandatory.

During prosthetic surgery and long bone repairs, the anesthesia care provider must monitor the patient for embolization of fat, marrow, and air. Signs and symptoms of embolization include a precipitous drop in end-tidal CO_2, a decrease in oxygen saturation, decreased pulmonary compliance, hypotension, tachycardia, increased central venous pressure, decreased pulmonary capillary wedge pressure, and increase in end-tidal N_2 (air embolism only), and petechiae on the chest (fat embolism only).

Hip Replacement Most often, both components, the acetabulum cup and femoral head and shaft, are manufactured in incremental standardized sizes and are selected to fit the patient and one another. The patient is placed in a supine position for an anterior or anterolateral approach, or a lateral decubitus position for a lateral or posterior approach. An incision is made over the joint. In a total hip arthroplasty (total hip replacement), the femoral head is dislocated from the acetabulum. The arthritic portions are then excised. A cemented or noncemented cup is inserted into the acetabulum in a reamed pocket. This cup is made of either plastic or metal. Then the femoral shaft is reamed and the femoral component, consisting of head and shaft, are inserted. This component may also be cemented or cementless. Then the joint is relocated and tissues are closed. The patient is usually placed into traction or positioning devices to prevent dislocation. Incremental mobility is gradually restored.[34]

There are several variations of this procedure. The first is to replace only the femoral stem and head. This is called a unipolar arthroplasty. In a bipolar arthroplasty, both the acetabular component and femoral component are inserted, but the acetabular component is not fixed to the pelvis.[34]

Revision procedures are more challenging because they usually require specialized equipment for extracting the existing prosthesis and its cement and rebuilding bone stock in the acetabulum or femoral shaft by allografts or autograft material. If the joint is infected, both the components may be removed, but not replaced for some time in a resection or excision arthroplasty.[34]

Anesthetic considerations include monitoring and maintaining intravascular volume because blood loss may be excessive. Lateral or posterolateral approaches can often present positioning challenges (see Chap. 10). Antibiotic coverage is indicated and a broad-spectrum cephalosporin is usually started preoperatively and continued for 24 hours. The number one complication associated with this procedure is a 50% risk of deep-vein thrombosis if no prophylactic measures are instituted. This incidence can be decreased to 10% to 20% with minidose heparin (or Coumadin), sequential compression devices, or antiembolism stockings. Other concerns include heterotopic ossification (3% to 50%, average 13%), urinary tract infection (7% to 14%), late aseptic loosening requiring revision (5% to 10%), major hematoma formation ($< 5\%$), pulmonary embolus without prophylaxis (1.8% to 3.4%), nerve injury (0.7% to 3.5%), and wound infection (1%).[34]

Knee Replacement An arthroplasty of the knee involves incising and exposing the knee joint, femur, patella, and tibia, and excising damaged cartilage and bone. In a supine position, the damaged portions are replaced by either metal or plastic components and may be cemented or cementless. Uni-compartmental knee replacements are performed if only one component is used. If the components need to be removed, a resection or excision arthroplasty is performed. In a revision procedure, one or more of the components of the old joint are replaced.[34]

A tourniquet can be used, and 300 to 500 mL of blood may still be lost. The most common complication of these procedures is deep-vein thrombosis without prophylaxis and can exceed 50% to 75% incidence. With prophylaxis (minidose heparin, Coumadin, sequential compression devices, antiembolism stockings) this incidence is reduced to 10% to 20%. Other concerns are postoperative subluxation/dislocation of the patella (35%), superficial wound necrosis (10% to 15%), wound infection (5% to 10% with history of primary rheumatoid, psoriatic arthritis, or diabetes), pulmonary embolism (1% to 7%), late aseptic loosening requiring revision (after 10 years, 5%), and peroneal nerve injury (1% to 5%).[34]

FEMUR OPEN REDUCTION AND INTERNAL FIXATION

Patients with proximal femoral fractures are usually either elderly, and have sustained their injury from a fall, or are younger victims of trauma. In the elderly, the fractures are most often in the intertrochanteric or subtrochanteric area. Displaced femoral neck fractures are usually treated with prosthetic replacement. Minimally displaced or nondisplaced fractures are treated with closed reduction and percutaneous pinning. Intertrochanteric and subtrochanteric fractures, whether displaced or nondisplaced, are usually treated by ORIF with a nail plate or nail-rod device. In the younger patient, proximal femoral fractures are almost always treated with ORIF with screws, plates, and intramedullary devices.[34]

The mortality rate for elderly patients with proximal femoral fractures can be as high as 10% to 30% in the first 12 months postoperatively. In younger patients, the mortality rate depends on other injuries sustained. Other serious complications in the elderly include dysrhythmias (50%), myocardial infarction (50%), respiratory failure (50%), urinary retention (50%), urinary tract infections (50%), thromboembolism (40%+), avascular necrosis and late segmental collapse (10% to 20%), infection (2% to 17%), septic arthritis (2% to 17%), nonunion (5% to 15%), and malunion ($< 10\%$).[34]

In distal femur fractures, an incision is made longitudinally along the femoral shaft, and a reduction is made with plates and screws under direct visualization. The number one complication is that of nonunion and malunion (4% to 31%), followed by infection (osteomyelitis, septic arthritis 1% to 20%), and vascular complications (2% to 3%).[34]

KNEE ARTHROSCOPY

Knee arthroscopy can be used to diagnose and treat internal derangements such as medial and lateral meniscus tears, condylar roughness, and loose bodies. The most common complication associated with this procedure is hemarthrosis (5% to 20%).[34] Anesthetic choices include regional, general, and local with intravenous sedation.

Local anesthesia with intravenous sedation compares favorably with the other techniques. Operative time is not increased, a wide variety of operative procedures can be successfully completed, recovery time is significantly shortened, and patient satisfaction remains high, improving cost effectiveness.[35]

ANTERIOR CRUCIATE LIGAMENT

Anterior cruciate ligament reconstruction is performed to improve stability to the joint after traumatic injury. An autologous graft is obtained and directly sutured or stapled/screwed into the bone. The knee is then immobilized after surgery with a long-leg splint. The procedure is often arthroscopically assisted, and a tourniquet is used. No preoperative antibiotic coverage is routinely recommended. Blood loss is usually minimal, and patients can usually be discharged the same day. The most common complications are thrombophlebitis ($< 5\%$) and infection (1%).[34]

☐ SPINAL AND EPIDURAL ANESTHESIA

Anesthesia for orthopedic surgery often lends itself to regional anesthetics.[8] Advantages of spinal and epidural anesthesia include reduced blood loss, airway control in patients with major airway problems secondary to rheumatoid arthritis, and reduced risk of postoperative deep-vein thrombosis and thromboembolism.

However, regional anesthesia is contraindicated in patients with coagulation derangements, and there is a risk of major spinal hematomas. The incidence of spinal hematomas increases with female gender, increased age, a history of excessive bruising/bleeding, hip surgery, continuous catheter anesthetic technique, large needle gauge, multiple needle passes, and moderate or difficult needle placement. There is always a chance for ineffective or incomplete regional blockade.

The use of antiplatelet medications (ASA and subcutaneous heparin) was not shown to be a significant risk factor.[36] There is also the concern of technical difficulties secondary to arthritic spinal changes and ineffective or spotty blockade.

SPINAL ANESTHESIA

Spinal landmarks are the spinous process and the iliac crests, which cross at the level of the fourth lumbar vertebrae. Punctures are usually made at the L3-4 or L4-5 interspaces by either the standard midline approach through the supraspinous ligament, intraspinous ligament, and ligamentum flavum, or by a paramedial (lateral) approach by passing possible calcified supraspinous and intraspinous ligaments, passing through only the ligamentum of flavum.

The injection level, potency, onset, degree of protein binding, and duration of the medication administered affect the quality of the block. The *level* obtained is most dependent on the *baricity* of the mixture and the patient's *position* and to a lesser extent on the volume and concentration of the drug and the speed of administration. The mixture can be hypertonic, isotonic, or hypotonic to the specific gravity of the cerebral spinal fluid (CSF) and used to an advantage. The majority of spinal blockades are accomplished with a hypertonic local anesthetic to which 5% dextrose has been added. The medication is distributed to dependent areas by gravity and is ideal when the spinal is administered to a patient in the sitting position or in the lateral position with the operative side down. For a patient with a hip fracture, it may be desirable to roll the fractured side up for patient comfort, in which case an isotonic or hypotonic spinal anesthetic should be administered.

The duration of the blockade depends on the drug selected and the addition of vasoconstrictive substances such as epinephrine or phenylephrine. The actions of these vasoconstrictors are more pronounced when using tetracaine than with lidocaine and bupivacaine. The *onset* of the local anesthetic is most dependent on the *pKa* of the solution and the pH of the fluid receiving the medication.

Complications   The most common complication associated with a subarachnoid block is hypotension that must be treated with fluids and systemic vasopressors. Other complications include postspinal headache caused by a CSF leak. This complication is best avoided by using the smallest possible spinal needle. Using a 25-gauge Whitacre spinal needle instead of a 22-gauge Whitacre spinal needle decreases the risk of spinal headache from 4% to 2% without changing the failure rate, patient satisfaction rate, or incidence of backache.[37] The incidence of postdural spinal headache was reported to be 0.8% with a Quincke needle and 0.5% with a Whitacre needle.[38] Both needles are associated with very low incidence of postdural puncture headache and an incidence of failed anesthesia of 5.5% to 8.5%.

Conservative treatment for postdural spinal headache includes keeping the patient in the supine position, hydration, and analgesics. Headaches that are unresolved can be treated with an epidural blood patch (90% to 95% effective).[39]

The incidence of intravascular injection can be minimized by aspiration till clear before any injection. If the spinal level is high enough to depress satisfactory respiratory effort, the patient must be intubated and ventilated, while appropriate vasopressors and fluids are being administered.

There are other concerns related to spinal anesthesia. Intrathecal morphine decreases gastric emptying status after spinal anesthesia.[40] There are two methods of administration, single-shot injections and continuous catheter infusions.

EPIDURAL ANESTHESIA

Continuous epidural anesthesia intraoperatively and reinforcement of blockade postoperatively can provide excellent analgesia. When administering an epidural anesthetic several aspects must be considered: the total number of segments and location of segments to be blocked; the drug used and its concentration; and the patient's age and condition (pregnant or nonpregnant). The average dose requirement of 2% lidocaine in a nonpregnant healthy adult is 1.5 mL per dermatome. In pregnant patients this decreases to 1 to 1.2 mL per dermatome.

Continuous epidural fentanyl has been helpful postoperatively in reducing pain and narcotic need. One study of 128 patients after lumbar laminectomy, comparing epidural fentanyl to patient-controlled analgesia (PCA) with morphine noted significantly lower pain and narcotic use. The patients in the PCA morphine group had an increased incidence of urinary retention and somnolence. There was no difference in the incidence of vomiting or pruritus. No patient developed respiratory depression or wound infection.[41]

The incidence of postdural puncture headaches was recently reported to be 7% for spinal and 4% for epidural anesthesia. Differences in failed blocks (5% each group) and patient satisfaction (97% and 93%) between the two anesthetic techniques were not statistically significant. The major advantage of spinal anesthesia was an increased onset of blockade, significantly lower incidence of postlumbar puncture backache (11% versus 30%), significantly lower incidence of incomplete sensory block at level L-5 to S-1, incomplete motor block, and pain during surgery.[42]

Continuous Postoperative Epidural Infusions Postoperative infusional continuous regional analgesia (PICRA) has been used successfully after surgery, drastically reducing the need for postoperative narcotic analgesics (60%).[34] Bupivacaine was delivered into peripheral nerve sheaths (axillary, lumbosacral trunk, femoral, and sciatic) through catheters placed intraoperatively. The anesthetic agent was administered through infusion pump.

☐ ANESTHETIC CONSIDERATIONS FOR PROCEDURES OF THE CALF, ANKLE, AND FOOT

TIBIA-FIBULA

An ORIF of the tibia (or fibula) or both after traumatic injury involves making a longitudinal incision along the lateral leg to the knee and reducing the fracture under direct visualization and applying plates and screws to stabilize the reduction. Homologous bone grafts may be necessary to bridge unions. These grafts are most often obtained in the iliac crest.[34]

Broad-spectrum cephalosporin coverage is indicated and should be started before the tourniquet is inflated. Blood loss is usually under 200 mL. Postoperative concerns include wound infection (7% to 15%), deep-vein thrombosis (3% to 5%), and peripheral nerve damage (3%).[34]

ANKLE

An ankle arthroplasty is performed by making an incision anterolaterally, midline, or anteromedially, then opening the joint capsule after carefully retracting the tendons and neurovascular structures. Then a debridement or ORIF can be performed. Antibiotics are often ordered. The most common complications include hemarthrosis (20%), thrombophlebitis (5%), and infection (1%). A fusion of ankle bones may need to be performed in patients with severe arthritis that limits function.[43]

☐ LOWER EXTREMITY BLOCKS

LATERAL FEMORAL CUTANEOUS BLOCK

The lateral femoral cutaneous nerve (L-1 to L-2) block by itself is advantageous for anesthetizing the thigh for muscle biopsies and to obtain skin grafts. It is often used in combination with the femoral and sciatic nerve blocks for lower extremity procedures and tourniquet pain. The patient is placed in a supine position. The lateral cutaneous nerve can be blocked just medially to the anterior superior iliac spine or 1 to 2 cm below it. Complications and side effects of this procedure are reported to be minimal.[44]

ANKLE BLOCK

An ankle block can be accomplished by anesthetizing the five nerves of the foot—the superficial peroneal nerve, the deep peroneal nerve, the saphenous nerve, the posterior tibial nerve, and the sural nerve (see also Chap. 13).

A pneumatic ankle tourniquet may be applied to the ankle region above the malleolar region to obtain a bloodless field for surgery of the foot used in conjunction with the regional ankle block without increased risk of neurovascular damage.

REFERENCES

1. Farfan HR. Major sports injury. *Clin Orthop.* 1982;164:2.
2. Schrader LL, McMillen MA, Watson CB, MacArthur JD. Is routine preoperative hemodynamic evaluation of nonagenarians necessary? *J Am Geriatr Soc.* 1991; 39(9):1–5.
3. Stoelting RK, Dierdorf SR. *Anesthesia and Co-Existing Disease.* 3rd ed. New York: Churchill Livingstone; 1993.
4. Smith G. Alterations in musculoskeletal function: rheumatic disorders. In: Copstead LED. *Perspectives on Pathophysiology.* Philadelphia: WB Saunders, 1995:1013.
5. Harris E. Pathogenesis of rheumatoid arthritis. In: Kelly W, Harris E, Ruddy S, Sledge D, eds. *Textbook of Rheumatology.* Philadelphia: WB Saunders, 1985:886–903.
6. Harris ED. Rheumatoid arthritis. Pathophysiology and implications for therapy. *N Engl J Med.* 1990; 332:1277–1288.

7. Campbell RS, Wou P, Watt I. A continuing role for pre-operative cervical spine radiography in rheumatoid arthritis? *Clin Radiol.* 1995;50(3):157–159.

8. Barash PG, Cullen BF, Stoelting RK. *Handbook of Clinical Anesthesia.* 2nd ed. Philadelphia: JB Lippincott; 1993.

9. Oishi CS, Carrion WV, Hoaglund FT. Use of parenteral prophylactic antibiotics in clean orthopedic surgery. A review of the literature. *Clin Orthop.* 1993;296:249–255.

10. Dierdorf SF. Rare and coexisting disease. In: Barash PG, Cullen BF, Stoelting RK. *Clinical Anesthesia.* 2nd ed. Philadelphia: JB Lippincott; 1992:577.

11. Charnley J. *Acrylic Cement in Orthopaedic Surgery.* Baltimore: Williams & Wilkins; 1970.

12. Ellis RH, Mulvein J. The cardiovascular effects of methylmethacrylate. *J Bone Joint Surg.* 1974; 56B:59.

13. Weissman BN, Sosman JL, Braunstein EM. Intravenous methylmethacrylate after total hip replacement. *J Bone Joint Surg.* 1984; 66A:44.

14. Bengston A, Larsson M, Gammer W. Anaphylatoxin release in association with methylmethacrylate fixation of hip prosthesis. *J Bone Joint Surg.* 1987; 69A:46.

15. Crout DHG, Corkill JA, James ML. Methylmethacrylate metabolism in man: the hydrolysis of methylmethacrylate to methacrylate acid during total hip replacement. *Clin Orthop.* 1974; 141:90.

16a. Smith TC. Anesthesia and orthopaedic surgery. In: Barash PG, Cullen BF, Stoelting RK. *Handbook of Clinical Anesthesia.* 2nd ed. Philadelphia: JB Lippincott, 1993.

16b. Levy J. Anaphylactic Reactions in Anesthesia and Intensive Care, 2nd ed. Boston: Butterworth-Heineman, 1992:111.

17. Zahrawi F. Microlumbar discectomy. Is it safe as an outpatient procedure? *Spine.* 1994; 19:1070–1074.

18. Barton CR, Weisburn Y, Castor S, Benson D, McVey J. Anaphylactic reaction to chymopapain injection: a review and anesthetic considerations. *American Association of Nurse Anesthetists Journal.* 1984; 52:280–295.

19. Jansen EF, Balls AK., Chymopapain: new crystalline proteinase from papaya latex. *J Biol Chem.* 1941; 137:459–460.

20. Smith L. Enzyme dissolution of the nucleus pulposus in humans. *JAMA.* 1964; 187:137–140.

21. Parkinson D, Shields C. Treatment of protruded lumbar intervertebral discs with chymopapain (Discase®). *J Neurosurg.* 1973; 39:203–208.

22. Watts C, Williams OB, Goldstein G. Sensitivity reactions to intradiscal injection of chymopapain during general anesthesia. *Anesthesiology.* 1976; 44:437–439.

23. Smith Laboratories. Chymodiactin® post marketing surveillance report, 1984.

24. Barton CR, Benson D, McVey J. Anaphylaxis and chemonucleolysis revisited. *American Association of Nurse Anesthetists Journal.* 1985; 53:95–100.

25. Roy CA, Barton CR. Intraoperative latex anaphylaxis compounded by atracurium sensitivity: a case report. *American Association of Nurse Anesthetists Journal.* 1991; 59:399–404.

26. Gokel E, Arkan A, Sagiroglu E, Karci A, Maltepe F. Focus on infusion: intravenous anaesthesia. Proceedings of intravenous anesthesia sessions held during a symposium in Cannes, France, April 28–29, 1991:180–183.

27. Newfield P, Cottrell JE. Neuroanesthesia. In: *Handbook of Clinical and Physiologic Essentials.* Boston: Little, Brown; 1992:361.

28. Ladd AI, Egan TD. Shoulder surgery. In: Jaffe RA, Samuels SI. *Anesthesiologist's Manual of Surgical Procedures.* New York: Raven Press; 1994:617–625.

29. Pollock RG, Duralde XA, Flatow EL, Bigliani LU. The use of arthroscopy in the treatment of resistant frozen shoulder. *Clin Orthop.* 1994; 304:30–36.

30. Braithwaite BD, Robinson GJ, Burge PD. Haemostasis during carpal tunnel release under local anesthesia: a controlled comparison of a tourniquet and adrenaline infiltration. *J Hand Surg.* 1993; 18:184–186.

31. Cousins MJ, Bridenbaugh PO, eds. Neural Blockade: *In Clinical Anesthesia and Management of Pain.* 2nd ed. Philadelphia: JB Lippincott; 1989.

32. Barnes CL, Blasier RD, Dodge BM. Intravenous regional anesthesia: a safe and cost-effective outpatient anesthetic for upper extremity fracture treatment in children. *J Pediatr Orthop.* 1992; 12:675–676.

33. Davison JK, Eckhardt WF, Perese DA, eds. *Clinical Anesthesia Procedures of the Massachusetts General Hospital.* 4th ed. Boston: Little, Brown; 1993:501.

34. Csongradi JJ, Goodman SB, Kosek PS, Mihm FG. Surgery of the lower extremities. In: Jaffe RA, Samuels SI. *Anesthesiologist's Manual of Surgical Procedures.* New York: Raven Press; 1994.

35. Shapiro MS, Safran MR, Crockett H, Finerman GA. Local anesthesia for knee arthroscopy. Efficacy and cost benefits. *Am J Sports Med.* 1995; 23:50–53.

36. Horlocker TT, Wedel DJ, Schroeder DR, et al. Preoperative antiplatelet therapy does not increase the risk of spinal hematoma associated with regional anesthesia. *Anesth Analg.* 1995; 80:303–309.

37. Lynch J, Krongs-Ernst I, Strick K, Topalidis K, Schaaf H, Fiebig M. Use of a 25-gauge Whitacre needle to reduce the incidence of postdural puncture headache. *Br J Anaesth.* 1991; 67:690–703.

38. Lynch J. Kasper SM, Strick K, et al. The use of Quincke and Whitacre 27-gauge needles in orthopedic patients: incidence of failed spinal anesthesia and postdural puncture headache. *Anesth Analg.* 1995; 80:124–128.

39. Szeinfeld M, Ihomeidan IH, Moser MM. Epidural blood patch: evaluation of the volume and spread of blood injected in to the epidural space. *Anesthesiology.* 1986; 64:820–822.

40. Petring OU, Dawson RJ, Blake DW, et al. Normal postoperative gastric emptying after orthopaedic surgery with spinal anaesthesia in i.m. ketorolac as the first postoperative analgesic. *Br J Anaesth.* 1995; 74:257–260.

41. Malawaer MM, Cuch R, Khurana JS, Garvey T, Rice L. Postoperative infusional continuous regional analgesia. A technique for relief of postoperative pain following major extremity surgery. *Clin Orthop.* 1991; 266:227–237.

42. Joshi GP. McCarroll SM, O'Rourke K. Postoperative analgesia after lumbar laminectomy: epidural fentanyl infusion versus patient-controlled intravenous morphine. *Anesth Analg.* 1995; 80:511–514.

43. Csongradi JJ, Goodman SB, Kosek, PS, Mihm, FG. Surgery of the lower extremities in Jaffe RA, Samuels SI, eds. *Anesthesiologist's Manual of Surgical Procedures,* New York: Raven Press; 1994, 681–5.

44. Cousins MJ, Bridenbaugh PO, eds. Neural Blockade: In *Clinical Anesthesia and Management of Pain,* 2nd. ed., Philadelphia: J. B. Lippincott Company: 429–31.

☐ QUESTIONS

1. Care must be taken when treating patients with rheumatoid involvement to prevent
   a. Subluxation of C-1 and C-2 (atlas-axis)
   b. Separation of the atlanto-odontoid articulation
   c. All of the above
   d. None of the above

2. Painless degeneration and atrophy of skeletal muscle is associated with
   a. Multiple sclerosis
   b. Muscular dystrophy
   c. Cerebral palsy
   d. None of the above

3. Muscular dystrophy can be associated with
   a. An exaggerated serum potassium elevation when succinylcholine is used
   b. A resistance to the effects of nondepolarizing neuromuscular blocking agents
   c. Gastrointestinal hypomotility
   d. All of the above
   e. a and c only

4. Common findings seen in the patient with scleroderma include all but which one of the following?
   a. Fibrosis of skin, viscera, and vasculature
   b. Systemic hypertension
   c. Narrowing of the mouth with limited mandibular motion
   d. Increased pulmonary compliance

5. The most common cause of death in the patient with scleroderma is
   a. Cardiac failure
   b. Renal failure
   c. Hepatic failure
   d. Pulmonary failure

6. Cefazolin is a first-generation cephalosporin and the antibiotic of choice for use in orthopedic surgery because of its coverage against
   a. Streptococcus
   b. Staphylococci
   c. Haemophilus bacillus
   d. E-coli

7. A laminar air flow system can provide up to _____ air exchanges per hour.
   a. 15
   b. 50
   c. 200
   d. 500
   e. 800

8. Hypothermia can cause all of the following *except*
   a. Impaired hemostasis
   b. Impaired leukocyte function
   c. Reduced cardiac output
   d. Increased stress hormone release

9. Rapid deflation of a tourniquet cuff can cause
   a. Transient metabolic acidosis
   b. Washout of potassium
   c. Elevation of Pa_{CO_2}
   d. All of the above
   e. a and c only

10. Tourniquets are generally considered _____ for use in patients with sickle cell disease or trait.
    a. Safe
    b. Unsafe
    c. Safe if there is an increased delivery of oxygen to tissues

11. Methylmethacrylate, when used to cement prosthesis into joints, is often associated with
    a. Hypotension
    b. Decreases in systemic vascular resistance
    c. Direct myocardiac depression
    d. All of the above
    e. a and b only

12. Often patients with scoliosis display
    a. Increased physiologic pulmonary shunting
    b. Increased Pa_{O_2} levels and increased work of breathing
    c. Right ventricular hypertrophy and cor pulmonale
    d. All of the above
    e. b and c only

13. A _____ minute advanced notice of the wake up test by the surgeon is ideal.
    a. 5–10
    b. 10–20
    c. 40–60
    d. 60–90

14. Open fractures should be debrided and irrigated within _____ hours if injury.
    a. 2
    b. 4
    c. 8
    d. 16

15. The risk of pneumothorax is greatest with
    a. Supraclavicular block
    b. Interscalene block
    c. Axillary block

16. Signs and symptoms of local anesthesia toxicity following the release of the tourniquet with Bier blocks include all of the following *except:*
   a. Tinnitus
   b. Dizziness and blurred vision
   c. Tachycardia
   d. Seizure activity

17. Signs of embolization of fat, marrow, or air during long bone repairs include all but which one of the following?
   a. Precipitous drop in end-tidal CO_2
   b. Decrease in oxygen saturation
   c. Hypertension
   d. Tachycardia
   e. Decreased pulmonary capillary wedge pressure

18. If there is no prophylactic treatment, the number one risk (50% incidence) of hip surgery is
   a. Urinary tract infection

   b. Deep-vein thrombosis
   c. Nerve injury
   d. Wound infection

19. The quality of a subarachnoid block is determined by
   a. The injection level
   b. The medication's potency
   c. Degree of protein binding
   d. All of the above
   e. a and c only

20. The two most common complications of spinal anesthesia in the order of occurrence are
   a. Hypotension, postspinal headache
   b. Postspinal headache, hypotension
   c. Intravascular injection, postspinal headache
   d. Hypotension, intravascular injection

☐ ANSWERS

1. c	5. b	9. d	13. c	17. c
2. b	6. b	10. b	14. c	18. b
3. e	7. d	11. d	15. a	19. d
4. d	8. d	12. d	16. c	20. a

CHAPTER 28

Geriatric Anesthesia

Laura Ricciardi

☐ PHYSIOLOGIC CHANGES IN THE ELDERLY

A geriatric patient is usually arbitrarily defined as one aged 65 or older. However, little correlation exists between physiologic and chronologic ages. *The geriatric patient undergoing anesthetic care is at risk for two reasons: a decline in organ function secondary to age and presence of concomitant diseases* (discussed later in this chapter). Pathology studies have shown that patients aged 81 years or older have a 92% incidence of at least one disease process.[1] Perioperative complications are associated more with a patient's ongoing diseases than with age. According to Gibson and colleagues,[2] mortality is four times more frequent in the elderly with a coexisting disease than in a healthy elderly patient. One explanation is that elderly patients who require emergency surgery may have advanced pathology and have delayed seeking health care, leading to a higher incidence of preoperative complications and death.

CENTRAL NERVOUS SYSTEM

Deterioration of the central nervous system (CNS) begins at age 50, affecting primarily frontal and temporal lobes. Brain weight decreases approximately 7% by age 80.[3] Axons degenerate, especially myelinated axons, causing alterations in the rate of impulse transmission. The actual numbers of synapses per neuron decrease. Cerebral blood flow in proportion to reduced brain mass and cerebral metabolism is reduced.[4] Neuronal processes dependent on Ca++ movement are inhibited because the ability to maintain calcium homeostasis is reduced (Table 28–1).[5]

Neurotransmitters The quantity of the neurotransmitters norepinephrine, dopamine, and serotonin is reduced.[6] In addition, the number of receptor sites available is diminished, which also contributes to the decline in neural function. Cardiovascular reflexes are blunted and cognitive and memory functions decline.[7] Depression in the elderly is thought to be related to diminished norepinephrine and serotonin levels. Both adrenergic and acetylcholine receptors are reduced. Interestingly, gamma-aminobutyric acid (GABA) receptor sites may be increased[8] and may be responsible for the increased sensitivity to GABA-mediated agents (i.e., benzodiazepines and barbiturates).

Changes in the neuroendocrine system of the geriatric patient affect the ability to maintain homeostasis. Some researchers feel it is the deterioration of the anterior hypothalamus[9] that leads to many diseases common to the elderly such as diabetes, atherosclerosis, and hypertension (Tables 28–2, 28–3).

Pathology
Dementia
Dementia is defined as a decline in all levels of mental functioning. Dementia can have many causes, the primary one being vascular disease. Metabolic causes may be renal failure, lupus erythematosus, adrenal insufficiency, and hypothyroidism.[7] A brief evaluation would be recall of name, address, date of birth, current president, the ability to count backward from 20, and recognition of two people.[10] Personality changes are common with dementia as opposed to the memory loss usually associated with aging.

Alzheimer's Disease
Alzheimer's disease is related to frontal and temporal lobe atrophy. The actual cause of Alzheimer's is unknown, but it

Table 28-1
CHANGES IN CELLULAR BIOCHEMISTRY AND PHYSIOLOGY

Decreased cerebral blood flow

Loss of vascular autoregulation and responsiveness to neuronal demand and hypercapnia

Decreased cellular oxygen and glucose metabolism

Altered sodium and potassium homeostasis

Alterations in calcium homeostasis

Table 28-3
BEHAVIORAL AND FUNCTIONAL CHANGES

Slowed reaction time

Dysfunction in learning

Reduced information retrieval (especially short-term memory)

Slower peripheral information acquisition time

Decrease in intelligence

Decline in language skills

Depression

Decreased sensory function

    Reduced visual sensitivity to short wavelengths

    High-frequency hearing loss

    Decreased proprioception and vibration

---

occurs in conjunction with cholinergic deficiencies.[11] The patient with dementia or Alzheimer's disease may be unable to cooperate and preoperative sedation that could exacerbate disorientation may be omitted. Central anticholinergic agents should be avoided in patients with Alzheimer's disease.

Parkinson's Disease

Parkinson's disease is a loss of dopaminergic fibers in the basal ganglia of the CNS. Dopamine inhibits the neurons that control the extrapyramidal motor system. Loss of dopamine results in unopposed firing of the extrapyramidal motor neurons, seen as involuntary tremors and akinesia. *Phenothiazines, butyrophenones (droperidol), and metoclopromide (Reglan) are avoided because of their ability to antagonize dopamine in the basal ganglia.* To increase levels of dopamine and decrease cholinergic function in the brain, levodopa, anticholinergics, amantidine, and bromocriptine are used. Halothane should be avoided in patients taking levodopa because the risk of cardiac dysrhythmias is increased.[12] Autonomic dysfunction such as dysphagia and orthostatic hypotension can result from levodopa treatment. Medications should be continued if possible to prevent recurrence of symptoms.

PERIPHERAL NERVOUS SYSTEM

Many disease entities lead to peripheral neuropathy. Those most commonly found in patients over age 55 are diabetes, cancer, hypertension, ethanol abuse, autoimmune dysfunction, and malnutrition. There is a loss of myelin as well as

Table 28-2
AUTONOMIC AND HOMEOSTATIC CHANGES

Decreased anterior hypothalamic activity

Decreased sensitivity of hypothalamus to inhibitory hormones

Increased threshold of vagal and sympathetic nerves

Altered sympathetic and parasympathetic function

Reduced control and responsiveness of cardiovascular tone

Reduced temperature regulation

Orthostatic hypotension

Chronic constipation

Decreased sympathetic function

    (slowed heart rate and decreased blood pressure)

---

fewer axons and synapses as discussed earlier. Conduction velocity is reduced.[13]

Respiratory

Physiologic Changes

The elderly show a decrease in vital capacity, forced exhaled volume in 1 second (FEV_1), forced vital capacity (FVC), and Pao_2. There is a significant loss of elastic recoil and a decrease in ventilatory and cardiovascular response to hypoxia and hypercarbia.[14] Reduced albumin and therefore decreased osmotic pressure places the geriatric patient at risk for pulmonary edema. The number of alveoli are decreased and many alveoli collapse due to reduced elasticity, resulting in higher closing volumes and air trapping.[15] Diminished muscle mass along with accumulations of interstitial water and air trapping make it difficult for the elderly to produce an effective cough. All of these changes put them at higher risk for postoperative atelectasis and pneumonia.

Pulmonary function studies as well as baseline arterial blood gas determination and chest x-ray are useful in assessing the geriatric patient's pulmonary status. Because of a reduced response to hypoxia, supplemental oxygen should be considered for 24 hours postoperatively along with aggressive pulmonary toilet (incentive spirometer, chest percussion, etc.).

Total lung capacity is reduced approximately 10% by age 70.[14] Kyphosis and scoliosis, as well as narrowing of the intervertebral spaces, reduce chest expansion. A 20-year-old patient can generate a maximum ventilation of 100 L/min, which equals approximately 15 times the basal metabolic requirements. By age 80 the same patient has a ventilation of 30 to 40 L/min, which is 7 times the requirement.[15] This would suffice in a healthy 80-year-old patient but may not be adequate for surgery, anesthesia, or infection.

Chronic Obstructive Pulmonary Disease

Chronic obstructive pulmonary disease (COPD) is often seen in the elderly with a history of long-term smoking. The changes that occur in the nonsmoking elderly patient actually mimic those that occur with COPD. For example, increased closing volumes, atelectasis, loss of elastic recoil, and reduced membrane permeability all result in increasing ventilation/perfusion (V/Q) mismatch. A simple equation to estimate a normal PaO_2 by age would be[16]:

$$PaO_2 = 100 - (.32 \times \text{age in years})$$

Patients with a history of long-term smoking will have a chronic productive cough and a reduced FEV_1. The diagnosis of COPD is based on a number of findings, including pulmonary function results, chest x-ray, blood gases, and clinical presentation of chronic dyspnea and a productive cough. Patients with COPD have airway narrowing secondary to inflammatory changes and secretions and loss of elastic recoil causing chronic hypoxia and polycythemia.[17] Treatment consists of preventing infections, maintaining hydration, using bronchodilators, and hopefully, quitting smoking. If necessary, glucocorticoids are added. COPD is generally irreversible and treatment goals are to halt the progression of respiratory failure.

Asthma

Asthma, a disease of the smaller airways, may or may not have a specific triggering agent. Bronchoconstriction may occur in association with an allergic reaction, an upper respiratory infection, or emotional stress. Clinical signs include tachypnea, tachycardia, hypoxia, and use of the accessory muscles to breathe. FEV_1, FVC, and FEV_1/FVC are decreased. IgE may be elevated and eosinophilia is seen. Active asthma is associated with eosinophil counts greater than 300 mm/h. Because of reduced cardiac and respiratory reserve, the elderly are less able to tolerate bronchospasm, resulting in dysrhythmias and possibly ischemia.[17]

Treatment goals are to increase cyclic adenosine monophosphate (cAMP). β-Adrenergic agonists are usually the first choice, particularly those with the fewest cardiac side effects. For acute episodes of asthma, epinephrine via nebulizer or subcutaneously is the drug of choice. Theophylline may also be used for non–life-threatening situations (5 mg/kg IV over 30 minutes as a loading dose and 0.5 mg/kg per hour to maintain a level). Serum levels should be closely monitored because theophylline clearance varies with age.[18] Tachydysrhythmias with ischemia can be seen with β-adrenergic drugs and theophylline treatment due to the endogenous release of catecholamines. Anticholinergics and ipratropium bromide are also effective bronchodilators. Ipratropium bromide is available in a metered inhaler and has the fewest cardiac side effects. Long-term steroids should be avoided in the elderly because of the possible complications of osteoporosis, diabetes, and congestive heart failure (CHF).

Pulmonary Hypertension

Pulmonary hypertension is seen in the elderly with ventricular septal defect, emboli, emphysema, or adult respiratory distress syndrome. Hypoxia with dyspnea is seen. Right ventricular hypertrophy with right axis deviation and right-sided failure may occur. Treatment is with supplemental oxygen. Currently nitric oxide is being studied for use as a pulmonary vasodilator.[19]

CARDIOVASCULAR

Many cardiovascular changes that were previously believed to be a normal consequence of aging are now thought to be related to the individual's life-style. Because cardiovascular diseases are more common in the elderly, it is difficult to ascertain which changes are due to the normal aging process and which to a disease state.

Myocardial Changes Left ventricular wall thickness increases by 30% from age 20 to age 70 because of an increase in myocyte size, which affects the intraventricular septal wall to the greatest extent.[20] Ventricular hypertrophy results in delayed diastolic filling and increased left ventricular end-diastolic pressure. The elderly heart is sensitive to small changes in preload similar to a patient with mitral stenosis. β-Adrenergic blockers, calcium channel blockers, and cardiovascular fitness can improve diastolic filling. Cardiac output decreases 1% for each year after age 30.[21] This will result in a delay in intravenous induction time. A test dose of Pentothal is a useful tool in both estimating onset of induction and hemodynamic response to a dose. Although intravenous induction time is slow in the elderly because of reduced cardiac output, inhalation time is more rapid. The uptake of inhaled anesthetics via alveolar perfusion is delayed, resulting in a higher partial pressure of anesthesia in the alveoli and, therefore, the heart and brain.

The intrinsic heart rate in the elderly is reduced. By age 75, the sinus node loses 80% of its pacing cells.[22] As the conduction system of the heart becomes fibrotic, left axis deviation may develop into left bundle branch block. The PR and QT intervals are also prolonged.[23] Responsiveness to exogenous and endogenous catecholamines is decreased with regard to inotropy and chronotropy. The elderly are capable of secreting catecholamines but apparently have a reduced response from the target organ. It is not known if this is due to a reduced number of receptor sites or simply a reduced response by the receptors. In addition, the aged are less capable of increasing the heart rate to improve cardiac output in response to increased oxygen requirements (i.e., infection, stress, hypovolemia, anemia). However, an increase demand (i.e., exercise) can be met by increasing end-diastolic volume to a greater extent than the end-systolic volume, resulting in an age-related increase in stroke volume. Consequently, this increase in filling pressures also predisposes the elderly to CHF.[24]

Peripheral Vascular Resistance Arterial elasticity is reduced, which increases total peripheral vascular resistance. This impedance to forward flow leads to increased systolic blood pressure, which in turn, causes left ventricular hypertrophy. Hypertension increases the risk of ischemic heart disease, stroke, CHF, and sudden death. Hypertension can be defined as a blood pressure greater than 160/95. Treatment is done in a step-wise fashion, beginning with diet and exercise, diuretics, β blockers, angiotensin-converting enzyme (ACE) inhibiters, calcium channel blockers, central α-adrenergic agents, and nitrates. Plasma volumes will be reduced with hypertension. Hypovolemia in elderly hypertensive patients leads to significantly labile blood pressure intraoperatively. The patient is unable to tolerate changes in position, fluid losses, or intrathoracic pressure. Degeneration at the capillary level may interfere with cellular respiration. Pulmonary artery pressures also increase with age. When assessing the aged heart, the clinical significance of elevated readings should not be misinterpreted.

Coronary Artery Disease   Coronary artery disease (CAD) is progressive and the patient may remain asymptomatic until critically ill. A history of angina or dyspnea cannot be relied on to assess CAD. Radionuclide imaging along with treadmill studies have shown people 70 years or older have a 50% incidence of CAD irrespective of any clinical symptoms. By age 70 incidence of myocardial infarction is equal between men and women.

Congestive Heart Failure   Congestive heart failure is a common diagnosis for patients over age 65. Once a diagnosis of CHF is made, a 50% 5-year survival is predicted. Reduced left ventricular compliance and increased peripheral vascular resistance with coronary ischemia predispose the elderly heart to CHF.[25] Failure caused by systolic dysfunction has a gradual onset of symptoms, associated with enlargement of the heart and a gradual decline in function. Treatment consists of diuresis, digitalization, vasodilators, and inotropic support. Diastolic dysfunction has an abrupt onset and is caused by increased circulating volume, impaired diastolic filling, (ischemia, tachycardia), or increased demand (sepsis, trauma). Goals of diastolic dysfunction treatment are to improve diastolic filling with β blockers, calcium channel blockers, or ACE inhibitors.

Dysrhythmias   Although all adults have ventricular dysrhythmias, the incidence increases with age; 50% of all adults as compared to 80% of all elderly have dysrhythmias. Bundle branch blocks occur with the fibrosis of the conduction system. A left bundle branch block carries a higher mortality rate. First-degree blocks are common; one study by Martin and coworkers[26] found atrial fibrillation in 17% of all patients over age 80. The aged are more sensitive to dysrhythmias that cause diastolic impairment (reduced filling and therefore reduced coronary perfusion) and have ongoing CAD. Because of decreased hepatic and renal function in the aged, any antidysrhythmic therapy must be closely monitored to prevent toxic drug levels.

RENAL/HEPATIC

By age 70, the kidneys decrease in weight by 20%. This loss in mass is both cortical and parenchymal and the renal tubules decrease in number.[27] Renal blood flow (RBF) drops 10% per decade after age 20. The glomerular filtration rate (GFR) is reduced 1 mL/min per year or 1% to 1.5% per year. This reduction in GFR is related to the reduced RBF. Creatinine levels may remain stable in a healthy aged patient in view of the reduced creatinine production with less skeletal mass.[28] Diminished renal function will lead to a reduced clearance of drugs and their metabolites. The elderly will also be less tolerate of fluid and electrolyte imbalances associated with medical and surgical problems. Renal failure that occurs as a result of hypovolemia, CHF, sepsis, or diabetes mellitus contributes significantly to mortality in the elderly. A urine output of 0.5 mL/kg per hour should be maintained. As RBF is reduced, glycosuria does not correlate as reliably with hyperglycemia.

The liver decreases about 25% in size from age 20 to 70.[29] A decrease in liver blood flow contributes to the delayed clearance of medications.[30] Liver function tests do not change with age despite functioning hepatic tissue loss of 40% to 50% by age 80. Any abnormalities in these tests should be investigated.

DIABETES MELLITUS

Approximately 18% of the elderly have diabetes mellitus. The World Health Organization[31] criteria for diabetes mellitus include a plasma glucose level of 200 mg/dL or higher after a 7.5-g oral glucose load or a fasting blood glucose level of 140 mg/dL or higher.[32] Patients with type I diabetes mellitus are insulin deficient and prone to ketoacidosis. Those with type II non–insulin-dependent diabetes are not prone to ketoacidosis and exhibit a degree of peripheral insulin resistance. The elderly frequently have type II disease and tend to be overweight. They are prone to develop a hyperglycemic, hyperosmolar, nonketotic (HHNK) state. Type II patients can secrete insulin but in inadequate amounts. They have an impaired beta cell response to glucose levels as well as a possible defect in the conversion of proinsulin to insulin.[33] Diabetic patients are at risk for many end-organ complications that require surgery. The surgical mortality rates are five times higher for diabetic compared to nondiabetic patients.[34]

Preoperative assessment should focus on system abnormalities known to be associated with diabetes; *the anesthetic goal is to preserve end-organ function*. It is important in the perioperative period to monitor the diabetic patient's individual requirements for fluid resuscitation, insulin supplementation, and electrolyte stability. Autonomic neuropathy associated with diabetes mellitus can lead to painless myocardial ischemia and infarction. Myocardial infarction is the most common cause of death in the elderly diabetic patients.[35] Cerebral vascular accidents often correlate with hyperglycemia and have a poor outcome.[36] Positioning of the diabetic patient is also important to prevent local tissue ischemia.

The diabetic patient is at increased risk for acute renal failure in the perioperative period. Reduced renal function superimposed with diabetes can lead to glomerulosclerosis and necrosis. Autonomic dysfunction of the bladder leads to urinary stasis and urosepsis. Metabolic decompensation can occur perioperatively and can lead to hyperglycemia, osmotic diuresis, and intravascular volume constriction. The goal is to maintain a blood glucose level in the 100 to 200 mg/dL range and hemodynamic stability. Hyperglycemia can cause a hyperosmolar crisis (serum osmolality > 350 mEq/L) and can be manifested as simple changes in mentation to coma. Hyperglycemia can cause electrolyte imbalances and hypovolemia leading to loss of perfusion to vital organs with thrombus formation. Many protocols can be used to manage diabetic patients, but the most important aspect of any protocol is frequent monitoring of the serum glucose concentration.

No anesthetic technique is specifically indicated for the diabetic patient. If any peripheral neuropathies are present it is important to document them before administering a regional anesthetic. Fluid support should be normal saline because lactate (in lactated Ringer's) can be converted in the liver to glucose, for which the patient may be unable to compensate. Emergency surgery is usually associated with increased infection. Tight control of serum glucose has been shown to improve wound healing. Delayed gastric emptying is seen in these patients. It may be helpful to empty the stomach before extubation and administer metaclopromide 10 mg IV in divided doses.

THERMOREGULATION

Normothermia can be difficult to maintain in the elderly because of their impaired thermoregulatory system,[37] which is related to a decrease in the basal metabolic rate of 1% per year after age 30.[38] An increased cardiac output with peripheral vasoconstriction can result in myocardial ischemia. General anesthesia results in profound peripheral vasodilation. The aged are less able to minimize such heat loss via peripheral vasoconstriction in the immediate postoperative period. Postoperative hypothermia can have a significant effect in the elderly. Shivering will increase oxygen consumption by 400% to 500%, stressing the cardiac and pulmonary systems. Every effort must be made to maintain normothermia; heated and humidified gases, fluid warmers, and external warming blankets are helpful.

☐ PHARMACOLOGY

PHARMACOKINETICS

Pharmacokinetics describe the absorption, distribution, hepatic transformation, and renal excretion of a medication. Multiple sites can influence the time of onset, peak effect, and duration of action of a drug. Drug absorption through the gastrointestinal tract is much less reliable than absorption after systemic administration. Changes in motility blood flow, emptying time, and even cellular transport mechanisms will slow absorption in the elderly patient.

Fluid Shifts Total body water decreases with age; other changes in body composition include a loss of skeletal mus-

cle and an increase in body fat. Total blood volume can decrease as much as 30%.

Volume of Distribution

The elderly have a *smaller* volume of distribution, which is calculated by dividing the total amount of drug by the drug concentration in plasma. The volume of distribution depends on lean body mass versus fat storage, total body water, and protein binding. Water-soluble agents will have a larger amount of medication available at active sites, whereas lipid-soluble drugs, which are stored in fatty tissue, will have less available agent at the site of action. Lipid-soluble agents can accumulate in the fat stores and be released at a slower rate, causing residual sedation in the elderly. An example of delayed sedation secondary to lipid storage is diazepam with an elimination half-time of 20 hours at age 20 and 90 hours at age 80.[39] A good estimation for diazepam is that the half-life in hours is approximately the same as the patient's age in years.

Protein Binding

Decreased protein binding and serum albumin levels in the elderly, compounded by the numerous medications that compete for protein-binding sites, put the geriatric patient receiving anesthesia at risk for higher plasma concentrations. The decrease in serum albumin leads to an increase in free agents available (e.g., phenytoin levels can be 20% higher in elderly patients). This has clinical significance when administering medications that are weak acids, such as meperidine, that depend on protein binding for clearance. At age 35, 75% of meperidine is protein bound versus 35% by age 75.[40]

Hepatic Clearance

Studies by Wynn demonstrate a *decrease* in liver blood flow by as much as 47% by age 91.[41] The rate at which the liver can metabolize an agent depends on the rate the drug is delivered to it via blood flow. The age-related reduction in hepatic blood flow correlates to an age-related drop in cardiac output and decrease in liver volume. The hepatic clearance of propranolol is reduced by 45% and morphine by 35%. Changes in metabolism seen in the elderly are primarily phase 1, oxidative metabolism.[42] Because midazolam is metabolized by oxidation, its clearance is reduced with age. A dose of 0.3 mg/kg will induce sleep in 100% of unpremedicated elderly patients. In contrast 0.5 mg/kg induces sleep in only 60% of young adults.[43]

Renal Clearance

Excretion of water-soluble agents occurs through the kidney. The extent of change in excretion is determined by the percentage of drug that is excreted by glomerular filtration. Therefore, agents that are excreted via GFR will be affected. By age 70, a 50% decrease in the clearance of gentamycin is seen.[44]

PHARMACODYNAMICS

Pharmacodynamics refer to the difference between the concentration of the agent at its end-organ site and the intensity of the effect it produces. The most apparent change seen in the elderly is the loss of neuronal substance. The loss of dopamine in the corpus striatum contributes to the side effects seen with neuroleptic agents, such as metaclopromide causing tardive dyskinesia.[45] Reduced chronotropy is seen in older patients when β stimulants are given (i.e., isoproterenol). Numerous studies have demonstrated both a reduced number of β receptor sites and reduced affinity. Evidence also indicates reduced α-adrenergic and cholinergic activities in the aged.[46] In general, a decrease in requirement and end-organ responsiveness can be expected in the elderly patient receiving anesthetic agents.

INHALATION AND INTRAVENOUS AGENTS

This section offers a brief systems review of the geriatric patient and discusses how these changes can alter anesthetic response. Inhalation agents are affected primarily by changes in respiratory and cardiac functions. The anatomic and physiologic changes seen in the elderly lung lead to V/Q mismatch, increased work of breathing, and air trapping. Due to a reduced total lung capacity and vital capacity with increased residual volumes, inhalation induction is rapid and emergence is delayed. Response to hypoxia and hypercarbia is impaired in the elderly; residual effects of anesthetic drugs and muscle relaxants can make extubation difficult.

As cardiac output is reduced and circulation time is prolonged, a more rapid inhalation induction is seen in the elderly. As renal function deteriorates, agents that are excreted by the kidneys should be avoided (e.g., enflurane with its potentially nephrotoxic metabolites). The minimum alveolar concentration (MAC) for each agent decreases approximately 4% for each decade after age 40. Recovery from inhalation agents is delayed, in part due to an increase in body fat. The newer inhalation agents, desflurane and sevoflurane, have lower blood gas partition coefficients (.45 for desflurane, .65 for sevoflurane). These agents should be eliminated more rapidly than the more soluble agents.

The same decrease in cardiac output and longer circulation time that leads to a more rapid inhalation induction also results in a delayed onset of intravenous agents. Because myocardial function is already reduced in the aged, any cardiac depressants will have an exaggerated response. Delayed renal excretion will increase the half-life and reduced liver blood flow will slow metabolism of intravenous agents. It is important to titrate intravenous agents to use the lowest dose possible to minimize untoward side effects. Agents with the shortest half-life would be best and prolonged sedation can be expected. Supplemental oxygen and careful assessment are important in the postoperative period (hemodynamic monitoring, pulse oximetry).

Neuromuscular Blockade Despite reduced skeletal muscle mass and impaired neuromuscular function associated with aging, the dose requirements of both depolarizing and nondepolarizing agents does not change with age. The duration of effect may be prolonged because of delayed me-

tabolism and excretion of agents. The exception to this is atracurium, which depends on Hoffmann elimination. Because of the increased circulation time, all neuromuscular blocking agents have a slower time of onset.

☐ ANESTHETIC MANAGEMENT

PREOPERATIVE ASSESSMENT

The preoperative visit is an excellent opportunity to evaluate a patient's physical and emotional status and prepare for a safe anesthetic. A preoperative visit is more reassuring than simply premedication. It is important to do a complete systems assessment to ascertain the need for any further consultation or treatment before administering an anesthetic.

The list of cardiac disease risk factors (Table 28–4) and accompanying flow chart (Figure 28–1) can be used as tools to assess the geriatric patient quickly. It is important to be patient when interviewing the elderly. They are often unaware of the significance of their symptoms. For a cardiovascular evaluation, examine the patient for adequate tissue perfusion (skin color) and determine any history of myocardial infarction, CHF, or angina. Neuropathy, especially in association with diabetes mellitus, may prevent angina from defining myocardial ischemia. A preoperative electrocardiogram (ECG) may need to be compared to a previous ECG to differentiate acute and chronic abnormalities. It can be helpful to contact the medical doctor for important information to differentiate an ongoing from an acute illness. A simple assessment tool is exercise tolerance. Can the patient walk a flight of stairs or a block without chest pain or shortness of breath? If there is any doubt as to the patient's cardiovascular stability, that is, hypertension, chest pain, jugular venous distention, rales, or an abnormal ECG that is not previously documented, a preoperative evaluation by a cardiologist is

Table 28–4
RISK FACTORS FOR CARDIAC DISEASE

Does the patient meet one or more of the following criteria?

1. Chest pain
2. Angina or anginal equivalents
3. Congestive heart failure symptoms or equivalents
4. History of high blood pressure
5. Diabetes
6. History of symptoms of dysrhythmia
7. History of shortness of breath
8. History of myocardial infarction
9. Age in males ≥ 40 or age in females ≥ 50
10. History of smoking
11. Patient not able to exercise without shortness of breath or chest pain
12. Patient needs vascular surgery

SOURCE: Reprinted with permission from Roizen MF: Preoperative patient evaluation. New Orleans Anesthesiology Comprehensive Review Course, June 1992.

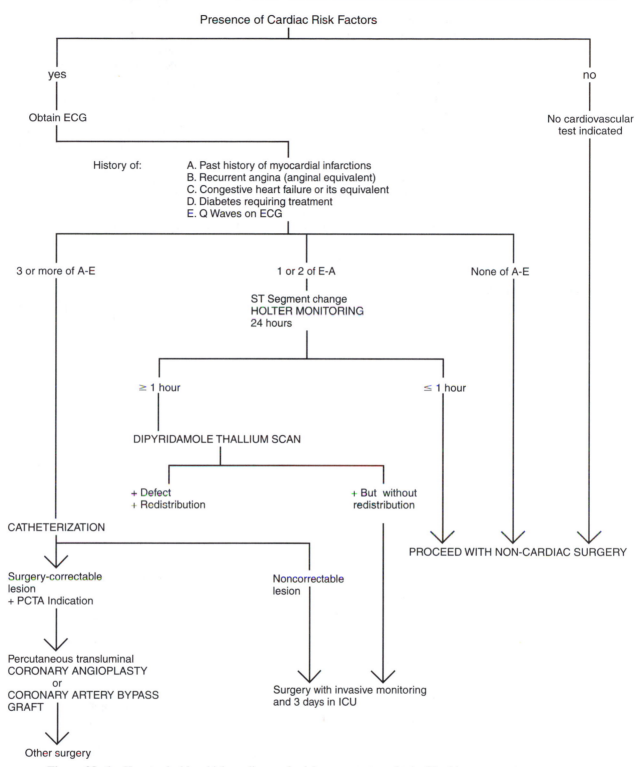

Presence of Cardiac Risk Factors

yes

no

Obtain ECG

No cardiovascular
test indicated

History of:
A. Past history of myocardial infarctions
B. Recurrent angina (anginal equivalent)
C. Congestive heart failure or its equivalent
D. Diabetes requiring treatment
E. Q Waves on ECG

3 or more of A-E

1 or 2 of E-A

None of A-E

ST Segment change
HOLTER MONITORING
24 hours

≥ 1 hour

≤ 1 hour

DIPYRIDAMOLE THALLIUM SCAN

+ Defect
+ Redistribution

+ But without
redistribution

CATHETERIZATION

PROCEED WITH NON-CARDIAC SURGERY

Surgery-correctable
lesion
+ PCTA Indication

Noncorrectable
lesion

Percutaneous transluminal
CORONARY ANGIOPLASTY
or
CORONARY ARTERY BYPASS
GRAFT

Surgery with invasive monitoring
and 3 days in ICU

Other surgery

Figure 28–1 How to decide which cardiovascular laboratory test to obtain. Use history to segregate patients. SOURCE: Adapted with permission from Roizen MF: Preoperative patient evaluation. *New Orleans Anesthesiology Comprehensive Review,* June 1992.

warranted. A thallium scan or exercise stress test can provide valuable information to the anesthetist. If the patient is taking antihypertensive or coronary vasodilators preoperatively, medications should be maintained up until the morning of surgery if possible.

The rate of infarction in a patient with a previous myocardial infarction is 5.9% if the procedure is less than 3 hours versus 15.9% if the procedure is longer than 3 hours. Mortality associated with reinfarction was 69%.[47] Stern and Tinker[48] felt this time correlation to be accurate when the surgery invaded a major body cavity (thoracic or abdominal). Warner and Hoskin[49] assessed postoperative mortality with regard to surgical site. The highest mortality, as expected, was seen with complex vascular, thoracic, and biliary procedures. Thoracic procedures had the highest mortality at 30 days (37.5%) versus vascular, which had the highest mortality at 48 hours (20%). Less invasive procedures such as a transurethral prostate resection and cataract surgery carried a zero mortality rate in this study.

Pulmonary assessment is important because the elderly frequently have a history of COPD. The anesthetist should be aware of a history of smoking, recent infections, or a productive cough. Has the patient ever been diagnosed as having asthma or emphysema? If so what treatments were required and when? Is the patient on supplemental steroids that would require steroid coverage during the perioperative period? Is the patient able to walk a flight a stairs without becoming short of breath? Is the patient taking bronchodilators that should be continued intraoperative? Pulmonary function studies are helpful in determining a patient's ability to tolerate the V/Q changes associated with surgery and anesthesia and to plan accordingly. A chest x-ray is useful as well. Arterial blood gas analysis along with pulmonary function studies are efficient and reliable indicators of a patient's pulmonary status. The pH may be altered by an underlying metabolic dysfunction (Table 28–5).

In Stephen's survey of preexisting complications found in geriatric patients, renal dysfunction occurred in 31% of patients, diabetes in 9%, and liver disease in 8.5%.[50] Because these pathologies may not present with overt symptoms, laboratory data and information obtained from the patient and the physician may be required. The elderly often live alone and may be malnourished. They have a diminished thirst response to dehydration and may be on diuretic treatment for hypertension. Neurologic changes from cerebral insufficiency, psychiatric disturbances, or medication side effects require thorough assessment to document the patient's level of orientation and comprehension. Premedication, used routinely in younger patients, may cause agitation, confusion or even somnolence in the aged.

Table 28–5
INDICATIONS FOR PREOPERATIVE EVALUATION OF PULMONARY FUNCTION

Planned thoracic surgery
Planned upper abdominal surgery
History of heavy smoking and cough
Marked obesity
Age > 70 years
History of pulmonary disease

SOURCE: Adapted and reprinted with permission from Tisi G: Preoperative identification and evaluation of the patient with lung disease. *Med Clin North Am* 71:399, 1987.

AIRWAY

It is important to evaluate the airway of geriatric patients, many of whom many have poor dentition or a prosthesis. Mobility of the head and neck may be reduced due to arthritic changes. Arthritis in the cervical spine can compromise an airway, necessitating a thorough assessment of the patient's ability to open the mouth and extend the head before induction. The anesthetist should be familiar with airway accessibility before induction to establish a safe plan of care. Laryngoscopy should be as brief and nontraumatic as possible; overextension of the neck can interrupt vertebrobasilar blood flow. Because protective airway reflexes are blunted in the elderly,[51] it is important to establish return of airway reflexes before extubation to minimize risk of aspiration. Older patients also have a less effective cough in terms of volume, flow, and force and with fewer cilia are less able to mobilize secretions.[52] Although tachycardia and hypertension due to laryngoscopy in the "lightly" anesthetized patient may be brief, this may precipitate myocardial ischemia, ventricular irritability, and left ventricular failure. It may be advantageous to administer additional narcotics or a short-acting antihypertensive before intubation. Clonidine, an α_2 agonist, can be used to minimize cardiovascular response to the stress of intubation. Clonidine also reduces the need for preoperative sedation (5 μg/kg).[53] Many other agents can also be used such as a combined α and β antagonist (labetolol) or esmolol (a β blocker). It is a challenge to avoid causing hypotension when inducing the elderly with propofol and other agents and yet prevent hypertension that can occur with laryngoscopy.

REGIONAL VERSUS GENERAL ANESTHESIA

No evidence definitely proves that one technique is superior in terms of long-term morbidity and mortality in the elderly. Advantages and disadvantages exist for both regional and general anesthesia. Combining regional and general anesthesia for certain procedures may be an option with many advantages intraoperatively and postoperatively. Anesthetic requirements will be reduced with this combined method. Some studies support regional anesthetics as beneficial in blocking the endocrine or "stress" response to surgery, for example, reducing epinephrine (T-2 to T-6) and cortisol (T-4 to S-5) secretions when these levels are blocked.[54] Postoperatively spinal or epidural narcotics can promote early ambulation, improve lung expansion, and reduce the disorientation that can accompany systemic narcotics. Regional anesthesia is also beneficial in reducing blood loss and the formation of thromboemboli. This is especially true with procedures involving the lower abdomen and orthopedic procedures of the lower extremities. Absolute contraindications for regional anesthesia are patient refusal or inability to cooperate, ester allergy, elevated intercranial pressure, infection at the site of entry, sepsis, hypovolemia, or a coagulopathy. Relative contraindications are more numerous and include neurologic dysfunction, certain cardiac lesions, and prior lumbar surgery. When adminstering a regional anesthetic to an elderly patient, it must be remembered that intervertebral spaces are narrowed and kyphosis is common, which leads to an increased "spread" of spinal or epidural agents reducing requirements. Although plasma levels of epinephrine and norepinephrine are higher in the aged, end-organ response is reduced. If a regional anesthetic inhibits catecholamines, volume expansion or vasoactive agents may be necessary.

Intravenous Anesthetic Sedation   The geriatric patient must be monitored closely whether the technique is intravenous sedation with or without regional anesthesia. The airway in an elderly patient has a tendency to obstruct due to poor dentition and reduced cough/gag reflexes. These patients also have a reduced response to hypoxia and hypercarbia. The increase in V/Q mismatch leads to early desaturation.

PERIOPERATIVE FLUID MANAGEMENT

The goal of fluid management is to sustain homeostasis including intravascular volumes, cardiac preload, cardiac output, and tissue perfusion. Fluid resuscitation of the elderly requires correlating the fluid requirements of the patient and amounts the cardiovascular and renal systems can accommodate. Fluids are traditionally classified as either crystalloid or colloid. Crystalloids augment the entire extracelluar space; colloids remain in the intravascular space. Isotonic fluids are generally used to support organ function. It is usually not necessary to administer solutions containing dextrose except with the diabetic patient receiving insulin.

Hyponatremia and water intoxication are possible when administering hypotonic fluids (D_5W). Colloids are beneficial in supporting circulatory volumes with minimal extravascular leakage.

The physiologic changes that occur in aging predispose the patient to fluid and electrolyte imbalances. Crystalloid infusion is monitored by urine output, blood pressure, and heart rate. Extreme caution should be used when administering large quantities of crystalloids because the elderly can easily become overloaded and develop CHF. When infusing colloids, a central venous pressure (CVP) or a pulmonary artery occlusion pressure (PAOP) monitor is safest. Most studies support the need to maintain an adequate colloid osmotic pressure with a colloid solution to prevent pulmonary edema.

The elderly depend on the Frank-Starling mechanism to increase cardiac output. They are unable to increase their heart rate to meet increased demands; therefore, they must increase contractility by increasing cardiac fiber length. This is done by increasing preload or venous return to increase end-diastolic volume of the heart. Each patient in a given clinical situation has an optimum preload that will give the best cardiac output. Obviously this value changes as the patient's clinical picture changes. Incremental boluses of fluid can be given and measurements of PAOP and cardiac index taken to establish the optimal state for a patient. This number is not a static value and may change as the case progresses.

Any evidence of inadequate tissue perfusion, such as hypotension or low urine output, requires prompt intervention. The limits of preload supplementation and vasoactive support must be tailored for each patient. Negative inotropes (volatile anesthetics, β blockers) may need to be discontinued and inotropic support may be necessary to sustain tissue perfusion.

REFERENCES

1. Haljamae T, Stefannsson T, Wickstrom I. Preanesthetic evaluation of the female geriatric patient with hip fracture. *Acta Anaesthesiol Scand.* 1982; 26:393.

2. Gibson JR, Mendelhall MK, Axel NJ. Geriatric anesthesia: minimizing the risk. In: Brindly GU, ed. *Clinics in Geriatric Medicine.* Philadelphia: WB Saunders; 1985:313.

3. Duckett S. The normal aging human brain. In: Duckett S, ed. *The Pathology of the Aging Human Nervous System.* Philadelphia: Lea & Febiger; 1991:1–19.

4. Strehler BL. Fundamental mechanisms of neuronal aging. In: Cervos-Navarro J, Sackander H-I, eds. *Brain Aging: Neuropathology and Neuropharmacology.* New York: Raven Press; 1983:75–95.

5. Smith DO. Cellular and molecular correlates of aging in the nervous system. *Exp Gerontol.* 1988; 23:399.

6. Rodgers J, Bloom FE. Neurotransmitter metabolism and function in the aging central nervous system. In: Finch CE, Schneider EL, eds. *Handbook of the Biology of Aging.* 2nd ed. New York: Van Nostrand Reinhold; 1985:645–691.

7. Long DM. Aging in the nervous system. *Neurosurgery.* 1985; 17:348.

8. Hubbard BM, Squier M. The physical aging of the neuromuscular system. In: Tallis R, ed. *The Clinical Neurology of Old Age.* Chichester, UK: John Wiley; 1989:3–26.

9. Frolkis V, Brezrukov W: Aging of the central nervous system. *Hum Physiol.* 1978; 78:478.

10. George J. The neurological examination of the elderly patient. In: Tallis R, ed. *The Clinical Neurology of Old Age.* Chichester, UK: John Wiley; 1989;67–88.

11. Samorajski T. Normal and pathological aging of the brain. In: Enna SJ, Samorajski T, Beer B, eds. *Brain Neurotransmitters and Receptors in Aging and Age-Related Disorders.* New York: Raven Press; 1981:991–1012.

12. Shipton EA, Roelofse JA. Anaesthesia in a patient with Parkinson's disease. *S Afr Med J.* 1984; 65:304.

13. Dorfman LJ, Bosley TM. Age related changes in peripheral and central nerve conduction in men. *Neurology.* 1979; 29:38.

14. Pontoppidan H, Geffins B, Lowenstein A. Acute respiratory failure in the adult. *N Engl J Med.* 1972; 287:690.

15. Smith TC. Respiratory effects of aging. *Semin Anesth* 1986; 5:14.

16. Raine JM, Bishop MJ: A-a differences in O_2 tensions and phys-

iological dead space in normal man. *J Appl Physiol.* 1963; 18: 284.

17. Hotchkiss RS. Perioperative management of the geriatric patient with chronic obstructive pulmonary disease. *Int Anesth Clin* 1988; 26(2):134.

18. Boush HA, Holtzman MJ, Sheller JR, Nadel JA. Bronchial hyperreactivity: state of the art. *Am Rev Respir Dis.* 1980; 121: 389.

19. Zehr BB, Hunninghake GW. Interstitial lung disease, hypersensitivity pneumonitis, and pulmonary vascular disease in the elderly. In: Hazzard WR, Andes R, Bierman EL, Blass JP, eds. *Principles of Geriatric Medicine and Gerontology.* 2nd ed. New York: McGraw-Hill; 1990:538–548.

20. Wei JY. Age and cardiovascular system. *N Engl J Med.* 1992; 327:1735.

21. Brandfonbrener M, Landowne M, Shock NW. Changes in cardiac output with age. *Circulation.* 1955; 12:557.

22. Arora RR, Machaa J, Goldman ME, et al: Atrial kinetics and left ventricular diastolic filling in the healthy elderly. *J Am Coll Cardiol.* 1987; 9:1255.

23. Wengwe NK. Cardiovascular disease in the elderly. *Curr Probl Cardiol.* 1992; 17:609.

24. Rodeheffer RJ, Gerstenblith G, Becker LC, et al. Exercise cardiac output is maintained with advancing age in human subjects: cardiac dilation and increased stroke volume compensate for a diminished heart rate. *Circulation.* 1984; 69:203.

25. Won WF, Gol S, Fukuyana O, Blanchette PL. Diastolic dysfunction in elderly patients with congestive heart failure. *Am J Cardiol.* 1989; 63:1526.

26. Martin A. Benbow LJ, Butrous GS, et al. Five year followup of 101 elderly subjects by means of long term ambulatory cardiac monitoring. *Eur Heart J.* 1984; 5:592.

27. Dunnhill MS, Halley W: Some observations on the quantitative anatomy of the kidney. *J Pathol.* 1973; 110:113.

28. Cockraft DW, Gault MH. Prediction of creatinine clearance from serum creatinine. *Nephron.* 1976; 16:31.

29. Calloway NO, Foley CF, Lagerbloom P. Uncertainties in geriatric data: II organ. *J Am Geriatr Soc.* 1965; 13:20.

30. Macklon AF, Barton M, James O, Rawlins MD. The effect of age on the pharmacokinetics of diazepam. *Clin Sci.* 1980; 59:479.

31. Harris MI, Holden WC, Knowler WC, Bennet PH. Prevalence of diabetes and impaired glucose tolerance and plasma glucose levels in the US population aged 20 to 74 years. *Diabetes* 1987; 36:523.

32. WHO Expert Committee on Diabetes Mellitus: Second Report. Geneva: WHO; 1980: *WHO Tech Rep Ser.* 646:1–80.

33. Minaker KL, Rowe JW, Tonin OR. Influence of age on clearance of insulin in man. *Diabetes* 1982; 31:851.

34. Mundth ED. Cholecystitis and diabetes mellitus. *N Engl J Med.* 1962; 267:642.

35. Ammon JR. Perioperative management of the diabetic patient. *ASA Annual Refresher Course Lectures.* 1994; 144:1–6.

36. Pulsinelli WA, Levy DE, Sigsbee B, et al. Increased damage after ischemic stroke in patients with hyperglycemia with or without established diabetes mellitus. *Am J Med.* 1983; 75:540.

37. Goldberg MJ, Roe F. Temperature changes during anesthesia and operations. *Arch Surg.* 1966; 93:365.

38. Roe CG, Goldberg MJ, Blair CS, et al. Influence of shivering on early post operative oxygen consumption. *Surgery* 1966; 60: 85.

39. Klotz U, Avant GR, Hoyumpa A, et al. The effect of age and liver disease on the disposition and elimination of diazepam. *J Clin Invest.* 1975; 55:347.

40. Mather LE, Tucker GT, Pflug AE, et al. Meperidine kinetics in man: intravenous injection in surgical patients and volunteers. *Clin Pharmacol Ther.* 1975; 17:21.

41. Wynne HA, Cope CH, James OFW, et al: The effect of age upon liver volume and apparent liver blood flow in healthy men. Hepatology 9:297, 1989.

42. O'Malley K, Crooke J, Duke E, et al. Effects of age and sex on human drug metabolism. *BMJ.* 1971; 3:607.

43. Reves JG, Fragen RJ, Vinik HR, et al. Midazolem: pharmacology and uses. *Anesthesiology* 1985; 62:310.

44. Matzke GR, Jameson JJ, Halstenson CE. Gentamycin disposition in young and elderly patients with various degrees of renal function. *J Clin Pharmacol* 1987; 27:216.

45. Feely J, Coakley D. Altered pharmacodynamics in the elderly. *Clin Geriatr Med.* 1990; 6:269.

46. Doherty JR. Aging and the cardiovascular system. *J Auton Pharmacol* 1986; 6:77.

47. Palmberg S, Hinjsjari E. Mortality in geriatric surgery. *Gerontology* 1979; 23:103.

48. Stern P, Tinker J. Myocardial reinfarction after anesthesia and surgery. *JAMA.* 1978; 239:2566.

49. Warner MA, Hoskin MP. Surgical procedures among those >90 years of age. *Ann Surg.* 1988; 207:380.

50. Stephen GR. The risk of anesthesia and surgery in the geriatric patient. In: Krechel S, ed. *Anesthesia and the Geriatric Patient.* New York: Grune & Stratton; 1984:231.

51. Pontoppidan H, Beecher HK. Progressive loss of protective reflexes in the airway in the patient with the advance of age. *JAMA.* 1960; 174:2209.

52. Spence AA. The lessons of CEPOD. *Br J Anaesth.* 1988; 60:753.

53. Maze M. Clinical use of alpha-2 agonists. ASA Annual Refresher Course Lectures. 1994; 162:1–6.

54. Kehlet H. Modification of Responses to Surgery by neural blockade: Clinical Implications. In: Cousins MJ, Bridenbaugh PO, eds. *Neural Blockade,* 2nd ed. Philadelphia: Lippincott; 1988:145–188.

☐ QUESTIONS

1. The elderly pulmonary system will exhibit:
    a. Increased vital capacity, increased forced expiratory volume in 1 second
    b. Increased vital capacity, reduced functional residual capacity
    c. Decreased vital capacity, increased Pao_2
    d. Decreased vital capacity, decreased Pao_2

2. Parkinson's disease is:
    a. Vascular insufficiency of the frontal lobe
    b. Inhibition of extrapyramidal motor system
    c. Associated with deficiency of neurotransmitters
    d. Loss of dopaminergic fibers in basal ganglia of the central nervous system

3. A patient with Parkinson's disease receiving anesthesia should:
    a. Have medications discontinued 2 weeks prior to surgery
    b. Be given a phenothiazine or butryphenone to inhibit nausea preoperatively
    c. Not be administered a central anticholingeric agent
    d. Should be induced using halothane

4. The elderly are prone to hypoxia because of:
    a. Decrease in compliance as well as a diminished cardiovascular and ventilatory response to hypoxia
    b. Increase in compliance as well as a diminished cardiovascular and ventilatory response to hypoxia
    c. Reduced minimum alveolar concentration requirements
    d. Shifting of the oxyhemoglobin dissociation curve due to reduced production of 2,3-diphosphoglycerate

5. GABA receptor sites in the elderly:
    a. Are reduced and may be responsible for increased sensitivity to benzodiazepines and barbiturates
    b. Are increased and may be responsible for increased sensitivity to benzodiazepines and barbiturates
    c. Are increased as are adrenergic and acetylcholine receptors
    d. Remain stable in number but are less responsive to stimulation

6. Chronic obstructive pulmonary disease in the elderly will demonstrate:
    a. Airway narrowing secondary to inflammation and loss of elastic recoil
    b. Left ventricular hypertrophy with left axis deviation
    c. Bronchospasm in association with atelectasis
    d. Precipitation of congestive heart failure

7. Treatment goals for the elderly asthmatic include:
    a. Long-term steroids
    b. Increase cyclic adenosine monosphosphate
    c. α-Adrenergic antagonists
    d. β-Adrenergic antagonists

8. Cardiac changes seen in the elderly:
    a. Decrease in preload that may precipitate hypotension with induction
    b. Decrease in left ventricular wall thickness increasing the risk of septal wall infarcts
    c. Reduced responsiveness to changes in preload
    d. Decreased cardiac output resulting in delayed IV induction time

9. The diagnosis of chronic obstructive pulmonary disease is based on the following:
    a. Tachypnea, hypoxia, and retracting
    b. Pulmonary function studies, chest x-ray, arterial blood gases, and clinical presentation of chronic dyspnea and productive cough
    c. Left axis deviation, left bundle branch block, nasal flaring and dyspnea
    d. Reduced total lung capacity, airway narrowing, and productive cough

10. Hypertension in the elderly is a concern intraoperatively because:
    a. Left ventricular hypertrophy leads to labile blood pressure
    b. Plasma volumes are increased precipitating congestive heart failure
    c. Plasma volumes are reduced leading to a labile blood pressure
    d. Plasma volumes are reduced requiring aggressive hydration

11. Intravenous induction time in the elderly is:
    a. Delayed due to a progressive decrease in cardiac output
    b. Delayed due to ventricular hypertrophy
    c. Delayed due to decreased GABA receptor sites
    d. Reduced due to constricted plasma volumes

12. Inhalation induction time in the elderly is:
    a. Delayed due to a progressive decrease in cardiac output
    b. Delayed due to pulmonary hypertension
    c. Reduced due to constricted plasma volumes
    d. Reduced due to a higher partial pressure of anesthetics in alveoli

13. A test dose of Pentothal is useful in the elderly as a tool to:
    a. Access for potential allergic reactions
    b. Treat acute hypertension prior to induction
    c. Estimate onset of induction and hemodynamic response to a dose
    d. Inhibit excessive catecholamine response to intubation

14. The elderly experience a loss of functioning hepatic tissue; liver function tests:
    a. Will increase by approximately 10% to 30%
    b. Will remain stable
    c. Will decrease by approximately 10% to 30%

15. An important consideration in managing the elderly diabetic patient is:
    a. Fluid support should be normal saline
    b. Fluid support should be ringer's lactate
    c. Fluid support must be aggressive, hyperglycemia causes dehydration
    d. Fluid support should be managed with central venous pressure or pulmonary artery occlusion pressure

16. Postoperative hypothermia leads to shivering, which can increase oxygen consumption by:
    a. 100% to 200%, stressing cardiac and pulmonary systems
    b. 200% to 300%, stressing cardiac and pulmonary systems
    c. 300% to 400%, stressing the cardiac and pulmonary systems

   d. 400% to 500%, stressing the cardiac and pulmonary systems

17. An example of altered pharmacokinetics in the elderly is diazepam with an elimination half-time of 20 hours at age 20 versus 90 hours at age 80. This occurs because:
   a. Cardiac output is reduced by 1% for each year after age 30
   b. Liver function is reduced by approximately 20% to 30% by age 80
   c. Lipid-soluble agents accumulating in adipose tissue are released at a slower rate
   d. Reduced renal function delays excretion of metabolites

18. The dose requirements for depolarizing and nondepolarizing agents in the elderly:
   a. Are increased due to impaired neuromuscular functioning
   b. Are decreased due to reduced total blood volume
   c. Are decreased due to reduced renal clearance
   d. Remain stable despite reduced muscle mass

19. The advantages of regional anesthesia in the elderly include:
   a. Avoidance of metabolite accumulation with reduced renal/hepatic function
   b. Reduction of blood loss and the formation of thromboemboli
   c. Reduction of preload improving coronary perfusion pressures
   d. Reduction of systemic vascular resistance in the hypertensive patient

20. Laryngoscopy in the elderly should be brief and nontraumatic. Overextension of the neck can:
   a. Cause interruption of vertebrobasilar blood flow
   b. Occlude carotid perfusion
   c. Precipitate a vasovagal response
   d. Occlude blood flow of the internal jugular

☐ ANSWERS

1. d		**5.** b		**9.** b		**13.** c	**17.** c
2. d		**6.** a		**10.** c		**14.** b	**18.** d
3. c		**7.** b		**11.** a		**15.** a	**19.** b
4. a		**8.** d		**12.** d		**16.** d	**20.** a

CHAPTER
29

Ambulatory Anesthesia

Laura Wild McIntosh

☐ HISTORY OF AMBULATORY ANESTHESIA

Initially, surgical procedures were routinely performed in a hospital setting with preoperative admission and testing, followed by a postoperative hospital stay. Anomalous to this idea was the outpatient Anesthesia Clinic in Sioux City, Iowa, as early as 1919.[1] Minor surgical and dental procedures were performed by Ralph Waters. At that time he predicted a successful future for outpatient procedures. Yet elective surgical procedures remained in the domain of the hospital even through the 1960s, when the University of California in Los Angeles formally opened the first hospital-based outpatient surgical unit.[2] It was not until the 1980s that significant numbers of elective surgical procedures gradually shifted from an inpatient to an outpatient basis. By 1985, approximately 34% of all elective surgical procedures were done on an outpatient basis, and in 1993, 60% of all elective surgeries were done in ambulatory surgical units.[2] As cost and efficiency have become modern dicta of our health care system, the ambulatory setting has become increasingly important in America. Twersky[3] has suggested that by the year 2000, nearly 70% of all elective procedures in the United States will be performed on an ambulatory surgical basis. This chapter discusses the goals of ambulatory anesthesia, appropriate ambulatory patient selection and preoperative assessment, surgical procedures suitable for same day surgery, the anesthetic management, and frequently seen complications. Finally, treatment of postoperative pain and criteria for patient discharge are discussed.

☐ GOALS IN AMBULATORY ANESTHESIA

The primary goal for ambulatory anesthesia is for a patient in optimal health to come in for surgery and return home the same day. On discharge the patient should be as close to presurgical function as possible, with a minimum of risk for the home recovery. Over the last 20 years the typical ambulatory patient has evolved from the predominately healthy American Society of Anesthesiologists (ASA) physical status I to now include a more complex patient of physical status II or even III. This assumes that the patient is in optimal health, despite any preexisting disease state. Although the typical ambulatory patient is still being defined, the goal for ambulatory surgery remains consistent with this goal. Using careful patient selection and communication, ambulatory surgery can be convenient for all involved. By the very nature of the ambulatory center it thrives on efficiency. The patient is one who must return to "street readiness" relatively soon, the anesthetic armamentarium is based on rapid recovery time, and the surgical procedures are those reserved for rapid recovery and minimal physical disruption. These combined factors provide a cost-effective setting where efficiency benefits all involved. A center that closes at 5 or 6 PM is more cost effective than the 24-hour-a-day facility. The benefits to the patient include decreased cost, decreased nosocomial infection, a familiar setting to recuperate in, and less anxiety from family separation. This final point is particularly important with children.

FUTURE GOALS

Future ambulatory surgery goals are to provide an optimally safe and efficient surgical experience as cost becomes an increasingly prominent factor in health care. This goal is becoming more realistic as surgical techniques improve and better anesthetic techniques and agents become available. Another important focus of improvement in the field of ambulatory anesthesia is the reduction in the cancellation rate through better preoperative screening. The role of the anesthetist in contributing to an efficient and safe ambulatory experience is critical.

☐ PREOPERATIVE EVALUATION

Crucial to the success of outpatient surgery is the preoperative assessment when a complete evaluation is performed to ensure optimal health preoperatively and an optimal postoperative outcome. Appropriate tests are done along with a routine history and physical. Preexisting disease is no longer uncommon in the patient presenting to outpatient centers. Studies have shown that existing diseases per se did not contribute to perioperative complications when the disease was well managed.[4] Furthermore, the Federated Ambulatory Surgery Association (FASA) published results of a survey involving 87,494 patients that concluded that there appears to be little or no cause and effect relationship between preexisting disease and incidence of complications.[5] However, no new health issues should be addressed or treated the day of surgery.

The preoperative evaluation should prepare the patient for surgery, both physically and psychologically. The patient should be given written instructions regarding preoperative medications, alcohol consumption restrictions, NPO protocol, the need to sign informed consent, accompaniment of a responsible adult, the need for notification of changes in physical status, and potential hospital admission.[6] A preoperative visit with the anesthetist should help to diminish anxiety regarding anesthesia. However, studies are inconclusive as to whether or not a preanesthetic meeting actually lowers a patient's level of anxiety.[7,8] A thorough preanesthetic assessment is a requirement of the Joint Commission on Accreditation of Healthcare Organizations (JCAHO) to ensure that each patient is an appropriate candidate for the planned anesthetic. Also required is a reevaluation immediately before anesthetic induction.[9]

LABORATORY STUDIES

Little is absolutely agreed on except the need for a complete history and physical examination along with a recent hemoglobin value in all outpatients. How each institution defines recent will vary; generally within 30 days is acceptable. There is much debate about the cost efficiency and efficacy of more in-depth laboratory studies. In the healthy young patient there is little evidence that additional tests provide new

information. The literature[10,11] supports that, in the asymptomatic healthy patient, the predictive value of additional tests can be low and the incidence of false-positive abnormal results can be relatively high. This puts a certain patient population at risk for unnecessary additional studies or even unnecessary postponement or cancellation of surgery. As age increases and disease becomes more prevalent, other tests such as a chemistry profile, coagulation studies, a chest x-ray, and an electrocardiogram (ECG) become more valuable diagnostic tools. However, Meyer and colleagues warn that age alone should not be used as a criterion for ordering batteries of screening laboratory tests.[12] Neither the JCAHO or the Accreditation Association for Ambulatory Health Care (AAAHC) mandates specific preoperative testing. It is up to the individual facility to establish a set of guidelines. In general, preoperative laboratory data will depend on the patient's history, physical examination, age, and current drug regimen. All patients should have a history and physical examination and recent hemoglobin determination. Due to the inevitable anesthetic exposure and the stress of surgery, regardless of how minor the procedure, women should be screened for pregnancy when appropriate. Chest x-rays and ECGs are of little value in the healthy patient under age 40. Risks associated with chest x-ray probably exceed the possible benefit provided the patient is relatively risk free, asymptomatic, and younger than 75 years.[13]

Electrolytes, glucose, and an ECG would be indicated accordingly if a person is being treated for a chronic disease such as hypertension or diabetes. Other suggestions are listed in Table 29–1. It is recommended that laboratory results be ordered in a sensibly prudent and cost-effective manner to enhance the quality of patient care. Until guidelines are mandated, each institution will follow its own guidelines to achieve this goal.

NPO STATUS

The standard of NPO after midnight remains somewhat controversial. Unfortunately, the goal of an empty stomach at the time of induction of anesthesia is not necessarily met by the NPO order. Recent literature supports the practice of clear liquid ingestion (clear gelatin, coffee, tea, apple juice, water) up to 2 hours before surgery in the non–high-risk outpatient.[14] It has been shown that recent intake of clear liquids can actually dilute acidic gastric secretions and enhance the rate of gastric emptying, decreasing gastric volume. Beyond 2 hours, gastric fluid volume and pH are not notably improved. Further benefits are decrease in hypovolemia, hypoglycemia, and potential anxiety from prolonged NPO. This is particularly important in the child having same day surgery. According to Patel and Hannallah,[15] NPO guidelines at the Children's Medical Center are the same for a healthy child as well as for one with systemic disease. Pediatric NPO guidelines are listed in Table 29–2. In the obese patient or those otherwise at risk for aspiration (hiatal hernia, diabetes, pregnancy, smokers) standard NPO orders should be followed with the prophylactic use of a premedication.

Table 29–1
SUGGESTED PREOPERATIVE LABORATORY GUIDELINES

Lab Study	Patient Selection
Complete blood count	All outpatients
Chemistry profile	Patients with significant systemic disease (hypertension, diabetes, renal disease, heart disease, electrolyte abnormalities)
	Patients on medications such as digoxin, potassium supplements, Lasix, dilantin, lithium, steroids and angiotensin-converting enzyme inhibitors
Urinalysis	May help in diabetic patients
	Rule out presence of infection
	False-positive results in menstruating females
Chest x-ray	Age 65 or above
	Existing cardiac or pulmonary indication (tuberculosis, cardiomegaly, history of smoking, recent bronchitis or pneumonia, etc.)
Electrocardiogram	Men > age 45
	Women > age 55
	Symptomatic patients of any age
Coagulation studies	Patients on anticoagulation therapy
	Patients with known or suspected coagulopathy or blood dyscrasia
Pregnancy test	Females of childbearing age

PREMEDICATION

Premedication goals for outpatient surgery are amnesia, analgesia, vagolysis, decreased anxiety, minimized intraoperative anesthetic requirements, and prophylaxis against emesis and aspiration. The most important requirement of premedication is that it not delay recovery time or contribute to unplanned hospital admission. For this reason not all providers of anesthesia routinely use premedication. However, if the proper drugs are used in the proper dosage and combinations, premedication need not prolong recovery room stay. Wetchler describes the use of preinduction that refers to the use of rapidly acting medications as a last minute premedication. The selected drugs and dosages should ensure a rapid onset of sedation with no delay of recovery time.[16] This is often the simplest method because it does not require the insertion of an intravenous catheter or an intramuscular injection before surgery. This is particularly important when continuous pre-

Table 29–2
PEDIATRIC NPO GUIDELINES FOR AMBULATORY PROCEDURES

Age	Guideline
< 6 mo	NPO 4 h before surgery
6–12 mo	NPO 6 h before surgery
> 12 mo	NPO 8 h before surgery

operative monitoring is not feasible. An exception is the pediatric outpatient who would clearly do well with some form of premedication. When working with the pediatric patient we are often dealing with the psychological upset of both the child and the parent when the parent is allowed in the operating room for induction, as is a common practice. This is probably the strongest indication for premedication of the child. A peaceful cooperative child makes for a more comforted parent than a child screaming and writhing during induction.

Anxiolytics and Hypnotics   Midazolam can be given either intramuscularly 30 to 60 minutes before surgery or intravenously immediately before surgery. Because of its rapid elimination and lack of significant side effects, midazolam has proven to be a superior agent in the outpatient setting. Other benzodiazepines such as diazepam, lorazepam, and temazepam are not recommended because of prolonged or unpredictable duration of action. Hannallah and Patel[17] have found ketamine 2 mg/kg intramuscular to be an acceptable preinduction sedative for infants and young children uncooperative for inhaled induction. Recovery time was not prolonged and delay of home discharge was minimal.

Analgesics   Opioid analgesics used as preinduction premedication are beneficial for the ambulatory patient. Hunt and coworkers[18] have found that a single dose of fentanyl, 75 to 125 µg, immediately before induction resulted in a statistically earlier recovery time. White and Chang agree that recovery times were decreased by narcotic premedication as a result of the deceased anesthetic requirement. Although it is reasonable to consider the potential for nausea and vomiting, the incidence seems unchanged.[19] Other indications for opioids include use before administration of regional blocks and for patients with painful conditions. It is probably better to avoid meperidine and morphine because of their long duration and prolonged recovery. Commonly used opioid premedication are found in Table 29–3. Of interest is the fact that the elimination half-life and clearance of alfentanil is prolonged in patients who have recently received erythromycin therapy.[20]

Anticholinergics   Use of anticholinergics as a routine preoperative medicine is no longer standard practice. Patients complain of excessive dryness of the mouth and report an increase of sore throats after general anesthesia. However, when excessive secretions may present a problem, such as in a sitting position for surgical access where secretions may interfere with the surgical site, anticholinergics are of value. Glycopyrrolate is preferred for drying secretions without crossing the blood–brain barrier. If bradycardia develops, it is best treated with intravenous atropine at that time.

Aspiration Prophylaxis   Outpatients, especially the high-risk patient, can benefit from prophylactic measures against aspiration. These drugs include premedication with the H_2 antagonists or gastrokinetic drugs. The combination

Table 29–3
COMMONLY USED OPIOID PREMEDICANTS IN THE SAME DAY SURGERY PATIENT

Drug	Dosage (μg/kg)	Onset (min)	Peak (min)	Duration (min)	Elimination Half-Time (min)
Alfentanil	5–10	1–2	1–2	20	70–98
Fentanyl	1–2	within 5	5–7	45–60	185–219
Sufentanil	0.15–0.2	1	3–4	Shorter than equipotent dose of fentanyl*	148–164

*Marshall BE, Longnecker DE. General anesthetics. In Gilman AG, Ralls TW, Nies AS, Taylor P, eds.: *Goodman and Gilman's The Pharmacological Basis of Therapeutics.* 8th ed. Pergamon Press; 1990:305.

of metoclopramide with an H_2 blocker given 30 minutes before induction provides greater protection against aspiration than either drug alone.[21] Sodium citrate may further decrease the risk. Particulate antacids are not recommend because of the potential for aspiration pneumonia if aspirated.

Antiemetic and Acid Aspiration Prophylaxis Drugs

These drugs are listed in Table 29–4.

Dopamine Antagonist

A major reason for discharge delay in ambulatory surgery is postoperative nausea and vomiting. Today many agents are used for prophylaxis. Droperidol, a butyrophenone, is an antiemetic that inhibits dopaminergic receptors in the chemoreceptor trigger zone of the medulla. In dosages of 2.5 mg or less, prolonged sedation and delayed discharge were unlikely.[22] When given preinduction, droperidol 20 μg/kg IV is a highly effective antiemetic for the female outpatient undergoing a laparoscopic procedure.[23] However, droperidol is not without side effects. Stoelting reports that as a dopaminergic antagonist, extrapyramidal reactions occur in about 1% of patients, and for this reason should not be given to patients being treated for Parkinson's disease.[24]

Metoclopramide is a dopamine antagonist acting primarily as a gastrokinetic agent. Gastrokinesis is achieved through cholinergic stimulation of the gastrointestinal tract via release of acetylcholine from cholinergic nerve endings. This leads to enhanced gastric emptying, increased lower esophageal tone, and lower gastric fluid volume, all of which produce an antiemetic effect. Other actions include secretion of prolactin

and extrapyramidal symptoms. However, metoclopramide does not affect gastric pH or acid secretion.

H_2 Antagonist

Other antiemetic premedicants important in the management of outpatients are the H^+ blockers, effective in acid aspiration prophylaxis. Best results are seen with a oral dose taken the night before surgery followed by a second dose the morning of surgery. Cimetidine is an H_2 antagonist that increases gastric pH without altering pH of gastric contents already in the stomach, emptying time, or lower esophageal tone. Cimetidine slows the metabolism of certain drugs such as propranolol, lidocaine, and diazepam via reduction of hepatic blood flow and inhibition of the hepatic mixed function P-450 oxidase system.[24] Ranitidine is a potent, selective H_2 antagonist lasting 8 to 12 hours. Stoelting reports that side effects are less likely, presumably because of minimal central nervous system involvement. This makes ranitidine preferable with the elderly population.[24] Famotidine is a potent long-acting H_2 blocker that suppresses gastric H^+ secretions for up to 12 hours. Hemodynamic side effects are minimal, unlike ranitidine and cimetidine.

Serotonin Antagonists

A newer class, the serotonin antagonists, ondansetron and dolasetron, have proved effective as both therapeutic and prophylactic antiemetics in the outpatient.[25] These agents seem to be devoid of the typical side effects seen in the dopamine antagonist class of antiemetics. However, at this time, cost is a prohibitive factor in routine use.

☐ PATIENT SELECTION

Who is an appropriate ambulatory surgical patient? Almost any medically stable patient who has a surgeon willing to do a certain procedure and an anesthetist comfortable with providing the needed anesthetic is eligible. One critical component to the successful ambulatory process is the patient. A person must be able to cooperate, or no procedure, however minor, can be done in the outpatient setting. It is perhaps more appropriate to speak in terms of what type of patients are *not* acceptable for same day surgery. Because there are no absolute guidelines it is often up to the comfort of those involved. Certain situations are probably best dealt with in an inpatient setting (Table 29–5).

Table 29–4
ANTIEMETIC AND ACID ASPIRATION PROPHYLAXIS DRUGS

Droperidol 10–20 μg/kg IV at induction of anesthesia
Metoclopramide 10 mg IV perioperatively (onset 1–3 min)
Ondansetron 4–8 mg IV intraoperatively
Ephedrine 25–50 mg IM intraoperatively or postoperatively
Hydroxyzine 25–50 mg IV, IM perioperatively
Cimetidine 300 mg IV preoperatively
Famotidine 20 mg IV preoperatively
Ranitidine 50 mg IV preoperatively
Bicitra 15 mL PO 10–15 min preoperatively

Table 29–5
INAPPROPRIATE PATIENT SELECTION FOR AMBULATORY PROCEDURES

1. Malignant hyperthermia susceptibility
2. Abnormal airway anatomy
3. Morbid obesity
4. Pyschosocial factors: unavailable home care, uncooperative patient
5. Uncontrolled seizure history
6. Unstable ASA patients (III, IV)
7. Acute substance abuse
8. High-risk pediatric population

ADVANCED AGED

Although ASA status is no longer a determinant as to who is an appropriate same day surgery candidate, there seems to be a weak correlation between age and postoperative outcome.[22] Yet Meridy[26] was unable to demonstrate advanced age as a predictor of postoperative complications or increase in recovery time. As a rule, the patient should have no unevaluated medical problems preoperatively. Gold and colleagues[27] were not able to identify any specific medical problems that increased the likelihood of hospital admission. Therefore there is probably no upper limit on the age of an appropriate same day patient. A suitable candidate must be willing to have surgery in an ambulatory facility and return home on the same day. The person should be reliable in following instructions or be accompanied by a responsible and intelligent adult. Other factors in patient selection to be considered are living within an hour's drive of the ambulatory center and knowing what to expect regarding postoperative pain and physical limitations. Pain medicine will be prescribed along with written instructions and a number to call if counseling is needed. If the patient is mentally or physically debilitated, a responsible adult must be present with the patient.

PEDIATRIC POPULATION

Overall, pediatric patients are good candidates for ambulatory surgery. The exception is the ex-premature infant because of an increased risk of apnea. The premature infant should be no less than 40 weeks postconceptional age and possibly even 60 weeks postconceptional age.[28,29] Postconceptual can be defined as the gestational age plus the postnatal age. A study by Steward indicated that preterm infants less than 10 weeks postnatal age developed apnea during anesthesia and up to a period of 12 hours postoperatively.[30] Infants born at term must be older than 4 weeks postnatal and more than 42 weeks gestational age. Other infants at increased risk are those who have had bronchopulmonary dysplasia or any other respiratory distress syndrome. Infants, in addition to immunosuppressed patients, benefit from having outpatient surgery because of the decreased risk of nosocomial infection.

SURGICAL PROCEDURE

As anesthetic drugs and surgical techniques continue to improve, the spectrum of cases that can be done in the ambulatory setting has expanded. Several factors exclude certain procedures or patients from successful outpatient surgery. For example, the degree of postoperative pain, nausea, and vomiting that might occur will depend on the patient and the procedure as well as the anesthetic, rather than one singular factor.

Although general guidelines were originally established in the 1970s, they no longer apply. More recently an accepted working definition concludes that "Any procedure that does not require a major intervention in the cranial vault, abdomen, or thorax can be considered acceptable."[31]

In fact, any surgical procedure that creates an actual or potential unstable airway should not be done in an outpatient setting. Because of the potential dire consequences, any such case should be monitored postoperatively during a hospital stay. The same situation exists where major fluid shifts or loss occurs, although potential for blood transfusion is no longer an absolute contraindication for outpatient surgery. Other situations unacceptable for same day surgery are emergency procedures and the presence of medically unstable disease, such as hypertension, diabetes, and noneuthyroid conditions. Finally, procedure suitability is integral to patient acceptance.

INTRAOPERATIVE ANESTHETIC MANAGEMENT

MONITORING

All ambulatory surgical patients should be monitored in accordance with the America Association of Nurse Anesthetists Patient Monitoring Standards. These standards of care are to be applied to all patients undergoing general, regional, or monitored anesthesia care. To ensure safe anesthetic care, continual monitoring of ventilation, oxygenation, and circulation as per heart rate and blood pressure should be documented at least every 5 minutes. Body temperature should be monitored continuously with general anesthesia and should be readily available for regional and monitored anesthesia care. The means for measuring neuromuscular function must also be available when neuromuscular blocking agents have been used.[32] For further discussion, please refer to Chapter 6 (Patient Monitoring).

ANESTHETIC TECHNIQUES

The decision of the anesthetic type will depend on the surgeon, the patient, and the anesthetist, including each person's level of comfort. Occasionally, either the patient or surgeon will choose general anesthesia in order to avoid any potential interaction. However, this may not always be the best choice given the risk–benefit ratio. Constant communication and a small amount of education regarding your preference can enhance the anesthesia and can make it the anesthetic of choice for all involved. Despite this, the final decision ultimately may not be made by the provider of anesthesia.

General General anesthesia by definition is that state in which the four following elements are present through administration of drugs: hypnosis, analgesia, amnesia, and muscle relaxation. Advantages of general anesthesia include a quiet surgical field, a protected airway when an endotracheal tube is used, and better success with the uncooperative patient. With the safe use of newer agents such as propofol, fentanyl, remifentanil, and desflurane, quick recovery is possible for ambulatory surgery. Potential disadvantages of general anesthesia include a slower return to the preanesthetic state and a potential for side effects such as myalgias and sore throat. General anesthesia can be delivered via *face mask, endotracheal tube,* and more recently via *laryngeal mask airway* (LMA). Each technique offers distinct advantages.

Face Mask

Face mask is best for shorter cases such as examination under anesthesia, dilatation and curettage, cone biopsies, superficial surgeries of the extremities, and hernia repairs. A face mask is appropriate when an airway problem is not anticipated and NPO status is ensured.

Endotracheal Tube

Placement of an endotracheal tube is necessary for ensured airway protection. Such cases include the obese patient undergoing general anesthesia or any condition that would predispose the patient to regurgitation or aspiration (e.g., Trendelenberg positioning, hiatal hernia, diabetes [gastroparesis], laparoscopic or high abdominal surgery). Often the prone position may be an indication for intubating the trachea.

Laryngeal Mask Airway

The use of the LMA has been steadily growing since 1992 when it was released in the United States. The LMA offers a practical alternative for airway management in the ambulatory surgical setting. However, there is no guaranteed airway protection from introduction of gastric contents. Fiberoptic bronchoscopy has shown a 6% to 9% incidence of esophageal visibility within the cuff of the secured LMA.[33] Because this may lead to gastric distension, the LMA has the same indications as a face mask would. Insertion is relatively easy and nontraumatic, eliciting minimal autonomic responses as compared to tracheal intubation. The morbidity associated with LMA insertion is approximately the same as with use of a face mask and oropharyngeal airway.[35] Proper insertion of the LMA is achieved by first lubricating the posterior aspect of the LMA, carefully avoiding the introduction of lubrication into the aperture of the mask. At this time the mask should be fully deflated to allow easy passage into the hypopharynx. For induction, propofol provides the best conditions for insertion of the LMA.[34,35] After induction the classical intubating position should be achieved. This sniffing

position allows for maximal alignment of the oral pharyngeal axis, as with tracheal intubation. The LMA should be held in one hand with the opening of the mask facing anteriorly. The mouth is then opened with the other hand and the lubricated posterior of the mask should be inserted midline and glide against the hard palate into the base of the hypopharynx until the tube can advance no farther. At all times the midline position should be maintained. At this point the cuff should be inflated until the tube pops slightly outward and a swelling of the cricoid and thyroid cartilages is seen as the cuff moves them anteriorly. The insertion can be assisted with a tongue blade by moving the tongue anteriorly. The placement is then confirmed by auscultation of breath sounds and the presence of end-tidal CO_2. Initial difficulties encountered on insertion may result from curling of the mask tip as it is moves down the hard palate against the esophageal sphincter. In this case the mask should be removed. Proper lubrication and head position should be confirmed and the mask should be reinserted midline. During insertion, resistance should not be felt initially. If malpositioning persists, rotation of the tube or application of the jaw-thrust maneuver may help. Insertion with a laryngoscope can also work although this is usually unnecessary. Once inserted properly, the LMA can be used for spontaneous, assisted, or controlled mechanical ventilation. Care should be taken to not exceed airway pressures of greater than 20 cm H_2O or 2 kPa related to potential gastric inflation.[36] Anesthetic maintenance can be achieved with a volatile agent or continuous propofol infusion. The LMA should be checked throughout the case for cuff overextension caused by nitrous oxide use, especially in longer procedures. On emergence, the LMA should be left in place until the patient is awake and can open the mouth to command. Once wakefulness is established, the LMA is then gently removed and only then should the oral pharynx be suctioned. However, the patient will be able to clear secretions at this point. The LMA in the same day surgical patient provides airway management with ease for those patients who do not necessarily require an endotracheal tube. For discussion of the LMA, refer to Chapter 9.

Regional Regional anesthesia in the outpatient population offers a simple and effective alternative to a general anesthetic in many cases. Advantages of regional anesthesia include preservation of mental status in the elderly population, postoperative analgesia, and diminished incidence of nausea and vomiting. Airway management difficulties such as laryngospasm and injured dentition can also be avoided. Potential setbacks include longer anesthetic time, prolonged return to function of blocked region, and possible need for heavy intraoperative sedation. However, in the cooperative patient where minimal or light sedation is tolerated, a regional block can result in rapid recovery and discharge. The initial time needed for insertion of regional anesthetic is often offset by the shortened recovery period. Regional anesthesia has a preemptive analgesic effect, thereby reducing both postoperative pain and analgesic requirements.[37] Local agents should be tailored to the surgical procedure and dura-

Table 29–6
INDICATIONS FOR SPINAL AND EPIDURAL ANESTHESIA

General Procedures	Orthopedic Procedures	Urologic Procedures	Gynecologic Procedures
Inguinal herniorrhaphy	Ankle and knee arthroscopy	Varicocelectomy	Dilation and Curettage
Hemorrhoidectomy	Removal of hardware; lower extremity	Cystoscopy	Hysteroscopy
Pilonidal cystectomy		Lithotripsy	Polypectomy

tion to avoid excessive stay in the postanesthesia care unit (PACU) and prolonged time until discharge. When a regional anesthetic is used, complete and detailed discharge information should be given to the patient regarding return of function and reasonable expectations for pain control. For a more comprehensive discussion on local anesthetics refer to Chapter 13.

Spinal and Epidural Anesthesia

Although spinal and epidural anesthesia may offer advantages especially in the elderly, younger patients are at particular risk for postpuncture headaches with spinals, which increase the likelihood of unplanned postoperative admissions. Other disadvantages include pain and anxiety during placement, urinary retention, backache, hypotension, and potential nerve damage, albeit rare. It may be reasonable to avoid a regional technique if large amounts of fluid are needed to correct hypotension related to sympathetic blockade. Indications for spinal and epidural anesthesia are given in Table 29–6.

Peripheral Nerve Blocks

The Bier block method is useful for producing analgesia and muscle relaxation in the extremities, usually the hand and wrist. In the awake patient the limb is exsanguinated after the insertion of an intravenous catheter. A double-cuff tourniquet is then applied to the upper arm and inflated to approximately twice the systolic pressure. Approximately 50 mL 0.5% lidocaine MPF plain is injected slowly into the cannulated vein. At this time it is wise to have an alert patient who can report symptoms should local toxicity occur. This technique is ideal for surgical procedures lasting an hour or less. The tourniquet should never be released sooner than 20 minutes from the time of local injection. If released in less than 40 minutes, the tourniquet should be deflated briefly, then reinflated while observing for signs and symptoms of toxicity before the final deflation. Nerve damage can occur if the tourniquet time exceeds 2 hours. Drawbacks of this technique include block failure, especially in the obese, potential for systemic toxicity from inadvertent tourniquet release, and tourniquet pain, which often leads to restless behavior. It can be preempted by switching from an inflated proximal cuff to an inflated distal cuff. Anesthetic agents should be limited to xylocaine because of the serious consequences related to toxicity with bupivacaine. In addition, patients with sickle cell anemia are not considered candidates, related to complications occurring from tourniquet application.

Upper and lower extremity nerve blocks may be ideal for patients in whom minimal systemic alterations are necessary

and prolonged analgesia is needed. However, the benefits may be outweighed by the potential of such complications as pneumothorax, as with the supraclavicular approach to a brachial plexus blockade. If the patient is to return home with residual anesthesia, complete instructions should be given as to the expected length of analgesia. The affected limb or area should also be well protected to avoid injury.

Local Anesthesia   Local anesthesia is the use of anesthetics infiltrated at the surgical site and is usually delivered by the surgeon. The benefit to the patient is absence of systemic residual effects postoperatively. Certain surgical procedures are amenable to this technique. Such procedures include the periorbital and retrobulbar blocks for cataract extraction, ilioinguinal iliohypogastric nerve block for hernia repairs, and local infiltration for superficial biopsies (e.g., breast, skin). This technique is usually combined with intravenous anesthetics such as propofol, ketamine, midazolam and a short-acting narcotic. Certain patients may benefit from a strict local technique when any depression with anesthetic agents would put the patient at an unacceptable risk. Under all circumstances, the anesthetist must know the maximum dose of local anesthesia allowable in milligrams per kilogram of lean body mass per hour and the toxic levels (Table 29–7).

Intravenous Sedation/Monitored Anesthetic Care   Often the most suitable anesthetic plan for the same day patient will be an intravenous sedation accompanying a local field block. Concerns include patient comfort (usually analgesia and amnesia) and a quiet surgical field, while maintaining an uncompromised airway. This technique is highly dependent on patient cooperation, surgical proce-

Table 29–7
ALLOWABLE DOSAGES OF LOCAL ANESTHETICS

Drug	Maximal Dose without Epinephrine (mg/kg)	Maximal Dose with Epinephrine (mg/kg)
lidocaine (Xylocaine)	5	7
bupivacaine (Marcaine)	3	5

dure, and level of provider comfort in the anesthetic management. Without the willingness of all involved, this technique has varied success.

ANESTHETIC TRENDS IN AMBULATORY ANESTHESIA

Much of the proliferation of ambulatory centers and undoubtable success can be attributed to the availability of a rapid, short-acting anesthetic armamentarium. These newer agents share a general profile of rapid onset and offset with minimal residual effects, while allowing adequate intraoperative anesthesia. Some of the newer anesthetics in the same day setting include induction agents such as propofol; opioid analgesics like alfentanil and remifentanil; volatile anesthetic agents like desflurane and sevoflurane; muscle relaxants such as mivacurium, cisatracurium, and rocuronium; and adjuvants that decrease common postoperative side effects (e.g., ondansetron).[25]

☐ FREQUENTLY SEEN COMPLICATIONS

Perioperative complications can result in prolonged recovery time, delayed discharge, or unanticipated hospital admission. Complications commonly seen are nausea, vomiting, pain, bleeding, urinary retention, postextubation croup, and more extensive surgery than anticipated. In general, major complications are more likely related to specific surgery type than to physical status or preexisting medical problems if well controlled.[4] Gold and coworkers[27] showed similar results and found that the likelihood of unanticipated admission is related more to the type of anesthesia and surgical procedure than to the patient's clinical characteristics.

The most frequently seen complication of general anesthesia is a sore throat.[38] If the ambulatory patient receives any form of general anesthesia, the anesthetist should warn of the possibility of a sore throat. Even mask anesthesia has a 15% to 20% incidence of postoperative sore throat when succinylcholine is used.[39] Unless necessary, succinylcholine should be avoided because outpatients are at particular increased risk of postoperative myalgias after its use.

Overall, complications in the outpatient are minor and manageable, due in part to the success of the preoperative interview. This screening process aids in proper patient selection and identifies who is an acceptable risk for ambulatory anesthesia. It is perhaps because of the preoperative screening process that the occurrence of death in the ambulatory surgical centers is extremely rare.

☐ POSTOPERATIVE PAIN MANAGEMENT

Anesthetic management of the ambulatory patient continues postoperatively until the time of discharge. This care includes ensuring patient comfort to ambulate and eventually to go home. Successful postoperative pain management is crucial to ambulatory surgery. Gold and coworkers found that pain is one of the most common reasons for unanticipated hospital admission in the outpatient.[27] Possibly the best approach begins with a thorough anesthetic plan that includes postoperative pain management from the onset. Therefore, a combination of carefully selected surgical procedures and meticulous attention to minimizing postoperative pain can be invaluable.

OPIOID ANALGESICS

The preoperative administration of opioids can result in less PACU discomfort with no delay in recovery time if used judiciously.[40] Fentanyl can decrease the need for intraoperative opioids and delay the need for PACU analgesia.[40,41] Although fentanyl is relatively short acting, it is not ideal for postoperative pain management due to high lipid solubility and prolonged elimination.

Alfentanil as a premedication results in quick recovery from anesthesia and sooner discharge. However, alfentanil has limited value in the PACU related to its short action. Likewise, the newer opioid remifentanil, which is eliminated via nonspecific ester hydrolysis, has virtually no postoperative value in pain management because of its brief duration.

Codeine is most commonly given postoperatively in the oral form due to its high bioavailability. Sedation and gastrointestinal side effects are common. Codeine is usually given as hydrocodone and oxycodone for moderate to severe pain. Opioids can be used in conjunction with nonsteroidal anti-inflammatory drugs (NSAIDs) to avoid complications such as sedation, nausea and vomiting, urinary retention, and decreased gastrointestinal motility.

NONSTEROIDAL ANTIINFLAMMATORY DRUGS

The NSAIDs produce analgesia peripherally through their ability to inhibit activity of cyclooxygenase enzyme, leading to a decrease in the synthesis and release of prostaglandins from cells.[24] Recent evidence suggests that these drugs may also act centrally as analgesics.[42] The use of NSAIDs perioperatively appears to be safe. However, it can be inappropriate in certain cases such as with aspirin-induced bronchial asthma, presence of nasal polyps,[43] bleeding dyscrasias, impaired renal function, and gastric ulcers. When used properly NSAIDs can be important adjuncts in decreasing narcotic requirement for acute moderate to severe postoperative pain. Although some authors have questioned the efficacy of ketorolac,[44,45] another study has shown 30 to 60 mg ketorolac to be as effective as morphine (6 to 12 mg) and meperidine (50 to 100 mg).[46] Green and associates[47] found that a combination of intraoperative fentanyl and ketorolac during diagnostic laparoscopy has a narcotic-sparing effect in the recovery room, whereas McLaughlin[48] showed that those laparoscopic patients who received Toradol were discharged an average of 30 minutes earlier than those who did not receive it. Although there is no value in the administration of Toradol for intraoperative pain relief, it performs well in providing postoperative analgesia related to incisional pain.[49] Care must be taken to not give NSAIDs intraoperatively when hemostasis is critical.

INTRA-ARTICULAR ANESTHETICS/ANALGESICS

Intra-articular analgesics offer a simple and excellent alternative means of pain control for surgical procedures involving the joint spaces. A key benefit is the avoidance of systemic side effects (primarily nausea, vomiting, urinary retention, and increased somnolence as seen with narcotics) that could jeopardize a timely recovery. For example, knee and shoulder arthroscopies can be followed with an intra-articular injection of local anesthetic such as bupivacaine or xylocaine, or opiates such as Duramorph, morphine, or fentanyl. Morphine has been used successfully alone and with bupivacaine to reduce postoperative pain. Stein and coworkers[50] found that low doses of intra-articular morphine can significantly reduce pain after knee surgery with maximal effect 3 to 6 hours after injection. Increased comfort leads to less sedation and quicker ambulation and general recovery.

LOCAL ANESTHETICS

Injection of local anesthetics is required for procedures where conscious sedation is used. If the surgical incision will be painful postoperatively the patient may benefit from the injection of bupivacaine at the incision at the time of closure. It is each practitioner's responsibility to understand the dosage, duration, and maximal allowed dosage for all local anesthetics.

All methods of pain control discussed share one goal for the anesthetist in the ambulatory setting: a more efficient and cost-effective experience through early patient mobility and decreased need for postoperative narcotics, reducing time to recovery and PACU discharge.

☐ DISCHARGE CRITERIA

Initial recovery from anesthesia lasts approximately 1 hour. The patient is monitored by a PACU nurse. During the recovery period, mental clarity, motor coordination, and gastrointestinal and urinary return to function are monitored. In addition, hemostasis, cardiovascular condition, and potential airway compromise (such as stridor or edema) are assessed during recovery. Presumably at the end of that time the ambulatory surgical patient has met all criteria to be discharged. In order to be discharged, the patient must demonstrate the ability to ambulate, tolerate liquids without nausea and vomiting, urinate, and be somewhat comfortable once narcotics have worn off and oral pain medicine has begun. A member of the anesthesia team then discharges the patient into the charge of a reliable adult who can follow instructions and be responsible. It is important to discharge the patient with a clear set of written instructions and a telephone number to call if problems should arise. The following day a call to the patient should address any concerns or questions that may have arisen, and should verify that home recovery has been uneventful.

REFERENCES

1. Waters RM. The down-town anesthesia clinic. *Am J Surg*, (*Anesth Suppl*) 1919; 33:71–73.
2. White PF, Smith I. Ambulatory anesthesia: past, present, and future. In: White PF, ed. *International Anesthesiology Clinics: Anesthesia for Ambulatory Surgery*. Boston: Little, Brown; 1994:1–16.
3. Twersky RS, ed. *The Ambulatory Anesthesia Handbook*. St. Louis: Mosby-Yearbook, 1995.
4. Natof HE. Pre-existing medical problems—ambulatory surgery. *Illinois Medical Journal* 1984; 166:101–104.
5. Federated Ambulatory Surgery Association. Special Study. Alexandria, VA: FASA; 1986.
6. McTaggart RA. Selection of patients for day care surgery. *Can Anaesth Soc J*. 1983; 30:543–545.
7. Rosenblatt MA, Bradford C, Miller R, et al. A preoperative interview by an anesthesiologist does not lower preoperative anxiety in outpatients. *Anesthesiology*. 1989; 71:A926.
8. Leigh JM, Walker J, Janaganathan P. Effect of preoperative anaesthetic visit on anxiety. *BMJ*. 1977; 2:987–989.
9. Everett LL, Kallar SK. Presurgical evaluation and laboratory testing. In: Twersky RF, ed. *The Ambulatory Anesthesia Handbook*. St. Louis: Mosby-Yearbook; 1995:1–34.
10. Narr BJ, Hansen TR, Warner M. Preoperative laboratory screening in healthy Mayo patients: cost-effective elimination of tests and unchanged outcomes. *Mayo Clin Proc*. 1991; 66: 155–159.
11. Roizen MF, Cohn S. Preoperative evaluation for elective surgery—what laboratory tests are needed? *Adv Anesth*. 1993; 10:25–47.
12. Meyer P, Thisted R, Roizen MF, et al. Is age a predictor of preoperative test requirements in asymptomatic patients? *Anesthesiology*. 1993; 79:A44.
13. Archer C, Levy AR, McGregor M. Value of routine preoperative chest x-rays: a meta-analysis. *Can J Anaesth*. 1993; 40: 1022–1027.
14. Hutchinson A, Maltby JR, Reid CRG. Gastric fluid volume and pH in elective inpatients. Part I: coffee or orange juice versus overnight fast. *Can J Anaesth*. 1988; 35:12–15.
15. Patel R, Hannallah R. Pediatric anesthetic techniques. In White PF, ed. *International Anesthesiology Clinics: Anesthesia for Ambulatory Surgery*. Boston: Little, Brown, 1994:37–53.
16. Wetchler BV. Outpatient anesthesia. In: Barash PG, Cullen BF, Stoelting RK, eds. *Clinical Anesthesia*. Philadelphia: JB Lippincott; 1992:1389–1416.

17. Hannallah RS, Patel RI. Low-dose intramuscular ketamine for anesthesia pre-induction in young children undergoing brief output procedures. *Anesthesiology.* 1988; 70:598–600.
18. Hunt TM, Plantevin OM, Gilbert FR. Morbidity in gynaecological day-case surgery: a comparison of two anaesthetic techniques. *Br J Anaesth.* 1979; 51:785–787.
19. White PF, Chang T. Effect of narcotic premedication on the intravenous anesthetic requirement. *Anesthesiology.* 1984; 61: A389.
20. Bartkowski RR, Larijani GE, Goldberg ME, Boerner TF. Erythromycin treatment inhibits alfentanil metabolism. *Anesthesiology.* 1988; 69:A590.
21. Gurkowski MA. Outpatient anesthesia. In: Bready LL, Smith RB, eds. *Decision Making in Anesthesiology.* 2d ed. St. Louis, Mosby-Yearbook; 1992:344–345.
22. Cohen SE, Woods WA, Wyner J. Antiemetic efficacy of droperidol and metoclopramide. *Anesthesiology.* 1984; 60:67–69.
23. Pandit SK, Kothary SP, Pandit UA, Randel F, Levy L. Dose-response study of droperidol and metoclopramide as antiemetics for outpatient anesthesia. *Anesth Analg.* 1989; 68:798–802.
24. Stoelting RK. *Pharmacology and Physiology in Anesthetic Practice.* 2d ed. Philadelphia: JB Lippincott; 1991.
25. Griffith KE. Preoperative assessment and preparation. In: White PF, ed. *International Anesthesiology Clinics: Anesthesia for Ambulatory Surgery.* Boston: Little, Brown; 1994:17–36.
26. Meridy HW. Criteria for selection of ambulatory surgical patients and guidelines for anesthetic management: a retrospective study of 1553 cases. *Anesth Analg.* 1982; 61:921–926.
27. Gold BS, Kitz DS, Lecky JH, Neuhaus JM. Unanticipated admission to the hospital following ambulatory surgery. *JAMA.* 1989; 262:3008–3010.
28. Naylor B, Radhakrishnan J, McLaughlin D. Postoperative apnea in infants. *J Pediatr Surg.* 1992; 27:955–957.
29. Kurth CD, Spitzer, Broennle AM, Downes JJ: Postoperative apnea in preterm infants. *Anesthesiology.* 1987; 66:483–488.
30. Stewart DJ. Preterm infants are more prone to complications following minor surgery than are term infants. *Anesthesiology.* 1982; 56:304–306.
31. Dawson B, Reed WA. Anaesthesia for adult surgical outpatients. *Can Anaesth Soc J.* 1980; 27:409–411.
32. Guidelines and Standards for Nurse Anesthesia Practice. *AANA.* 1992; 60:137–138.
33. Pennant JH, White PF. The laryngeal mask airway, its uses in anesthesiology. *Anesthesiology.* 1993; 79:144–163.
34. McGoldrick KE. The laryngeal mask airway. *The Day Surgery Patient.* 1993; 2:3.
35. Brown GW, Patel N, Ellis FR. Comparison of propofol and thiopentone for laryngeal mask insertion. *Anaesthesia.* 1991; 46:771–772.
36. Gensia Pharmaceuticals, Inc. *Instruction Manual.* Dr. AIJ Brain. 1992:19.
37. Seltzer J, Greek R, Maurer P, et al. The preemptive analgesic effect of regional anesthesia for shoulder surgery. *Anesthesiology.* 1993; 79:A815.
38. Fuller PB. The relationship between preintubation lidocaine and postanesthesia sore throat. *AANA.* 1992; 60:374–378.
39. Capan LM, Bruce DL, Patel KP, et al. Succinylcholine-induced postoperative sore throat. *Anesthesiology.* 1983; 59:202–206.
40. Kiss I, Kilian M. Does opiate premedication influence postoperative analgesia? A prospective study. *Pain.* 1992; 48:157–158.
41. Tverskoy M, Ox Y, Isakson A, Finger J, Bradley EL, Kissin I: Preemptive effect of fentanyl and ketamine on postoperative pain and wound hyperalgesia. *Anesth Analg.* 1994; 78: 205–209.
42. Malmgrem AB, Yaksh TL. Hyperalgesia mediated by spinal glutamate or substance P receptor blocked by spinal cyclooxygenase inhibition. *Science.* 1992; 257:1276–1279.
43. Haddow FR, Riley E, Isaacs R, McSharry R. Ketorolac, nasal polyposis, and bronchial asthma: a cause for concern. *Anesth Analg.* 1993; 76:420–422.
44. Chaumont J, VanderCar D, Farrell C. Intraoperative ketorolac does not reduce postoperative pain. *Anesthesiology.* 1993; 79: A42.
45. Higgins M, Givogre J, Marco A, Blumenthal P, Furman N: Recovery from outpatient laparoscope tubal ligation is not improved by preoperative administration of ketorolac or ibuprofen. *Anesth Analg* 1994; 79:274–280.
46. O'Hara DA, Fragen RJ, Kinzer M, et al: Ketorolac tromethamine as compared with morphine sulphate for treatment of postoperative pain. *Clin Pharmacol Ther.* 1987;41: 556–559.
47. Green CR, Pandit SK, Kothary SP, Schork MA, Tait AR. A combination of intraoperative fentanyl and ketorolac during diagnostic laparoscopy has a narcotic sparing effect in the recovery room. *Anesthesiology.* 1993; 79:A43.
48. McLaughlin ME. The intraoperative administration of ketorolac tromethamine in evaluating length of stay in a same day surgery unit. *AANA.* 1994; 62:433–436.
49. Schoneboom BA. Ketorolac tromethamine: a nonsteroidal anti-inflammatory analgesic used as an adjunct for general anesthesia. *AANA.* 1992; 60:304–306.
50. Stein C, Comisel K, Haimeri E, et al. Analgesic effect of intraarticular morphine after arthroscopic surgery. *N Engl J Med.* 1991; 325:1123–1126.

☐ QUESTIONS

1. What is the maximum allowable dose (in mg/kg) of incisionally infiltrated bupivacaine without epinephrine in a 70-kg patient?
   a. 3 mg/kg
   b. 12 mg/kg
   c. 2.5 mg/kg
   d. 7 mg/kg

2. All of the following are true regarding cimetidine *except:*
   a. Prolongs the action of propanolol
   b. Causes inhibition of the hepatic mixed function P-450 oxidase system
   c. Increases lower esophageal tone
   d. Categorically a H$_2$ antagonist

3. Which statement best describes Toradol (ketorolac) for the ambulatory patient?
   a. Is contraindicated in the asthmatic with nasal polyps
   b. Should be given at the beginning of a laparoscopic tubal ligation
   c. In doses of 30 to 60 mg is as effective for postoperative pain as 5 to 7 mg morphine sulfate
   d. Leads to an increase in the synthesis and release of prostaglandins from cells

4. What is *not* a common cause for unanticipated hospital admission in the same day patient?
   a. Vomiting
   b. Pain

   c. Cardiovascular changes

   d. Extensive surgery

5. When is it safe for an ex-premature infant to have outpatient surgery?
   a. 10 weeks postnatal
   b. Not appropriate for these infants to have outpatient surgery
   c. 30–40 weeks postconceptional
   d. 40–60 weeks postconceptional

6. What is the best aspiration prophylaxis regimen for the same day patient at risk?
   a. Particulate antacids
   b. Standard NPO protocol
   c. 20 mg IM Reglan 1 hour preoperatively
   d. Combination of a gastrokinetic drug with an H_2 blocker given 30 minutes prior to surgery

7. Which statement is true regarding NPO status?
   a. An 8-hour fast results in lower residual gastric volume and increased pH.
   b. Adults and pediatric patients should follow the same NPO guidelines.
   c. In the non–high-risk patient, clear liquids up to 2 hours before surgery can dilute acidic gastric secretions and enhance the rate of gastric emptying.
   d. Breast milk is not considered a clear liquid.

8. The most appropriate same day surgical candidate would be:
   a. A 32-year-old with a childhood history of asthma for a possible ectopic pregnancy
   b. Cataract extraction in a patient with a blood pressure 195/100 the morning of surgery without a previous history
   c. Hernia repair in a 3-month-old term infant with a hematocrit of 28%
   d. Healthy 72-year-old woman scheduled for breast biopsy; recent ECG shows new St segment changes

9. All are appropriate anesthetic plans suited for the outpatient *except:*
   a. Supraclavicular approach to a brachial plexus block in a emphysemic patient
   b. Axillary approach to a brachial plexus block for hand surgery
   c. An intravenous sedation technique with local infiltrate for a 90-kg healthy women undergoing a hernia repair who refused regional or general anesthesia
   d. A laryngeal mask airway general anesthetic in a spontaneously breathing 42-year-old man having hardware removed from lower leg

10. Discharge criteria for the ambulatory patient include which true statements:
    1. Ability to count from 20 to 10 backward on discharge
    2. Ambulation with assistance 60 minutes postoperatively
    3. Adequate pain control 10 minutes postoperatively
    4. Ability to tolerate clear liquids 45 minutes postoperatively
       a. 1,3
       b. 1,2,3
       c. 2,4
       d. All are true.

11. A preoperative assessment for a 17-year-old man scheduled for adenoidectomy and tonsillectomy on an outpatient basis would include all *except:*
    a. A responsible adult to care for patient at home
    b. A recent hematocrit and hemoglobin
    c. A recent chest x-ray
    d. A complete history and physical

12. Benefits of ambulatory procedures include all *except:*
    a. Less family separation and personal disruption
    b. Lower cost
    c. Lower risk of nosocomial infection
    d. Decreased anesthetic requirement

13. Which anesthetic agent may be the *least* appropriate in the same day surgical patient?
    a. Mivacurium
    b. Succinylcholine
    c. Zemuron
    d. Propofol

14. Which statement is false regarding ambulatory anesthesia?
    a. By the year 2000, a projected 70% of all elective surgical procedures in the United States will be in the outpatient setting.
    b. The overwhelming majority of ambulatory surgical patients are healthy ASA I or II patients.
    c. A key element in the success of outpatient surgery is preoperative screening process.
    d. Deaths in the surgical outpatient is extremely rare.

15. Anesthetic goals in the ambulatory surgical patient receiving intravenous sedation/monitored anesthetic care include all elements *except:*
    a. A quiet surgical field
    b. An amnestic surgeon
    c. An uncompromised airway
    d. Patient comfort

16. Advanced age is a reliable indicator of postoperative complications in the same day surgical setting. True or False?
    a. True
    b. False

17. An 80-year-old woman 6 months after aortic valve replacement presents for inguinal hernia repair. Medications include coumadin and digoxin. What is the best postoperative pain management plan?
   a. 30 mg IV Toradol
   b. 25 μg Fentanyl
   c. 6 mg IM morphine sulfate
   d. Incisional infiltration of 0.25% bupivacaine plain

18. What is the least desirable pharmacologic characteristic in an anesthetic agent for ambulatory anesthesia?
   a. Metabolism via nonspecific ester hydrolysis
   b. Large V_d
   c. High FA/FI ratio
   d. High lipid solubility

19. All situations are probably unsuitable for ambulatory surgery *except:*
   a. Sickle cell anemia trait
   b. Strong family history of malignant hyperthermia
   c. Young child with history of severe asthma
   d. Patient on monamine oxidase inhibitors recently on suicide precautions

20. Premedication with opioids decreases postoperative need for analgesia in the same day surgical patient. True or False?
   a. True
   b. False

☐ ANSWERS

1.	a	**5.**	d	**9.**	a	**13.**	b	**17.**	d
2.	c	**6.**	d	**10.**	c	**14.**	b	**18.**	b
3.	a	**7.**	c	**11.**	c	**15.**	b	**19.**	a
4.	c	**8.**	c	**12.**	d	**16.**	b	**20.**	a

Anesthesia for the Trauma Patient

Charles R. Barton

Trauma is the principal cause of death in individuals below the age of 45 years in the United States. It is the fourth leading cause of death, following heart disease, cancer, and cerebrovascular disease, when patients of all ages are included in the overall mortality rate. In contrast to heart disease, cancer, and cerebrovascular disease, trauma occurs mainly between the ages of 1 and 44. Recognizing the tremendous loss of life and high rates of residual disability associated with traumatic injury, a group of concerned anesthesia professionals were inspired to form the International Trauma Anesthesia and Critical Care Society (ITACCS) in 1988. Actually, trauma is a "disease" that humankind has battled through the ages, especially during times of war. The pathophysiologic responses to injury are so invariable that it is appropriate to use the term traumatic disease.[1,2] Trauma has been characterized as the neglected disease of modern society. The term "trauma system" denotes a consolidated approach to the care of the critically injured patient. The ideal system includes: (1) triage and in-field treatment, (2) a communications network, (3) transportation by air and ground, (4) patient management within the hospital, (5) education of paramedical personnel and the public on trauma care and accident prevention, and (6) evaluation of care.

Trauma patients are hospitalized 20 million days annually—more than the total for all heart patients and four times the days required for cancer patients.[3] Because the incidence of trauma is projected to continue increasing and because emergency medical care is improving dramatically, the number of severely injured trauma patients admitted to trauma facilities will continue to rise.

☐ PRIMARY AND SECONDARY SURVEY OF THE TRAUMA PATIENT

PRIMARY SURVEY

Traditionally, trauma patients have been initially evaluated with the ABCs, indicating assessment of the *airway, breathing,* and *circulation* status. The advanced trauma life support (ATLS) course has extended the customary ABCs to ABCDE (Table 30–1). The D is used to designate *disability,* which is indicated by evaluation of the neurologic status that can be assessed initially with the Glasgow Coma Scale (Table 30–2) and then with a more detailed neurologic examination. The E is used to designate *exposure,* which is to indicate the need to completely undress the trauma patient to assess the patient in a thorough manner.

Airway Providing or confirming a patent airway is the first area of the ABCs that needs to be addressed. If the patient is able to verbalize clearly, the airway can be considered patent. In contrast, in the patient who is obtunded or unconscious or who has significant maxillofacial or neck trauma, ventilatory support may be needed to various degrees from the time of initial assessment. In such patients, the possibility of a cervical spine injury should be assumed. Establishment of adequate airway patency should always take priority over neck injury, but the cervical spine can be protected during airway manipulations with the use of *in-line axial stabilization* of the cervical spine during intubation.[4] Although the majority of trauma patients can have their trachea intubated

Table 30–1
PRIMARY SURVEY OF THE TRAUMA PATIENT

A = airway (patency)
B = breathing (ventilation)
C = circulation (perfusion)
D = disability (neurologic status)
E = exposure (undress to assess)

by conventional means, the preparation for cricothyroidotomy or trachestomy should always be made in these situations (Table 30–3).

Breathing   Following the establishment of an adequate airway, breathing is the second priority that needs to be addressed in the primary survey. The patient is assessed for breathing problems by observing the respiratory rate, depth, and pattern of exchange. If the alert patient can take a deep breath without significant discomfort, the probability of significant respiratory dysfunction is remote.[5] The patient should be observed for use of accessory muscles, paradoxical chest wall motion, presence of a flail chest, sounds of a sucking chest wound, or presence of tracheal shift. The patient should be evaluated for the presence of a pneumo- or hemopneumothorax, diaphragmatic rupture, and pulmonary contusion. Low oxygen saturation values as observed with pulse oximetry will often be an early indicator of inadequate respiratory exchange and pulmonary dysfunction. Occlusive dressings are applied to sucking chest wounds, needle or tube thoracotomies are placed to treat pneumothorax, and sandbags are placed to help stabilize flail chest segments. Appropriate mechanical ventilation in the patient with an intubated trachea is often augmented with sedation, analgesia, and paralysis of skeletal muscles as indicated by the individual patient's status.

Table 30–2
THE GLASGOW COMA SCALE

Best verbal response	
None	1
Incomprehensible sound	2
Inappropriate words	3
Confused	4
Oriented	5
Eyes open	
None	1
To pain	2
To speech	3
Spontaneously	4
Best motor response	
None	1
Abnormal extensor	2
Abnormal flexion	3
Withdraws	4
Localizes	5
Obeys	6
Total coma scale	

Table 30–3
NEEDLE CRICOTHYROIDOTOMY KIT FOR JET VENTILATION

- 14-gauge or larger plastic IV catheter
- Tuberculin syringe barrel
- 6 feet of noncompliant tubing (e.g., suction tubing)
- Y connector

Directions: Assemble the above materials in advance. Remove the IV stylet and connect to tuberculin syringe barrel. Place the Y connector in line with one port to the oxygen source, one port to the cricothyroidectomy needle, and one port open. Connect the tubing to an oxygen source having 15 L/min or more delivery capability. Place the IV catheter through the cricothyroid membrane. Place thumb on the open port on the Y connector to jet ventilate the patient.

Circulation   Following the establishment of a patent airway and adequate breathing, the circulation is the third priority to be addressed. Quick initial assessment of the circulation should include the presence and quality of peripheral pulses, adequacy of capillary refill, and measurement of the arterial blood pressure. The patient is examined for any external bleeding that needs to be controlled. The patient should be assessed for adequacy of the intravascular volume and for signs of pump failure. The patient is observed for flat or collapsed neck veins that suggest hypovolemia. Conversely, distended neck veins may indicate a pump problem, for example, myocardial contusion or infarction or pericardial tamponade.

Disability   The neurologic status of the trauma patient is the fourth concern in the primary survey. The ATLS course uses the simple AVPU method to determine the patient's initial neurologic status (Table 30–4).

Both the AVPU assessment and the Glascow coma score will give initial information about the patient's neurologic status, although they must be viewed as a crude measurement of consciousness and should be followed with a more detailed neurologic examination.

Exposure   To properly assess the trauma patient, all clothing is removed. When indicated, clothing should be cut away to avoid motion that may endanger spinal stability, exacerbate bleeding, or precipitate pain. Care should be taken to keep the patient warm during this time.

Table 30–4
AVPU METHOD

A = alert
V = responds to verbal stimuli
P = responds to painful stimuli
U = unresponsive

Table 30-5
SECONDARY SURVEY OF TRAUMA PATIENTS

Head Exam: observation and palpation of the scalp; pupillary size and reactivity; ocular abnormalities, auditory canals and tympanic membranes, observing for blood or cerebrospinal fluid from ears and nose; observe for bulging over the mastoid area (Battles's sign) or in the periorbital soft tissue (raccoon eyes).

Neck Exam: inspection and careful palpation of the neck with the head in neutral alignment and with the patient on a long spine board with a cervical collar in place; observe for penetrating wounds, crepitance, tracheal alignment, and the status of neck veins

Chest Exam: observation of breathing pattern; observe electrocardiogram pattern; auscultation of heart and breath sounds; palpation of the sternum, clavicles, and all of the ribs

Abdominal Exam: local exploration of penetrating wounds; peritoneal lavage or computed tomography scan for blunt trauma; placement of a nasogastric tube or orogastric tube if a cribriform fracture is suspected

Rectal Exam: observe for blood, prostate injury, rectal injury, lack of sphincter tone, and pelvic fractures

Extremities Exam: observe and palpate for soft-tissue injuries and hematoma, palpate pulses, check capillary refill, and observe for venous stasis; inspect for dislocations

Neurological Exam: assess hemispheric function, brain stem function, spinal cord motor activity, sensation, and bulbocavernosus reflex

SECONDARY SURVEY

Whereas the primary survey is used to provide basic physiologic support, the secondary survey is used to prepare a complete problem list that in turn leads to an orderly treatment plan. The secondary survey is used to examine the patient carefully and comprehensively (Table 30-5).

☐ PRINCIPAL DRUGS USED DURING RESUSCITATION

The following drugs are commonly used in cardiopulmonary resuscitation (CPR) situations, as well as in postresuscitative periods.

EPINEPHRINE

This historic cardiovascular stimulant is still unsurpassed by other sympathomimetic amines for use during cardiac arrest and CPR because of its combined strong α- and β-receptor stimulation effects. It increases systemic peripheral vascular resistance without constricting the coronary and cerebral vessels and raises systolic and diastolic pressures during cardiac compressions, which thereby improves myocardial and cerebral blood flow, which, in turn, facilitates the return of spontaneous cardiac contractions. The combined α and β effects give a high initial cardiac output and arterial pressure at the beginning of spontaneous reperfusion, which may benefit cerebral and other vital organ systems' blood flow.

In asystole, epinephrine helps restart spontaneous cardiac action as it elevates perfusion and increases myocardial contractility. In pulselessness with bizarre electrocardiographic (ECG) complexes (electromechanical dissociation), epinephrine often restores a spontaneous pulse. After restoration of spontaneous circulation, a continuous intravenous infusion of epinephrine (1 mg/250 mL) may be used to increase and sustain arterial pressure and cardiac output.

LIDOCAINE

All antidysrhythmic drugs are cardiac depressants and, therefore, harmful. Lidocaine is the antidysrhythmic agent of choice for the treatment of premature ventricular complexes (PVCs) and for preventing progression to ventricular tachycardia (VT) or ventricular fibrillation (VF). In established VF, however, antidysrhythmic drugs should be withheld until several attempts at electric defibrillation have failed because these drugs depress ventricular ectopy and make initial defibrillation more difficult. In equipotent antidysrhythmic doses, lidocaine produces less myocardial depression than do other antidysrhythmic drugs.

Lidocaine alone cannot convert VF to a stable rhythm, but might convert VT. In intractable VF, lidocaine should be used in conjunction with electric defibrillation attempts and, if ineffective, should be replaced by bretylium. Side effects of lidocaine include myocardial depression, which is more likely to be apparent in the presence of cardiogenic shock. In such cases, the normal bolus dose may be reduced by half.

PROCAINAMIDE HYDROCHLORIDE (PRONESTYL)

This drug preceded lidocaine historically for the suppression of PVCs. It is indicated when lidocaine is contraindicated. In the presence of spontaneous circulation, it is more likely than lidocaine to produce hypotension and reduce conduction, even with a normal myocardium. The recommended dose of procainamide is about the same as that of lidocaine, but to a maximum of 1 g.

BRETYLIUM (BRETYLOL)

An antidysrhythmic agent that raises the VF threshold, bretylium decreases the joules required. By contrast, the joules required for defibrillation seem to be raised by lidocaine and quinidine. It facilitates subsequent electric defibrillation and helps prevent recurrent VT or VF in patients with very sick hearts. The effects of bretylium are unpredictable. It is presently recommended as a second line of defense in the control of VT or VF, when countershocks and lidocaine have not been effective or when VF has recurred despite use of lidocaine.

SODIUM BICARBONATE

This is the third drug to be given during CPR (after epinephrine and lidocaine), in an initial dose of approximately

1 mEq/kg intravenously, but only after prolonged arrest or CPR time. The purpose of administering sodium bicarbonate is to neutralize the fixed acids coming from ischemic tissues after circulatory arrest and during the borderline perfusion produced by CPR. Severe acidemia (arterial pH < 7.2)—actually tissue acidosis—should be reversed because it causes vasodilation, capillary leakage, myocardial depression, conduction block, and a decrease in fibrillation threshold. Acidemia and tissue acidosis reduce the efficacy of epinephrine, but intravenous epinephrine in large enough doses is effective without sodium bicarbonate.

Excessive sodium bicarbonate (metabolic alkalemia) results in impaired oxygen release from hemoglobin, reduced ionized (effective) unionized calcium ratio, a potassium shift from serum into cells, VT and VF, and sustained cardiac contraction (stone heart). Sodium bicarbonate may also be injurious by producing hypernatremia with hyperosmolality.

CARDIAC STIMULANTS

Vasopressors and cardiac stimulants do not seem to have significant advantages over epinephrine for use during CPR. Sympathomimetic amines with primary α-receptor stimulating properties, such as norepinephrine and metaraminol, and drugs that are pure α-receptor stimulants, such as phenylephrine or methoxamine, also are effective in raising diastolic arterial pressure during cardiac compressions and in facilitating restoration of spontaneous circulation in asystole. They do not, however, provide the additional cardiac inotropic (β-receptor stimulating) effect, which also might be desirable. Pure β-receptor stimulating sympathomimetic amines, such as isoproterenol, low-dose dopamine, dobutamine, and calcium, do not aid in the restoration of spontaneous circulation because they lack the ability to increase diastolic arterial pressure and coronary reperfusion during cardiac compressions. Often, CPR stabilization of cardiovascular parameters with vasoactive agents with or without cardiac-stimulating effect are indispensable. All potent vasoactive infusions should be titrated, if possible, with the aid of direct intra-arterial pressure monitoring, use of microdrips, infusion pumps, or in some situations with the use of a pulmonary artery catheter.

Norepinephrine   A naturally occurring catecholamine, norepinephrine is primarily an α-receptor stimulant. During CPR, prior to restoration of spontaneous circulation, norepinephrine may be given in the same doses as epinephrine and is effective in helping to restore spontaneous circulation. When norepinephrine is given to the point of excess, vasoconstriction and renal and mesenteric blood flow are compromised and severe metabolic acidosis may develop. The heart rate may slow as a result of carotid baroreceptor reflex, if hypertension occurs. Prolonged administration of norepinephrine in hypovolemia is contraindicated. In the presence of spontaneous circulation with reduced peripheral resistance and hypotension, norepinephrine is given by titrated intravenous infusion.

Dopamine   This sympathomimetic amine is a biologic precursor of norepinephrine and epinephrine. It exerts dose-dependent cardiac inotropic action (β-receptor stimulant) in low doses and vasoconstrictor action (α-receptor stimulant) in high doses. Response differs among individuals and with dose and rate of administration. Its vasopressor potency is less than that of norepinephrine.

The principal use of dopamine is in the support of perfusion pressure in cardiogenic or septic shock, using infusion rates of 2 to 20 μg/kg/min. The infusion rate is increased until arterial pressure and urine flow respond. In CPR cases after restoration of spontaneous circulation, dopamine is useful for supporting arterial perfusion pressure after the more potent norepinephrine is no longer required. Frequently dopamine is used as the first choice vasopressor when the epinephrine effects begin to wear off. As in administering any vasopressor, normovolemia or even slight expansion of blood volume should be established.

Dobutamine   A synthetic derivative of isoproterenol with predominantly β-receptor stimulating (inotropic and vasodilating) effects, dobutamine has proved useful in the treatment of heart failure. Its α-receptor (vasoconstrictor) effect, even with large doses, is minimal. In high doses, dobutamine can produce VT.

Ephedrine   This is the oldest natural sympathomimetic amine. It increases arterial pressure indirectly by causing a release of norepinephrine from tissue stores. In addition, ephedrine has a direct cardiac stimulating effect that does not depend on release of norepinephrine. Ephedrine produces not only vasoconstriction and tachycardia, but also central nervous system (CNS) arousal. It is not recommended for prolonged use or in intermittent doses because its effect fades due to *tachyphylaxis.*

Isoproterenol   This drug is a synthetic sympathomimetic amine with pure β-receptor stimulation. Because of its lack of peripheral vasoconstricting action, it does not increase arterial pressure and thereby does not selectively enhance cerebral and coronary perfusion during CPR. As a result, isoproterenol does not by itself enhance restoration of spontaneous circulation. Although isoproterenol exerts a potent chronotropic and inotropic effect on the heart, resulting in increased cardiac output, it increases myocardial oxygen requirements. For these reasons, isoproterenol has no place during cardiac compressions, except in severe atropine-resistant bradycardia and heart block pending pacemaker insertion. Even in these cases, however, epinephrine is preferred during CPR for restarting the heart.

Atropine   The classic parasympatholytic drug, atropine, which *reduces vagal tone,* enhances atrioventricular conduction. And, despite normally producing tachycardia, atropine reduces the likelihood of VF triggered by the myocardial hypoperfusion associated with extreme bradycardia. It may increase the heart rate in sinus bradycardia and in high-degree atrioventricular block with bradycardia, but not in complete atrioventricular block where isoproterenol is indicated. Therefore, atropine essentially has no place during cardiac arrest and CPR except possibly in refractory asystole. During spontaneous circulation, however, when the heart rate decreases to below 50 beats/min or when there is bradycardia with PVCs or hypotension, atropine is indicated.

Calcium A physiologically important cation that is essential for excitation-contraction coupling in muscle, calcium has been recommended for the treatment of electromechanical dissociation when epinephrine has failed to restart spontaneous cardiac action. It can cause coronary spasm and also increased myocardial irritability. Excessive doses may cause the heart to stop in contraction, particularly in the fully digitalized patient. The usefulness of calcium in resuscitation is limited, and it may even be contraindicated, considering the myocardial and cerebral preservation effects of calcium entry blockers. It may be more appropriate to use calcium than sympathomimetic amines in cardiac depression resulting from certain drugs, such as barbiturates and other anesthetic agents, but conclusive evidence is lacking.

VASODILATORS

Vasodilators have no place during CPR, when efforts must be directed at increasing diastolic arterial pressure. After restoration of spontaneous circulation, however, control of arterial normotension—important for cerebral recovery—and reduction of systemic vascular resistance to reduce myocardial oxygen demand may require individualized, titrated infusion of combinations of vasodilator and vasoconstrictor agents. Vasodilators reduce both arterial pressure (i.e., afterload) and venous return and central venous right atrial–left atrial pressures (i.e., preload). If diastolic arterial pressure is sustained at the same time (important for coronary perfusion), the heart should benefit. Nitroprusside and nitroglycerin, both direct vasodilators, may not be the agents of choice for the post-CPR state with coma, because they bring about cerebral vasodilation and increased intracranial pressure (ICP). The ganglionic blocker *trimethaphan* seems a better choice for control of hypotension during coma.

Nitroprusside A rapidly acting potent peripheral vasodilating agent, nitroprusside is very controllable because of its brief effect. It dilates arteries and veins directly. Although nitroprusside has no role during cardiac arrest and cardiac compressions, it has become a valuable adjunct for the reduction of peripheral vascular resistance and venodilation in protracted myocardial failure (to increase cardiac output) and for the control of hypertensive crises.

Nitroglycerin This classic direct vasodilator, used for relief of angina pain, also is now being used for the reduction of preload and afterload by peripheral venous and, to a lesser degree, arterial dilation. Nitroglycerin also *dilates* coronary

vessels and is beneficial in heart failure resulting from myocardial infarction. Nitroglycerin has no role during cardiac compressions.

PROPRANOLOL

A β-adrenergic receptor blocking drug that decreases automaticity, conduction, and contractility of the heart, propranolol has no place in emergency resuscitation during cardiac compressions because it may make the heart unresuscitable. Its principal use is in the patient with spontaneous circulation accompanied by recurrent PVCs or atrial tachydysrhythmias. VT and VF occasionally may respond to a β-blocker. β-receptor blockers are hazardous when myocardial contractility is depressed and are relatively contraindicated in *asthmatics*.

ESMOLOL

This drug appears to be a better choice for β-blockade because of its extremely short half-life. Esmolol is particularly attractive to treat hypertensive episodes during anesthesia because of its rapid onset and short duration of action.

FUROSEMIDE AND ETHACRYNIC ACID

These drugs inhibit the reabsorption of sodium in the loop of Henle. Furosemide has an additional venodilating effect in pulmonary edema. Diuresis starts within 20 minutes after intravenous administration, peaks at about 30 minutes, and lasts for several hours. The diuretic action of these drugs is indicated in pulmonary edema. Furosemide and ethacrynic acid also may reduce intracranial hypertension caused by postanoxic or posttraumatic cerebral edema, partly because of a reduction in cerebrospinal fluid (CSF) production and increase in CSF clearance.

BARBITURATES

The barbiturates have been used primarily because of their CNS depressant effects. Anesthesia primarily is accomplished with larger doses of ultrashort-acting agents such as thiopental. After restoration of normotension, the intravenous titration of thiopental or pentobarbital is effective in controlling convulsions and restlessness. Safety is provided by controlled ventilation and blood pressure support, as needed. A reasonably safe anesthesia induction dose for the normovolemic person with a healthy cardiovascular system is about 3 to 4 mg/kg. Convulsions are best controlled initially by intravenous thiopental or diazepam in titrated does, which are then followed up for long-term suppression of seizures by phenytoin by intravenous infusion. Control of seizures usually is achieved with phenytoin plasma concentrations of 10 μg/mL. Because of its membrane-stabilizing effect, phenytoin also may have a resuscitation effect on cerebral neurons after ischemia.

PHENYTOIN

This is the drug of choice for the long-term treatment of seizure disorders. Phenytoin decreases membrane ion fluxes, similar to local anesthetics, and thereby *stabilizes excitable membranes*. Although phenytoin is used effectively in titrated fashion for convulsions and cardiac dysrhythmias, its intravenous administration in excessive doses can cause cardiac dysrhythmias, hypotension, and CNS depression.

☐ PATHOPHYSIOLOGIC CHANGES EVOLVING FROM TRAUMATIC INJURY

Cell injury can be defined as an alteration of normal homeostasis that leads to unfavorable consequences for the organism.[6] Depending on the severity of cell injury, various changes can be seen morphologically and biochemically. After traumatic injury, these changes may lead to eventual restoration of the cell or to ultimate cell death. When shock and hypoxia are involved, injured tissues with high oxygen consumption are more vulnerable to injury and subsequent death.

The body's response to trauma and shock has been described as a complex series of neural and hormonal reflexes induced by injury and resulting in an integrated attempt by the organism to preserve oxygen delivery, mobilize energy substrates, and reduce pain.[7]

Trauma causes the body to call on many physiologic mechanisms. These defense responses include fever, immune system activation, leukocytic and reticuloendothelial cell changes, metabolic effects, responses by the brain and autonomic nervous system, the release of various hormones, and sometimes the activation of the coagulation, complement, and kinin systems.[8] These responses include a general acceleration of body metabolism, a catabolic degradation of skeletal muscle protein, the production of needed extra energy substrates from endogenous sources, and the production of new body cells and molecular products as needed for host defense and the healing process. In addition, other responses include certain transient derangements in electrolyte and water metabolism, a redistribution of certain minerals and trace elements, a need for the elimination of toxic waste products and metabolites, and the direct participation of body cells in defensive mechanisms such as inflammatory processes, immune responses, and tissue repair.

When trauma results in hemorrhagic blood loss or sequestration of extracellular fluid in the injured tissues, the loss of circulating volume triggers a response by low-pressure baroreceptors in the right atrium and by high-pressure baroreceptors in the carotid arteries and aorta.[9,10] When the blood volume is reduced, the venous return and cardiac output are similarly diminished. This, in turn, results in a neuroendocrine response of increased secretion of adrenocorticotropic hormone (ACTH), vasopressin, and growth hormone through central pathways and in the secretion of epinephrine, norepi-

nephrine, renin, and glucagon via peripheral sympathetic pathways. In turn, some of these hormones stimulate a further hormonal response of inhibition of pancreatic secretion of insulin by epinephrine or stimulation of adrenocortical secretion of aldosterone by ACTH and renin-angiotensin.[11] Pain, which is an almost universal finding following traumatic injury, stimulates a neuroendocrine response. Pain causes activation of nociceptive fibers resulting in the release of endogenous opiates, vasopressin, ACTH, catecholamines, and other hormones.[12,13]

☐ PROFILE OF THE TRAUMA PATIENT

Trauma patients often present to surgery and anesthesia with many differences compared with the general surgical population. These differences are not always immediately apparent to a cursory evaluation. Frequently trauma patients will present in an obtunded state and will be unable to supply information about past medical history, possible allergies, or previous response to anesthesia. The trauma patient frequently has a "full stomach" and is at high risk for developing *aspiration pneumonitis*. In trauma, medical personnel are frequently dealing with an acute disease process occurring in a previously healthy patient. Compensatory mechanisms cannot often be established as often happens in chronic disease processes. In contrast to elective surgery, postponement of anesthesia and surgery in the trauma patient generally is not possible if an optimal outcome is to be achieved. The compensatory mechanisms, which evolve during the shock state, may eventually cause death.

☐ LEVELS OF CARE IN TRAUMA SYSTEMS

Trauma centers are classified into three levels to make the best possible use of community resources. The practice of taking the severely injured patient to the nearest hospital is no longer acceptable.

Death resulting from trauma has a trimodal distribution.[14] The initial peak in deaths is within seconds or minutes of injury. Invariably, these deaths are the result of lacerations of the brain, brain stem, upper spinal cord, heart, aorta, or other large vessels. Few of these patients can be saved.

The second peak in deaths occurs within the first 2 hours after injury. Death is usually caused by subdural and epidural hematomas, hemopneumothorax, ruptured spleen, lacerations of the liver, fractured femur, or multiple injuries associated with significant blood loss. These patients, whose numbers are significant and who can usually be saved, benefit most from regionalized trauma care.

The third peak in deaths occurs days or weeks after the injury and is usually the result of sepsis and multiple organ failure. These patients can benefit also from a trauma center where the concentration of expertise of surgeons, anesthesia professionals, and other specialists allows for a rational therapeutic approach that positively affects patient outcomes.

LEVEL I AND II TRAUMA CARE

The goals of the Committee on Trauma of the American College of Surgeons are: (1) improved care of the injured patient, (2) education for all personnel involved in trauma care, and (3) research in trauma. In keeping with these goals, the committee believes that the commitment to quality of patient care should be identical in the level I and II hospital. Level I hospitals have training and research programs as an essential part of their facilities.

Injuries can be divided into three general categories: severe, urgent, and nonurgent. Severe injuries are those that are immediately life-threatening. Although they represent only 5% of all injuries, they account for 50% of all trauma deaths. Urgent injuries are those that are not immediately life-threatening but may become so or result in significant disability. Urgent injuries account for approximately 10% to 15% of all injuries. Nonurgent injuries account for 80% of all trauma. These injuries are not immediately life-threatening nor do they present a risk of permanent disability.

LEVEL III TRAUMA CARE

The level III hospital generally serves communities that do not have resources for a level I or II institution. However, a level III hospital reflects a maximum commitment to trauma care commensurate with resources. Planning care for the injured in small community or suburban settings usually calls for transfer agreements and protocols for the most severely injured.

In the ideal system, the capability of the hospital and its personnel matches precisely the severity of the injury. Improved care for the seriously injured, with maximum efficiency and minimal costs in terms of life, disability, and dollars, depends on the appropriate use of trained personnel, specific facilities, and equipment.

☐ INITIAL RESUSCITATION AND STABILIZATION

At the scene of an accident, emergency medical technicians attempt to stabilize the patient. The resuscitation efforts should occur in minutes as team members move rapidly to perform their duties. Speed is essential. Prompt, appropriate treatment provided during the first 60 minutes after a severe traumatic injury will often determine whether a patient will survive. Certainly not all trauma patients are in shock, but for patients who are in hemorrhagic shock the time to adequate resuscitation is critical. If the effects of shock are not sufficiently corrected within the first 60 to 90 minutes, the mortality rate rises substantially. The term "golden hour" denotes the principles developed by R. Adams Cowley, MD, founder of the University of Maryland Shock Trauma Center. This principle demonstrates that as more time elapses between the moment that a trauma patient develops hemorrhagic shock and the beginning of resuscitation, the percentage of surviving patients decreases.[15(pp100–132)] The highest rate of mortality culminates at approximately 60 minutes. Awareness of the "golden hour" concept encourages trauma care providers to begin aggressive resuscitation efforts at the earliest possible moment.

Because trauma patients are susceptible to infection, vascular lines placed in the field under less-than-ideal conditions are replaced at the trauma center when possible. Arterial, central venous, and pulmonary artery catheters are inserted using an aseptic approach. Fluid status is monitored and appropriate fluid replacement continued.

☐ INITIAL AIRWAY MANAGEMENT AT THE TRAUMA CENTER

Rapid control of the airway and ventilation with oxygen are critical for traumatic shock resuscitation. Although in certain critical situations tracheal intubation must be accomplished immediately, intubation conditions are generally closer to optimal after initial fluid resuscitation and general stabilization. If the patient can maintain adequate spontaneous respiration, the cervical spine is radiographed before intubation to help evaluate possible cervical spine injuries. Arterial blood gases (ABG) are drawn immediately after the patient arrives and the results are used to guide subsequent airway interventions. Placing the patient on a known fraction inspired oxygen (FIO_2) before the ABG measurement is advantageous so that the adequacy of oxygen exchange can be evaluated.

With a Philadelphia cervical collar in place and the patient on a long spinal board, well maintained axial stabilization of the head (in-line stabilization with the head in the neutral position) should be performed in all trauma patients with suspected or confirmed cervical spine injuries. An awake nasal intubation, while being ideal in patients with cervical spine injuries, is often difficult to carry out in the inebriated, obtunded, frightened, or confused trauma patient. This unprepared emergency patient who frequently has a "full stomach" will often be uncooperative and thrash about during attempts at awake intubation. Local and topical anesthesia can obtund protective laryngeal reflexes and promote the possibility of pulmonary aspiration. Additionally, head-injured patients with suspected basilar skull fractures (raccoon eyes, battle signs, CSF from the nose or ears) should have oral intubations to avoid penetration of the *cribriform plate* with subsequent entry of foreign material into the brain through the fracture site.

Fiberoptic-guided nasal intubation should be attempted only in very cooperative patients. Overall, oral intubation is preferable to nasal intubation in the trauma patient.

Many trauma patients have inadequate respiratory function and are hypoxic on arrival at the trauma center. Until the trachea can be intubated, they are ventilated continuously with a mask. Maintaining continuous ventilation (with cricoid pressure) will prevent further hypoxic insults that can otherwise occur during the apneic period between the administration of a neuromuscular blocking agent and completed intubation. Sellick demonstrated the efficacy of cricoid pressure to prevent regurgitation of stomach contents during the induction of anesthesia while the patient is continuously ventilated with a mask.[16] If an intubation attempt fails, cricoid pressure is continued and mask ventilation is resumed before the next attempt.

Lawes has demonstrated that applying sufficient pressure to the cricoid ring to press the esophagus firmly against the anterior vertebral bodies to seal the esophagus against possible regurgitation is important.[17] *Testing the airway* is a term used to describe the checking of the ability to ventilate the patient before the use of muscle relaxants. Muscle relaxants should not be administered before the airway is opened and ventilation ensured by visible rising of the chest. This gives the anesthetist the knowledge that the patient can be adequately ventilated if intubation attempts fail.[18] Early intubation often prevents potential long-term problems such as those caused by aspiration or hypoxic insult.

If endotracheal intubation is not possible due to severe facial injuries or other causes and ventilatory effort is poor or absent due to partial or complete obstruction, either an emergency cricothyroidotomy, tracheostomy, or a percutaneous tracheal catheter should be placed to allow oxygenation. (See Chapter 9.) Emergency supplies and equipment need to be readily available for this possibility. General anesthesia may be required after intubation for further diagnostic workup with or without subsequent surgery.

Release of cricoid pressure can be concluded following observation of appropriate end-tidal CO_2 ($ETCO_2$) concentrations with normal waveform morphology. Use of this technique will verify endotracheal placement. Verification by $ETCO_2$ is now considered the gold standard for ensuring proper placement of an endotracheal tube in the trachea. $ETCO_2$ values also serve as a guide to adequate ventilation, in conjunction with ABGs. It should be noted that during cardiac arrest, the endotracheal tube can be in the correct place and yet *no carbon dioxide* will be observed by the capnography unit. With no perfusion, carbon dioxide cannot be delivered to the lungs. As perfusion improves, the carbon dioxide levels will again begin to rise. Conversely, the endotracheal tube can be placed in the esophagus and carbon dioxide may be initially detected. This can be caused by the patient previously swallowing "air" or by the prior ingestion of a carbonated beverage. Generally the waveform observed in that situation will be flattened and generally will be essentially nonexistent after a few attempts at ventilation are completed.

Following intubation, ventilation is controlled using a large tidal volume and low respiratory rate. In patients with impaired gas exchange due to aspiration, adult respiratory distress syndrome, or fluid overload, distending ventilatory pressures such as positive end-expiratory pressure (PEEP) or continuous positive airway pressure should be applied with the level titrated according to PaO_2 and hemodynamic response.[19]

☐ MONITORING OF THE TRAUMA PATIENT

Initial noninvasive monitoring procedures should include continuous temperature measurements, pulse oximetry, and continuous $ETCO_2$ monitoring, end-tidal agent measurements, and placement of automatic blood pressure cuffs. Insertion of an indwelling urinary catheter should also be done in this initial period.

Arterial, central venous, and pulmonary artery catheters are inserted as indicated using an aseptic approach. Fluid status should be continuously assessed as appropriate fluid resuscitation is accomplished. Initially, volume replacement should be guided by monitoring of mean arterial pressure, pulse rate, central venous pressure (CVP), urinary output, and peripheral oxygen saturation (SaO_2) values. Measurements of cardiac output and derived hemodynamic variables will help guide fluid and vasoactive drug management. Restoration of these values to normal ranges is a major goal of resuscitation. The ECG should be monitored for heart rate, dysrhythmias, and ST-T segment abnormalities. The urinary output should be monitored for volume, concentration, and color.

Initial laboratory screening should include a complete blood count, coagulation profile, electrolytes, blood sugar, toxicology screen, blood alcohol and serum osmolality, and an ABG analysis. An upright chest radiograph is obtained to screen for acute pathology including pneumothorax, hemothorax, pulmonary contusion, and widening of the mediastinum that could suggest cardiac or major vascular injury.

☐ CARDIOTHORACIC INJURIES

Blunt chest trauma often results from unbelted drivers hitting the steering wheel during a motor vehicle accident. Penetrating and blunt trauma to the chest may injure several structures and thus compromise optimal resuscitation. These structures include the chest wall, the lungs and airways, the heart and pericardium, and the great vessels of the thorax. Injuries to these structures will also compromise anesthesia care by affecting gas exchange and cardiac output.

Several life-threatening conditions require immediate interventions in patients with certain chest injuries. A *tension pneumothorax* develops when the pleural cavity is punctured, creating a one-way valve that controls flow of air into this cavity. With each breath, more air becomes trapped in this space, increasing intrapleural pressure to the point that it eventually exceeds all other intrathoracic pressures. The enlarging pleural cavity will then collapse the ipsilateral lung, as well as shift structures of the mediastinum (trachea, great vessels, heart) into the opposite hemithorax and thereby compress the contralateral lung. The size of a pneumothorax rapidly increases during positive-pressure ventilation, especially if nitrous oxide is used in the field for analgesia or during anesthesia in the trauma facility. Patients with a pneumothorax will often present with hypotension, subcutaneous emphysema of the neck or chest, a unilateral decrease in breath sounds, diminished chest wall motion, hyperresonance to percussion of one hemithorax, distended neck veins, or tracheal shift. An upright expirational chest radiograph provides definite information if the problem is significant. However, if the trauma patient is unstable, a large-bore intravenous catheter should be inserted into the second intercostal space along the midclavicular line. A "hissing" sound may be created by the escaping air under pressure. The catheter can then be attached to an intravenous line extension tube and placed under "water seal" by placing it in a bottle of sterile water that is kept beneath the level of the patient.

Many thoracic injuries can be life-threatening. *Massive hemothorax,* which can be caused by bleeding from the heart and great vessels, and *pericardial tamponade,* which restricts filling of the cardiac chambers during diastole and produces a fixed low cardiac output, need to be treated immediately if survival is likely. *Cardiac rupture* without pericardial tamponade is seldom associated with survival because exsanguination is extremely rapid. *Traumatic aortic rupture,* if complete, is usually fatal; but with an intimal tear with dissecting aneurysm, the patient can be saved if the diagnosis and repair are done promptly during well managed fluid resuscitation and anesthesia care. Management of these cases requires rapid and accurate assessment and appropriate surgical and anesthesia intervention. *Partial disruption of the trachea or major bronchi* can be handled in many cases through securing the airway by intubation or tracheostomy and surgical correction. *Total disruption of the trachea* is frequently fatal unless there is rapid surgical retrieval of the distal disrupted airway segment, thereby allowing lifesaving mechanical ventilation.

☐ TRAUMA-INDUCED SHOCK

The term *choc* was coined in 1743 by H. G. Le Dran, a French physician, to note a sudden collapse in the clinical status of a patient after a serious traumatic episode.[20] In 1867 an English physician, E. A. Morris, first used the term *shock.*[21]

Shock is a generalized state of severe circulatory inadequacy caused by reduced perfusion and inadequate delivery of oxygen and nutrients to tissues. Shock results in a profound and sustained loss of effective circulating blood volume. It leads to hypoperfusion of peripheral tissues and to a deficit in transcapillary exchange function.[22] Traumatic shock following severe hemorrhage inevitably leads to depression of physiologic systems in multiple organs. The sooner emergency intervention begins, the greater the patient's chances for survival. Rapid control of the airway and ventilation with oxygen and appropriate fluid replacement is critical for traumatic shock resuscitation. During CPR, placement of a 16-gauge or larger catheter in the largest accessible peripheral vein is preferred. Ideally the antecubital veins should be used for drug administration during CPR.[23] Insertion of a central line would hamper CPR. When possible after restoration of

spontaneous circulation, a central venous catheter should be placed. Attempts at cannulating subclavian or internal jugular veins for central line placement are contraindicated during CPR because of the danger of inducing pneumothorax when these measures are attempted in the patient who is being bounced by cardiac compressions.[24] It is advantageous to have at least one large-bore intravenous catheter above and below the diaphragm when there are injuries to the abdomen or pelvis. If injuries to the superior or inferior vena cava are present, venous return will be ineffective from catheters placed distal to the vena caval disruptions. Use of lower extremity veins is generally not suitable because the veins are often smaller and may be occluded from chronic venous stasis. As well, military antishock trousers (MAST suits) may impede venous drainage.

THREE PHASES OF SHOCK[25]

Stage I of shock is often called nonprogressive shock or compensated shock. A negative feedback control mechanism of the circulation attempts to return the cardiac output and arterial pressure to normal levels. This is mediated through the baroreceptor reflexes, CNS ischemic responses, contraction of blood vessels, release of vasopressin (antidiuretic hormone), formation of angiotensin, and compensation mechanisms that tend to return the blood volume back toward normal by mobilization of fluids from other spaces of the body.

Stage II of shock is also known as progressive shock. A positive feedback mechanism comes into play with this phase of shock. When shock becomes severe enough, components of the cardiovascular system start to deteriorate. Cardiac depression is due to ischemia, vasomotor failure, thrombosis of small vessels, increased capillary permeability, release of endotoxins by ischemic tissues, and generalized cellular deterioration.

Stage III of shock is also called irreversible shock. This occurs when adenosine triphosphate reserves are depleted. Death will follow as the natural consequence of not successfully halting progressive shock.

FLUID MANAGEMENT AND RESUSCITATION

The mortality rate for shock is approximately 50% if treatment is initiated at 30 minutes from the onset, and rises to 90% if 1 hour is allowed to elapse.[15(p101)] This is the basis for initiation of fluid resuscitation in the field. Red blood cells must be replaced to provide adequate oxygen-carrying capacity. Shed blood should be replaced with 1:1 volume of packed red blood cells and a 3:1 volume of crystalloids. Evaluation of the patient's fluid status can be accomplished in part with CVP or pulmonary artery catheter monitoring and by observation of the clinical signs for a return of the heart rate and blood pressure to normal levels.

Colloids usually allow rapid restoration of intravascular volume, but can contribute to a later episode of pulmonary edema in some patients. Balanced electrolyte solutions should be given to help maintain the CVP level between

1 and 15 mm Hg (8 to 10 mm Hg in anesthetized patients). Up to 1500 mL of 5% plasma protein fraction (Plasmanate) or hetastarch (Hespan®) can be used initially to restore intravascular volume in unstable patients. Fresh-frozen plasma is indicated in single or multiple coagulation deficiencies. It should not be used for volume replacement or any other nonspecific use.

Dextrose-containing solutions are generally *undesirable* for use in initial resuscitation fluids. Rapid determination of blood glucose levels is critical in diabetics and in children. Traumatized infants and children in shock may rapidly consume their gluconeogenic substrate allowing significant hypoglycemia to occur.[26] Although it is more common for patients to become hyperglycemic following traumatic injury, hypoglycemia can occur. On the other hand, significant hyperglycemia is associated with further neurologic injury.[27]

Dilutional thrombocytopenia is the most common cause of coagulopathy in the trauma patient, followed by hypofibrinogenemia.[28] These should be treated with pooled platelets, fresh-frozen plasma, or cryoprecipitate, as indicated. Cryoprecipitate is the most concentrated source of fibrinogen. *Cryoprecipitate* should also be given when fibrinogen or von Willebrand factor is needed. Consider giving supplemental platelets when the values for platelets go below 50,000 mm^3 or below 70,000 mm^3 if there are signs of unaccountable bleeding during surgical procedures. Autotransfusion is an excellent alternative to homologous transfusion, considering the risks associated with bank blood (e.g., type and crossing mismatches or transmission of infectious diseases). *Autotransfusion* blood has several advantages, including a higher oxygen-carrying capacity and elimination of incompatibilities and disease transmission. Use of micropore blood filters should be considered. Standard blood administration sets have 170 μm filters. Although these filters trap a notable share of cellular debris from blood transfusions, some of the materials will bypass these standard pore size filters and become lodged in the lungs. Micropore filters, with pore sizes of 20 to 40 μm, will filter out a greater portion of cellular debris. Although the literature is inconsistent on this issue, if massive transfusions are given, use of micropore filters probably provides some benefits.[29,30]

The MAST suits can be placed temporarily to improve cardiac and venous filling until fluid resuscitation is effective. Inflated MAST suits will compress the arterial inflow to the legs and effectively raise both the arterial resistance and blood pressure, measured in the arms.[15] Complications observed with the use of MAST suits include ischemia of the skin and superficial tissues, acidosis, hyperkalemia, ventilatory embarrassment from pressure on the abdomen, muscle damage, increased capillary permeability, coagulopathy, and elevated levels of thrombolytic products.[31]

☐ MECHANISM OF INJURY

Understanding the mechanism of injury is critical because it determines the pattern of injuries that can be anticipated from a given type of traumatic insult. Lack of understanding of these injury mechanisms can result in inadequate or inappropriate anesthesia care.

At the earliest feasible time in the assessment/intervention of the trauma patient, a careful history of the sequence of physical events leading to the traumatic injury should be obtained. This information may be obtained from a variety of sources, including the patient (if conscious and coherent), paramedics, other rescue workers, and eyewitnesses.

Blunt trauma is caused by high- or low-velocity impact from generally dull objects. Penetrating trauma usually results from the piercing of tissue by sharp objects such as stab wounds or projectiles like bullets. Mixed blunt and penetrating injuries can be seen in impalement injuries. Falls from substantial heights can cause vertical high-velocity injuries. Burns are caused by thermal, electrical, or chemical exposures. Airway burns and smoke inhalation injuries are often associated with carbon monoxide poisoning. Chemical, biologic, and nuclear injuries are other forms of trauma that have a known basis. Environmental injuries can be caused by such things as poisonous insect bites, animal bites, or snake venom.

CLASSIFICATIONS OF TRAUMA

Penetrating injuries can range from a simple pinprick to high-velocity projectiles. The extent of damage depends on three interactive factors[32]:

1. Type of wounding instrument—knife, missile, fragment
2. Velocity at time of impact
3. Characteristics of tissue through which it passes (e.g., bone, muscle, fat, vessels, nervous tissues, organs)

The crush component of penetrating injuries disrupts by fraying tissues as they are stretched to accommodate the wounding instrument (e.g., a car falling onto leg of individual working under it). The blunter the penetrating instrument, the greater the crushing.

If perforating trauma occurs, the amount of energy deposited in the tissues equals the difference between the amount of energy that a missile had before it entered the body and the energy it retains after it leaves the body. In penetrating trauma, all of the energy that the missile possesses at the time of impact is transferred to the body. Low- and high-velocity bullets differ in the amount and pattern of damage they create. Low-velocity bullets usually cut and crush tissues to form a "drill" hole known as a permanent cavity that approximates the same diameter as the missile. A high-velocity bullet creates a temporary cavity in addition to the permanent cavity. The temporary cavity forms in the wake of the high-velocity bullet that creates a shock wave with a series of rapid tissue expansions followed by collapse. This "cavitation effect" causes a stretching and tearing of tissues as far as 10 cm from the permanent cavity.

High-velocity bullets will "pulp" less elastic organs such

as the liver, spleen, kidney, brain, or heart due to the temporary cavity effect. More elastic tissues such as the lung, bowel, skin, and muscle will tend to sustain less damage from high-velocity missiles.

PENETRATING INJURIES TO SPECIFIC STRUCTURES

With *neck penetration injuries* large arteries and veins, nerves, and the vertebral column can be damaged from either direct impact or by the effects of cavitation. The airway can be damaged by either effect, as well. With *penetrating head injuries,* cavitation within the brain from a high-velocity missile can cause massive damage if not instant death. Transmitted energy from a tangential missile injury can cause skull fractures, brain contusions, or lacerations.

Penetration of the chest cavity can cause a variety of severe injuries. A high-velocity missile can shatter the heart causing instantaneous death. Low-velocity missiles may cause small holes in the heart that are usually repairable if tamponade or hemorrhage is not excessive. Major vessel penetration will frequently cause death unless tamponade is sufficient to contain the hemorrhagic state. Isolated lung injuries often can be treated by placement of a chest tube. Significant major airway or blood vessel damage may necessitate lobectomy. A high-velocity missile may rupture the diaphragm and cause damage to the upper abdominal organs from cavitation effect. Patients with a pneumothorax should have a chest tube placed before placement of an endotracheal tube (or immediately after tracheal intubation) to prevent the significant problems that can develop from progression of a tension pneumothorax as the result of positive-pressure ventilation.

Penetrating injuries to the abdomen by high-velocity bullets cause temporary cavitation and "pulps" the liver, spleen, and kidney. Low-velocity bullets generally produce less severe "drill hole" injuries unless blood vessels are directly hit.

An injury from a high-velocity missile can produce trauma of the entire extremity. Low-velocity missiles will cause "drill hole" injuries through muscle, bone, and subcutaneous tissues. The presence or absence of a pulse distal to an injury is not a reliable indicator of vascular integrity.

BLUNT TRAUMA

Direct impact, deceleration, continuous pressure, shearing forces, and rotary forces may all contribute to the end result of blunt trauma. These factors are associated with high levels of energy, such as may result from high-speed collisions and falls from marked heights. Newton's first law can explain most trauma: an object tends to remain in motion until affected by an outside force. Abrupt deceleration creates negative gravitational forces. As the human body decelerates, the internal organs continue forward at the original velocity. The organs that continue to move forward are torn from their attachments through rotary and shearing forces. These forces often cause disruption of connective tissue, blood vessels, and nerves.

MOTOR VEHICLE ACCIDENTS

The five types of motor vehicle accidents are classified as head-on, rear impact, side impact, rotational impact, or rollover. A complete understanding of the factors involved in a particular traumatic injury can allow health care providers to see the "complete picture" instead of being limited to seeing only the "second half" of an otherwise "mysterious" picture.

☐ ABDOMINAL TRAUMA

Use of diagnostic peritoneal catheter for lavage and analysis of the obtained fluid can help in the prevention of unnecessary exploratory laparotomy. The incidence of false-positive lavages is less than 2%.[33,34] This procedure can be done under local anesthesia with intravenous analgesia as appropriate. Peritoneal washings can be analyzed for the presence of red blood cells, white blood cells, amylase, bacteria, feces, or bile. Peritoneal lavage is unreliable in patients sustaining gunshot wounds of the lower chest and abdomen, where false-negative rates may reach 25%.[35,36] In stable trauma patients sustaining abdominal injuries, CT scans, magnetic resonance imaging, or angiographic studies may help in the diagnosis of specific injuries. Extremely unstable patients with abdominal trauma need immediate surgery.

Anesthetic problems with abdominal trauma include hemorrhage, hypothermia, sepsis, and interference with ventilation. Major hemorrhage is associated with fractures of solid organs, liver, spleen, and kidney, and with vascular injuries. The patient with significant abdominal trauma should have an indwelling arterial line to allow close monitoring of blood pressure as well as provide a route for sampling blood for blood gases, hematology, and chemistry. Placement of a central line facilitates CVP measurements for volume assessment and provides a route for drawing venous blood samples.

Hypothermia is a frequent complication of abdominal trauma surgery because of both increased heat loss through the open mesentery and reduced heat production as a consequence of shock and anesthesia. Warming all intravenous fluids with an efficient system and guarding against factors that tend to encourage heat loss are mandatory. Use of heat moisture exchangers in the airway circuit are beneficial in all trauma patients to prevent dry and cool gases from being delivered directly to the lungs.

☐ HEAD-INJURED PATIENTS

Head-injured patients will sustain initial damage from trauma that is beyond response to treatment. The goal of care is then to prevent secondary brain damage that results from intracranial complications that are aggravated by intracranial bleeding, edema, and resultant increased ICP. Common extracranial causes of death in the head-injured patient are hypoxia and shock. Anesthesia management of the head-injured patient should include early control of the airway, establishment of cardiovascular stability, and avoidance of intracranial hypertension. Baseline evaluation of the patient's Glascow coma score, pupillary reactivity, and motor function should be carefully documented prior to therapeutic maneuvers. Early oral endotracheal intubation with hyperventilation is helpful in reducing hypercarbia and hypoxemia and favors reduction of the ICP. Judicious use of induction agents and neuromuscular blocking agents can facilitate a straightforward intubation. Attempts to perform an awake intubation in an obtunded semicomatose patient may promote coughing, bucking, and thrashing about of the head-injured patient with concomitant increases in the ICP, which carries the risk of tentorial herniation. Nasal intubation is not recommended in the head-injured patient because of possible basilar skull fractures that can facilitate contamination and ultimate sepsis from nasal microorganisms introduced into the cranial vault. Late sepsis can also occur from a sinus infection caused by prolonged nasal tracheal intubation. Levine tubes are placed orally in head-injured patients for these same reasons.

Patients with a suspected open or closed head injury should be placed in a head-up position to help promote venous drainage and reduce ICP. Placement of an ICP measurement device may be indicated to monitor changes in ICP. In addition, hyperventilation to a $PaCO_2$ of 25 to 30 mm Hg will help reduce increased ICP. The Committee on Trauma Research has declared that "the most important topic to be addressed with regards to treatment of trauma patients is control of swelling of the brain; improvement could substantially reduce injury mortality." [37]

A judicious dose of thiopental usually is suitable in the preparation of the head-injured patient for intubation. Although succinylcholine has been traditionally used to facilitate intubation in these patients, data indicate succinylcholine may increase the ICP, especially if the ICP is already elevated. [38,39] When the use of succinylcholine is contraindicated, nondepolarizing neuromuscular blocking agents should be used because they do not cause rises in the ICP. The use of higher doses (0.28 mg/kg) of vecuronium will allow rapid intubation conditions (60 to 80 seconds) without potentiation of further rises in the ICP. [40] The newer steroidal structured nondepolarizing muscle relaxant rocuronium has an even faster onset than vecuronium. At a dose of 0.6 mg/kg, rocuronium can facilitate good to excellent intubation conditions in 60 seconds with a duration of approximately 30 minutes. [41] Using a higher dose of 1.2 mg/kg of rocuronium will allow good intubation conditions in 45 seconds with a duration of approximately 60 to 70 minutes. Rapid recovery from neuromuscular blockade allows early neurologic evaluation of the head-injured patient.

Patients with significant head injuries will benefit from the placement of an arterial line in addition to the standard monitoring, which should include capnography and pulse oximetry. The placement of an ICP monitoring device will facilitate the observation of changes in ICP dynamics in relation to drug administration and other manipulations that influence ICP. *Intracranial hypertension* exists when the ICP is at a sustained elevation above 15 mm Hg.

An anesthetic technique with fentanyl and a halogenated inhalation agent, following appropriate hyperventilation with oxygen, has been found satisfactory for management of the head-injured patient. The safety of isoflurane in maintaining autoregulation at 1.4% end-tidal concentration has been demonstrated. [42] Avoidance of nitrous oxide is recommended due to the aggravation of potential pneumocephalus and pneumothorax in the traumatized patient. Ketamine should be avoided in the head-injured patient to prevent increased ICP. Temporary reduction of the ICP can often be accomplished by small incremental doses of thiopental, hyperventilation, use of furosemide or mannitol for diuresis, and by elevation of the patient's head in relationship to the heart for beneficial gravitational influence. Etomidate has been advocated to control elevation of ICP. [43] No studies have been made to compare etomidate with barbiturates in situations in which ICP could not be controlled by the standard methods of hyperventilation, diuretics, and steroids. It has unfortunately been demonstrated that etomidate is a potent inhibitor of adrenal steroid production, which blocks the normal response to stress. [44] This effect may last for up to 4 hours after a single dose. [45] Even though no significant effects have been reported from single doses of etomidate, long-term use may be associated with increased mortality in patients with multiple trauma. [46] Until conclusive evidence of the safety of etomidate is established regarding the benefits gained versus the possible hazards, it would seem prudent to avoid its use in head-injured patients. [47] Propofol has been used in a small number of head-injured patients with promising results. [48,49] If evidence is found that propofol is able to control severe increases in ICP, it may become a satisfactory alternative to barbiturates in those situations.

☐ EVALUATION AND MANAGEMENT OF THE SPINAL CORD–INJURED PATIENT

More than 11,000 spinal cord injuries occur to individuals in the United States each year. Approximately 4200 of those injured die before they can be transported to a treatment facility and another 1150 die during hospitalization. The leading cause of death in spinal cord victims at the scene is aspiration pneumonia. The majority of injuries occur in young men in the second and third decades of life. The spinal cord injuries are usually sustained as a result of falls, motor vehicle accidents, diving injuries, penetrating missiles, and sport injuries. Few severe injuries have as devastating physical and psychological effects as those that can be caused by spinal cord injuries. Eventual outcome following acute spinal cord injury is basically dependent on three factors: (1) severity of the acute injury; (2) prevention of exacerbation of the injury during rescue, transport, and hospitalization; and (3) avoidance of hypoxia and systemic hypotension that can further compromise neural function.[50]

Cervical spinal cord injury should be assumed in any patient sustaining trauma to the head or face, in any unconscious trauma patient, and in any patient who complains of pain before or after careful palpation of the cervical spine. The anesthetist should be aware of the six conditions that are highly correlated with spinal cord injuries: paralysis, pain, position, parathesias, ptosis, and priapism.

If spinal cord injury is suspected, care should be taken to prevent further extension of the injury. A properly fitted cervical collar should be carefully placed before the patient is moved or extricated.

Precautions should be taken to prevent further extension of actual or potential neurologic deficits. Spinal immobilization should be completed before the patient is moved. The patient should be placed on a long spinal back board before movement.

All suspected spinal cord–injured patients must be assessed for adequacy of a patent airway. Care should be used to avoid extension, flexion, or rotation of the neck in attempting to open the airway. A gentle "chin lift" maneuver may be adequate to secure a patent airway without disturbing the neutral neck position. Oxygen by mask should be initiated immediately in the patient with a secured airway at the scene. Hypoxia and hypercarbia can further accentuate the extent of damage in spinal cord injuries. These injuries at the C-1 or C-2 level will result in complete respiratory paralysis. Death will ensue within a few minutes if artificial ventilation is not begun immediately.

If the spinal cord–injured patient arrives breathing spontaneously, the anesthetist needs to evaluate the adequacy of ventilation. If the patient is not able to protect the airway (due to being unconscious or semiconscious, absent or diminished gag reflex or cough, intraoral or facial injuries with significant edema or bleeding), rapid intubation will be needed. An adequate evaluation must include all seven cervical vertebrae because C-7 is the *most common* site of injury.[51] In the stable cooperative patient, awake nasal intubation is the method of choice.[52] The nasal intubation can be accomplished blindly with the use of an Endotrol® tube, which has a trigger device that allows the tip of the endotracheal tube to be positioned with relative ease. The tube can also be guided with use of a direct fiberoptic laryngoscope. Sedation may be accomplished by use of small doses of midazolam and fentanyl. Topical anesthesia can also be useful but transtracheal injection should be avoided when a full stomach is anticipated. In younger pediatric patients and uncooperative adults or in situations where awake intubation fails, a carefully selected dose of thiopental and a neuromuscular blocking agent are used to induce general anesthesia for the intubation.[53] These patients have the best chance of recovery if hypoxia, hypercarbia, and hypotension are avoided or rapidly corrected if encountered. ABG values indicating suboptimal ventilation should be corrected by intubation and mechanical ventilation.

USE OF MUSCLE RELAXANTS IN THE SPINAL CORD–INJURED PATIENT

Succinylcholine may precipitate *cardiac arrest* in patients who have sustained massive muscle injury or denervation, such as seen in patients sustaining spinal cord injuries, crush injuries of muscles, or burns.[54] The basis for this problem involves supersensitivity of the neuromuscular junction to the depolarizing effect of both acetylcholine and succinylcholine. This results in the release of large quantities of potassium during contraction of muscles. Normal depolarization results in a small potassium flux across the muscle cell membrane. *If a muscle is crushed, burned, or denervated, acetylcholine receptors proliferate around the injured cell, so that when the muscle is depolarized the flux of potassium is increased 33 to 34 times.*[55] The problem in response to succinylcholine is thought to develop about *5 to 15 days* after the injury. Succinylcholine is not recommended for intubation of the acute spinal cord–injured patient because muscle fasciculation may exacerbate the cord injury.[47] A conservative approach to caring for spinal cord-injured patients would be to avoid succinylcholine by using nondepolarizing muscle relaxants that do not cause these problems. The inadvertent use of succinylcholine in patients susceptible to hyperkalemia can be managed with intravenous calcium, glucose, and insulin in conjunction with CPR.[18] CPR should be continued to support the circulation until the serum potassium falls to normal levels consistent with normal cardiac function.

SPINAL SHOCK

A triad of hypotension, bradycardia, and hypothermia frequently results from a relative *sympathectomy* in spinal cord–injured patients. The spinal shock is progressively intensified as the segment of injury is progressively more cephalad at the involved level. Injury at the T-6 level or higher will severely impair CNS function. Sympathetically medicated cardioaccelerator responses will no longer oppose vagal innervation so that the heart rate will frequently slow dramatically. Loss of sympathetic tone allows vasodilation, pooling of the peripheral circulation, and decreased venous return to the heart. This results in a decreased cardiac output and hypotension. The spinal cord injury also interrupts sympathetic pathways from the hypothalamus (temperature control center) to peripheral blood vessels. The spinal shock patient is unable to constrict vessels or shiver to produce heat or to dilate vessels to dissipate heat. The patient's body temperature has a tendency to migrate toward the environmental level.

Treatment of Spinal Shock The patient in spinal shock will be hypotensive and bradycardic with warm pink extremities. In contrast, patients with hemorrhagic shock tend to be hypotensive and tachycardic with cold clammy skin. To properly care for spinal cord–injured patients (especially with high cervical lesions) invasive monitoring is critical to conduct fluid resuscitation and appropriate vasoactive drug intervention. An indwelling arterial catheter is mandatory in managing the acute phase of spinal shock. In addition, ABG assessments will be facilitated by an indwelling arterial catheter. In these patients, it is preferable to use the femoral or pedal artery rather than the radial artery. Paraplegic patients will be at a severe disadvantage if they lose use of either hand due to ischemic injuries that can occur as an aftermath of an indwelling radial, brachial, or axillary artery catheter.

A pulmonary artery catheter is helpful in managing fluid and drug therapy. It allows for measurement of the cardiac output and derived hemodynamic variables that are needed for proper therapy. Patients can readily develop pulmonary edema if their fluids and vasoactive drug therapy are not guided by the variables derived from use of a pulmonary artery.

A general principle in any therapeutic protocol must be aimed at preventing the worsening of neurologic status following acute spinal cord injury. In severe spinal cord injuries, electrical conduction through the injured cord segment ceases due to direct tissue disruption from the trauma as well as from the secondary concussion effect. Vasomotor reactivity of the injured cord is lost, leading to changes in the spinal cord flow. These local injury changes in the microcirculation may be compounded by cardiovascular instability secondary to the trauma itself. To maintain adequate arterial blood pressure and cord perfusion, pressor therapy is usually initiated. Dopamine is titrated to obtain a positive inotropic effect at a low-dose β range and to improve vascular tone if given in higher α-adrenergic doses. Generally dopamine is started in the 4 to 5 μg/kg/min range.

OTHER CONSIDERATIONS

Patients with spinal cord injury should be extubated as soon as possible after spinal stabilization surgery. If the patient requires intubation due to associated pulmonary injuries or dysfunction, then a weaning program is started as soon as tolerated by the patient. With frequent assessment, this is usually done within the first few days. Useful guidelines for assessing adequacy of spontaneous ventilation include measurement of the tidal volume ($>$ 5 mL/kg), negative inspiratory force (minus 20 to 25 cm H_2O pressure — needed for adequate cough), and vital capacity ($>$ 15 mg/kg). Patients with high spinal cord injury often lose innervation of the intercostal and abdominal musculature.

Therefore, continued assessment of adequate diaphragmatic innervation, needed to generate adequate ventilation, will be mandatory. Some patients will require tracheostomies. Oral or nasogastric tubes are placed to decompress the stomach. This facilitates diaphragmatic excursion for improved ventilation and reduces the risk of aspiration. Peptic ulceration in the high spinal cord–injured patient with loss of sympathetic innervation is a well described complication especially in patients receiving steroids. Therefore, gastric pH is

controlled early in the hospitalization by use of antacids and H_2 blockers such as cimetidine or ranitidine.

SURGICAL INTERVENTION AND ANESTHESIA APPROACH

The neurosurgeon and anesthesia team should document the current neurologic status and note any deficits before the start of anesthesia and intubation. When performing an awake intubation, the patient should be assessed prior to and following endotracheal tube placement and after the patient is positioned for surgery.

Whether an anterior or posterior surgical approach is used in cervical injury depends on the nature of the injury. Internal fixation devices are frequently placed in the acute phase to stabilize lower cord injuries. At times, these procedures can be associated with significant surgical blood loss.

In patients who are deferred for elective spinal stabilization procedures, awake nasal intubations are performed. In controlled conditions, this allows use of local, topical, and transtracheal anesthesia without the concern of pulmonary aspiration that is present in emergency procedures.

Anesthetic techniques that avoid hypotension and provide good cardiovascular stability are recommended. Generally baseline analgesia is provided with a narcotic (fentanyl or sufentanil). Muscle relaxation is provided with a nondepolarizing neuromuscular blocking agent such as vecuronium or rocuronium to promote cardiovascular stability. Nitrous oxide should be avoided because many of these patients may have a known or unknown head injury or possible pneumothorax. Ketamine can be useful as an induction agent in unstable patients, but it is contraindicated if there is any question of a head-associated injury because it increases the ICP. A low concentration of isoflurane is useful to supplement anesthesia and provide amnesia. Isoflurane in low concentrations has minimal cardiovascular depressant effects.

Anesthetic Management Shock trauma patients arriving in the admitting area are frequently unable to provide reliable information about their past medical history. The anesthetist may have no knowledge of the patient's possible allergies or previous response to anesthesia. Moreover, 30% to 50% of trauma patients are intoxicated, usually with alcohol and sometimes with illicit "street drugs." These substances may alter a patient's response to drugs administered during anesthesia; postoperative hallucinations or delayed recovery from anesthesia may occur. In shock trauma patients, maintenance of cardiovascular stability is the major criterion in formulating a safe plan for anesthesia management.

Non nitrous oxide techniques are often preferable in trauma patients due to many problems that can occur if nitrous oxide is used. Because of its affinity for diffusing into closed spaces, nitrous oxide is contraindicated if a pneumothorax, a closed head injury with possible pneumocephalus, or a bowel injury is probable. Isoflurane has an ideal cardiovascular profile because it reduces systemic vascular resistance before causing significant cardiac depression. Although isoflurane provides good amnesia in lower doses, it also can be used to control hypertensive responses that frequently occur in otherwise young, healthy trauma patients after fluid resuscitation is accomplished. Anesthesia can be maintained with isoflurane and a mixture of oxygen and air to achieve an appropriate FIO_2 concentration. Vecuronium and rocuronium are two steroidal muscle relaxants that are useful during the induction and maintenance of anesthesia in the trauma patient. Both can be used as a bolus or an infusion. Neither drug tends to promote histamine release often associated with the benzoisoquinolinium muscle relaxants. Rocuronium has the advantage over vecuronium in that it has a faster onset and shorter duration of action. A mild mean heart rate increase from 82 to 94 has been observed in children following the use of rocuronium.[56] In contrast, in a recent study, the heart rate increase in adults following rocuronium was small (7% to 8%) compared to succinylcholine (10% to 15%).[57]

During the preoperative phase, midazolam in small doses is helpful during insertion of invasive monitoring lines to provide consistent amnesia. A narcotic such as fentanyl or sufentanil can be used to supplement the induction and maintenance of anesthesia. The use of standard doses of thiopental in stable patients and reduced doses in unstable trauma patients is useful as an induction agent. Thiopental is useful in patients with brain injuries because it tends to reduce cerebral metabolic rate, ICP, and cerebral blood flow. Ketamine should be avoided in any patient with suspected head injury to avoid the risk of ICP. Propofol and etomidate have limited value in the acute anesthetic management of trauma patients.

Depolarizing Neuromuscular Blocking Agent

For years succinylcholine has been considered the agent of choice for rapid endotracheal intubation; however, it is not the ideal blocking agent for shock trauma patients because it increases intracranial, intraocular, and intragastric pressures. Additionally, succinylcholine can cause rises in serum potassium to dangerous levels, with resultant cardiac arrest in certain patients who have sustained burns, massive trauma, spinal cord lesions, and paraplegia, and in specific neurologic diseases. Hyperkalemia caused by succinylcholine is thought to start occurring approximately 24 to 48 hours after the time of injury. Pretreatment with a nondepolarizing neuromuscular blocking agent does not stop the hyperkalemia response.

Nondepolarizing Neuromuscular Blocking Agents

The ideal nondepolarizing neuromuscular blocking agent for the severely injured frequently unstable trauma patient should have several characteristics. Primarily, it should have a high specificity of action; that is, it should provide prompt neuromuscular block with minimal or no side effects. It should not cause nontherapeutic cardiovascular conditions such as hypotension, hypertension, tachycardia, bradycardia, or cardiac dysrhythmias. Because many trauma patients are obtunded or inebriated, it is often impossible to obtain a history of past medical conditions, response to previous anesthesia, or allergies. For this reason, the ideal agent should not promote histamine release that could cause hypotension in the hypovolemic trauma patient or bronchospasm in the atopic or asthmatic patient. It should have a rapid onset and it should be capable of pharmacologic reversal in a relatively short time span. Finally, it should not possess the known detrimental side effects of succinylcholine.

Pancuronium is a longer-acting nondepolarizing neuromuscular blocking agent that unfortunately may cause undesirable cardiovascular stimulation resulting in tachycardia and hypertension. These cardiovascular alterations can be confused with hemodynamic instability, hypovolemia, and inadequate analgesia. Pipecuronium and doxacurium are generally more suited for patients requiring long periods of neuromuscular blockade.

High-dose vecuronium (250 to 300 μg/kg) allows rapid endotracheal intubation in shock trauma patients and avoids the many problems associated with succinylcholine. In contrast to pancuronium, which often causes tachycardia, high-dose vecuronium produces no clinically significant hemodynamic alterations.

Atracurium generally has not been suitable for rapid endotracheal intubation because rapid injection of recommended doses or administration of high doses often causes clinically significant histamine release and hypotension.

Rocuronium (ORG-9426) is a new, short-acting, steroidal nondepolarizing neuromuscular blocking agent that has a faster onset of action than other currently available agent in its class.[59] Rocuronium has pharmacologic properties and a safety profile that are similar to vecuronium. Specifically, rocuronium has minimal potential for clinically significant adverse hemodynamic effects or release of histamine. A major advantage of rocuronium over vecuronium is a significantly more rapid onset when compared at equipotent doses. One of the most remarkable features of rocuronium is the brief time it requires to cause detectable twitch depression or "lag time."[60] This effect may be augmented by rocuronium's relatively low plasma binding that allows three times greater free plasma concentration compared to vecuronium.[61]

In many anesthesia situations involving the trauma patient, the speed of drug onset can be critical. A technique known as facilitation can enhance the onset time of drugs significantly. For example, by injecting 10 mL of intravenous fluid as a flush following the injection of a muscle relaxant, approximately 15 seconds can be saved on the onset time.

Cisatracurium is a new nondepolarizing neuromuscular relaxant that is a curariform drug without the side effects of histamine release seen with most other drugs in this class. Cisatracurium appears to be a good choice for longer trauma procedures and in the management of ventilatory-dependent patients. Its cardiovascular profile is similar to that of vecuronium. Because it has the Hoffmanns pathway of elimination, it appears that this will be a useful drug in the management of patients with significant renal or hepatic dysfunction.

Postoperative Analgesia

Shock trauma patients frequently experience severe postoperative pain. Intravenous narcotics such as fentanyl and sufentanil are often helpful to alleviate that pain. Patient-controlled analgesia systems can also maintain a stable level of pain relief. Alternatively, morphine can be administered via continuous epidural catheters. Continuous intercostal catheter techniques can be used to inject local anesthetic agents in patients with chest injuries.

Extubation   Patients should be extubated only after they have demonstrated that they are awake and alert, have an adequate tidal volume, vital capacity, and minute volume, and are able to cough effectively (i.e., negative inspiratory force of 25 cm H_2O). Patients with long bone fractures resulting from high-energy blunt trauma are less likely to develop the fat embolism syndrome if they are maintained on mechanical ventilation for several hours postoperatively. Finally, patients who have sustained multiple traumatic injuries, especially of the abdomen and chest, usually have an improved postoperative course if they are maintained on mechanical ventilation for one or more days.

☐ AUTONOMIC HYPERREFLEXIA (MASS REFLEX)

Trauma centers frequently deal with post acute trauma patients during the initial hospitalization or for future related surgery. In this post acute setting, the anesthesia plan needs to address certain implications of autonomic hyperreflexia. Hyperreflexia is seen in 85% of spinal cord–injured patients with lesions above T-5. The incidence is progressively less if the lesion level is lower than T-5. Signs and symptoms of this condition can include paroxysmal hypertension, bradycardia, dysrhythmias, cutaneous vasodilation below, and vasoconstriction above the level of injury, severe headaches, seizures, and loss of consciousness. Hyperreflexia is not observed until after the spinal shock phase has passed. It is therefore usually seen when patients return to surgery for procedures like cystoscopy that are done later in their recovery phase. The condition is caused by stimulation below the level of the lesion. It is typically precipitated by distension of the bladder or rectum caused by bladder distension, defecation, childbirth, and even cutaneous stimulation. It can occur intraoperatively with local, spinal and nitrous oxide narcotic general anesthesia. No episodes have been reported with the use of potent inhalation anesthetics. Bradycardia should be treated with atropine or glycopyrrolate.

☐ SUBSTANCE ABUSE/OVERDOSE

Ethanol is the most common intoxicating substance seen in trauma patients. Trauma patients are often under the influence of illicit drugs or ethanol at the time of their injury. Illicitly used drugs can include cocaine, heroin, amphetamines, narcotics, barbiturates, benzodiazepines, lyseric acid diethylamide (LSD), and cannabis (marijuana and hashish). Stress,

Table 30–6
ANESTHESIA PROBLEMS IN SUBSTANCE ABUSERS

Sclerosis of peripheral and deep veins in IV drug abusers
Acute disturbances caused by drugs taken prior to injuries
Occurrence of cardiovascular stimulation with amphetamines and LSD
Acute and chronic medical problems secondary to drug abuse
Pharmacokinetics of digitalis, warfarin, and phenytoin are altered in the drug addict

fatigue, and hemorrhage in addition to trauma and subsequent surgery may modify these responses when ethanol and illicit drugs are present (Tables 30–6 and 30–7). Trauma centers routinely measure ethanol and drug levels, but often these measurements are not available until after the induction of anesthesia.

Several potential anesthetic problems are related to acute ethanol intoxication or drug abuse.

☐ ORGAN HARVESTING FROM BRAIN DEAD PATIENTS FOR TRANSPLANTATION

A consolation to the tragedy of death in the trauma patient can be the donation of organs that can be transplanted to other individuals to improve and extend their lives. Trauma patients who were previously healthy and who sustain isolated brain death are ideal candidates for organ donation. Protocols are established to guide the organ harvesting procedure. Relative contraindications to organ harvesting may be somewhat variable. Generally absolute contraindications will include advanced age, septicemia, many malignancies, and transmissible diseases that are not readily amenable to treatment with antibiotics. A wide surgical incision midline

Table 30–7
EFFECTS OF SPECIFIC ABUSED DRUGS

Narcotics: mood changes, dysphoria, nausea and vomiting, repiratory depression, apnea, miosis, convulsions, hypotension, syncope, pulmonary edema, hypothermia
Barbiturates and benzodiazepines: somnolence, respiratory depression, hypotension, hypothermia
Amphetamines: anxiety, psychosis, hyperreflexia, hypertension, tachycardia, dysrhythmias, palpitations, sweating, hyperthermia, acidosis, ketoacidosis
Cocaine: dysphoria, agitation paranoia, delirium, tremors, seizures, hypertension, dysrhythmias causing sudden death, hyperpyrexia, nausea and vomiting, respiratory arrest
LSD: hallucinations, tremor, hyperreflexia, convulsions, respiratory arrest, hypertension, tachycardia, increased temperature
Cannabis (marijuana and hashish): somnolence, tachycardia, orthostatic hypotension

from the sternal notch to the pubis is generally done because several organs may be harvested. The estimated blood loss is approximately 1000 mL, and blood transfusions for the donor may be required.

As part of the preoperative preparation, hemoglobin and hematocrit, coagulation profile, and serum electrolytes are obtained. Confirmation of brain death is done by a physician other than the transplant surgeon. Because the criteria for brain death vary depending on the state, region, hospital, and other factors, a neurologist confirms the diagnosis of brain death. Guidelines for making the diagnosis of brain death generally include several of the following criteria:

Complete lack of response to stimuli, loss of gag reflex, corneal reflex, and pupillary reflex

Cause of death not related to toxic-metabolic causes or hypothermia

Electroencephalogram and brain stem auditory evoked potential consistent with brain death

Because spinal reflexes may remain intact, neuromuscular blocking agents are used to prevent reflex body movements. Brain death donors are nonresponsive, so no anesthetic agents are needed. To maintain adequate perfusion pressures for maximal preservation of organs, it is helpful to place an indwelling arterial line and a central venous line. Donors should always have endotracheal intubation performed to prevent aspiration and to facilitate mechanical ventilation before and during the harvesting procedure. The anesthetists should determine from the surgeon which organs are being harvested and the estimated time of the procedures. The surgical time is generally between 2 and 4 hours. Dopamine is often used to maintain adequate perfusion, but because it may cause depletion of norepinephrine stores in the donor heart, the surgeon should be consulted about its potential use. Heparin is generally administered prior to the harvesting of the heart. Hemodynamic instability and coagulopathies may develop within 24 to 48 hours after brain death.

☐ BURN INJURIES

Burn injuries may be due to heat, chemical exposure, radiation, or electricity. Burns are classified according to the depth and extent of tissue damage. Three categories are used to categorize the tissue damage. First-degree (superficial) burns consist of destruction of the epidermis tissues that causes pain and erythema and is represented by an intense sunburn. Second-degree (partial thickness) burns cause both epidermal and dermal destruction, but the basement membrane remains intact and the architectural integrity of the skin is preserved. Second-degree burns are characterized by vesicle formation and pain. A third-degree (full thickness) burn results in destruction of all of the layers of the skin, including the epidermis, dermis, and the dermal appendages. Third-degree burns

Table 30–8
RULE OF NINES*

Head and neck—9%
Upper extremities—9% each
Chest (ant. & post.)—9% each
Abdomen—9%
Lower back—9%
Lower extremities—18% each
Perineum—1%

*Modified in children due to head and neck being proportionally larger than in adults.

extend into the subcutaneous fat, will not heal spontaneously, and require skin grafting. Coagulation and deep-vein thrombosis may occur in third-degree burns. Third-degree burns will develop a leather-like eschar that is not associated with pain due to destruction of nerve endings.

The quantification of burn area is usually expressed as a percentage and can be calculated by the "rule of nines" in adults (Table 30–8) with some modification in children (see Chap. 25, section on pediatric burns).

The major cause of early death in burns is asphyxia and the major cause of late mortality is septic complications. Several prominent pathophysiologic changes occur during the acute and subacute phases of thermal injury. The capillary beds in the burn area are damaged or destroyed so that leakage of protein-rich fluid occurs with sequestration in the interstitial spaces. This loss of fluid results in hemoconcentration and hypovolemia. There is an increased release of antidiuretic hormone that causes renal conservation with a resultant drop in the urinary output. Alterations in the permeability of vascular beds may also occur distal to the area of burn injury. This can lead to increased permeability in the vascular beds of the lungs that can lead to severe, potentially fatal pulmonary edema.

Inhalation injuries should be assumed to occur if the burn patient displays signs of respiratory distress or gives a history of sustaining burns in a closed space. Signs of possible inhalation injury include burns to the face and neck, perioral soot, carbonaceous sputum, and respiratory distress. The presence of stridor, dyspnea, and wheezing warrants close examination of the airway. Because the pharynx and upper trachea have a large capacity for cooling gases, direct thermal injury below the cords is rare except for steam exposure. Because the thermal capacity of water is 4000 times that of air, steam injuries cause significantly greater damage and can reach structures deep into the tracheobronchial tree.

Potential airway problems present in burn patients as in multiple trauma patients. Glottic edema usually does not present an immediate problem but may become severe several hours after the burn is sustained. Patients displaying signs of respiratory depression with carbon dioxide retention are considered to be strong candidates for prompt tracheal intubation. Careful monitoring of the burn patient is needed to assess the adequacy of resuscitation.

Table 30–9
PARKLAND FORMULA

Initial 24 h
4 mL/kg/% total body surface area (TBSA) burned
Composition: isotonic crystalloid, e.g., Ringer's lactate, normal saline)
Infuse $\frac{1}{2}$ calculated amount over first 8 h with $\frac{1}{4}$ each next 8 h
Maintain urine output at 0.5–1 mg/kg/h
Second 24 h
D_5W to maintain urinary output (adults); in children, add $\frac{1}{2}$ normal saline to avoid hyponatremia
Colloid solutions, e.g., albumin proportional to burn—generally 0.3–0.5 mL of 5% albumin solution/kg/percentage of TBSA burned (see below)
30–50% burn: 0.3 mL/kg/% burn
50–70% burn: 0.4 mL/kg/% burn
>70% burn: 0.5 mL/kg/% burn

FLUID RESUSCITATION

Massive capillary leakage is one of the earliest pathophysiologic changes seen in burned skin. This allows the loss of fluid from the intravascular space to the extracellular space. A variety of fluid replacement formulae have been developed for management of the burn patient. The Parkland Hospital Formula (Table 30–9) and close variations are frequently used to guide fluid replacement. Each case requires careful evaluation of fluid replacement and adjustments to clinical and laboratory parameters.

PREOPERATIVE EVALUATION OF THE BURN PATIENT

The burn patient is evaluated like other patients for signs of significant disturbances to the cardiac, pulmonary, hepatic, and renal systems. Additionally, a number of other factors need to be considered in the anesthetic management of the burn patient.

ANESTHETIC MANAGEMENT OF THE BURN PATIENT

Providing anesthesia for the burn patient requires careful planning for and meticulous administration of anesthesia. The burn patient's care can be complicated by multiple trauma injuries that were sustained with the burn injuries (Table 30–10).

☐ CONCLUSION

Trauma care is a critical area in modern anesthesia practice. Organization of trauma care in the United States has substan-

Table 30–10
ANESTHETIC MANAGEMENT FOR THE BURN PATIENT

Anesthesia drugs and techniques—should provide adequate sedation, analgesia, amnesia, lack of movement, and hemodynamic stability
Succinylcholine—should be strictly avoided in the burn patient after the initial 24 h following injury to avoid severe hyperkalemic responses; rapid-acting nondepolarizing neuromuscular blocking agents can be used to secure the airway, e.g., rocuronium in a 1 mg/kg dose will allow for rapid sequence intubation in approximately 45 s
High-dose opioid techniques—generally provide substantial analgesia and good cardiovascular stability; midazolam helps provide sedation and amnesia; N_2O with minimal concentrations of potent inhalation agents may be useful to supplement the opioid technique
Propofol—can be especially useful in short procedures in the stable burn patient who needs to undergo frequent debridements, minor skin grafting, and other short procedures; the wake-up tends to be quicker and more pleasant and nausea and vomiting appears less likely than when sodium pentothal is used
Ketamine—can be useful in the hemodynamically unstable patient who needs short and repeated procedures; midazolam helps reduce the psychomimetic effects of ketamine

tially improved survival and quality of outcome for traumatically injured patients. The role of the anesthetist should begin as soon as the patient reaches the trauma facility. The major concern is to evaluate the patient's airway and maintain ventilation until endotracheal intubation can be performed. The principles for successful management of the trauma patient are based on organization and preparation, assessment of the patient's injuries, proper priority for therapeutic interventions, achievement and maintenance of a patent airway, fluid resuscitation, application of appropriate continuous invasive and noninvasive monitoring, correction of acid–base and electrolyte disturbances and careful titration of anesthetic and adjunctive agents. The degree of functional outcome of trauma patients is largely dependent on the early involvement of sound principles of anesthesia care in the resuscitation and overall anesthetic management during the perioperative period. In a well managed team approach, assessment and treatment are carried out in rapid succession or even simultaneously.

There are various ways to achieve the goals of anesthesia care for the trauma patient, but the importance of providing the highest level of care by anesthesia providers is imperative. Most anesthetists work outside major trauma facilities; however, life-threatening traumatic-injured patients may arrive at a general hospital's emergency department at any time. Anesthetists at those facilities must have an adequate knowledge base to manage these compromised patients effectively.

REFERENCES

1. Booij LH. Pitfalls in anaesthesia for multiply injured patients. *Injury.* 1982; 14:81.
2. Gann DS, Lilly MP. The neuroendocrine response to multiple trauma. *World J Surg.* 1983; 7:101.
3. Tenzer ML. The spectrum of myocardial contusion: a review. *J Trauma.* 1985; 25:620.
4. Grande CM, Barton CR, Stene JK. Appropriate techniques for airway management of emergency patients with suspected spinal cord injury. *Anesth Analg.* 1988; 67:714.
5. Markison RE, Trunkey DD. Establishment of care priorities. In: Capan LM, Miller SM, Turndorf H., eds. *Trauma Anesthesia and Intensive Care.* Philadelphia: JB Lippincott; 1991:30.
6. Marzella LL, Trump BF. Cell injury and its meaning in shock and resuscitation. In: Siegel JH, ed. *Trauma: Emergency Surgery and Critical Care.* New York: Churchill Livingstone; 1987:35–36.
7. Gann DS, Amaral JF. Pathophysiology of trauma and shock. In: Zuidema GD, Rutherford RB, Ballinger WF, eds. *The Management of Trauma.* 4th ed. Philadelphia: WB Saunders; 1985:37–103.
8. Beisel WR. Humoral mediators of cellular response and altered metabolism. In: Siegel JH, ed. *Trauma: Emergency Surgery and Critical Care.* New York: Churchill Livingstone; 1987:57–78.
9. Baertschi AJ, Ward DG, Gann DS. Role of atrial receptors in the control of ACTH. *Am J Physiol.* 1976; 231:692.
10. Gann DS, Cryer GL, Pirkle JC. Physiological inhibition and facilitation of adrenocortical response to hemorrhage. *Am J Physiol.* 1977; 232:R5.
11. Reid IA, Ganon WF. Control of aldosterone secretion. In: Genest J, Koiw E, Kuchel O, eds. *Hypertension.* New York: McGraw-Hill; 1977:265.
12. Cochrane JP, Forsling ML, Gow NM. Arginine vasopressin following surgical operations. *Br J Surg.* 1981; 68:209.
13. Pflug AE, Halter JB. Effect of spinal anesthesia on adrenergic tone and the neuroendocrine response to surgical stress in humans. *Anesthesiology.* 1981; 55:120.
14. Trunkey DD. Trauma. *Sci Am.* 1983; 249(2):28–35.
15. Stene JK, Grande CM, Giesecke A. Shock resuscitation. In: Stene JK, Grande CM, eds. *Trauma Anesthesia.* Baltimore: Williams & Wilkins; 1991.
16. Sellick BA. Cricoid pressure to control regurgitation of stomach contents during induction of anaesthesia. *Lancet.* 1961; 2:404–406.
17. Lawes EG, Campbell I, Mercer D. Inflation pressure, gastric insufflation and rapid sequence induction. *Br J Anaesth.* 1987; 59:315–318.
18. Stene JK. Anesthesia for trauma. In: Miller RD, ed. *Anesthesia.* 3rd ed. New York: Churchill Livingstone; 1990:1991–1999.
19. Capan LM, Gottlieb G, Rosenberg A. General principles of anesthesia for major acute trauma. In: Capan LM, Miller SM, Turndorf H, eds. *Trauma Anesthesia and Intensive Care.* Philadelphia: JB Lippincott; 1991:264.
20. Le Dran HG. A treatise, or reflections drawn from practice on gunshot wounds. London: Clark; 1743.
21. Morris EA. A practical treatise on shock after operations and injuries. London: Hardwicke; 1867.
22. Altura BM, Lefer AM, Schumer W. Historical perspective of shock. In: Altura BM, Befer AM, Schumer W, eds. *Handbook of Shock and Trauma.* New York: Raven Press; 1983:1–2.
23. American Heart Association. Guidelines for cardiopulmonary resuscitation and emergency cardiac care. III: adult advances cardiac life support. *JAMA.* 1992; 268:2199–2241.
24. Safar P. *Cardiopulmonary Cerebral Resuscitation.* Stavanger, Norway: Laerdal; 1981:95. (Distributed by WB Saunders, Philadelphia.)
25. Guyton AC, Hall JE. Circulatory shock and physiology of its treatment. In: Guyton AC, ed. *Textbook of Medical Physiology,* 9th ed. Philadelphia: WB Saunders; 1996:285–293.
26. Kliegman RM, Fanaroff AA. Developmental metabolism and nutrition. In: Gregory GA, ed. *Pediatric Anesthesia.* New York: Churchill Livingstone; 1983; 1:169–251.
27. Pulsinelli WA, Waldman S, Rawlinson D, Plum F, et al. Moderate hyperglycemia augments ischemic brain damage: a neuropathologic study in the rat. *Neurology* 1982; 32:1239–1246.
28. Coursin DB, Cicala RS. Perioperative care of the trauma patient. In: Barash PG, ed. *Refresher Courses in Anesthesiology.* Philadelphia: JB Lippincott, 1992; 20:40.
29. Reul GJ, Greenberg SD, Lefrak EA. Prevention of post-traumatic pulmonary insufficiency with fine screen filtration of blood. *Arch Surg.* 1973; 106:386.
30. Grindlinger GA, Vegas AM, Churchill WH. Is respiratory failure a consequence of blood transfusion? *J Trauma.* 1980; 20:627.
31. Schwab CW, Gore D. MAST: medical antishock trousers. In: Nyhus L, ed. *Surgery Annual.* East Norwalk, Conn. Appleton-Century-Crofts; 1983; 15:41–59.
32. Grande CM. Mechanisms and patterns of injury: the key to anticipation in trauma management. In: *Critical Care Clinics: Trauma Anesthesia and Critical Care.* Philadelphia: WB Saunders; 1990; 6:25–35.
33. Pachter HL, Hofstetter SR. Open and percutaneous paracentesis and lavage for abdominal trauma: a randomized prospective study. *Arch Surg.* 1981; 116:318.
34. Parham AM, Smith DE, Asher WM. Effectiveness of peritoneal lavage in blunt abdominal trauma. *Ann Surg.* 1975; 181:255.
35. Thal ER, May RA, Beesinger D. Peritoneal lavage: its unreliability in gunshot wounds of the lower chest and abdomen. *Arch Surg.* 1980; 115:430.
36. Cox EF, Siegel JH. Blunt trauma to the abdomen. In: Siegel J, ed. *Trauma: Emergency Surgery and Critical Care.* New York: Churchill Livingstone; 1987:883.
37. Committee on Trauma Research. Injury in America: A continuing public health problem. Washington, DC: National Academy Press; 1985.
38. Lanier WL, Iaizzo PA, Midle JH. Cerebral function and muscle afferent activity following intravenous succinylcholine in dogs anesthetized with halothane: the effects of pretreatment with a defasciculating dose of pancuronium. *Anesthesiology.* 1989; 71:87–95.
39. Lanier WL, Midle JH, Michenfelder JD. Cerebral stimulation following succinylcholine in dogs. *Anesthesiology.* 1986; 64:551–559.
40. Stene JK, Barton CR, Grande CM, Bowman-Bell N, Burns B. Time course of relaxation from high-dose (0.28 mg/kg) vecuronium. 9th World Congress of Anaesthesiologists, Washington, DC: 1988. (Abstract).
41. Bartkowski RR, Witkowski TA, Azad S, Lessin J. Rocuronium onset of action: a comparison with atracurium and vecuronium. *Anesth Analg.* 1993; 77:574–578.
42. McPherson RW, Traystman RJ. Effects of isoflurane on cerebral autoregulation. *Anesthesiology.* 1987; 67(suppl 3A):A576.
43. Dearden NM, McDowall DG. Comparison of etomidate and althesin in the reduction of increased intracranial pressure after head injury. *Br J Anaesth.* 1985; 57:361.
44. Wagner RL, White PF. Etomidate inhibits adrenocortical function in surgical patients. *Anesthesiology.* 1984; 61:647.

45. Fragen RJ, Shanks CA, Molteni A. Effects of etomidate on hormonal responses to surgical stress. *Anesthesiology.* 1984; 61: 652.

46. Ledingham I McA, Watt I. Influence of sedation on mortality in critically ill multiple trauma patients. *Lancet.* 1983; 1:1270.

47. Miller SM. Management of central nervous system injuries. In: Capan LM, Miller SM, Turndorf H, eds. *Trauma Anesthesia and Intensive Care.* Philadelphia: JB Lippincott; 1991.

48. Wright PJ, Murray RJ. Penetrating cerebral airgun injury. *Anaesthesia.* 1989; 44:219.

49. Farling PA, Johnston IR, Coppel DL. Propofol infusion for sedation of patients with head injury in intensive care. *Anaesthesia.* 1989; 44:222.

50. Kopaniky DR. Pathophysiology and management of spinal cord trauma. In: Frost E, ed. *Clinical Anesthesia in Neurosurgery.* 2nd ed. Boston: Butterworth-Heinemann; 1991.

51. Parks RE, Livoni JP. Detection of cervical spine injury in the multi-trauma patient. In: Blaisdell FW, Trunkey DD, eds. *Trauma Management III: Cervical Thoracic Trauma.* New York: Theime; 1986:56.

52. Fraser A, Edmonds-Seal J. Spinal cord injuries: a review of problems facing the anaesthetist. *Anaesthesia.* 1982; 37:1084.

53. Grande CM, Barton CR, Stenes JK. Emergency airway management in trauma patients with a suspected cervical spine injury: in response. *Anesth Analg.* 1989; 68:416–418.

54. Gronert GA, Theye RA. Pathophysiology of hyperkalemia induced by succinylcholine. *Anesthesiology.* 1975; 43:89.

55. Sommer RM, Bauer RD, Errico TJ. Cervical spine injuries. In: Capan LM, Miller SM, Turndorf H, eds. *Trauma Anesthesia and Intensive Care.* Philadelphia: JB Lippincott; 1991: 447–480.

56. Vuksanaj D. Pharmacokinetics and pharacodynamics of intubating doses of ORG 9426 (rocuronium) in children. *Anesthesiology.* 1995; 82(5):1104–1110.

57. Robertson EN, Hull JM, Vanlinthout LEH, Booij LHDJ. Pharmacodynamics of rocuronium and succinylcholine and their effects on BP, HR, and IOP. *Anesthesiology.* 1994;81:A1071.

☐ QUESTIONS

1. Which one of the following is a false statement? Spinal cord injured patients have the best chance of recovery if:
   a. Hypoxia is avoided
   b. Hypercarbia is avoided
   c. Rapid fluid expansion is accomplished
   d. Hypotension is avoided

2. Awake nasal intubation is the best way to secure the airway in uncooperative or obtunded patients with suspected acute cervical spinal cord trauma. True or false?
   a. True
   b. False

3. Spinal shock is best treated with which one of the following?
   a. Generous fluid administration
   b. Dopamine in the 2–5 micrograms/kg/minute
   c. Isuprel infusion
   d. Epinephrine bolus of .01 mg / kg

4. If surgery is indicated for a significant head, chest, or extremity injury, the diagnosis of possible abdominal injury is best accomplished by
   a. CT scan of the abdomen
   b. Diagnostic peritoneal lavage
   c. MRI of the abdomen
   d. Emergent exploratory laparotomy

5. Spinal shock is composed of a triad of all but which one of the following clinical signs?
   a. Hypotension
   b. Hypoxia
   c. Bradycardia
   d. Hypothermia

6. Patients with burns tend to become _____ NMBAs.
   a. More resistant to
   b. More sensitive to
   c. About the same degree of sensitivity to

7. Poikilothermia in the acute spinal cord injured patient is caused by all but one of the following mechanisms?
   a. The interruption of sympathetic pathways from the hypothalamus to peripheral blood vessels
   b. Inability to constrict blood vessels
   c. Inability to shiver
   d. Being phylogenetically evolved from reptilian species

8. If there is significant doubt about the need to intubate a burn patient with inhalation injury, it is probably best to
   a. Hold off on elective intubation as long as possible
   b. Have a low threshold for deciding to intubate

9. Signs and symptoms of hyperreflexia include
   a. Paroxysmal hypertension
   b. Bradycardia and dysrhythmias
   c. Cutaneous vasoconstriction below the level of the lesion
   d. All of the above
   e. a and c only

10. Second-degree burns affect both epidermal and dermal destruction and the basement membrane is intact. True or false?
    a. True
    b. False

11. Hyperreflexia has been observed with
    a. Local anesthesia
    b. Spinal anesthesia
    c. Potent inhalation anesthesia
    d. a and b

12. Rapid sequence oral intubation with cricoid pressure and in-line axial stabilization is the best approach to the uncooperative, obtunded, or inebriated spinal cord injured patient. True or false?
  a. True
  b. False

13. In general, the treatment and recovery following _____ trauma to the abdomen is relatively straightforward as compared to the alternative type of trauma listed.
  a. Penetrating
  b. Blunt

14. Pancreatic injuries
  a. Rarely hemorrhage enough to be detected by diagnostic peritoneal lavage or contrast enhanced CT scan
  b. Will cause autodigestion of abdominal tissues
  c. Can be observed without celiotomy most of the time
  d. a and b only

15. Through fluoroscopic/contrast dye studies, Dr. Sellick indicated that which one of the following is true in the patient with stomach contents at the induction of anesthesia?
  a. Positive pressure ventilation should not be used with cricoid pressure.
  b. Positive pressure ventilation can be safely used with cricoid pressure.

16. Anesthetic preparation for major abdominal trauma should generally include all but which one of the following options
  a. Two or more large-bore IV catheters
  b. Type and crossmatch for appropriate amount of blood
  c. Effective warming and infusion device
  d. Pulmonary artery catheter
  e. Indwelling arterial line

17. Hyperreflexia is caused by stimulation
  a. Above the level of the lesion
  b. Below the level of the lesion
  c. All of the above

18. Weaning from mechanical ventilation for the spinal cord injured patient should be accomplished
  a. As soon as tolerated by the patient
  b. After several days of stabilization
  c. After 2–3 days of intensive pulmonary therapy

19. Fluid shift from the intravascular space is _____ to the extent of the burn and the patient's size
  a. Proportional
  b. Variable
  c. Inversely proportional
  d. No good correlation

20. Bradycardia in the spinal cord injured patient is due to which one of the following mechanisms?
  a. Increased sympathetically mediated cardioaccelerator responses
  b. Decreased sympathetically mediated cardioaccelerator responses
  c. Increased vagal tone
  d. Decreased vagal tone

☐ ANSWERS

1. c	**5.** b	**9.** d	**13.** a	**17.** b
2. b	**6.** a	**10.** a	**14.** d	**18.** a
3. b	**7.** d	**11.** d	**15.** b	**19.** a
4. b	**8.** b	**12.** a	**16.** d	**20.** b

Complications During Anesthesia

Nancy A. Smilen

The goal of every anesthetic, whether general, regional, or monitored care, is the safe disposition of the stable patient to the recovery room or other postoperative facility. Despite the extensive vigilance of the anesthetist, complications do arise during the course of some of these anesthetics. Although some complications can be anticipated, many others arise unexpectedly. Therefore, the anesthetist must promptly recognize and treat any complication that develops, to ensure the best possible outcome and minimize postoperative sequelae for the patient.

☐ ANAPHYLAXIS

DETECTION

Drug-induced anaphylaxis occurs in the United States once in every 3000 patients.[1] In addition, drug-induced anaphylaxis is responsible for more than 500 deaths each year.[2] Therefore, anaphylactic reactions present a substantial threat to the patient undergoing anesthesia.

Anaphylaxis can be defined as a severe life-threatening allergic reaction that is mediated by the immune system. It is an immediate hypersensitivity reaction that occurs after exposure to an antigen, which stimulates production of IgE antibodies specific to that antigen. The IgE antibodies interact with mast cells throughout the body, resulting in the release of chemical mediators such as histamine, slow reactive substance of anaphylaxis, kinins, and prostaglandins, which cause a generalized systemic immunologic response. Manifestations of this response include, but are not limited to, peripheral vasodilation, hypotension, cardiovascular collapse, urticaria, bronchospasm, and upper airway edema (Table 31–1). In addition, once anaphylaxis occurs, the immuno-

logic response is reproducible after reexposure to the offending antigen.

Another type of hypersensitivity reaction virtually indistinguishable from anaphylaxis, except for its pathophysiology, is the anaphylactoid reaction. In the *anaphylactoid reaction* the release of chemical mediators is not IgE dependent but rather the direct effect of a substance on mast cells and basophils. In addition, because this response is not antigen–antibody dependent, it can occur without previous exposure to the offending substance. Many anesthetics and their adjuncts have been implicated in anaphylactoid reactions. Drugs such as morphine, vancomycin, *d*-tubocurarine, and atracurium cause histamine release, the degree of which depends on the speed of administration.

When anaphylaxis occurs in the anesthetized patient, as in all sensitized patients, the onset is almost always immediate. However, reactions may be delayed for as long as half an hour to $2\frac{1}{2}$ hours after parenteral administration of an antigen.[3] Although anaphylaxis is not a common occurrence in the operating room, many substances and drugs used for anesthetic and surgical purposes have been implicated as causative agents and should be familiar to all anesthesia personnel (Table 31–2).

TREATMENT

Although prevention of all anaphylactic reactions would be the ideal, it is not always possible without a prior history of hypersensitivity. Therefore, early recognition and prompt treatment are the goals of therapy. Because the manifestations of anaphylaxis can range from mild generalized pruritis to full-blown cardiovascular collapse, the anesthetist must be fully prepared to deal with this medical emergency (Table 31–3). Mortality due to anaphylaxis is a direct result of se-

Table 31–1
SIGNS AND SYMPTOMS OF ANAPHYLACTIC REACTIONS

Cardiovascular
   Tachycardia
   Dysrhythmias
   Peripheral vasodilation, hypotension
   Cardiovascular collapse
   Cardiac arrest
Respiratory
   Bronchospasm, wheezing
   Increased peak airway pressure
   Arterial hypoxemia
   Pulmonary edema/hypertension
Other
   Urticaria, flushing due to histamine release
   Pharyngeal/laryngeal edema

Table 31–3
MANAGEMENT OF ANAPHYLAXIS

Acute Therapy
1. Stop administration of causative agent (known or potential)
2. Administer 100% oxygen via secured airway
3. Discontinue all anesthetic agents (potentiate hypotension)
4. Intravascular volume expansion: secure IV access and administer 2–4 mL/kg isotonic crystalloid
5. Administer epinephrine
   For hypotension: 0.05–0.1 mg IV—titrate to effect
   For cardiovascular collapse: 0.1–0.5 mg IV as needed followed by IV infusion 2–20 µg/min—titrate to effect

Adjunct Therapy
1. Antihistamines—Benadryl 0.5–1.0 mg/kg
2. Aminophylline 5–6 mg/kg over 20 min
3. Steroids—hydrocortisone 0.25–1.0 g
4. Sodium bicarbonate—titrate based on arterial blood gases

Extubation only after careful airway evaluation

vere hypotension, bronchospasm, and upper airway edema, which makes ventilation and oxygenation impossible.

The initial treatment of anaphylaxis is aimed at providing adequate oxygenation and combating the profound hypotension. *Epinephrine* is the drug of choice in anaphylaxis because of its potent α- and β-adrenergic effects. In addition, the administration of all anesthetics and potential causative agents should be discontinued and the patient's airway secured before laryngeal or upper airway edema makes emergency tracheostomy the only alternative.

Once cardiovascular stability is achieved, secondary treatment is aimed at halting the immunologic response by blocking further release of chemical mediators and their remaining unoccupied receptor sites. This is achieved through the use of antihistamines and corticosteroids. Other resuscitative therapies are used as needed, based on the patient's condition. It is important to recognize that after an anaphylactic reaction occurs, patients should be monitored in an intensive care setting because chemical mediators are released for up to 48 hours after an initial response, posing a potential risk for re-

currence of symptoms. Extubation should be considered only after a complete airway evaluation and only in the presence of personnel trained in emergency airway management.

PREVENTION AND ANESTHETIC CONSIDERATIONS

In the patient with a known history of severe allergic reaction to an anesthetic agent or other drug, measures must be taken to prevent reexposure to that agent. A careful, detailed history that focuses on the clinical manifestations and sequence of events surrounding the allergic reaction should be obtained from the patient and previous records made available. Strict avoidance of the offending agent(s), as well as other related substances, is required at all times during the hospitalization. These patients should be instructed to obtain and wear a Medic Alert bracelet in case emergency medical treatment is ever needed.

Prophylactic treatment with H_1 and H_2 blockers or corticosteroids should be considered in the patient with severe drug allergies to prevent or decrease the severity of an anaphylactic reaction if one should occur. In patients with a history of allergy, use of known histamine-releasing agents should be avoided as well. Common anesthetics in this category include induction agents such as thiopental, etomidate, and ketamine; narcotics such as demerol and morphine; nondepolarizing muscle relaxants such as atracurium, pancuronium, and gallamine; and the ester local anesthetics. Use of the agents may worsen or initiate an allergic response. Anesthetic agents considered safe are those with a low incidence of causing histamine release and include midazolam, fentanyl, vecuronium, and the inhalational agents.

Latex Anaphylaxis Latex has long been used in the manufacture of medical and anesthetic equipment. However, only recently has latex hypersensitivity become a recognized etiology of anaphylactic reactions. In fact, the first cases of true latex anaphylaxis were not reported until 1989.[4] It is

Table 31–2
AGENTS IMPLICATED IN ANAPHYLAXIS

Anesthetics	Other Agents
Barbiturates	Antibiotics
Etomidate	Penicillin
Ester local anesthetics	Cephalosporins
Muscle relaxants	Vancomycin
Succinylcholine	Methylmethacrylate
Gallamine	Protamine
Pancuronium	Radiocontrast dye
Metocurine	Colloid volume expanders
d-Tubocurarine	Dextrans
Atracurium	Hetastarch (Hespan)
Narcotics	Albumin
Demerol	Protein fractions
Morphine	

now recognized that latex allergy can produce a range of reactions from contact dermatitis and rhinitis to fulminant life-threatening anaphylaxis.

Little information is currently available on the incidence of latex hypersensitivity in the population at large. However, studies have shown that the incidence of latex hypersensitivity to surgical gloves among physicians to be 7.5%, nurses 5.6%, and hospital employees 1.3%, as compared with 0.8% among nonmedical personnel.[5] In addition, recent studies report an unusually high incidence of IgE antibodies specific for latex in approximately 34% of patients who undergo repeated surgical and medical procedures such as those with spina bifida.[6] These studies suggest that repeated exposure to latex products is necessary to put the individual at risk for developing latex hypersensitivity. In addition, the most severe anaphylactic reactions have been reported in patients after contact of rubber gloves with disrupted vaginal, peritoneal, and bucosal membranes where large surface areas for absorption exist.[7] In these cases contact with intact skin may have been insufficient to precipitate anaphylaxis, but once large surface areas for absorption of allergen were available, severe immunologic responses were precipitated. This may help to explain why the occurrence of latex anaphylaxis is unpredictable and so few cases have actually been reported to date.

Although the treatment of latex anaphylaxis does not differ regardless of the antigen, specific precautions must be taken to prevent a response in the latex-sensitive individual. A thorough preoperative assessment of patients with known or suspected latex allergy is essential. Special focus should be placed on documenting any itching, rash, or wheezing that occurs after exposure to a latex-containing product (i.e., latex gloves or a rubber balloon). If time is available, preoperative radioallergosorbent testing for latex-specific IgE may be helpful in confirming the diagnosis. In the case of emergency surgery where latex allergy is suspected, all latex-containing products should be avoided.

The presence of latex in medical supplies and anesthesia equipment is well known (Table 31–4). Avoidance of exposure to these products during the perioperative period is the goal. Alternatives to standard medical and anesthesia supplies are available for the latex-sensitive individual. Examples include vinyl surgical gloves, silicon urinary catheters, replacement of multidose medication vials with single-dose ampules, and non-latex based blood pressure cuffs. Detailed guidelines for care of the latex-sensitive patient have been outlined by the American Association of Nurse Anesthetists and are presented in Appendix 31–1.

Even when all preventive measures are instituted, latex allergy should be suspected if unexplained anaphylactic reactions occur after the start of a surgical procedure without an obvious temporal relationship to the administration of any drug.[8] Most cases of drug-induced anaphylaxis develop within minutes of induction, whereas cases of latex anaphylaxis take 40 minutes or longer to occur.[9] All patients shown to have a true IgE-mediated sensitivity should be instructed to carry epinephrine and wear a Medic Alert bracelet because

Table 31–4
LATEX-CONTAINING ANESTHESIA AND MEDICAL EQUIPMENT

Anesthesia Equipment	Medical/Surgical Equipment
Endotracheal tubes	Latex surgical gloves
Face masks	Adhesive tape
Oral/nasal airways	Urinary catheters
Bite blocks	Wound drains/IV tourniquets
Blood pressure cuffs	Nasogastric tubes
Rubber breathing bags	Protective rubber pads
Ventilator hoses/bellows	Elastic ACE bandages
Electrocardiogram electrodes	
Latex injection ports on IV tubing/vials	
Rubber tips on syringe plungers	

of the potential life-threatening consequences of latex exposure.

☐ MALIGNANT HYPERTHERMIA

DETECTION

Malignant hyperthermia (MH) is a rare clinical syndrome that occurs during the administration of general anesthesia and is primarily triggered by the volatile anesthetics and succinylcholine. MH is characterized by a loss of intracellular calcium from the sarcoplasmic reticulum in susceptible individuals. An elevated intracellular calcium level leads to unopposed skeletal muscle contraction and activation of all metabolic processes, resulting in excessive production of heat, carbon dioxide, and lactic acid, as well as excessive consumption of intracellular adenosine triphosphate (ATP). Cellular integrity is lost, rhabdomyolosis occurs, and intracellular contents such as creatine phosphokinase (CPK), K^+, Ca^{++}, and myoglobin are released into the general circulation.

The derangement of skeletal muscle metabolism seen in MH exhibits an autosomal dominant pattern of inheritance and is believed to be the result of a defective gene located on chromosome 19. This gene is linked to the ryanodine receptor, which is responsible for transferring the wave of depolarization from the transverse tubule to the sarcoplasmic reticulum during skeletal muscle contraction.[10] Despite the genetic link, no specific screening test exists and therefore susceptibility is currently based on family history, patient history, and the results of skeletal muscle biopsy.

Studies reporting the overall incidence of MH vary depending on the patient population, type of anesthetic administered, and the definition of MH used for inclusion. A recent study from Denmark estimates the overall incidence of MH (both mild and fulminant cases) to be 1/16,000 and for fulminant cases alone 1/250,000. In addition, when considering cases where volatile agents and succinylcholine were used exclusively, the incidence increases to 1/62,000.[11] Early reports on the mortality from MH have been estimated to be as high as 70%. However, with the introduction of dantrolene in 1979 and early detection, this rate has dropped to less than 5%.[12]

Differential diagnosis of MH can be difficult. Many disorders exhibit similar signs and symptoms, and early signs may be masked by the depth of anesthesia or delayed until emergence. In addition, MH can occur at any time during an anesthetic as well as several hours after.

In the MH patient, as hypermetabolic processes take over, oxygen consumption, carbon dioxide production, and lactic acid production dramatically increase. In the presence of controlled ventilation, end-tidal carbon dioxide ($ETCO_2$) levels will rise and respiratory acidosis will become apparent. In patients who are spontaneously breathing, tachypnea will occur as the patient tries to compensate for the increased carbon dioxide load. Central venous oxygen and carbon dioxide levels change more dramatically than do arterial levels and are a more accurate reflection of body carbon dioxide production.[13] In addition, the patient will exhibit unexplained tachycardia, cardiac dysrhythmia, cyanosis, masseter muscle rigidity, increased temperature (1°C/5 min), sweating, and generalized muscle rigidity. Hyperkalemia, myoglobinemia, myoglobinuria, and elevated CPK levels result as cellular destruction occurs. If untreated, MH can lead to renal failure, disseminated intravascular coagulation, pulmonary and cerebral edema, cardiovascular collapse, and death (Table 31–5).

Masseter Muscle Rigidity   Masseter muscle rigidity has been identified as a possible early sign of MH. It is defined as jaw muscle rigidity in association with limb muscle flaccidity that occurs after the administration of succinylcholine.[14] Once considered to be a completely pathologic occurrence, it is now believed to be a unique property of the masseter muscle in healthy individuals. A spectrum of

responses to succinylcholine exists. Most patients exhibit a normal rise in masseter muscle tension, but a small subset exhibits an extreme rise in muscle tension manifested by complete inability to open the mouth. It is only this extreme group that shows a greater than 50% incidence of being susceptible to MH. Rigidity of other muscle groups in addition to masseter muscle spasm makes the association with MH certain. Anesthesia should be halted at once and treatment of MH begun. In other cases, treatment of masseter muscle rigidity is controversial. The decision should be made on a case-by-case basis.

TREATMENT

Once the diagnosis of MH is made a treatment plan must be instituted immediately. The Malignant Hyperthermia Association of the United States has been established to assist the anesthetist 24 hours a day in dealing with an MH crisis (Hotline number: 209-634-4917). Mortality during the early stages of MH is usually the result of fatal dysrhythmias secondary to the metabolic changes occurring in the skeletal muscle.[15] Discontinuation of all triggering agents and hyperventilation with 100% O_2 is the first priority in the management plan to control hypercarbia and acidosis. Dantrolene is the drug specific for the treatment of MH. *It inhibits the release of calcium from the sarcoplasmic reticulum without interfering with its reuptake,* thus blocking the rate-limiting step in the hypermetabolic process.[16] An initial intravenous dose of 1.0 to 2.5 mg/kg is administered and may be repeated to a total dose of 10 mg/kg if symptoms persist. Dantrolene should be repeated at a dose of 1 mg/kg every 6 hours for at least 12 hours after the acute episode depending on the patient's clinical course. The drug is supplied in crystal form in 20-mg vials and must be reconstituted with sterile water prior to administration. Dantrolene in high doses does not produce paralysis. At the therapeutic doses muscle weakness may occur with preservation of muscle strength for effective coughing and deep breathing. Further treatment is guided by the specific signs of MH manifested by the patient and is outlined in Table 31–6.

PREVENTION AND ANESTHETIC CONSIDERATIONS

Prevention of MH is based on identifying high-risk individuals and avoiding triggering agents in this population. Preoperative evaluation of susceptibility to MH involves obtaining a personal and family history of any myopathies or a history of any unusual reaction or unexplained death as a result of anesthesia. Because MH is a disease of the muscle, an association has been made with a wide range of anomalies including Duchenne's muscular dystrophy, club foot, central core disease, ptosis, strabismus, kyphoscoliosis, and pediatric hernias. If any of the above conditions are elicited from the history and a known MH-susceptible patient is in the family, serum CPK levels should be determined. An elevated CPK level is considered consistent with susceptibility. If CPK val-

Table 31–5
SIGNS AND SYMPTOMS OF MALIGNANT HYPERTHERMIA

Early
  Tachycardia
  Tachypnea
  ↑ end-tidal CO_2 (nonspecific but sensitive early sign)
  Skeletal muscle rigidity
  Cyanosis, mottling
  Masseter muscle rigidity
  Sweating
  Dysrhythmias, unstable blood pressure
Late
  Fever
  Metabolic/respiratory acidosis
  Central venous desaturation/hypercarbia
  Hyperkalemia
  Myoglobinemia, myoglobinurea
  ↑ Creatine phosphokinase

Table 31–6
TREATMENT OF MALIGNANT HYPERTHERMIA

1. Stop anesthesia—discontinue all triggering agents; volatile anesthetics, succinylcholine. Discontinue surgery, if possible change all circuits, anesthesia machine.
2. Hyperventilate with 100% O_2
3. Administer dantrolene 1.0–2.5 mg/kg IV; repeat every 5 min to total dose 10 mg/kg.
4. Correct acidosis—HCO_3 1–2 mg/kg initially, then guided by ABGs.
5. Correct hyperkalemia—glucose 0.5 g/kg and regular insulin 0.15 U/kg
6. Cool patient: iced saline IV, surface cooling, stomach, bladder lavage
7. Treat dysrhythmias—procainamide 15 mg/kg IV
8. Monitor urinary output—maintain 2 mL/kg/h, administer mannitol 12.5 g IV and Lasix 50 mg IV as needed.
9. Monitor patient in intensive care unit
10. Labs as needed: ABGs, SMA_6, venous blood gases, PT, PTT, platelets, urine myoglobin, etc.
11. Oral dantrolene—when stable—1 mg/kg Po every 6 h for 24–48h.
12. Counsel patient and family—need for Medic Alert bracelet, muscle biopsy, etc.

ABG, arterial blood gas; PT, prothrombin time; PTT, partial thromboplastin time; SMA, Sequential Multiple Analysis

ues are normal then skeletal muscle biopsy and a contracture test are recommended. All patients are encouraged to wear Medic Alert bracelets and carry cards identifying themselves as MH-susceptible individuals.

Anesthesia for the known MH-susceptible patient is based on the avoidance of triggering agents and the administration of "safe" anesthetics such as nitrous oxide, barbiturates, propofol, opiates, benzodiazepines, and nondepolarizing muscle relaxants (Table 31–7). Clean MH-designated anesthesia equipment should be used to prevent contamination of the anesthesia circuit. Regional anesthesia is considered safe and may be preferred for many procedures. Amide anesthetics were once considered dangerous in MH-susceptible patients because they induce or worsen contractures in vitro as

Table 31–7
CLASSIFICATION OF ANESTHETIC DRUGS IN MALIGNANT HYPERTHERMIA

Triggering Agents	"Safe" Anesthetics
All volatile anesthetics	Benzodiazepines
Halothane	Opiates
Enflurane	Barbiturates
Isoflurane	Propofol
Desflurane	Ketamine
Sevoflurane	Nondepolarizing muscle relaxants
Depolarizing muscle relaxants	Dantrolene
Succinylcholine	Ester and amide local anesthetics

a result of increased Ca^{++} release in the sarcoplasmic reticulum.[16] However, recent studies have demonstrated that they can be used safely.[17]

The controversy concerning the pretreatment of the MH-susceptible patient with dantrolene still exists. Although its use in humans is safe, it does have disadvantages. Dantrolene causes phlebitis, weakness and lethargy, prolonged neuromuscular blockage, postpartum uterine atony, and prenatal weakness due to placental transfer. The current trend is against dantrolene prophylaxis in the MH-susceptible patient because the avoidance of triggering agents has been shown to be sufficient. Regardless, an MH cart containing dantrolene and all other necessary supplies should be readily available.

It is the responsibility of the anesthetist to discuss all possible anesthetic options with the MH-susceptible individual to alleviate unnecessary anxiety and make the patient as comfortable as possible. It is important to let the patient know that with appropriate preparations and precautions anesthesia can be administered safely.

☐ CARDIAC ARREST

DETECTION

Cardiovascular complications during anesthesia range from those that are minor and well tolerated by the anesthetized patient to those resulting in patient death. Anesthesia personnel play an integral role in reducing cardiovascular complications in the perioperative period. Cardiac arrest is the most life-threatening of the complications and must be identified and treated quickly for a positive outcome. A wide range of potential causes of intraoperative cardiac arrest have been identified (Table 31–8). However, airway problems resulting in inadequate ventilation and drug overdose are the primary

Table 31–8
MAJOR CAUSES OF INTRAOPERATIVE CARDIAC ARREST

Factors affecting cardiac conduction
1. Ventricular tachycardia
2. Ventricular fibrillation
3. Asystole
4. Complete heart block
5. Severe bradycardia

Factors altering myocardial contractility
1. Ischemia, myocardial infarction
2. Hypoxia
3. Severe metabolic acidosis
4. Electrolyte abnormalities, i.e., hyperkalemia
5. Drug overdose

Factors altering venous return and cardiac output
1. Hypovolemia
2. Pericardial tamponade
3. Pulmonary embolism
4. Aortocaval compression

causes.[18] During cardiac arrest, organ perfusion is impaired, resulting in tissue hypoxia, anaerobic metabolism, and compromised organ function. *Permanent* organ damage develops within 4 to 5 minutes unless adequate circulation is reestablished.

During an anesthetic, basic monitoring (i.e., blood pressure, pulse oximetry, capnography) provides the anesthetist with a continuous picture of the patient's condition and therefore immediate knowledge of any deviations from baseline. The signs of cardiac arrest must be detected with certainty because resuscitative measures are not without their own risk. Artifact and equipment malfunction must be ruled out before therapy is initiated.

The identification of major cardiac dysrhythmias such as asystole or ventricular fibrillation is highly suggestive of a cardiac arrest. Confirmation is based on the absence of a detectable blood pressure or palpable pulse in any major vessel. Pulse oximetry will fail to register a wave because of the loss of pulsatile blood flow. Capnography will show a complete absence or a rapid decline in $ETCO_2$ levels, and cyanosis may be seen with a lack of bleeding at the surgical site.

TREATMENT

The anesthetist must be capable of treating all aspects of a cardiac arrest. This involves proficiency in both basic and advanced cardiac life support as well as an understanding of postresuscitative care. Basic life support involves the provision of adequate ventilation through the use of established airway management techniques (i.e., mask ventilation followed by endotracheal intubation) and the performance of external chest compressions to provide effective circulation and vital organ perfusion. Table 31–9 outlines basic life support guidelines for adult, pediatric, and infant resuscitation. In addition to basic life support measures, all anesthetics should be discontinued, the patient placed on 100% O_2, and surgery halted or canceled until the patient's condition is stabilized.

Advanced cardiac life support is used in conjunction with these basic lifesaving techniques. It involves the use of electrocardiographic (ECG) monitoring and interpretation, drug therapy, defibrillation, and the establishment of intravenous access to stabilize the patient's condition. If advanced cardiac life support is to be optimally beneficial, measures must be instituted within 10 minutes of the onset of cardiac arrest. Because it is beyond the scope of this chapter to discuss these treatment modalities in depth, please refer to the algorithms for the treatment of cardiac dysrhythmias as presented in the *Textbook of Advanced Cardiac Life Support,* published by the American Heart Association.

PREVENTION

Prevention of intraoperative cardiac arrest, while not always possible, is based on identifying those patients at risk for an intraoperative cardiac event. Because the primary cause of cardiac arrest in the perioperative period is related to inadequate ventilation, preventive measures must be aimed at providing appropriate airway management during every anesthetic administered. Patients with anticipated difficult airways should have the airway secured before the start of a surgical procedure using techniques appropriate for the particular situation rather than waiting until the need for intubation becomes emergent. Thus, the difficult airway may be considered a relative contraindication for the use of regional anesthesia because the potential exists for failed or inadequate anesthesia requiring emergency intubation. Regardless of the anesthetic technique used, careful monitoring of $ETCO_2$ levels and arterial oxygenation will alert the anesthetist to changes in patient status before actual or potential problems arise.

Identification of patients with a prior history of cardiac disease is also important in predicting adverse outcome in the perioperative period. Multiple studies have demonstrated that preoperative myocardial infarction significantly increases the risk for postoperative myocardial reinfarction depending on the time interval between infarction and surgery. Goldman and colleagues[19] and Steen and coworkers[20] have demonstrated that myocardial infarction during the 6-month period before surgery is the most critical predictor of adverse cardiac outcomes (i.e., reinfarction or death). *Postponement of surgery until after the critical 6-month period is advisable to reduce perioperative morbidity.* When surgery is absolutely necessary an individualized anesthetic plan is rec-

Table 31–9
BASIC LIFE SUPPORT

1. Establish absence of respiration—establish airway (mask, endotracheal tube, etc.), give 2 full breaths
2. Establish absence of pulse—carotid, brachial, or radial and begin chest compressions:

Compression/Ventilation Ratio	Adult (rate 80–100 beats/min)	Pediatric >4 y (rate 80–100 beats/min)	<4 y (rate 100 beats/min)	Infant(rate 100–120 beats/min)
1 rescuer	15:2	5:1	5:1	5:1
2 rescuers	5:1	5:1	5:1	5:1
Depth of compressions (inches)	1.5–2	1.5–2	1.0–1.5	0.5–1.0

3. Reassess for return spontaneous ventilation and cardiac activity after first 4 cycles and then every few minutes thereafter.

ommended because no convincing data support the choice of a well-conducted regional versus general anesthetic. Although studies on the benefit of invasive monitoring in these patients have been controversial, its utilization is recommended based on the patient's presenting clinical condition (i.e., congestive heart failure, cardiac dysrhythmias, and so on).

PULMONARY COMPLICATIONS

INTRAOPERATIVE PULMONARY RISK: DETECTION AND PREVENTION

Pulmonary complications are a leading cause of perioperative morbidity and mortality. Both anesthesia and surgery induce major alterations in lung function. Patients with no preexisting disease experience a 6% to 10% incidence of postoperative pulmonary complications.[21] Few data support the claim that the anesthetic technique used plays a major role in determining outcome. A high spinal can be more detrimental to the patient than a well-conducted general anesthetic. Thus, it is difficult to determine exactly which patients will develop postoperative problems and which will not.

Several factors have consistently been shown to be associated with an increased risk for developing pulmonary complications. Advanced age, preexisting pulmonary disease, including reactive airway disease, smoking, and morbid obesity bring an already compromised patient to the operating room where additional demands will be placed on the respiratory system. Forced vital capacity (FVC), forced expiratory volume (FEV), and functional residual capacity (FRC) are all reduced in these patients, sometimes to alarmingly low levels. When FEV and FVC are abnormally low and improve in response to bronchodilator therapy, surgery should be delayed until optimal pulmonary function can be achieved through the use of bronchodilator therapy, antibiotics, cessation of smoking, and chest physiotherapy, as indicated. Patients with morbid obesity demonstrate an increased risk for developing deep-vein thrombosis and an increased incidence of hiatal hernia and esophageal reflux. They are likely to experience pulmonary emboli and aspiration of gastric contents as a result.

Factors related to the surgical intervention also play a large role in determining morbidity. *Thoracic and upper abdominal* incisions are associated with a higher incidence of postoperative pulmonary complications. These result from postoperative pain and the patient's inability to fully expand the lungs due to "splinting." In these patients, atelectasis occurs with an associated increase in ventilation/perfusion mismatch and hypoxia. Adequate postoperative pain management is a priority. In addition, because most thoracic procedures are required for primary lung pathology, resection may result in respiratory failure making surgical intervention incompatible with survival. Complete preoperative testing, including pulmonary function tests, arterial blood gases, and prediction of postoperative pulmonary values must be carried out to identify patients most likely to benefit from surgical intervention.

ANESTHETIC CONSIDERATIONS

Even with thorough preoperative assessment and identification of patients at risk, pulmonary complications will arise. They include, but are not limited to, bronchospasm, aspiration, pulmonary embolism, and pneumothorax. The key to successful management of these life-threatening complications is prompt recognition and treatment.

Bronchospasm   Bronchospasm is a form of lower airway obstruction characterized by smooth muscle contraction and increased resistance to airflow through the bronchial tree. Bronchospasm is commonly seen in patients with hyperreactive airway disease as well as in response to local airway irritation from physical, pharmacologic, and chemical stimuli. During anesthesia, tracheal intubation and airway manipulation, light anesthesia, carinal irritation from the endotracheal tube, aspiration, and allergic reactions may all precipitate an episode of severe bronchospasm.

In the anesthetized individual, bronchospasm can be detected by the presence of wheezing on both inspiration and expiration, as well as an increase in peak respiratory pressure due to decreased lung compliance. In the awake individual marked tachypnea and dyspnea may be present. If bronchospasm is severe, air trapping, hypoxemia, hypercarbia, impaired venous return, and decreased cardiac output may occur.

Prevention and Treatment

The primary goal of anesthetic management is the prevention of intraoperative bronchospasm. A smooth, deep induction of general anesthesia with minimal airway manipulation and attempts at laryngoscopy is desirable. Rapid sequence intubations should be reserved for emergency/full stomach situations when the benefits outweigh the risks. Avoidance of histamine-releasing drugs (i.e., magnesium sulfate, demerol, curare, atracurium, and barbiturates) and β-adrenergic blockers is also recommended because they may worsen bronchoconstriction. Pretreatment of susceptible patients with aerosolized bronchodilators and intravenous lidocaine, 1 to 2 mg/kg, may help to blunt airway reflexes as well.

When measures to prevent intraoperative bronchospasm fail, the cause should be identified and treatment initiated promptly. Airway patency and tube position must be assessed. The repositioning of an endotracheal tube may be all that is required if carinal irritation is the cause. If "light anesthesia" is suspected, deepening the anesthetic level with either inhalational or intravenous agents may completely reverse the episode. Extrinsic causes such as aspiration and anaphylaxis must also be sought because the course of therapy in these situations is different.

If brochospasm does not resolve even with these measures, inhaled bronchodilator and intravenous therapy is then indi-

Table 31–10
DRUG THERAPY FOR THE TREATMENT OF INTRAOPERATIVE BRONCHOSPASM

1. Inhaled β-adrenergic agonists
   A. Albuterol (Proventil/Ventoline): 2 puffs every 3–4 h
   B. Metaproterenol (Alupent): 2 puffs every 3–4 h
2. Intravenous/subcutaneous agents
   A. Sympathomimetics
      1. Epinephrine: 0.25–1.0 μg/min (at low doses β_2 effects predominate)
      2. Terbutaline: 0.25 mg subcutaneously (may be repeated in 15 min × 1 dose, not to exceed 0.5 mg in a 4-h period)
   B. Methylxanthines—aminophylline: 5 mg/kg over 30 min loading dose, followed by IV drip 0.5–1.0 mg/kg/h to maintain serum levels 10–20 μg/mL
3. Corticosteroids
   Solumedrol: 30–60 mg/kg IV every 6 h

Table 31–11
RISK FACTORS ASSOCIATED WITH PULMONARY ASPIRATION

Loss of protective airway reflexes
  • Coma
  • Intrinsic neurologic disease
  • Anesthesia and drug overdose
Recent ingestion of food—"full stomach"
Obesity
Pregnancy
Hiatal hernia, gastroesophageal reflux
Disruption of gastroesophageal junction—nasogastric tube in place
Airway trauma, anatomic anomalies (i.e., laryngectomy)
Difficult intubation

cated (Table 31–10). Inhaled β-agonist bronchodilators are the first line of treatment. They are well tolerated by patients because of limited systemic absorption and therefore minimal cardiovascular effects. Intravenous and subcutaneous agents are used when inhaled bronchodilators fail or the bronchospasm episode is so severe as to prevent delivery of the drug to the bronchial tree. The intraoperative use of aminophylline is controversial because of its narrow therapeutic window and altered metabolism under certain clinical conditions. This makes toxicity an issue requiring careful monitoring of serum blood levels. It is recommended that systemic sympathomimetics be tried before initiating aminophylline therapy. Corticosteroids, while helpful, are used only as a supplement to therapy during the acute phase of treatment. Beneficial effects of steroid therapy can take hours to manifest.

Aspiration of Gastric Contents Pulmonary aspiration of gastric contents is one of the most devastating complications that can occur during anesthesia. The syndrome has been reported in the literature for thousands of years, but was finally scientifically delineated by Curtis Mendelson in 1946 with a report of 66 cases of aspiration in the obstetric patient.[22] His experiments outlined the differences between acid and nonacid aspiration, as well as the benefit of neutralizing the acidity of stomach contents.

The incidence of aspiration during anesthesia has been difficult to determine. Reports of mortality range from 3% to 70% depending on the type and quantity of material aspirated and the aggressiveness of therapy.[22-24] The more severely gas exchange is impaired, the greater the risk of adverse sequelae. Clinically significant cases of aspiration are associated with aspirates whose volumes exceed 25 mL and have a pH less than 2.5.[25] Aspirates containing food particles as opposed to clear liquid cause the most severe forms of tissue damage.

Many factors place the patient at risk for pulmonary aspi-

ration (Table 31–11). However, the loss of protective airway reflexes, whether as a result of obstructive airway disease, trauma, coma, or drug administration, poses the most significant threat. Other conditions of particular concern are pregnancy, obesity, hiatal hernia, and gastroesophageal reflux. These cause impairment of gastric motility and gastroesophageal sphincter tone rendering the patient at risk for passive regurgitation. All patients at risk for aspiration are considered to have a full stomach regardless of the time interval since the last ingestion of food.

Detection of pulmonary aspiration can be difficult in the anesthetized patient. Although the classic picture involves the presence of gastric contents in the oropharynx, wheezing, cyanosis, dyspnea, tachypnea, hypoxemia, and pulmonary edema, many or all of these symptoms may be absent. This is especially true in cases of silent aspiration. If stomach contents cannot be suctioned from the oropharynx or trachea, the diagnosis of pulmonary aspiration can only be presumed. The earliest and most reliable sign of aspiration is *hypoxemia,* which occurs even with minute aspirates. Abnormal arterial blood gases indicating hypoxemia, hypercarbia, and acidosis may help to confirm the diagnosis. Additionally, 90% of all patients who aspirate will have abnormal chest radiographs with the right lower lobe being the most common site of involvement. In severe cases, bilateral pulmonary infiltrates may be seen mimicking the picture seen in adult respiratory distress syndrome (ARDS).

Prevention and Treatment
Treatment of pulmonary aspiration is costly both to the patients and the health care system. Many believe that the most effective means of preventing aspiration is to avoid general anesthesia and use regional techniques. However, heavy sedation that obtunds airway reflexes can be more dangerous than a well-planned general anesthetic in the patient at risk. With this in mind, specific measures can be taken to decrease the incidence and severity of pulmonary aspiration.

When planning the anesthetic care for the patient at risk of pulmonary aspiration, NPO status should be maintained whenever possible to decrease gastric volume. Extensive research has been conducted to quantify the length of time necessary for a patient to be NPO. In the adult, 6 hours before surgery is the current accepted rule. Pretreatment with nonparticulate antacids (i.e., Bicitra) within 1 hour prior to induction, histamine (H_2) blockers, and metoclopramide is recommended. These drugs work by raising gastric pH, decreasing stomach acid production, and promoting gastric emptying, respectively. If general anesthesia is planned, the airway must be protected by a cuffed endotracheal tube because the most dangerous time for aspiration is during induction and emergence. This is achieved through the performance of a rapid sequence induction and the maintenance of cricoid pressure until confirmation of tube placement is made. During induction, patients should be placed in the reverse Trendelenberg position, which decreases the incidence of regurgitation through gravity. After successful placement, the stomach should be decompressed to decrease the risk of aspiration at the time of emergence. Extubation should be performed only when the patient is fully awake, with airway reflexes intact, and able to respond appropriately to commands.

Despite the best efforts of the anesthesia provider, pulmonary aspiration can still occur. Therapy is primarily supportive. Treatment modalities are initiated depending on the severity of the aspiration and the symptoms exhibited by the patient. Whether aspiration occurs on induction or emergence from anesthesia, the trachea should be intubated and the endotracheal tube suctioned before ventilation to avoid pushing gastric contents further down the bronchial tree. Supplemental oxygen, mechanical ventilation, positive endexpiratory pressure (PEEP), or continuous positive airway pressure is used as needed to maintain PaO_2 above 60 to 70 mm Hg. When aspiration of particulate matter (e.g., peanuts) is suspected, bronchoscopy and lavage may be indicated to remove the foreign body (see Chapter 24).

Pharmacologic treatment of aspiration is governed by the individual patient situation. The use of steroids and antibiotics is not routinely recommended because they have no effect on the course of the disease. Steroids may actually interfere with the healing process, and antibiotics alter the normal flora of the respiratory tract making the patient more susceptible to infection.[26,27] Antibiotics are reserved for patients who exhibit actual signs of superimposed pulmonary infection.

Pulmonary Embolism   Pulmonary embolism is a leading cause of morbidity and mortality in the United States. It is estimated that 630,000 cases occur each year resulting in some 67,000 deaths.[28] Pulmonary emboli can result from any substance present within the vascular system that is capable of obstructing pulmonary blood flow. Of greatest concern are thromboembolism, fat embolism, air embolism, and amniotic fluid embolism. However, only the first three will be discussed here. Predisposing factors for pulmonary embolism vary greatly depending on the offending substance as does the size of the embolism and the severity of the disease process. Early recognition and intervention are essential to prevent devastating consequences.

Thromboembolism

The majority of thromboemboli arise in the deep venous system of the lower extremities as a result of venous stasis, vessel wall anomalies, and alterations in coagulation. Pregnancy and obesity are two conditions familiar to the anesthetist that put the patient at risk. When deep-vein thrombi mobilize and travel to the lung, a wide range of nonspecific symptoms can occur. These include chest pain, dyspnea, tachypnea, tachycardia, hypoxemia, hypercarbia, and pulmonary edema. Hypoxemia may develop as a result of increased dead space ventilation and loss of the hypoxic pulmonary vasoconstriction reflex intrinsic to the lung. ECG anomalies may develop but are not considered diagnostic. These include anterior T wave inversion, right axis deviation caused by right ventricular overload, and the development of an incomplete or complete right bundle branch block.

When thromboembolism occurs during anesthesia, treatment is completely supportive. The primary goal is to maintain cardiovascular stability and pulmonary function. Volume expansion is used in an attempt to increase right ventricular preload and subsequently cardiac output. Sympathomimetic therapy is used when volume expansion alone is not effective. Oxygenation is optimized by increasing the fraction of inspired oxygen (FIO_2) and using mechanical ventilation with PEEP. Systemic heparinization and thrombolytic therapy are not routinely used in the operating room because of the risk of hemorrhage. However, in life-threatening situations heparin therapy may be necessary.

Prevention of thromboembolism is difficult. Many studies advocate the use of regional anesthesia techniques for lower extremities and prostate surgery because they lower the incidence of deep-vein thrombosis and pulmonary embolization possibly by improving blood flow to the lower extremities.[29,30] However, in most cases anesthetic technique plays little role. Sequential inflation TED stockings are commonly used as prophylaxis. They improve venous return and decrease the incidence of deep-vein thrombosis. They do not affect the severity of thromboembolitic disease should it occur.

Fat Embolism

Fat embolism is commonly associated with severe trauma, orthopedic surgery, and fractures of the leg bones, pelvis, and ribs where bone marrow can be released into the circulation. Following leg bone fractures, fat embolism occurs in 100% of the patients, but clinically significant embolization appears to occur in less than 3% of these patients.[31] Initial signs and symptoms are the result of mechanical obstruction of the pulmonary vasculature and mimic those seen with thromboembolism and other forms of ARDS. However, as free fatty acids are released from bone marrow, destruction of the capillary endothelium occurs causing hemorrhagic exudates in the lungs and brain. Pulmonary edema and mental status changes occur as a result of these exudates. Characteristic petechiae develop on the upper chest, axilla, and conjunctiva. Although the presence of fat globules in the urine and diffuse pulmonary infiltrates are nonspecific, they help to confirm the diagnosis.

Prevention of pulmonary fat embolism by the anesthesia providers is next to impossible because its occurrence is primarily the result of trauma and surgical manipulation. Because most cases of fat embolism occur within 24 to 48 hours of the insult, early fixation may be useful to halt the release of fat globules, although this is controversial. Early detection and treatment of pulmonary embolism may be the most the anesthetist can do in these cases. As with pulmonary thromboembolization, therapy is completely supportive. In mild cases supplemental oxygen may be all that is necessary. In severe cases, mechanical ventilation and cardiovascular support may be required. With appropriate fluid management, adequate ventilation, and the prevention of hypoxemia, outcome in cases of pulmonary fat embolism is excellent.

Venous Air Embolism

Venous air embolism (VAE) is a form of pulmonary embolization that is unique to anesthesia and surgery. Most cases occur during intracranial surgery in the sitting position where venous sinuses are open and negative intravascular pressures, relative to atmospheric pressures, exist. VAE has also been described in head and neck surgery, open cardiac procedures, insufflation associated with laparoscopy, or any surgical procedure where a pressure gradient between open vessels and the heart develops. Reports of the incidence of VAE vary significantly depending on the monitoring techniques used. Early detection with Doppler has increased the reported incidence but has not helped to decrease the occurrence of clinically significant emboli.[32]

Diagnosis of VAE depends on the monitoring devices used by the anesthetist. Transesophageal echocardiography and precordial Doppler over the right atrium are most sensitive, being able to detect air entrainment as small as 0.1 to 0.25 mL/kg/min.[33] Continuous respiratory gas monitoring will detect decreases in $ETCO_2$ and increases in end-tidal nitrogen with entrainments 0.25 to 5 mL/kg/min.[33] These changes are indicative of increasing dead space ventilation and diffusion of nitrogen across capillary membranes. It is not until alterations in central venous pressure, pulmonary artery pressure, and arterial blood are seen that significant entrainment occurs. Once the classic mill-wheel murmur is audible through the precordial or esophageal stethoscope, VAE is present (1.5 mL/kg/min), requiring immediate intervention.

As with fat embolization, little can be done to prevent VAE in the anesthetized patient because it is primarily a surgical complication. Nevertheless, when the risk for VAE is present, a combination of monitoring devices as described above is desirable. Invasive monitoring including an arterial line and central venous catheter or pulmonary artery catheter is also required.

When VAE is suspected, treatment follows a distinct sequence of events (Table 31–12). Nitrous oxide should be discontinued and 100% O_2 administered to the patient. Nitrous oxide is more soluble than nitrogen; therefore, it will diffuse into a VAE faster than nitrogen can leave, causing expansion of the bubble. The surgical field should next be

Table 31–12
TREATMENT OF VENOUS AIR EMBOLISM

1. Discontinue N_2O, administer 100% O_2
2. Flood surgical field with saline
3. Aspiration of air from central line/pulmonary artery catheter
4. Trendelenberg position with left side down
5. Intravascular volume expansion
6. Inotropic support

flooded with saline to limit air entrainment and attempts at aspiration of air through central venous catheters made. If cardiovascular instability has occurred as a result of massive embolism volume expansion, supportive inotropic therapy and mechanical ventilation may be required. The use of PEEP in the setting of VAE is controversial. It may help to limit air entrainment by raising central venous pressure but at the expense of venous return and cardiac output.

Pneumothorax Pneumothorax is a fairly uncommon complication of anesthesia, but when it occurs, the consequences can be life-threatening. It is caused by air entrance into the pleural space as a result of external trauma to the chest wall, rupture of the visceral pleura during vascular cannulation or nerve block, or direct rupture of alveoli either spontaneously or secondary to positive-pressure ventilation.[34] Once air enters the pleural space, pressure rises above subatmospheric, collapsing the lung and overexpanding the rib cage. In some cases of spontaneous pneumothorax the communication between the lung and the pleural space acts as a check valve through which air can enter but not exit the thorax. This is known as a tension pneumothorax and is considered a medical emergency. Intrathoracic pressures may rise well above atmospheric pressure and interfere with venous return to the heart.

The overall incidence of pneumothorax in anesthesia is unknown. In a series of 10,000 intercostal nerve blocks reported by Moore and Bridenbaugh, the incidence was reported at 0.073%.[35] The statistics, however, are clearly influenced by the skill and experience of the practitioner. Patients considered at risk include, but are not limited to, those with chronic obstructive pulmonary disease, blebs, or requiring high-pressure mechanical ventilation (Table 31–13).

When pneumothorax occurs during the administration of anesthesia, it is of special concern because of the frequent use of positive-pressure ventilation and nitrous oxide. These two factors predispose to the development of life-threatening tension pneumothorax. As previously discussed, nitrous oxide will diffuse into an air bubble, causing a dramatic increase in size and therefore the pressure in a confined space. Depending on the concentration of nitrous oxide and the duration of its use, this phenomenon can occur very rapidly. Manifestations of pneumothorax largely depend on the size and cause of the collapse. Early diagnosis can be difficult be-

Table 31–13
RISK FACTORS ASSOCIATED WITH THE DEVELOPMENT OF PNEUMOTHORAX

1. Preexisting lung disease
   - Chronic obstructive pulmonary disease
   - Emphysematous blebs
   - Necrotizing pneumonia
2. Chest trauma
3. Operative procedures
   - Tracheostomy
   - Laparoscopy
   - Rib resection
4. Traumatic intubation/endoscopy resulting in tracheal or esophageal perforation
5. Nerve blockade (i.e., intercostal, interscalene)
6. Positive-pressure ventilation/positive end-expiratory pressure
7. Continuous positive airway pressure

cause many signs and symptoms can be masked by the administration of anesthesia. Tachypnea, wheezing, increased peak airway pressures, and diminished breath sounds on the side of the pneumothorax will be present early on. If tension pneumothorax develops, hypotension and decreased cardiac output may occur as a result of compression of the great vessels. If untreated, cardiac arrest will ensue. Arterial blood gas analysis will demonstrate hypoxemia and hypercarbia as a result of both pulmonary shunting and alveolar hypoventilation. Chest x-rays are diagnostic but can be of limited use in the acute operating room setting.

Treatment of pneumothorax, like its manifestations, depends on the size and cause. When a small pneumothorax occurs and is hemodynamically insignificant, a "wait and see" approach can be taken. Many small pneumothoraces will resolve spontaneously. However, when a tension pneumothorax or other collapse occurs, the primary treatment is the immediate insertion of a chest tube to decompress the thorax and reexpand the lung. In an emergency situation needle aspiration with a 14-gauge Jelco may be necessary for acute relief and diagnosis. This is, however, not a substitute for a chest tube, which should be placed as soon as possible. If nitrous oxide is being used, it should be discontinued and replaced with 100% O_2 to prevent expansion of the air mass. Additionally, the delivery of high tidal volumes and very high airway pressures during mechanical ventilation must be minimized especially in the case of tension pneumothorax, until the pneumothorax can be decompressed. In these cases cardiac compromise will be more of a problem than alveolar hypoventilation and, therefore, must be dealt with first. If necessary, neuromuscular blockade can be used to allow ventilation of patients at lower airway pressures.

Although prevention of pneumothorax would be the ideal, it is usually not possible because of the pathogenesis of the condition. Efforts can be made to identify patients at risk and then avoid interventions known to predispose to pneumothorax. These include the use of nitrous oxide and high-pressure

mechanical ventilation. Minimizing delivered tidal volumes and respiratory rate may also aid in this endeavor. In most cases, the best that can be expected is early detection and intervention to avoid adverse sequelae.

☐ AIRWAY EMERGENCIES: LARYNGOSPASM

DETECTION

Upper airway obstruction is one of the most common complications seen in anesthesia practice. Although its causes are many, laryngospasm is by far the most life-threatening. Laryngospasm is the result of reflex closure of the vocal cords from sensory stimulation of the superior laryngeal nerve, causing partial or total obstruction of the glottic opening in response to some form of noxious stimulation during a light plane of anesthesia. It most often occurs during induction and emergence. Common causes include surgical manipulation, laryngoscopy, airway placement, and the presence of secretions, blood, or vomitus in the oropharynx.

When airway obstruction occurs, the anesthesia provider will observe the use of accessory muscles, sternal retractions, and the presence of a tracheal tug in the patient. With partial laryngospasm stridor will be audible with each respiratory effort. When obstruction is total, respiratory efforts will be present, but no air movement will be detectable. The patient will exhibit a characteristic "rocking" pattern of ventilation in which chest retraction and abdominal expansion occur on inspiration. Laryngospasm can be differentiated from other forms of upper airway obstruction by the placement of an oral or nasal airway. With laryngospasm, the obstruction will not improve.

If laryngospasm is left untreated hypoxia, hypercarbia, and acidosis will develop. This will be manifested in the patient with hypertension and tachycardia. Unless ventilation is restored within minutes, ventricular dysrhythmias and hypotension leading to cardiac arrest will ensue. Children are more prone to these complications than are adults because of their small FRC, high oxygen requirements, and limited respiratory reserve. Early intervention is therefore crucial.

TREATMENT

Treatment of laryngospasm is aimed at removing the noxious stimuli and deepening the anesthetic level whenever possible. This in itself may be sufficient to resolve an episode of laryngospasm. If the laryngospasm is not relieved by these measures, continuous positive airway pressure (10 to 20 cm H_2O) by face mask with 100% O_2 will help to distend the pharynx and vocal cords, causing them to open.[36] If still unsuccessful, a small dose of succinylcholine (10 to 20 mg/70 kg) will relax the skeletal muscle of the larynx, abduct the vocal cords, and allow the patient to be ventilated. Once the airway is reestablished, either the anesthetic level should be deepened or the patient should be allowed to awaken depending on when the laryngospasm occurred. If time permits, the patient's stomach should be decompressed to prevent regurgitation from distention during positive-pressure ventilation.

PREVENTION AND ANESTHETIC CONSIDERATIONS

Although not all episodes of laryngospasm can be prevented, it is unlikely to occur if laryngoscopy, airway manipulation, and/or extubation are attempted during deep surgical planes of anesthesia, when response to noxious stimulation is blunted. When deep extubation is attempted, patients should be transported to the recovery room in the lateral Sims' position (side-lying, head-down position) to facilitate drainage of secretions away from the larynx. If deep extubation is not possible, extubation should not be attempted until the patient is fully awake with all airway reflexes intact.

REFERENCES

1. Boston Collaborative Drug Surveillance Program. Drug induced anaphylaxis. *JAMA.* 1973; 224:613–615.
2. Wasserman SI, Marquardt DL. Anaphylaxis. In: Middelton E Jr, Reed CE, Ellis EF, Adkinson NF Jr, Yunginger JW, eds. *Allergy: Principles and Practice.* Vol. 2. St. Louis: CV Mosby; 1995:1365–1376.
3. Roizen MF. Anesthetic implications of concurrent diseases. In: Miller RD, ed. *Anesthesia.* Vol. 1, 4th ed. New York: Churchill Livingstone; 1994:962–963.
4. Slater JE. Rubber anaphylaxis. *N Engl J Med.* 1989; 320: 1126–1130.
5. Turjanmaa K. Incidence of immediate allergy to latex gloves in hospital personnel. *Contact Dermatitis.* 1987; 17:270–275.
6. Slater JE, Mostello LA, Shaer C. Rubber specific IgE in children with spina bifida. *J Urol.* 1991; 146:578–579.
7. Sethra NF, Sockin SM, Holzman RS, Slater JE. Latex anaphylaxis in a child with a history of multiple anesthetic drug allergies. *Anesthesiology.* 1992; 77:372–375.
8. Gerber AC, Jorg W, Zbinden S, Seger RA, Dangel PH. Severe intraoperative anaphylaxis to surgical gloves: latex allergy, an unfamiliar condition. *Anesthesiology.* 1989; 71:800–802.
9. Gold M, Swartz JS, Brande BM, Dolovich J, Shandling B, Gilmour RF. Intraoperative anaphylaxis: an association with latex sensitivity. *J Allergy Clin Immunol.* 1991;87: 662–666.
10. Maclennan DH, Duff C, Zorzato F, et al. Ryanodine receptor gene as a predisposition to malignant hyperthermia. *Nature.* 1990; 343:559–561.
11. Ording H. Incidence of malignant hyperthermia in Denmark. *Anesth Analg.* 1985; 64:700–704.
12. Ellis FR, Halsall PJ, Christian AS. Clinical presentation of suspected malignant hyperthermia during anesthesia in 402 probands. *Anaesthesia.* 1990; 45:838–841.
13. Verburg MP, Oerlemans FTJ, van Bennekom CA, et al. In vivo induced malignant hyperthermia in pigs. I: physiological and biochemical changes and the influence of dantrolene sodium. *Acta Anaesthesiol Scand.* 1984; 28:1–8.
14. Gronert GA, Antognini JF. Malignant hyperthermia. In: Miller RD, ed. *Anesthesia.* Vol. 1, 4th ed. New York: Churchill Livingstone; 1994:1075–1093.
15. Heffron JJA. Malignant hyperthermia: biochemical aspects of the acute episode. *Br J Anaesth.* 1988; 60:274–278.
16. Gronert GA. Malignant hyperthermia. *Anesthesiology.* 1980; 53:395–423, 427.
17. Berkowitz A, Rosenberg H. Femoral nerve blockade with mepivacaine for muscle biopsy in malignant hyperthermia patients. *Anesthesiology.* 1985; 62:651–652.
18. Keenan RL, Boyan CP. Cardiac arrest due to anesthesia. *JAMA.* 1985; 253:2373–2377.
19. Goldman L, Caldera DL, Nussbaum SR, et al. Multifactorial index of cardiac risk in noncardiac surgical procedures. *N Engl J Med.* 1977; 297:845–850.
20. Steen PA, Tinker JH, Tarhan S. Myocardial reinfarction after anesthesia and surgery. *JAMA.* 1978; 239:2566–2570.
21. Boysen PG. Pulmonary disease. In: Brown DL, ed. *Risk and Outcome in Anesthesia.* 2nd ed. Philadelphia: JB Lippincott; 1992:77.
22. Mendelson CL. The aspiration of stomach contents into the lungs during obstetric anesthesia. *Am J Obstet Gynecol.* 1946; 52:191–205.
23. Cameron JL, Mitchell WH, Zuidema GD. Aspiration pneumonia: clinical outcome following documented aspiration. *Arch Surg.* 1973; 106:49–52.
24. Arms RA, Dines DE, Tintsman TC. Aspiration pneumonia. *Chest.* 1974; 65:136–139.
25. Roberts RB, Shirley MA. Reducing the risk of acid aspiration during cesarean section. *Anesth Analg.* 1974; 53:859–868.
26. Wynne JW, Reynolds JC, Hood CI, et al. Steroid therapy for pneumonitis induced in rabbits by aspiration of foodstuff. *Anesthesiology.* 1979; 51:11–19.
27. Wynne JW, Modell JH: Respiratory aspiration of stomach contents. *Ann Intern Med.* 1977; 87:466–474.
28. Spence TH, Mehra MR, Bode FR. Pulmonary embolism. In: Civetta JM, Taylor RW, Kirby RR, eds. *Critical Care.* Philadelphia: JB Lippincott; 1992:1293–1301.
29. MacLaren AD, Stockwell MC, Reid VT. Anesthetic techniques for surgical correction of fractured neck of femur: a comparative study of spinal and general anesthesia in the elderly. *Anesthesia.* 1978; 33:10–14.
30. Modig J, Maripuu E, Sahlstedt B. Thromboembolism following total hip replacement: a prospective investigation of 94 patients with emphasis on the efficacy of lumbar epidural anesthesia in prophylaxis. *Reg Anesth.* 1986; 11:72.
31. Gossling HR, Pellegrini VD. Fat embolism syndrome: a review of the pathophysiological basis of treatment. *Clin Orthop.* 1982; 165:68–82.
32. Shapiro HM, Drummond JC. Neurosurgical anesthesia. In: Miller RD, ed. *Anesthesia.* Vol. 2, 4th ed. New York: Churchill Livingstone; 1994:1897–1946.
33. Pashayan AG. Monitoring the neurosurgical patient. In: Gravenstein N, ed. *Monitoring Problems in Anesthesia.* Philadelphia: JB Lippincott; 1987:104.
34. Kirby RR. Respiratory system. In: Gravenstein N, ed. *Manual of Complications During Anesthesia.* Philadelphia: JB Lippincott; 1991:346.
35. Moore DC, Bridenbaugh LD. Pneumothorax: its incidence following intercostal nerve block. *JAMA.* 1960; 174:842–847.
36. Gammage GW. Airway. In: Gravenstein N, ed. *Manual of Complications During Anesthesia.* Philadelphia: JB Lippincott; 1991:175.

☐ QUESTIONS

1. Anaphylaxis is a generalized systemic immunologic response characterized by all of the following *except*:
   a. The release of chemical mediators such as histamine as a result of a direct effect of an antigen on mast cells and basophils
   b. Reproducibility on reexposure to the antigen, "sensitization"
   c. Peripheral vasodilation, hypotension, and tachycardia
   d. Bronchospasm and upper airway edema

2. Treatment of anaphylaxis in the acute phase includes all of the following *except*:
   a. Epinephrine 0.05 to 0.1 mg IV
   b. Benadryl 0.5 to 1.0 mg/kg
   c. Emergency intubation and the administration of 100% O_2
   d. Intravascular volume expansion

3. The drug of choice for the treatment of anaphylaxis is:
   a. Benadryl
   b. Ephedrine
   c. Epinephrine
   d. Corticosteroids

4. Patient populations considered at high risk for the development of latex anaphylaxis include all of the following *except*:
   a. Spina bifida patients
   b. Patients requiring repeated bladder catheterizations
   c. Patients with a history of hypersensitivity after touching rubber balloons
   d. Patients with a history of mild latex glove contact dermatitis

5. Malignant hyperthermia is associated with all of the following *except*:
   a. Loss of intracellular calcium control in skeletal muscle leading to unopposed skeletal muscle contraction
   b. Autosomal recessive pattern of inheritance linked to chromosome 19
   c. Excessive production of heat, carbon dioxide, and lactic acid
   d. Increased incidence in patients with known or unknown neuromuscular disorders

6. Early signs and symptoms of malignant hyperthermia include all of the following *except*:
   a. Tachycardia
   b. Fever
   c. Skeletal muscle rigidity
   d. Hypercarbia

7. The first step in the treatment of malignant hyperthermia involves:
   a. Administration of dantrolene 1.0 to 2.5 mg/kg
   b. Internal and external cooling of the patient
   c. Discontinuation of all triggering agents
   d. Hyperventilation with 100% O_2

8. All of the following are considered "safe" in the anesthetic management of the malignant hyperthermia patient *except*:
   a. Propofol
   b. Amide local anesthetics
   c. Magnesium sulfate
   d. Sevoflurane

9. Dantrolene:
   a. Is recommended for routine prophylaxis in all malignant hyperthermia-susceptible patients
   b. Has no known side effects
   c. Inhibits the release of calcium from the sarcoplasmic reticulum in skeletal muscle
   d. Is not required after the acute phase of malignant hyperthermia

10. The number one cause of intraoperative cardiac arrest is:
    a. Intraoperative cardiac dysrhythmias
    b. Hypoxia and inadequate pulmonary ventilation
    c. Myocardial infarction
    d. Hemorrhage

11. Factors associated with increased risk for the development of pulmonary complications include all of the following *except*:
    a. Morbid obesity
    b. Presence of preexisting pulmonary disease
    c. Lower abdominal surgery
    d. History of smoking

12. Prevention of intraoperative bronchospasm involves all of the following *except*:
    a. Pretreatment with aerosolized bronchodilators
    b. Lidocaine 1 to 2 mg/kg IV
    c. Minimal airway manipulation
    d. The use of magnesium sulfate, atracurium, and thiopental for the induction and maintenance of anesthesia

13. The use of aminophylline for the treatment of intraoperative bronchospasm is reserved for cases unresponsive to sympathomimetics for all the following reasons *except*:
    a. Its onset of action is too long to be useful in the operative setting.
    b. Aminophylline has a narrow therapeutic window.

c. The metabolism of aminophylline is altered under many clinical conditions causing potential toxicity.

d. It requires careful monitoring of serum blood levels.

14. All of the following statements are true regarding aspiration of gastric contents *except*:
    a. Clinically significant cases of aspiration are associated with aspirates greater than 25 mL in volume and pH less than 2.5.
    b. Clear liquid aspirates cause more severe forms of tissue damage than aspirates of particulate matter.
    c. Pregnancy, obesity, hiatal hernia, and gastro-esophageal reflux are all conditions that increase the patient's risk for aspiration.
    d. Hypoxemia is the earliest and most diagnostic sign of aspiration.

15. Treatment of pulmonary aspiration involves:
    a. Routine use of corticosteroids and antibiotics
    b. Supplemental oxygen, mechanical ventilation, or continuous positive airway pressure to maintain PaO_2 greater than 80 mm Hg
    c. Tracheal intubation and suctioning
    d. Bronchoscopy and pulmonary lavage regardless of the aspirate involved

16. All of the following statements are true concerning pulmonary thromboemboli *except*:
    a. Symptoms are nonspecific and include dyspnea, tachycardia, hypoxemia, and pulmonary edema.
    b. Hypoxemia is caused by an increase in dead space ventilation and a loss of hypoxic pulmonary vasoconstriction reflex.
    c. Electrocardiographic changes include left axis deviation and anterior T wave inversion.
    d. Systemic heparinization is not used except in life-threatening circumstances because of the risk of hemorrhage.

17. The most sensitive diagnostic tool for the detection of venous air embolism is:
    a. Respiratory gas monitoring, end-tidal carbon dioxide, nitrogen
    b. Swan-Ganz catheter
    c. Precordial stethoscope
    d. Precordial Doppler

18. The first therapeutic measure instituted when venous air embolism is detected is:
    a. Aspiration of air from central line/pulmonary artery catheter
    b. Flooding of the surgical field with saline
    c. Discontinuation of nitrous oxide and the administration of 100% O_2
    d. Intravascular volume expansion

19. Pneumothorax is of special concern in the anesthetized patient for all of the following reasons *except*:
    a. Positive-pressure ventilation predisposes to the development of life-threatening tension pneumothorax.
    b. The administration of nitrous oxide can cause rapid expansion of a pneumothorax resulting in cardiovascular compromise.
    c. Early diagnosis can be difficult because signs and symptoms can be masked by the administration of anesthesia.
    d. Treatment of pneumothorax is more difficult in the anesthetized patent.

20. Complete laryngospasm can be differentiated from partial laryngospasm by:
    a. The use of accessory muscles and the presence of sternal retractions during normal breathing
    b. Presence of stridor
    c. A characteristic "rocking" pattern of ventilation
    d. Resolution with the presence of an oral airway

☐ ANSWERS

1. a	5. b	9. c	13. a	17. d
2. b	6. b	10. b	14. b	18. c
3. c	7. c	11. c	15. c	19. d
4. d	8. d	12. d	16. c	20. c

American Association of Nurse Anesthetists Latex Allergy Protocol

This latex allergy protocol was developed by the AANA Infection/Environmental Control Task Force and was approved by the AANA Board of Directors in April 1993.

Introduction

In the past four to five years, latex allergy has been recognized as a significant problem for specific patients (e.g., patients with spina bifida requiring multiple surgeries) and healthcare workers.[1]

Approximately 0.8% of the population is latex sensitive. However, patients and/or healthcare workers who have frequent exposure to latex devices such as gloves, catheters, and drains may be sensitized.[2] It has been reported that 6-7% of surgical personnel and 18-40% of spina bifida patients are latex sensitive.[3] It is estimated that 7.5% of surgeons and 5.6% of nurses are sensitive to latex or the chemicals used in processing latex.[2] Latex, the sap of the rubber tree *Hevea Brasiliensis*, contains low molecular weight soluble proteins which are the likely allergy cause. New rubber products, especially very soft ("dipped") products contain the greatest proportion of these soluble proteins.[3]

Immediate hypersensitivity reactions to latex vary from contact urticaria to systemic anaphylaxis that requires lifesaving intervention.

Anaphylactic reactions have complicated a variety of common medical procedures including surgery (particularly of the genito-urinary tract) and anesthesia, as well as oral, vaginal, and rectal examinations utilizing latex gloves. In most cases, there has been contact between latex products and mucous membranes. However, in some exquisitely sensitive individuals, exposure through inhalation of aerosolized latex or through intravenous administration has led to severe reactions. The type of reactions is similar to immediate drug reactions or stinging insect venom and may be associated with rapidly progressive anaphylaxis and death.[1]

The most reliable screening test for predicting an anaphylaxic reaction to latex is a medical history, as sensitive and specific reagents for testing for latex allergy are not commercially available at this time.[1]

Population Considered High Risk for Developing Latex Allergy

Individuals considered high risk for developing latex allergy should be labeled *latex risk*, and those that have known or suspected allergy to latex should be labeled *latex allergy*.

Patients (particularly of the pediatric age group) who are considered *high risk* include:

■ Those with neural tube defects —
   Myelomeningocele/meningocele
   Spina bifida
   Lipomyelomeningocele
■ Patients requiring chronic bladder catheterizations —
   Spinal cord trauma
   Exstrophy of the bladder
   Neurogenic bladder
■ Patients that have multiple operations
■ Those with a history of atopy and multiple allergies
■ Patients with occupational exposure to latex —
   Workers in latex industry
   Healthcare workers
■ Those with a history of allergic reaction after touching balloons, rubber gloves or powder from rubber gloves, dental dams, latex consumer products, and medical devices; especially atopic patients
■ Those with a history of having experienced anaphylactic reaction during surgery, urinary catheterization, rectal or vaginal examination, and/or bladder stimulation
■ Healthcare personnel and others who wear latex gloves, due to the generalized usage of universal precautions, may become sensitized.
■ Healthcare providers or other workers who give a history of mild latex glove eczema rarely have anaphylactic events. However, a

history of severe or worsening latex glove induced eczema, urticaria, or work-related conjunctivitis, rhinitis, asthma, or urticaria may indicate allergic sensitization and increase the risk for more severe reactions in the future.

Latex Avoidance Precautions

By touching any latex object, the healthcare worker can transmit the allergen by hand to the patient. Caution should be taken to keep the powder from the gloves away from the patient because the powder will act as a carrier for the latex protein. Therefore, in order to reduce the possibility of the latex protein becoming airborne, care must be taken not to snap gloves on and off.

Patients should be identified as being *latex sensitive*. The room needs to be labeled *latex free* to avoid personnel from bringing rubber products (wrist bands, chart labels, bed, room signs, etc.) into the room.

A readily available master list of *latex-free* devices and products should be developed.*

Establish a latex consultant in your institution; an allergist is recommended.

Develop programs to educate healthcare workers in the care of *latex-sensitive* patients.

Develop educational programs for patients and their families in the care and precautions that should be taken to prevent latex exposure. This should encompass a first-aid protocol in the event a severe reaction should arise.

Encourage *latex-sensitive* patients to obtain and carry with them, at all times, some type of identification such as a medical alert bracelet.

---

*A sample letter to manufacturers requesting latex information and resource articles regarding latex allergy are available in a *Latex Packet* from the Practice Department, American Association of Nurse Anesthetists, 222 South Prospect Avenue, Park Ridge, IL 60068-4001. Phone: (708) 692-7050, ext. 305

Recommendations for Patient Care — Patients with Latex Allergy or Latex Risk[1,4,5]

Schedule *latex-allergy* and/or *latex-risk* patients as the first case(s) in the morning. This will allow latex dust (from the previous day) to be removed overnight.

The Operating Room

■ Remove all latex products from the operating room.
■ Bring a *latex-free* cart (if available) into the room.
■ Use a *latex-free* reservoir bag. If not available, cover the existing one with a plastic bag and secure with tape.
■ Use a *non-latex* circuit with plastic mask and bag.
■ Ventilator bellows must be a *non-latex* bellows.
■ Place all monitoring devices, cords/tubes (oximeter, blood pressure, ECG wires) in stockinet and secure with tape.

Intravenous Line Preparation

■ Use intravenous (IV) tubing without latex ports.
■ If unable to obtain IV tubing without latex ports, cover latex ports with tape.
■ Cover all rubber injection ports on IV bags with tape and label in the following way: *Do not inject or withdraw fluid through the latex port.*

Operating Room Patient Care

■ Use *non-latex* gloves. (Use caution when selecting non-latex gloves. Not all substitutes are equally impermeable to bloodborne pathogens; care and investigation should be taken in the selection of substitute gloves.)

- Use *non-latex* tourniquets/may use *non-latex* examination glove or polyvinyl chloride tubing.
- Draw medication directly from opened multidose vials (remove stoppers) if medications are not available in ampoules.
- Draw up medications just prior to the beginning of the case. The rubber allergen could leach out of the plunger of the syringe causing a reaction.
- Glass syringes are another alternative.
- Use stopcocks to inject drugs rather than latex ports.
- Minimize mixing/agitating lyophilized drugs in multidose vials with rubber stoppers.
- Notify Pharmacy and Central Supply that the patient you are caring for is latex sensitive so that these departments can use the appropriate procedure when preparing preparations for the patient.

Signs and Symptoms of Allergic Reactions to Latex[6]

Symptoms usually occur within 30 minutes from anesthesia induction. However, the time of onset can range from 10-290 minutes.

Awake Patient	*Anesthetized Patient*
Itchy eyes	Tachycardia
Generalized pruritus	Hypotension
Shortness of breath	Wheezing
Feeling of faintness	Bronchospasm
Feeling of impending doom	Cardiorespiratory arrest
Nausea	Flushing
Vomiting	Facial edema
Abdominal cramping	Laryngeal edema
Diarrhea	Urticaria
Wheezing	

Management

All the following should be done to manage a latex allergic reaction:

- Remove latex agents, if possible. **Do not delay immediate emergency therapy.**
- Stop treatment/procedure.
- Support airway—administer 100% oxygen.*
- Start intravascular volume expansion with **Ringer's lactate*** or **normal saline.***
- Administer **epinephrine*** 0.5-1.0 µg/kg bolus (10 µg/mL dilution). May need to repeat dose or give subcutaneously or by continuous infusion.

Secondary Treatment:

- **Diphenhydramine*** 1 mg/kg IV (maximum dose 50 mg).
- **Methylprednisolone*** 2 mg/kg IV (maximum dose 125 mg).
- **Ranitidine*** 0.5 mg/kg IV every 6 hours for 2-4 doses (maximum dose 50 mg).

*These drugs and fluids should be readily available for timely administration.

Recommended Premedication Prior to Procedure[5,6]

The use of preoperative prophylaxis may not change the rate of anaphylaxis but may lessen the severity of a reaction. All of the following are recommended:

Outpatient
- **Prednisone:** 1mg/kg by mouth every 6 hours (maximum dose 40 mg/dose) for 12-24 hours prior to the patient arriving at the hospital and 1 hour prior to the induction of anesthesia
- **Hydroxyzine:** 0.7 mg/kg by mouth every 6 hours (maximum dose 50 mg/dose) for 12-24 hours prior to the patient arriving at the hospital and 1 hour prior to the induction of anesthesia

Inpatient
- **Methylprednisolone:** 1 mg/kg IV every 6 hours for 2-4 doses (maximum dose 125 mg)
- **Diphenhydramine:** 1mg/kg IV every 6 hours for 2-4 doses (maximum dose 50 mg)

- **Ranitidine:** 0.5 mg/kg IV every 6 hours for 2-4 doses (maximum dose 50 mg)

Medication may be discontinued postoperatively if there is no evidence of an allergic reaction intraoperatively or postoperatively.

Inpatients with known *latex allergy* should be continued on the inpatient protocol for 24 hours postoperatively.

Common Latex Medical Devices Used in the Hospital[4-6]
- Mattresses found on stretchers
- Rubber gloves
- Adhesive tape
- Urinary catheters
- Electrode pads
- Wound drains
- Stomach and intestinal tubes
- Condom urinary collection devices
- Protective sheets
- Enema tubing kits
- Dental cofferdams
- Rubber pads
- Fluid circulating warming blankets
- Hemodialysis equipment
- Ambu bags
- Bulb syringes
- Elastic bandages, Ace™ wraps
- Medication vial stoppers
- Stethoscope tubing
- Band-Aids™ and other similar products
- Gloves — examination and sterile
- Patient controlled analgesia syringes
- Tourniquets

Anesthesia Equipment Containing Latex
- Rubber masks
- Electrode pads, e.g., electrocardiogram, peripheral nerve stimulator
- Head straps
- Rubber tourniquets
- Rubber nasal-pharyngeal airways
- Rubber oral-pharyngeal airways
- Teeth protectors
- Bite blocks
- Blood pressure cuffs (inner bladder and tubing)
- Rubber breathing circuits
- Reservoir breathing bags
- Rubber ventilator hoses
- Rubber ventilator bellows
- Rubber endotracheal tubes
- Latex cuffs on plastic tracheal tubes
- Latex injection ports on intravenous tubing
- Certain epidural catheter injection adapters
- Multidose vial stoppers
- Patient controlled analgesia syringes
- Rubber suction catheters
- Injection ports on intravenous bags

REFERENCES

(1) *Interim Recommendations to Health Professionals and Organizations Regarding Latex Allergy Precautions.* Palatine, Illinois: American College of Allergy and Immunology. March 1992.

(2) Latex Allergies: Anesthesia Concerns. *AANA NewsBulletin/Anesthesia Quality Plus.* 1992;46(9)(suppl):3.

(3) U.S. Food and Drug Administration. Allergic reactions to latex-containing medical devices. *FDA Medical Bulletin.* 1991; 21:2.

(4) Holzman R. *Latex-Free Environment Precautions for Patients with a Latex Allergy/Patients at High Risk for Latex Allergy.* Boston, Massachusetts: Boston Children's Hospital (Departmental Policy). 1992.

(5) Pasquariello CA. Lowe DA. *Protocol for the Management of Patients with Allergy and Risk for Allergy to Latex Products.* Department of Anesthesia and Critical Care, St. Christopher's Hospital for Children, Philadelphia, Pennsylvania. 1992.

(6) Roy CA, Barton CR. Intraoperative latex anaphylaxis compounded by atracurium sensitivity: A case report. *AANA Journal.* 1991;59:399-404.

SEVEN

Anesthesia Outside the Operating Suite

CHAPTER 32

Anesthesia for Specialty Areas

Colleen T. Ober

As health care continues to change with the emergence of a greater number of outpatient surgical centers, new less invasive specialty procedures, and more technical diagnostic procedures, the anesthetist is required to spend more time away from the main operating suite. These procedures are often performed in remote hospital locations and present unique problems such as lack of personnel and equipment and special environmental considerations. This chapter reviews basic anesthesia for patients undergoing electroshock wave lithotripsy (ESWL), electroconvulsive therapy (ECT), and diagnostic procedures; issues facing patients in the postanesthesia care unit (PACU) and critical care are discussed. Finally, the chapter concludes with a discussion of the care of the cancer patient with a focus on antineoplastic agents, surgical procedures, and pain management.

☐ ELECTROSHOCK WAVE LITHOTRIPSY

The surgical removal of urinary calculi is becoming obsolete since the advent of ESWL in the early 1980s. ESWL is a noninvasive method that uses shock waves to disintegrate urinary calculi. Although newer second-generation lithotripters produce less pain than earlier models,[1] anesthesia is needed to maintain analgesia, immobility, and support of vital functions.

This procedure occurs in a special operating room with a large tub filled with demineralized water. The patient is placed in the semi-Fowler's position with arms secured over the head. At the base of the tub within an elliptical cone, a high-energy spark (18,000 to 20,000 V) creates an underwater bubble that compresses surrounding water. Body tissues have a density equivalent to the water; therefore, there is little impedance to a shock wave of 15,000 psi generated and transmitted to a focal point 23 cm above the floor of the tub. Patient placement (Figure 32–1) is such that the target stone is located at a 1.5 cm³ focal point; this focal point is obtained by the use of two fluoroscopy units at right angles, which results in a three-dimensional image of the stone.[2] Crystalline objects that lie above the focal point will be shattered.

Shocks generated by the lithotripters are synchronized to occur 20 milliseconds after the R wave on an electrocardiogram (ECG). Over a 30- to 60-minute period, a series of 1000 to 2000 shocks may be delivered to eliminate the stone. Remaining stone fragments will pass with normal urine flow over several days.[3]

ANESTHETIC MANAGEMENT

Adequate preoperative evaluation should include routine laboratory tests such as urinalysis, hematocrit, electrolytes, and a coagulation profile. Careful assessment of cardiopulmonary status is imperative because these systems are greatly affected by physical changes produced by immersion into the water bath. Patients with permanent pacemakers are questionable candidates because shock waves may interfere with pacemaker function.

Monitoring should include blood pressure monitoring and a five-lead ECG. ECG leads and wires should be covered with a bio-occlusive dressing to minimize interference. The distance between the anesthetist and patient is relatively far. Therefore, pulse oximetry and end-tidal CO_2 ($ETCO_2$) monitoring are necessary to ensure adequate airway support and to detect possible disconnects and accidental extubation.

General anesthesia with conventional mechanical and jet

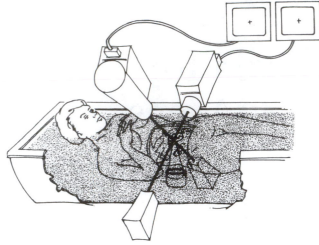

Figure 32–1 Positioning for beam during ESWL.

Table 32–1
CONTRAINDICATIONS TO ELECTROSHOCK WAVE LITHOTRIPSY

Absolute

- Aortic aneuyrsm
- Orthopedic implants in the lumbar region
- Pregnancy
- Coagulation disorders
- Morbid obesity
- Hemangioma in the vertebral canal

Relative

- Cardiac disease
- Cardiac pacemaker

---

ventilation or regional and monitored sedation techniques have all been used successfully for patients undergoing ESWL. Regional anesthesia is an attractive choice because the patient may be moved in and out of the tub to radiology to confirm stone dissolution. Movement is easier in an awake patient. Epidural is preferred to spinal anesthesia because the exact duration of the procedure will vary from patient to patient. An anesthetic level to dermatome T-6 is required for ESWL.[2] Disadvantages of this technique include a precipitous drop in blood pressure from sympathetic blockade and relative hypovolemia. Blood pressure effects can be attenuated with adequate intravenous (IV) fluid replacement and immersion in the tub. The hydrostatic compression of the lower extremities will increase central venous pressure (CVP).[3] Chest wall excursion from spontaneous respiration can cause stone movement, making ablation more difficult. In addition, pain radiating from the shock site may not be attenuated by regional blockade.

General anesthesia provides adequate anesthesia and analgesia as well as a secure airway. Reduction in functional residual capacity (FRC) from hydrostatic pressure is attenuated by mechanical ventilation. However, caudad movement of the diaphragm from large tidal volumes may move the stone from the target focus. The use of high-frequency jet ventilation with IV agents has been suggested. Overall, minimal stone movement from diaphragm movement has not altered the success rate of ESWL[4]; therefore, jet ventilation is undesirable because of the added necessary equipment and the potential for barotrauma. Disadvantages of general anesthesia include the potential for brachial plexus injury from arm positioning, endobronchial intubation from extreme head flexion, and airway disconnects.

ANESTHETIC CONCERNS

Cardiovascular considerations include the potential for dysrhythmias and alterations in CVP and systemic pressure. Shock waves triggered on the R wave can produce premature ventricular contraction (PVC), tachycardia, and atrioventric-

ular (AV) dissociation. Be prepared to treat dysrhythmias with lidocaine, verapamil, or atropine as needed. Immersion into warm water causes vasodilation with a drop in systemic blood pressure and increased CVP. Increased venous return may be poorly tolerated by patients with preexisting congestive heart failure or valvular dysfunction. Assess the need for CVP or pulmonary artery pressure monitoring.

Hypoxemia from atelectasis and ventilation/perfusion (V/Q) mismatch is produced by the *reduction in FRC* from hydrostatic forces against the chest wall. This can be attenuated by mechanical ventilation with 10 to 15 cc/kg tidal volume.

Other concerns include potential nerve injury, hematoma at the stone site, and temperature alterations from the water bath.[5]

Contraindications are listed in Table 32–1.[6]

☐ ELECTROCONVULSIVE THERAPY

Electroconvulsive therapy became a routine procedure to treat psychiatric patients in the 1940s. Today, ECT remains a staple in the treatment of patients with severe acute depression, suicidal tendencies, and no response to antidepressant pharmaceutical regimes. The exact mechanisms responsible for the therapeutic effect of ECT remain unknown.

PROCEDURE

Conduction electrodes are attached to the patient's head over one or both cerebral hemispheres. Although bilateral lead placement is frequently used, unilateral lead placement on the nondominant hemisphere causes less memory disturbance and preserves language function.[7] These electrodes are then connected to a machine that generates an electrical stimulus.

The ECT machines produce brief electrical pulses of 60 Hz, with a duration of 0.75 seconds, which are combined with periods of electrical inactivity.[8] The induced seizures consist of a tonic phase that occurs 2 to 3 seconds after stimulation and lasts 10 to 12 seconds. A 30- to 50-second clonic phase immediately follows the first phase.[9] To produce the clinically desired effects, seizure duration should be at least 30 seconds.[10]

Treatments are given two to three times a week until a clinical effect is achieved or until the patient receives no further benefit.

PHYSIOLOGIC EFFECTS

Central Nervous System   There is marked increase in cerebral metabolism and cerebral oxygen consumption from ECT-produced seizures. These increased metabolic needs are met by a sevenfold increase in cerebral blood flow that follows an initial period of cerebrovascular constriction, which occurs as the electrical stimulus passes through brain tissue.[8] This rapid increase in cerebral blood flow correlates with an increase in intracranial pressure. Therefore, patients with increased intracranial pressure and fixed intracranial lesions are not candidates for ECT.

Cardiovascular System   Electroconvulsive therapy produces an overall Valsalva effect from the stimulation of the vagus nerve. An initial cholinergic discharge inhibits the sinoatrial node, producing bradycardia, ventricular escape beats, AV dissociation, and possible asystole. The cholinergic phase is followed by an increase in sympathetic (adrenergic) discharge with subsequent hypertension, increased systemic vascular resistance (SVR), and sinus tachycardia with rates up to 120 to 200 beats/min.[9]

Cholinergic effects can be attenuated by preoperative treatment with atropine. IV atropine is more effective than intramuscular and glycopyrrolate may be as effective with less increase in heart rate.[11]

Sympathetic effects can be ameliorated by preoperative β blockade, phenoxybenzamine, or intraoperative sodium nitroprusside. Dysrhythmias can be treated by ensuring adequate ventilation, perioperative beta-blocking agents such as propranalol, or dysrhythmic agents such as lidocaine.

Respiratory System   Increases in cerebral oxygen consumption, tachycardia, and muscle activity produced by ECT lead to greater metabolic oxygen needs. Oxygen therapy and maintenance of adequate ventilation before and immediately after the electrical stimulus is required to avoid hypoxemia.[12] The airway should be secured with an endotracheal tube if the patient is at risk for aspiration. A bite block may be inserted to prevent damage to teeth.

ANESTHETIC CONSIDERATIONS

Anesthetic management must consider the patient's underlying physiologic disease and concomitant drug therapy. Preoperative evaluation should consider possible underlying intracranial pathology and cardiac and pulmonary disease. A baseline ECG should be performed. It is extremely important to note history of angina and cardiovascular disease because *cardiopulmonary dysfunction* accounts for 85% of the deaths attributed to ECT.[7] ECT is contraindicated in patients with a history of recent myocardial infarction (within 6 to 12 months). Permanent pacemakers are not contraindicated; however, a chest x-ray should be obtained to ensure that the pacemaker generator and leads are intact. Synchronous AV pacers should be changed to a fixed rate to prevent possible misfires.

Premedication is not desirable because it may prolong postoperative sedation or alter seizure threshold.

Induction Agents   The ideal agent used for ECT should have a rapid onset and short duration, without altering seizure threshold. Methohexitol has been the drug of choice for ECT because of its rapid induction and faster recovery compared to sodium thiopental. Drawbacks of methohexitol include decreased duration of seizures produced by ECT, central nervous system (CNS) excitement, hiccoughs, and involuntary muscle movements.

Thiopental offers little advantage as an induction agent and prolongs recovery time when compared to methohexitol. There is an increased incidence of postictal ECG anomalies including PVCs, atrial dysrhythmias, heart block, and ST wave changes in patients with preexisting coronary artery disease receiving thiopental for ECT.[8]

Propofol appears to be an ideal agent for ECT. However, recent studies suggest that propofol has anticonvulsive effects and that seizure duration is reduced to less than the recommended 25 to 30 seconds.[13] Although the actual exhibited clinical effect may not be changed,[14] propofol decreases blood pressure to a greater degree on induction when compared to methohexitol.

Ketamine is a poor choice for ECT because of increases in intracranial pressure, myoclonus, and myocardial oxygen consumption.

The cardiovascular stability of etomidate may make it a logical choice in patients with a significant cardiac history. However, prolonged recovery, myoclonus, and activation of seizure foci are deterrents. In addition, etomidate is associated with a high degree of postoperative nausea and vomiting.

Succinylcholine remains the muscle relaxant of choice to prevent damage to teeth, fractures, and damage to limbs from electrically induced seizures. The optimal dose to reduce risk of fractures and decrease duration of postseizure apnea is 0.5 mg/kg.[11] To determine the presence of seizure activity, in addition to the use of electroencephalography, an extremity can be isolated by the use of a tourniquet. The tourniquet is inflated to occlude arterial circulation before succinylcholine is injected; muscle tremors can be detected in the isolated limb.

Electroconvulsive Therapy and Psychotropic Drugs

Antipsychotics

Drugs included in this class are phenothiazines, thioxanthenes, and butyrophenones. Their therapeutic action is through the antagonism of dopamine at receptor sites.

Dopaminergic blockade can lead to a decrease in blood pressure as well as a potentiation in sedative effects of barbiturates, narcotics, and other sedative hypnotics.[15] Phenothiazines may decrease serum pseudocholine and prolong the neuromuscular effects of succinylcholine.[9]

TRICYCLICS

Tricyclics interfere with the reuptake of norepinephrine and serotonin in postganglionic symptomatic nerve endings. Continuation of tricyclics in the perioperative period is considered safe, but there are several drug reactions of importance. There is a two- to tenfold increase in pressor response when intraoperative hypotension is treated with indirect-acting sympathomimetic drugs such as ephedrine. It is best to treat intraoperative hypotension with phenylephedrine or methoxamine. Anticholinergic effects of tricyclics are additive and preoperative treatment with atropine increases postoperative disorientation.[16]

MONOAMINE OXIDASE INHIBITORS

There has been a resurgence in the use of monoamine oxidase inhibitors (MAOIs) to treat depression. MAOIs include phenelzine, isocarboxazid, iproniazid, tranylcypromine, pargyline, clorgyline, and selegiline. These pharmaceuticals inhibit the enzyme monoamine oxidase, which is the primary intraneural enzyme precursor to the neurotransmitters norepinephrine, epinephrine, dopamine, and serotonin. It is the increase in these neurotransmitters (dopamine, serotonin) that produces the antidepressant effects.

Discontinuation of MAOIs 2 weeks before anesthesia has been standard practice in many institutions. However, this may not be possible in the acutely depressed patient presenting for ECT. A recent study implies that patients on chronic MAOI therapy for greater than 3 weeks do not exhibit cardiovascular instability perioperatively.[17]

Treat perioperative hypotension with direct-acting sympathomimetics such as phenylephrine. As with tricyclics, exaggerated sedative effects develop from opioids and barbiturates and their doses should be decreased by 25%. Meperidine is contraindicated. The combination of meperidine and MAOIs can lead to a hypermetabolic state that presents as hypertension, CNS excitability, convulsions, and hyperpyrexia. Increased IV fluid and acidification of urine with lysine hydrochloride with production of a large urine output may facilitate meperidine excretion.[16] Treatment of MAOI crisis is supportive. Treat symptoms with cooling to decrease temperature, oxygen to meet metabolic demand, and sodium nitroprusside or phentolamine to lower blood pressure.

LITHIUM

Lithium is used for the treatment of mania. Alteration in gamma-aminobutyric acid, dopamine, serotonin, or acetylcholine may be responsible for the effects of lithium. (Normal blood levels should range from 0.75 to 1.5 mEg/L.) Lithium toxicity is common; the therapeutic window is small. Lithium toxicity is precipitated by factors that increase proximal tubular resorption of sodium such as dehydration, decreased sodium intake, and diuretics.[18]

Table 32–2
CONTRAINDICATIONS TO ELECTROCONVULSIVE THERAPY

Absolute

- Recent myocardial infarction—6–12 mo
- Recent cerebrovascular accident
- Intracranial mass lesion

Relative

- Severe pulmonary disease
- Congestive heart failure
- Glaucoma
- Retinal detachment
- Thrombophlebitis—prior treatment with minidose heparin
- Severe osteoporosis
- Angina
- Cardiac pacemaker—change to asynchronous mode

SOURCE: Reproduced by permission from Selvin.[10]

Lithium acts as a poor substitute for sodium ions. It is the effects on sodium channels that is of significance to the nurse anesthetist. Lithium ion substitution for the sodium ion alters the resting membrane potential at the neuromuscular junction and reduces the height of the action potential.[19] Action of depolarizing and nondepolarizing muscle relaxants can be prolonged and use of a nerve stimulator is recommended to adequately titrate neuromuscular blocking agents.

CONTRAINDICATIONS

Contraindications to ECT are listed in Table 32–2.[10] Pregnancy is relatively contraindicated. However, it may be less risky in severe acute depression to treat the parturient with ECT than antidepressant drugs that would cross the placenta and affect the fetus.[10]

MALIGNANT NEUROLEPT SYNDROME

Malignant neurolept syndrome occurs in 0.5% to 1% of all patients receiving antipsychotic medication. The exact mechanism of neurolept malignant syndrome is unknown. Dopamine antagonism in the brain[20] or dysfunction in skeletal muscle similar to malignant hyperthermia[21] may produce the muscular rigidity, confusion, hypermetabolism, and autonomic symptoms associated with the syndrome. Predisposing factors are exhaustion, dehydration, and concurrent brain disease.

Treatment of a malignant neurolept syndrome is symptomatic with dantrolene, carbidopa/levodopa combination, and bromocriptine.[20] Use of a nondepolarizing muscle relaxant such as curare will help with a differential diagnosis. *Malignant hyperthermia is postsynaptic in origin, whereas neurolept malignant syndrome is presynaptic* and these patients will respond to neuromuscular blockade with flaccid muscle paralysis.[22]

☐ MAGNETIC RESONANCE IMAGING AND COMPUTED TOMOGRAPHY

COMPUTED TOMOGRAPHY SCAN

Computed tomography (CT) scans are used to detect intracranial, intrathoracic, and abdominal pathology. CT scans can also be used to diagnose spinal, long bone, and pelvic fractures and intervertebral disk herniation or compression.

Computed tomography uses a standard x-ray beam within a tube. The x-ray beams that pass through the patient are detected by two sensory devices that constantly point to the x-ray source. The image produced by the scan rotates by 1° with each image and this continues for a full 180°.[23]

Sedation or general anesthesia is used to decrease movement during imaging. CT scanning does not interfere with routine monitoring devices and poses little interference with anesthetic management. Problems with CT scanning are the inaccessibility of the patient to the anesthetist, decreased patient visualization, exposure to ionizing radiation, and allergic reactions to radiographic contrast dyes.

MAGNETIC RESONANCE IMAGING

In the body, the nucleus of certain atoms, principally hydrogen nuclei (protons), sodium, and carbon, when placed in a magnetic field, absorb or emit radiation. Nuclei with an odd number of protons are responsive to magnetic resonance imaging (MRI). In the presence of the magnetic field the protons in the body act like magnets and align themselves with the magnetic field produced by the MRI in the long axis of the patient. Radiofrequent pulses are used by means of a coil surrounding the patient in the MRI and rotate the protons into the transverse plane, thus producing the image.[23]

Patient immobility is crucial; even slight changes in position reduce the consistency of the magnetic field, which in turn will result in a distorted MRI signal and an inferior final image.

Anesthesia is used frequently in pediatric and adult patients during MRI. Unfortunately, the unique properties of the MRI scanner make monitoring patients and the administration of anesthetic agents an arduous task.

Monitoring and the Magnet Standard monitoring of patients receiving either sedation or general anesthesia is a requirement. However, monitoring devices can act as radiofrequency antennae and distort images. In addition, objects made of ferrous magnetic material become projectile when the magnet is activated. Anesthesia and monitoring equipment must be located beyond the 30 to 50 gauss line (actual distance in feet depends on field strength and shielding), or must be made of nonferrous materials to avoid flying objects in the MRI suite.[24]

Anesthetic Equipment Within the magnetic field, ECG leads and cables can produce an altered ECG reading, which may resemble hyperkalemia or pericarditis. In addition, rapidly changing magnetic fields produce energy changes across loops of ECG leads and may resemble tachycardia on the ECG.[24]

To minimize ECG interference avoid twisting ECG cables; place leads close to the magnetic center and in close proximity to one another. Fiberoptic cables and electrodes can be used; the magnetic field does not interfere with these tracings.[25]

Blood pressure monitoring with noninvasive oscillometric devices or invasive arterial pressures does not alter images produced by MRI. However, when using disposable or nondisposable cuffs it is important to ensure that these monitors are free of metal connectors and that leads from all invasive arterial and venous catheters pass through a radiofrequency filter.

Pulse oximetry provides an indirect assessment of a patient's respiratory status. Unfortunately, within the magnetic field both oxygen saturation (SaO_2) and MRI signals can be altered. In addition, pulse oximetry has produced burns on some patients, possibly caused by heat generated by electrical currents passing through electrical oximetry lead wires. To avoid these complications, SaO_2 detectors should be placed as far away from the magnetic core as possible (e.g., place on the toe if scanning the head); avoid looping cable wires and place padding between the wires and the patient's skin.[26]

Burns have also been associated with the use of esophageal stethoscope probes to monitor axillary temperature. Again, avoid wire loops and unnecessary skin contact or switch to intermittent sampling.[27]

Anesthesia With a patient located within a narrow magnetic tube, airway management can become impossible. When providing monitored sedation it is vital to have SaO_2 and $ETCO_2$ monitoring. $ETCO_2$ monitoring can be provided by use of a nasal cannula with a special adapter or by improvising with an IV catheter attached to restrictive tubing placed through the nasal cannula. MRI does not interrupt $ETCO_2$ sampling although end-tidal values may be *decreased* from long extension tubing. Oxygen therapy should be administered from wall sources or from aluminum tank sources.

General anesthesia in the MRI suite can be provided with the patient spontaneously breathing or paralyzed with controlled ventilation. A laryngeal mask airway (LMA) can be used to provide general anesthesia in children and adults. LMAs contain no ferromagnetic materials and special spring-free models (standard models contain metallic springs in the pilot valve) are available for MRI so there is no interference with scanning. A disadvantage that must be remembered is that the LMA does not provide a water-tight seal and does not ensure against the risk of aspiration. LMAs should not be used to maintain general anesthesia in patients with hiatal hernia, obesity, gastric obstruction, or a high potential for gastric aspiration.[28]

When providing general anesthesia through an endotracheal tube it is important to avoid the use of anode tubes because of their metal components. When intubating, the anesthetist should use laryngoscopes with lithium paper-covered batteries or disposable plastic laryngeal scopes, or intubate outside the magnetic field. Laryngeal scopes themselves do not contain ferromagnetic materials but the batteries inside make them highly projectile.[24]

Connection of the endotracheal tube to a modified Ayres T piece or Bain's system using IV agents and maintaining spontaneous ventilation has been suggested. You may also use long tubing connected to a ventilator outside of the magnetic field. Ohmeda manufactures a machine for MRI with aluminum oxygen and nitrogen tanks and a stainless steel frame. This machine, with Tec 4 vaporizors, can be used within the field without interference in MRI image or alteration in inspired concentration of volatile agents. MRI will not affect the concentration of inhalation agents in these vaporizors.[29]

Most often you will be sedating or anesthetizing children for MRI. The agents used should be safe and ensure immobility with rapid recovery. Intramuscular pediatric cocktails consisting of meperidine, promethazine, secobarbitol, and atropine have been used in the past; however, they have been associated with ineffective sedation[25] and greater amounts of respiratory depression.[30] Oral chloral hydrate has also been used (75 to 80 mg/kg), but it does not provide adequate sedation in 15% of pediatric patients.[25]

All IV agents for sedation and anesthesia in the MRI suite have some undesirable effects. Ketamine increases intracranial pressure and its use is inappropriate in pediatric patients with brain masses, artiovenous malformation, or hydrocephalus.

Methohexitol decreases response to pain and agitation; however, it is associated with greater amounts of oropharyngeal secretions, which can lead to laryngeal spasm. Rectal methohexitol has variable absorption and sedative effects.

Propofol can be advantageous in the pediatric population; it allows quick sedation, easy titration, and swift recovery. Presently, propofol is not recommended for use in pediatric patients for sedation or use in children under 3 years of age.[31] There have also been reports of tolerance in some patients undergoing repeated procedures.[32]

Laryngeal mask airways can be used to provide general anesthesia. Remove the LMA carefully at the end of the procedure after adequate oropharyngeal suctioning. There is an increased incidence of laryngeal spasm with LMA removal in children.[28]

Contraindications Magnetic resonance imaging is not recommended for use in female patients in the first trimester of pregnancy. Permanent pacemakers should be placed in demand mode because the MRI field can induce electrical currents and may inhibit pacemaker function. Intracranial clips may move if they are made of ferromagnetic material. In addition, large metallic implants may generate heat, producing pain and discomfort.

Finally, the anesthetist should leave digital watches, credit cards, scissors, identification tags, and stethoscopes at home. All can be erased or drawn to the magnet.[23]

MONITORED ANESTHESIA CARE

Many surgical and diagnostic procedures today are performed under local anesthetic blocks with anesthesia standing by for monitoring IV sedation and emergency airway management. Monitored sedation should provide the patient with amnesia and analgesia. This should render patients anxiety and pain free so they will better tolerate the operative environment and surgical procedure. Muscle relaxation and anesthesia *are not* included in monitored sedation. The patient should be easily arousable to verbal and tactile stimuli. There is a fine line between sedation and general anesthesia. The anesthetist is the key monitor to gauge an adequate level of sedation without passing into a level of general anesthesia.

Types of procedures appropriate for monitoring sedation include cataract extraction, peripheral biopsies, hernia repairs, Mediport/Broviac insertion, bone marrow biopsies, MRI and CT scan, and cardiac catheterization. IV sedation may also be given to supplement regional anesthetic blocks. Therapeutic agents most frequently used for sedation are short-acting medications. Choice of agents should include an anxiolytic, such as midazolam, an opioid such as alfentanil, and an amnestic such as thiopental, propofol, or ketamine. Oxygen supplementation via nasal cannula is vital.

Along with sedation, monitored anesthesia care includes monitoring. A vigilant anesthetist is the best monitor. Routine monitoring equipment should include a blood pressure cuff, ECG, pulse oximetry, precordial stethoscope, and a temperature probe. Some form of $ETCO_2$ monitoring is also desirable if available.

There are several important aspects to remember during monitored sedation. First, be prepared with oral/nasal airways, endotracheal tubes, and suctioning and induction agents, in the event that you need to rapidly maintain the airway or proceed to general anesthesia. Second, maintain a constant rapport with the patient to alleviate anxiety and monitor the depth of sedation. Finally, communicate with the surgeon. Know the amount of local anesthetic given and notify the surgeon if the patient feels noxious stimuli. Patients may move because of discomfort, dysphoria, or prolonged surgical time. Reassure the patient, ensure that an adequate block has been given, and if movement continues and the surgeon is unable to attain adequate exposure, proceed with a general anesthetic.

☐ POSTOPERATIVE CARE UNIT/CRITICAL CARE

The standards of the American Association of Nurse Anesthetists (AANA) for care in the PACU are listed in the appendix.

Perhaps the most critical episodes you will address as a nurse anesthetist will occur in the immediate postoperative period or when you are called to an emergency situation requiring rapid airway management.

Problems most frequently occurring in the postoperative period include alterations in respiratory status, hypertension, hypotension, cardiac dysrhythmias, pain, decreased urine output, and emergence delirium.

PULMONARY CHANGES

Significant alterations occur in oxygenation and elimination of carbon dioxide during general anesthesia. Alterations such as increased right-to-left shunt, increased alveolar dead space, altered oxygen delivery, alterations in cardiac output, and decreased FRC (secondary to the cephalad movement of the diaphragm with increased closing capacity leading to an increase in pulmonary artery-alveolar gradient) may occur.[33] Regardless of the cause, all factors may lead to a greater potential for V/Q mismatch and postoperative hypoxemia.

Reduction in Pa_{O_2} after general anesthesia is greatest within the first 3 hours after surgery, but may last for days depending on the surgical site and the patient's premorbid condition. Patient factors that increase the risk of postoperative respiratory events include age over 60 years, male gender, underlying cardiopulmonary disease, diabetes, obesity, thoracoabdominal incisions, narcotic overdose, and emergency surgery.[34]

Postoperative factors that lead to hypoxia are decreased ventilation from anesthetic agents and narcotic overdose, decreased chest wall excursion from surgical site discomfort and residual muscle relaxants, upper airway obstruction from soft tissue relaxation, laryngeal edema, and aspiration. In addition, nitrous oxide exchange with nitrogen leads to decreased oxygen content in the blood and diffusion hypoxia.[35] Tachycardia, hyperventilation, decreasing Pa_{O_2} on increasing fraction inspired oxygen (FI_{O_2}), SVR may be indicative of hypoxia.

Anesthetic Interventions   To prevent postoperative hypoxemia and untoward respiratory events, the first action should be to evaluate whether the patient adequately meets extubation criteria (Table 32–3).[36] After extubation, all patients should receive supplemental oxygen, and Sa_{O_2} should be monitored as per AANA standards (see Chapter 6, Patient Monitoring). The most common cause of alteration in ventilation is upper airway obstruction by the tongue. Nasal/oropharyngeal airways and jaw thrust may relieve obstruction. Obstruction related to laryngeal edema may be treated with nebulized racemic epinephrine and humidified oxygen. As a final measure, reintubation may become necessary.

Secretions in the upper airway can lead to laryngeal spasm, which can lead to obstruction and decreased ventilation. Treatment of laryngeal spasm is with positive-pressure mask ventilation, or if the patient cannot be ventilated, give succinylcholine 20 to 40 mg. Laryngeal spasm can lead to acute pulmonary edema secondary to the negative transpulmonary pressure caused by inspiration against obstruction, which rapidly progresses to arterial oxygen desaturation. Immediate treatment is with intubation, controlled ventilation,

Table 32–3
CLINICAL CRITERIA FOR RESPIRATORY FAILURE

Clinical Criteria	Normal Value	Intubate
Respiratory rate	12–20/min	> 35/min
Vital capacity	65–75 mL/kg	< 15 mL/kg
Forced expiratory volume in 1s	50–60 mL/kg	< 10 mL/kg
Inspiratory force	$(-)75-(-)100$ cm H_2O	< $(-)25$ cm H_2O
Pa_{O_2}	75–100 mmHg (room air)	≤ 70 mm Hg with O_2
Aa D_{O_2} (after 10 min 100%/O_2)	25–65 mm Hg	> 0.6 mm Hg
Pa_{CO_2}	35–45 mm Hg	> 55 mm Hg (except chronic obstructive pulmonary disease)

Reproduced by permission from Pontoppidan and colleagues.[36]

and diuresis. Table 32–4 presents other causes of postoperative hypoxia.[37]

CARDIAC ALTERATIONS

Hypotension is a common postoperative complication due to inadequate perioperative fluid replacement, third-space losses, and undiscovered hemorrhage. Treat hypotension with fluid boluses to maintain a urine output of 0.5 to 1

Table 32–4
CAUSES OF POSTOPERATIVE HYPOXIA

I. Impaired delivery
  • No O_2 administration—empty O_2 tank
II. Alveolar ventilation
  • ↑Pa_{CO_2} or Pa_{N_2O}
  • Mainstem bronchus intubation
  • Bronchospasm
  • Pneumothorax
III. Increased O_2 requirements
  • Shivering
  • Seizures
  • Fever
  • Airway obstruction
  • Distended abdomen
  • Respiratory depressant drugs/muscle paralysis
  • Hypothyroidism
  • Malignant hyperthermia
  • Hyperdynamic septic shock
IV. Altered O_2 transfer
  • Aspiration/pulmonary embolism
V. Cardiac
  • Pulmonary edema
  • Myocardial infarction
  • Hypervolemic shock
VI. Hematologic
  • Anemia
  • Oxyhemoglobin curve shifts

SOURCE: Reproduced by permission from Reed and Kaplan.[37]

mL/kg and check hematocrit to determine necessity of blood transfusion. Inotropes such as dopamine, epinephrine, dobutamine, or amrinone may be necessary to treat hypotension produced by low cardiac output.

Cardiac dysrhythmias seen in the postoperative period may be related to underlying cardiac disease or perioperative cardiac ischemia. ECG and cardiac enzymes should be performed to rule out ischemia. Tachycardia occurs most frequently and can be related to hypoxia, hypovolemia, and pain.

Hypertension in the postoperative stage is frequently seen in clients with essential hypertension. Patients receiving short-acting β blockers such as propanolol may experience rebound hypertension with abrupt cessation of drug treatment. Therefore, β blockers should be continued in the perioperative period.[38]

Multiple pharmaceutical agents can be used to treat perioperative hypertension. Labetalol lowers blood pressure through α blockade and reflex tachycardia from vasodilation is blocked by concomitant β blockade.[39] Sublingual nifedipine promptly decreases blood pressure through calcium channel blockade. Nifedipine does not produce tachycardia and there is some beneficial coronary vasodilation.[40]

Severe hypertension may require rapid control with IV agents such as sodium nitroprusside, nitroglycerin, or nicardipine.

POSTOPERATIVE OLIGURIA

Diminished cardiac output or insufficient volume are predisposing factors for postoperative oliguria. Hypovolemia is a dominant cause of prerenal oliguria. If fluid resuscitation is not provided, prerenal oliguria may rapidly progress to renal failure. Oliguria in normovolemic patients may be related to increased antidiuretic hormone (ADH) secretion. Because pain and stress are associated with increased secretion of ADH, maintenance fluids should be titrated to achieve an hourly urine output of 0.5 mL/kg. It is important to ensure adequate pain relief. If oliguria persists in the normovolemic patient, initial treatment is with loop diuretics such as IV furosemide. Low-dose dopamine at 0.5 to 2 mg/kg increases renal blood flow, decreases peripheral vascular resistance, decreases plasma renin activity, and increases urine output.[41]

EMERGENCE DELIRIUM

Commonly seen in the postoperative period, emergence delirium has multiple etiologies including hypoxemia, urinary retention, and gastric distension. Premedication with anticholinergics has been associated with an increase in emergence delirium. Delirium from anticholinergics can be treated with physostigmine 15 to 45 μg/kg with glycopyrrolate.

POSTOPERATIVE PAIN

Inadequate pain relief in the postoperative period precipitates alterations in respiration, circulation, and initiation of cate-

cholamine response. The release of catecholamines with subsequent increases in blood pressure and heart rate produces an increase in SVR, myocardial work, and oxygen consumption. This may lead to myocardial ischemia and hypoxemia; therefore, adequate pain relief is vital in the postoperative period. Pain relief can be achieved through the use of parenteral narcotics or local or regional blocks.

☐ ANESTHESIA AND CANCER CARE

Cancer remains one of the leading causes of death in adults and children in the United States. It is estimated that 25% of the population will develop some type of cancer in their lifetime. Genetic mutations within individual cells cause uncontrolled proliferation and growth of these cells, thus invading normal body tissues; we define this as cancer.

The causes of cell mutations are vast and include alterations by ionizing radiation, chemical and physical irritants, heredity, and immunosuppression.

TREATMENT MODALITIES

Radiotherapy Radiotherapy is used for curative treatment in small localized tumors as well as adjuvant treatment after surgery to prevent local metastatic tumor spread. Radiation is also used palliatively to control malignant growth in end-stage disease to reduce pain from tumor encroachment on nerves and viscera.[42]

The radiosensitivity of tumor cells parallels that of the normal cell of the tissue of origin with lymphoid tissue being the most sensitive. Responsiveness of a tumor depends on tumor size, vascularity, and growth rate.[43]

Anesthesia is not usually provided for routine radiotherapy treatments. Yet, it is imperative that the anesthesia provider comprehend the effects of radiation on the patient. Complications vary from minor fatigue, weakness, and nausea to the more serious ones including bone marrow suppression, skin breakdown, pericarditis, pneumonitis, tissue necrosis, and fistula formation.

Airway management and intubation may become difficult in patients with head and neck radiation due to glottic edema and immobility of the larnyx and epiglottis. In addition, breakdown in mucosal membranes leads to bleeding and ulcerations that may obscure the view of airway structures.

Direct radiation of lung fields is associated with radiation pneumonitis, which may be related to ionizing particles, vassoactive substances, or oxygen free radicals.[43] Be aware of potential perioperative hypoxemia and development of adult respiratory distress syndrome (ARDS).

Bone marrow suppression and decreases in lymphocytes, leukocytes, and platelets increase the risk of infection and hemorrhage. Use strict aseptic technique during surgery and check platelet counts before surgery.

Pericarditis may develop after chest radiation, especially if the dose is greater than 4000 rads.[43] Pericarditis or pericardial effusion will evolve in the first couple of years after radiotherapy. Later cardiac changes are myocardial fibrosis, ischemic heart disease, valvular dysfunction, and pericardial constriction. Adequate cardiac work-up is mandatory in patients with a history of chest radiation. The work-up should include an ECG, chest radiograph, and echocardiograph. Physical examination should note indications of pericardial effusion such as neck vein distention, shortness of breath, tachycardia, and hypotension. Be prepared to treat patients for emergency pericardial window or pericardiocentesis.

Chemotherapy After World War I, discovery of the effects of nitrogen mustard gas on white blood cells (producing leukopenia) gave rise to the development of these chemical agents to combat neoplasms. Antineoplastic agents act by interfering with the cell enzyme activity or on enzyme substrates, ultimately altering function of tumor cell DNA leading to destruction of the cell. The goal of chemotherapy is to destroy all malignant cells. This is best achieved by the use of a combination of chemotherapeutic agents over short periods of time. A constant percentage of cells is killed by a given therapeutic dose of an agent; combination chemotherapy is most effective to eradicate greater than 100% of tumor cells, prevent tumor resistance, and ameliorate adverse effects of each individual agent.[44] Details on various antineoplastic drugs are presented in Table 32–5.[45]

Alkylating Agents

Alkylating agents form covalent linkages (alkylation) with various nucleic acid substances, thereby disturbing mechanisms responsible for cell growth, mitosis, differentiation, and function.[44] Bone marrow suppression is the dose-limiting factor as well as tumor resistance. Drugs in this class include mechlorethamine, cyclophosphamide, busulfan, thiotepa, and chlorambucil (Leukeran).

Adverse effects include hemolytic anemia and increased skin pigmentation. Inhibition of plasma cholinesterase may occur in patients receiving cyclophosphamide, thiotepa, and mechlorethamine and may prolong effects of succinylcholine.[46] Rapid destruction of purine may progress to uric acid nephropathy.

Table 32–5
ANTINEOPLASTIC AGENTS

Agent	Disease Most Often Treated	Toxicity
Alkylating Agents mechlorethamine, cyclophosphamide, busulfan, thiotepa, chlorambucil	cyclophosphamide for Ewing's sarcoma, CLL, small-cell lung carcinoma, non-Hodgkin's lymphoma, neuroblastoma, busulfan for chronic granulocytic leukemia	hemolytic anemia, increased skin pigmentation (thiotepa), inhibition of plasma cholinesterase, hemorrhagic cystitis (cyclophosphamide)
Antimetabolites (folic acid analogues) methotrexate (purine analogues) mercaptopurine, azathioprine, thioguanine (pyridamine analogues) fluorouracil (5-FU), cytarabine	methotrexate for cancer of head and neck, ALL, CML, non-Hodgkin's lymphoma, CNS lymphomas mercaptopurine for ALL 5-FU for colorectal, gastric, pancreatic cancer	bone marrow suppression, hemorrhagic enteritis, confusion, ataxia, meningeal irritation with intrathecal methotrexate
Plant Alkaloids vincristine, vinblastine	vincristine/vinblastine for rhabdomyosarcoma, ALL, non–small cell lung, Burkitt's lymphoma, myeloma, Wilms' tumor	neurotoxicity dose-limiting factor with vincristine, peripheral neuropathies, SIADH, adynamic ileus; no cross tolerance
Antibiotics doxorubicin/daunorubicin bleomycin mitomycin C mithramycin	doxorubicin for sarcomas, endometrial, metastatic breast, lung small cell, Hodgkin's disease, retinoblastoma; bleomycin for testicular, Hodgkin's, ovarian disease; mitomycin for gastric adenocarcinoma; mithramycin for metastatic bone tumors	*doxorubicin = cardiotoxicity,* bone marrow suppression, pancytopenia, hepatic dysfunction *bleomycin = pulmonary toxicity,* noncardiogenic pulmonary edema *mitomycin* C = *glomerular damage, renal failure,* mithramycin impairs clotting, hemorrhagic diathesis, prolonged PT/PTT
Nitrosureas carmustine (BCNU), lomustine, streptozocin	BCNU for myeloma, lomustine for brain neoplasm, streptozocin for pancreatic cancer	BCNU hepatoxicity, pulmonary fibrosis, myelosuppression, thrombocytopenia, streptozocin hypoinsulinemia
Enzymes L-asparaginase	L-asparaginase for ALL	L-asparaginase severe coagulation defects, CNS effects
Synthetics cisplatin procarbazine	cisplatin for metastatic testicular, ovarian, head and neck, lung non–small cell carcinoma procarbazine for Hodgkin's disease	Cisplatin renal toxicity dose-limiting factor, ototoxicity procarbazine has synergistic effects with opioids and barbiturates

ALL, acute lymphocytic leukemia; CLL, chronic lymphocytic leukemia; CML, chronic myelogenous leukemia; PT/PTT, prothrombin time/partial thromboplastin time; SIADH, syndrome of inappropriate antidiuretic hormone.

Cyclophosphamide is well absorbed orally and is activated by cytochrome P-450. It produces hepatotoxicity, thrombocytopenia, and inappropriate ADH secretion. The major adverse effect is hemorrhagic cystitis, which occurs in 5% to 10% of patients.[47] It is recommended to adequately hydrate with IV fluids, give allopurinol, and alkalinize the urine with sodium bicarbonate.[48] Anesthetic considerations include cautious use of neuromuscular relaxants, use of twitch monitor and avoidance of hepatotoxic agents.

Antimetabolites

Antimetabolites interfere with normal cell metabolites that are necessary for cell function, such as synthesis of RNA and DNA. Three subcategories of antimetabolites are (1) folic acid analogues—methotrexate; (2) purine analogue—mercaptopurine, azathoprine, thioguanine; and (3) pyridamine analogues—fluorouracil (5-FU), cytarabine.

METHOTREXATE

Methotrexate is a poorly soluble folic acid derivative. It prevents formation of tetrahydrofolic acid cofactors that provide single carbon group transfer necessary for the synthesis of RNA and DNA.[44] Methotrexate is used to treat acute lymphocytic leukemia in children and it is used intrathecally for cerebral involvement and choriocarcinoma. Adverse effects are bone marrow suppression, hemorrhagic enteritis of the intestinal tract, and hepatic dysfunction. After IV administration, the patient may develop encephalopathic symptoms that present as confusion, ataxia, tremors, slurred speech, and possible seizures. When given intrathecally, methotrexate causes meningeal irritation in 60% of patients.[49]

Anesthetic concerns include avoiding the use of rectal probes and cautiously inserting esophageal stethoscopes. Do a complete neurologic examination on patients who have received intrathecal methotrexate before surgery.

AZATHIOPRINE

Azathioprine has potent immunosupressive effects and is used most frequently after organ transplantation to prevent rejection.[50] A major anesthetic concern is to adhere to strict aseptic techniques.

FLUOROURACIL

Fluorouracil is used most frequently to combat gastrointestinal and colorectal cancers and for palliative treatment in breast cancer. Alterations in mucosal membranes in the mouth and gastrointestinal tract are the most common adverse effects. 5-FU has been associated with myocardial ischemia and infarction in 17% of patients treated with this drug.[49]

Plant Alkaloids

Vincristine and vinblastine are chemotherapeutic agents derived from the periwinkle plant. Cytotoxic action is produced by the ability to bind with microtubule proteins, thereby stopping mitosis. A unique characteristic of this class of drugs is that there is no cross tolerance between individual vinca alkaloids.[47] Neurotoxicity is the dose-limiting factor with cranial nerve palsies occurring in 10% of patients.[49] Manifestations of neurotoxicity include loss of Achilles' ten-

don reflex, peripheral neuropathies, encephalopathy, syndrome of inappropriate antidiuretic hormone (SIADH), and adynamic illeus.[51]

Antibiotics

The antibiotics used to treat cancer are highly toxic and are associated with significant cardiac and pulmonary compromise. These drugs are doxorubicin, daunorubicin, bleomycin, plicamycin, mitomycin C, and mithramycin.

DOXORUBICIN/DAUNORUBICIN

Doxorubicin and daunorubicin are anthrax antibiotics whose interaction with the DNA helix impairs template activity and further cell replication.[51] Daunorubicin is used to treat breast, bladder, osteogenic, metastatic thyroid, and oat cell cancer. Unlike the vinca alkaloids these drugs possess cross tolerance. Doxorubicin is commonly called the "red devil"; urine is discolored red 2 to 3 days after treatment.

Adverse effects of doxorubicin and daunorubicin are bone marrow suppression, pancytopenia, hepatic dysfunction, radiation recall in previously irradiated areas, and significant cardiotoxicity. Prior mediastinal radiation, prior cardiac disease, increasing age, total dose of doxorubicin of 550 mg/m^2, and adjunct treatment with cyclophosphamide have been associated with an increased occurrence of cardiomyopathy.[51]

Two forms of cardiomyopathy are produced by daunorubicin and doxorubicin. The acute form presents in 10% of all patients and is characterized by ECG changes such as sinus tachycardia, nonspecific ST-T wave changes, premature atrial contractions, PVCs, and low voltage ECG with left axis deviation. The ECG changes are not associated with total dose and usually return to baseline within 2 months of treatment.[47] The second form presents with an insidious onset of a dry, nonproductive cough that rapidly progresses to congestive heart failure. Incidence of cardiomyopathy is 0.4% to 9% of patients treated with doxorubicin with over 60% mortality and 79% mortality in those treated with daunorubicin.[51] Initial symptoms may be treated with diuretics, nitroglycerin, and angiotensin-converting enzyme inhibitors. Digoxin levels should be checked frequently because of the increased incidence of drug toxicity.[49] In later stages the cardiac dilatation and ventricular failure are refractory to inotropic and mechanical intervention.

BLEOMYCIN

Bleomycin produces fragmentation of the DNA and is used most frequently in conjunction with vinblastine and surgery to treat testicular cancer. Pulmonary toxicity with interstitial pulmonary fibrosis in a similar pattern to ARDS has been demonstrated in patients treated with bleomycin.

Pulmonary toxicity is related to cumulative doses with patients receiving more than 500 U at increased risk. Precipitating factors include prior pulmonary radiation, increasing age, and renal impairment (leads to decreased clearance of bleomycin).[52]

Using high inspired concentrations of oxygen and volume replacement with crystalloids increases pulmonary damage from bleomycin with destruction of type I and II pneumocytes leading to ARDS.[53] Maintenance of anesthesia should be with the lowest FIO_2 to maintain adequate oxygenation (FIO_2 <30%) and replacement of third-space and blood loss should be with colloid solutions such as 5% albumin, hetastarch, or blood products as required.

Pulmonary effects of bleomycin can occur at any point after treatment. Some patients may not be able to tolerate low inspired concentrations. Several studies have used higher FIO_2 and crystalloid replacement without an increased incidence of ARDS.[54] As an anesthetist it is imperative to maintain adequate oxygenation and circulating volume first and foremost.

Pulmonary toxicity and lesions and noncardiogenic pulmonary edema have been associated with mitomycin, methotrexate, VM-26, cyclophosphamide, carmustine, and busulfan. Pulmonary effects from busulfan may present 3 to 4 years after treatment and are unrelated to total dose. Toxic effects of carmustine may present in 9 days or up until 12 years after treatment.[49]

Mitomycin C

Mitomycin C is used to treat gastric and pancreatic cancer. Mitomycin inhibits synthesis of DNA. Mitomycin produces dose-dependent renal toxicity in 4% to 10% of patients. Studies indicate that a total dose of mitomycin C, less than 50 mg/m^2, significantly decreases the occurrence of nephrotoxicity.[55]

Mithramycin

Mithramycin produces cytotoxic activity by inhibiting RNA synthesis. Mithramycin is used infrequently because of its highly toxic effects on bone marrow and potential for hepatorenal dysfunction. Mithramycin impairs clotting factors; therefore, it is not unusual for patients to present with thrombocytopenia, epistaxis, prolonged prothrombin time (PT), partial thromboplastin time (PTT), and increased fibrolytic activity with fatal hemorrhagic diathesis in 1% to 5% of patients.[45] A primary anesthetic consideration is the potential for large blood loss in these patients. Examine the patient for ecchymosis, bruising, and overt bleeding. In addition, check the coagulation profile with bleeding time before surgery. During surgery, ensure availability of blood and blood products.

Nitrosureas

Cytotoxic action of nitrosureas is from inhibition of RNA and DNA synthesis by alkylation and carboxylation. These drugs are highly lipid soluble and can permeate the blood–brain barrier. Carmustine (BCNU), lomustine, and streptozocin are drugs in this class. Multiple adverse effects include hepatotoxicity, pulmonary fibrosis, and damage to renal tubules. Profound myelosuppression leads to leukopenia and thrombocytopenia, which develop 6 weeks after treatment.

Streptozocin

Streptozocin is used primarily to combat pancreatic cancer and malignant carcinoid syndrome. This agent has a high affinity for pancreatic islet beta cells. This drug leads to hepatic and renal toxicity as well as hypoinsulinemia in 67% of patients.[45] It is important to check glucose and electrolyte levels throughout the perioperative period.

Enzymes

L-Asparaginase

The antineoplastic action of L-asparaginase occurs by depleting malignant cells of extracellular supplies of asparagine through the catalytic conversion of asparagine to aspartic acid and ammonia. Major adverse effects include severe coagulation defects with prolongation of PT/PTT and vitamin K-dependent factors, hemorrhagic pancreatitis, CNS depression or hyperexcitability, and anaphylaxis.[48]

Synthetics

Cisplatin

Cisplatin acts by cross-linking DNA and disrupting the DNA helix. It is cell cycle nonspecific and is used to treat metastatic testicular, squamous head and neck, and ovarian cancer. Renal toxicity is the dose-limiting factor with azotemia occurring in 25% to 30% of patients after a single dose of 50 mg/m^2.[43]

To attenuate renal side effects it is prudent to adequately hydrate patients with oral and IV fluids with or without osmotic diuretics such as mannitol to maintain a urine output equivalent to 100 mL/h. Allopurinol is also used to remove uric acid deposits to prevent hyperuricemia. Other effects are electrolyte disturbances, anaphylaxis, and ototoxicity.[56]

Procarbazene

Procarbazene halts DNA synthesis and is used for the treatment of Hodgkin's disease. Procarbazene demonstrates sedative effects and has a *synergism* with narcotics, barbiturates, and antihypertensive drugs. This drug exhibits weak monamine oxidase inhibition and it is wise to treat intraoperative hypotension with direct-acting sympathomimetic agents.[47]

Adjunct Agents

Multiple agents are used in combination with antineoplastic agents to slow or prevent tumor growth. Agents used are hormones, such as androgens and estrogens, and antihormones, such as tamoxifen and steroids. It is important to note prior corticosteroid use and the necessity for supplements in the intraoperative period. Most authorities recommend corticosteroid supplementation if corticosteroids were used for more than 1 week in the past 6 to 12 months.

Cancer Surgery This section reviews some types of surgery used to resect primary malignant tumors and their anesthetic considerations. Brain neoplasms are addressed in Chapter 22 and lung resection is addressed in Chapter 21.

Several unique conditions must be considered when preparing the patient for cancer surgery. The patient may appear relatively healthy; many patients will be young, without evidence of prior illness. However, when caring for these patients, keep in mind that you only see the "tip of the iceberg." Tumors may be wrapped around major vessels or compress the mediastinum and upper airway, increasing the technical difficulty of both surgical and anesthetic management. Large

Table 32–6
CANCER SURGERY—GENERAL CONSIDERATIONS

1. Preop testing to include CBC—special attention to WBC count, platelet count.
2. Electrolytes. Liver function tests—hepatic dysfunction, coagulation anomalies
3. X-ray/MRI/CT scan—note location/size of mass
4. ECG—note anomalies related to chemotherapy. Possible echocardiography if ECG changes—history prior adriamycin/chest radiation therapy
5. Strict asepsis
6. Large-bore IV at least 18 gauge—CVL and multiple PVL per surgical procedure
7. Ensure availability of blood and blood products as surgery begins
8. Hetastarch/albumin for third-space loss
9. Question surgeon to possible extent of operation—limited versus total resection
10. Multiple endotracheal tubes, jet ventilation, bronchoscope available for head or neck tumors/upper airway tumors, mediastinal masses

CBC, complete blood count; CVL, central venous line; PVL, peripheral venous line; WBC, white blood count.

tumors are associated with large blood and third-space losses. Wide areas of tissue may need to be resected to ensure tumor-free margins. The anesthetist must always be prepared for flexible and modified surgical approaches (Table 32–6).

Head and Neck Surgery

The patient undergoing head and neck surgery presents the anesthetist with many challenges. These patients frequently have a significant history of tobacco and alcohol use that influences metabolism of anesthetic agents as well as the potential for underlying pulmonary, cardiac, and hepatic disease.

Airway management is of paramount importance. Tumors may encroach anywhere on the upper or lower airway including nasopharyngeal, glottic, and subglottic masses. Know the location of the mass, have several endotracheal tubes of different sizes available, and prepare for possible fiberoptic bronchoscopy. In addition to the tumor mass, prior radiation may stiffen the epiglottis and larynx making it immobile, which may make laryngoscopy difficult or impossible.[57]

Overall thyroid surgery, radical neck dissection, and node biopsies are relatively nonstimulating and do not require large doses of narcotics. Blood loss is small; however, there is potential for large losses due to the dissection around major vessels. Maxillectomy, mandibulectomy, and resection of large tumor masses are associated with continued slow blood loss.

Mastectomy

Patients undergoing mastectomy vary in age and health status; however, we are seeing an increase in younger women. These patients are understandably anxious, necessitating the need for generous premedication. IV access and noninvasive

blood pressure cuffs should be placed on the unaffected side or on one of the lower extremities. An 18-gauge IV is usually adequate. Use a larger-bore IV in patients who have had prior breast radiation. Radiation produces scarring and tissue becomes friable, thereby increasing the difficulty of surgical exposure and estimated blood loss. Use of a muscle relaxant is questionable when performing axillary node dissection; surgeons will be testing the *long thoracic nerve*. Accidental transection of the long thoracic nerve will lead to a condition known as winged scapula.

Mastectomy may be followed by immediate reconstruction with either a saline tissue expander, transverse rectus abdominus muscle (TRAM), or free flap. TRAM and free tissue flaps are prolonged procedures with a potential for increased estimated blood loss. Discuss use of nitrous oxide with the surgeon; abdominal distention may increase the difficulty with harvesting of the rectus abdominus muscle and of abdominal wound closure.

Intra-abdominal Cancer

Intra-abdominal cancers are associated with alterations in intravascular and third-space fluids with or without ascites. These cases are arduous, with high estimated blood loss because of tumor encroachment on other abdominal organs, possible adhesions, and the microvascular blood supply. The tumor may also cause obstruction anywhere along the gastrointestinal tract. For this reason consider the patient a "full stomach" and intubate with cricoid pressure. Use of invasive monitoring should be based on the patient's premorbid condition.

Blood loss during colon or gastric resection should be replaced with crystalloid and colloids as necessary. There has been much debate over transfusion of allogenic blood and decreased survival rates in patients undergoing gastrointestinal tumor resection. It is theorized that allogenic blood transfusion produces immunosuppression and an increase in tumor recurrence.[58] Techniques to diminish blood loss such as hypotensive anesthesia and use of epidural anesthesia should be considered. In addition, if transfusion is needed based on alterations in cardiovascular status, the use of autologous blood is most desirable because it does not produce the immunosuppressive effects associated with allogenic transfusion.[59]

Lung Cancer Surgery

Eaton-Lambert syndrome is associated with small-cell cancer of the lung. *Eaton-Lambert* presents as weakness of proximal limb muscles, which affects the lower more than the upper extremities. Skeletal muscle weakness is not reliably reversed with anticholinesterase drugs as in myasthenia gravis, and exercise improves strength. Muscle weakness is believed to be caused by a reduced number of quanta of acetylcholine released per nerve impulse with normal end-plate sensitivity. Calcium access through voltage-operated channels is reduced with subsequent decrease in calcium-dependent acetylcholine release through presynaptic membranes.[60]

Anesthetic management should include judicious use of muscle relaxant, with either decreased doses or no muscle relaxant, in any patient presenting for lung resection, bronchoscopy, or mediastinoscopy. Patients with Eaton-Lambert syndrome are extremely *sensitive* to both nondepolarizing and depolarizing muscle relaxants.

Mediastinal Mass

Anesthetizing a patient with a mediastinal mass can be a great challenge. Relaxation of the thorax and upper airway with anesthetic agents and muscle relaxation can lead to *total airway occlusion* and lung collapse, thus producing cardiovascular collapse and death. Intrathoracic complications are common in patients with Hodgkin's and non-Hodgkin's lymphoma. Fifty percent of pediatric patients with Hodgkin's disease present with a mediastinal mass.[61]

Preoperative tests should include a current chest radiograph to determine location and extent of mass and an ECG to note evidence of pulsus paradoxus and signs and symptoms similar to pericardial tamponade. Echocardiography should be performed to determine cardiac output. Encasement of the heart by tumor mass can lead to a fixed cardiac output, which is aggravated by the supine position. Pulmonary function tests in both the upright and supine positions are necessary before the induction of anesthesia. Intrathoracic airway obstruction will present with reduction in forced expiratory volume in 1 second (FEV_1) and peak flows in the supine position[62] (Table 32–7).

Cancer Surgery in Pediatric Patients

Leukemias and lymphomas are the most common cancers in the pediatric population. However, the patients may present to the operating room for the removal of solid mass tumors such as osteogenic sarcomas, mediastinal masses, teratomas, and neuroblastomas. In addition, they frequently present for diagnostic tests such as bone marrow aspiration, liver and node biopsies, and insertion of venous access devices.

Pediatric cancer patients tend to have severe leukopenia, thrombocytopenia, and coagulopathies. Strict aseptic technique is necessary in preparing anesthetic agents. Transfusion of platelets or fresh-frozen plasma before each procedure may be required.

Be prepared for alteration in drug requirements in the pediatric oncology population. Physiologic changes from chemotherapy with alteration in drug metabolism and distribution may occur. In addition, frequent anesthetics and use of opioids may increase dose requirements. Pediatric patients with neuroblastoma have increased catecholamine concentration and may have increased anesthetic requirements.[63] Hypertensive patients who present for neuroblastoma resection should be treated similarly to those with pheochromocytoma. Anesthetic care includes an adequate anesthetic level to blunt hypertensive response to stimuli, increased intraoperative volume, control of hypertension with α-adrenergic blockade, and avoidance of histamine-releasing drugs that may precipitate hypertension.

Bone Marrow Harvest

The cancer patient is frequently given high doses of chemotherapy or irradiation to destroy the bone marrow. Afterward bone marrow stem cells from either allogenic or autologous donation are infused. Patients receiving bone marrow transfusion exhibit severe immunodeficiency for 6 to 12 months after treatment with interstitial pneumonitis and pulmonary infection occurring in approximately 40% of patients.[64]

Anesthetic management, whether an autologous donation or an anonymous donor bone marrow harvest, is a simple procedure lasting 1 to 3 hours. Average bone marrow harvested is 15 mL/kg for the recipient. General anesthesia is required with endotracheal intubation because the patient will be prone during harvesting from the posterior iliac crest. Replacement therapy should consist of 3cc's of crystalloid, colloid, or autologous blood transfusion for each 1 cc of bone marrow aspirated. Tachycardia and hypotension are frequent complications due to hypovolemia. The use of nitrous oxide is controversial because of adverse effects on bone marrow. Opioids or ketorolac to ameliorate postoperative pain is prudent. Although bone marrow harvest is relatively noninvasive, patients experience pain and soreness from 24 to 72 hours postoperatively.

Cancer Pain With all the advances that have been made in the surgical, chemical, and radiologic treatment of invasive neoplasms the treatment of the pain associated with cancer still needs to be reinforced. In the past, cancer pain was routinely undertreated because of fear of addiction, side effects of opioids, and the complexity of cancer pain syndromes.

Cancer pain varies in origin. The pain produced may be related to direct tumor involvement into viscera with compres-

Table 32–7
ANESTHETIC CONSIDERATIONS FOR MEDIASTINAL MASS

Preoperative Evaluation

- Assess for signs and symptoms: shortness of breath, dyspnea, increased pulse rate, wheezing
- Chest x-ray, CT scan
- Pulmonary function tests with flow volume loops in supine and upright position
- Echocardiography upright and supine
- ECG

Induction of Anesthesia

- Avoid general anesthesia, if possible.
- Insert arterial and central venous lines.
- Cardiopulmonary bypass on standby
- Thoracic surgeon available
- Awake fiberoptic intubation (possible passage of endotracheal tube beyond mediastinal mass)
- Inhalation induction with patient in semi-Fowler's position
- Maintain spontaneous ventilation.
- Avoid muscle relaxants.
- Turn in lateral decubitus position or prone if airway compromised.
- Standby rigid bronchoscope

sion of organs and nerves, or be related to new metastases into bone. In addition pain is produced by chemotherapy, radiation, and surgical resection.

Types of Pain

Nociceptive pain occurs from identifiable somatic or visceral lesions with coexisting tissue damage. Inflammation and the subsequent release of chemical mediators activate peripheral nociceptors. When nociceptors are activated, the individual perceives pain.[65]

Neuropathic pain is often described as a burning sensation or dysesthesia. Neuropathic pain involves aberrant signals of peripheral or central afferent neural pathways. This pain is not attributed to continued tissue damage and is less responsive to opioid drugs.[66]

Idiopathic pain is usually used to describe pain that is in excess to the actual disease process. This pain is most likely related to psychological factors such as depression.[65]

Pain Treatment Plan

Before any analgesic intervention is started, it is important to be familiar with types of pain and to determine each patient's pain source. The World Health Organization has set up a tier program for the treatment of cancer pain. Initially, pain should be treated with nonsteroidal anti-inflammatory drugs. For moderate to severe pain, codeine and analogues such as Percocet should be used. Morphine, hydromorphone, and methadone should be saved for treatment of severe pain.[65]

When treating cancer pain it is advisable to use the easiest, least invasive method first, such as oral or rectal routes. Oral opioids can be given in large doses and provide more consistent serum blood levels when compared to intramuscular and subcutaneous routes.[66] If the patient is unable to take oral narcotics, rectal morphine suspension is successful in relieving cancer pain with a faster onset and less tolerance.[67] Transdermal patches such as fentanyl are also useful to provide continuous pain management.

It is imperative to adequately medicate with opioids and titrate until pain is relieved. Most opioid tolerance occurs in the first few weeks of therapy and this can be mediated by titrating to effect.[68] If tolerance occurs, or increasing doses lead to increased adverse effects, rotating equipotent doses of different opioids may attenuate side effects and decrease tolerance.[69]

When parenteral narcotics are no longer effective, spinal and epidural blocks can be used to treat pain. Spinal and epidural blocks are more effective for lower extremity and trunk pain, with low-dose opioids providing adequate pain relief. Complications of spinal and epidural blocks include lack of pain relief, infection, and catheter dislodgment. Use of epidural percutaneous injection ports has reduced epidural catheter complications.[70] If a patient continues to have pain with spinal and epidural opioids, small doses of a local anesthetic such as bupivacaine have been effective.[71]

Adjunct drugs such as benzodiazepams, tricyclics, steroids, and anticonvulsants are used to potentiate the effects of analgesics. In addition, use of relaxation techniques and transcutaneous electrical stimulation units should not be overlooked.

Neurolytic blocks are usually reserved for pain management in patients with end-stage cancer. They have limited use because sympathetic and motor function of blocked nerves is lost before sensory blockade to relieve pain is achieved and malignancies often protrude outside the blocked area.[72] However, celiac plexus blocks have been used most successfully for treating pancreatic cancer.

In general, nerve blocks are more successful when blocking continuous C fiber-mediated pain as opposed to intermittent pain produced by A delta fibers. Alcohol solution (50%) is a commonly used neurolytic agent. Neurolytic agents affect posterior nerve roots of the spinal cord causing permanent anesthesia in responding dermatomes.[72]

Surgical intervention such as cordotomy can be used for unilateral pain with multifocal location. A cordotomy interrupts the spinothalamic tract in the spinal cord and pain in the lower extremities, thorax, and upper extremities has been successfully treated with open or percutaneous cordotomy. Cordotomy is effective in controlling somatic and visceral pain and is usually reserved for patients with end-stage disease.[66]

REFERENCES

1. Knudsen F, Jorgensen S, Bonde J, Andersen JT, Morgensen P. Anesthesia and complications of extracorporeal shock wave lithotripsy of urinary calculi. *J Urol.* 1992;148:1030–1033.
2. Duvall J, Griffith D. Epidural anesthesia for extracoporeal shock wave lithotripsy. *Anesth Analg.* 1985;64:544–546.
3. London R, Kudiak J, Riehle R. Immersion anesthesia for extracorporeal shock wave lithotripsy. *Urology.* 1986;28:89–63.
4. Zeitlin GL, Roth R. Effects of three anesthetic techniques on the success of extracorporeal shock wave lithotripsy in nephrolithiasis. *Anesthesiology.* 1988;68:272–276.
5. Stoelting RK, Miller RD. *Basics of Anesthesia.* 2nd ed. New York: Churchill Livingstone; 1988.
6. Lui WS, Wong KC. Anesthesia for genitourinary surgery. In: Barash P, ed. *Anesthesia.* Philadelphia: J.B. Lippincott; 1990: 1105–1115.
7. Crowe R. Electroshock therapy — a current perspective. *N Engl J Med.* 1984;311:163–166.
8. Gaines GY, Rees I. Electroconvulsive therapy and anesthetic consideration. *Anesth Analg.* 1986;65:1345–1356.
9. Elliot DL, Linz D, Kane J. Electroconvulsant therapy, pretreatment medical evaluation. *Arch Intern Med.* 1982;142:979–981.
10. Selvin BL. Electroconvulsive therapy — 1987. *Anesthesiology.* 1987;67:367–385.
11. Marks LJ. Electroconvulsive therapy: physiological and anesthetic considerations. *Can Anaesth Soc J.* 1984;31:541–548.
12. Lew J, Eastley R, Hanning C. Oxygenation during electroconvulsant therapy. *Anaesthesia.* 1986;41:1092–1097.
13. Fear CF, Littlejohns CS, Rouse E, McQuail P. Propofol anesthesia in electroconvulsive therapy; reduced seizure duration may not be relevant. *Br J Psychiatry.* 1994;165:506–509.

14. Mårtensson B, Bartfai A, Mallén B, Hellström C, Junthè T, Olander M. A comparison of propofol and methohexital as anesthetic agents for ECT: effects on seizure duration, therapeutic outcome, and memory. *Biol Psychiatry*. 1994;35: 179–189.

15. Stoelting RK. Drugs used in the treatment of psychiatric disease. In: *Pharmacology and Physiology in Anesthetic Practice*. 2nd ed. Philadelphia: JB Lippincott; 1991:365–382.

16. Janowsky EC, Risch C, Janowsky D. Effects of anesthesia on patients taking psychotropic drugs. *J Clin Psychopharmacol*. 1981;1:14–18.

17. El-Ganzales AR, Ivankovich AD, Braveman B, McCarthy R. Monoamine oxidase inhibitors: should they be discontinued preoperatively? *Anesth Analg*. 1985;64:596–596.

18. Price LM, Meninger GR. Lithium in the treatment of mood disorders. *N Engl J Med*. 1994;331:591–597.

19. Hill GE, Wong KC, Hodges MR. Lithium carbonate neuromuscular blocking agents. *Anesthesiology*. 1977;46:122–126.

20. Granato JE, Stern BJ, Ringel A. Neurolept malignant syndrome: successful treatment with dantrolene and bromocriptine. *Ann Neurol*. 1983;14:89–90.

21. Caroff SN, Rosenberg H, Fletcher JE, Heinner-Patterson TD, Mann SC. Malignant hyperthermia susceptibility in neurolept malignant syndrome. *Anesthesiology*. 1987;67:20–25.

22. Guze BH, Baxter LR. Malignant neurolept syndrome. *N Engl J Med*. 1985;313:163–165.

23. Weston G, Struvin L, Amundson GM. Imaging for anaesthetists: a review of methods and anaesthetic implications of diagnostic imaging techniques. *Can Anaesth Soc J* 1985;32: 552–561.

24. Penden CJ, Menson DK, Hall AS, Sargentoni J, Whitwam JG. Magnetic resonance for the anaesthetist: Part II: anesthesia and monitoring in MR units. *Anaesthesia*. 1992;47:508–517.

25. Kuharik MA. Sedation, anesthesia and patient monitoring. In: Cohen MD, Edwards MK, eds. *Magnetic Resonance Imaging of Children*. Philadelphia: BC Decker; 1990:75–80.

26. Bastrein G, Syrovy G. Burns associated with pulse oximetry during magnetic resonance imaging. *Anesthesiology*. 1991;75: 382.

27. Hall SC, Stevenson GW, Suresh S. Burns associated with temperature monitoring during magnetic resonance imaging. *Anesthesiology*. 1992;76:152.

28. McEwan AJ, Mason DG. The laryngeal mask airway. *J Clin Anesth*. 1992;4:252–257.

29. Rao C. Anesthesia machine for use during magnetic resonance imaging. *Anesthesiology*. 1990;73:1054–1055.

30. Mitchell A, Louik C, Lacouture P, Slone D, Goldman P, Shapiro S. Risk to children from computed tomographic scan premedication. *JAMA*. 1982;247:2385–2388.

31. Panning B, Leuwer M. Propofol for children undergoing magnetic resonance imaging—editorial reply. *Anesthesiology*. 1994;80:1401.

32. Deer TR, Rich GF. Propofol tolerance in a pediatric patient. *Anesthesiology*. 1992;77:828–829.

33. Rehder K, Sessler A, Marsh H. General anesthesia and the lung. *Am Rev Respir Dis*. 1975;112:541–557.

34. Rose DK, Cohen M, Wigglesworth DF, DeBoer D. Critical respiratory events in the postanesthesia care unit. *Anesthesiology*. 1994;81:410–418.

35. Marshall BE, Wyche M. Hypoxemia during and after anesthesia. *Anesthesiology*. 1972;37:178–201.

36. Pontoppidan H, Geffin B, Lowenstein E. Acute respiratory failure in the adult. *N Engl J Med*. 1972;287:690, 743, 799.

37. Reed A, Kaplan J. Hypoxia. In: *Clinical Cases in Anesthesia*. New York: Churchill Livingstone; 1989:3–13.

38. Craig D, Bose D. Drug interactions in anaesthesia: chronic antihypertensive therapy. *Can Anaesth Soc J*. 1984;31:580–588.

39. Leslie J, Kalayjian V, Sirgo M, Plachetka J, Wathens W. Intravenous labetalol for treatment of postoperative hypertension. *Anesthesiology*. 1987;67:413–416.

40. Adler A, Leahy J, Cressman M. Management of perioperative hypertension using sublingual nifedipine. *Arch Intern Med*. 1986;146:1927–1930.

41. DiSesa V. The rational selection of inotropic drugs in cardiac surgery. *J Card Surg*. 1987;2:385–406.

42. Burns N. Radiotherapy. In: *Nursing and Cancer Care*. Philadelphia: WB Saunders; 1982:123–145.

43. Howland W. Cancer—an overview. In: *Manual of Anesthesia in Cancer Care*. New York: Churchill Livingstone; 1986:chap 1.

44. Calabresi P, Chabner B. Antineoplastic agents. In: Gilman AG, Rall TW, Nies AS, Taylor P, eds. *Goodman & Gilman's—The Pharmacological Basis of Therapeutics*. 8th ed. New York: Pergamon Press; 1990:1202–1257.

45. Selvin B. Cancer chemotherapy: implication for the anesthesiologist. *Anesth Analg*. 1981;60:425–432.

46. Zsigmond EK, Robins G. The effect of a series of anticancer drugs on plasma cholinesterase activity. *Can Anaesth Soc J*. 1972;19:75–82.

47. Stoelting R, Dierdorf S, McCammon R. eds. Cancer. In: *Anesthesia and Co-existing Disease*. 2nd ed. New York: Churchill Livingstone; 1988:chap 30.

48. Abramowicz M, ed. *The Medical Letter on Drugs and Therapeutics*. 1995;37:945.

49. Lema M. Cancer chemotherapy drugs and the patient. *ASA Refresher Course* #164, 1994.

50. Stoelting R. Chemotherapeutic drugs. In: *Pharmacology and Physiology in Anesthetic Practice*. 2nd ed. Philadelphia: JB Lippincott; 1991.

51. Howland WS. Complications of chemotherapy. In: *Manual of Anesthesia in Cancer Care*. New York: Churchill Livingstone; 1986.

52. Douglas M, Coppin C. Bleomycin and subsequent anesthesia: a retrospective study at Vancouver General Hospital. *Can Anaesth Soc J*. 1980;27:449–451.

53. Goldiner P, Carlon G, Cvitkovic E, Schweizer O, Howland W. Factors influencing postoperative morbidity and mortality in patients treated with bleomycin. *BMJ*. 1978;1:1664–1667.

54. LaMantia K, Glick J, Marshall B. Supplemental oxygen does not cause respiratory failure in bleomycin-treatment surgical patients. *Anesthesiology*. 1984;60:65–67.

55. Valavaara R, Nordman E. Renal Complications of mitomycin C therapy with special reference to the total dose. *Cancer* 1985;55:47–50.

56. Einhorn LH, Williams SD. The role of cis-platinum in solid tumor therapy. *N Engl J Med*. 1979;300:289–291.

57. Dougherty TB, Nguyen DT. Anesthetic management of the patient scheduled for head and neck cancer surgery. *J Clin Anesth*. 1994;6:74–82.

58. Rustover JJ. Blood transfusion and cancer: clinical studies. In: Singal DP, ed. *Immunological Effects of Blood Transfusion*. Boca Raton, Fla: CRC Press; 1994.

59. Schriemer PA, Longnecker DE, Mintz PD. The possible immunosuppressive effects of perioperative blood transfusion in cancer patients. *Anesthesiology*. 1988;68:422–428.

60. Miller JD, Lee C. Muscle diseases. In Katz J, Benumof J, Kadis LB, eds. *Anesthesia and Uncommon Diseases*. Philadelphia: WB Saunders; 1990.

61. Prakash UB, Abel MD, Hubmayr RD. Mediastinal mass and tracheal obstruction during general anesthesia. *Mayo Clin Proc*. 1988;63:1004–1011.

62. Neuman GG, Weingarten AE, Abramowitz RM, Kushins LG, Abramson AL, Ladner W. Anesthetic management of the patient with anterior mediastinal mass. *Anesthesiology*. 1984; 60:144–147.

63. Haberkern CM, Coles PG, Morray JP, Kennard SC, Sawin RS. Intraoperative hyypertension during surgical excision of neuroblastoma. *Anesth Analg*. 1992;75:954–958.

64. Howland W. Special considerations in the cancer patient. In: *Manual of Anesthesia in Cancer Care*. New York: Churchill Livingstone; 1986.

65. Portenoy RK. Cancer pain: pathophysiology and syndromes. *Lancet.* 1992;339:1026–1031.

66. Ashburn MA, Lipman AG. Management of pain in the cancer patient. *Anesth Analg.* 1993;76:401–416.

67. DeConno F, Ripanonti C, Saita L, Maclachern T, Brue E. Role of rectal route in treating cancer pain. *J Clin Oncol.* 1995;13:1004–1008.

68. Long SP. Management of acute pain in the postoperative and nonoperative environments. *New York State Anesthesia Review Lecture.* June, 1992.

69. Hanks GW, Justin S. Cancer pain: management. *Lancet.* 1992;339:1031–1035.

70. deJong PC, Kan Sen PJ. A comparison of epidural catheters with or without subcutaneous injection ports for treatment of cancer pain. *Anesth Analg.* 1994;78:94–100.

71. Sjöberg M, Nitescu P, Appelgren L, Curelaru I. Long-term intrathecal morphine and bupivacaine in patients with refractory cancer pain. *Anesthesiology.* 1994;80:284–297.

72. Arnér S. The role of nerve blocks in the treatment of cancer pain. *Acta Anaesth.* 1982;74:104–108.

☐ QUESTIONS

1. A 56-year-old woman presents for electroshock wave lithotripsy. Past medical history includes heart murmur, mitral valve disease, and ejection fraction of 40%. Medications are digoxin, captopril, and furosemide. Prior to induction of general anesthesia vital signs are 130/70, heart rate 76, CVP 12. General anesthesia is maintained with isoflurane and vecuronium. As the procedure begins, her pressure drops to 100/50, heart rate 88, CVP 22. The *most likely* precipitating cause of these vital sign changes is:
   a. Overhydration with IV fluids
   b. Deep anesthesia from inhalation agent producing hypotension and myocardial depression
   c. A normal occurrence from repetitive shock waves from the lithotriptors that will cease when shock waves are discontinued
   d. A normal occurrence from immersion into the warm water bath and hydrostatic pressure on peripheral vasculature

2. A 64-year-old, 80-kg man is scheduled for a small-bowel resection. History includes smoking, hypertension treated with hydrochlorothiazide, and manic depression treated with lithium. Cefotetan is given for prophylaxis. Vecuronium (total 6 mg over 3 hours) is given as a muscle relaxant, with the last dose given 45 minutes before the end of the procedure. After an adequate reversal with neostigmine and glycopyrrolate, the patient has residual muscle blockade. This may be related to:
   a. Overdosage of vecuronium
   b. Neuromuscular relaxant blockade enhancement from preoperative antibiotic
   c. Neuromuscular relaxant blockade enhancement from increased sodium ion excretion
   d. Neuromuscular relaxant blockade enhancement from increased lithium ion excretion

3. A 30-year-old man is scheduled for a clamshell thoracotomy for mediastinal mass. He has a history of testicular cancer that has been treated with cisplatin and bleomycin. He arrives to the operating room with blood pressure 108/90, heart rate 112, respiratory rate 36, wheezing, and shortness of breath that is exacerbated in the supine position. Anesthetic should include:

   a. General anesthesia with thiopental/succinylcholine induction and direct laryngoscopy; maintenance with inhalation agent, 100% O_2, and narcotic
   b. Awake fiberoptic intubation; then IV induction with thiopental and a nondepolarizing muscle relaxant maintenance with inhalation agent, O_2/N_2O 50/50
   c. Awake fiberoptic intubation with patient in semi-Fowler's position; maintenance with deep inhalation agent, spontaneous respiration with $FIO_2 < 30\%$
   d. Induction with thiopental and nondepolarizing muscle relaxant; maintenance with inhalation agent with $FIO_2 < 30\%$

4. A 6-year-old, 20-kg patient presents for MRI to diagnose a possible brain neoplasm. General anesthesia is maintained with a LMA, O_2/N_2O, propofol, and alfentanil. Spontaneous respirations are maintained. During the case, the $ETCO_2$ drops from 27 to 19. The most likely cause of the drop in $ETCO_2$ is:
   a. Light anesthesia leading to patient hyperventilation
   b. Decreased $ETCO_2$ values from long extension tubing
   c. Normal interruption of $ETCO_2$ sampling from MRI scanner
   d. Air embolism

5. Cardiovascular changes seen during ECT include:
   a. Bradycardia
   b. Sinus tachycardia with rates of up to 120 to 200
   c. Asystole
   d. All of the above

6. All are relative contraindications for ECT *except:*
   a. Intracranial mass lesions
   b. Recent myocardial infarction
   c. Severe osteoporosis
   d. Obesity

7. A 46-year-old woman presents for a laparoscopic cholecystectomy. Past medical history is significant for depression treated with isocarboxazid. Considerations for intraoperative care of patients on MAOIs include all of the following *except:*
   a. Treat intraoperative hypotension with direct-acting sympathomimetics.

b. Do not treat postoperative pain with meperidine.

c. Increase doses of opioids and barbiturates by 25%.

d. If possible discontinue medication 2 weeks before elective surgery.

8. Generalized muscle rigidity, hyperthermia, and tachycardia are symptoms of both malignant neurolept syndrome and malignant hyperthermia. To aid a differential diagnosis the anesthetist should:

   a. Give dantrolene; malignant hyperthermia patients will respond with a decrease in symptoms and neurolept malignant patients will not.

   b. Give a nondepolarizing muscle relaxant such as pancuronium; patients with malignant neurolept syndrome will respond with flaccid muscle paralysis.

   c. Give labetalol; only patients with malignant hyperthermia will have a decrease in heart rate.

   d. There is no discernible difference and both should be treated with active cooling, hyperventilation, and avoidance of triggering agents.

9. Factors that increase the risk of postoperative pulmonary dysfunction include all *except:*

   a. Underlying cardiopulmonary disease

   b. Thoracoabdominal incisions

   c. Use of low-dose narcotics

   d. Emergency surgical cases

10. Thirty minutes after an abdominal peritoneal resection, the patient in the PACU has a blood pressure drop to 80/50; heart rate is 110, and respiratory rate is 18. Urine output has been 15 mL for the last half hour. The most likely cause of these changes is:

    a. Narcotic overdose that should be treated with Narcan

    b. Hypovolemia from lack of fluid replacement that should be treated with crystalloid

    c. Impending cardiac failure that should be treated with inotropes such as dopamine

    d. Normal from rewarming and vasodilatation, no treatment necessary

11. Monitored anesthesia care is suitable for cataracts, localized peripheral biopsies, and many diagnostic procedures. The most important monitor to have during anesthesia is:

    a. A vigilant anesthetist

    b. Oxygen saturation pulse oximetry

    c. Electrocardiograph

    d. $ETCO_2$

12. Chemotherapeutic agents associated with a reduction in pseudocholinesterase are:

    a. Plant alkaloids, vincristine and vinblastine

    b. Bleomycin

    c. Alkylating agents, cyclophosphamide and chlorambucil

    d. L-Asparaginase

13. A 36-year-old woman with metastatic breast cancer initially had a lumpectomy with follow-up tamoxifen and radiation. When tumor recurrence was discovered, chemotherapy with doxorubicin was begun. She presents for mastectomy. Chest x-ray was within normal limits, ECG demonstrated nonspecific ST-T wave change with left axis deviation. Recently, she has had a dry, nonproductive cough. Thirty minutes after the start of surgery, peak airway pressures increase from 20 to 32, pink frothy sputum is noted in the endotracheal tube, blood pressure decreases to 90/60, and heart rate increases to 110 beats/min. Anesthetic management should include:

    a. Decrease volatile anesthetic, decrease fluids, start nitroglycerin drip, and give IV diuretics. Begin central pressure monitoring.

    b. Increase volatile anesthetic, give metered-dose β_2-agonist inhaler, and begin aminophylline drip.

    c. Suction endotracheal tube and send off sputum specimen.

    d. Discontinue volatile anesthetic, switch to balance technique with high-dose narcotics.

14. A 72-year-old man is admitted for a pancreatic bypass for pancreatic cancer. Past medical history is significant for alcoholism, chronic obstructive pulmonary disease, and hypertension. Preoperative chemotherapy included streptozocin. Anesthetic intraoperative considerations include:

    a. Control of blood pressure and adequate replacement of large blood loss

    b. Control of blood pressure, maintenance of adequate ventilation, and frequent blood glucose and electrolyte level checks during the procedure

    c. Control of blood pressure and heart rate with short-acting β blockers

    d. Use of balanced technique to avoid myocardial depression from volatile anesthetics and preparation for postoperative mechanical ventilation

15. Anesthetic considerations for the patient undergoing head and neck cancer surgery include all of the following *except:*

    a. Be prepared for fiberoptic bronchoscopy or emergent tracheotomy

    b. Have several different endotracheal tubes in various sizes

    c. Insert large-bore IV line for potential blood loss

    d. Insert central venous monitoring because of large fluid shifts

16. Anesthetic management for the patient with an anterior mediastinal mass includes all of the following *except:*

    a. Availability of fiberoptic and rigid bronchoscopes

    b. Rapid sequence induction with thiopental and succinylcholine

    c. Availability of cardiopulmonary bypass and a thoracic surgeon before the induction of anesthesia

   d. Preoperative pulmonary function tests in supine and upright positions, chest x-ray, CT scan, and ECG

17. A 68-year-old man underwent a left thoracotomy and left upper lobe resection for adenocarcinoma. He has a two-pack per day smoking history. Postoperatively he develops shortness of breath with respiratory rate 36, Sao_2 90% on 100% non-rebreather. Clinical criteria for reintubation include:
   a. Respiratory rate greater than 35 and vital capacity less than 15 mL/kg
   b. Pao_2 less than 70 mm Hg with oxygen
   c. $Paco_2$ greater than 50 mm Hg
   d. a and b only
   e. a, b, and c

18. Chemotherapeutic agents that produce pulmonary toxicity include:
   a. Vincristine, busulfan, and cisplatin
   b. Bleomycin, doxorubicin, and fluorouracil
   c. Thiotepa, azothaprine, vinblastine
   d. Busulfan, bleomycin, and mitomycin

19. The World Health Organization advocates the use of these drugs for first-line management in treating cancer pain:
   a. Ketorolac, acetaminophen, and ibuprofen
   b. Ibuprofen, codeine, and Percocet
   c. Oral morphine and codeine
   d. Oral morphine and methadone

20. Celiac plexus blocks have been effective in treating pancreatic cancer pain. Unfortunately, neurolytic blocks are often unsuccessful in treating cancer pain because:
   a. Sympathetic and motor nerves are blocked before pain relief is achieved.
   b. Tumors are localized in the neurolytic block area only.
   c. They do not block continuous C fiber-mediated pain successfully.
   d. They are often used to treat pain early in the disease process and do not work later on.

☐ ANSWERS

1. d	**5.** d	**9.** c	**13.** a	**17.** d
2. c	**6.** d	**10.** b	**14.** b	**18.** d
3. c	**7.** c	**11.** a	**15.** d	**19.** a
4. b	**8.** b	**12.** c	**16.** b	**20.** a

Index